Early Praise for *Machine Learning in Elixir*

There is no better person to teach Machine Learning in Elixir than the person who started it all: Sean Moriarity. Regardless, if you are new to Elixir or new to Machine Learning, this book has you covered with plenty of concepts, examples, and tools.

➤ **José Valim**
Creator of Elixir, Dashbit

Machine Learning in Elixir is a superbly structured dive into the world of ML in Elixir. Sean has put tremendous care into making the learning experience as streamlined and engaging as possible. I found myself eagerly following along with practical examples in Livebook that made the information jump off the page and into my hands.

➤ **Brooklin Myers**
Elixir Instructor, DockYard

From basic concepts to building real-world applications, *Machine Learning in Elixir* guides you through the complex world of AI, with practical insights to make you a proficient developer in today's AI market.

➤ **Nicholas Franck**
Software Developer, Independent

Machine Learning in Elixir

Learning to Learn with Nx and Axon

Sean Moriarity

The Pragmatic Bookshelf

Dallas, Texas

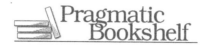

For our complete catalog of hands-on, practical, and Pragmatic content for software developers, please visit *https://pragprog.com*.

Contact *support@pragprog.com* for sales, volume licensing, and support.

For international rights, please contact *rights@pragprog.com*.

The team that produced this book includes:

Publisher:	Dave Thomas
COO:	Janet Furlow
Executive Editor:	Susannah Davidson
Development Editor:	Tammy Coron
Copy Editor:	Corina Lebegioara
Indexing:	Potomac Indexing, LLC
Layout:	Gilson Graphics

ISBN-13: 979-8-88865-034-9
Book version: P1.0—September 2024

To Riley, Weston, and Indy.

Contents

Mayo Clinic Gastroenterology and Hepatology Board Review

Sixth Edition

Mayo Clinic Gastroenterology and Hepatology Board Review

SIXTH EDITION

Editor-in-Chief

Stephen C. Hauser, MD

*Emeritus Member, Division of Gastroenterology and Hepatology,
Mayo Clinic, Rochester, Minnesota; Emeritus Professor of Medicine,
Mayo Clinic College of Medicine and Science*

Associate Editors

Seth R. Sweetser, MD

*Consultant, Division of Gastroenterology and Hepatology, Mayo
Clinic, Rochester, Minnesota; Associate Professor of Medicine, Mayo
Clinic College of Medicine and Science*

Michael D. Leise, MD

*Consultant, Division of Gastroenterology and Hepatology, Mayo
Clinic, Rochester, Minnesota; Associate Professor of Medicine, Mayo
Clinic College of Medicine and Science*

Karthik Ravi, MD

*Consultant, Division of Gastroenterology and Hepatology, Mayo
Clinic, Rochester, Minnesota; Associate Professor of Medicine, Mayo
Clinic College of Medicine and Science*

David H. Bruining, MD

*Consultant, Division of Gastroenterology and Hepatology, Mayo
Clinic, Rochester, Minnesota; Associate Professor of Medicine, Mayo
Clinic College of Medicine and Science*

MAYO CLINIC SCIENTIFIC PRESS

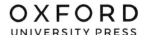

MAYO
CLINIC

The triple-shield Mayo logo and the words MAYO, MAYO CLINIC, and MAYO CLINIC SCIENTIFIC PRESS
are marks of Mayo Foundation for Medical Education and Research.

OXFORD
UNIVERSITY PRESS

Oxford University Press is a department of the University of Oxford. It furthers
the University's objective of excellence in research, scholarship, and education
by publishing worldwide. Oxford is a registered trade mark of Oxford University
Press in the UK and certain other countries.

Published in the United States of America by Oxford University Press
198 Madison Avenue, New York, NY 10016, United States of America.

© Mayo Foundation for Medical Education and Research 2024

Library of Congress Cataloging-in-Publication Data
Names: Hauser, Stephen C., editor. | Sweetser, Seth R., editor. |
    Leise, Michael D., editor. | Ravi, Karthik, editor. | Bruining, David H.,
    editor. | Mayo Foundation for Medical Education and Research,
    issuing body.
Title: Mayo Clinic gastroenterology and hepatology board review /
    Stephen C. Hauser, editor-in-chief ; Seth R. Sweetser, Michael D. Leise,
    Karthik Ravi, David H. Bruining, associate editors.
Other titles: Gastroenterology and hepatology board review
Description: Sixth edition. | New York, N.Y. : Oxford University Press ;
    [Rochester, Minn.?] : Mayo Foundation for Medical Education and
    Research, [2024] | Includes bibliographical references and index.
Identifiers: LCCN 2023034282 (print) | LCCN 2023034283 (ebook) |
    ISBN 9780197679753 (paperback) | ISBN 9780197679777 (epub) |
    ISBN 9780197679784
Subjects: MESH: Gastrointestinal Diseases | Liver Diseases |
    Examination Questions
Classification: LCC RC801 (print) | LCC RC801 (ebook) | NLM WI 18.2 |
    DDC 616.3/3—dc23/eng/20231004
LC record available at https://lccn.loc.gov/2023034282
LC ebook record available at https://lccn.loc.gov/2023034283

DOI: 10.1093/med/9780197679753.001.0001

Mayo Foundation does not endorse any particular products or services, and the reference to any products or
services in this book is for informational purposes only and should not be taken as an endorsement by the
authors or Mayo Foundation. Care has been taken to confirm the accuracy of the information presented and
to describe generally accepted practices. However, the authors, editors, and publisher are not responsible for
errors or omissions or for any consequences from application of the information in this book and make no
warranty, express or implied, with respect to the contents of the publication. This book should not be relied
on apart from the advice of a qualified health care provider.

The authors, editors, and publisher have exerted efforts to ensure that drug selection and dosage set forth in
this text are in accordance with current recommendations and practice at the time of publication. However,
in view of ongoing research, changes in government regulations, and the constant flow of information
relating to drug therapy and drug reactions, readers are urged to check the package insert for each drug
for any change in indications and dosage and for added wordings and precautions. This is particularly
important when the recommended agent is a new or infrequently employed drug.

Some drugs and medical devices presented in this publication have US Food and Drug Administration
(FDA) clearance for limited use in restricted research settings. It is the responsibility of the health care
providers to ascertain the FDA status of each drug or device planned for use in their clinical practice.

Printed by Integrated Books International, United States of America

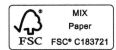

To the many persons who have taught, encouraged, and inspired us so that we can provide the best care for our patients and help educate our colleagues to do the same.

Preface

Gastroenterology and hepatology encompass a vast anatomical assortment of organs that have diverse structure and function and potentially are afflicted by a multiplicity of disease processes. We have designed the Mayo Clinic Gastroenterology and Hepatology Board Review course and the revised sixth edition of this book to assist both physicians-in-training who are preparing for the gastroenterology board examination and the increasing number of gastroenterologists awaiting recertification. *Mayo Clinic Gastroenterology and Hepatology Board Review* is not intended to replace the many more encyclopedic textbooks of gastroenterology, hepatology, pathology, endoscopy, nutrition, and radiology now available. Nor is this book intended to serve as an "update" to physicians looking for the newest advances in the science and art of gastroenterology and hepatology. Instead, this book provides a core of essential knowledge in gastroenterology, hepatology, and integral related areas of pathology, endoscopy, nutrition, and radiology. Clinical knowledge related to diagnostic and therapeutic approaches to patient management is emphasized. Case-based presentations and short board examination–type, single-best-answer multiple-choice questions with annotated answers are featured. The text is also intended to be used by medical students and residents during their clerkships in internal medicine and gastroenterology and by gastroenterology fellows in training. Physicians in practice should find this book to be a practical review for consolidating their knowledge in gastroenterology.

The book is organized by subspecialty topics, including esophageal disorders, gastroduodenal disorders, small-bowel disease and nutrition, colonic disorders, pancreaticobiliary disease, liver disease, and miscellaneous disorders. Numerous color and black-and-white figures support the text. Each subspecialty section concludes with a chapter containing board examination–type, single-best-answer multiple-choice questions with annotated answers. (The content of the questions and answers is not included in the index.) The faculty responsible for the book (at the time it was produced) all are Mayo Clinic gastroenterologists and hepatologists who spend the majority of their time caring for patients but have a commitment to teaching medical students, house officers, fellows, nurses, and physicians. Most of the faculty have particular interests in subspecialty areas of clinical gastroenterology and hepatology, which provides broad expertise.

We want to thank the staffs of Scientific Publications and Media Support Services at Mayo Clinic and the Mayo Clinic School of Continuous Professional Development for their contributions. The support of Mayo Clinic Scientific Press and our publisher, Oxford University Press, are also greatly appreciated. We want to give special thanks to Barb Hinrichs and to Darrell S. Pardi, MD, for his ongoing enthusiasm and support for our faculty and teaching mission.

Stephen C. Hauser, MD
Editor

Table of Contents

Contributors

Andres J. Acosta, MD, PhD
Consultant, Division of Gastroenterology and Hepatology, Mayo Clinic, Rochester, Minnesota; Associate Professor of Medicine, Mayo Clinic College of Medicine and Science

Jeffrey A. Alexander, MD
Consultant, Division of Gastroenterology and Hepatology, Mayo Clinic, Rochester, Minnesota; Professor of Medicine, Mayo Clinic College of Medicine and Science

Alina M. Allen, MD
Consultant, Division of Gastroenterology and Hepatology, Mayo Clinic, Rochester, Minnesota; Associate Professor of Medicine, Mayo Clinic College of Medicine and Science

Amindra S. Arora, MB, BChir
Consultant, Division of Gastroenterology and Hepatology, Mayo Clinic, Rochester, Minnesota; Professor of Medicine, Mayo Clinic College of Medicine and Science

Adil E. Bharucha, MBBS, MD
Consultant, Division of Gastroenterology and Hepatology, Mayo Clinic, Rochester, Minnesota; Professor of Medicine, Mayo Clinic College of Medicine and Science

David H. Bruining, MD
Consultant, Division of Gastroenterology and Hepatology, Mayo Clinic, Rochester, Minnesota; Associate Professor of Medicine, Mayo Clinic College of Medicine and Science

Vinay Chandrasekhara, MD
Consultant, Division of Gastroenterology and Hepatology, Mayo Clinic, Rochester, Minnesota; Associate Professor of Medicine, Mayo Clinic College of Medicine and Science

Victor G. Chedid, MD, MS
Consultant, Division of Gastroenterology and Hepatology, Mayo Clinic, Rochester, Minnesota; Assistant Professor of Medicine, Mayo Clinic College of Medicine and Science

Angela C. Cheung, MD
Fellow in Gastroenterology and Hepatology, Mayo Clinic School of Graduate Medical Education, Mayo Clinic College of Medicine and Science, Rochester, Minnesota; now with the University of Ottawa Department of Medicine, Ottawa, Ontario, Canada

Chamil C. Codipilly, MD
Senior Associate Consultant, Division of Gastroenterology and Hepatology, Mayo Clinic, Rochester, Minnesota; Assistant Professor of Medicine, Mayo Clinic College of Medicine and Science

Nayantara Coelho-Prabhu, MBBS
Consultant, Division of Gastroenterology and Hepatology, Mayo Clinic, Rochester, Minnesota; Associate Professor of Medicine, Mayo Clinic College of Medicine and Science

Jaime De La Fuente, MD
Fellow in Gastroenterology and Hepatology, Mayo Clinic School of Graduate Medical Education, Mayo Clinic College of Medicine and Science, Rochester, Minnesota; now with Eagan Endoscopy Center & Clinic, Eagan, Minnesota

John E. Eaton, MD
Consultant, Division of Gastroenterology and Hepatology, Mayo Clinic, Rochester, Minnesota; Associate Professor of Medicine, Mayo Clinic College of Medicine and Science

Derek W. Ebner, MD
Senior Associate Consultant, Division of Gastroenterology and Hepatology, Mayo Clinic, Rochester, Minnesota; Assistant Professor of Medicine, Mayo Clinic College of Medicine and Science

Khushboo S. Gala, MBBS
Fellow in Gastroenterology, Mayo Clinic School of Graduate Medical Education, Mayo Clinic College of Medicine and Science, Rochester, Minnesota

Stephanie L. Hansel, MD, MS
Consultant, Division of Gastroenterology and Hepatology, Mayo Clinic, Rochester, Minnesota; Associate Professor of Medicine, Mayo Clinic College of Medicine and Science

Moira Hilscher, MD
Fellow in Gastroenterology and Hepatology, Mayo Clinic School of Graduate Medical Education, Mayo Clinic College of Medicine and Science, Rochester, Minnesota; now with Perelman Center for Advanced Medicine, University of Pennsylvania, Philadelphia, Pennsylvania

Robert C. Huebert, MD
Consultant, Division of Gastroenterology and Hepatology, Mayo Clinic, Rochester, Minnesota; Associate Professor of Medicine and of Regenerative Medicine, Mayo Clinic College of Medicine and Science

Sumera I. Ilyas, MBBS
Consultant, Division of Gastroenterology and Hepatology, Mayo Clinic, Rochester, Minnesota; Associate of Medicine and Assistant Professor of Immunology, Mayo Clinic College of Medicine and Science

Prasad G. Iyer, MD
Consultant, Division of Gastroenterology and Hepatology, Mayo
Clinic, Rochester, Minnesota; Professor of Medicine, Mayo Clinic
College of Medicine and Science

Laurens P. Janssens, MD
Fellow in Gastroenterology, Mayo Clinic School of Graduate
Medical Education, Mayo Clinic College of Medicine and Science,
Rochester, Minnesota

Amrit K. Kamboj, MD
Fellow in Gastrointestinal and Esophageal Disease, Mayo Clinic
College of Graduate Medical Education and Instructor in Medicine,
Mayo Clinic College of Medicine and Science, Rochester,
Minnesota; now with Cedars-Sinai Hospital, Los Angeles,
California

Sunanda V. Kane, MD
Consultant, Division of Gastroenterology and Hepatology, Mayo
Clinic, Rochester, Minnesota; Professor of Medicine, Mayo Clinic
College of Medicine and Science

Sahil Khanna, MBBS, MS
Consultant, Division of Gastroenterology and Hepatology, Mayo
Clinic, Rochester, Minnesota; Professor of Medicine, Mayo Clinic
College of Medicine and Science

John B. Kisiel, MD
Consultant, Division of Gastroenterology and Hepatology, Mayo
Clinic, Rochester, Minnesota; Professor of Medicine, Mayo Clinic
College of Medicine and Science

Tasha B. Kulai, MD
Fellow in Transplant Hepatology, Mayo Clinic School of Graduate
Medical Education, Mayo Clinic College of Medicine and Science,
Rochester, Minnesota; now with Dalhousie University Department
of Medicine, Halifax, Nova Scotia, Canada

Michael D. Leise, MD
Consultant, Division of Gastroenterology and Hepatology, Mayo
Clinic, Rochester, Minnesota; Associate Professor of Medicine,
Mayo Clinic College of Medicine and Science

Shounak Majumder, MD
Consultant, Division of Gastroenterology and Hepatology, Mayo
Clinic, Rochester, Minnesota; Associate Professor of Medicine,
Mayo Clinic College of Medicine and Science

Harmeet Malhi, MBBS
Consultant, Division of Gastroenterology and Hepatology, Mayo
Clinic, Rochester, Minnesota; Professor of Medicine and of
Physiology, Mayo Clinic College of Medicine and Science

Daniel B. Maselli, MD
Fellow in Gastroenterology and Hepatology, Mayo Clinic School
of Graduate Medical Education, Mayo Clinic College of Medicine
and Science, Rochester, Minnesota; now with Vanderbilt Health,
Nashville, Tennessee

Omar Y. Mousa, MBBS, MD
Chair for Gastroenterology, Mayo Clinic Health System –
Southwest Minnesota region, Mankato, Minnesota; Assistant
Professor of Medicine Mayo Clinic College of Medicine and
Science, Rochester, Minnesota

Joseph A. Murray, MD
Consultant, Division of Gastroenterology and Hepatology, Mayo
Clinic, Rochester, Minnesota; Professor of Medicine, Mayo Clinic
College of Medicine and Science

Amy S. Oxentenko, MD
Consultant, Division of Gastroenterology and Hepatology, Mayo
Clinic, Rochester, Minnesota; Professor of Medicine, Mayo Clinic
College of Medicine and Science

Darrell S. Pardi, MD
Chair, Division of Gastroenterology and Hepatology, Mayo Clinic,
Rochester, Minnesota; Professor of Medicine, Mayo Clinic College
of Medicine and Science

Gopanandan Parthasarathy, MBBS
Associate Consultant, Division of Gastroenterology and
Hepatology, Mayo Clinic, Rochester, Minnesota

John J. Poterucha, MD
Supplemental Consultant, Division of Gastroenterology and
Hepatology, Mayo Clinic, Rochester, Minnesota; Emeritus Professor
of Medicine, Mayo Clinic College of Medicine and Science

David O. Prichard, MB, BCh, PhD
Research Collaborator in Gastroenterology and Hepatology, Mayo
Clinic School of Graduate Medical Education, Mayo Clinic College
of Medicine and Science, Rochester, Minnesota

Kevin P. Quinn, MD
Research Collaborator in Gastroenterology, Mayo Clinic School of
Graduate Medical Education, Mayo Clinic College of Medicine and
Science, Rochester, Minnesota; now with Park Nicollet Clinic, St.
Louis Park, Minnesota

Laura E. Raffals, MD
Consultant, Division of Gastroenterology and Hepatology, Mayo
Clinic, Rochester, Minnesota; Professor of Medicine, Mayo Clinic
College of Medicine and Science

Karthik Ravi, MD
Consultant, Division of Gastroenterology and Hepatology, Mayo
Clinic, Rochester, Minnesota; Associate Professor of Medicine,
Mayo Clinic College of Medicine and Science

Lewis R. Roberts, MB, ChB, PhD
Consultant, Division of Gastroenterology and Hepatology, Mayo
Clinic, Rochester, Minnesota; Professor of Medicine, Mayo Clinic
College of Medicine and Science

William Sanchez, MD
Consultant, Division of Gastroenterology and Hepatology, Mayo
Clinic, Rochester, Minnesota; Associate Professor of Medicine,
Mayo Clinic College of Medicine and Science

Tarek Sawas, MD
Fellow in Gastroenterology, Mayo Clinic School of Graduate Medical
Education, Mayo Clinic College of Medicine and Science, Rochester,
Minnesota; now with UT Southwestern Medical Center, Dallas, Texas

Vijay H. Shah, MD
Chair, Department of Internal Medicine, Mayo Clinic, Rochester,
Minnesota; Professor of Medicine and of Physiology, Mayo Clinic
College of Medicine and Science

Douglas A. Simonetto, MD
Consultant, Division of Gastroenterology and Hepatology, Mayo
Clinic, Rochester, Minnesota; Associate Professor of Medicine,
Mayo Clinic College of Medicine and Science

Andrew C. Storm, MD
Consultant, Division of Gastroenterology and Hepatology, Mayo
Clinic, Rochester, Minnesota; Associate Professor of Medicine,
Mayo Clinic College of Medicine and Science

Seth R. Sweetser, MD
Consultant, Division of Gastroenterology and Hepatology, Mayo Clinic, Rochester, Minnesota; Associate Professor of Medicine, Mayo Clinic College of Medicine and Science

Prowpanga Udompap, MD
Resident in Gastroenterology, Mayo Clinic School of Graduate Medical Education, Mayo Clinic College of Medicine and Science, Rochester, Minnesota

Kornpong Vantanasiri, MD
Resident in Gastroenterology, Mayo Clinic School of Graduate Medical Education, Mayo Clinic College of Medicine and Science, Rochester, Minnesota

Eric J. Vargas Valls, MD, MS
Senior Associate Consultant, Division of Gastroenterology and Hepatology, Mayo Clinic, Rochester, Minnesota; Assistant Professor of Medicine, Mayo Clinic College of Medicine and Science

Priya Vijayvargiya, MD
Fellow in Gastroenterology, Mayo Clinic School of Graduate Medical Education, Mayo Clinic College of Medicine and Science, Rochester, Minnesota; now with Erlanger Gastroenterology, Chattanooga, Tennessee

Xiao Jing (Iris) Wang, MD
Consultant, Division of Gastroenterology and Hepatology, Mayo Clinic, Rochester, Minnesota; Assistant Professor of Medicine, Mayo Clinic College of Medicine and Science

Esophagus

1

Gastroesophageal Reflux Disease[a]

AMRIT K. KAMBOJ, MD

JOSEPH A. MURRAY, MD

Gastroesophageal reflux is the reflux of gastric contents other than air into or through the esophagus. *Gastroesophageal reflux disease* (GERD) refers to reflux that produces frequent symptoms or results in damage or dysfunction to the esophageal mucosa or contiguous organs of the upper aerodigestive system.

> ✓ **Gastroesophageal reflux disease**—reflux that produces frequent symptoms or results in damage or dysfunction to the esophagus and occasionally the respiratory tract

Etiology

Gastroesophageal reflux results from several factors that lead to symptoms or injury of the esophageal mucosa by reflux of corrosive material from the stomach (Box 1.1). These factors include a weak or defective sphincter, transient lower esophageal sphincter (LES) relaxation (TLESR), hiatal hernia, poor acid clearance from the esophagus, impaired esophageal peristalsis, diminished salivary flow, decreased mucosal resistance to injury, increased acid production, delayed gastric emptying, and obstructive sleep apnea (Figure 1.1). The relative contribution of these varies from patient to patient.

Box 1.1.   Etiologic Factors of Gastroesophageal Reflux Disease

Motility disorders

Transient lower esophageal relaxations[a]

Weak lower esophageal sphincter[a]

Weak esophageal peristalsis

Scleroderma and CREST syndrome

Delayed gastric emptying

Damaging factors

Increased gastric acid production

Bile and pancreatic juice

Resistance factors

Reduced production of saliva and bicarbonate

Diminished mucosal blood flow

Growth factors, protective mucus

Others

Obesity[a]

Hiatal hernia[a]

Obstructive sleep apnea

Abbreviation: CREST, calcinosis cutis, Raynaud phenomenon, esophageal dysfunction, sclerodactyly, and telangiectasia.

[a] Major or common factor.

---

[a] Portions of this chapter were adapted from Szarka LA, DeVault KR, Murray JA. Diagnosing gastroesophageal reflux disease. Mayo Clin Proc. 2001 Jan; 76(1):97-101; used with permission.

Abbreviations: CMV, cytomegalovirus; CREST, calcinosis cutis, Raynaud phenomenon, esophageal dysfunction, sclerodactyly, and telangiectasia; EGD, esophagogastroduodenoscopy; EoE, eosinophilic esophagitis; GERD, gastroesophageal reflux disease; H_2, histamine; HSV, herpes simplex virus; LA, Los Angeles; LES, lower esophageal sphincter; PPI, proton pump inhibitor; SAP, system association probability; TLESR, transient lower esophageal sphincter relaxation

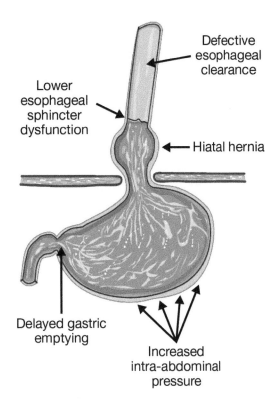

Figure 1.1. Causes of Increased Exposure of the Esophagus to Gastric Refluxate. (Adapted from AstraZeneca Pharmaceuticals LP [Internet]. Wilmington [DE]. From: http://www.astrazeneca.com; used with permission.)

Factors Contributing to GERD

Barrier Function of the LES

The LES and its attached structures form a barrier to reflux of material across the esophagogastric junction and are the central protection against pathologic reflux of gastric contents into the esophagus. This barrier has several components, including the smooth muscle LES, the gastric sling fibers, and the striated muscle crural diaphragm. The LES maintains tone at rest and relaxes with swallowing and gastric distention as a venting reflex, constituting a TLESR. In persons with mild reflux disease, acid liquid contents (instead of only air) are vented, resulting in many episodes of acid reflux. In patients with severe reflux, the resting pressure of the LES is often diminished and easily overcome.

The presence of hiatal hernia is important in defective barrier function both by removing the augmentation that the crural diaphragm provides the LES and by lowering the threshold for TLESR to occur.

Acid Clearance

The clearance of acid from the esophagus is a combination of mechanical volume clearance (gravity and peristalsis) and chemical neutralization of the lumen contents (saliva and mucosal buffering). This may be delayed in patients with GERD because of either impaired esophageal peristalsis or reduced buffering effects of swallowed saliva. The defective peristalsis can be a primary idiopathic motor disorder or, occasionally, it can result from a connective tissue disorder such as limited scleroderma associated with calcinosis cutis, Raynaud phenomenon, esophageal

dysfunction, sclerodactyly, and telangiectasia (CREST). Drugs and Sjögren syndrome can decrease salivary flow. Normally, salivary flow is decreased at night; thus, if reflux occurs during the night when the person is supine, acid will not be cleared by either gravity or saliva. Consequently, episodes of reflux at night are long-lasting and have a greater chance of causing severe injury to the mucosa.

Intrinsic Mucosal Factors

The mucosa of the esophagus has intrinsic factors that protect the esophageal lining against acid damage. These include the stratified squamous mucosa, intercellular tight junctions, growth factors, buffering blood flow, and production of mucin, bicarbonate, and epidermal growth factors. When these factors are overcome, GERD causes reflux esophagitis (Figure 1.2).

Gastric Factors

Delayed gastric emptying or increased gastric production of acid is a less frequent part of GERD. Reflux esophagitis is rarely a manifestation of Zollinger-Ellison syndrome. The availability of corrosive gastric contents in the cardia of the stomach is necessary for reflux to occur during TLESRs or when a defective LES is overcome during recumbency or abdominal

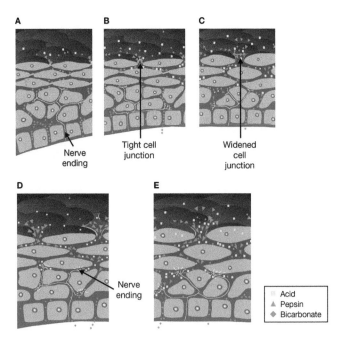

Figure 1.2. Mechanism of Action of Refluxate in Gastroesophageal Reflux Disease. The sequence of events hypothesized to lead to symptoms and tissue damage in gastroesophageal reflux disease is as follows: A and B, Acid-peptic attack weakens cell junctions. C, The cell gaps widen, thus allowing acid penetration. Exposure to gastric acid and pepsin can cause microscopic damage to the esophageal mucosa; even though the damage may not be visible endoscopically, it may still result in heartburn. D, Penetration of acid and pepsin into the mucosa allows contact of acid with epithelial nerve endings (which may result in heartburn). E, Additional influx of acid and pepsin into the mucosa triggers a cascade of events, ultimately leading to cell rupture and mucosal inflammation. (Adapted from AstraZeneca Pharmaceuticals LP [Internet]. Wilmington [DE]. From: http://www.astrazeneca.com; used with permission.)

straining. The cardia is often submerged under liquid gastric contents when a person is recumbent, especially in the right lateral decubitus position. It has been suggested that what differentiates patients with GERD from healthy patients is not the number of actual reflux events but the reflux of acidic gastric contents instead of the release of air alone. The timing of reflux is also important. Because gastric acid is buffered by food during the first hour after eating, normal physiologic reflux that may occur during maximal gastric distention is not as harmful as the reflux that occurs later after the stomach pH has again decreased. Any obstruction of the outflow from the stomach increases the propensity to reflux, although this is often associated with nausea and vomiting. Pure bile reflux may occur in patients who have had gastric surgery. More common is pathologic reflux associated with a restrictive bariatric procedure such as vertical banded gastroplasty. If too much acid-producing mucosa is present above the restriction, pathologic reflux may occur.

Obesity and Obstructive Sleep Apnea

Obesity has been established as a risk factor for GERD. An increased body mass index is also associated with Barrett esophagus and reflux esophagitis. In addition, obesity is associated with an increased risk of adenocarcinoma of the distal esophagus. Moreover, a strong correlation exists between obstructive sleep apnea and GERD. One proposed mechanism is that obstructive sleep apnea generates negative intrathoracic pressure, which leads to more episodes of acid reflux.

Helicobacter pylori and GERD

Whether chronic *Helicobacter pylori* infection protects against GERD is controversial. Duodenal ulcers and distal gastric cancer (both caused by *H pylori* infection) are becoming rare in high-income countries, and adenocarcinoma of the proximal stomach and esophagus is becoming more common as the carriage rates of *H pylori* decrease. Patients with GERD symptoms may be less likely to carry *H pylori* than patients without GERD symptoms. Reports that symptoms of GERD developed after the eradication of *H pylori* have led to a reexamination of those treatment trials of duodenal ulcers, which included *H pylori* eradication, for the new development of GERD symptoms. The evidence is conflicting as to whether the symptoms of GERD are more common in those in whom *H pylori* eradication has been successful or in those with persistent infection. In some persons, *H pylori* infection may cause chronic atrophic gastritis that affects the corpus of the stomach, resulting in diminished acid secretion. It is this relative hypochlorhydria that is thought to protect against GERD. Indeed, it has been suggested that acid suppression heals reflux esophagitis faster in patients with *H pylori* infection (Figure 1.3).

Connective Tissue Disease

Scleroderma, CREST syndrome, and mixed connective tissue diseases are rare causes of reflux, but these should be considered in young women who have Raynaud phenomenon or subtle cutaneous features of scleroderma in the hands or face. Occasionally, GERD may be the first manifestation of these disorders. Esophageal manometry characteristically demonstrates a low-pressure LES and decreased amplitude of contractions in the esophagus (Figure 1.4).

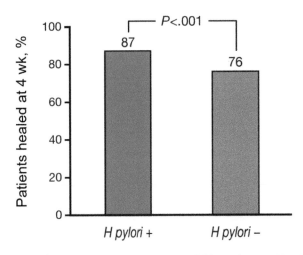

Figure 1.3. Efficacy of Proton Pump Inhibitor Therapy. The efficacy may be greater in patients with gastroesophageal reflux disease who are positive for *Helicobacter pylori* (*H pylori* +) than in those negative for *H pylori* (*H pylori* –).

Mechanism for Extraesophageal Symptoms

The mechanism for extraesophageal manifestations of GERD, such as wheeze or cough, may not always be direct aspiration or damage of mucosa in the respiratory tract but a vagally mediated reflex triggered by acidification of the distal esophageal mucosa. However, establishing a causative relationship is challenging, and in many cases GERD may instead coexist with suspected extraesophageal symptoms. Subglottic stenosis and granuloma of the vocal cords are serious consequences of reflux caused by direct contact injury of the delicate mucosa of the airway, resulting in stridor, cough, or dysphonia (Figure 1.5).

✓ Gastroesophageal reflux can result from several factors, including the following:
- A weak or defective sphincter
- TLESRs
- Hiatal hernia
- Poor acid clearance from the esophagus
- Impaired esophageal peristalsis
- Diminished salivary flow
- Reduced mucosal resistance to injury
- Increased acid production
- Delayed gastric emptying
- Obesity and obstructive sleep apnea

✓ Causes of extraesophageal symptoms (ie, cough) due to GERD:
- Direct aspiration and mucosal damage in the respiratory tract
- A vagally mediated reflex due to acidification of the distal esophagus

---

Epidemiology of GERD

GERD can be defined as the abnormal reflux of gastric contents causing troublesome symptoms (typically heartburn or acid regurgitation) with or without esophageal damage. GERD is one of the most prevalent diseases of the gastrointestinal tract in the US, and its prevalence has increased over the past 3 to 4 decades. Symptoms suggestive of GERD are common: In the US, up to 40% of adults report that they have heartburn and regurgitation on a regular basis (Figure 1.6), 18% report that it occurs weekly, and GERD accounts for approximately 4.7 million health care visits annually in the US. GERD becomes more common as

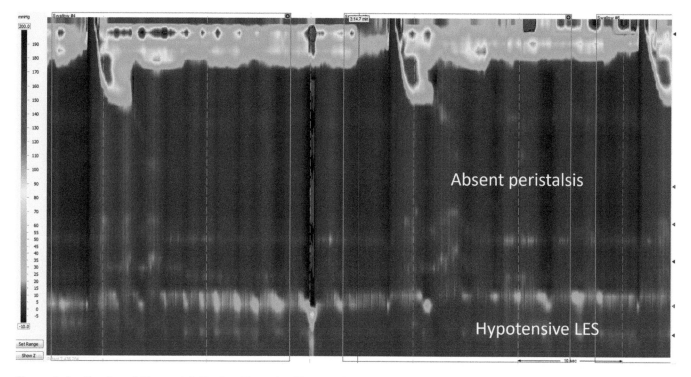

Figure 1.4. **Esophageal Manometric Tracing.** The tracing illustrates the complete absence of peristalsis and the hypotonicity of lower esophageal sphincter (LES) pressure consistent with esophageal involvement in scleroderma.

people age (Figure 1.7). Previously, GERD and its complications were rare in China, Japan, and other Asian countries, but this is changing rapidly with the adoption of a Western diet worldwide. A protective role of *H pylori*–induced hypochlorhydria has been suggested as a protective influence in countries with high carriage rates of infection.

Esophageal damage from GERD is observed less frequently, however, and less than 50% of patients who present for medical attention for reflux symptoms have esophagitis. Among patients who undergo endoscopy for GERD, 10% have benign strictures, 3% to 4% have Barrett esophagus, and an extremely small

percentage have esophageal adenocarcinoma. Complications of GERD may be more common in persons who are male, White, or older. Whether reflux is becoming more common is not clear, but it certainly is diagnosed more frequently than in the past. Also, because of direct-to-consumer advertising and public education campaigns, the public is more aware of GERD.

For patients with GERD, the quality of life may be impaired even more than for those with congestive heart failure or angina pectoris (Figure 1.8). GERD is associated with considerable health care costs related to its widespread prevalence, its effect on patients' quality of life, and the frequent need for long-term therapy, such as with proton pump inhibitors (PPIs).

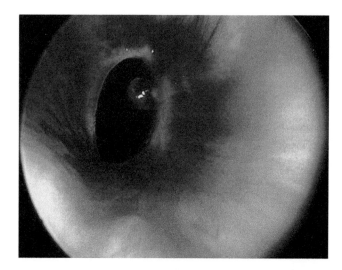

Figure 1.5. **Endoscopic View of Laryngeal Stenosis.** (Courtesy of Dana M. Thompson, MD, Department of Otorhinolaryngology, Mayo Clinic, Rochester, Minnesota; used with permission.)

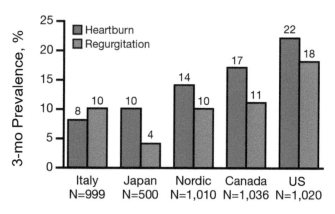

Figure 1.6. **Three-Month Prevalence of Gastroesophageal Reflux Disease Worldwide.** The prevalence varies markedly from country to country, largely because of differences in physicians' awareness and understanding of the condition. Nordic countries include Denmark, Finland, Norway, and Sweden.

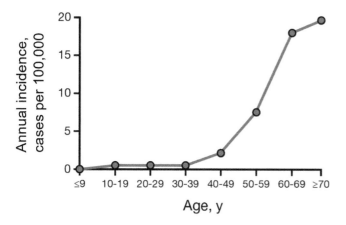

Figure 1.7. **Annual Incidence of Gastroesophageal Reflux Disease With Age.** The incidence increases markedly after age 40 years. (Adapted from Brunnen PL, Karmody AM, Needham CD. Severe peptic oesophagitis. Gut. 1969 Oct;10[10]:831-7; used with permission.)

Symptoms

The classic symptoms of GERD, that is, heartburn and acid regurgitation, are common in the general population and usually readily recognized. GERD may be manifested in a wide array of esophageal and extraesophageal symptoms (Box 1.2), and it may contribute to many clinical syndromes, either as a common factor or as a rare culprit.

✓ **Heartburn**—retrosternal burning that ascends toward the neck
✓ **Acid regurgitation**—the unpleasant return of gastric contents to the pharynx

---

Esophageal Symptoms

The cardinal symptoms of GERD are *heartburn* (defined as retrosternal burning ascending toward the neck) and *acid regurgitation* (the unpleasant return of sour or bitter gastric contents to the pharynx). These should be differentiated from the nonacid (bland) regurgitation of retained esophageal contents in an obstructed esophagus, as occurs in achalasia, or the effortless regurgitation of recently swallowed food that is remasticated and swallowed, typifying rumination. Patient symptoms of *GERD*, *reflux*, and *heartburn* should be differentiated from the burning epigastric sensation of dyspepsia.

Patients may report relief of symptoms with antacids or milk. The symptoms of heartburn and acid regurgitation are suggestive for GERD and can warrant empirical medical therapy. Objective confirmation, however, is required before consideration is given to endoscopic or surgical management of GERD.

Although regurgitation of acid is a specific symptom highly suggestive of GERD, *heartburn* may have many different meanings for patients, and, indeed, patients may use different and imprecise terms to describe their symptoms, such as *indigestion*, *upset stomach*, or *sour stomach*. Less common symptoms suggestive of GERD, but not diagnostic of GERD, include *water brash* (hypersalivation associated with an episode of esophageal acid exposure), *dysphagia* (difficulty swallowing), *odynophagia* (painful swallowing), and chest discomfort not identified as heartburn. Given the broad differential diagnosis for causes of dysphagia, odynophagia, and chest discomfort, if these symptoms are present, additional evaluation may be required before medical therapy is empirically started.

Reflux is more common after eating. Although reflux symptoms can occur at any time, they tend to occur most frequently 1 to 3 hours after eating, when acid production overcomes

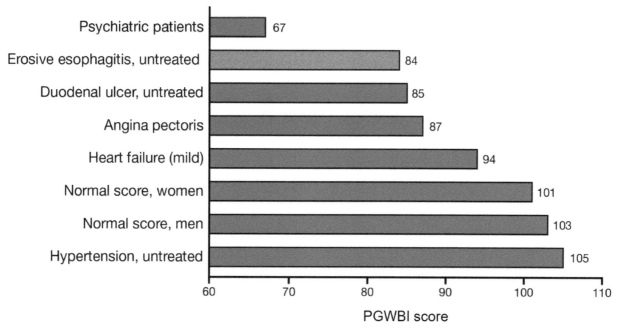

Figure 1.8. **Gastroesophageal Reflux Disease (GERD) and Quality of Life.** GERD has a greater effect on quality of life than other common diseases. Quality of life, assessed by the Psychological General Well-being Index (PGWBI), was compared between patients with untreated GERD and those with other disorders. For example, the mean PGWBI score for patients with untreated erosive esophagitis is similar to that for patients with untreated duodenal ulcer and lower (ie, worse) than that for patients with angina pectoris or mild heart failure. Normal scores are 101 for women and 103 for men, but they vary slightly from country to country. (Data from Dimenas E. Methodological aspects of evaluation of quality of life in upper gastrointestinal diseases. Scand J Gastroenterol Suppl. 1993;199:18-21.)

---

the buffering effects of food (Figure 1.9). It has been reported that a layer of acid may remain unbuffered on the surface of the gastric meal contents. Reflux may occur also at night or when a person with a weak LES is supine or, especially, in the right lateral decubitus position.

Esophageal Chest Pain

GERD is the most common esophageal cause of noncardiac chest pain. The pain may be referred to any point on the chest, anteriorly or posteriorly, with radiation to the neck, arms, or back. It may be indistinguishable from cardiac-related pain.

Because cardiac-related pain may be fatal, a patient who has chest pain from an unclear cause must have a cardiac investigation before an esophageal investigation. Frequently, patients who have both cardiac and esophageal diseases cannot distinguish between reflux-associated pain and real angina. GERD may decrease the threshold for coronary ischemia, further confusing the clinical picture. Therefore, it is especially important to first investigate the heart and then, when appropriate, other vital structures.

Extraesophageal Symptoms

GERD may contribute to symptoms originating in other areas of the upper aerodigestive system. These symptoms, which can occur without the classic symptoms of heartburn and acid regurgitation, include cough, wheeze, hoarseness, sore throat, repetitive throat clearing, postnasal drip, neck or throat pain, globus, apnea, and otalgia. They are not specific for GERD. Indeed, GERD is only 1 of many causes of most of these symptoms. Cough and wheezing are very common and likely to coexist with GERD by chance alone. Whether these symptoms are due to GERD needs to be confirmed by investigation (if typical esophageal symptoms are absent) or by the response to an empirical trial of potent acid-blocking therapy (if typical esophageal symptoms are concomitantly present). Ideally, the demonstration of a pathologic degree of GERD and a response of the atypical symptoms to an adequate antireflux regimen are needed to conclude that GERD is the cause. GERD may produce extraesophageal symptoms in 1 of 2 ways: 1) by direct irritation or inflammation of the delicate mucosa of the larynx, trachea, or bronchi or 2) by reflex-mediated changes in function. Both mechanisms may operate in some patients.

Establishing a Diagnosis

A proposed algorithm for the diagnosis of GERD when typical symptoms are present is shown in Figure 1.10.

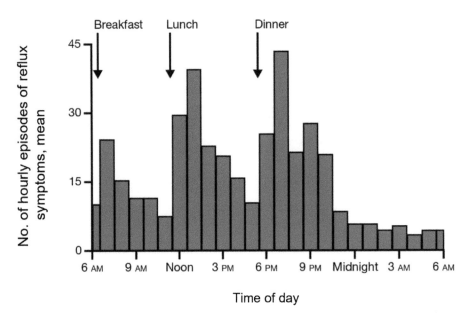

Figure 1.9.   Temporal Distribution of Symptoms of Gastroesophageal Reflux Disease. Distribution of the mean number of episodes of reflux symptoms over 24 hours is shown for 105 patients who ate their main meals at the same time of day. Food intake was associated with a marked increase in the number of episodes, and relatively few episodes occurred during the night. (Adapted from Johnsson L, Adlouni W, Johnsson F, Joelsson B. Timing of reflux symptoms and esophageal acid exposure. Gullet. 1992;2:58-62; used with permission.)

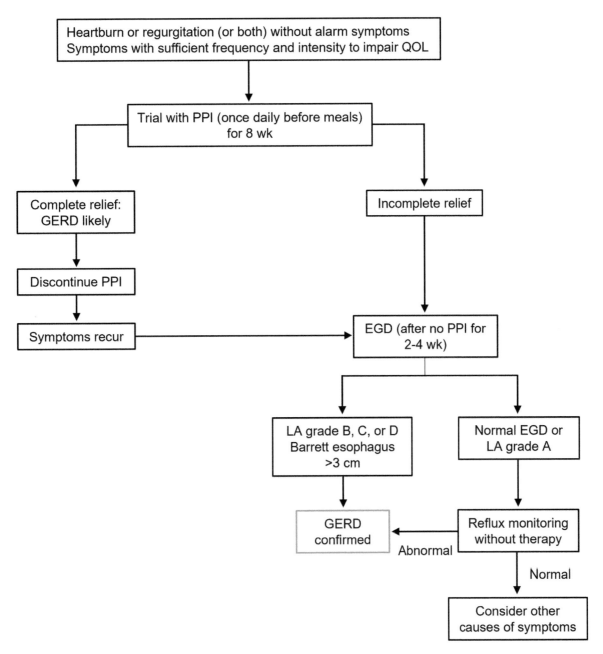

Figure 1.10. **A Proposed Algorithm for the Diagnosis of Gastroesophageal Reflux Disease (GERD) When Typical Symptoms Are Present.** EGD indicates esophagogastroduodenoscopy; LA, Los Angeles; PPI, proton pump inhibitor; QOL, quality of life. (Adapted from Katz PO, Dunbar KB, Schnoll-Sussman FH, Greer KB, Yadlapati R, Spechler SJ. ACG clinical guideline for the diagnosis and management of gastroesophageal reflux disease. Am J Gastroenterol. 2022 Jan 1;117[1]:27-56; used with permission.)

Typical Symptoms of GERD

Patients who present with typical symptoms of GERD without alarm symptoms should be given acid-suppressive therapy, typically for 8 weeks. Complete resolution of the symptoms with treatment and relapse when treatment is discontinued confirms the diagnosis and suggests the need for a long-term management strategy. However, even in these patients, the specificity of a response to potent acid suppression is not specific for GERD because other acid peptic disorders respond to acid-suppressive therapy. If symptomatic improvement is limited, either an increase in dose or additional diagnostic testing is needed. If the patient has little or no symptomatic improvement with acid-suppressive therapy, further investigation is indicated.

✓ If patients have typical symptoms of GERD (heartburn or acid regurgitation or both) and no alarm symptoms, an 8-week trial of acid suppression therapy is appropriate

✓ If symptoms resolve completely with acid suppression but return when treatment is discontinued, the patient may have GERD but probably requires esophagogastroduodenoscopy for further evaluation of recurrent symptoms when PPI therapy has been held for 2 to 4 weeks

✓ If the patient has little or no response to acid suppression, further investigation is needed

Atypical Symptoms of GERD

GERD may cause or contribute to many different clinical syndromes. The more common or dangerous causes of these syndromes should be evaluated first. For example, patients with chest pain should be evaluated for coronary artery disease; patients with chronic cough, for asthma; and patients with hoarseness, for laryngeal neoplasm. If GERD is considered a possible cause, options include trying a therapeutic trial of acid suppression or performing additional testing. A trial of acid suppression is a reasonable next step if patients have symptoms that are both typical and atypical. However, if the patient has only atypical symptoms, additional testing (eg, a pH monitoring study while medication is held) would be the best next test.

The acid-suppression test uses a potent regimen of acid suppression, such as PPIs (eg, omeprazole, 20 mg in the morning and 20 mg in the evening). If the symptoms resolve, the patient should receive long-term treatment, with an attempt at dose reduction or cessation. Atypical symptoms may have had alternative causes that resolved spontaneously. However, if reversible factors are altered and if GERD is the major cause, the symptoms will probably recur when therapy is discontinued. If the symptoms do not resolve completely, further evaluation with upper endoscopy or 24-hour ambulatory esophageal pH monitoring with symptom-reflux correlation (or both) is indicated. Ideally, the test should be conducted when the patient is not taking a PPI, so that acid regurgitation can be assessed.

If GERD is confirmed, long-term acid-suppressive therapy is indicated. If symptoms persist, ambulatory esophageal pH monitoring may be repeated to document that the esophagus is no longer exposed to acid.

Diagnostic Tests for GERD

Diagnostic tests are unnecessary for most persons with GERD. Investigations should be conducted if patients have alarm symptoms (ie, dysphagia, odynophagia, hematemesis, vomiting, or unintentional weight loss), equivocal results on a treatment trial, recurrent symptoms after completion of a treatment trial, or atypical symptoms of sufficient importance to warrant confirmation of GERD. Investigations should also be conducted if patients are undergoing surgical or endoscopic therapy for GERD. For most patients, the endoscopic demonstration of severe esophagitis is sufficient proof of GERD, and further investigation is unnecessary. However, up to 70% of patients with symptoms typical of GERD have normal endoscopic findings, with so-called *nonerosive reflux disease*, and additional tests are required to identify increased esophageal exposure to acid. This is typically done with ambulatory pH monitoring (Box 1.3).

✓ Diagnostic testing for GERD is not necessary if patients have typical symptoms (heartburn or regurgitation or both) of short duration and no alarm symptoms
✓ Diagnostic testing for GERD should be performed if patients have any of the following:
  • Alarm symptoms
  • Long-standing symptoms (>5 years)
  • An equivocal or poor response to an acid-suppression trial
  • Recurrence of symptoms after completion of a PPI trial
  • Atypical symptoms that warrant confirmation of GERD
  • A need for endoscopic or surgical management of GERD

Endoscopic Examination

Endoscopic examination with esophagogastroduodenoscopy (EGD) allows direct visualization of the esophageal mucosa. Reflux esophagitis is characterized by mucosal erosions in the

---

Box 1.3.   Uses of Diagnostic Tests for GERD

Endoscopy
  Differentiate reflux esophagitis from other causes of esophagitis (eg, eosinophilic or infectious)
  Biopsy for Barrett esophagus or adenocarcinoma
  Dilate strictures
  Provide endoscopic therapy (if desired)

Contrast radiography (not recommended for GERD diagnosis)
  Identify hiatal hernia
  Identify strictures
  Reproduce reflux of barium (not sensitive)

Ambulatory 24-h pH studies
  Quantify acid reflux in the absence of esophagitis
  Determine temporal correlation between gastroesophageal reflux and atypical symptoms

---

Abbreviation: GERD, gastroesophageal reflux disease.

---

distal esophagus. These usually start at the esophagogastric junction and extend proximally for various distances. By their appearance alone, these erosions usually are readily differentiated from rarer infectious, allergic (eosinophilic), or corrosive causes of inflammation. If the diagnosis is in question, biopsy specimens should be obtained, not primarily to confirm reflux but to identify alternative pathologic conditions, such as eosinophilic esophagitis (EoE). Given that the presence of these findings may be influenced by PPI intake, endoscopy should be done when the patient has not received PPI therapy for 2 to 4 weeks if this is feasible and if therapy can be held safely without dramatically worsening the patient's symptoms.

Several grading schemes, generally based on the extent of involvement, have been used for reflux esophagitis. The Los Angeles (LA) classification system, the one most commonly used worldwide, grades esophagitis on a scale from *A* (least severe) to *D* (most severe) (Figure 1.11). It is generally accepted that the presence of LA grade C or D esophagitis establishes a diagnosis of GERD. With the considerable interobserver variability for a diagnosis of LA grade A esophagitis, this finding by itself is not considered diagnostic of GERD. However, the finding of LA grade B esophagitis in a patient with typical symptoms and a response to PPI therapy does confirm a diagnosis of GERD. Severe esophagitis (ie, LA grade C or D) may occasionally be unrelated to reflux (eg, patients with bulimia who have severe, repeated episodes of vomiting or, rarely, patients who have pill esophagitis). Erythema and increased vascularity are nonspecific features, and a break in the mucosa is required to make the diagnosis of reflux esophagitis. Careful scrutiny of the esophagogastric junction with adequate air insufflation is needed to examine the mucosa in its entirety.

Endoscopy is also used to identify the potential esophageal complications of GERD, including esophageal ulceration and peptic stricture, Barrett esophagus, and esophageal adenocarcinoma. Alarm symptoms that suggest these complications include long duration (>5 years) of typical symptoms, dysphagia, hematemesis or melena, and weight loss. The presence of these alarm symptoms is a strong indication for diagnostic testing, especially endoscopy. Male sex, middle age, and nocturnal heartburn may be associated with a higher risk of esophagitis and its complications.

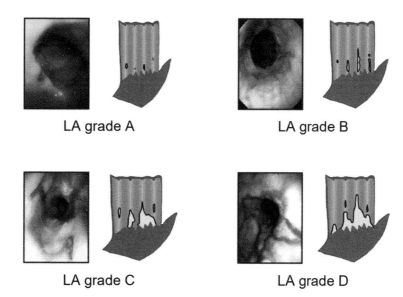

LA grade A   LA grade B

LA grade C   LA grade D

Figure 1.11. **Summary of Los Angeles (LA) Classification for Erosive Esophagitis.** *LA grade A* indicates 1 or more mucosal breaks with maximal length 5 mm or less; *LA grade B*, 1 or more mucosal breaks with maximal length more than 5 mm but not continuous between the tops of 2 mucosal folds; *LA grade C*, mucosal breaks that are continuous between the tops of 2 or more mucosal folds but involve less than 75% of the esophageal circumference; *LA grade D*, mucosal breaks that involve at least 75% of the esophageal circumference. (Adapted from AstraZeneca Pharmaceuticals LP [Internet]. Wilmington [DE]. From: http://www.astrazeneca.com; used with permission.)

✓ **Los Angeles classification system**—commonly used to grade erosive esophagitis as follows:
  • Grade A: 1 or more mucosal breaks, less than 5 mm long and not continuous between the tops of 2 mucosal folds
  • Grade B: 1 or more mucosal breaks, 5 mm or longer and not continuous between the tops of 2 mucosal folds
  • Grade C: mucosal breaks that are continuous between the tops of 2 mucosal folds and involve less than 75% of the esophageal circumference
  • Grade D: mucosal breaks that involve at least 75% of the esophageal circumference

---

✓ LA grade C or D esophagitis is consistent with severe esophagitis, confirms a diagnosis of GERD, and warrants treatment with a PPI twice daily for 6 to 8 weeks with follow-up EGD to assess for healing of esophagitis and to rule out the presence of underlying Barrett esophagus
✓ Long-term acid suppression is typically indicated for patients with LA grade C or D esophagitis, usually at the lowest effective dose to control symptoms, given the high risk for recurrence of symptoms and associated complications without medical therapy
✓ When severe erosive esophagitis (LA grade C or D) or long-segment Barrett esophagus is seen on endoscopy, the diagnosis of GERD is established and pH monitoring should not be performed to determine whether GERD is present

Barium Upper Gastrointestinal Tract Series

Although the barium contrast study is a readily available test, it is of limited usefulness in the evaluation of patients with GERD and is no longer recommended for the diagnosis of GERD. Its major utility in GERD is for identifying strictures and large hiatal hernias. It is insensitive for detecting erosions or superficial mucosal changes. The ability to reflux barium while at rest or in response to a provocative maneuver or postural change is not a sensitive test for GERD because in most patients the LES pressure is normal. The contrast study has limited value for the detection of mucosal changes other than the most pronounced

inflammation, which requires a double-contrast study. The sensitivity for GERD is only 20%. With the addition of provocative maneuvers, the sensitivity increases but the specificity decreases greatly. A barium contrast study may also be useful for the delineation of postoperative anatomical relationships and for evaluation of whether an antireflux repair is intact.

✓ Although a barium contrast study (esophagram) should not be used for the diagnosis of GERD, it can be helpful for evaluation of large hiatal hernias and strictures

---

Prolonged Ambulatory Esophageal pH Monitoring Studies

Ambulatory pH monitoring of the esophageal lumen, a well-established test, was introduced in the early 1970s. It provides objective evidence of the degree of GERD and its timing. This test is not needed for most patients with typical symptoms of GERD and for whom the diagnosis is not in doubt (ie, presence of severe erosive esophagitis or Barrett esophagus on endoscopy). The indications for ambulatory esophageal pH monitoring are listed in Box 1.4.

Box 1.4. Indications for Ambulatory Esophageal pH Monitoring

Atypical symptoms affecting the respiratory tract, ear, nose, or throat

Frequent atypical chest pain

Refractory symptoms in well-established GERD[a]

Preoperative confirmation of GERD

Abbreviation: GERD, gastroesophageal reflux disease.

[a] Esophageal pH monitoring is done during acid blockade.

The test is performed with a probe that has a pH sensor at its tip. The tip is placed 5 cm above the proximal border of the LES. Accurate location of this sphincter is critical because normal values for acid exposure apply only if the distance between the pH probe and the sphincter is 5 cm. The position of the LES usually is determined manometrically with a standard esophageal manometry study or with a single-pressure transducer in combination with the pH probe, which can locate accurately the proximal border of the sphincter. Endoscopic measurement and pH step-up on withdrawal are not sufficiently accurate for the placement of the nasoesophageal probe. The pH is recorded by a small portable recorder, and study duration is 24 hours.

Alternatively, wireless pH monitoring uses a wireless pH capsule that is pinned to the distal esophagus 6 cm above the endoscopically determined squamocolumnar junction. It transmits the pH measurements to a recorder worn on the chest. Its advantages are that it can record for prolonged periods and patients may eat without the discomfort of the nasal tube. Patients should maintain their usual diet, activity, and habits during the study to allow the assessment of findings in relation to their normal lifestyle. The recorders have a patient-activated event button (or buttons) to indicate meals, changes in posture, and symptom events. A typical wireless pH study is 48 hours in duration and can be extended up to 96 hours to potentially increase diagnostic yield.

Ambulatory reflux studies are analyzed initially by visual inspection of the graphs and then by computer-assisted quantitative analysis of the number and duration of reflux episodes and the relation to any symptoms the patient may have recorded. *Reflux of acid* is defined as a sudden decrease in intraesophageal pH to less than 4.0 that lasts longer than 5 seconds. *Acid exposure time* is the percentage of time that the esophageal pH is less than 4.0 during the ambulatory reflux study. An acid exposure time less than 4% is considered definitively normal (GERD is absent); acid exposure time greater than 6% is considered definitively abnormal (GERD is present); and values in between are considered indeterminate or inconclusive. Another important strength of ambulatory reflux monitoring is that it allows determination of whether a temporal relation exists between the patient's recorded symptoms and acid reflux. This determination is made initially by examining the tracing on which the symptom events have been marked and then performing a semiquantitative analysis.

Several measures have been used to calculate the correlation between symptoms and reflux, including the *symptom index* (ie, the percentage of symptom events that are associated with a gastroesophageal reflux event). A symptom index greater than 50% is considered positive. The *symptom sensitivity index* is the percentage of reflux events associated with symptoms. A symptom sensitivity index greater than 5% usually is regarded as indicating an association between symptoms and acid reflux. The *symptom association probability* (SAP) is the likelihood that symptoms occurring in association with gastroesophageal reflux are true associations and not the result of chance. The SAP uses a 2×2 Fisher exact test that compares time periods with and without symptoms and with and without reflux events. A positive SAP is greater than 0.95. Ultimately, however, the ability to determine whether a temporal association exists is dependent on patients recording their symptoms diligently and accurately during the study.

The 24-hour ambulatory esophageal pH monitoring test has limitations. Absolute values for sensitivity and specificity have been estimated because no standards exist for comparison with prolonged ambulatory pH monitoring. Also, pH monitoring may give false-negative results in 17% of patients with proven erosive esophagitis. This may reflect day-to-day variability in reflux, or patients may have limited their diet or activities that would lead to reflux. Even simultaneous recording of pH from adjacent sensors may give different results in 20% of patients. Some patients have a physiologic degree of acid reflux but have a strong correlation between the short-lived reflux events and symptoms. This may be due to a hypersensitive esophagus. Patients who frequently have symptoms of heartburn without corresponding reflux may have *functional heartburn.*

Generally, pH monitoring is performed when the patient is not taking any acid-suppressive medication. However, occasionally and for specific indications, pH monitoring may be performed when a patient is taking these medications. These indications include frequent typical reflux symptoms that are refractory to what should be adequate acid-suppressive therapy with usual doses of PPIs. Another indication is persistent extraesophageal symptoms despite high-dose PPI therapy in patients with confirmed reflux disease. If pH monitoring is performed while the patient is receiving treatment, a usual prerequisite is that the diagnosis of GERD is fairly certain, and the intent is to verify that the suppression of acid reflux is complete.

A secondary aim of the study may be to establish a temporal correlation between symptoms and acid reflux events. However, heartburn and regurgitation may occur in the absence of acid reflux. This may be due to nonacid reflux, gastric dyspepsia, rumination, or an unrelated process. Often, gastric pH is measured simultaneously to assess the degree of gastric acid suppression. Approximately one-third of patients receiving regular doses of PPIs have marked production of acid in the stomach at night, but this breakthrough acid production does not always produce symptoms or actual esophageal acid reflux.

✓ **Acid exposure time**—percentage of time that the esophageal pH is less than 4.0 during the pH monitoring study
✓ **Symptom index**—percentage of symptom events that occur immediately after an acid reflux event (>50% is considered meaningful)
✓ **Symptom sensitivity index**—percentage of reflux events associated with symptoms (>5% is considered meaningful)

✓ Acid exposure time less than 4%—normal (ie, GERD most likely absent)
✓ Acid exposure time greater than 6%—abnormal (ie, GERD most likely present)
✓ For diagnosis or confirmation of GERD, pH monitoring should be performed when the patient has not been receiving acid-suppressive medication (PPI therapy should be stopped for ≥7 days before the study)
✓ In certain clinical scenarios, pH monitoring with or without impedance may be performed while the patient is receiving acid-suppressive medications (eg, when the diagnosis of GERD is fairly certain, and testing is used to verify that acid reflux has been completely suppressed with medication)

Detection of Nonacid Reflux

The main limitation of standard esophageal pH monitoring is the detection of weakly acidic reflux, which may also contribute to symptoms. This limitation is addressed with technology that uses a single probe to provide multilumen impedance sensor measurements and pH measurements (Figure 1.12). It is useful especially for explaining persistent or recurrent symptoms in patients who are already receiving potent acid blockade therapy. Intraluminal impedance uses an array of electrodes spaced along the length of a catheter positioned transnasally across the esophagus.

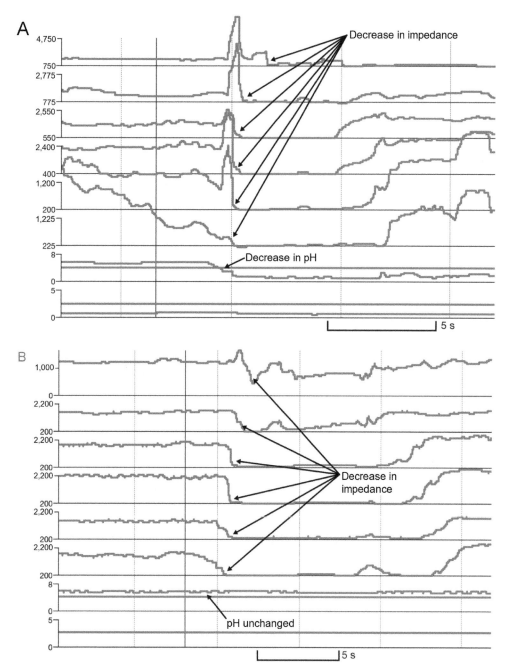

Figure 1.12. Typical Traces From Multichannel Intraluminal Impedance and pH Measurements. A, Acid reflux event. B, Nonacid reflux or weakly acidic reflux event. (Adapted from Wise JL, Murray JA. Utilising multichannel intraluminal impedance for diagnosing GERD: a review. Dis Esophagus. 2007; 20[2]:83-8; used with permission.)

Intraluminal movement of esophageal contents is detected by decreased or increased impedance moving antegrade or retrograde within the esophagus according to the conductivity of the esophageal contents. In the event of gastroesophageal reflux, the highly conductive liquid gastric contents result in a retrograde decrease in esophageal impedance, illustrating a gastroesophageal reflux event. Impedance relies on the differences in the impedance to the flow of electrical current in a medium according to its conductivity.

Although this technology has been used for several years, its sensitivity for true reflux is probably about 90% with the use of computer-based algorithms for detection of reflux. It has not been validated as well as the 24-hour pH test. The reflux events detected with impedance tend to be much shorter in duration than

the actual change in pH; this relates to the volume of clearance of the refluxate from the esophagus. So-called volumetric clearance occurs much faster, whereas the change in pH tends to be slower because actual buffering is required. The most robust measure of abnormality of nonacid reflux is based on the frequency of the events, but the system has limitations. For example, meals must be excluded. If patients already have esophagitis or Barrett esophagus or retained secretions, the baseline impedance in the esophagus may be abnormally low, which may preclude the detection of further decreases. Placement of the probe is especially crucial since intermittent movement of the catheter into a hiatal hernia may result in spurious reflux. In addition, patients who are not receiving acid blockade therapy may have a normal number of events, but the probe may not detect the delayed clearance at night when patients have nocturnal or supine reflux.

The major strength of this technology and its greatest utility are in looking with high fidelity at symptom-reflux correlations. The most common symptom association is regurgitation. Scoring systems have not yet evolved as they have with 24-hour pH monitoring; rather, determining the number of reflux events and the correlation with actual symptoms is the most appropriate use of this technology. It is also necessary to manually review the tracing to ensure that events identified as reflux by the monitoring system are true reflux events. Otherwise, chaotic tracings that occur after swallowing, for example, may be spuriously identified as reflux. A further limitation is the lack of a reliable diagnostic threshold for GERD; most experts suggest a threshold of 80 impedance-detected reflux events when a patient is receiving PPI therapy. However, impedance-detected reflux events are considered a supportive diagnostic tool and should not be used in isolation to diagnose GERD in clinical practice.

Other Tests

Gastroesophageal scintigraphy is used rarely to demonstrate gastroesophageal reflux or aspiration. The technique involves feeding the patient a technetium Tc 99m sulfur colloid–labeled meal and obtaining postprandial images with a gamma camera. Delayed images obtained the following morning may show scintigraphic activity within the lung fields, demonstrating aspiration (usually only gross aspiration is apparent). The Bernstein test is largely of historical interest.

Treatment

Patient- or physician-initiated empirical therapy for presumed GERD has become commonplace. Indeed, guidelines for primary care have supported this approach for patients who have typical symptoms without alarm symptoms. Treatment options for GERD are summarized in Table 1.1. In general, an 8-week trial of PPIs is recommended. Potent acid suppression with PPIs is effective and heals reflux esophagitis after only a few weeks of therapy. This has resulted in a shift in the disease as it appears

Table 1.1. Summary of Treatment Options for Gastroesophageal Reflux Disease

Treatment	Options	Healing rate, %
Lifestyle modifications	Elevate the head of the bed	20-30
	Avoid eating within 3 h before going to bed	
	Eat meals of moderate size and fat content	
	Lose excess weight	
	Decrease intake of caffeine and chocolate	
	Stop smoking	
Acid neutralization	Antacids	20-30
	Chewing gum	
	Alginate preparations	
Acid suppression	Histamine blockers	50
	Proton pump inhibitors	≥80
Prokinetics	Metoclopramide (not useful)	30-40
Mechanical prevention of reflux	Laparoscopic surgery	≥80
	Endoscopic therapies	≥50

to endoscopists. It is rare to find severe disease in patients who have been treated with PPIs. This practice poses a problem when symptoms do not resolve as expected or when they improve only partially. Even if the diagnosis of GERD was suggested at the time of presentation and initiation of PPI therapy, the disease cannot be confirmed by the usual method without stopping the medications for a substantial time, and this may not be acceptable to patients in whom PPIs have healed the esophagitis. A careful reexamination of the pretreatment symptoms may show that what the patient thought was GERD may have been something else, such as dyspepsia.

Acid-suppressive therapy is the cornerstone of GERD treatment. It provides excellent healing and relief of symptoms in patients with esophagitis or classic heartburn. The relief appears to be related directly to the degree of acid suppression achieved.

If symptoms resolve after an 8-week course of PPIs, an attempt should be made to discontinue PPI therapy. However, before therapy is discontinued, lifestyle modifications should be emphasized to the patient and the patient should implement them. Lifestyle modifications alone may produce remission in 25% of patients with symptoms, but only a few patients are compliant with the restrictions. Consequently, long-term maintenance therapy is needed for most patients since symptoms often recur when PPI therapy is discontinued. The same principles that apply to short-term therapy apply also to long-term therapy: Less acid equals less recurrence.

Proton Pump Inhibitors

PPIs are absorbed rapidly and taken up and concentrated preferentially in parietal cells. They irreversibly complex with the hydrogen-potassium-ATPase pump, which is the final step in acid production. To produce acid, parietal cells must form new pumps, a process that takes many hours. PPIs are more potent than histamine (H_2) blockers as suppressors of acid reflux. The healing of esophagitis and the relief of chronic symptoms occur more rapidly with PPIs than with H_2 blockers. With PPI therapy, esophagitis heals within 4 weeks in more than 80% of patients and in virtually 100% by 8 weeks. However, the rate of complete relief from symptoms is less than the rate of healing. Patients must understand that PPIs should be taken 30 to 60 minutes before meals and not with food or at bedtime.

In general, if GERD is causing bothersome symptoms, the initial step in treatment often involves use of PPIs to maximize the degree of acid suppression. It is well established that sometimes therapy can be gradually decreased successfully after treatment with a PPI or switched to on-demand therapy, but this is rarely suitable for patients with substantial complications of GERD.

Although routine doses of PPIs (eg, esomeprazole 40 mg daily, lansoprazole 30 mg daily, omeprazole 20 mg daily, pantoprazole 40 mg daily, and rabeprazole 20 mg daily) are adequate for most patients with GERD, some patients may require higher or more frequent dosing to suppress GERD completely. If patients do not have a response to a PPI, switching to another PPI may be reasonable. Data have demonstrated that standard PPI dosing may be limited by nocturnal breakthrough of gastric acid suppression. In patients with resultant nocturnal GERD symptoms, escalation of the PPI dose to twice daily or addition of a nighttime dose of an H_2 blocker can be considered.

Inadequate response to PPI therapy may be the result of differences in metabolism by cytochrome P450 2C19 isozyme or bioavailability. Optimal timing of PPI administration is also an important consideration because PPIs such as omeprazole are

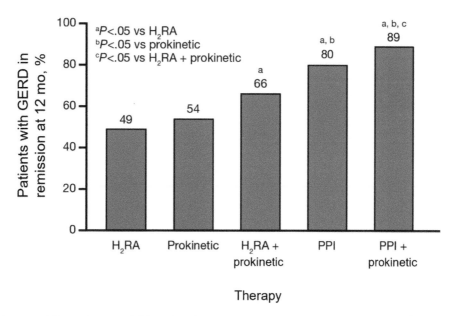

Figure 1.13. **Effectiveness of Proton Pump Inhibitors (PPIs).** PPIs are the most effective drugs for maintenance therapy of gastroesophageal reflux disease (GERD). Although the remission rate was slightly higher with PPI in combination with prokinetic therapy than with PPI alone, the difference was not significant. H_2RA indicates histamine-receptor antagonist. (Data from Vigneri S, Termini R, Leandro G, Badalamenti S, Pantalena M, Savarino V, et al. A comparison of five maintenance therapies for reflux esophagitis. N Engl J Med. 1995 Oct;333[17]:1106-10.)

most effective if the stomach parietal cells are stimulated. This is achieved by having patients eat within an hour after taking the medication. Variable-release PPIs that are now available can alter the pattern of release. They may be useful if stable preprandial dosing is not practical for a patient.

With maintenance PPI therapy, the rate of relapse of esophagitis is 20% or less, which is lower than with H_2 blockers (Figure 1.13). Also, maintenance PPI therapy is more effective than H_2 blockers in decreasing the need for redilatation in patients with reflux-associated benign strictures.

PPI therapy causes a clinically insignificant increase in the serum level of gastrin. However, no risk of carcinoid has been realized. The increase in serum levels of gastrin and parietal cell mass may lead to rebound acid secretion after the therapy is stopped.

Potential Adverse Effects of PPIs

It is well accepted that the benefits of PPIs, when medically indicated, outweigh their potential adverse effects. The most common adverse effects of PPIs include headache, abdominal pain, nausea, diarrhea, and constipation. Epidemiologic studies have raised the possibility of an association between PPI therapy and multiple potential adverse events, including osteoporosis, pneumonia, dementia, and chronic kidney insufficiency. However, by virtue of their retrospective design and use of large databases, these studies are limited by confounders that are amplified by statistically weak associations identified. Further, they are hampered by protopathic bias, the concept that the identified association is the result of the PPI being given in the context of the presumed adverse event and not precipitating it. For these reasons, current guidelines recommend long-term PPI use when clinically indicated without the need for routine monitoring.

H_2-Receptor Blockers

H_2-receptor blockers act by blocking the histamine-induced stimulation of gastric parietal cells. H_2 blockers provide moderate

benefit when given in moderate doses (eg, cimetidine 400 mg twice daily, famotidine 20 mg twice daily, nizatidine 150 mg twice daily, or ranitidine 150 mg twice daily) and heal esophagitis in 50% of patients. Higher doses suppress acid more rapidly. Lower doses are less effective, and nighttime-only dosing misses all the daytime reflux that predominates. A particular role for H_2 blockers may be to augment PPIs when given at night to block nocturnal acid breakthrough; however, tachyphylaxis may develop if H_2 blockade is used daily for more than 4 weeks.

Prokinetics

The idea that a motility disorder is the genesis of GERD made a prokinetic approach intellectually enticing. Drugs such as metoclopramide and, formerly, cisapride, which increase the tone of the LES and esophageal clearance and accelerate gastric emptying, have been used to treat reflux. However, the healing rate and safety of these drugs have been questioned. Cisapride has been effectively withdrawn from use in the US, and the long-term use of metoclopramide is associated with a risk of irreversible tardive dyskinesia, limiting its use in clinical practice. Further, evidence of the efficacy of prokinetics in the management of GERD is lacking. Drugs that target the TLESRs also have been used, including baclofen, which has been shown to reduce the total number of gastroesophageal reflux events, but its use in clinical practice is limited by its lack of tolerability.

> ✓ PPIs produce more acid suppression than H_2 blockers because they irreversibly complex with the hydrogen-potassium-ATPase pump rather than block histamine-induced stimulation of parietal cells alone
> ✓ Long-term use (>4 weeks) of daily H_2 blockers can result in tachyphylaxis or diminished effectiveness with successive dosing of the medication
> ✓ Unless they are indicated otherwise (eg, for gastroparesis), prokinetics should generally not be used in the treatment of GERD because of their adverse effect profile and limited efficacy

Refractory Reflux Disease

Refractory reflux disease can be defined as symptoms of GERD that are refractory to treatment with regular dosages of PPIs. The many common causes of refractory reflux symptoms are listed in Box 1.5. In patients with refractory reflux, PPI dosing and administration should first be optimized (taken ≥30 minutes before meals), and patient adherence to therapy should be assessed. If patients have negative results on a pH monitoring study while PPIs are being held, GERD is unlikely, and PPI therapy should be discontinued. In refractory cases when patients have persistent, bothersome symptoms despite having an initial evaluation, additional testing may be indicated, such as esophageal manometry to exclude a motility disorder (eg, achalasia) and EGD with biopsy (while PPIs are held) to exclude EoE. Other considerations for refractory reflux include nonesophageal conditions (eg,

---

Box 1.5. Causes of Refractory Reflux Symptoms in Patients Receiving Proton Pump Inhibitor Therapy

Incorrect initial diagnosis

    Nonreflux esophagitis—pill injury, skin diseases, eosinophilic esophagitis, infection

    Heart disease

    Chest wall pain

    Gastric pain

Additional diagnoses

    Dyspepsia

    Delayed gastric emptying

    Gastritis

    Peptic ulcer disease

    Nonulcer dyspepsia

Inadequate acid suppression

    Noncompliance

    Rapid metabolizers of proton pump inhibitors

    Dose timing

    Insufficient dose

    Zollinger-Ellison syndrome

    Nonacid reflux

Adenocarcinoma in Barrett esophagus

    Postoperative reflux

        Partial gastrectomy

        Vertical-banded gastroplasty

Esophageal dysmotility

    Spasm

    Achalasia

    Nutcracker esophagus

Functional chest pain

    Hypersensitive esophagus

    Somatic features of depression

    Functional heartburn

Free regurgitation

    Absence of lower esophageal sphincter tone

    Large hiatal hernia

    Achalasia

    Rumination

---

rumination or gastroparesis) or functional conditions (eg, functional heartburn).

> ✓ **Refractory reflux disease**—GERD symptoms that are refractory to treatment with PPIs

Functional Chest Pain

Many patients who describe having severe reflux often have very little reflux on 24-hour pH monitoring and have no endoscopic features of reflux. This condition has been termed *functional heartburn*. As with other functional gastrointestinal tract problems, female patients are overrepresented. Features of anxiety, panic, hyperventilation, and somatization may be clues to the diagnosis. Antacid therapies may help decrease the frequency of the symptoms, but they rarely relieve them completely. Therapies aimed at decreasing visceral hypersensitivity may be helpful (eg, a low dose of an antidepressant).

> ✓ **Functional heartburn**—a sensation of heartburn that has no correlation with esophageal acid exposure

Surgical and Endoscopic Antireflux Procedures

What is the role of laparoscopic and endoscopic methods of therapy? Medical therapy has been reduced to acid neutralization or suppression of acid production. Surgeons and endoscopists have focused on the role of the mechanical or functional failure of the antireflux barrier, and this has become the prime target of various approaches for preventing the reflux of gastric contents into the esophagus. However, most surgical and endoscopic antireflux procedures are considered irreversible, so patients must be selected carefully to maximize chances of long-term success without adverse outcomes.

For many years, antireflux surgery was performed through a transabdominal or transthoracic approach, but morbidity was considerable. Surgical treatment was reserved for intractable reflux that the available medical therapy could not cure.

With the advent of PPIs, even severe degrees of reflux could be well controlled, although the therapy can be expensive. With the advent of minimally invasive surgery, surgical treatment has had a renaissance. The laparoscopic antireflux procedure, namely Nissen fundoplication, has become a staple of the community surgeon, and outcomes are similar to those of the open approach. With well-chosen patients and experienced surgeons, a success rate of 80% to 90% is expected. The success rate decreases remarkably if patients have symptoms refractory to PPI therapy, patients have atypical symptoms other than heartburn or acid regurgitation, there is poor documentation of objective evidence of reflux disease, or the procedure is performed by less experienced surgeons. A substantial number of these patients resume taking acid-blocking medications after surgery, often for unclear reasons.

Preoperatively, it is important to verify that the patient's symptoms are indeed due to reflux. This is accomplished by documenting severe reflux esophagitis (LA grade C or D) and a response to PPI therapy or by confirming the pathologic degree of reflux with a 24-hour pH assessment while the patient is not receiving therapy. Patients who belch frequently should be informed that belching may not be possible after the operation and that gas bloat may result. Preoperative esophageal manometry should also be performed to rule out achalasia or an important motility disorder. It can identify a severe motility disturbance such as achalasia or connective tissue disease, and some surgeons want confirmation of a weak LES (if present).

Postoperatively, 20% of patients have some dysphagia, but this persists in only 5%. Gas bloat, diarrhea, and dyspepsia may occur or become more evident postoperatively and may be troubling to patients. As many as one-third of patients may still require PPI therapy postoperatively for persistent reflux or dyspepsia. Patients who have respiratory symptoms, free regurgitation, or simple but severe heartburn without gastric symptoms seem to have the best response to antireflux surgery. Female sex, lack of objective evidence of pathologic reflux, and failure to respond to PPI therapy all predict a poor response to surgery. Patient selection and operator experience appear to be the main determinants of a favorable surgical outcome. Reflux surgery is superior to long-term treatment with H_2 blockers to maintain the healing of GERD; however, follow-up for more than 10 years has shown an unexplained increase in mortality, predominantly due to cardiovascular disease, in the surgical group.

Newer surgical techniques, such as the use of a band consisting of multiple permanent magnets, have been developed and shown to have potential benefit. Magnetic sphincter augmentation helps to augment the LES with magnets. Implantation of the magnetic sphincter can be performed with laparoscopic or robotic techniques, but patients must be selected carefully to identify those that are most likely to benefit from the surgery. This procedure should be avoided in those with large hiatal hernias, severe esophagitis, Barrett esophagus, obesity (body mass index >35), and esophageal dysmotility.

In patients with both obesity and GERD who desire surgical management, Roux-en-Y gastric bypass can be helpful for both conditions. During this surgery, the creation of a small gastric pouch results in considerably less acid exposure to the esophagus. In patients with obesity, Nissen fundoplication alone risks poor outcomes, such as fundoplication disruption or herniation, due to continued elevated intra-abdominal pressure after surgery.

Patients Who Are Not Surgical Candidates

If a patient has symptoms that are refractory to PPIs, the wisdom of recommending surgical therapy should be reconsidered carefully. A hypersensitive esophagus or gastric dysmotility may be worse after fundoplication. Also, symptoms of irritable bowel syndrome may worsen postoperatively.

Endoscopic Methods of Therapy

Several endoscopic methods have been tried or are in development for the treatment of GERD. Endoscopic methods to alter the shape or to tighten the esophagogastric junction are in various stages of development. These consist of inserting sutures or other devices into the gastric wall to create a mechanical barrier to reflux (the barrier acts like a speed bump). Some endoscopic procedures are an attempt to replicate the mechanical barrier provided by fundoplication. Although some of these methods have been in clinical use, evidence for long-term efficacy is lacking.

Transoral incisionless fundoplication also requires upper endoscopy and creates a full-thickness, serosa-to-serosa plication and partial fundoplication with fastener fixations that extend longitudinally 3 cm and circumferentially 200° to 300°. For this procedure, patients should be selected carefully, and those with a large hiatal hernia, severe esophagitis, Barrett esophagus, or

motility disorder are not considered good candidates. The Stretta procedure requires upper endoscopy with radiofrequency energy delivered to the LES. This technique may be considered for patients who have chronic heartburn or regurgitation (or both), have a partial or complete response to acid-suppressive therapy, and have decided against surgical management. Patients who have large hiatal hernias, LES pressure that is very low, or poor response to acid suppression therapy are not good candidates for this procedure. Although early studies of these endoscopic procedures for management of GERD show promising results with good safety profiles, additional studies are necessary to understand the long-term clinical course after these procedures.

Eosinophilic Esophagitis

The most common cause of esophagitis has been acid reflux disease; however, since the late 1990s, a truly emerging disorder, EoE, has come to the fore. This typically occurs in adults with dysphagia and a history of food impaction. It occurs in young adults and children and more frequently in men than in women. In children, typical symptoms are vomiting and regurgitation in addition to dysphagia. Most patients with this disorder have a history of atopy or a family history of atopy. Many have other atopic illnesses, including allergic rhinitis and asthma. Many patients have identified reactions to foods, although this is documented better in children than in adults. In addition to the classic history of episodic dysphagia or food impaction, adults who present with EoE may or may not have symptoms suggestive of reflux disease.

Diagnosis

The diagnosis can be suspected endoscopically by finding concentric rings, linear fissures or furrows, edema, strictures, or white plaque in the esophagus (Figure 1.14). These may occur in the proximal, middle, or distal esophagus. Occasionally, abrupt fissuring or cracking of the esophageal mucosa is reported during endoscopy. Although this can be alarming, it rarely is associated with true esophageal perforation. Rare cases have been reported of Boerhaave syndrome (ie, spontaneous esophageal rupture) or dilatation-induced perforation. An esophagus with a normal appearance, however, does not rule out the possibility of EoE. Radiographic findings also can include concentric rings or so-called feline esophagus or tapered narrowing. The diagnosis is confirmed by examination of 6 to 8 biopsy samples from the esophagus. An increased number of eosinophils (>15 per high-power field) in the esophagus is required for diagnosis.

It has become apparent that *eosinophilia of the esophagus*, a more encompassing term than *EoE*, does not solely represent EoE; rather, this is a clinicopathologic condition that also requires symptoms of esophageal dysfunction for the diagnosis. In addition, patients with gastroesophageal reflux can also have esophageal mucosal eosinophilia that responds to vigorous acid blockade. In these patients, reflux is the primary cause of the eosinophilia and likely symptoms, and often the recommendation is to treat patients who have acid suppression and then retest them after 12 weeks of therapy. However, the diagnosis of EoE does not require an unsuccessful PPI treatment trial.

✓ **Eosinophilic esophagitis**—a common cause of dysphagia; diagnosis requires the finding of more than 15 eosinophils per high-power field on esophageal biopsies

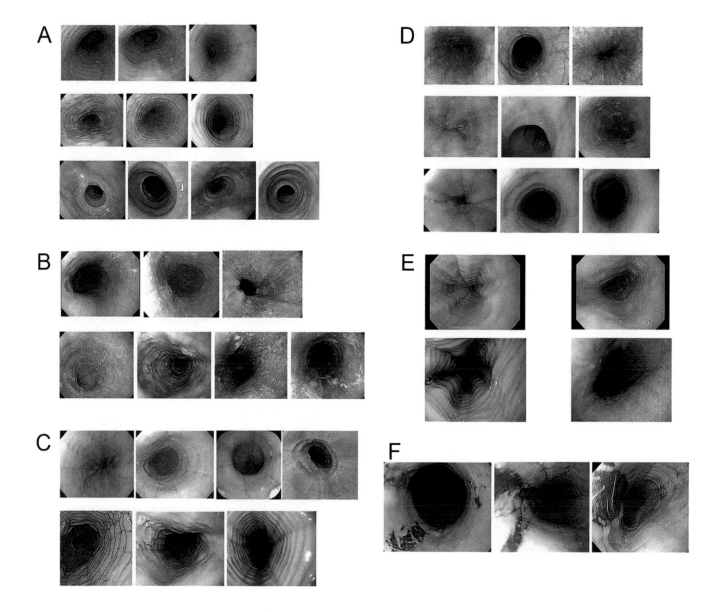

Figure 1.14.   Endoscopic Features of Eosinophilic Esophagitis Showing Spectrum of Severity. A, Fixed rings. Top row, Mild case shows subtle circumferential ridges with esophageal distention. Middle row, Moderate-severity case shows distinct rings that do not occlude passage of a diagnostic endoscope. Bottom row, Severe case shows distinct rings that do not permit passage of a diagnostic endoscope. B, Exudates. Upper row, Mild case has white lesions occupying less than 10% of the esophageal surface area. Lower row, Severe case has white lesions occupying 10% or more of the esophageal surface area. C, Furrows. Upper row, In this mild case, the vertical lines do not have visible depth. Lower row, In this severe case, the vertical lines are clearly indented into the mucosa. D, Edema. Top row, Normal findings include distinct vasculature. Middle row, Mild case shows decreased vascular clarity. Bottom row, In this severe case, the vessels cannot be appreciated. E, Transient rings. Two examples (upper row and lower row) show the esophagus without insufflation (images on left) and with insufflation (images on right). F, Crepe paper esophagus. (Adapted from Hirano I, Moy N, Heckman MG, Thomas CS, Gonsalves N, Achem SR. Endoscopic assessment of the oesophageal features of eosinophilic oesophagitis: validation of a novel classification and grading system. Gut. 2013 Apr;62[4]:489-95; used with permission.)

✓ EoE can be accompanied by various endoscopic findings, including rings, furrows, exudates, stricture, and edema; however, an esophagus with a normal appearance does not exclude the possibility of EoE

Treatment

Although treatment of EoE is often focused on symptomatic improvement, endoscopic and histologic remission should also be documented. The various treatment options include pharmacologic and nonpharmacologic therapies. PPIs, topical corticosteroids, and dupilumab are considered to be first-line pharmacologic therapies. Although all 3 therapies may be effective, PPIs are often used initially given their generally favorable side-effect profile and long track record. However, topical corticosteroids are generally also considered safe and are not accompanied by the adverse effects of systemic corticosteroids. Dupilumab, a monoclonal antibody that inhibits interleukin-4 and interleukin-13 signaling, has been shown to be effective and safe and is the first medication approved by the US Food and Drug Administration for EoE. However, where dupilumab fits in the treatment algorithm for EoE still needs to be fully established.

The mainstay of nonpharmacologic therapy is the 6-food elimination diet, whereby patients initially eliminate dairy products, wheat, eggs, soy, seafood, and nuts from their diet. More recently, 2-food and 4-food elimination diets have been proposed, which also show a favorable response rate, albeit lower than that observed with the 6-food elimination diet. In general, with elimination diets, the food items are eliminated for 6 to 8 weeks, and then the patient is evaluated with endoscopy and biopsies to monitor for histologic remission. If the eosinophil count has improved, the food items are slowly introduced 1 at a time (over 4-6 weeks), and follow-up endoscopy with biopsies is performed with the goal of identifying the food allergen(s).

The use of intermittent dilatation has also been supported, particularly in adults, although many physicians restrict the use of dilatation to dominant strictures that have resisted or have not responded to treatment with topical corticosteroids. Other agents, including experimental biologic therapies, have been tried with the hope of decreasing the infiltration of eosinophils, and several clinical trials are underway to identify other novel therapies.

The potential overlap between EoE and reflux esophagitis is considerable. Reflux esophagitis can be associated with occasional infiltration of eosinophils in the esophagus. In contrast, EoE is associated with at least 15 eosinophils per high-power field. Sampling variation may also be a consideration because in some patients, eosinophilic infiltration sometimes involves only specific locations. In general, biopsies should be taken from both the distal and the proximal or middle esophagus for evaluation of EoE.

Clinicians should be able to recognize the typical clinical scenario. For example, a young male patient who has a history of food impaction has concentric rings or fissuring in the esophagus in a radiographic or endoscopic image. The diagnosis is made by finding a substantial number of eosinophils (>15 per high-power field) in esophageal biopsy specimens (Figure 1.15).

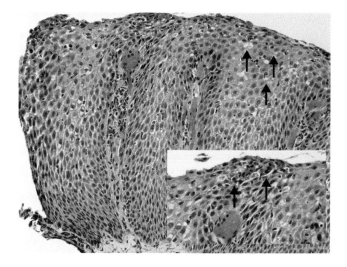

Figure 1.15. Hyperplastic Squamous Esophageal Epithelium. Many intraepithelial eosinophils are present (arrows). The superficial distribution is characteristic of eosinophilic esophagitis. Inset, A collection of eosinophils (arrows) is close to the surface (hematoxylin-eosin). (Courtesy of Thomas C. Smyrk, MD, Department of Laboratory Medicine and Pathology, Mayo Clinic, Rochester, Minnesota; used with permission.)

> ✓ Mainstay of treatment of EoE—PPIs, topical corticosteroids, and dietary therapy (6-food elimination diet); clinicians and patients should discuss these options and determine the best initial therapy
> ✓ Six-food elimination diet
> • Initial elimination of 6 food groups (dairy foods, wheat, eggs, soy, seafood, and nuts) for 6 to 8 weeks
> • After initial elimination period, reevaluation with upper endoscopy and biopsies
> • If eosinophil count has improved, food allergens are introduced individually
> • Subsequent upper endoscopy with biopsies is used to identify the culprit food allergen

Infectious Esophagitis

Infections are the third leading cause of esophagitis, behind reflux esophagitis and EoE. Patients with infectious esophagitis classically present with odynophagia. The most common causes include *Candida*, herpes simplex virus (HSV), and cytomegalovirus (CMV) (Figure 1.16). Infection with *Candida* is the most common cause of infectious esophagitis. The characteristic finding on endoscopy is thick, white plaques in the esophagus. Topical antifungals (eg, nystatin) are acceptable treatment of oropharyngeal candidiasis, but the mainstay of therapy for esophageal candidiasis is systemic antifungal therapy, typically with oral fluconazole.

While esophageal candidiasis and HSV esophagitis may be present in immunocompetent and immunocompromised patients, esophagitis secondary to CMV is generally present only in immunocompromised patients. The classic endoscopic and histologic appearance of HSV esophagitis is multiple, small lesions with a punched-out, volcano-like appearance and multinucleated giant cells with nuclear molding and nuclear chromatin. In contrast, the characteristic endoscopic and histologic findings of CMV esophagitis are linear, deeper ulcerations with nuclear and cytoplasmic inclusions known as owl's eyes. The mainstay of therapy is acyclovir for HSV esophagitis and ganciclovir for CMV esophagitis. Consultation with an ophthalmologist is also recommended to rule out CMV retinitis in these patients.

> ✓ Common causes of infectious esophagitis—*Candida*, HSV, and CMV
> ✓ Endoscopic and histologic findings in infectious esophagitis
> • Esophageal candidiasis—thick, white plaques
> • HSV esophagitis—multiple, small, punched-out ulcers with a volcano-like appearance; multinucleated giant cells
> • CMV esophagitis—linear, deeper ulcerations; owl's eyes cytoplasmic inclusions
> ✓ Treatment of infectious esophagitis
> • Esophageal candidiasis—systemic (not topical) antifungals
> • HSV esophagitis—acyclovir
> • CMV esophagitis—ganciclovir or valganciclovir

Pill-Induced Esophagitis

Pill-induced esophagitis is a common cause of odynophagia and dysphagia. Although many medications have been implicated with pill-induced esophagitis, commonly implicated medications include oral bisphosphonates, nonsteroidal anti-inflammatory drugs, potassium, iron, quinidine, and antibiotics such as tetracycline and clindamycin. The most common site of injury is the middle esophagus, which may be affected

Type of esophagitis	Pathologic findings
Candida	
HSV	
CMV	

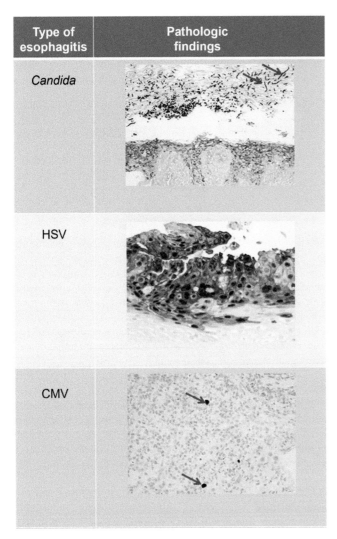

Figure 1.16. Infectious Esophagitis. Characteristic pathologic findings are shown for esophagitis caused by *Candida*, herpes simplex virus (HSV), and cytomegalovirus (CMV). Top, Grocott methenamine-silver stain shows numerous yeast forms, including pseudohyphae (arrows) consistent with *Candida* species. Middle, HSV immunohistochemical stain shows nuclear and granular cytoplasmic positivity in infected cells. Bottom, CMV immunohistochemical stain shows intranuclear and cytoplasmic positivity (arrows) in infected cells. (Adapted from Hoversten P, Kamboj AK, Katzka DA. Infections of the esophagus: an update on risk factors, diagnosis, and management. Dis Esophagus. 2018 Dec 1;31[12]; used with permission.)

by extrinsic compression from the aortic arch or left atrium, resulting in mild luminal narrowing and allowing for medication to lodge in this area. Most cases resolve within a few days with discontinued use of the medication. Rarely, strictures develop. When possible, use of culprit medications should be discontinued; otherwise, they should be taken with precautions. In general, potentially offending medications should be taken with at least 250 mL (about 8 oz) of water, and patients should sit in the upright position for a minimum of 30 minutes after taking the medication. While the diagnosis is primarily based clinically on the history and presence of a culprit medication, EGD may be considered if patients have severe or alarm symptoms or symptoms that last beyond 1 week after use of the medication was discontinued.

Suggested Reading

Chang KJ, Bell R. Transoral incisionless fundoplication. Gastrointest Endosc Clin N Am. 2020 Apr;30(2):267–89.

Dent J. Patterns of lower esophageal sphincter function associated with gastroesophageal reflux. Am J Med. 1997 Nov 24;103(5A):29S-32S.

DeVault KR, Castell DO; The Practice Parameters Committee of the American College of Gastroenterology. Updated guidelines for the diagnosis and treatment of gastroesophageal reflux disease. Am J Gastroenterol. 1999 Jun;94(6):1434–42.

Elliott EJ, Thomas D, Markowitz JE. Non-surgical interventions for eosinophilic esophagitis. Cochrane Database Syst Rev. 2010 Mar 17;(3):CD004065.

El-Serag HB, Sweet S, Winchester CC, Dent J. Update on the epidemiology of gastro-oesophageal reflux disease: a systematic review. Gut. 2014 Jun;63(6):871–80.

Fass R, Cahn F, Scotti DJ, Gregory DA. Systematic review and meta-analysis of controlled and prospective cohort efficacy studies of endoscopic radiofrequency for treatment of gastroesophageal reflux disease. Surg Endosc. 2017 Dec;31(12):4865–82.

Fletcher J, Wirz A, Young J, Vallance R, McColl KE. Unbuffered highly acidic gastric juice exists at the gastroesophageal junction after a meal. Gastroenterology. 2001 Oct;121(4):775–83.

Furuta GT, Katzka DA. Eosinophilic esophagitis. N Engl J Med. 2015 Oct 22;373(17):1640–8.

Furuta T, Ohashi K, Kosuge K, Zhao XJ, Takashima M, Kimura M, et al. CYP2C19 genotype status and effect of omeprazole on intragastric pH in humans. Clin Pharmacol Ther. 1999 May;65(5):552–61.

Ganz RA, Edmundowicz SA, Taiganides PA, Lipham JC, Smith CD, DeVault KR, et al. Long-term outcomes of patients receiving a magnetic sphincter augmentation device for gastroesophageal reflux. Clin Gastroenterol Hepatol. 2016 May;14(5):671–7.

Ganz RA, Peters JH, Horgan S, Bemelman WA, Dunst CM, Edmundowicz SA, et al. Esophageal sphincter device for gastroesophageal reflux disease. N Engl J Med. 2013 Feb 21;368(8):719–27.

Genval Workshop Report. An evidence-based appraisal of reflux disease management. Gut. 1999 Apr;44 Suppl 2:S1–16.

Gillen D, Wirz AA, Ardill JE, McColl KE. Rebound hypersecretion after omeprazole and its relation to on-treatment acid suppression and Helicobacter pylori status. Gastroenterology. 1999 Feb;116(2):239–47.

Gonsalves N. Dietary therapy for eosinophilic esophagitis. Gastroenterol Hepatol (N Y). 2015 Apr;11(4):267–76.

Gyawali CP, Kahrilas PJ, Savarino E, Zerbib F, Mion F, Smout AJPM, et al. Modern diagnosis of GERD: the Lyon Consensus. Gut. 2018 Jul;67(7):1351–62.

Hirano I, Dellon ES, Hamilton JD, Collins MH, Peterson K, Chehade M, et al. Efficacy of dupilumab in a phase 2 randomized trial of adults with active eosinophilic esophagitis. Gastroenterology. 2020 Jan;158(1):111–22.

Hirano I, Moy N, Heckman MG, Thomas CS, Gonsalves N, Achem SR. Endoscopic assessment of the oesophageal features of eosinophilic oesophagitis: validation of a novel classification and grading system. Gut. 2013 Apr;62(4):489–95.

Hogan WJ, Shaker R. Supraesophageal complications of gastroesophageal reflux. Dis Mon. Mar 2000;46(3):193–232.

Holtmann G, Cain C, Malfertheiner P. Gastric *Helicobacter pylori* infection accelerates healing of reflux esophagitis during treatment with the proton pump inhibitor pantoprazole. Gastroenterology. 1999 Jul;117(1):11–6.

Hoversten P, Kamboj AK, Katzka DA. Infections of the esophagus: an update on risk factors, diagnosis, and management. Dis Esophagus. 2018 Dec 1;31(12).

Kahrilas PJ, Shi G, Manka M, Joehl RJ. Increased frequency of transient lower esophageal sphincter relaxation induced by gastric distention in reflux patients with hiatal hernia. Gastroenterology. 2000 Apr;118(4):688–95.

Katz PO, Dunbar KB, Schnoll-Sussman FH, Greer KB, Yadlapati R, Spechler SJ. ACG clinical guideline for the diagnosis and management of gastroesophageal reflux disease. Am J Gastroenterol. 2022 Jan 1;117(1):27–56.

Katz PO, Gerson LB, Vela MF. Guidelines for the diagnosis and management of gastroesophageal reflux disease. Am J Gastroenterol. 2013 Mar;108(3):308–28.

Katzka DA. Eosinophilic esophagitis. Curr Opin Gastroenterol. 2006 Jul;22(4):429–32.

Katzka DA, Paoletti V, Leite L, Castell DO. Prolonged ambulatory pH monitoring in patients with persistent gastroesophageal reflux disease symptoms: testing while on therapy identifies the need for more aggressive anti-reflux therapy. Am J Gastroenterol. 1996 Oct;91(10):2110–3.

Klauser AG, Schindlbeck NE, Muller-Lissner SA. Symptoms in gastro-oesophageal reflux disease. Lancet. 1990 Jan 27;335(8683):205–8.

Klinkenberg-Knol EC, Nelis F, Dent J, Snel P, Mitchell B, Prichard P, et al. Long-term omeprazole treatment in resistant gastroesophageal reflux disease: efficacy, safety, and influence on gastric mucosa. Gastroenterology. 2000 Apr;118(4):661–9.

Labenz J, Jaspersen D, Kulig M, Leodolter A, Lind T, Meyer-Sabellek W, et al. Risk factors for erosive esophagitis: a multivariate analysis based on the ProGERD study initiative. Am J Gastroenterol. 2004 Sep;99(9):1652–6.

Locke GR, 3rd, Talley NJ, Fett SL, Zinsmeister AR, Melton LJ, 3rd. Prevalence and clinical spectrum of gastroesophageal reflux: a population-based study in Olmsted County, Minnesota. Gastroenterology. May 1997;112(5):1448–56.

Orlando RC. Why is the high grade inhibition of gastric acid secretion afforded by proton pump inhibitors often required for healing of reflux esophagitis? An epithelial perspective. Am J Gastroenterol. Sep 1996;91(9):1692–6.

Peery AF, Crockett SD, Murphy CC, Jensen ET, Kim HP, Egberg MD, et al. Burden and cost of gastrointestinal, liver, and pancreatic diseases in the United States: update 2021. Gastroenterology. 2022 Feb;162(2):621–44.

Richter JE, Rubenstein JH. Presentation and epidemiology of gastroesophageal reflux disease. Gastroenterology. 2018 Jan;154(2):267–76.

Shaheen NJ, Falk GW, Iyer PG, Souza RF, Yadlapati RH, Sauer BG, et al. Diagnosis and management of Barrett's esophagus: an updated ACG guideline. Am J Gastroenterol. 2022 Apr 1;117(4):559–87.

Shay S, Tutuian R, Sifrim D, Vela M, Wise J, Balaji N, et al. Twenty-four hour ambulatory simultaneous impedance and pH monitoring: a multicenter report of normal values from 60 healthy volunteers. Am J Gastroenterol. 2004 Jun;99(6):1037–43.

Stanghellini V. Three-month prevalence rates of gastrointestinal symptoms and the influence of demographic factors: results from the Domestic/International Gastroenterology Surveillance Study (DIGEST). Scand J Gastroenterol Suppl. 1999;231:20–8.

Tobey NA. How does the esophageal epithelium maintain its integrity? Digestion. 1995;56 Suppl 1:45–50.

Tobey NA. Systemic factors in esophageal mucosal protection. Digestion. 1995;56 Suppl 1:38–44.

Trad KS, Fox MA, Simoni G, Shughoury AB, Mavrelis PG, Raza M, et al. Transoral fundoplication offers durable symptom control for chronic GERD: 3-year report from the TEMPO randomized trial with a crossover arm. Surg Endosc. 2017 Jun;31(6):2498–508.

Triadafilopoulos G. Stretta: a valuable endoscopic treatment modality for gastroesophageal reflux disease. World J Gastroenterol. 2014 Jun 28;20(24):7730–8.

Vakil N, Kahrilas P, Magner D, Skammer W, Levine J. Does baseline Hp status impact erosive esophagitis (EE) healing rates? [Abstract]. Am J Gastroenterol. 2000;95(9):2438–9.

Vigneri S, Termini R, Leandro G, Badalamenti S, Pantalena M, Savarino V, et al. A comparison of five maintenance therapies for reflux esophagitis. N Engl J Med. 1995 Oct 26;333(17):1106–10.

Wise JL, Murray JA. Utilising multichannel intraluminal impedance for diagnosing GERD: a review. Dis Esophagus. 2007;20(2):83–8.

Wu ZH, Yang XP, Niu X, Xiao XY, Chen X. The relationship between obstructive sleep apnea hypopnea syndrome and gastroesophageal reflux disease: a meta-analysis. Sleep Breath. 2019 Jun;23(2):389–97.

Zografos GN, Georgiadou D, Thomas D, Kaltsas G, Digalakis M. Drug-induced esophagitis. Dis Esophagus. 2009;22(8):633–7.

2

Barrett Esophagus and Esophageal Cancer

PRASAD G. IYER, MD

KORNPONG VANTANASIRI, MD

Barrett Esophagus

Definitions

Barrett esophagus (BE) is an acquired condition characterized by the replacement of the squamous epithelium lining the esophagus by partially intestinalized columnar epithelium. It is thought to be a complication of gastroesophageal reflux and may reflect an adaptive response to reflux of gastric contents into the esophagus. It is the strongest known risk factor for esophageal adenocarcinoma (EAC) and increases the risk of EAC by 30- to 50-fold. Endoscopic and pathologic criteria must be met to make the diagnosis of BE.

The endoscopic criterion is the presence of columnar-appearing mucosa in the tubular esophagus (Figure 2.1), extending at least 1 cm above the proximal extent of the gastric folds, which is the anatomical landmark for the esophagogastric junction (EGJ). A population-based study from Olmsted County, Minnesota, published in 2011, showed that patients with specialized intestinal metaplasia of the EGJ have a significantly lower risk for EAC compared with patients who have BE. The most commonly used endoscopic grading system for BE, the Prague C & M criteria, was developed to help promote the use of standardized reporting systems to uniformly determine the endoscopic length and appearance of BE with good interobserver agreement.

The pathologic criterion is the presence of intestinal metaplasia with goblet cells (ie, specialized intestinal metaplasia) in the endoscopic biopsy specimens (Figure 2.2). This criterion is based on evidence that columnar metaplasia with goblet cells in the esophagus is associated with an increased risk of progression to esophageal adenocarcinoma.

BE has been classified into *long-segment BE* (length of visible columnar mucosa in the esophagus ≥3 cm) and *short-segment BE* (length of visible columnar mucosa in the esophagus <3 cm). *Intestinal metaplasia of the cardia* or *intestinal metaplasia of the EGJ* refers to the histologic finding of intestinal metaplasia with goblet cells at a squamocolumnar junction in the normal location and with a normal appearance (Figure 2.3). Given this distinction, a normal-appearing and normally located squamocolumnar junction should not be biopsied.

> ✓ Diagnosis of BE—endoscopic evidence of at least 1 cm of columnar mucosa in the tubular esophagus *and* histopathologic evidence of intestinal metaplasia with goblet cells on biopsy specimens

Pathophysiology

BE is thought to be a reparative response to the epithelial damage caused by chronic reflux of gastric contents into the distal esophagus. In the US, approximately 10% of patients with chronic gastroesophageal reflux symptoms have evidence of BE on endoscopy. Patients who have BE have longer durations of esophageal acid exposure, larger hiatal hernias, decreased lower esophageal sphincter pressures, evidence of decreased esophageal motility, and decreased esophageal sensitivity to acid reflux compared with patients who do not have gastroesophageal reflux and those who have gastroesophageal reflux but without

Abbreviations: BE, Barrett esophagus; BMI, body mass index; CT, computed tomography; EAC, esophageal adenocarcinoma; EGJ, esophagogastric junction; EMR, endoscopic mucosal resection; ESD, endoscopic submucosal dissection; GERD, gastroesophageal reflux disease; HGD, high-grade dysplasia; LGD, low-grade dysplasia; PET, positron emission tomography; RFA, radiofrequency ablation; SCC, squamous cell carcinoma

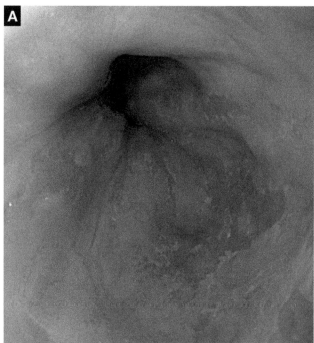

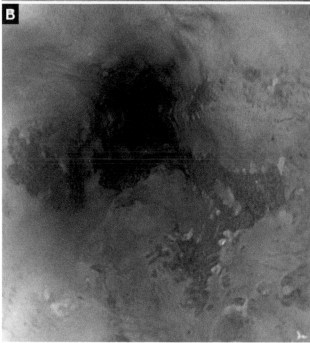

Figure 2.1. Endoscopic Appearance of Barrett Esophagus. A, Columnar mucosa in the distal esophagus is shown with white light imaging. B, This corresponding image was obtained with narrow band imaging (tongues and islands of pink mucosa are present amid pale white squamous mucosa).

BE. Control of acid reflux (when documented with ambulatory pH studies) in patients with BE is more difficult than in patients without BE. Resolution of acid reflux symptoms correlates poorly with control of acid reflux in patients with BE. Persistent acid reflux (documented with 24-hour pH studies) occurs in 26% to 40% of patients with BE who are asymptomatic while receiving proton pump inhibitor therapy. Predictors of persistent acid reflux despite symptom control in patients with BE are not well described.

Epidemiology

An autopsy study from Olmsted County, Minnesota, published in 1990 documented that the prevalence of long-segment BE in Olmsted County was 376 cases per 100,000 population. This study also highlighted that the prevalence of long-segment BE when assessed by autopsy was almost 20-fold the prevalence when assessed by clinically indicated endoscopy (22 cases per 100,000 population), indicating that most cases of BE in the community are not diagnosed.

Data from 2 population-based studies from Europe have shed additional light on the population prevalence of BE. In a Swedish study, 1,000 participants living in 2 counties underwent endoscopy; 16 of the participants (prevalence, 1.6%) were identified as having BE (with endoscopic evidence of columnar mucosa in the esophagus and histologic confirmation of intestinal metaplasia). The prevalence of BE in those with symptomatic reflux (2.3%) and those without (1.8%) was not statistically different. In a second study, performed in Italy, 1,033 participants with and without reflux symptoms had endoscopy and 1.3% were found to have BE. The generalizability of these study estimates to the US is not clear. In both studies the prevalence of BE may have been underestimated because of the low rate of confirmation of intestinal metaplasia in patients with endoscopically suspected BE; this may have been due to differences in the number and size of biopsy specimens. In addition, the threshold of the length of suspected BE for biopsy acquisition was not specified. Compared with the US population, the population studied was younger and had a higher prevalence of *Helicobacter pylori* infection (37%) and a lower prevalence of obesity (only 16% had a body mass index [BMI] >30 [calculated as weight in kilograms divided by height in meters squared]).

A recent systematic review and meta-analysis reported that the prevalence of BE was 0.8% in low-risk populations overall and slightly higher (1.1%) in Western populations. The prevalence increases with the increasing number of additional risk factors, such as age older than 50 years, male sex, gastroesophageal reflux disease (GERD), family history of BE or EAC, and obesity.

Different studies have reported that the incidence of the diagnosis of BE is increasing in conjunction with the increasing incidence of EAC both in older patients and in younger patients (<50 years old). A recent study showed that the incidence of young-onset EAC has been rapidly increasing, and patients have been presenting with more advanced stages. A study from Olmsted County, Minnesota, showed a parallel increase in the number of endoscopic examinations performed (Figure 2.4). However, a study from Europe showed that the increase in the incidence of BE persisted even after adjustment for the number of endoscopic examinations.

Risk Factors

Age

BE is an acquired disorder. The prevalence of long-segment BE increases with age, particularly after the fifth decade. The mean age at the time of clinical diagnosis was 63 years in 1 population-based study. Long-segment BE is rare in children.

Male Sex

BE is more prevalent among male patients. In a Mayo Clinic study of patients who had endoscopy between 1976 and 1989, long-segment BE was twice as common in male patients as in

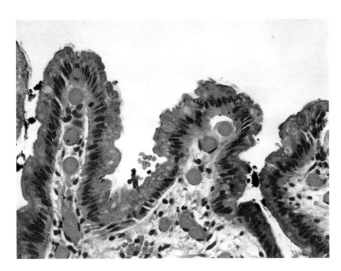

Figure 2.2. Intestinal Metaplasia With Goblet Cells. (Hematoxylin-eosin, original magnification ×400.)

female patients. This finding has been corroborated in other studies as well. In a large multicenter Italian study (patients were enrolled from 1987-1989), BE was 2.6 times more common in male patients than in female patients. In the 2005 Swedish population-based study, the male to female ratio of biopsy-proven BE was 1.5:1.

Geography and Ethnicity

BE has been described frequently in countries in North America, Europe, and Australia, but it appears to be less common in other countries, such as Japan. However, recent reports from China, Singapore, and other Asian countries have appeared. In a recent single-center US retrospective cross-sectional cohort study of 2,100 people (11.8% Black, 22.2% Hispanic, and 37.7% White) who had endoscopy from 2005 to 2006, White persons (6.1%) were more likely to have BE of any length than Black (1.6%, $P=$ .004) or Hispanic persons (1.7%, P <.001).

Reflux Symptoms

BE has been described in 2% to 20% of patients with symptoms of gastroesophageal reflux (higher estimates are from referral center studies and lower estimates are from population-based studies). The duration of reflux symptoms (>5-10 years, compared with shorter durations) appears to predict the presence of BE better than the severity or frequency of symptoms. Short-segment BE is twice as prevalent as long-segment BE in patients with reflux symptoms. However, it is important to note that a substantial proportion of patients with BE (as many as 40%-50%) do not have frequent symptoms of gastroesophageal reflux. Recent studies have reported that the association of reflux symptoms with BE is strong for long-segment BE and weak for short-segment BE.

Obesity

The association of BMI with BE has been investigated by multiple authors, but the results have been conflicting (some studies have shown an association with increased BMI and others have not). A systematic review clarified this: BMI was not significantly different between patients with BE and controls with GERD, but it was higher for patients with BE than for healthy controls. This led the authors to conclude that increased BMI may contribute to an increased risk of BE by causing increased gastroesophageal reflux, but it may not increase the risk of BE in patients with GERD. In addition, the strong male and White predominance of BE and esophageal carcinoma is not explained by increasing obesity (as measured by BMI), which afflicts both sexes and all ethnic groups.

Visceral adiposity (in contrast to BMI as a measure of overall adiposity) may provide a better explanation for the male and White predilection of BE. The distribution of body fat is more visceral than truncal in groups at high-risk for BE (male and

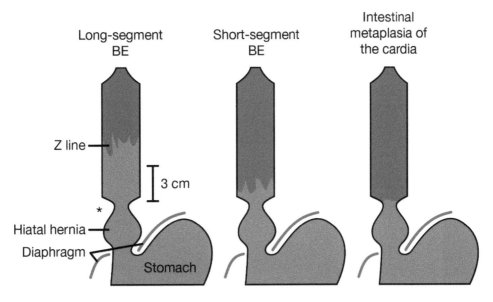

Figure 2.3. **Barrett Esophagus (BE) Compared With Intestinal Metaplasia of the Cardia.** Patients with long-segment or short-segment BE have columnar mucosa extending into the tubular esophagus. Biopsy specimens show intestinal metaplasia with goblet cells. If intestinal metaplasia with goblet cells is found at a normally located Z line, the patient has intestinal metaplasia of the cardia, which confers a lower cancer risk. Asterisk indicates end of tubular esophagus and beginning of stomach.

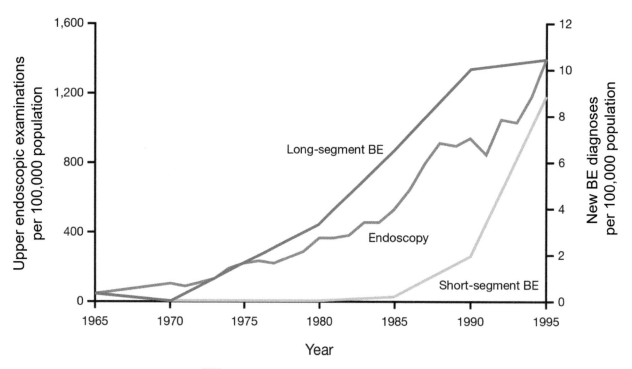

Figure 2.4. Incidence of Diagnosed Barrett Esophagus (BE) and Number of Upper Endoscopic Examinations Performed Annually in Residents of Olmsted County, Minnesota, From 1965 to 1995. (Adapted from Conio M, Cameron AJ, Romero Y, Branch CD, Schleck CD, Burgart LJ, et al. Secular trends in the epidemiology and outcome of Barrett's oesophagus in Olmsted County, Minnesota. Gut. 2001 Mar;48[3]:304-9; used with permission.)

White) compared to others (female and Black). Also, abdominal diameter (independent of BMI) is associated with symptoms of gastroesophageal reflux in White persons but not in Black or Asian persons. Several authors have reported an association between visceral adiposity (measured as waist circumference) and BE. A population-based case-control study found an association between increased waist circumference and the diagnosis of BE, independent of BMI (odds ratio, 2.24), when compared with population controls. This study reported an increased risk for persons with a waist circumference greater than 80 cm. The study did not find an association between BMI and BE. Another clinic-based case-control study reported that an increased waist to hip ratio, a measure of central adiposity, was associated with the diagnosis of BE (odds ratio, 2.8). The association between BMI and BE was attenuated when both waist to hip ratio and BMI were modeled together. This association is strengthened further by studies that found that abdominal obesity (measured by waist circumference) is associated with increased postprandial intragastric pressure, disruption of the EGJ (leading to the formation of hiatal hernia), and increased transient lower esophageal sphincter relaxations in the postprandial state. A reflux-independent systemic effect of abdominal fat on esophageal inflammation and neoplasia has been postulated, mediated by proinflammatory factors, adipokines produced by visceral fat, and insulin or insulin growth factors.

Family History

Familial aggregation of BE and esophageal adenocarcinoma has been reported in multiple studies. Studies have reported the presence of confirmed BE or esophageal adenocarcinoma in first- or second-degree relatives in 7% of probands with BE or esophageal adenocarcinoma. Increased prevalence of reflux

symptoms in relatives of probands with BE or esophageal adenocarcinoma has been reported, although data are not definitive for an increased risk of BE in relatives of probands with BE. BE is probably a complex genetic disease influenced by environmental factors. Research into identifying gene loci that may influence the risk of BE is continuing.

Cigarette Smoking

Several studies have shown that cigarette smoking is a strong risk factor for BE and significantly increases the risk of progression of BE to EAC. A study analyzing data from the Barrett's and Esophageal Adenocarcinoma Consortium showed that cigarette smoking is a risk factor for BE, and the association strengthened with increased smoking exposure. Another population-based study (from Northern Ireland) showed that tobacco smoking doubled the risk of progression of BE to high-grade dysplasia (HGD) or EAC, compared to patients with BE who were nonsmokers.

Intestinal Metaplasia of the Cardia or EGJ

In various studies, the prevalence of intestinal metaplasia of the EGJ has been reported to range from 6% to 15%. Compared with patients who have BE, patients with intestinal metaplasia appear to have a lower prevalence of reflux symptoms, no evidence of male predominance, and a higher prevalence of *H pylori* infection. Also, the prevalence of dysplasia among patients with intestinal metaplasia of the EGJ has been reported to be lower than that among patients with BE. The natural history of intestinal metaplasia of the EGJ was described in 2 studies, which found substantially lower rates of prevalent or incident dysplasia among patients who had intestinal metaplasia of the EGJ compared with patients who had BE. However, because intestinal metaplasia is more common than BE, it is likely that the rate of progression to adenocarcinoma would be much lower than for patients with BE.

Cancer Risk

Among patients with BE, the rate of progression to esophageal adenocarcinoma in the absence of prevalent dysplasia was estimated to be 5 to 6 per 1,000 patient-years of follow-up. More recent European studies have reported a lower risk of progression, and a recent meta-analysis reported that the risk of progression in patients with nondysplastic BE was 3.3 per 1,000 patient-years of follow-up. The risk of progression in patients with low-grade dysplasia (LGD) is debated, with estimates ranging from 0.6% to 1.2% per year. A recent meta-analysis reported that the rate of progression to esophageal adenocarcinoma in persons with LGD was 16.98 per 1,000 person-years compared with 5.98 per 1,000 person-years for persons with no dysplasia, although there was considerable heterogeneity between the studies. The estimated rate of progression among patients with HGD is the highest: 65.8 per 1,000 patient-years of follow-up.

Screening

Screening for BE in patients with symptomatic gastroesophageal reflux or in the general population is a matter of controversy. However, there is growing evidence and support from major gastrointestinal societies to consider BE screening in high-risk patients with multiple risk factors. Endoscopic evaluation of patients thought to be at high risk for BE may be considered on an individual basis after discussing the pros and cons with patients. Arguments in favor of screening include the large number of undiagnosed cases of BE in the community and the progression of BE from gastroesophageal reflux to metaplasia, dysplasia, and adenocarcinoma (which can be detected at an early stage with a screening and surveillance program). Furthermore, retrospective studies have found that adenocarcinomas diagnosed in surveillance programs were earlier-stage adenocarcinomas and were associated with improved survival compared with adenocarcinomas diagnosed after the onset of symptoms. However, arguments against screening include the following: The presence of symptomatic gastroesophageal reflux has poor accuracy for predicting or excluding the absence of BE on endoscopy, surveillance poses challenges, and there is a lack of strong prospective evidence that screening and surveillance may improve survival of patients who have esophageal adenocarcinoma.

Current American College of Gastroenterology guidelines suggest that BE screening should be considered for patients who have chronic GERD (>5 years) or frequent gastroesophageal reflux symptoms (at least weekly) and at least 3 risk factors (male sex, White race, age >50 years, central obesity, current or past history of cigarette smoking, and confirmed history of BE or EAC in a first-degree relative). For female patients, the yield from BE screening may be low because they have a significantly lower risk of EAC, but screening can be considered, after a discussion of the risks and benefits, if they have multiple risk factors.

Conventional high-definition upper endoscopy is the gold standard for screening and diagnosis of BE. However, the use of novel minimally invasive screening methods may make screening high-risk populations more accessible and cost-effective. Several options are available, such as unsedated transnasal endoscopy and swallowable esophageal cell collection devices (encapsulated polyurethane foam spheres and inflatable balloons) in combination with biomarkers (trefoil factor 3 or methylated DNA markers). A recent randomized trial demonstrated substantially higher rates of BE detection with the use of a swallowable cell collection device in combination with a protein biomarker. Analysis of exhaled volatile organic compounds may have a potential role in BE screening.

✓ Endoscopic screening for BE should be considered for patients who have chronic reflux symptoms and at least 3 risk factors (age >50 years, male sex, White race, central obesity, current or past history of smoking, and family history of BE or EAC)
✓ Endoscopic screening after only 1 negative endoscopic evaluation is not recommended
✓ Patients with erosive esophagitis (Los Angeles grade B, C, or D) should have another endoscopic evaluation after 8 to 12 weeks of proton pump inhibitor therapy to assess for underlying BE and healing of esophagitis

---

Surveillance

Surveillance of patients with known BE is endorsed by all major gastrointestinal societies. The goal of surveillance is the early detection of dysplasia or carcinoma so that therapeutic intervention may be applied to improve patient outcomes. Surveillance has several limitations, including the following:

1. Poor interobserver agreement between pathologists on the grade of dysplasia (particularly LGD)
2. Variable natural predictive value of dysplasia, with variable progression rates reported for different cohorts for the same grade of dysplasia
3. Patchy and subtle distribution of advanced dysplasia, so that sampling error is likely during surveillance

Despite these limitations, the grade of dysplasia (no dysplasia, LGD, or HGD) is the primary clinical risk-stratification tool (Figure 2.5). Patients with long-segment BE and patients with short-segment BE should undergo similar surveillance because the primary predictor of progression is the grade of dysplasia.

Surveillance should be offered to patients with reasonable life expectancy so that therapy for progression (if detected) would be tolerated and would benefit the patient. Optimization of the acid-suppressive regimen titrated to control symptoms and to heal esophagitis should be undertaken to minimize confounding the interpretation of dysplasia grade by reactive atypia (which can occur from inflammation caused by uncontrolled reflux). Diagnoses of LGD and HGD should be confirmed by expert gastrointestinal pathologists because community pathologists may tend to overcall LGD (and report false-positive results). There is some evidence that the risk of progression in patients with LGD confirmed by expert gastrointestinal pathologists may be higher.

Surveillance biopsies should be performed after careful inspection of the segment of BE with high-resolution endoscopy to identify any visible lesions that may indicate a higher grade of dysplasia. The use of narrow band imaging (Figure 2.1B) or other imaging techniques that enhance superficial mucosal and vascular patterns may improve detection rates of focal abnormalities (such as nodules and ulcers) and advanced dysplasia. These areas should be biopsied separately and sent for histopathologic study in specifically labeled bottles. The remaining BE mucosa should be biopsied in a 4-quadrant manner every 2 cm, with tissue being submitted in separate bottles at each 2-cm level. For patients with HGD, surveillance should be

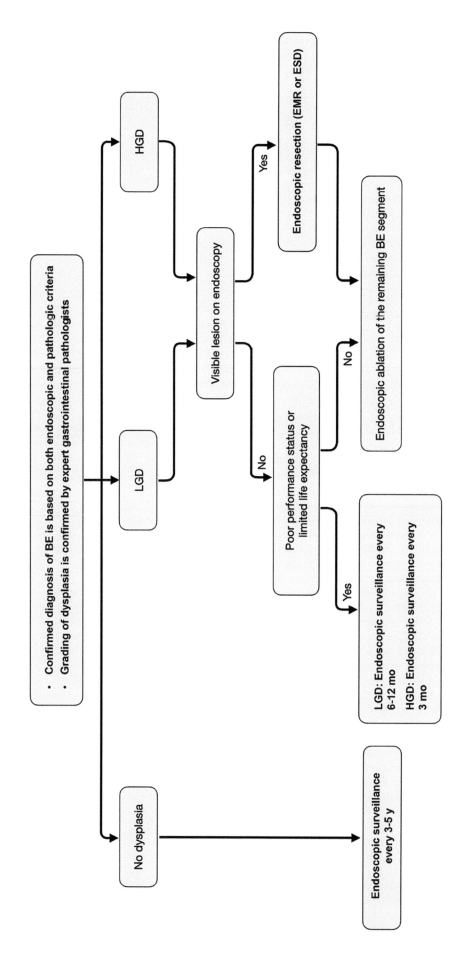

Figure 2.5. Algorithm for Management of Nondysplastic and Dysplastic Barrett Esophagus (BE). EMR indicates endoscopic mucosal resection; ESD, endoscopic submucosal dissection; HGD, high-grade dysplasia; LGD, low-grade dysplasia.

performed every 1 cm in a 4-quadrant fashion to exclude prevalent carcinoma.

No Dysplasia and LGD

Patients with no dysplasia should undergo endoscopic surveillance every 3 to 5 years to exclude prevalent dysplasia. Patients with LGD (Figure 2.6) should have the diagnosis of LGD confirmed by a pathologist who has expertise in BE pathology. If LGD is confirmed, endoscopic ablation should be considered as a first-line treatment option. In a multicenter randomized control trial from Europe, endoscopic ablation significantly decreased the rate of neoplastic progression to HGD or EAC over a 3-year follow-up period. However, endoscopic surveillance every 6 to 12 months is also an acceptable strategy, particularly for patients who have poor performance status or life-limiting comorbidities. If no dysplasia is detected in 2 successive years, the surveillance frequency can be changed to every 3 to 5 years. The natural history of LGD is somewhat

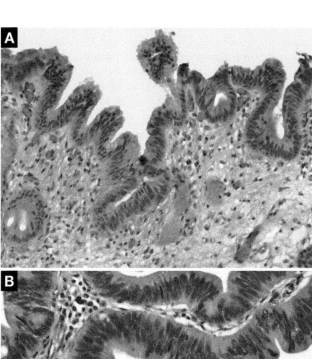

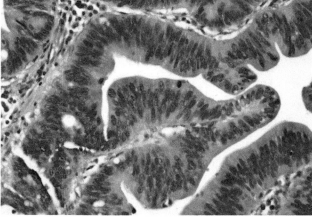

Figure 2.6. Low-Grade Dysplasia in Barrett Esophagus. A, Nuclei show evidence of stratification; they are longer, darker, and more crowded than when dysplasia is absent (Figure 2.2) (hematoxylin-eosin, original magnification ×200). B, Nuclei retain polarity toward the basement membrane and are not pleomorphic (hematoxylin-eosin, original magnification ×400). (Courtesy of Jason T. Lewis, MD, Department of Laboratory Medicine and Pathology, Mayo Clinic, Rochester, Minnesota; used with permission.)

variable and is characterized, in most cases, by reversion to no dysplasia or stability at LGD.

High-Grade Dysplasia

If HGD is detected (Figure 2.7), it should be confirmed by an expert gastrointestinal pathologist because therapeutic decisions may need to be made on the basis of the confirmation. In a multicenter randomized study for photodynamic therapy, the diagnosis of HGD made by a community pathologist was overruled by an expert pathologist in two-thirds of cases.

Diagnosis should be followed by careful endoscopic evaluation, with the use of high-resolution or high-definition endoscopes (with dye-based or virtual chromoendoscopy and the use of techniques such as narrow band imaging), to assess for the presence of any visual abnormality. Also, endoscopic ultrasonography may be performed to exclude the presence of a coexisting invasive neoplasm (which may be present in 10%-12% of patients treated with esophagectomy). Any visible lesion should be removed by endoscopic resection. Endoscopic resection techniques include cap-assisted endoscopic mucosal resection (EMR) and endoscopic submucosal dissection (ESD).

In EMR, a submucosal injection is used to lift a mucosal lesion that is then resected by use of either a plastic cap with a snare or band ligation with subsequent snare excision. The technique allows precise staging of the depth of invasion into the mucosa or submucosa (with better interobserver agreement between pathologists in grading dysplasia than with biopsies) and the assessment of margins, and it may be therapeutic if lateral and deep margins are clear (Figure 2.8). Studies have shown that EMR of visible lesions may show that the grade of dysplasia is higher in as many as 30% of patients with HGD.

In ESD, specialized endoscopic knives are used to dissect the lesion in the submucosal plane after being lifted with submucosal injection. ESD is recommended for larger lesions (>15 mm), for lesions that may be invading the submucosa, and for lesions with fibrosis. ESD has been shown to achieve a substantially higher rate of en bloc and histologic resection compared to EMR, but ESD requires a steep learning curve and carries a higher complication rate.

Options for the management of HGD can be divided into 2 approaches:

1. *Endoscopic eradication therapy* includes EMR or ESD to remove any visible lesions with subsequent ablation of the remaining segment of BE. Ablation is based on the concept that destruction of the metaplastic mucosa, with subsequent control of reflux, leads to regrowth of squamous epithelium. Several published studies have shown comparable outcomes for patients treated endoscopically or surgically. Treatment options for ablation include *radiofrequency ablation* (RFA), which involves the use of thermal energy delivered with balloon-based and over-the-scope catheters to destroy BE mucosa. It is the most commonly used ablation modality for treatment of dysplastic BE. In a randomized controlled trial, RFA was found to be superior to sham procedure in eliminating dysplasia and metaplasia at 1 year and in decreasing the risk of progression to EAC. Multiple studies have reported variable rates of recurrent intestinal metaplasia after successful ablation. Other techniques such as cryotherapy, which involves the use of cryogens (liquid nitrogen and carbon dioxide) to damage the metaplastic mucosa, are being studied as alternatives, with preliminary observational reports showing efficacy comparable to that of RFA.

2. *Endoscopic surveillance* involves careful endoscopic evaluation every 3 months, with surveillance biopsy samples taken at every centimeter along the segment of BE. If a focal abnormality

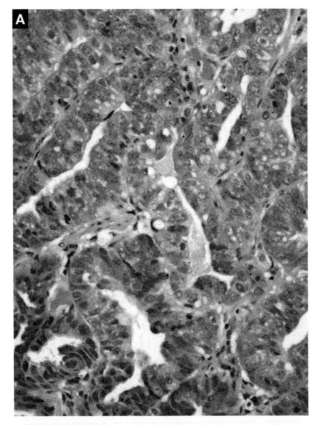

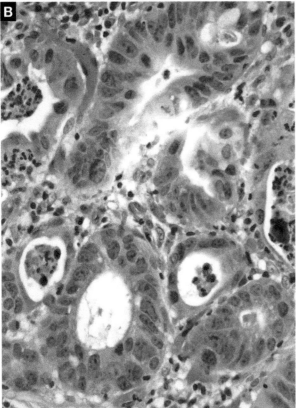

Figure 2.7.   High-Grade Dysplasia in Barrett Esophagus. A, Nuclei are rounded and oriented haphazardly (not perpendicular to basement membrane), unlike in low-grade dysplasia (Figure 2.6). B, Nuclei are pleomorphic (ie, with different shapes and sizes) (hematoxylin-eosin, original magnification ×400). (Courtesy of Jason T. Lewis, MD, Department of Laboratory Medicine and Pathology, Mayo Clinic, Rochester, Minnesota; used with permission.)

is visualized, the patient undergoes additional EMR or ESD. This option is reserved for patients with limited life expectancy.

✓ Patients with reasonable life expectancy who have dysplastic BE (confirmed by an expert gastrointestinal pathologist) should undergo endoscopic resection (with EMR or ESD) of all visible lesions and subsequent endoscopic ablation of residual flat BE mucosa
✓ Goal of endoscopic eradication therapy—complete eradication of all intestinal metaplasia

---

Risk Stratification of BE

The histologic finding of dysplasia (LGD or HGD) is the best clinical tool for identifying patients at risk for progression to EAC. However, it is challenging to predict the trajectory of neoplastic progression on the basis of the histologic grade of dysplasia alone in a real-world practice setting, given that in some patients HGD does not progress to EAC. To help bridge this gap, risk stratification tools have been developed on the basis of clinical parameters (eg, male sex, cigarette smoking, older age, and length of BE segment). Moreover, the use of clinical biomarkers to determine the risk of progression to EAC in patients with BE has been studied and has shown potential to improve risk stratification of patients with BE. One of the most studied biomarkers for BE is p53 oncoprotein. Aberrant expression of p53 oncoprotein is associated with increased risk of neoplastic progression in patients with BE.

Esophageal Cancer

Epidemiology

Squamous cell carcinoma (SCC) (Figure 2.9A) and adenocarcinoma (Figure 2.9B) are the most common types of esophageal cancer. Esophageal carcinoma is the seventh leading cause of death in the world. SCC accounts for most cases of esophageal cancer throughout the world and is more common in Asia and resource-limited countries; esophageal adenocarcinoma is more common in industrialized countries.

In the US, approximately 18,000 cases of esophageal carcinoma are diagnosed annually, with the proportion of esophageal adenocarcinoma increasing to more than 50% since 2000. The incidence of esophageal adenocarcinoma in the US has been increasing exponentially since the 1970s (from 1.0 new cases per 100,000 persons per year in the 1970s to 5.69 new cases per 100,000 persons per year in 2004 for White men, and from 0.17 new cases per 100,000 persons per year in the 1970s to 0.70 new cases per 100,000 persons per year in 2004 for White women). However, the incidence of SCC in the US has decreased from 3.8 new cases per 100,000 persons per year in the 1970s to 1.90 new cases per 100,000 persons per year in 2004 for White men, with a similar trend for White women. In contrast, in certain regions of China, India, and Iran, SCC is exceedingly common, occurring in 132 new cases per 100,000 persons per year.

Overall, neoplasms of the esophagus carry a poor prognosis, particularly if they are diagnosed after the patient has symptoms. In the US, the number of deaths from esophageal carcinoma closely approximates the number of new cases per year, and the overall 5-year survival rate is less than 20%.

Risk Factors for SCC

Several types of factors increase the risk for SCC: geographic, dietary, preexisting diseases, and smoking and alcohol consumption. In the US, the incidence rates for SCC are higher in urban

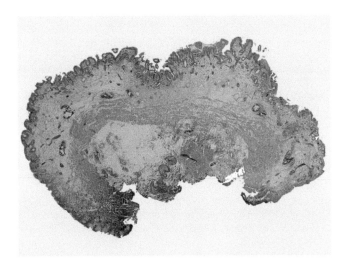

Figure 2.8. Endoscopic Mucosal Resection Specimen. This technique enables visualization of the mucosa, lamina propria, muscularis mucosa, and submucosa, thus allowing an accurate determination of the depth of invasion of malignant lesions (hematoxylin-eosin, original magnification ×12.5).

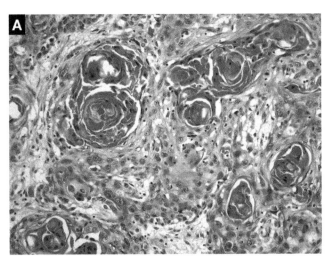

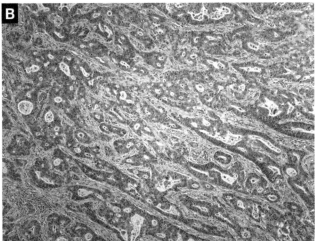

Figure 2.9. Histologic Features of Esophageal Carcinoma. A, Squamous cell carcinoma. Irregular nests of malignant squamous cells show abnormal production of keratin (hematoxylin-eosin, original magnification ×200). B, Adenocarcinoma. Infiltrative adenocarcinoma glands have complex architecture (hematoxylin-eosin, original magnification ×100). (Courtesy of Tsung-Teh Wu, MD, PhD, Department of Laboratory Medicine and Pathology, Mayo Clinic, Rochester, Minnesota; used with permission.)

areas and in low-income areas. The higher incidence rates in parts of Asia (China, India, and Iran) may be influenced by dietary and environmental issues. Dietary risk factors include foods with *N*-nitroso compounds (which can cause DNA damage); betel nuts (when chewed); selenium, zinc, vitamin C, and folate deficiencies; and intake of hot liquids. Preexisting esophageal diseases that are recognized risk factors include lye-induced strictures and achalasia; systemic diseases include tylosis. The risk of SCC increases with increasing use of tobacco and alcohol.

Risk Factors for Adenocarcinoma

The risk factors for esophageal adenocarcinoma mirror the risk factors for BE, and BE is the strongest risk factor for esophageal adenocarcinoma. Other established risk factors for esophageal adenocarcinoma are older age, male sex, chronic reflux of gastric contents, White race, obesity (particularly central or male pattern obesity), and smoking. Heartburn and acid regurgitation, especially if present for more than 12 years, are also risk factors. As many as 40% to 50% of patients who have esophageal adenocarcinoma do not have symptoms of frequent gastroesophageal reflux. Debate continues on the role of *H pylori* infection in the increasing incidence of esophageal adenocarcinoma. Some reports suggest that an inverse correlation exists (with atrophic gastritis from *H pylori* infection decreasing gastric acid output and, hence, decreasing reflux of gastric contents and protecting against esophageal adenocarcinoma), but other studies do not.

Signs and Symptoms

The symptoms of esophageal cancer include progressive solid food dysphagia that progresses to dysphagia with soft solids and then with liquids. Unintentional weight loss is commonly reported with late-stage disease. Other than the skin changes of tylosis or lichen planus in patients with SCC, there are no specific signs of esophageal cancer. In most patients, the physical examination findings are normal. With late-stage disease or disease of the proximal esophagus, supraclavicular lymphadenopathy or hepatomegaly can be palpated, indicating the possibility of metastatic disease.

Diagnosis and Staging

Diagnosis of esophageal carcinoma requires endoscopy with biopsy. Although the diagnosis may be suspected from the results of a barium study or other imaging tests, tissue to confirm a diagnosis is obtained best from endoscopy. After histologic confirmation of the diagnosis, attention should be directed toward staging.

The goal of staging is to classify the tumor as *early* or *localized to the esophagus*, *locally advanced*, or *metastatic*. Tools available for staging include positron emission tomography (PET), which is best suited and most sensitive for detecting distant metastatic disease. It has greater sensitivity than computed tomography (CT) and can be used to detect unsuspected metastatic disease in 10% to 15% of patients who have no evidence of disease on CT. The use of PET has been shown to lead to a change in management in 10% to 20% of patients. However, PET is expensive and may not be widely available. Usually CT is performed first to exclude metastatic disease before PET (if available) is performed to exclude any metastatic lesions missed with CT. Endoscopic ultrasonography is used to perform locoregional staging for assessing the T (tumor) stage (invasion into the esophageal wall) and the N (node) stage. Endoscopic ultrasonography is most sensitive for staging locally advanced disease (T2 or T3), with

Table 2.1. TNM Staging System for Esophageal
Adenocarcinoma

Stage	Description
Primary tumor (T)	
T1	Tumor invades lamina propria, muscularis mucosae, or submucosa
T1a	Tumor invades lamina propria or muscularis mucosae
T1b	Tumor invades submucosa
T2	Tumor invades muscularis propria
T3	Tumor invades adventitia
T4	Tumor invades adjacent structures
T4a	Resectable tumor is invading pleura, pericardium, diaphragm
T4b	Unresectable tumor is invading aorta, vertebral body, trachea
Regional lymph nodes (N)[a]	
N0	No regional lymph node metastasis
N1	Metastasis in 1 or 2 regional lymph nodes
N2	Metastasis in 3-6 regional lymph nodes
N3	Metastasis in ≥7 regional lymph nodes
Distant metastasis (M)	
M0	No distant metastasis
M1	Distant metastasis present

[a] The 2010 edition of the staging recommendations eliminated emphasis on the location of lymph nodes and replaced it with the number of lymph nodes involved (because the number of lymph nodes has been shown to be more prognostic of survival).

Adapted from Edge SB, Byrd DR, Compton CC, Fritz AG, Greene FL, Trotti A 3rd, eds; American Joint Committee on Cancer. AJCC cancer staging manual. 7th ed. New York (NY): Springer; 2010:109; used with permission.

modest accuracy for staging early disease (mucosal or submucosal), and for establishing the N stage (particularly with the use of fine-needle aspiration of enlarged lymph nodes). Metastatic involvement of celiac lymph nodes is detected best with endoscopic ultrasonography. The current TNM staging criteria for esophageal adenocarcinoma are listed in Table 2.1.

In early-stage disease (T1N0M0), endoscopic mucosal resection is an accurate tool to distinguish between mucosally confined disease (T1a) and submucosally invasive disease (T1b). This distinction is important because endoscopic therapy may be considered for T1a disease, given the low risk of metastatic lymphadenopathy (2%) compared with submucosal disease, for which the risk of metastatic lymphadenopathy is 20% to 30%, and the therapy of choice is esophagectomy (which allows lymph node dissection and removal) in operative candidates.

Treatment options depend on the stage of the disease. Endoscopic therapy (with endoscopic mucosal resection and additional ablative techniques) may be considered for T1a disease; recent reports have documented excellent overall 5-year survival outcomes in comparison with outcomes after surgery. More invasive disease is treated by esophagectomy with lymph node dissection (T2 or N0 disease) or neoadjuvant chemoradiotherapy, with subsequent restaging and esophagectomy (for T3 or N1 disease). This treatment strategy is based on limited data from studies that reported a modest survival advantage with neoadjuvant chemoradiotherapy when results from neoadjuvant chemoradiotherapy and subsequent surgery were compared with results from surgery alone. Metastatic disease can be managed with a combination of palliative chemoradiotherapy, esophageal stent placement, and nutritional support (administered orally with supplements or with percutaneously placed enteric tubes).

Suggested Reading

Abrams JA, Fields S, Lightdale CJ, Neugut AI. Racial and ethnic disparities in the prevalence of Barrett's esophagus among patients who undergo upper endoscopy. Clin Gastroenterol Hepatol. 2008 Jan;6(1):30–4.

Codipilly DC, Sawas T, Dhaliwal L, Johnson ML, Lansing R, Wang KK, et al. Epidemiology and outcomes of young-onset esophageal adenocarcinoma: an analysis from a population-based database. Cancer Epidemiol Biomarkers Prev. 2021 Jan;30(1):142–9.

Coleman HG, Bhat S, Johnston BT, McManus D, Gavin AT, Murray LJ. Tobacco smoking increases the risk of high-grade dysplasia and cancer among patients with Barrett's esophagus. Gastroenterology. 2012 Feb;142(2):233–40.

Conio M, Cameron AJ, Romero Y, Branch CD, Schleck CD, Burgart LJ, et al. Secular trends in the epidemiology and outcome of Barrett's oesophagus in Olmsted County, Minnesota. Gut. 2001 Mar;48(3):304–9.

Cook MB, Shaheen NJ, Anderson LA, Giffen C, Chow WH, Vaughan TL, et al. Cigarette smoking increases risk of Barrett's esophagus: an analysis of the Barrett's and Esophageal Adenocarcinoma Consortium. Gastroenterology. 2012 Apr;142(4):744–53.

Desai TK, Krishnan K, Samala N, Singh J, Cluley J, Perla S, et al. The incidence of oesophageal adenocarcinoma in non-dysplastic Barrett's oesophagus: a meta-analysis. Gut. 2012 Jul;61(7):970–6.

El-Serag H. Role of obesity in GORD-related disorders. Gut. 2008 Mar;57(3):281–4.

Fitzgerald RC, di Pietro M, O'Donovan M, Maroni R, Muldrew B, Debiram-Beecham I, et al. Cytosponge-trefoil factor 3 versus usual care to identify Barrett's oesophagus in a primary care setting: a multicentre, pragmatic, randomised controlled trial. Lancet. 2020 Aug 1;396(10247):333–44.

Iyer PG, Taylor WR, Johnson ML, Lansing RL, Maixner KA, Hemminger LL, et al. Accurate nonendoscopic detection of Barrett's esophagus by methylated DNA markers: a multisite case control study. Am J Gastroenterol. 2020 Aug;115(8):1201–9.

Jung KW, Talley NJ, Romero Y, Katzka DA, Schleck CD, Zinsmeister AR, et al. Epidemiology and natural history of intestinal metaplasia of the gastroesophageal junction and Barrett's esophagus: a population-based study. Am J Gastroenterol. 2011 Aug;106(8):1447–55.

Lagergren J, Bergstrom R, Lindgren A, Nyren O. Symptomatic gastroesophageal reflux as a risk factor for esophageal adenocarcinoma. N Engl J Med. 1999 Mar 18;340(11):825–31.

Peters Y, Schrauwen RWM, Tan AC, Bogers SK, de Jong B, Siersema PD. Detection of Barrett's oesophagus through exhaled breath using an electronic nose device. Gut. 2020 Jul;69(7):1169–72.

Prasad GA, Wang KK, Buttar NS, Wongkeesong LM, Krishnadath KK, Nichols FC 3rd, et al. Long-term survival following endoscopic and surgical treatment of high-grade dysplasia in Barrett's esophagus. Gastroenterology. 2007 Apr;132(4):1226–33.

Prasad GA, Wu TT, Wigle DA, Buttar NS, Wongkeesong LM, Dunagan KT, et al. Endoscopic and surgical treatment of mucosal (T1a) esophageal adenocarcinoma in Barrett's esophagus. Gastroenterology. 2009 Sep;137(3):815–23.

Qumseya BJ, Bukannan A, Gendy S, Ahemd Y, Sultan S, Bain P, et al. Systematic review and meta-analysis of prevalence and risk factors for Barrett's esophagus. Gastrointest Endosc. 2019 Nov;90(5):707–17.

Reid BJ, Li X, Galipeau PC, Vaughan TL. Barrett's oesophagus and oesophageal adenocarcinoma: time for a new synthesis. Nat Rev Cancer. 2010 Feb;10(2):87–101.

Sharma P, Dent J, Armstrong D, Bergman JJ, Gossner L, Hoshihara Y, et al. The development and validation of an endoscopic grading system for Barrett's esophagus: the Prague C & M criteria. Gastroenterology. 2006 Nov;131(5):1392–9.

Sharma P, McQuaid K, Dent J, Fennerty MB, Sampliner R, Spechler S, et al; AGA Chicago Workshop. A critical review of the diagnosis and management of Barrett's esophagus. Gastroenterology. 2004 Jul;127(1):310–30.

Spechler SJ, Fitzgerald RC, Prasad GA, Wang KK. History, molecular mechanisms, and endoscopic treatment of Barrett's esophagus. Gastroenterology. 2010 Mar;138(3):854–69.

Vakil N, van Zanten SV, Kahrilas P, Dent J, Jones R; Global Consensus Group. The Montreal definition and classification of gastroesophageal reflux disease: a global evidence-based consensus. Am J Gastroenterol. 2006 Aug;101(8):1900–20.

van Soest EM, Dieleman JP, Siersema PD, Sturkenboom MC, Kuipers EJ. Increasing incidence of Barrett's oesophagus in the general population. Gut. 2005 Aug;54(8):1062–6.

Wang KK, Sampliner RE; Practice Parameters Committee of the American College of Gastroenterology. Updated guidelines 2008 for the diagnosis, surveillance and therapy of Barrett's esophagus. Am J Gastroenterol. 2008 Mar;103(3):788–97.

Wani S, Puli SR, Shaheen NJ, Westhoff B, Slehria S, Bansal A, et al. Esophageal adenocarcinoma in Barrett's esophagus after endoscopic ablative therapy: a meta-analysis and systematic review. Am J Gastroenterol. 2009 Feb;104(2):502–13.

3

Esophageal Motility

CHAMIL C. CODIPILLY, MD

KARTHIK RAVI, MD

The esophagus is the conduit for oral contents to pass from the oropharynx into the stomach. An intricate network of neuro-muscular processes allows for the propulsion of food into the stomach while avoiding the passage of boluses into the respiratory system and inhibiting the reflux of gastric contents into the esophagus. Esophageal dysmotility manifests mainly as dysphagia or gastroesophageal reflux disease (GERD), although in rare instances it may also result in chest pain and discomfort. This chapter reviews the normal physiology of swallowing and discusses the pathophysiology, diagnostic evaluation, and management of esophageal motility disorders.

Anatomy

The esophagus is a tubular structure that passes through the posterior mediastinum. The proximal esophagus acts as a funnel, shuttling oral contents from the pharynx, with passage controlled by the upper esophageal sphincter (UES), which at rest is typically contracted to prevent the reflux of esophageal or gastric contents into the mouth and airways. The distal esophagus attaches to the proximal stomach; the lower esophageal sphincter

(LES), which is also tonically contracted at rest, prohibits the reflux of gastric contents into the esophagus.

Each of the distinct layers of the esophagus is vital to proper functioning of the organ (Figure 3.1). The innermost layer, the *mucosa*, is normally composed of squamous epithelium and provides a measure of protection from oral contents. The *submucosa* provides nourishment to the mucosa and contains mucus-secreting glands; mucus eases the passage of food boluses. The *muscularis propria* consists of 2 layers: The inner layer contains muscle arranged circularly around the esophagus, and the outer layer includes longitudinal muscle running the length of the esophagus. Coordinated contraction of the 2 layers allows for peristalsis of contents down the esophagus. The outermost layer of the esophagus, the *adventitia*, provides connective tissue and structure to the organ.

In the upper third of the esophagus, the muscular layer (the muscularis propria) is made of striated skeletal muscle; the lower two-thirds is made of smooth muscle. A transition zone near the level of the aortic arch marks the change in muscle type, although this landmark cannot typically be identified on endoscopy. The proximal striated muscle innervation is carried by cranial nerves IX (glossopharyngeal nerve) and X (vagus nerve), while the smooth muscle is innervated mainly by input from cranial nerve X.

Normal Physiology

The initiation of swallowing is a voluntary process that, once started, cannot be halted under normal circumstances. Swallowing begins with movement of the tongue cephalad to the hard palate, which pushes the food bolus into the pharynx. This triggers the involuntary swallowing reflex, in which the tongue and soft palate seal off the nasopharynx and oral cavity, while the epiglottis

Abbreviations: CDP, contraction deceleration point; DCI, distal contractile integral; DES, distal esophageal spasm; DI, distensibility index; DL, distal latency; EGD, esophagogastroduodenoscopy; EGJ, esophagogastric junction; EGJOO, esophagogastric junction outflow obstruction; FLIP, functional lumen imaging probe; GERD, gastroesophageal reflux disease; HRM, high-resolution manometry; IRP, integrated relaxation pressure; LES, lower esophageal sphincter; LHM, laparoscopic Heller myotomy; PD, pneumatic dilation; POEM, peroral endoscopic myotomy; PPI, proton pump inhibitor; RYGB, Roux-en-Y gastric bypass; UES, upper esophageal sphincter; VFSS, videofluoroscopic swallow study

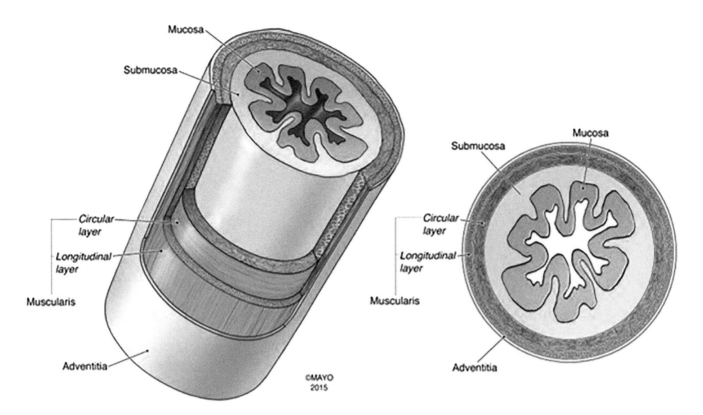

Figure 3.1. Layers Within the Wall of the Esophagus.

everts to prevent food from entering the laryngeal (and by extension, pulmonary) spaces. Shortening of the pharynx removes
the recesses formed by the valleculae and piriform sinuses, and
peristalsis of the pharyngeal muscles pushes the bolus posteriorly to the UES, which mainly consists of the cricopharyngeus
muscle. The UES relaxes, allowing the bolus to enter the proximal esophagus, but quickly contracts again after the bolus has
passed. Peristalsis of the esophageal body then propels the food
toward the stomach. Relaxation of the LES allows passage of the
bolus into the stomach; with contraction of the LES afterward, a
reflux barrier is formed.

This process is mediated by the competing effects of nitric
oxide and acetylcholine. Excitatory input, resulting in peristalsis,
is mediated by acetylcholine, while relaxation of the sphincters is
mediated by the inhibitory effect of nitric oxide.

Oropharyngeal Dysphagia

Symptoms of oropharyngeal dysphagia, which may be distinct from those of esophageal body dysphagia, may include
difficulties with formation of food boluses, transfer of food
boluses, coughing, and choking. Patients may localize symptoms
to the neck superior to the sternal notch.

Patients frequently have a history of neuromuscular or systemic diseases, or mechanical obstruction. Causes of oropharyngeal dysphagia are shown in Table 3.1. Neurologic deficits
may affect other functions that are controlled by the same nerves
involved in the initial steps of swallowing, and concurrent
difficulties with speaking, tongue movement, oral bolus retention, and laryngeal protection may be elicited from the history
or physical examination. Expectedly, patients with oropharyngeal dysphagia may present with recurrent aspiration pneumonia,

hoarseness, and regurgitation (particularly through the nose if the
seal between the tongue and soft palate is ineffective).

Structural or mechanical abnormalities may also cause oropharyngeal dysphagia. Causes include malignancy, thyromegaly,
prominent cricopharyngeal bar (Figure 3.2), tonsillar enlargement, and cervical osteophytes. Erosion or migration of anterior
cervical spine hardware may also result in oropharyngeal dysphagia. Zenker diverticulum (Figure 3.2) can form in the Killian
triangle, an area of relative pharyngeal weakness due to high
pressure from the cricopharyngeus muscle, and result in dysphagia and retention with resultant regurgitation of food. Patients
with proximal esophageal body obstruction may also have oropharyngeal symptoms.

Physical examination findings may include weakness
involving cranial nerves. Patients may not be able to retain oral
contents in the mouth without drooling. Coughing may occur
with swallowing. Patients may need to swallow 2 or 3 times to
clear small boluses (such as a sip of water). Halitosis may be
present in patients with a Zenker diverticulum.

A videofluoroscopic swallow study (VFSS), done in conjunction with a speech and swallowing pathologist, is the best test
to evaluate oropharyngeal dysphagia. Functions assessed include
the following:

- Tongue coordination—an uncoordinated tongue impairs transmission of the bolus
- Soft palate elevation—dysfunction of the soft palate can lead to
nasopharyngeal regurgitation
- Laryngeal closure—failure of laryngeal closure can lead to
aspiration
- Pharyngeal peristalsis—poor pharyngeal peristalsis results in
residue in the valleculae or piriform sinuses, requiring multiple
swallows and often leading to aspiration

Table 3.1. Causes and Treatment of Oropharyngeal Dysphagia

Cause	Therapy
Neuromuscular	
Cerebrovascular accident	Swallowing rehabilitation
Trauma	
Peripheral neuropathy	
Amyotrophic lateral sclerosis	
Muscular dystrophy	
Poliomyelitis	
Multiple sclerosis	Treatment of underlying medical
Myasthenia gravis	condition; swallowing rehabilitation
Parkinson disease	if needed
Polymyositis, dermatomyositis	
Guillain-Barré syndrome	
Hypothyroidism	
Lymphadenopathy	
Tardive dyskinesia	
Obstructive	
Zenker diverticulum	Bougienage, dilation; cricomyotomy
Prominent cricopharyngeus muscle	
Proximal esophageal strictures, webs	Bougienage, dilation; assessment for iron deficiency anemia and treatment
Thyromegaly	Treatment of underlying medical
Malignancy (head, neck, or esophageal cancer)	condition
Migration of anterior cervical hardware	Conservative measures and reassurance; if severe, possibly
Tonsillar enlargement	surgery
Cervical osteophytes	

Multifaceted therapeutic approaches are used in the management of oropharyngeal dysphagia. Patients should be counseled to carefully focus on eating and to chew food well to avoid aspiration events. Soft or pureed foods may be recommended. Certain

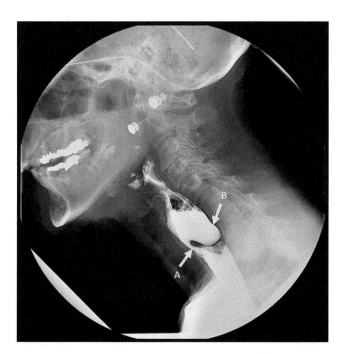

Figure 3.2. Obstructive Causes of Oropharyngeal Dysphagia. Barium esophagram shows a prominent cricopharyngeal bar (A) that is obstructing the esophageal lumen by more than 75% and a concomitant Zenker diverticulum (B).

maneuvers, such as the chin tuck, can improve swallowing mechanics and help the patient avoid aspiration, and the maneuvers can be tailored on the basis of the VFSS findings. Swallowing rehabilitation may improve oropharyngeal dysphagia even in patients with structural abnormalities. However, in patients with structural abnormalities, endoscopic or surgical intervention (or both) may improve symptoms. Dysphagia due to a proximal cricopharyngeal bar or hypertensive UES may respond to bougienage or myotomy, particularly if radiographic evidence confirms obstruction at the level of the cricopharyngeus muscle.

As previously mentioned, many patients with oropharyngeal dysphagia have underlying neuromuscular disease processes that result in symptoms. Therefore, in appropriate patients, evaluation may include laboratory assessment (creatine kinase and antinuclear antibody) and imaging (magnetic resonance imaging of the brain). These patients should be evaluated and treated in a multidisciplinary manner with input from neurologists, otorhinolaryngologists, rheumatologists, and gastroenterologists. Targeted pharmacologic therapies should be administered in appropriate patients (eg, carbidopa-levodopa in patients with Parkinson disease), but in these patients dysphagia is frequently progressive. Swallowing rehabilitation may delay the need for enteral or parenteral feeding.

✓ Videofluoroscopic swallow study—diagnostic test of choice when patients present with symptoms of oropharyngeal dysphagia
✓ Oropharyngeal dysphagia may be a manifestation of an underlying neuromuscular condition; a multidisciplinary approach for evaluation should be considered

Esophageal Dysphagia

In contrast to oropharyngeal dysphagia (characterized by patients choking, coughing, or aspirating with swallowing), esophageal dysphagia is characterized by the sense that swallowed boluses get "stuck" or "hung up" after the swallow is initiated, and symptoms can be localized anywhere from the neck to the lower chest. Patients may have pain or discomfort when the bolus is delayed in the esophagus. They may report having symptoms at a level that differs from the actual site of obstruction.

Obstruction is the major cause of esophageal dysphagia, and the usual evaluation includes a barium esophagram and esophagogastroduodenoscopy (EGD). Solid food dysphagia alone typically implies an obstructive process, although a rapidly growing lesion will eventually cause dysphagia with both solids and liquids. However, the onset of both solid and liquid dysphagia may indicate a motility disorder.

It can be helpful to have the esophagram done before the EGD so that therapies, such as dilation of a subtle esophageal stricture, can be planned and performed during the endoscopy. In appropriate patients who do not have clear structural abnormalities, random esophageal biopsies (from the proximal and distal esophagus) should be performed to rule out eosinophilic esophagitis.

Rapidly progressive symptoms accompanied by weight loss are concerning for esophageal cancer, although patients with secondary causes of achalasia (which may also include malignancy) can present similarly. Evaluation of these patients should be expedited to establish the diagnosis. Notably, the sense of dysphagia from a cancer typically implies that it is deeper than a T2 lesion (invading at least into the muscularis propria).

If obstruction and inflammatory disorders of the esophagus are ruled out, esophageal high-resolution manometry (HRM) is usually the best next step in the evaluation of dysphagia.

Esophageal HRM

During esophageal HRM, a thin, flexible catheter is inserted through the nares and traverses the entire length of the esophagus into the stomach. Solid-state pressure transducers are positioned every centimeter along the catheter length to allow for simultaneous assessment of the entire esophagus during swallowing and at rest. Further, this allows creation of a color-coded pressure topographic image, a *Clouse plot*, in which high pressures are represented by red and orange, while low pressures are displayed in blue and green. The Clouse plot eases study interpretation and has been shown to improve interobserver agreement compared to conventional line tracings. The length of the esophagus is shown along the y-axis, while time is along the x-axis. After a baseline landmark phase is captured, the patient is instructed to drink 10 swallows of water (5 mL water in each swallow) typically in the supine position and another 5 swallows in the upright position. Standard esophageal HRM can be supplemented with adjunctive tests such as the multiple rapid swallow sequence, during which a patient is instructed to swallow water every 2 seconds for 5 swallows to assess inhibitory input and peristaltic reserve, and a rapid drink challenge to assess functional obstruction at the esophagogastric junction (EGJ).

During a normal swallow (Figure 3.3), relaxation of the UES can be seen as a decrease in the tonic contraction of the UES with a subsequent peristaltic wave traveling distally to the LES, which is represented as a change in color that indicates increased esophageal pressure propagating from the proximal esophagus to the distal esophagus. When the UES opens, the LES pressure also decreases, as indicated by a change in color that represents the deglutitive window.

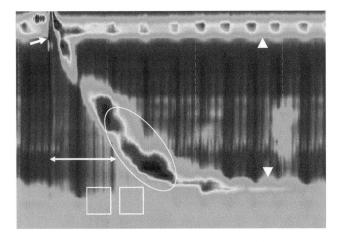

Figure 3.3. Normal Swallow on High-Resolution Esophageal Manometry. At the initiation of the swallow (white arrow), the upper esophageal sphincter (upper arrowhead) relaxes, and the waveform moves toward the lower esophageal sphincter (LES) (lower arrowhead) in a peristaltic fashion. The distal latency (DL) (double arrow) is normal (ie, >4.5 s); a short DL would indicate spasm. The oval shows where the distal contractile integral, a measure of peristaltic vigor (normally 450-8,000 mm Hg·cm·s), is assessed. The 2 boxes indicate measurement of the integrated relaxation pressure (IRP), which is a composite of the lowest 4 seconds of pressure (not necessarily contiguous seconds) in the first 10 seconds after initiation of the swallow. An increased IRP indicates nonrelaxation of the LES during swallowing.

Assessment of HRM With the Chicago Classification Version 4.0

Currently in its fourth iteration, the Chicago Classification was developed to standardize the interpretation of HRM tracings. Although it is a valuable tool for gastroenterologists, this classification system is not all-encompassing, and clinicians need to carefully consider HRM findings in the appropriate clinical context.

The Chicago Classification uses 3 metrics to interpret an HRM study. The *integrated relaxation pressure* (IRP), which is a marker of deglutitive LES relaxation, is the lowest mean LES pressure for 4 noncontiguous seconds in the first 10 seconds after a swallow. The reference range for median IRP is less than 15 mm Hg as measured from 10 swallows in the supine position. A second metric is *distal latency* (DL), a measure of esophageal inhibitory input. Normal esophageal peristalsis is defined by graded inhibitory and excitatory input such that there is relatively more inhibitory input in the distal esophagus than in the proximal esophagus. The *contraction deceleration point* (CDP) is the point at which the velocity of the peristaltic wave slows, marking the end of the stripping peristaltic segment of esophageal body emptying. The DL is simply the time from when a swallow begins (ie, the opening of the UES) until the CDP. A short CDP indicates that distal esophageal contraction occurred earlier than expected, reflecting loss of inhibitory input, and is used to define a spastic contraction. The reference range is greater than 4.5 seconds. A third metric is the *distal contractile integral* (DCI), which is the product of the amplitude, length, and time of the peristaltic wave and is a measure of peristaltic vigor.

The current version of the Chicago Classification can be used to broadly categorize esophageal motility disorders as either *disorders of EGJ outflow* or *disorders of peristalsis* (Figure 3.4). The first step in the classification process is to assess the IRP.

If the median IRP is abnormally high (≥15 mm Hg in the supine position), the interpretation follows the pathway for disorders of EGJ outflow. If peristalsis is absent in 100% of swallows, the manometric diagnosis of achalasia is made. If peristalsis is present in any swallows, LES relaxation is then assessed in another position with at least 5 swallows. If the median IRP is consistently high (≥12 mm Hg in the upright position) *and* results are abnormal from a timed barium esophagram or functional lumen imaging probe planimetry (or from both) in the appropriate clinical context, the manometric diagnosis is EGJ outflow obstruction (EGJOO).

If the median IRP is normal, the interpretation follows the pathway for disorders of peristalsis in a hierarchal fashion. *Absent contractility* is diagnosed from 100% failed peristalsis. *Distal esophageal spasm* is the diagnosis when 20% or more of the swallows have premature contraction (ie, DL <4.5 s). *Hypercontractile esophagus* is diagnosed when 20% or more of the swallows show hypercontractility (DCI >8,000 mm Hg·cm·s). *Ineffective esophageal motility* is characterized by more than 70% ineffective swallows (DCI <450 mm Hg·cm·s or transition zone defect >5 cm) or more than 50% failed swallows (DCI <100 mm Hg·cm·s). If none of these criteria are met, the swallow is considered normal. Table 3.2 provides diagnostic criteria for select motility disorders.

Functional Lumen Imaging Probe Planimetry

The functional lumen imaging probe (FLIP) is a recent addition to the armamentarium of esophageal motility testing. FLIP

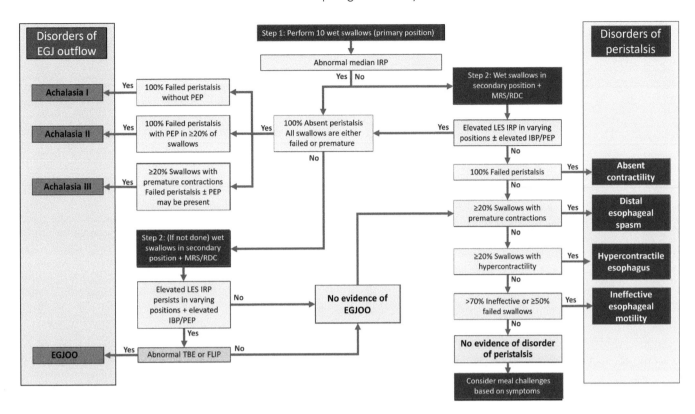

Figure 3.4. **Chicago Classification Version 4.0.** EGJ indicates esophagogastric junction; EGJOO, esophagogastric junction outflow obstruction; FLIP, functional lumen imaging probe; IBP, intrabolus pressurization; IRP, integrated relaxation pressure; LES, lower esophageal sphincter; MRS, multiple rapid swallow; PEP, panesophageal pressurization; RDC, rapid drink challenge; TBE, timed barium esophagram. (Adapted from Yadlapati R, Kahrilas PJ, Fox MR, Bredenoord AJ, Prakash Gyawali C, Roman S, et al. Esophageal motility disorders on high-resolution manometry: Chicago classification version 4.0(c). Neurogastroenterol Motil. 2021 Jan;33[1]:e14058; used with permission.)

planimetry uses impedance planimetry to measure pressure and esophageal luminal cross-sectional area. In addition, real-time FLIP planimetry allows for the assessment of esophageal contractility through dynamic changes in esophageal diameter.

FLIP planimetry, performed immediately after the patient has undergone endoscopy with sedation, involves placement of a transoral catheter with impedance electrodes along its length surrounded by an infinitely compliant balloon, which is positioned

Table 3.2. Diagnostic Criteria and Therapeutic Options for Select Esophageal Motility Disorders

Disorder	Manometric diagnostic criteria	Treatment
Achalasia (IRP ≥15 mm Hg)		
Type I	Absent peristalsis (100% of swallows)	Definitive treatment, types I and II:
Type II	Panesophageal pressurization in ≥20% of swallows (pressure >30 mm Hg with isobaric contour tool) and 100% failed swallows	POEM is equivalent to HM with fundoplication HM with fundoplication is equivalent to PD, but PD is associated with higher perforation rate (2%)
Type III	≥20% spastic swallows (DL <4.5 s) without evidence of peristalsis	Recommendation: HM with fundoplication or POEM according to clinical scenario Definitive treatment, type III: POEM is preferred to HM with fundoplication, so myotomy length can be tailored to length of spastic component on manometry Temporary treatment for poor surgical candidates: Botulinum toxin injection into LES
Distal esophageal spasm	DL <4.5 s and DCI ≥450 mm Hg·cm·s with normal IRP	PPI therapy Botulinum toxin injection into LES Long myotomy tailored to spastic component (in refractory cases)
Hypercontractile esophagus	DCI >8,000 mm Hg·cm·s in ≥20% of swallows with normal IRP	PPI therapy CCBs or nitrates (poor-quality evidence) Botulinum toxin injection into LES
Ineffective esophageal motility	Normal IRP, but ≥70% weak swallows (DCI 100-450 mm Hg·cm·s) or ≥50% failed swallows (DCI <100 mm Hg·cm·s)	Assess and treat underlying medical condition (connective tissue diseases) PPI therapy Lifestyle modifications if considerable reflux burden

Abbreviations: CCB, calcium channel blocker; DCI, distal contractile integral; DL, distal latency; HM, Heller myotomy; IRP, integrated relaxation pressure; LES, lower esophageal sphincter; PD, pneumatic dilation; POEM, peroral endoscopic myotomy; PPI, proton pump inhibitor.

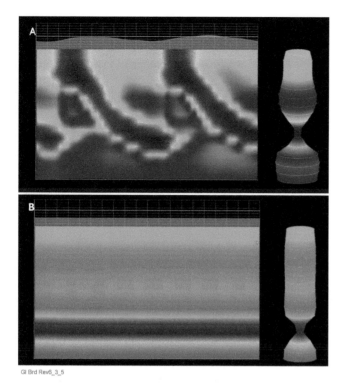

GI Brd Rev6_3_5

Figure 3.5. **Functional Luminal Imaging Probe (FLIP). An infinitely compliant balloon is used to assess distensibility and secondary contractions.** A, Repetitive anterograde contractions are present in a patient with normal motility. B, FLIP in a patient with achalasia shows the lack of peristalsis and the poorly distensible esophagogastric junction marked by the red band.

with the distal 2 to 3 cm in the stomach. The balloon is sequentially filled with a liquid of known conductivity, and, with use of the Ohm law, the cross-sectional area at each impedance electrode can be determined along with pressure within the balloon itself. If the ratio of the cross-sectional area at the EGJ and the pressure within the balloon have been determined, the distensibility index (DI) can be calculated. The DI can be predictive of disordered LES relaxation. In addition, real-time diameter changes from distention-induced secondary peristalsis are plotted topographically and allow for assessment of esophageal contractility. A low DI and smaller diameter at the EGJ in addition to disordered or absent contractility are predictive and can confirm achalasia (Figure 3.5). Overall, FLIP planimetry is safe and well tolerated.

> ✓ A motility disorder of the esophagus should be considered after an obstructive or mechanical cause of dysphagia is ruled out with esophagogastroduodenoscopy and possibly a barium esophagram
> ✓ Chicago classification—an algorithmic approach to interpreting high-resolution manometry by first assessing esophagogastric junction relaxation (integrated relaxation pressure) and potential achalasia and subsequently assessing potential abnormalities of esophageal body peristalsis in a hierarchal manner

Achalasia

Achalasia (from the Greek prefix *a-* denoting absence and the Greek word for relaxation, *chalasis*) is defined by failure of LES relaxation along with the absence of esophageal peristalsis. Although achalasia was thought to be rare, recent publications have highlighted an incidence rate of more than 25 per 100,000

in the Medicare population. The diagnosis tends to be more common among older patients; although achalasia can occur at any age, onset of symptoms before the age of 20 years is uncommon. No sex or racial predilection is apparent.

Achalasia can be categorized as *primary* (idiopathic) or *secondary* (pseudoachalasia). Secondary achalasia is most commonly caused by malignant compression or infiltration of the distal esophagus, and this must be considered, particularly during assessment of older patients who present with rapid onset of symptoms and marked weight loss (>10 kg) within a short time (<6 months). Less commonly, secondary achalasia may indicate a paraneoplastic phenomenon typically associated with lung cancer. Nonmalignant causes of secondary achalasia include amyloid deposition, benign tumors, peripheral neuropathy, and central nervous system disorders. Iatrogenic causes of secondary achalasia include tight fundoplications, lap band surgery, and antireflux rings. In endemic regions (Central and South America), Chagas disease, due to infection with *Trypanosoma cruzi,* can result in achalasia and can be accompanied by megacolon, cardiomegaly, and neurologic dysfunction.

Pathophysiology

The underlying pathogenesis of achalasia is loss of esophageal peristaltic activity coupled with a lack of LES relaxation, which impedes bolus transit through the esophagus and results in dysphagia. Histologic analysis shows degeneration of myenteric plexus ganglion cells associated with lymphocytic infiltration. The possibility of an autoimmune or inflammatory reaction to infection or another trigger naturally arises from this finding, but no clear link has been established.

Diagnosis

Patients universally complain of dysphagia, often to both solids and liquids and may describe a stacking phenomenon, in which food can accumulate in the chest during a meal. Patients may also have chest pain and discomfort. Regurgitation may be associated with relief of symptoms, and some patients may find regurgitated contents on their pillow upon awakening. Patients with achalasia may describe themselves as slow eaters, and they often use adaptive behaviors such as extending the torso and "power drinking" liquids. Consequently, primary achalasia has an average diagnostic delay of 2 years from symptom onset and is typically associated with minimal weight loss. The Eckardt score (Table 3.3) is a validated assessment tool that incorporates patient symptoms.

The diagnostic evaluation for achalasia involves a single-contrast esophagram with barium, which may show the characteristic birdbeak sign with a smooth tapering of the dilated distal esophagus as it approaches the tonically contracted LES (Figure 3.6). If the esophagram is timed, a distinct retained column may be present at 1 and 5 minutes after the swallow.

Table 3.3. Eckardt Score for Assessment of Achalasia

Score[a]	Dysphagia	Regurgitation	Retrosternal pain	Weight loss, kg
0	None	None	None	0
1	Occasional	Occasional	Occasional	<5
2	Daily	Daily	Daily	5-10
3	With every meal	With every meal	Several times daily	>10

[a] Scores of 4 or more typically indicate more severe symptoms.

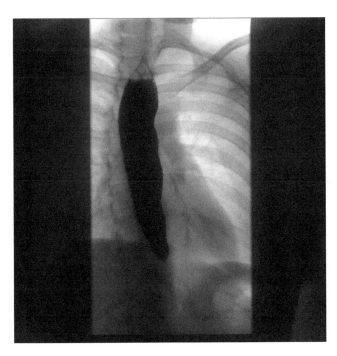

Figure 3.6. Esophagram From Patient With Achalasia. The bird-beak sign is apparent where the esophagus tapers distally as it approaches the esophagogastric junction.

Findings on EGD include a dilated esophagus (frequently filled with food), a puckered EJG (Figure 3.7), and resistance to passage of the scope through the EJG. However, the absence of these findings does not rule out achalasia. Endoscopic evaluation is required for ruling out secondary causes of achalasia as outlined above. However, patients with particularly concerning clinical histories may require further evaluation with computed tomography of the chest or endoscopic ultrasonography before malignancy can be ruled out.

HRM can be considered the gold standard for diagnostic testing. According to the Chicago Classification version 4.0 criteria, achalasia is diagnosed when the median IRP is high (≥15 mm Hg) and peristalsis is 100% absent or has failed. Achalasia can be stratified

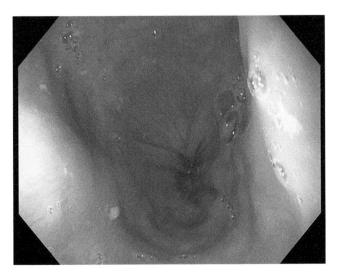

Figure 3.7. Endoscopic Image From a Patient With Achalasia. The esophagogastric junction has a puckered appearance.

further into 3 subtypes (Figure 3.8). As outlined above, FLIP planimetry can be confirmatory in select cases.

Therapy

There are currently no medications or procedures that specifically address the lack of peristalsis in achalasia. As a result, all therapies involve some disruption (either physically or pharmacologically) of the LES. Although multiple oral medications have been used for achalasia (eg, nitrates, calcium channel blockers, and nitric oxide donors), none have demonstrated efficacy. Furthermore, the use of these medications is limited by their adverse effects. Consequently, medical therapies are not typically used in achalasia management.

Botulinum toxin injection into the LES is another effective therapeutic option in achalasia. The therapeutic effect lasts for an average of 3 to 6 months. The injection must be administered into the muscle, not the submucosa, at approximately 1 to 2 cm above the endoscopic EGJ. Repeated botulinum toxin injections can make future surgical or endoscopic myotomy more complicated because of fibrosis, and the injections may lose efficacy over time. Consequently, this therapy is typically reserved for patients who have serious comorbidities and thus are not candidates for more invasive treatment.

For all other patients with achalasia, 3 durable therapeutic options can be used: pneumatic dilation (PD) with a balloon, laparoscopic Heller myotomy (LHM) with partial fundoplication, and peroral endoscopic myotomy (POEM). Randomized controlled trials have shown equivalence in therapeutic efficacy between PD and LHM and between LHM and POEM.

PD involves the use of the Rigiflex balloon dilator (Boston Scientific Corp), which is available in various sizes (30-mm, 35-mm, and 40-mm diameters) and uses pneumatic pressure rather than hydrostatic pressure. Under fluoroscopic guidance, the balloon is typically positioned across the EGJ and inflated until the waist (ie, a narrowing at the muscular ring of the LES) is obliterated, which signals disruption of the muscle at the LES. The main risk of this procedure is perforation, which is reported to occur in up to 2% of patients. Therefore, patients who undergo PD should be candidates for major surgery in case a perforation occurs, and the procedure should not be considered for patients who are not appropriate candidates. Although a 30-mm balloon is typically used first, durable success may require sequential dilation with a 35-mm and a 40-mm balloon.

LHM typically involves an anterior myotomy, which is usually extended 2 cm into the gastric cardia. Given that the ensuing patulous EGJ affords no protection from gastroesophageal reflux, LHM is performed in combination with either an anterior (Dor) or a posterior (Toupet) partial fundoplication, which improves control of gastroesophageal reflux without adversely affecting the improvement in dysphagia. However, approximately 10% of patients may still have reflux symptoms.

POEM is an endoscopic procedure in which a submucosal tunnel is created to access the muscular layer of the esophagus and then carefully dissected with electrosurgical knives. The approach can be either anterior or posterior. Advantages of POEM include its minimally invasive nature and the ability to complete a long myotomy, which is limited by vascular structures with LHM. However, because POEM does not involve an antireflux procedure, up to 50% to 60% of patients who undergo POEM have reflux symptoms, positive results on acid reflux testing, or erosive esophagitis at 3 to 6 months, although most patients have good results with proton pump inhibitor

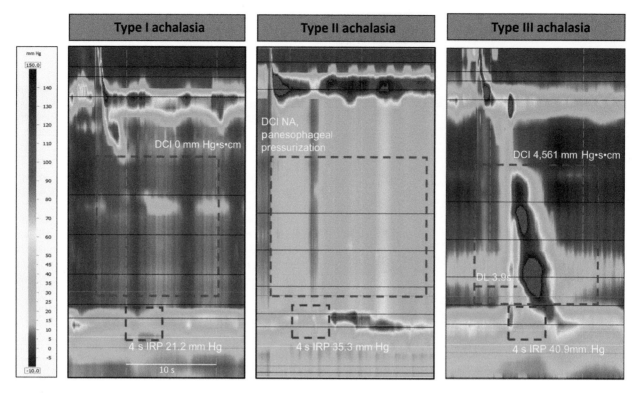

Figure 3.8. **Manometry Tracings of Subtypes of Achalasia.** In all 3 subtypes, the integrated relaxation pressure (IRP) is increased (IRP ≥15 mm Hg). Left, In type I achalasia, peristalsis is absent. The large dashed rectangle indicates a distal contractile integral (DCI) of 0 mm Hg·s·cm; the small dashed square, an integrated relaxation pressure (IRP) of 21.2 mm Hg. Center, Type II achalasia shows panesophageal pressurization. The DCI (large dashed square) is not applicable (NA); the IRP (small dashed square) is 35.3 mm Hg. Right, Type III achalasia has a spastic wave (distal latency <4.5 seconds). The DCI (large dashed square) is 4,561 mm Hg·s·cm; the IRP (small dashed square) is 40.9 mm Hg; and the distal latency (DL) (small dashed rectangle) is 3.9 seconds. (Adapted from Yadlapati R, Kahrilas PJ, Fox MR, Bredenoord AJ, Prakash Gyawali C, Roman S, et al. Esophageal motility disorders on high-resolution manometry: Chicago classification version 4.0(c). Neurogastroenterol Motil. 2021 Jan;33[1]:e14058; used with permission of University of California San Diego Center for Esophageal Diseases.)

(PPI) therapy. PD, LHM, and POEM are largely considered equivalent therapeutic options for type I or II achalasia, with type II achalasia representing an early form of achalasia with a greater therapeutic response rate than the other achalasia subtypes. POEM is considered superior for type III achalasia because it allows for a longer myotomy in patients who have spastic esophageal body contraction.

✓ Secondary achalasia related to malignancy should be suspected in an older patient with rapidly progressive dysphagia and marked weight loss

✓ Three subtypes of achalasia—type II has the best response to treatment, and type III is preferentially treated with peroral endoscopic myotomy

---

EGJ Outflow Obstruction

Patients with EGJOO have an increased median IRP (≥15 mm Hg supine and ≥12 mm Hg upright), but peristalsis is preserved (unlike in patients with achalasia) (Figure 3.9). Patients may present with regurgitation, dysphagia, chest discomfort, or reflux or a combination of these symptoms, but the high IRP may also be an incidental manometric finding. Consequently, the latest iteration of the Chicago Classification (version 4.0) mandates further testing to make this diagnosis (in contrast to earlier versions). The recommendation is that swallows be assessed in an alternate position (supine and upright), with the median IRP remaining high in both positions. Further, a clinically relevant diagnosis of EGJOO requires symptoms of dysphagia or chest pain (or both) along

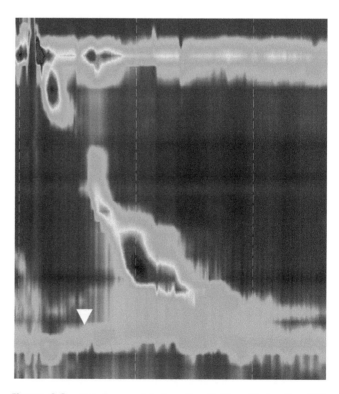

Figure 3.9. **Esophagogastric Junction Outflow Obstruction.** This manometry tracing shows preserved peristalsis but lack of relaxation of the lower esophageal sphincter (arrowhead). This patient presented with dysphagia after placement of an antireflux ring.

with findings on timed barium esophagram or FLIP (or both) that support obstruction.

Before EGJOO is diagnosed, mechanical causes must be ruled out (eg, a tight fundoplication, benign obstruction or stricture, esophageal antireflux ring device, or laparoscopic gastric band). If patients present with the possibility of coexistent malignancy, they may need to undergo cross-sectional imaging or endoscopic ultrasonography. However, that imaging is not indicated otherwise because the diagnostic yield is low. Finally, chronic opioid use can have important effects on esophageal motility, including increased contractile vigor and impaired LES relaxation; the possibility of this condition, *opioid-induced esophageal dysfunction*, must be considered.

Hypercontractile Esophagus

Hypercontractile esophagus is defined by a normal IRP but increased peristaltic vigor reflected by a DCI of at least 8,000 mm Hg·cm·s (Figure 3.10). Symptoms may be nonspecific, but patients may complain of intermittent chest pain or dysphagia (or both). However, the clinical significance of this finding is unclear, and in many patients the finding does not reliably correspond with symptoms and may be an incidental finding. As noted above, chronic opioid use can be associated with hypercontractile esophagus and should be considered. Further, in some patients hypercontractile esophagus may be associated with GERD, and PPI therapy can be considered. However, for most patients, conservative treatment is often considered (eg, use of peppermint oil or neuromodulators).

Distal Esophageal Spasm

Distal esophageal spasm (DES) is defined by a shortened DL (<4.5 s) with a normally relaxing LES (median IRP <15 mm Hg) and a DCI greater than 450 mm Hg·cm·s. Clinically, patients with DES have intermittent onset of chest pain and dysphagia, often

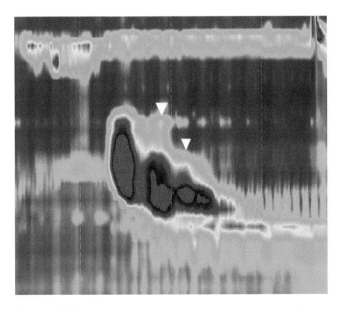

Figure 3.10. Hypercontractile Esophagus. Multiple peaks are shown (white arrowheads) with a distal contractile integral greater than 8,000 mm Hg·cm·s, which is consistent with jackhammer esophagus (a subset of hypercontractile esophagus) according to the Chicago Classification version 4.0.

precipitated by the ingestion of contents that are extremely cold or hot. Although esophageal spasm is a frequently proposed diagnosis for noncardiac chest pain, results from only 1% of all manometry studies support this finding. The esophagram may show a corkscrew appearance (which may also be seen on endoscopy), but frequently the appearance is normal.

The pathophysiology of spasm is also unclear but may be a reflex for clearing esophageal contents in persons with acid reflux. Confirmed DES is rare, so evidence-based treatment options are lacking. However, case reports have described the use of smooth muscle relaxants, such as calcium channel blockers and nitrates, and endoscopic and surgical options such as POEM or LHM.

Absent Contractility

Patients with absent contractility may present with dysphagia, regurgitation, and classic heartburn symptoms. Absent contractility is confirmed by the absence of peristasis on all swallows but with preserved LES relaxation. Absent contractility may be present in patients with connective tissue diseases, and the diagnostic evaluation may include assessment of autoantibody profiles to exclude diseases such as limited scleroderma.

Management is not well determined. Patients with connective tissue disease such as scleroderma may have a patulous EGJ, so PPI therapy is recommended to prevent the formation of strictures, Barrett esophagus, and other complications that can arise from long-term exposure to acid reflux. Diagnostic evaluation of new-onset dysphagia mandates an EGD to assess for treatable GERD-related complications, such as erosive esophagitis, peptic stricture, and esophageal malignancy. If patients have dysphagia without complications, conservative measures are instituted to decrease symptom burden. These measures include adequate fluid intake, elevation of the head of the bed, remaining upright for 3 to 4 hours after eating, and slow, careful eating.

Postfundoplication Motor Disorders

Patients with postfundoplication motor disorders may present with dysphagia, and the usual cause is a fundoplication that is too tight, although a slipped or herniated fundoplication should also be ruled out. An esophagram with a 13-mm barium tablet may illustrate these issues, particularly if the tablet becomes lodged at the level of the fundoplication. Results from manometry may be nonspecific, but the findings could be consistent with achalasia or EGJOO, with increased LES pressure or increased IRP (or both). Dilation, potentially with a pneumatic balloon, may be required to relieve symptoms, but in severe cases fundoplication may need to be redone.

Post–Obesity Surgery Esophageal Dysfunction

Post–obesity surgery esophageal dysfunction is an uncommon but increasingly recognized cause of dysphagia in patients who have had bariatric surgery, such as Roux-en-Y gastric bypass (RYGB) or sleeve gastrectomy. The underlying pathology most likely stems from the high pressures of the gastric pouch in an RYGB or low compliance of the stomach after sleeve gastrectomy. Stenosis at the gastrojejunal anastomosis after RYGB may also result in compatible symptoms. The diagnosis can be suspected from findings on a barium esophagram. Potential therapeutic options are dilation, myotomy, botulinum toxin injection, and surgical revision.

Opioid-Induced Esophageal Dysmotility

Long-term opiate use can result in dysphagia with nonspecific abnormalities on esophageal manometry. Common findings include increased IRP, shortened DL, and absent (or weak) peristalsis. FLIP planimetry has also been used to identify aberrations in secondary peristalsis. If patients have dysphagia and chronic opiate use, the use of opiates should be discontinued.

✓ Esophagogastric junction outflow obstruction—clinically relevant diagnosis requires fulfillment of manometric criteria, symptoms of dysphagia or chest pain (or both), and findings supportive of obstruction with timed barium esophagram or functional lumen imaging probe (or both)

✓ Absent contractility can be a manifestation of connective tissue disease (specifically, limited scleroderma)

✓ Long-term opioid use can cause esophageal manometric abnormalities

---

Summary

The differential diagnosis of dysphagia is broad. Clinicians must first differentiate between oropharyngeal dysphagia and esophageal dysphagia from the history and physical examination. If obstruction is ruled out, esophageal HRM may be used to elucidate the underlying motility disorder and allow for appropriate therapeutic management.

Suggested Reading

Ahuja NK, Clarke JO. Scleroderma and the esophagus. Gastroenterol Clin North Am. 2021 Dec;50(4):905–18.

Balko RA, Codipilly DC, Ravi K. Minor esophageal functional disorders: are they relevant? Curr Treat Options Gastroenterol. 2020 Jan 17. [Epub ahead of print]

Jansson-Knodell CL, Codipilly DC, Leggett CL. Making dysphagia easier to swallow: a review for the practicing clinician. Mayo Clin Proc. 2017 Jun;92(6):965–72.

Kahrilas PJ, Bredenoord AJ, Fox M, Gyawali CP, Roman S, Smout AJPM, et al; International Working Group for Disorders of Gastrointestinal Motility and Function. Expert consensus document: Advances in the management of oesophageal motility disorders in the era of high-resolution manometry: a focus on achalasia syndromes. Nat Rev Gastroenterol Hepatol. 2017 Nov;14(11):677–88.

Miller AT, Matar R, Abu Dayyeh BK, Beran A, Vela MF, Lacy BE, et al. Postobesity surgery esophageal dysfunction: a combined cross-sectional prevalence study and retrospective analysis. Am J Gastroenterol. 2020 Oct;115(10):1669–80.

Ponds FA, van Raath MI, Mohamed SMM, Smout A, Bredenoord AJ. Diagnostic features of malignancy-associated pseudoachalasia. Aliment Pharmacol Ther. 2017 Jun;45(11):1449–58.

Vaezi MF, Pandolfino JE, Yadlapati RH, Greer KB, Kavitt RT. ACG clinical guidelines: diagnosis and management of achalasia. Am J Gastroenterol. 2020 Sep;115(9):1393–411.

Yadlapati R, Kahrilas PJ, Fox MR, Bredenoord AJ, Prakash Gyawali C, Roman S, et al. Esophageal motility disorders on high-resolution manometry: Chicago classification version 4.0(c). Neurogastroenterol Motil. 2021 Jan;33(1):e14058.

Yazaki E, Sifrim D. Anatomy and physiology of the esophageal body. Dis Esophagus. 2012 May;25(4):292–8.

Questions and Answers

Questions

Abbreviations used:

BE,	Barrett esophagus
CT,	computed tomography
EAC,	esophageal adenocarcinoma
EGD,	esophagogastroduodenoscopy
EGJ,	esophagogastric junction
EMR,	endoscopic mucosal resection
EoE,	eosinophilic esophagitis
EUS,	endoscopic ultrasonography
FLIP,	functional lumen imaging probe
GERD,	gastroesophageal reflux disease
HGD,	high-grade dysplasia
LES,	lower esophageal sphincter
LGD,	low-grade dysplasia
POEM,	peroral endoscopic myotomy
PPI,	proton pump inhibitor
RFA,	radiofrequency ablation
TLESR,	transient lower esophageal sphincter relaxation

Multiple Choice (choose the best answer)

I.1. A 42-year-old woman presents with cough and frequent throat clearing without any heartburn, regurgitation, dysphagia, or vomiting. She took omeprazole 20 mg twice daily, but her symptoms did not improve. Both her parents were told that they had GERD, although their primary symptom was heartburn. The patient is convinced that her symptoms are secondary to GERD, so she came to the gastroenterology clinic for further evaluation. What is the best next test in her management?

   a. EGD
   b. A pH monitoring study when omeprazole therapy has been held
   c. A pH monitoring study during omeprazole therapy
   d. CT of the neck

I.2. A 65-year-old man presents with a 10-year history of heartburn. He has symptoms multiple times per week, and the symptoms are worse at night. He has had some relief by managing the heartburn with over-the-counter antacids as needed. He has never taken a PPI or a histamine blocker. Over the past 6 months, he has also had occasional dysphagia and nausea. He has not had any weight loss. His comorbidities include obesity, type 2 diabetes, and hypertension. His medications include metformin, amlodipine, and lisinopril. He describes occasional use of alcohol and tobacco. What is the best next step in management?

   a. EGD
   b. A pH monitoring study
   c. A 2-week trial of oral omeprazole twice daily
   d. Referral to a thoracic surgeon for Nissen fundoplication

I.3. A 25-year-old man with a history of asthma and eczema presents for evaluation of intermittent solid food dysphagia over the past year. He has solid food dysphagia approximately once every 2 weeks and, rarely, he has a mild food impaction that clears in 1 to 2 minutes. He cannot recall any food triggers, and he does not have difficulty swallowing liquids. He has not had to visit an emergency department for food impaction. On EGD, his esophagus appears normal; esophageal biopsy specimens have 35 eosinophils per high-power field. What is the best next step in management?

   a. Dietary modifications with small, frequent meals consisting primarily of liquids
   b. Begin therapy with infliximab 5 mg/kg every 8 weeks
   c. Begin therapy with omeprazole 20 mg twice daily
   d. Begin a prednisone taper starting at 40 mg daily and decreasing by 5 mg every week

I.4. A 68-year-old man presents with a 3-month history of odynophagia. The symptoms are worse with solid foods, but they occur intermittently with liquids. He does not report any nausea, vomiting, or weight loss. His comorbidities include intermittent asthma, which is treated with albuterol as needed; heartburn, which is treated with once-daily omeprazole; and osteoarthritis that requires frequent use of acetaminophen and ibuprofen several times weekly. Examination of his oral cavity shows mild thrush. EGD shows 2 superficial ulcerations located opposite one another in the middle esophagus. Otherwise, the esophagus does not have rings, furrows, exudates, strictures, or inflammation. What is the most likely cause of the patient's odynophagia?

a. Medication-induced esophagitis
b. Infectious esophagitis
c. Erosive esophagitis due to GERD
d. EoE

I.5. A 55-year-old man with a history of tobacco use presented for further evaluation of long-standing heartburn that had continued for more than 7 years. He underwent upper endoscopy, which showed a 3-cm segment of circumferential, salmon-colored mucosa proximal to the EGJ and a 1-cm nonulcerated, raised lesion within the area of columnar metaplasia. The rest of the esophagus looked normal. Which of the following would be the most appropriate next step?

a. Perform RFA
b. Perform EUS
c. Perform targeted biopsies or EMR of the visible lesion
d. Start PPI therapy and have the patient return for endoscopic follow-up in 3 years

I.6. Which of the following patients should undergo endoscopic screening for BE?

a. A 45-year-old White woman with a history of tobacco use who has had GERD symptoms for more than 7 years
b. A 55-year-old White man with a history of alcohol use disorder and *Helicobacter pylori*–associated peptic ulcer disease
c. A 70-year-old Hispanic man with a family history of BE in a first-degree relative who is being treated with a daily PPI for functional dyspepsia
d. A 65-year-old Asian man with a history of tobacco use who has weekly GERD symptoms

I.7. A 60-year-old White man with obesity and chronic GERD symptoms underwent upper endoscopy and was found to have a 6-cm segment of salmon-colored mucosa proximal to the EGJ without any focal lesions seen on a good-quality endoscopic evaluation. Biopsies were consistent with BE with HGD. Which of the following is the most appropriate next step?

a. Repeat the upper endoscopy with biopsies in 6 months
b. Repeat the upper endoscopy with biopsies in 12 months
c. Start twice-daily PPI therapy and continue indefinitely
d. Perform RFA in 1 to 2 months
e. Consult a thoracic surgeon about the possibility for antireflux surgery

I.8. A 52-year-old man with long-standing GERD underwent upper endoscopy for BE screening at his community hospital and was found to have a 2-cm columnar-lined segment in the distal tubular esophagus. Biopsies showed intestinal metaplasia with LGD. Which of the following is the most appropriate next step?

a. Repeat the upper endoscopy with biopsies in 6 months
b. Confirm the dysplasia with a gastrointestinal pathologist who has expertise in BE pathology
c. Start twice-daily PPI therapy and repeat the upper endoscopy with biopsies in 1 year
d. Perform EUS
e. Repeat the upper endoscopy with biopsies in 3 to 5 years

I.9. A 72-year-old man presents with a 3-month history of solid food and liquid dysphagia. He reports food sticking in his midchest and describes a stacking phenomenon that occurs during meals. In the past 3 months, he has lost approximately 20 kg. His medical comorbidities include high blood pressure and type 2 diabetes, and he is a current smoker with a history of more than 50 pack-years. On upper endoscopy, the esophageal lumen is dilated and there is moderate resistance to passage of the endoscope through the EGJ, but the findings are normal otherwise. An esophagram shows distal tapering of the esophagus as it approaches the EGJ and poor opening of the junction itself. High-resolution esophageal manometry results confirm the diagnosis of type II achalasia. Which of the following is the best next step?

a. No further evaluation is required, but he should be advised to chew his food carefully and to eat slowly
b. No further evaluation is required, but arrangements should be made for enteral nutrition access
c. He should be referred for either Heller myotomy with fundoplication or POEM
d. He should undergo CT of the chest
e. He should receive an injection of botulinum toxin into the LES

I.10. A 53-year-old woman presents with a 10-year history of heartburn symptoms, and in the past 2 to 3 years progressive solid food dysphagia has developed. Her heartburn had been well controlled with once-daily omeprazole, but in the past 6 months she has had difficulty controlling the symptoms even though she has increased the PPI dosage. Upper endoscopy shows grade C esophagitis and a patulous EGJ. Esophageal biopsy findings are unremarkable. An esophagram shows mild dysmotility without other abnormalities. The results of high-resolution esophageal manometry are shown below:

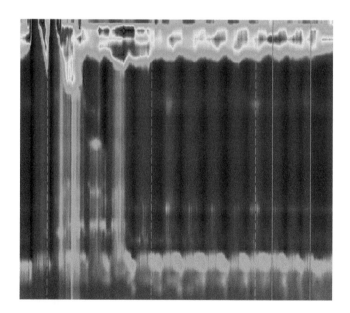

Which of the following is the best next step?

a. Proceed with FLIP planimetry
b. Discontinue PPI therapy and initiate twice-daily histamine-receptor antagonist therapy
c. Test for anticentromere and anti–Scl-70 antibodies
d. Arrange for botulinum toxin injection into the LES
e. Perform 24-hour pH-impedance testing when she is not receiving PPI therapy

I.11. **Which of the following may result in excess gastric acid exposure in the esophagus?**

    a. Increased number of TLESRs

    b. Diminished activity of nitric oxide on esophageal sphincter receptors

    c. Diminished visceral body fat

    d. Rapid gastric emptying

    e. Increased rate of secondary contractions in the esophagus

I.12. **A 65-year-old man presents with a 5-year history of slowly progressive dysphagia. He reports that food, particularly meats and dry breads, hang at the top of his chest. He describes nocturnal regurgitation of food that he had eaten earlier in the day. His wife remarks that he has always been a slow eater. He has hypertension that is controlled well with once-daily hydrochlorothiazide. A representative swallow from high-resolution esophageal manometry is shown below:**

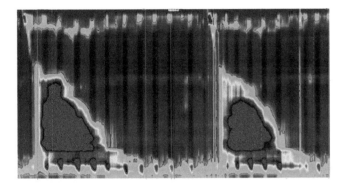

The integrated relaxation pressure is 28.3 mm Hg, and distal latency is 2.3 seconds. Which of the following would be the definitive therapeutic option for this patient?

    a. Calcium channel blockers

    b. Botulinum toxin injection into the LES

    c. Heller myotomy with fundoplication

    d. Pneumatic dilation

    e. POEM

Answers

I.1.   Answer b.

The patient presents with atypical, extraesophageal symptoms that can sometimes be associated with GERD. However, she has had no response to acid-suppressive therapy, so GERD is less likely. To determine whether she has GERD, she should undergo a pH monitoring study when omeprazole therapy has been held. She does not have any alarm symptoms such as nausea, vomiting, dysphagia, odynophagia, hematemesis, or unintentional weight loss, so EGD would not be the best next test. A pH monitoring study should be performed during therapy with a PPI when the diagnosis of GERD is certain, but the patient has not had a response to acid-suppressive therapy. CT of the neck is used to evaluate for structural causes of oropharyngeal symptoms and may be considered after an evaluation has been completed for GERD, which is the patient's primary concern.

I.2.   Answer a.

The patient presents with long-standing symptoms typical of GERD. However, recently he has had alarm symptoms, including dysphagia and nausea. Therefore, additional evaluation is needed

to rule out a structural cause for his symptoms before the administration of empirical medical therapy with a PPI. EGD would allow for assessment of complications due to long-standing GERD such as erosive esophagitis, peptic stricture, Barrett esophagus, and esophageal adenocarcinoma. The patient has a typical symptom of GERD and a positive response to antacids, which is suggestive of GERD; therefore, pH monitoring should not be the next test. A referral for surgery without an appropriate evaluation would not be recommended.

I.3.   Answer c.

This young man with a history of atopic conditions (asthma and eczema) presents with dysphagia, and this scenario is characteristic of a patient with EoE. The diagnosis is confirmed with the esophageal biopsies showing more than 15 eosinophils per high-power field. Notably, sometimes the esophagus does appear normal in EoE. First-line treatment of EoE includes PPIs, topical (not systemic) corticosteroids, and a food-elimination diet. Dietary modifications with small, frequent meals of primarily liquids are not a good long-term option and may be more appropriate for a patient with gastroparesis. Infliximab is not a good initial choice, but it may be considered rarely for patients with truly refractory disease. Oral corticosteroids may be effective but are associated with adverse effects and are not a good long-term option for this young patient. The use of topical corticosteroids would be reasonable and would avoid the adverse effects of systemic corticosteroids.

I.4.   Answer a.

The most common causes of odynophagia include medication-induced esophagitis and infectious esophagitis. This patient takes ibuprofen, which is associated with medication-induced esophagitis. Additionally, the EGD shows kissing ulcers in the middle esophagus, which is also suggestive of this condition. The aortic arch is near the middle esophagus, and medications often become lodged in this area when patients do not take pills with water or take them in the supine position. This can result in ulceration on opposite walls of the esophagus. In patients with medication-induced esophagitis, commonly implicated medications include oral bisphosphonates, nonsteroidal anti-inflammatory drugs, potassium, iron, and antibiotics such as tetracycline. Endoscopic findings from this patient did not show thick, white exudates that are characteristic of esophageal candidiasis. The presence of thrush in the oral cavity does not necessarily indicate the presence of esophageal candidiasis. Patients with erosive esophagitis from GERD most commonly present with erosions, inflammation, or ulcerations in the distal esophagus instead of involvement of only the middle esophagus. EoE would not be likely because patients usually have dysphagia, and this patient did not have the typical endoscopic features of this condition (ie, rings, furrows, exudates, strictures, or edema).

I.5.   Answer c.

EMR should be performed in patients who have visible mucosal abnormalities within the underlying Barrett mucosa to rule out invasive adenocarcinoma and obtain a precise histologic diagnosis. EMR provides larger specimens, decreases interobserver variability among pathologists, and leads to upstaging of the histologic diagnosis (compared to biopsies) in 30% to 40% of cases. In the absence of EMR expertise, targeted biopsies from the lesion (placed in a separate appropriately labeled jar) may be acceptable. If histologic examination from the EMR shows dysplasia or intramucosal carcinoma with negative deep and lateral margins, the remaining flat BE mucosa should be treated with ablative therapy to eradicate the residual Barrett mucosa given the risk of metachronous dysplasia within the remaining Barrett segment. EUS would not be indicated in the absence of confirmed invasive adenocarcinoma.

I.6.   Answer d.
Current American College of Gastroenterology guidelines suggest that BE screening should be considered for patients who have chronic GERD (>5 years) or frequent gastroesophageal reflux symptoms (at least weekly) and have at least 3 risk factors (male sex, White race, age >50 years, central obesity, current or past history of cigarette smoking, and confirmed history of BE or EAC in a first-degree relative).

I.7.   Answer d.
If HGD is detected in patients without limited life expectancy, endoscopic eradication therapy should be performed. This includes endoscopic resection to remove any visible lesions with subsequent endoscopic ablation of the remaining BE segment. For nonnodular BE, endoscopic ablative therapy such as RFA should be performed to ensure complete eradication of Barrett mucosa and to prevent further progression to EAC. Antireflux surgery is not indicated if HGD has been confirmed by an expert gastrointestinal pathologist and medical therapy has controlled the gastroesophageal reflux (symptomatically with confirmation by the absence of esophagitis or stricturing). Confirmed HGD is unlikely to reverse by optimizing antireflux therapy and is an actionable diagnosis.

I.8.   Answer b.
The presence of LGD or HGD should be confirmed by a gastrointestinal pathologist before the treatment strategy is finalized. Studies have shown that most cases of LGD reported in the community are downgraded to "no dysplasia" after they are reviewed by academic or expert pathologists. This is most likely due to the lack of experience in the diagnosis of BE dysplasia in the community and the overcalling (ie, providing false-positive results) of inflammation-related reactive atypia as dysplasia (particularly LGD). Given that current recommendations are to consider endoscopic ablation in patients with LGD (on the basis of evidence from randomized controlled trials), it is critically important that all diagnoses of dysplasia (LGD and HGD) be confirmed by an expert gastrointestinal pathologist. After LGD is confirmed, ablative therapy can be discussed with the patient, and both surveillance (at 6 months, 12 months, and annually thereafter) and endoscopic ablative therapy are reasonable options. Additionally, evaluation at an expert BE center (after optimization of the PPI dose) leads to upstaging to HGD or carcinoma in almost 25% of these patients. In the absence of EAC, EUS is not indicated and surveillance in 3 to 5 years is recommended for patients without dysplasia.

I.9.   Answer d.
This patient presents with typical symptoms of achalasia. However, his symptom onset was quite rapid. Secondary achalasia must be ruled out given his age and comorbidities (smoking history) and the considerable weight loss over a short time. Therefore, further evaluation is required. Definitive therapy for achalasia (with Heller myotomy or POEM) would not be the best next step before secondary causes of achalasia are ruled out

because the dysphagia may improve with treatment of the primary issue. Temporary therapy with a botulinum toxin injection would not be appropriate because evaluation of the cause of secondary achalasia has not been initiated. CT of the chest is the best next step because of the patient's smoking history. An underlying pulmonary malignancy should be ruled out as a cause of his secondary achalasia.

I.10.   Answer c.
This patient has gastroesophageal reflux and dysphagia, and endoscopic findings include a patulous EGJ. Results from manometry show essentially an absence of peristalsis and weak LES pressures. The overall clinical picture is consistent with connective tissue disease, and testing should proceed for anticentromere and anti–Scl-70 antibodies to assess for scleroderma. FLIP planimetry will not provide further information. Given the patulous EGJ seen on endoscopy, the distensibility index of the EGJ is probably high, but management would not be changed. PPIs are more effective than histamine-receptor antagonists, so PPI therapy should not be discontinued. Botulinum toxin injection will not improve dysphagia and would probably worsen this patient's reflux because her LES is already weak. The presence of grade C esophagitis confirms the presence of reflux disease, and pH-impedance testing may be helpful to assess the degree of gastric acid suppression when the patient is receiving PPI therapy, but if this testing were performed when she was not receiving PPI therapy, the results would not be clinically useful.

I.11   Answer a.
TLESRs allow for the release of increased pressure within the stomach. While this can allow for air to escape, TLESRs may allow for acid to reflux into the esophagus, and a higher number of TLESRs has been hypothesized to be a cause of reflux disease and excess acid exposure. Nitric oxide mediates sphincter relaxation; therefore, diminished activity may result in less acid reflux owing to fewer sphincter relaxations. Excess visceral body fat can increase pressure on the stomach, resulting in heightened reflux events, and may explain why obesity is a risk factor for reflux and reflux-related complications. However, diminished visceral body fat would not be expected to increase esophageal acid exposure. Similarly, gastroparesis can result in excess acid exposure because of increased gastric pressures, but rapid emptying would not be expected to cause excess gastric acid exposure. Secondary contractions in the esophagus would allow for clearance of refluxate, so increased numbers of contractions should decrease esophageal acid exposure.

I.12.   Answer e.
This patient has classic symptoms of achalasia. Results of manometry are consistent with a diagnosis of type III achalasia. Lack of relaxation of the LES and a spastic component (distal latency <4.5 seconds) are hallmarks of this diagnosis. Calcium channel blockers are poorly effective in management of achalasia. Botulinum toxin injection would probably provide some symptomatic improvement, but the effects would not last long, and symptoms would probably return in 3 to 6 months. For patients with type III achalasia, POEM is preferred because the length of the myotomy can be tailored to that of the spastic component as identified on manometry. Therefore, POEM would be preferred for definitive management over Heller myotomy with fundoplication or pneumatic dilation.

II

Stomach

4

Peptic Ulcer Disease

STEPHANIE L. HANSEL, MD, MS

A *peptic ulcer* is a persistent break in the gastrointestinal mucosa of the stomach or duodenum that is at least 5 mm and penetrates through the muscularis mucosa. At endoscopy, an ulcer with perceivable depth should be readily apparent. Smaller, shallower mucosal breaks are erosions. Most peptic ulcers are due to *Helicobacter pylori* infection or the administration of nonsteroidal anti-inflammatory drugs (NSAIDs). The term *peptic ulcer disease* (PUD) refers to ulceration that depends in part on the acid and peptic (ie, with pepsins) activity of gastric juice. Most peptic ulcers occur in the stomach or duodenal bulb.

> ✓ **Peptic ulcer**—a persistent break in the gastrointestinal mucosa of the stomach or duodenum that is at least 5 mm and penetrates through the muscularis mucosa
> ✓ *Helicobacter pylori*—a gram-negative, urease-producing bacterium that lives in the mucous layer of the gastric epithelium; the major infectious cause of peptic ulcer disease

Epidemiology

PUD is a common condition worldwide and occurs in persons of all ages. In resource-limited countries, most children are infected with *H pylori* before they are 10 years old, and they may carry a chronic infection into adulthood. Children living in resource-rich countries are unlikely to be infected with *H pylori*. The overall prevalence in the US is approximately 30%. In the US,

Abbreviations: COX-2, cyclooxygenase 2; ECL, enterochromaffin-like; EGD, esophagogastroduodenoscopy; GERD, gastroesophageal reflux disease; H₂, histamine; NSAID, nonsteroidal anti-inflammatory drug; PPI, proton pump inhibitor; PUD, peptic ulcer disease

the infection rate is lower in the non-Hispanic White population and higher in other racial and ethnic groups.

Pathophysiology

Peptic ulcers result from an imbalance between processes that damage the gastrointestinal mucosa and mechanisms that protect it. Acid secretion occurs through gastric proton pumps located in parietal cells. These are hydrogen-potassium-ATPase pumps, which use adenosine triphosphate to transport hydrogen across the cell membrane into the gastric lumen and to transport potassium in the opposite direction. At rest, these pumps are located intracellularly. Stimulation of parietal cells by a combination of acetylcholine (vagus nerve), gastrin (antral G cells), and histamine (enterochromaffin-like [ECL] cells) translocates the proton pumps to the apical secretory canalicular (luminal) membrane, where they become functional (Figure 4.1). During the cephalic phase of meal-stimulated acid secretion, vagal activity stimulates ECL cells, G cells, and parietal cells. During the gastric phase, distention of the stomach augments vagal output, and short peptides, amino acids, calcium, and alkaline pH stimulate gastrin release by G cells. Gastrin release is inhibited by a gastric pH less than 3. Acid pH also stimulates somatostatin-producing D cells in the antrum and body of the stomach, with somatostatin inhibiting gastrin release from G cells and acid secretion from parietal cells.

The normal mucosal defense mechanisms against gastric acid include the surface mucous layer; the secretion of bicarbonate, mucus, and phospholipid by gastroduodenal epithelial surface mucous cells; the epithelial barrier; mucosal blood flow; epithelial cell restitution; and epithelial cell renewal (Figure 4.2). Many of these defense mechanisms are prostaglandin dependent.

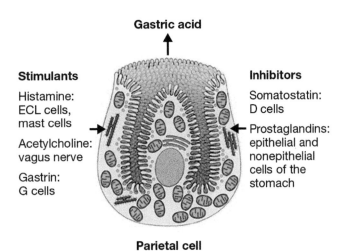

Figure 4.1. Physiology of the Parietal Cell. ECL indicates enterochromaffin-like.

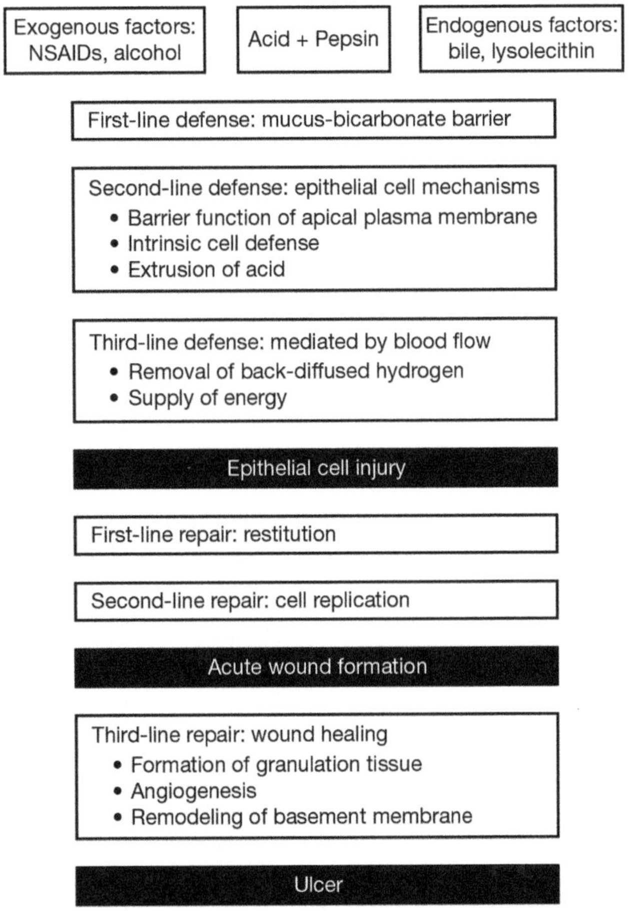

Exogenous factors: NSAIDs, alcohol | Acid + Pepsin | Endogenous factors: bile, lysolecithin

First-line defense: mucus-bicarbonate barrier

Second-line defense: epithelial cell mechanisms
- Barrier function of apical plasma membrane
- Intrinsic cell defense
- Extrusion of acid

Third-line defense: mediated by blood flow
- Removal of back-diffused hydrogen
- Supply of energy

Epithelial cell injury

First-line repair: restitution

Second-line repair: cell replication

Acute wound formation

Third-line repair: wound healing
- Formation of granulation tissue
- Angiogenesis
- Remodeling of basement membrane

Ulcer

Figure 4.2. Cascade of Mucosal Defense and Repair Mechanisms. Damaging effects on epithelial cells of exogenous and endogenous factors are amplified by peptic acid activity. If the 3 lines of defense fail, epithelial cell injury occurs. Repair is by restitution and cell replication. If these repair mechanisms fail, an acute wound forms. Ulcers form only with the failure of acute wound healing mechanisms. NSAID indicates nonsteroidal anti-inflammatory drug. (Adapted from Soll AH. Peptic ulcer and its complications. In: Feldman M, Sleisenger MH, Scharschmidt BF, editors. Sleisenger & Fordtran's gastrointestinal and liver disease: pathophysiology, diagnosis, management. Vol 1. 6th ed. Philadelphia [PA]: WB Saunders Company; c1998. p. 620-78; used with permission.)

Etiology

As stated above, the most common causes of PUD are *H pylori* infection and use of NSAIDs, including low-dose aspirin. Less common causes of PUD include hypersecretory states, viral infections (cytomegalovirus and herpes simplex virus 1 infections), drug exposure (cocaine), ischemia, radiotherapy, and infiltrative disorders (malignancy, sarcoidosis, and Crohn disease). Cirrhosis, chronic obstructive pulmonary disease, kidney failure, and organ transplant are associated with PUD, but the pathophysiologic mechanisms are unclear. When stress-related ulcerations of the stomach occur in critically ill patients, ischemia is the most likely mechanism.

H pylori Infection

Worldwide, *H pylori* infection is the main cause of both gastric ulcers (60%) and duodenal ulcers (up to 90%). More than half of all persons in the world are infected with *H pylori*, but ulcers develop in only 10% of them. In resource-limited countries, many children (>70%) are infected with *H pylori* before the age of 10 years, and more than 90% of adults are infected by the age of 50 years. In the US, *H pylori* infection is uncommon in persons born after 1945—improved sanitation and the increased use of antibiotics during childhood may be largely responsible. Persons born before 1945 are more likely to have been infected with *H pylori* (60% of them were infected by age 60 years). Having a lower socioeconomic status, residing in a crowded household, and living with someone infected with *H pylori* are known risk factors for *H pylori* infection. In the US, people of Hispanic or East Asian ethnicity have the highest rates of *H pylori* infection. The infection rates are similar between men and women. The mode of transmission is believed to be from person to person through oral-oral and fecal-oral routes.

H pylori is a gram-negative, spiral-shaped microaerophilic bacterium with multiple flagella. The organisms exist as dormant coccoid forms in culture and survive only on gastric-type mucosa in the stomach or metaplastic gastric-type epithelium in the duodenum or small bowel (Meckel diverticulum). In the stomach, *H pylori* lives within the mucous layer, surviving the acidic pH of the stomach in part by its urease activity, which converts urea (ubiquitous) to ammonia, and by its motility, its ability to adhere to epithelial cells, its microaerophilic properties, and its proteases, which may digest mucus (Figure 4.3). Often *H pylori* does not survive in an alkaline environment in the stomach (eg, after gastroenterostomy).

Gastric-type mucosa is damaged by *H pylori* through its production of ammonia, proteases, lipases, phospholipases, and mucinases and by its induction of a local immune response (chemotactic factors for neutrophils and monocytes and a host T-cell response). Virulence factors specific for *H pylori* and associated with ulcer disease include a *cag* pathogenicity island, whose product (CagA) enters host epithelial cells, and certain *vacA* loci that encode a bacterial toxin (VacA). In many persons infected with *H pylori*, gastrin levels are higher than normal because of antral-predominant, active chronic gastritis that decreases the number of antral D cells and the level of somatostatin; the result is an increased rate of gastric acid secretion and a greater likelihood of the development of a duodenal ulcer. Abnormally high levels of gastric acid secretion may damage the duodenum and result in gastric metaplasia, allowing *H pylori* to colonize the duodenum. This pattern of duodenal ulcers appears to be more common in persons who are infected with *H pylori* later in life. In contrast, persons infected with *H pylori* early in life have a

4. Peptic Ulcer Disease **53**

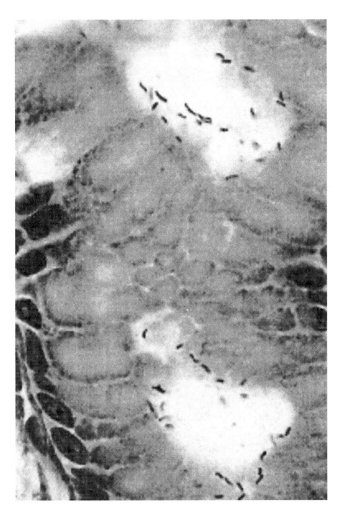

Figure 4.3. Section of Stomach Showing *Helicobacter pylori*. The bacteria are the black rods (Wenger-Angritt stain). (Adapted from Emory TS, Carpenter HA, Gostout CJ, Sobin LH. Atlas of gastrointestinal endoscopy & endoscopic biopsies. Washington [DC]: Armed Forces Institute of Pathology, American Registry of Pathology; c2000.)

multifocal and pan-gastric gastritis. These patients have parietal cell damage, decreased production of acid, and a greater risk for gastric ulcer.

Eradication of *H pylori* eliminates gastric and duodenal ulcers and prevents recurrence. In the US, the recurrence rate of infection with *H pylori* is less than 3% per year.

Nonsteroidal Anti-inflammatory Drugs

NSAIDs constitute approximately 5% of all prescribed medications worldwide. PUD has been estimated to develop in up to 15% of long-term NSAID users, and a complication such as bleeding or perforation may develop in up to 4% of them. When ingested orally, NSAIDs cause damage to the gastric epithelium topically and cause systemic damage by inhibiting the production of prostaglandins by gastroduodenal epithelial cells. Risk factors for NSAID-related gastrointestinal tract ulceration and its complications include age older than 60 years; previous history of PUD (especially if complicated); the first 30 to 90 days of NSAID therapy; use of high-dose NSAIDs or simultaneous use of multiple NSAIDs; concomitant use of corticosteroids, use of other antiplatelet drugs, alendronate, or anticoagulants; history of comorbid conditions; and *H pylori* infection.

The risk of injury to the gastroduodenal mucosa by aspirin is dose-related and can occur even with administration of low-dose aspirin. Because of the antiplatelet effects of aspirin and other NSAIDs, complications such as ulceration with bleeding or perforation can occur throughout the gastrointestinal tract. Cyclooxygenase 2 (COX-2) selective inhibitors have been associated with a decreased risk of clinically apparent PUD, including complications, but as with nonselective NSAIDs, cardiovascular risks are a concern. PUD may develop in up to 5% of patients who take COX-2 inhibitors, and ulceration may heal slowly in persons who continue to ingest COX-2 inhibitors. COX-2 activity appears to be important for ulcer healing. Persons who take both low-dose aspirin and a COX-2 inhibitor have an increased risk for PUD and its complications compared with those who take either drug alone. Antiplatelet agents such as clopidogrel have been linked to a high rate of complications, such as gastrointestinal tract bleeding, particularly in patients who previously have had gastrointestinal tract complications, whether the antiplatelet agents were taken alone or with NSAIDs. Platelet activity, like COX-2 activity, appears to be important for ulcer healing.

> ✓ Most common causes of PUD—NSAIDs and *H pylori* infection
> ✓ PUD may develop in up to 15% of long-term users of NSAIDs; up to 4% of those patients may have a complication such as bleeding or perforation

H pylori Infection and NSAIDs

The relationship between NSAID use and *H pylori* infection is complex and controversial. Patients who are infected with *H pylori* and have increased levels of gastric acid secretion and patients who have active or subclinical PUD are most likely to be at increased risk for PUD and its complications after initiation of NSAID therapy. These risks are decreased if *H pylori* infection is eradicated before treatment with NSAIDs. In contrast, persons who take NSAIDs long-term and who have a history of complicated PUD and are infected with *H pylori* are not protected from additional PUD complications after eradication of *H pylori* infection. Ongoing ingestion of NSAIDs perpetuates the increased risk of additional complications.

Hypersecretion of Gastric Acid

Mild hypersecretion of gastric acid occurs in many but not all patients who have PUD and are infected with *H pylori*, especially in those who have duodenal ulcers. Zollinger-Ellison syndrome is a rare cause of hypersecretion of gastric acid. In most patients who have the syndrome, upper gastrointestinal tract ulceration occurs, often involving the esophagus, stomach, and duodenum and including ulceration of the duodenum beyond the duodenal bulb. Gastric acid hypersecretion with PUD occurs in about one-third of patients who have systemic mastocytosis because of the increased release of histamine by mast cells. Increased release of histamine, acid hypersecretion, and PUD have been identified also in patients who have basophilic leukemia and chronic myelogenous leukemia with basophilia. Uncommonly, antral G-cell hyperplasia has been found in patients who do not have Zollinger-Ellison syndrome (according to negative secretin test results) but do have PUD with gastric acid hypersecretion due to hypergastrinemia. Many of these patients also have *H pylori* infection, and their PUD and gastric acid hypersecretion resolve when *H pylori* is eradicated. Gastric outlet or duodenal obstruction due to various causes can produce gastric distention,

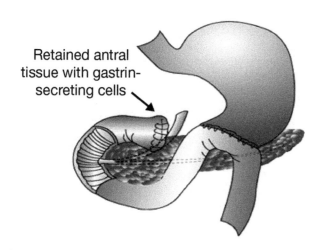

Retained antral
tissue with gastrin-
secreting cells

Figure 4.4.   Retained Antrum After Billroth II Operation. (Adapted from Tringali A, Loperfido S, Costamagna G, Familiari P. Endoscopic retrograde cholangiopancreatography (ERCP) after Billroth II reconstruction [Internet]. In: Howell DA, editor. UpToDate: Waltham [MA]. c2020. [updated 2020 Dec 18; cited 2022 Sep 8]. Available from: http://www.uptodate.com/; used with permission.)

hypergastrinemia, hypersecretion of acid, and ulceration proximal to the obstruction. Severe PUD, hypersecretion of gastric acid, and hypergastrinemia are common in the few patients in whom retained gastric antrum syndrome occurs after a Billroth II operation, when a small cuff of gastric antrum is left as part of the afferent limb (Figure 4.4). In patients who undergo substantial small-bowel resection, postoperative complications can include hypergastrinemia, hypersecretion of gastric acid, and severe PUD because of the sudden loss of inhibitors of gastrin and acid secretion.

Miscellaneous Conditions

Ulceration of the gastroduodenal area rarely occurs with infections other than those caused by *H pylori*. In immunocompromised patients, cytomegalovirus infection may cause ulceration, often producing large, deep, and multiple ulcers that are frequently complicated by bleeding, perforation, or obstruction. Rarely, ulceration can occur from infections such as syphilis or tuberculosis (often antral), after radiotherapy, and from sarcoidosis, Crohn disease, vasculitis, and ischemia. Gastric ulceration can be due to malignancy, including adenocarcinoma, lymphoma, sarcoma, gastrointestinal stromal tumors, and metastatic malignancies.

Among persons who smoke cigarettes, compared with nonsmokers, PUD is more common and is more likely to be complicated, to require surgery, to be slow to heal, and to recur. Although alcohol can directly damage the gastroduodenal mucosa and stimulate acid secretion, there is no evidence that alcohol is a risk factor for PUD. Similarly, there is no clear link between either diet or psychologic factors and ulcer disease.

Clinical Features

The presentation of patients with PUD varies. Many patients present with dyspeptic symptoms, but some are asymptomatic, and others present with perforation. Ulcerlike dyspepsia is one of the most common symptoms. Classically, patients with duodenal ulcers present with epigastric burning or a hunger sensation, especially 1 to 3 hours after a meal or during the night. The pain improves after the ingestion of food, antacids, or antisecretory agents. Thus, these patients tend to gain weight. In contrast, persons with gastric ulcers are more likely to feel discomfort after eating and may have weight loss. Patients who have nonulcer dyspepsia can have the same symptoms as those with PUD, and many persons with PUD have atypical symptoms. Also, the overlap of symptoms between patients with gastroesophageal reflux disease (GERD) and those with PUD is considerable. The differential diagnosis for PUD includes functional dyspepsia, GERD, biliary pain, gastric or duodenal malignancy, medication adverse effect, pancreatitis, and ischemia.

Diagnosis

Diagnosis of PUD is difficult from the history and physical examination alone given the wide variation in presentation. The definitive diagnosis can be established with esophagogastroduodenoscopy (EGD). It is sensitive for detecting small ulcerations and is the best method for determining the location and severity of the ulceration. In addition, biopsies can be obtained to assess for the cause of PUD, or endoscopic therapy can be applied if the ulcer is bleeding.

Diagnosis of *H pylori* Infection

Many tests are available for diagnosing *H pylori* infection (Table 4.1). However, testing should be ordered only if the patient will be offered treatment if the results are positive. No single test is considered the criterion standard for the diagnosis of *H pylori*. Two categories of test are available: noninvasive and invasive (or endoscopic). The decision as to which test to order should be based on the clinical circumstances, the pretest probability, and the cost and availability of the test. In patients who have PUD without an obvious cause, a second test for *H pylori* should be conducted because false-negative results are possible. Many tests (culture, histology, breath and stool antigen tests, and urease testing) depend on the number of organisms, and false-negative results are frequent if the patient has been exposed recently to antibiotics, bismuth, or a proton pump inhibitor (PPI). Before testing, patients should not receive treatment with antibiotics or bismuth for 4 to 6 weeks or with PPIs for 2 weeks before testing (histamine [H$_2$]-receptor blockers can be taken).

Serologic Tests

Serologic testing for *H pylori* should be avoided because it has low accuracy in low-prevalence populations (such as in the US)

Table 4.1.   Diagnostic Tests for *Helicobacter pylori*

Test	Sensitivity, %	Specificity, %
Nonendoscopic tests		
In-office antibody test	88-94	74-88
ELISA on serum	85	79
Stool antigen test	94	97
Urea breath test	88-95	95-100
Endoscopic tests		
Biopsy urease test	90	95
Histology	95	98
Culture	80-98	100

Abbreviation: ELISA, enzyme-linked immunosorbent assay.

and would result in inappropriate treatment of many patients. If serologic testing is performed, it should be confirmed with additional testing for *H pylori*, such as the stool antigen test or urea breath test.

> ✓ Serologic testing for *H pylori* should be avoided because it has poor accuracy where the prevalence is low, such as in the US

Stool Antigen Test

The *H pylori* stool antigen test is rapid, highly sensitive, and highly specific. In contrast to serologic testing, it can be used to evaluate both active infection and response to therapy; thus, it is cost-effective. This test is affected by recent use of bismuth compounds, antibiotics, and PPIs.

Urea Breath Test

Because *H pylori* is practically the only infectious organism in the upper gastrointestinal tract capable of producing urea via urease, urea labeled with carbon 13 or carbon 14 can be administered as a breath test. The urea breath test is rapid, highly sensitive, and highly specific. Like stool antigen testing, it is a highly reliable method for confirming eradication of *H pylori* after treatment.

Rapid Urease Tests

Biopsy specimens obtained during endoscopy can be tested for urease with rapid urease testing. These tests are rapid, highly sensitive, and highly specific. False-positive results can occur with small intestinal bacterial overgrowth (from urease-producing *Proteus*) and from *Helicobacter* species other than *H pylori*. Gastrointestinal tract bleeding can cause false-negative results.

Histologic Examination

Histologic examination is highly sensitive and highly specific but expensive. Biopsy specimens (5 or 6) should be taken from the antrum, fundus, and incisura. Silver staining is recommended to facilitate the detection of *H pylori*.

Culture

Culture for *H pylori* after endoscopic biopsy is not widely available, is not rapid, and is less sensitive than noninvasive tests and histologic examination. Culture may be used best to determine antimicrobial sensitivity for patients who have resistant *H pylori* infections.

Treatment

With improved understanding of the pathogenesis of PUD, appropriate treatment has been developed. PPIs are a mainstay of therapy and are critical to ulcer healing independently of the cause. PPI therapy is superior to antacids, H$_2$-receptor antagonists, sucralfate, and prostaglandins. Additional treatment depends on the cause of the ulcer.

Treatment of *H pylori* Infection

Patients who test positive for *H pylori* should be given therapy to eradicate it because *H pylori* is classified as a carcinogen. Therapy is also indicated for patients who have *H pylori* infection and extranodal marginal zone B-cell lymphoma or gastric adenocarcinoma. In addition, first-degree relatives of patients who have *H pylori* infection and gastric adenocarcinoma should receive treatment.

The optimal therapeutic regimen for *H pylori* infection has not been defined, but the guidelines for first-line therapy for eradication of *H pylori* require 14 days of therapy. If a patient with an active infection has been exposed to macrolides or the local rates for clarithromycin resistance exceed 15%, bismuth-based quadruple therapy should be prescribed. Quadruple therapy includes a PPI, bismuth, metronidazole, and tetracycline.

Patients may be offered triple therapy if they have not been exposed to macrolides and if the local clarithromycin resistance rates are low. Triple therapy includes a PPI in combination with clarithromycin and amoxicillin (metronidazole is used instead of amoxicillin for patients allergic to penicillin) (Table 4.2).

Although metronidazole resistance may occur, the use of metronidazole in combination with other agents (PPI, bismuth, or tetracycline) besides clarithromycin and the use of a higher dose (500 mg twice daily) can diminish the rate of treatment failure. Resistance to amoxicillin, tetracycline, or bismuth is rare.

If a patient has a persistent *H pylori* infection, the choice of therapy should be guided by the prior treatment regimen. For example, if triple therapy was given, quadruple therapy should be prescribed. If quadruple therapy was given, a levofloxacin-based

Table 4.2. American College of Gastroenterology First-Line Regimens for *Helicobacter pylori* Eradication

Patients	Regimen
Patients who are *not* allergic to penicillin and have *not* previously received a macrolide	Bismuth subsalicylate 300 mg orally 4 times daily, metronidazole 250-500 mg orally 4 times daily, tetracycline 500 mg orally 4 times daily, and standard-dose PPI twice daily for 10-14 d
Patients who are *not* allergic to penicillin and *have* previously received a macrolide	Bismuth subsalicylate 300 mg orally 4 times daily, metronidazole 250-500 mg orally 4 times daily, tetracycline 500 mg orally 4 times daily, and standard-dose PPI twice daily for 10-14 d
Patients who *are* allergic to penicillin and have *not* previously received a macrolide or cannot tolerate bismuth quadruple therapy	Standard-dose PPI twice daily, clarithromycin 500 mg twice daily, and metronidazole 500 mg twice daily for 10-14 d
Patients who *are* allergic to penicillin and *have* previously received a macrolide	Bismuth subsalicylate 300 mg orally 4 times daily, metronidazole 250-500 mg orally 4 times daily, tetracycline 500 mg orally 4 times daily, and standard-dose PPI twice daily for 10-14 d

Abbreviation: PPI, proton pump inhibitor.

Data from Chey WD, Leontiadis GI, Howden CW, Moss SF. ACG clinical guideline: Treatment of Helicobacter pylori infection. Am J Gastroenterol. 2017 Feb;112(2):212-39.

regimen could be offered. In discussions with the patient, the clinician should assess for medication nonadherence and reinforce the importance of completing the regimen. Eradication of *H pylori* should be confirmed after treatment.

Treatment of NSAID Ulcers

If possible, a patient who has active ulceration should stop taking all NSAIDs, especially if the patient is losing blood. If NSAID therapy cannot be discontinued, the use of a decreased NSAID dose should be considered. In addition, PPI therapy should be started and the patient should be monitored.

Antacids

Antacids can heal ulcers by binding bile, inhibiting pepsin, and promoting angiogenesis. However, ulcer healing requires high doses of antacids, which often cause adverse effects. Thus, antacids are rarely used to treat PUD.

H$_2$-Receptor Antagonists

Three H$_2$-receptor antagonists (cimetidine, nizatidine, and famotidine) are available. All 3 are highly effective for the treatment of PUD. Cimetidine is rarely prescribed because it has a short half-life, several drug-drug interactions, and adverse effects. Cimetidine binds to cytochrome P450 and may affect the metabolism of certain drugs, such as warfarin, lidocaine, theophylline, and phenytoin. It also has dose-dependent adverse effects that include gynecomastia, breast tenderness, and impotence. Nizatidine and famotidine are longer acting, and famotidine has the longest duration of action. (Ranitidine was recalled from the US market in April 2020.) Healing of ulceration can be accomplished with an 8-week regimen of single dosing at bedtime with any H$_2$-receptor blocker. H$_2$-receptor blockers do not have activity against *H pylori*.

Proton Pump Inhibitors

PPIs are the most potent antisecretory agents available. They are enteric coated or combined with sodium bicarbonate to protect them from acid inactivation. After being absorbed in the upper small bowel, PPIs are taken up by parietal cells and secreted into the canalicular (luminal) space, where they are converted to a metabolite that binds covalently with proton pumps and irreversibly inactivates them. These proton pumps must be active, and the parietal cells must be stimulated for the PPI–proton pump interaction to occur. Thus, PPIs should be taken 15 to 30 minutes before a meal. They are not as effective if administered while acid secretion is being inhibited by H$_2$-receptor blockers. Several PPIs are available, including omeprazole, lansoprazole, pantoprazole, rabeprazole, esomeprazole, and dexlansoprazole. All PPIs are capable of healing duodenal ulcers in 4 weeks. Gastric ulcers, depending on size, may require a considerably longer duration of treatment.

> ✓ First-line therapy for *H pylori* infection—quadruple therapy with a PPI, bismuth, metronidazole, and tetracycline

Follow-up and Maintenance Therapy

Patients who have uncomplicated duodenal ulcers without *H pylori* infection do not require follow-up endoscopy after therapy if they do not have recurrent or persistent symptoms. The decision to perform follow-up endoscopy for gastric ulcers to exclude malignancy is made on a case-by-case basis depending on the level of concern. However, about 95% of gastric cancers associated with gastric ulceration can be diagnosed at initial endoscopy when an adequate number of biopsy specimens are obtained from the edge of the ulcer (≥4) and from the base (≥1). Patients at high risk for gastric cancer or gastric ulcers with worrisome features at endoscopy should undergo follow-up endoscopy to document complete healing of the ulcer. Patients with gastric or duodenal ulcers without an obvious cause (ie, idiopathic ulcers) should receive maintenance PPI therapy to prevent ulcer relapse.

Prevention of PUD

Persons about to be prescribed aspirin or NSAIDs for long-term therapy should be tested for *H pylori* and treated if infected. If they are at high risk for PUD, prophylactic therapy with misoprostol or a PPI should be considered. H$_2$-receptor blockers have not been useful for these patients. Patients at highest risk are those who have a previous history of ulcer disease; the elderly; patients who are also receiving treatment with warfarin, corticosteroids, or other antiplatelet agents; and those who have clinically important comorbid conditions.

PUD in Pregnancy

The occurrence of PUD in pregnant patients is uncommon. The focus of treatment during pregnancy is acid suppression. Medications that are considered safe include sucralfate and antacids, particularly the magnesium-containing antacids in the second and early third trimesters and aluminum-containing antacids in the second and third trimesters. H$_2$-receptor antagonists can be given because they are considered relatively safe, and PPI therapy is also considered to be low risk in pregnancy. Misoprostol is contraindicated and should be avoided because it increases the risk of major birth defects. If patients have severe symptoms or have symptoms refractory to treatment, EGD examination can be considered for confirmation of the diagnosis. Clear communication is necessary between the obstetrician, gastroenterologist, and patient about the benefits and risks of the procedure. If *H pylori* is present, treatment is typically delayed until after delivery.

Suggested Reading

Bindu S, Mazumder S, Bandyopadhyay U. Non-steroidal anti-inflammatory drugs (NSAIDs) and organ damage: A current perspective. Biochem Pharmacol. 2020 Oct;180:114147.

Chey WD, Leontiadis GI, Howden CW, Moss SF. ACG clinical guideline: Treatment of Helicobacter pylori infection. Am J Gastroenterol. 2017 Feb;112(2):212–39.

Kamboj AK, Cotter TG, Oxentenko AS. Helicobacter pylori: The past, present, and future in management. Mayo Clin Proc. 2017 Apr;92(4):599–604.

Kavitt RT, Lipowska AM, Anyane-Yeboa A, Gralnek IM. Diagnosis and treatment of peptic ulcer disease. Am J Med. 2019 Apr;132(4):447–56.

Lanas A, Chan FKL. Peptic ulcer disease. Lancet. 2017 Aug;390(10094): 613–24.

Sonnenberg A, Turner KO, Genta RM. Low prevalence of Helicobacter pylori-positive peptic ulcers in private outpatient endoscopy centers in the United States. Am J Gastroenterol. 2020 Feb;115(2): 244–50.

Waskito LA, Salama NR, Yamaoka Y. Pathogenesis of Helicobacter pylori infection. Helicobacter. 2018 Sep;23 Suppl 1:e12516.

5

Gastritis and Gastropathy

STEPHANIE L. HANSEL, MD, MS

Inflammation of the stomach can manifest itself as gastritis or gastropathy. *Gastritis* is a histologic diagnosis referring to inflammatory processes of the stomach. Patients with gastritis may or may not have identifiable endoscopic findings or clinical symptoms. *Gastropathy* refers to epithelial damage with little or no inflammation.

There are several classifications of gastritis and gastropathy. Most of them distinguish between acute and chronic disease and the predominant inflammatory infiltrate seen in biopsy specimens. The etiology of the gastritis or gastropathy is also an important factor in the classification, as is the topography or specific areas of involvement in the stomach. The updated Sydney System (Table 5.1) often is used to classify gastritis. To ensure proper mucosal sampling, the diagnosis and classification of gastritis require a total of 6 biopsy specimens: 2 from the antrum, 2 from the body, and 2 from the incisura (Figure 5.1). Sometimes duodenal biopsies may assist in the overall diagnosis of a disease, such as celiac disease in patients with lymphocytic gastritis, Crohn disease in patients with granulomatous gastritis, and eosinophilic gastroenteritis in patients with eosinophilic infiltration of the antrum.

✓ **Gastritis**—histologic diagnosis of acute or chronic inflammation of the stomach
✓ **Gastropathy**—epithelial damage to the stomach with little or no inflammation

---

Abbreviations: CMV, cytomegalovirus; HLA, human leukocyte antigen; NSAID, nonsteroidal anti-inflammatory drug

Gastritis

Acute Gastritis

Acute *gastritis* is an acute inflammatory process that involves the stomach with a predominantly neutrophilic infiltration. It may or may not have features of intramucosal hemorrhage, superficial mucosal sloughing, or erosion. Most often, acute gastritis is related to use of aspirin or other nonsteroidal anti-inflammatory drugs (NSAIDs), excess alcohol intake, uremic toxins, heavy use of tobacco, therapy with cancer chemotherapeutic drugs, ischemia, or infection.

Acute gastritis due to *Helicobacter pylori* infection is rarely identified. Abdominal pain, nausea, or vomiting may develop. Endoscopic findings such as erythema or erosion are absent or nonspecific. Biopsy specimens show mucosal neutrophilic infiltration in the antrum, with or without desquamation and erosions. In most persons acutely infected with *H pylori*, an active chronic gastritis develops.

Aspirin and other NSAIDs can cause acute injury to the gastric mucosa. With gastritis, endoscopic findings range from minimally visible changes to erythema, petechial hemorrhages, or erosions. Histologically, there can be evidence of superficial lamina propria hemorrhage, mucosal sloughing, neutrophilic infiltration, and mucosal necrosis. The changes are limited to the mucosa and do not extend into the muscularis mucosa. Clinical symptoms such as abdominal pain, nausea, vomiting, or gastrointestinal tract bleeding may or may not be present as well. Similar findings occur after the ingestion of large amounts of alcohol and other toxic substances and after ischemia (Figure 5.2). All these insults impair mucosal barrier function by affecting prostaglandin synthesis (NSAIDs) or mucosal blood flow (alcohol or ischemia) or by direct injury to the surface mucosal cells

Table 5.1.   Sydney System for Classification of Gastritis

Type of gastritis	Etiologic factors	Synonyms
Nonatrophic	Helicobacter pylori	Superficial
		Diffuse antral
		Chronic antral
		Interstitial follicular
		Type B
Atrophic-autoimmune	Autoimmunity	Type A
	H pylori	Diffuse corporeal
		Pernicious anemia
Atrophic-multifocal	H pylori	Type B
		Environmental
		Metaplastic
		Atrophic pangastritis
		Progressive intestinalizing pangastritis
Chemical/radiation	Bile	Reactive
	NSAIDs	Reflux
	Alcohol or other agents (possibly)	Radiation
	Radiation	
Lymphocytic	Idiopathic	Varioliform
	Autoimmune	Celiac disease–associated
	Gluten	
	H pylori	
Granulomatous	Crohn disease	Isolated granulomatous
	Sarcoidosis	
	Granulomatosis with polyangiitis	
	Infectious	
Eosinophilic	Food sensitivities	Allergic
	Allergies	
	Idiopathic	
Infectious	Bacteria	Phlegmonous
	Viruses	Cytomegalovirus
	Fungi	Anisakiasis
	Parasites	

Abbreviation: NSAID, nonsteroidal anti-inflammatory drug.

Adapted from Dixon MF, Genta RM, Yardley JH, Correa P. Classification and grading of gastritis: The updated Sydney System. International Workshop on the Histopathology of Gastritis, Houston 1994. Am J Surg Pathol. 1996 Oct;20(10):1161-81; used with permission.

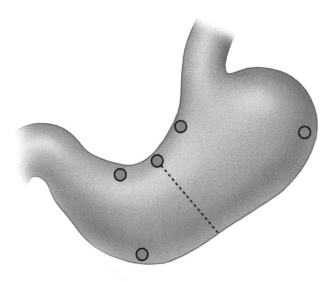

Figure 5.1. Gastric Biopsy Protocol to Diagnose Gastritis. Biopsy specimens (circles) should be obtained from the greater and lesser curvatures of the body and the antrum and from the incisura (dotted line).

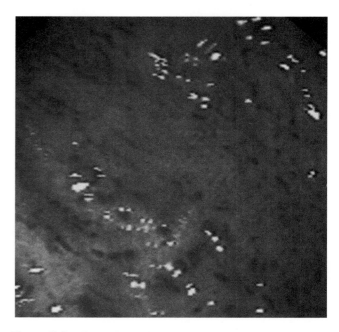

Figure 5.2. Acute Hemorrhagic Gastritis. (Adapted from Emory TS, Carpenter HA, Gostout CJ, Sobin LH. Atlas of gastrointestinal endoscopy & endoscopic biopsies. Washington, DC: Armed Forces Institute of Pathology, American Registry of Pathology; c2000. p. 101.)

(NSAIDs, other drugs, or infection). Treatment of acute gastritis includes management of the underlying condition, withdrawal of any offending drug or toxin, and acid-suppression therapy with a proton pump inhibitor.

Chronic Gastritis

Chronic gastritis is classified as nonatrophic, atrophic, or special forms. Mucosal injury occurs in all forms of chronic gastritis. The atrophic forms of chronic gastritis can be autoimmune or multifocal, and, subsequently, metaplasia, dysplasia, and carcinoma may develop.

Nonatrophic Chronic Gastritis

Nonatrophic chronic gastritis is typical in persons who have *H pylori* infections with acute gastritis and who do not clear the infection (Figure 5.3). Endoscopic findings include gastric mucosal erythema, erosions, granularity, and nodularity. Nonatrophic chronic gastritis usually is most evident in the antrum. Histologic findings include a marked lymphoplasmacytic and neutrophilic infiltrate. Lymphoid aggregates or germinal centers may be seen. Gastric atrophy, metaplasia, and dysplasia are not seen. However, this type of active chronic gastritis due to *H pylori* infection does increase the risk of duodenal ulcer disease.

Atrophic Chronic Gastritis

Multifocal Atrophic Gastritis. Multifocal atrophic gastritis may develop in persons infected with *H pylori*. This type of active chronic gastritis includes the loss of glands and metaplastic change principally involving the body and antrum of the stomach (Figure 5.4). Inflammation consists of both acute and chronic inflammatory cells. Affected persons have an increased risk of gastric ulcer disease and gastric adenocarcinoma with this type of gastritis.

✓ Aspirin and NSAIDs—common causes of gastropathy
✓ *H pylori* can cause acute or chronic gastritis

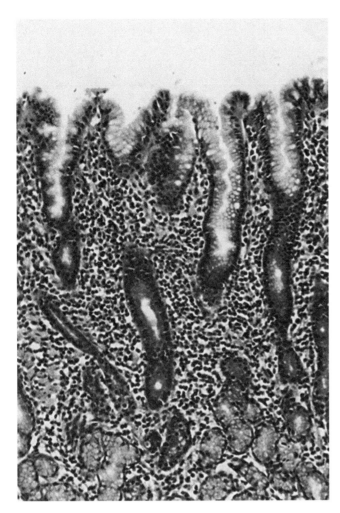

Figure 5.3. **Active (Nonatrophic) Chronic Gastritis of the Antrum of the Stomach.** Stain is hematoxylin-eosin. (Adapted from Emory TS, Carpenter HA, Gostout CJ, Sobin LH. Atlas of gastrointestinal endoscopy & endoscopic biopsies. Washington, DC: Armed Forces Institute of Pathology, American Registry of Pathology; c2000. p. 90.)

✓ *H pylori*—the most common cause of chronic gastritis
✓ Persons with antral gastritis due to *H pylori* are more prone to duodenal ulcers, whereas persons with multifocal atrophic gastritis due to *H pylori* are more prone to gastric ulceration

---

Autoimmune Atrophic Gastritis. Patients with autoimmune atrophic gastritis can present with abdominal discomfort or pain, weight loss, and pernicious anemia. This type of gastritis is an autosomal dominant condition and is responsible for less than 5% of all cases of chronic gastritis (Figure 5.5). It involves the body and fundus of the stomach, sparing the antrum. Endoscopic findings include a loss of gastric folds and prominence of the submucosal vasculature. Laboratory findings include autoantibodies to parietal cells and intrinsic factor, elevated serum gastrin level, and low vitamin B_{12} level. Hypochlorhydria, achlorhydria, iron deficiency, or pernicious anemia may develop in some patients. Histologically, the abnormal findings are limited to the body and fundic mucosa. A typical finding is the loss of oxyntic glands (chief and parietal cells) and a prominent lamina propria lymphocytic and plasma cell infiltration directed at the fundic glands. Patients do have a small risk of gastric carcinoids (<10%) and

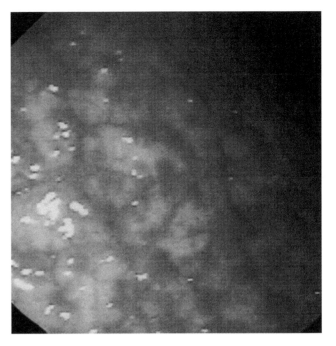

Figure 5.4. **Multifocal Atrophic Gastritis.** (Adapted from Emory TS, Carpenter HA, Gostout CJ, Sobin LH. Atlas of gastrointestinal endoscopy & endoscopic biopsies. Washington, DC: Armed Forces Institute of Pathology, American Registry of Pathology; c2000. p. 93.)

gastric adenocarcinoma (<3%). Patients or their relatives may have other autoimmune disorders, including Hashimoto thyroiditis, Graves disease, Addison disease, diabetes, and vitiligo. There is also an association with human leukocyte antigen (HLA)-B8 and HLA-DR3.

Special Forms of Gastritis

Infectious Gastritis. Bacterial gastritis is most often caused by *H pylori* (see Chapter 4, "Peptic Ulcer Disease"). However, other species of bacteria may be found in the stomach after antrectomy or in association with achlorhydria. Organisms such as *Streptococcus, Staphylococcus, Lactobacillus, Bacteroides, Klebsiella,* and *Escherichia coli* have all been cultured from gastric juice but rarely have clinical significance. These organisms likely represent oral flora that has been swallowed. In circumstances of ischemia or immunosuppression, these organisms may produce marked morbidity.

Mycobacterium tuberculosis is an important cause of bacterial gastritis in resource-limited countries. Patients present with weight loss, anorexia, night sweats, and fevers and can have symptoms of gastric outlet obstruction. Biopsies from ulcerated or nodular areas with stains for acid-fast bacilli and cultures for *M tuberculosis* are necessary for diagnosis. Secondary or tertiary syphilis can also involve the stomach, especially the antrum.

Phlegmonous gastritis is a rare, life-threatening condition associated with full-thickness purulent necrosis of the gastric wall. Multiple bacteria are responsible, and it usually occurs in immunocompromised patients, including alcoholics and patients with diabetes. Invasive procedures may trigger the onset; fever, chills, abdominal pain, and hypotension are common. If gas-forming organisms are involved, emphysematous changes may be apparent on imaging studies. The mortality rate is high, and surgery may be required to remove the necrotic portion of the stomach.

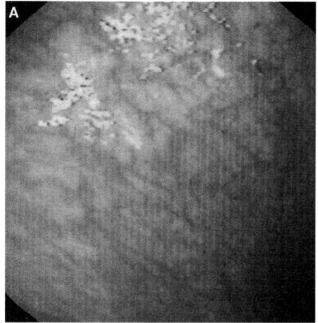

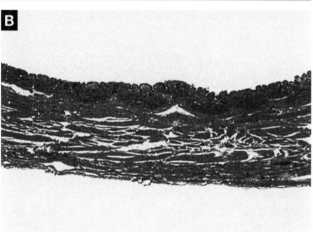

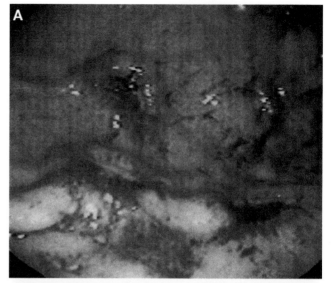

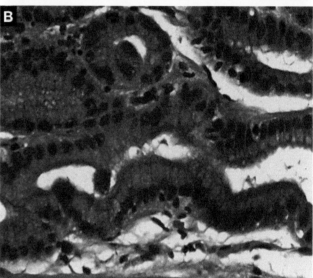

Figure 5.5. Chronic Autoimmune Atrophic Gastritis. A, Gross appearance. B, Section through the body of the stomach (hematoxylin-eosin stain). (Adapted from Emory TS, Carpenter HA, Gostout CJ, Sobin LH. Atlas of gastrointestinal endoscopy & endoscopic biopsies. Washington, DC: Armed Forces Institute of Pathology, American Registry of Pathology; c2000. p. 94.)

Figure 5.6. Cytomegalovirus (CMV) Infection of the Stomach. A, Gross appearance of CMV ulcers. B, CMV gastropathy (hematoxylin-eosin stain). (Adapted from Emory TS, Carpenter HA, Gostout CJ, Sobin LH. Atlas of gastrointestinal endoscopy & endoscopic biopsies. Washington, DC: Armed Forces Institute of Pathology, American Registry of Pathology; c2000. p. 123.)

Cytomegalovirus (CMV) infection is the most recognized viral infection of the stomach (Figure 5.6). This infection may or may not have endoscopic findings that include edema, erythema, erosions, or ulcers. Patients with CMV infection of the stomach may or may not have symptoms, such as fever, abdominal pain, nausea, vomiting, or bleeding, and they usually are immunosuppressed. Biopsy specimens from macroscopically involved and apparently normal areas may show typical CMV cells and inclusions. When ulceration is present, biopsy specimens from the center of the ulcer are more likely to be diagnostic than specimens from the edge because of vascular endothelial involvement of this virus. If the diagnosis is in doubt, immunohistochemistry enhances the diagnostic yield.

Fungal and parasitic infections of the stomach are uncommon. In immunosuppressed patients, gastric infections may be caused by *Histoplasma, Candida, Aspergillus, Cryptococcus,*

or mucormycosis. Ingestion of raw fish can result in anisakiasis. *Cryptosporidium* and *Strongyloides* infections can rarely involve the stomach in immunosuppressed patients.

Noninfectious Granulomatous Gastritis. In the absence of infection, granulomatous gastritis (Figure 5.7) occurs most commonly with Crohn disease (52%). The differential diagnosis includes isolated granulomatous gastritis (25%), foreign body granuloma (10%; eg, suture, food), tumor-associated granuloma, sarcoidosis, infection (*H pylori* infection, tuberculosis, histoplasmosis, syphilis), and vasculitis-associated granulomas. Most often, an antral inflammatory infiltration is found. Many patients with granulomatous gastritis are asymptomatic. In a few patients, particularly those with Crohn disease or sarcoidosis, symptoms of gastric outlet obstruction due to ulceration and scarring of the antrum and pylorus can develop. Nonspecific treatment, such as

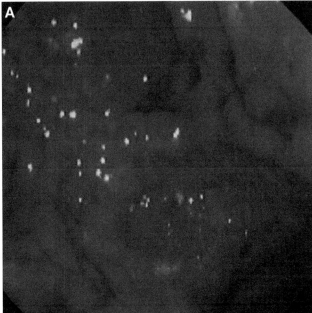

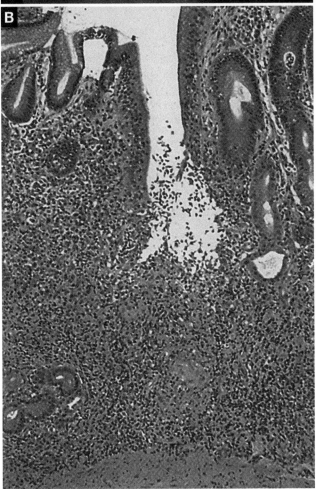

Figure 5.7. Granulomatous Gastritis. A, Gross appearance. B, Histologic appearance of granuloma (hematoxylin-eosin stain). (Adapted from Emory TS, Carpenter HA, Gostout CJ, Sobin LH. Atlas of gastrointestinal endoscopy & endoscopic biopsies. Washington, DC: Armed Forces Institute of Pathology, American Registry of Pathology; c2000. p. 98, 99.)

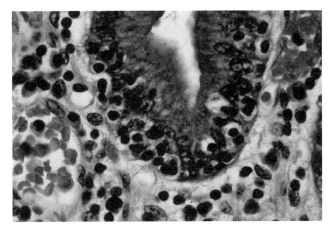

Figure 5.8. Lymphocytic Gastritis. Intraepithelial lymphocytes can be seen without any destruction of surrounding epithelial cells (hematoxylin-eosin stain). (Adapted from Owen DA. Gastritis and carditis. Mod Pathol. 2003 Apr;16[4]:325-41; used with permission.)

acid-reduction therapy, or therapy directed toward the underlying disorder usually is indicated.

Lymphocytic Gastritis. Lymphocytic gastritis is uncommon and often is asymptomatic. If symptoms do occur, dyspepsia is most common. On endoscopy, mucosal nodules, erosions, and enlarged gastric folds may be seen. Histologic findings include active chronic pangastritis with epithelial infiltration by mature lymphocytes, which are usually T lymphocytes (Figure 5.8). The lamina propria is expanded by the lymphocytes and plasma cells. Most often, when found in patients with celiac disease, lymphocytic gastritis is antral predominant. However, when lymphocytic gastritis occurs in patients with *H pylori* infection, it tends to be gastric body predominant and often has polymorphonuclear cells. Staining for *H pylori* should be performed in every case of lymphocytic gastritis. Patients with microscopic colitis or Ménétrier disease may also have lymphocytic gastritis. Therapy is directed toward the underlying condition.

Eosinophilic Gastritis. Various disorders are associated with eosinophilic infiltration of the stomach, including parasitic infestation, hypereosinophilic syndrome, gastric Crohn disease, gastric carcinoma, lymphoma, connective tissue disorder, peptic ulcer disease, mast cell disease, and Churg-Strauss vasculitis. *Eosinophilic gastritis* is a rare inflammatory condition. Patients generally have a history of allergy, asthma, food intolerance, eczema, drug sensitivities, or peripheral eosinophilia and increased serum levels of immunoglobulin E. On endoscopy, the gastric mucosa ranges from normal to erosions and erythema. In the most common mucosa-predominant form, biopsy specimens typically show patchy but dense eosinophilic infiltration (Figure 5.9). The antrum is typically involved. Less commonly, full-thickness or open biopsy may be necessary for diagnosis if only the muscle or serosa layers are affected. Corticosteroids are used for treatment.

✓ Autoimmune atrophic gastritis is characterized by hypochlorhydria and hypergastrinemia with autoantibodies to parietal cells and intrinsic factor

✓ Pernicious anemia due to autoimmune atrophic gastritis is the most common cause of vitamin B_{12} deficiency

✓ *H pylori* infection and celiac disease—the 2 main causes of lymphocytic gastritis

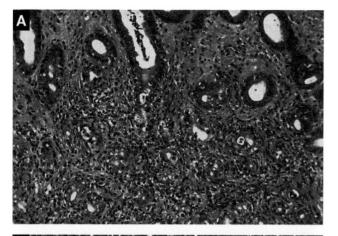

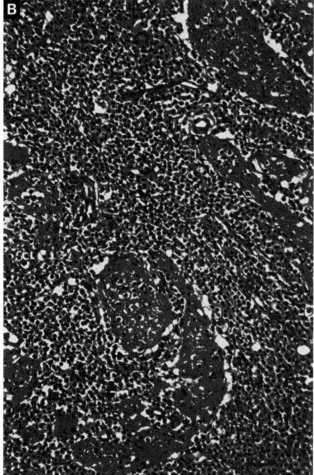

Figure 5.9. Eosinophilic Gastritis. Note the marked eosinophilic infiltration. A, High-power view. B, Low-power view. (Adapted from Emory TS, Carpenter HA, Gostout CJ, Sobin LH. Atlas of gastrointestinal endoscopy & endoscopic biopsies. Washington, DC: Armed Forces Institute of Pathology, American Registry of Pathology; c2000. p. 97.)

Gastropathy

Chemical Gastropathy

Long-term exposure to substances that can damage the gastric mucosa can result in chronic gastropathy. Other common names for this condition include reactive gastritis, reactive gastropathy, and bile reflux gastritis or gastropathy. The etiology includes aspirin

or other NSAIDs, bile reflux, and alcohol. Endoscopic findings include edema, erythema, erosions, and visible bile in the stomach. Most involvement is in the antrum, and biopsy specimens show foveolar hyperplasia, loss of mucin, proliferation of lamina propria smooth muscle, and vascular congestion in the lamina propria. Bile reflux gastropathy usually follows surgical intervention, such as gastroenterostomy, vagotomy, or pyloroplasty, but can occur in persons with gastric emptying disorders or in stomachs that have not had a surgical procedure. Symptoms such as epigastric discomfort, nausea, and vomiting do not correlate well with endoscopic or histologic findings. Treatment of chemical gastropathy includes discontinued use of the offending agent if possible and use of acid-reducing medication and ursodiol if bile acid is the most likely cause. Cholestyramine, sucralfate, and aluminum-containing antacids have been prescribed for bile acid gastropathy but have mostly been unsuccessful. Ursodiol has been shown to decrease symptoms without improving histologic findings. A surgical Roux-en-Y revision to divert bile from the stomach in patients with previous gastroenterostomy and symptomatic bile reflux gastropathy has been found to reduce symptoms in 50% to 90% of patients.

Vascular Gastropathies

Vascular gastropathies are defined as abnormalities of the gastric vasculature affecting mucosal blood vessels, with little or no inflammation. Typical examples include congestive gastropathy from congestive heart failure, portal hypertensive gastropathy, and gastric vascular ectasia (ie, *watermelon stomach*).

In patients with portal hypertension, dilatation and sclerosis of small mucosal and submucosal venules and capillaries can produce an endoscopically recognizable mucosal mosaic pattern, usually most prominent in the fundus and body of the stomach (Figure 5.10). Nodularity and punctate erythema also may be seen. Clinically, patients may have iron deficiency anemia or melena. Treatment involves attempts to decrease portal pressure; endoscopic therapy is not effective (see Chapter 27, "Vascular Diseases of the Liver").

Patients with gastric vascular ectasia develop dilated mucosal capillaries with fibrin thrombi and fibromuscular hyperplasia of the lamina propria with minimal or no inflammation. Endoscopic findings typically include linear or nodular erythematous streaks without a mosaic pattern, usually involving the antrum but sometimes extending into the gastric body (Figure 5.11). Gastric vascular ectasia tends to occur in patients who have an array of underlying conditions, including pernicious anemia, collagen vascular disease, cirrhosis, kidney failure, bone marrow transplant, and antral mucosal trauma (as in pyloric prolapse). Like patients with portal hypertensive gastropathy, patients may have iron deficiency anemia or melena. Endoscopic therapy with argon plasma coagulation can diminish blood loss in patients with anemia (see Chapter 10, "Nonvariceal Gastrointestinal Tract Bleeding"). Liver transplant can benefit patients with gastric vascular ectasia who have cirrhosis, but transjugular intrahepatic portosystemic shunts are not helpful (see Chapter 27, "Vascular Diseases of the Liver").

Hypertrophic Gastropathy

Hypertrophic gastropathy refers to a group of conditions with giant enlargement of the rugal folds. This group includes some cases of chronic gastritis from *H pylori* infection or lymphocytic gastritis, Zollinger-Ellison syndrome, infiltrative disorders (sarcoidosis and malignancy), and Ménétrier disease. Patients with Ménétrier

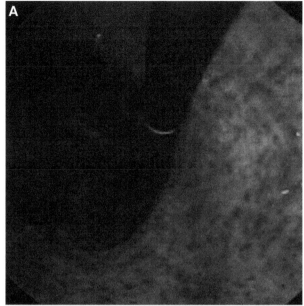

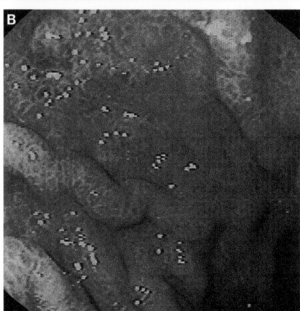

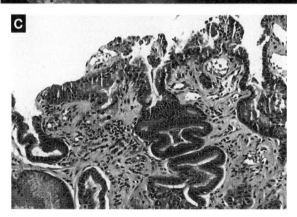

Figure 5.10. Portal Hypertensive Gastropathy. A and B, Gross specimens show mosaic mucosal pattern. C, Histologic section show dilated, tortuous blood vessels (hematoxylin-eosin stain). (Adapted from Emory TS, Carpenter HA, Gostout CJ, Sobin LH. Atlas of gastrointestinal endoscopy & endoscopic biopsies. Washington, DC: Armed Forces Institute of Pathology, American Registry of Pathology; c2000. p. 116.)

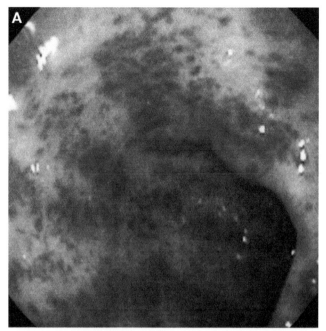

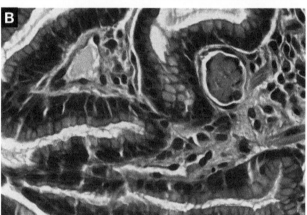

Figure 5.11. Watermelon Stomach (Antrum). A, Gross specimen. B, Histologic section shows thick-walled, ectatic vessels (hematoxylin-eosin stain). (Adapted from Emory TS, Carpenter HA, Gostout CJ, Sobin LH. Atlas of gastrointestinal endoscopy & endoscopic biopsies. Washington, DC: Armed Forces Institute of Pathology, American Registry of Pathology; c2000. p. 118.)

disease often have such symptoms as epigastric pain, nausea, vomiting, diarrhea, edema, and weight loss. Many patients have evidence of a protein-losing gastropathy manifested by low serum level of albumin and increased stool clearance of α_1-antitrypsin. Endoscopically, giant gastric rugal folds and a cobblestone pattern are present but may spare the antrum. A full-thickness gastric biopsy specimen or endoscopic snare biopsy specimen from an enlarged fold usually is necessary to make the diagnosis. Histologic examination shows extreme surface mucous cell hyperplasia with deeper glandular atrophy. Often, gastric hypochlorhydria or achlorhydria is present together with excessive secretion of mucus. The driver of the histologic changes is increased levels of transforming growth factor-α signaling through epidermal growth factor receptor on surface mucous cells. Treatment with agents to counteract the effects of transforming growth factor-α, such as cetuximab, has been successful. Patients with Ménétrier disease most likely have an increased risk for gastric adenocarcinoma.

- ✓ Gastric vascular ectasia often manifests as iron deficiency anemia
- ✓ Ménétrier disease—a rare hypertrophic, protein-losing gastropathy due to increased mucosal levels of transforming growth factor-α

Suggested Reading

Annibale B, Esposito G, Lahner E. A current clinical overview of atrophic gastritis. Expert Rev Gastroenterol Hepatol. 2020 Feb;14(2):93–102.

Bacha D, Walha M, Ben Slama S, Ben Romdhane H, Bouraoui S, Bellil K, et al. Chronic gastritis classifications. Tunis Med. 2018 Jul;96(7):405–10.

Bhattacharya B. Non-neoplastic disorders of the stomach. In: Iacobuzio-Donahue CA, Montgomery E, eds. Gastrointestinal and liver pathology. 2nd ed. Elsevier/Saunders; 2012. p. 65–141

Chen PH, Anderson L, Zhang K, Weiss GA. Eosinophilic gastritis/gastroenteritis. Curr Gastroenterol Rep. 2021 Jul;23(8):13.

Dixon MF, Genta RM, Yardley JH, Correa P. Classification and grading of gastritis: The updated Sydney System. International Workshop on the Histopathology of Gastritis, Houston 1994. Am J Surg Pathol. 1996 Oct;20(10):1161–81.

Gala K, Luckett RT, Shah N. Gastric sarcoidosis presenting as dyspepsia. Cureus. 2020 Feb;12(2):e7139.

Shah SC, Piazuelo MB, Kuipers EJ, Li D. AGA clinical practice update on the diagnosis and management of atrophic gastritis: expert review. Gastroenterology. 2021 Oct;161(4):1325–32.

Yee EU, Kuo E, Goldsmith JD. Pathologic features of infectious gastritis. Adv Anat Pathol. 2018 Jul;25(4):238–53.

6

Gastric Neoplasms and Gastroenteric and Pancreatic Neuroendocrine Tumors[a]

SETH SWEETSER, MD

Gastric neoplasms are an important contributor to cancer-related mortality. Of the various neoplasms that can affect the stomach, adenocarcinoma is the most common and accounts for up to 85% of gastric neoplasms, with 15% due to lymphomas, gastrointestinal stromal tumors (GISTs), neuroendocrine tumors (NETs), and metastatic disease involving the stomach (Table 6.1). This chapter considers the epidemiology, pathogenesis, clinical manifestation, diagnostic evaluation, treatment, and prognosis of these neoplastic diseases.

Gastric Adenocarcinoma

Epidemiology

Gastric adenocarcinoma is the third most frequent cause of cancer-related death worldwide. Gastric cancer is rare in persons younger than 40 years, but its incidence increases steadily thereafter, peaking in the seventh decade of life.

The incidence of gastric cancer varies by geographic location, with 60% of gastric cancers occurring in resource-limited countries. The highest incidence rates are in Japan, China, Chile, and Ireland. Incidence rates are lower in industrialized nations. Regardless of region, gastric cancer is more common in men than in women.

In the US, gastric cancer is diagnosed in approximately 28,000 patients annually, and over 10,000 are expected to die of gastric cancer each year. Although gastric cancer is relatively infrequent in North America, its contribution to the burden of cancer deaths is substantial: It is the third most common gastrointestinal tract malignancy, after colorectal and pancreatic cancer, and the third most lethal neoplasm overall.

The worldwide incidence of gastric cancer has decreased since the middle of the 20th century. Part of the decrease in gastric cancer in the US may be due to the recognition and alteration of certain risk factors, such as the identification and treatment of *Helicobacter pylori* infection and changes in dietary trends. The increasingly widespread use of refrigerators was likely the initial turning point for the decrease in the incidence of gastric cancer. Refrigeration decreased bacterial and fungal contamination of

[a] Portions of this chapter were adapted from Ravi K, Sweetser S. Persistent nausea and vomiting in pregnancy. Gastroenterology. 2014 Jan;146(1):33, 323; used with permission.

Abbreviations: CgA, chromogranin A; CHOP, cyclophosphamide, doxorubicin, vincristine, and prednisone; CT, computed tomography; DLBCL, diffuse large B-cell lymphoma; EGJ, esophagogastric junction; ENMZL, extranodal marginal zone B-cell lymphoma; EUS, endoscopic ultrasonography; 5-HIAA, 5-hydroxyindoleacetic acid; GIM, gastric intestinal metaplasia; GIST, gastrointestinal stromal tumor; GNET, gastroenteric neuroendocrine tumor; HDGC, hereditary diffuse gastric cancer; MALT, mucosa-associated lymphoid tissue; MEN, multiple endocrine neoplasia; MRI, magnetic resonance imaging; NET, neuroendocrine tumor; PET, positron emission tomography; PNET, pancreatic neuroendocrine tumor; SEER, Surveillance, Epidemiology, and End Results; SRS, somatostatin receptor scintigraphy; VIP, vasoactive intestinal polypeptide

Table 6.1. Frequency of Different Types of Gastric Neoplasms

Tumor type	Percentage of gastric neoplasms
Adenocarcinoma	85
Lymphomas (diffuse large B cell and extranodal marginal zone B cell), gastroenteric and pancreatic neuroendocrine tumors, gastrointestinal stromal tumors, and metastatic disease to the stomach	15

food, increased the availability of fresh fruits and vegetables (which provide protective antioxidants), and lessened the need for salt-based preservation—all of which may have reduced some of the most important risk factors for gastric cancer. Although the incidence of gastric cancer overall is decreasing, the absolute number of new cases annually is increasing because the world population is increasing and aging. Consequently, gastric cancer will continue to be an important cause of cancer and cancer-related death for the foreseeable future.

Pathogenesis

Much effort has been made to understand the etiology of gastric adenocarcinoma. It is widely held that there is no single cause but rather multiple causative factors, including diet, exogenous substances, infectious agents, and genetic factors.

Gastric adenocarcinomas are subdivided into 2 pathologically defined categories: 1) an intestinal type, which is characterized by cohesive neoplastic cells that form glandular structures, and 2) a diffuse type in which cellular cohesion is absent, so that individual cells infiltrate the stomach wall without forming a discrete mass. In addition, these 2 types of gastric adenocarcinoma have distinct molecular genetic profiles and appear to have separate pathogenetic pathways. A key difference is the presence or absence of intercellular adhesion molecules produced when there is expression of the cell adhesion protein E-cadherin encoded by the *CDH1* gene (OMIM 192090).

In the diffuse type of gastric adenocarcinoma, an initial carcinogenic event is the loss of expression of *CDH1*, the tumor suppressor gene encoding for the protein E-cadherin that is critical for establishing intercellular connections and maintaining the organization of epithelial tissues. Without this protein, individual tumor cells tend to invade surrounding tissues without forming typical epithelial glands. The diffuse type of gastric cancer tends to invade and then broadly extend along the gastric wall. Occasionally, the stomach is infiltrated extensively, giving it a rigid, fixed appearance, a condition known as *linitis plastica*. Diffuse-type tumors are highly metastatic and are characterized by rapid disease progression and generally a poor prognosis.

In contrast, intercellular adhesion molecules are well preserved in intestinal-type gastric adenocarcinomas, and the tumor cells tend to occur in tubular or glandular formations, similar in appearance to adenocarcinomas in the colorectum and small intestine. The pathogenesis appears to follow a multistep progression that usually results from *H pylori* infection. The first stage is chronic gastritis, when there are fluctuating periods of greater or lesser inflammatory infiltrates. In some patients, this process results in *atrophic gastritis*, sometimes referred to as *gastric atrophy*, which is the multifocal disappearance of gastric glands within the epithelium. When multifocal atrophy is present, glands that mimic intestinal epithelial glands may appear. This represents intestinal metaplasia. As atrophy and metaplasia become more extensive, the chance of dysplasia developing increases. Dysplastic

cells are precancerous and undergo increasing degrees of nuclear atypia and cellular disorganization, evolving from low-grade to high-grade dysplasia, which increases the risk of an invasive, intestinal-type adenocarcinoma.

Intestinal-type gastric adenocarcinoma does not develop de novo. Whether the cause is autoimmune or from environmental factors or *H pylori* infection, gastritis is usually the first step in cancer induction. A sequence of pathologic changes occurs: Inflammation is followed by intestinal metaplasia and then dysplasia, as genetic variations occur in rapidly dividing cells, and, finally, intestinal-type cancer. This model of gastric carcinogenesis is commonly referred to as the Correa cascade (Figure 6.1), named after the gastrointestinal pathologist who first described this sequence of tissue changes leading to cancer.

Gastric intestinal metaplasia (GIM) is a premalignant condition and an intermediate step in the progression to intestinal-type adenocarcinoma. Patients with GIM have up to a 9-fold risk for gastric cancer irrespective of race. For progression, high-risk groups include patients who have a family history of gastric cancer or who are members of ethnic populations at high risk, patients who smoke tobacco, patients who have extensive and multifocal GIM, and patients who have dysplasia on biopsies. The finding of GIM confers a risk such that approximately 1 in 40 patients would be expected to have gastric adenocarcinoma develop within 20 years after index endoscopy. Therefore, if extensive or multifocal GIM is identified, a reasonable approach would be to monitor with endoscopic surveillance every 3 years to detect the development of dysplasia or gastric cancer.

✓ The 2 histologic types of gastric adenocarcinoma differ in pathogenesis
  • Intestinal type has cohesive neoplastic cells that form glandular structures
  • Diffuse type lacks cellular cohesion; individual cells infiltrate the stomach wall without forming a discrete mass
✓ Correa cascade—multistep process leading to intestinal-type gastric adenocarcinoma

---

Risk Factors

Diet

Epidemiologic studies have documented an association between diet and gastric cancer. Although dietary factors have been shown to influence the development of gastric cancer, specific substances have not been isolated. The most consistent association is the ingestion of nitroso compounds. Nitroso compounds are formed from nitrates, which are found naturally in foods such as vegetables and potatoes but are also used as preservatives for meats, cheeses, and pickled foods. These preservatives were common in foods before the era of refrigerators. The incidence of gastric cancer is higher in regions where nitrate-based fertilizers are used.

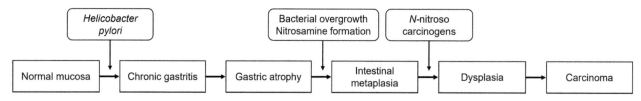

Figure 6.1.   **Correa Cascade of Gastric Adenocarcinoma Carcinogenesis.**

Diets high in salt also have been linked with an increased incidence of gastric cancer. In animal models, high salt intake has been associated with atrophic gastritis. Diets low in uncooked fruits (particularly citrus fruits) and vegetables and high in processed meat, fried food, and alcohol are associated with an increased risk of gastric cancer. The protective effect from fruits and vegetables is thought to be from their vitamin C content, which may decrease the formation of nitroso compounds inside the stomach.

Tobacco Use

Smoking increases the risk of gastric cancer, especially in men, at least 1.5-fold. This risk decreases after 10 years of smoking cessation. Socioeconomic status also affects the risk of gastric cancer. Distal cancer is 2-fold higher among patients of low socioeconomic status, and proximal gastric cancer is more likely among those of higher socioeconomic status.

Gastric Surgery

Patients who have had gastric surgery have a higher risk of gastric cancer. This risk is greatest 15 to 20 years after the operation. Billroth II surgery carries a higher risk than Billroth I surgery, most likely because a Billroth II operation increases the reflux of bile and pancreatic juices into the stomach, which is thought to be instrumental in the development of gastric cancer. Because this risk is low, patients who have had a partial gastric resection do not warrant endoscopic screening.

Infection

The most important risk factor for the development of gastric adenocarcinoma is *H pylori* infection of the stomach. Although several viral infections cause cancer, *H pylori* infection was the first bacterial infection linked to a human cancer. In 1994, the World Health Organization classified *H pylori* as a group 1 human carcinogen for gastric adenocarcinoma. *H pylori* is also a key factor in the development of gastric extranodal marginal zone lymphoma of the mucosa-associated type. As reviewed above, *H pylori* infection causes inflammation that results in atrophy and may progress to intestinal metaplasia, dysplasia, and cancer. Although gastric cancer develops in a minority of individuals with *H pylori* infection (<1%), 90% of those with gastric cancer have evidence of *H pylori* infection.

The precise mechanism by which *H pylori* infection leads to gastric cancer is not understood clearly. It is well established that *H pylori* infection leads to chronic gastritis. The inflammation associated with chronic gastritis reduces the mucous layer overlying mucosal cells and exposes these cells to mutagenic compounds (eg, nitroso compounds and free radicals). Chronic infection with *H pylori* can result in the destruction of the gastric mucosa, leading to atrophic gastritis. *H pylori* infection has been associated most strongly with cancers in the distal portion of the stomach and does not seem to be associated with cancers involving the gastroesophageal junction and cardia regions. First-degree relatives of persons with gastric cancer should be tested for *H pylori* infection and treated if infected.

Genetics

Genetic predisposition to the development of gastric cancer has been identified. An inactivating germline sequence variation in

> **Box 6.1. Genetic Testing Criteria for Hereditary Diffuse Gastric Cancer Syndrome[a,b]**
>
> DGC when younger than 50 y
>
> DGC at any age with a personal or family history of cleft lip or cleft palate
>
> History of DGC and LBC when younger than 70 y
>
> Bilateral LBC or LCIS when younger than 70 y
>
> Gastric biopsy with in situ SRCs or pagetoid spread of SRCs when younger than 50 y
>
> ≥2 Cases of gastric cancer in family (at any age), with ≥1 confirmed case of DGC[c]
>
> ≥2 Cases of LBC in family members when younger than 50 y[c]
>
> ≥1 Case of DGC any age and ≥1 case of LBC when younger than 70 y in different family members[c]
>
> ---
>
> Abbreviations: DGC, diffuse gastric cancer; LBC, lobular breast cancer; LCIS, lobular carcinoma in situ; SRC, signet ring cell.
>
> [a] Germline testing for *CDH1* mutations is recommended when 1 of the criteria listed below has been met.
>
> [b] All diagnoses of DGC and LBC must be confirmed with histology.
>
> [c] Family members must be first- or second-degree blood relatives of each other.
>
> Adapted from Blair VR, McLeod M, Carneiro F, Coit DG, D'Addario JL, van Dieren JM, et al. Hereditary diffuse gastric cancer: updated clinical practice guidelines. Lancet Oncol. 2020 Aug;21(8):e386-e97; used with permission.

the cadherin 1 tumor suppressor gene (*CDH1*) causes an autosomal dominantly inherited form of the diffuse type of gastric adenocarcinoma, *hereditary diffuse gastric cancer* (HDGC), which is characterized by high penetrance and young age at onset. Female carriers of this mutation are also at greater risk for development of lobular breast cancer. Established diagnostic criteria for cadherin 1 (*CDH1*) genetic testing for HDGC are outlined in Box 6.1.

It is recommended that identification of a germline pathogenic variant in the cadherin 1 gene (*CDH1*) should prompt prophylactic total gastrectomy by age 20 years. Annual endoscopic surveillance incorporating multiple, nontargeted gastric biopsies is an alternative for surveillance for those who decline risk reduction surgery. However, endoscopy is associated with low sensitivity for occult cancer detection.

Although the principal familial gastric cancer syndrome is HDGC caused by germline pathogenic variants in *CDH1*, several other hereditary cancer syndromes have been associated with gastric cancer (Table 6.2). These syndromes include Lynch syndrome, familial adenomatous polyposis, Li-Fraumeni syndrome, and hamartomatous polyposis syndromes (juvenile polyposis and Peutz-Jeghers syndrome). In addition, gastric adenocarcinoma and proximal polyposis of the stomach is caused by point mutations in the *APC* gene (OMIM 619182) promoter 1B and carries an overall high lifetime risk for gastric adenocarcinoma of approximately 15%.

Persons with blood group A have a higher incidence of gastric cancer, which may be related to differences in mucous secretion that lead to altered mucosal protection from carcinogens.

Table 6.2.   Hereditary Cancer Syndromes Associated With Gastric Cancer

Syndrome	Gene(s)	Lifetime gastric cancer risk, %	Surveillance
Lynch	Mismatch repair	5	Upper endoscopy every 3-5 y
FAP and *MUTYH*-associated polyposis	*APC* and *MYH*	5	Upper endoscopy according to Spigelman classification
Li-Fraumeni	*TP53*	5	Upper endoscopy every 2-5 y
Peutz-Jeghers	*STK11*	30	Upper endoscopy every 2-3 y
Juvenile polyposis	*SMAD4* and *BMPR1A*	20	Upper endoscopy every 1-3 y
GAPPS	*APC* promoter 1B	15	No guidelines

Abbreviations: FAP, familial adenomatous polyposis; GAPPS, gastric adenocarcinoma and proximal polyposis of the stomach.

Gastric Disorders

Persons with atrophic gastritis have an increased risk for gastric cancer. Gastric polyps also may increase the risk of gastric cancer depending on histologic type. The most common type of gastric polyp is the cystic fundic gland polyp, which does not have neoplastic potential unless it occurs with familial adenomatous polyposis. Hyperplastic gastric polyps are common and should be removed because they have a small risk of malignant transformation when they are relatively large (>1 cm). Adenomatous gastric polyps are less common but may give rise to or coexist with gastric adenocarcinoma. Adenomatous polyps usually occur in areas of chronic atrophic gastritis. Because they have malignant potential, all gastric adenomas should be completely excised.

Hypertrophic gastropathy (Ménétrier disease) is a rare, idiopathic condition characterized by rugal fold enlargement and protein-losing gastropathy. Gastric cancer reportedly occurs in up to 10% of patients with this disease. The major risk factors for gastric cancer are listed in Box 6.2.

✓ *H pylori* infection—the most important risk factor for gastric adenocarcinoma

✓ HDGC is the principal familial gastric cancer syndrome and is caused by pathogenic germline mutations in the *CDH1* gene

---

Clinical Features

Weight loss and persistent midepigastric pain are the most common symptoms at initial presentation, but for many patients the symptoms are so vague that the diagnosis is delayed. Patients may complain of early satiety, abdominal bloating, meal-induced dyspepsia, nausea, or anorexia. Abdominal pain in the epigastric area may be mild and intermittent initially but more severe and constant as the disease progresses. Patients with cancer involving the distal antrum or pylorus may have persistent vomiting due to gastric outlet obstruction. Occult or overt bleeding may occur in early- or late-stage cancers. Dysphagia is a prominent symptom in lesions of the gastric cardia or gastroesophageal junction.

Patients who have a diffuse cancer called *linitis plastica*, which is characterized by poor distensibility of the stomach, may present with nausea and early satiety. Occult gastrointestinal tract bleeding with or without iron deficiency anemia is not uncommon, while overt bleeding (eg, hematemesis) is seen infrequently.

A pseudoachalasia syndrome may occur as the result of tumor involvement of the gastric cardia and gastroesophageal junction area. For this reason, gastric malignancy must always be considered when older patients present with symptoms suggestive of achalasia.

Gastric cancer spreads by direct extension through the stomach wall to perigastric tissue, and it invades adjacent structures, including the pancreas, colon, spleen, kidney, and liver. Lymphatic metastases occur early, and local and regional nodes are the first to be involved. The disease then spreads to more distant intra-abdominal lymph nodes and to the supraclavicular region (Virchow node), periumbilical area (Sister Mary Joseph nodule), left axilla (Irish node), or peritoneal cul-de-sac (Blumer shelf palpable on rectal or vaginal examination), or it may result in peritoneal carcinomatosis with malignant ascites. The liver is the most common site of hematogenous spread; other sites are the lungs, bones, and brain.

Patients with gastric cancer occasionally present with paraneoplastic syndromes such as acanthosis nigricans, the sign of Leser-Trélat (sudden onset of diffuse seborrheic keratoses on the trunk), migratory thrombophlebitis, and microangiopathic hemolytic anemia.

Tumor Features

Location

Endoscopically, gastric adenocarcinoma may appear as an exophytic, polypoid mass or as an irregular, infiltrating lesion with surface nodularity or ulceration. The location of the primary tumor in the stomach has etiologic and prognostic significance. Proximal lesions are biologically more aggressive and carry a worse prognosis, stage for stage, than distal cancers—a finding that suggests that the pathogenesis differs from that of cancers

---

Box 6.2.   Risk Factors for Gastric Adenocarcinoma

Helicobacter pylori infection

Chronic atrophic gastritis

Intestinal metaplasia

Dysplasia

Adenomatous gastric polyps

Cigarette smoking

History of gastric surgery (especially Billroth II operation)

Genetic factors

Ménétrier disease

Data from Zali H, Rezaei-Tavirani M, Azodi M. Gastric cancer: prevention, risk factors and treatment. Gastroenterol Hepatol Bed Bench. 2011 Fall;4(4):175-85.

arising in other parts of the stomach. Distal cancers may be related closely to chronic *H pylori* infection, whereas cardia and gastroesophageal junction cancers may have a different cause, such as chronic gastroesophageal reflux. A contributing factor to the persistently high mortality rate among persons with gastric cancer may be that since the 1980s the distribution of cancers has changed from the body and antrum to the proximal stomach. The incidence of cancers involving the proximal stomach and gastroesophageal junction has increased steadily at a rate exceeding that of any other cancer except melanoma and lung cancer. The reasons for this are unclear. Distal cancers (in the gastric body or antrum) are more common in populations with a high incidence of gastric cancer, whereas cardia cancers are more prevalent in populations with a low incidence of gastric cancer.

Infiltration

Linitis plastica, the diffusely infiltrating form of gastric adenocarcinoma, occurs in 5% of gastric adenocarcinomas. The tumor may extend over a broad region of the gastric wall, resulting in a rigid, thickened stomach. The presence of this lesion at the time of diagnosis is usually associated with locally advanced or metastatic disease and portends a worse prognosis.

Histology

The most widely used histologic classification of gastric adenocarcinoma divides these tumors into 2 types: intestinal and diffuse. Intestinal-type gastric adenocarcinoma has epithelial cells that form discrete glands, microscopically resembling colonic adenocarcinoma. Typically, the intestinal type is better circumscribed than the diffuse type, and it may be polypoid or ulcerated or both. The intestinal type is the more frequent variety in populations with a high incidence of gastric adenocarcinoma. It often arises within an area of intestinal metaplasia. This pathologic variant generally carries a better prognosis than the diffuse type.

Diffuse-type gastric adenocarcinoma is characterized by sheets of epithelial cells. Glandular structure is rarely present. The diffuse type extends widely, with no distinct margins. Mucus-producing signet ring cells are often present (Figure 6.2). The diffuse type occurs more commonly in younger persons, is less likely to be associated with intestinal metaplasia, tends to be infiltrating and poorly differentiated, and is less likely to be associated with *H pylori* infection; generally, the prognosis is poor.

> ✓ Mucus-secreting signet ring cells—the hallmark histologic feature of diffuse gastric cancer

Staging

Most patients with gastric cancer who are symptomatic already have advanced, incurable disease at the time of their initial presentation. The most important aspect of staging is determination of whether the cancer is resectable. Clinical stage is determined preoperatively, whereas pathologic staging is based on findings during surgical exploration and examination of the pathology specimen. The TNM staging system of the American Joint Committee on Cancer, updated in 2017, is used most frequently (Table 6.3). The 2017 update changes the definition of the boundary between esophageal and gastric cancers. Tumors that involve the esophagogastric junction (EGJ) with the tumor

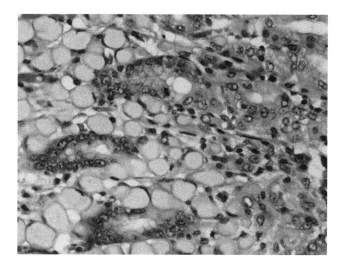

Figure 6.2. Diffuse Type of Gastric Adenocarcinoma With Mucus-Producing Signet Ring Cells. (Stain is hematoxylin-eosin.) (Courtesy of Thomas C. Smyrk, MD, Anatomic Pathology, Mayo Clinic; used with permission.)

epicenter no more than 2 cm into the proximal stomach are staged as esophageal cancers rather than gastric cancers. In contrast, EGJ tumors with their epicenter located more than 2 cm into the proximal stomach are staged as gastric cancers.

Preoperative staging for patients with gastric cancer begins with physical examination. Next, computed tomography (CT) of the chest (for proximal lesions), abdomen, and pelvis is usually the initial imaging test. CT is widely available and is suitable for evaluating widely metastatic disease, especially hepatic involvement, and for assessing ascites or distant nodal spread. Patients who have CT-defined visceral metastatic disease (biopsy proven) can often avoid unnecessary surgery. However, peritoneal metastases are frequently missed with CT.

Table 6.3.   The TNM Staging System for Gastric Adenocarcinoma

Stage	Description
Tumor (T)	
TX	Primary tumor cannot be assessed
T0	No evidence of primary tumor
Tis	Carcinoma in situ (intraepithelial tumor without invasion of the lamina propria; high-grade dysplasia)
T1	Tumor invades lamina propria or submucosa
T2	Tumor invades muscularis propria or subserosa
T3	Tumor penetrates serosa without invasion to adjacent structures
T4	Tumor invades adjacent structures
Nodal (N)	
NX	Regional nodes cannot be assessed
N0	No regional node metastasis
N1	Metastasis in 1 or 2 regional lymph nodes
N2	Metastasis in 3-6 regional lymph nodes
N3	Metastasis in ≥7 regional lymph nodes
Metastasis (M)	
MX	Presence of distant metastasis cannot be assessed
M0	No distant metastasis
M1	Distant metastasis or positive peritoneal cytology

Adapted from Ajani J, In H, Sano T, Gaspar L, Erasmus J, Tang L, et al. Stomach. In: Amin MB, Edge SB, American Joint Committee on Cancer, eds. AJCC cancer staging manual. Eighth ed. American Joint Committee on Cancer; 2017:203-20; used with permission.

Another limitation of CT is determination of the depth of tumor invasion, particularly with small tumors. CT is accurate for assessment of the T stage of the primary tumor in about 50% to 70% of cases. Endoscopic ultrasonography (EUS) is the best nonsurgical method for estimating accurately the depth of invasion, particularly for early (T1 or T2) lesions. Although the accuracy of EUS for nodal staging is only slightly better than with CT, EUS-guided fine-needle aspiration of suspicious nodes and regional areas adds to the accuracy of EUS nodal staging; however, this added feature is operator dependent. Positron emission tomography (PET) or combined PET/CT is more sensitive than CT alone for the detection of distant metastases, but its sensitivity for detecting peritoneal carcinomatosis appears to be limited.

Treatment and Prognosis

Surgery is the mainstay of therapy for gastric cancer. Complete surgical removal of a gastric tumor, with resection of the adjacent lymph nodes, offers the only chance for cure. However, two-thirds of patients present with advanced disease, which is incurable by surgery alone. This problem is complicated further by a recurrence rate of 50% among patients who had resection with curative intent.

For patients with potentially resectable noncardia gastric cancer, there are data to support several approaches, including adjuvant chemoradiotherapy, perioperative chemotherapy, and adjuvant chemotherapy, over surgery alone. Most experts recommend a combined modality therapy over surgery alone for patients with stage T2 or higher gastric cancer. An optimal therapeutic approach of multimodality therapy has not been established. In addition, the best approach to patients with locally advanced, unresectable but nonmetastatic disease is unclear. A common approach is to attempt downstaging with chemotherapy or chemoradiotherapy with subsequent restaging.

✓ Surgery is the mainstay of therapy for localized gastric cancer

Gastric Lymphoma
Epidemiology

The stomach is the most frequent site of extranodal lymphoma. Primary gastric lymphoma is uncommon and accounts for 2% of all lymphomas and up to 15% of gastric neoplasms. Although these are rare tumors, the incidence of primary gastric lymphoma has increased in frequency during the past 35 years.

Risk Factors

There are several risk factors for the development of gastric lymphoma. They include *H pylori*–associated chronic gastritis, autoimmune diseases, immunodeficiency syndromes, long-term immunosuppressive therapy, and celiac disease.

Clinical Features

The clinical features of gastric lymphoma are nonspecific and frequently include abdominal discomfort, anorexia, early satiety, and weight loss as well as gastric outlet complaints due to obstruction or impairment of gastric motility and also anemia due to blood loss from ulceration. Systemic B symptoms (fever and night sweats) are present in only about 12% of patients.

Diagnostic Evaluation

Endoscopically, gastric lymphoma has a broad range of appearances—from large, firm rugal folds to eroded nodules to exophytic ulcerated masses. Enlarged folds, if present, are due to the subepithelial infiltrative growth pattern of lymphomas.

When the disease is suspected, standard endoscopic biopsy specimens may not be adequate or the histologic findings may be equivocal, especially when the involvement is primarily submucosal without affecting the mucosa. Deeper biopsy or snare biopsy specimens from a polypoid mass or large rugal fold may be needed to make the diagnosis.

CT of the abdomen and chest is useful for identifying involvement of regional lymph nodes, extension of the tumor into surrounding structures, and distant metastases. If there is no evidence of metastatic disease, EUS is accurate for determining the extent of gastric wall infiltration and can provide useful information for treatment planning.

Tumor Features

The vast majority of gastric lymphomas are of B-cell origin. More than 90% of gastric lymphomas are approximately equally divided into 2 histologic subtypes: low-grade *extranodal marginal zone B-cell lymphoma* (ENMZL) of mucosa (gut)-associated lymphoid tissue (MALT) and *diffuse large B-cell lymphoma* (DLBCL).

Extranodal Marginal Zone B-Cell Lymphoma

ENMZLs of the MALT type, formerly known as MALT lymphoma, constitute a group of low-grade neoplasms that have similar clinical, pathologic, immunologic, and molecular features and arise in the context of preexisting prolonged lymphoid proliferation in mucosal sites. ENMZLs occur most often in the gastrointestinal tract but have been described in various extranodal sites, including the ocular adnexa, salivary glands, thyroid, lungs, thymus, and breast.

Like gastric adenocarcinoma, infection with *H pylori* increases the risk for gastric lymphoma in general and ENMZLs in particular. Gastric ENMZLs are associated with *H pylori* infection in as many as 90% of cases. In health, the stomach does not have much lymphoid tissue. *H pylori*–induced gastritis leads to an aggregation of CD4$^+$ lymphocytes and B cells in the gastric lamina propria. Antigen presentation occurs, followed by T-cell activation, B-cell proliferation, and lymphoid follicle formation. As these follicles become prominent, they develop B-cell monoclonal populations that appear to be sustained by stimuli that come from *H pylori*–sensitized T cells. As the monoclonal B-cell populations proliferate, they begin to spill into the gastric epithelium and invade gastric glands, forming lymphoepithelial lesions that are characteristic of ENMZLs (Figure 6.3).

The best evidence supporting the role of *H pylori* in ENMZL in the stomach is remission of the tumor after eradication of *H pylori* infection with antibiotic therapy. Several clinical studies have documented complete remission in approximately 50% of patients with ENMZL and in 80% if the tumor is in an early clinical stage. A lack of response to antimicrobial treatment has been linked to a specific chromosomal abnormality, the translocation t(11;18).

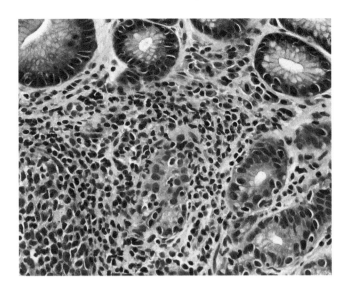

Figure 6.3. Lymphoepithelial Lesion of Mucosa-Associated Lymphoid Tissue Lymphoma With Neoplastic Lymphocytes Infiltrating Gastric Gland. (Stain is hematoxylin-eosin.)

Diffuse Large B-Cell Lymphoma

DLBCL describes a heterogenous group of non-Hodgkin lymphoma. DLBCL may occur de novo, but it also may occur as a high-grade transformation from a low-grade B-cell lymphoma such as an ENMZL. Transformation from indolent ENMZL to DLBCL has been described repeatedly in the course of the disease, and some investigators believe that all DLBCLs of the stomach are due to transformation of an ENMZL.

Staging

The staging systems for primary gastric lymphoma are complicated (a variant of the standard staging by lymph node involvement). Generally, stage I disease is limited to the stomach, and stage II disease implies localized involvement of the lymph nodes within the abdomen. In stage III disease, lymph nodes are involved on both the thoracic and the abdominal sides of the diaphragm. Stage IV disease is disseminated disease.

Treatment

First-line therapy for gastric ENMZL in patients infected with *H pylori* is antibiotics to eradicate *H pylori*. Only patients with localized, mucosal, or submucosal flat lesions and without metastatic disease, lymphadenopathy, or frank DLBCL are candidates for antimicrobial therapy alone. For patients who do not meet these criteria, therapy for *H pylori* eradication should be administered in conjunction with conventional therapy.

When treatment of *H pylori* infection has been administered, eradication of the organism must be proved. Histologic regression requires several months after the infection has been cured with antibiotics, and patients require endoscopic follow-up at frequent intervals. If the response to antibiotics is incomplete or the disease recurs, standard therapies for lymphoma, such as systemic chemotherapy, radiotherapy, or surgery, should be administered. Patients who do not initially have a response to anti–*H pylori* therapy or who have disease relapse after therapy still have a high cure rate.

Conventional therapy for DLBCL depends primarily on the tumor stage. Exploratory laparotomy and partial gastrectomy

may be indicated when stage I disease is suspected. For stage II, III, or IV disease, the primary therapy is systemic chemotherapy. Radiotherapy generally is used to reduce the size of large lesions and to control localized disease.

Rituximab (a chimeric monoclonal antibody targeting the CD20 epitope present on virtually all B cells) is effective therapy for patients with various lymphomas, including ENMZL and DLBCL. It is commonly used in combination with cyclophosphamide, doxorubicin, vincristine, and prednisone (CHOP).

Prognosis

The 5-year survival rate for all patients with gastric lymphoma is 50%. Patients with stage I or II tumors less than 5 cm in diameter have a 10-year survival rate greater than 80%.

✓ Stomach—the most frequent extranodal site for lymphoma
✓ Like gastric adenocarcinoma, *H pylori* infection increases the risk for gastric lymphoma
✓ The 2 most common types of primary gastric lymphoma are ENMZL and DLBCL
✓ Eradication treatment with antibiotics for *H pylori* infection is the first-line therapy for ENMZL

Gastrointestinal Stromal Tumors

Stromal or mesenchymal neoplasms affecting the gastrointestinal tract include GISTs, lipomas, hemangiomas, schwannomas, leiomyomas, and leiomyosarcomas. The most common of these tumors is the GIST.

Epidemiology

GISTs are the most common mesenchymal tumor involving the gastrointestinal tract. The true incidence and prevalence of GISTs are unknown because most of them are found incidentally.

Surveillance, Epidemiology, and End Results (SEER) analysis of histologically confirmed GISTs showed an incidence of 0.68 per 100,000. In autopsy series of patients with gastric cancer, the frequency of incidental subcentimeter GISTs is much higher, which suggests that only a few microscopic tumors grow to a clinically relevant size.

Pathogenesis

The cellular origins of GISTs are the interstitial cells of Cajal, the gastrointestinal pacemaker cells, which form an interface between the autonomic innervation of the bowel wall and the smooth muscle. GISTs almost universally express the CD117 antigen, which allows differentiation from leiomyomas and other subepithelial tumors of the gastrointestinal tract.

The CD117 molecule is part of the c-kit receptor, a membrane tyrosine kinase that is a product of the *c-kit* or *KIT* proto-oncogene (OMIM 164920). In 80% of cases, c-kit activation is the result of an activating *KIT* variant. The majority (>90%) of mesenchymal tumors arising within the gastrointestinal tract are GISTs.

Clinical Features

Patients with GISTs are often asymptomatic, and the tumors are found incidentally at endoscopy or at surgery. Patients with large GISTs may present with vague symptoms, as with all cancers of the upper gastrointestinal tract, or with gastrointestinal tract bleeding. Cases have been reported of patients with GISTs who present with hypoglycemia due to paraneoplastic production of insulinlike growth factor 2 by the tumor.

Tumor Features

GISTs can arise anywhere in the gastrointestinal tract, but they are most common in the stomach and proximal small bowel. The biologic behavior of GISTs is variable, and all GISTs have the potential for malignant behavior. Tumor site, size, and mitotic rate are used for stratifying lesions for risk of recurrence and metastasis. Small intestinal primary site, tumor size larger than 5 cm, and mitotic rate greater than 5 per 50 high-power fields are poor prognostic factors that indicate an increased risk of malignant behavior. When GISTs metastasize, metastasis is usually hematogenous to the liver and peritoneum. Lymphatic spread of GISTs, like other sarcomas, is unusual.

Staging

Staging of GISTs involves primarily endoscopy and imaging studies. Many GISTs occur in the upper gastrointestinal tract and are discovered incidentally. A common manifestation is gastrointestinal tract bleeding secondary to tumor ulceration (Figure 6.4). Endoscopic biopsy specimens obtained with standard techniques typically are not sufficient for definite diagnosis. Although EUS-guided biopsy may not yield sufficient tissue, specific sonographic features may distinguish GIST from other submucosal lesions. The characteristic EUS feature of a GIST is a hypoechoic lesion arising from the muscularis propria. CT is the imaging method of choice to characterize large GISTs and to identify metastatic disease. On CT, a GIST appears as a solid mass that enhances brightly with an intravenous contrast agent.

If noninvasive methods are unsuccessful for correctly defining a GIST when it is suspected, preoperative biopsy may not be necessary if the tumor appears to be resectable and the patient is otherwise a surgical candidate. GISTs frequently metastasize to liver and peritoneum and rarely to regional lymph nodes. However, if metastatic disease is present, surgical biopsy may be necessary to confirm the diagnosis if chemotherapy is a consideration.

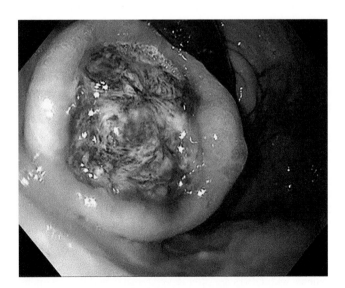

Figure 6.4. Endoscopic Image of an Ulcerated Gastrointestinal Stromal Tumor in the Proximal Portion of the Stomach.

Treatment

Surgical resection is the treatment of choice for potentially resectable tumors, and the recommendation is to resect all GISTs that are 2 cm or larger. The management of smaller GISTs is controversial because their natural history is unknown. Imatinib mesylate (Gleevec), a potent inhibitor of KIT signaling, is often used in neoadjuvant and adjuvant therapy.

Prognosis

Prognosis is influenced by tumor site (small intestine is worse than stomach), tumor size (if larger, the prognosis is worse), the ability to resect the tumor completely, and the response to imatinib in advanced disease.

✓ GISTs
  • Most common mesenchymal tumor of the gastrointestinal tract
  • Originate from the interstitial cells of Cajal and most frequently occur in the stomach
✓ CD117 antigen is the immunostain marker for GISTs
✓ Risk factors for malignant behavior of GISTs include larger size, greater number of mitotic figures, and location other than stomach

---

Gastroenteropancreatic NETs

Neuroendocrine cells occur throughout the body; for example, they cluster together in small groups called islets throughout the pancreas. NETs can be classified by their site of origin: Those that develop from pancreatic endocrine cells are referred to as pancreatic neuroendocrine tumors (PNETs), and those that originate in the stomach or gut, as gastroenteric neuroendocrine tumors (GNETs).

Further classification of NETs is complex since they arise from many locations, their histologic features are quite varied, and they have a wide range of clinical behaviors. In general, they are separated into 2 major categories:

1. *Poorly differentiated neuroendocrine carcinomas* are high-grade carcinomas that resemble small cell or large cell neuroendocrine carcinoma of the lung. They are associated with a rapidly progressing downhill clinical course and, in general, a poor prognosis.
2. *Well-differentiated NETs of the digestive tract* traditionally include both gastrointestinal tumors and PNETs.

Although both tumor types have similar histologic characteristics, morphology alone does not allow prediction of the clinical course associated with these tumors. They are not a clinically homogeneous group, and while most are slow growing and have a relatively indolent course, they display a wide spectrum of biologic and clinical behavior. Up to 40% of patients with GNETs present with liver metastases at the time of diagnosis, but many patients survive for many years even with advanced-stage disease; overall 5-year survival is about 67%.

Epidemiology

Both GNETs and PNETs are relatively rare; however, the incidence of both has been increasing in the US and elsewhere; data from the SEER program showed a 5-fold increase since the 1980s. The reasons are not clear, but the increase may largely result from increased detection on cross-sectional imaging, such as CT or magnetic resonance imaging (MRI), and during endoscopy.

Pathogenesis

Most NETs occur sporadically, although some may appear as part of an autosomal dominant inherited multiple endocrine neoplasia (MEN) syndrome. All NETs can be associated with MEN-1, which is characterized by pituitary, parathyroid, and pancreatic hyperplasia or tumors. In addition, PNETs can occur as part of 3 other inherited disorders: von Hippel-Lindau disease, neurofibromatosis 1 (von Recklinghausen disease), and the tuberous sclerosis complex.

Clinical Features

NETs are usually diagnosed in the sixth or seventh decade of life. Because they develop from neuroendocrine cells, they may secrete various peptides and hormones simultaneously. Secretion of some of these will not result in clinical symptoms, whereas others, if produced in large enough quantities, will result in the appearance of a clinical syndrome.

NETs and Carcinoid Syndrome

NETs (previously termed carcinoid tumors) most commonly occur in the gastrointestinal tract (about two-thirds), while about one-fourth arise in the bronchopulmonary system. They can occur anywhere in the alimentary tract, with the ileum and rectum being the most common sites. The clinical manifestation varies from an asymptomatic incidental finding to symptomatic tumors from local invasion, metastases, or production of bioactive amines causing the classic carcinoid syndrome.

Clinical and Tumor Features

Most NETs are found incidentally; thus, at the time of diagnosis, most patients are asymptomatic. If symptoms are present, they often are nonspecific and associated with the location and extent of the tumor. Symptoms due to the direct effects of a tumor in the gastrointestinal tract may be abdominal pain, intestinal obstruction, nausea, weight loss, or intestinal bleeding. Many patients have vague or mild symptoms for years and are sometimes thought to have irritable bowel syndrome or other functional disorders of the gastrointestinal tract for years before the correct diagnosis is made.

Most NETs do not produce noticeable symptoms since the metabolic products are efficiently metabolized by the liver. However, when secreting tumors metastasize to the liver (the most common site of metastasis), substances are released directly into the systemic circulation, circumventing hepatic metabolism.

Carcinoid syndrome, which is the primary clinical manifestation, occurs in a subset of patients with NETs (10% of patients). When the syndrome is present, it is associated most commonly with tumors in the small bowel; these are the most common and frequently metastasize.

Carcinoid syndrome is due to peptides released by the tumor into the systemic circulation. As many as 40 secretory products have been identified; the common ones are histamine, kallikrein, prostaglandins, serotonin, and tachykinins. The liver is capable of inactivating these peptides, which is why carcinoid syndrome primarily occurs in association with liver metastases: The bioactive products are secreted directly into the hepatic veins.

The most common symptoms of carcinoid syndrome are diarrhea and facial flushing; others are cramping abdominal pain, skin telangiectasia, peripheral edema, and wheezing. The most common physical finding is hepatomegaly. Intermittent facial flushing occurs in up to 85% of patients. The flush usually starts suddenly and can last from 30 seconds to 30 minutes. The typical flush is red or violaceous and appears on the face, neck, and upper chest. Flushes can be associated with hypotension and tachycardia. Several inciting factors are known for the flushing associated with carcinoid syndrome: eating, alcohol ingestion, the Valsalva maneuver, increased emotional states, trauma or pressure on the liver (including on physical examination), and anesthesia. Anesthesia can provoke long episodes of flushing that can result in life-threatening hypotension known as *carcinoid crisis*. Carcinoid crisis can be prevented by the administration of octreotide before anesthesia.

Diarrhea occurs in 80% of patients with carcinoid syndrome and can be quite severe. It is a secretory diarrhea, and patients may pass as many as 30 stools per day. Although the diarrhea usually is unrelated to the flushing episodes, the associated dehydration can contribute to the hypotension from flushing.

Wheezing is a common component of carcinoid syndrome and is due to bronchospasm and right-sided valvular heart disease. Unlike diarrhea, wheezing and dyspnea are worse during flushing episodes. Of importance, wheezing associated with carcinoid syndrome should not be treated like bronchial asthma: Treatment with β-agonists can incite prolonged vasodilation and severe hypotension. Hypertension usually is not present in carcinoid syndrome but, as stated above, the syndrome can cause paroxysmal and clinically important hypotension.

Aside from carcinoid syndrome, the clinical presentation, tumor features, treatment recommendations, and prognosis related to NETs vary by the location of the primary tumor. Characteristics of NETs based on location are outlined in Table 6.4.

Table 6.4. Characteristics of Neuroendocrine Tumors Based on Location

Location	Secretory products	Carcinoid syndrome	Clinical characteristics
Foregut			
Stomach, duodenum, pancreas, bronchus	Serotonin, histamine	Atypical (with type 3)	Indolent except for type 3
Midgut			
Jejunum, ileum, appendix, ascending colon	Serotonin, prostaglandins, polypeptides	Classic, but present in only 10% of cases	Often multiple; usually in ileum
Hindgut			
Transverse, descending, and sigmoid colon and rectum	None	Rare	Usually indolent

Stomach

Gastric NETs tend to occur in the body of the stomach. They may be single or multiple, and, to endoscopists, they may appear to be an ordinary ulcer, polyp, or tumor mass. They are often round and gray or yellow.

Gastric NETs occur most frequently in patients with hypergastrinemia caused by atrophic gastritis and achlorhydria. They also occur in patients with MEN-1–associated Zollinger-Ellison syndrome. Any condition in which serum levels of gastrin are increased for a prolonged period should alert clinicians to the possible presence of gastric NETs.

Gastric NETs are classified into 3 types, each of which has a different behavior and prognosis (Table 6.5).

Type 1

Up to 80% of all gastric NETs are type 1. They are associated with pernicious anemia or chronic atrophic gastritis. The tumors are derived from enterochromaffin-like cells and are thought to develop from long-standing stimulation by increased serum levels of gastrin. Type 1 NETs usually are diagnosed in patients aged 60 to 70 years. As with chronic atrophic gastritis and pernicious anemia, type 1 NETs are more common in women than in men. These tumors are usually small and multiple. Metastatic disease is rare and occurs in less than 10% of tumors 2 cm or smaller but in as many as 20% of larger tumors. These tumors generally are indolent and often are considered benign.

Type 2

NETs of the stomach due to hypergastrinemia from MEN-1–associated gastrinomas are classified as type 2 NETs. They are rare (5% of gastric carcinoids) and, like type 1 NETs, they are typically small, multiple, slow growing, and indolent and have little malignant potential.

For gastric NET types 1 and 2 smaller than 1 cm, the treatment of choice is endoscopic resection, if possible. Because the patients often have sustained hypergastrinemia, endoscopic surveillance every 12 months has been recommended, but progression to malignant disease and death is unusual.

For patients with multiple tumors or advanced disease that is not appropriate for resection, antrectomy or medical therapy aimed at decreasing the serum levels of gastrin has been advocated. Antrectomy decreases hypergastrinemia by removing much of the gastrin-producing cell mass in the stomach.

Type 3

Type 3 gastric NETs are sporadic and do not appear to be associated with hypergastrinemia. Of all gastric NETs, 15% are type 3. They are the most aggressive of the gastric NETs, and 65% of patients have local or liver metastases when the tumor is discovered. Type 3 is the only type of gastric NET that is associated with an atypical carcinoid syndrome; these tumors can produce histamine that results in flushing. Because sporadic gastric carcinoids (type 3) are more aggressive, they usually are treated with partial or total gastrectomy with local lymph node resection.

Small Intestinal NETs

Clinically, small intestinal NETs are the most important NETs because patients are more likely to present with intestinal symptoms and carcinoid syndrome, which occurs in up to 10% of these patients. Abdominal pain or bowel obstruction can be caused by the direct mechanical effect of the tumor and an associated fibroblastic reaction, intussusception, or mesenteric ischemia due to tumor-associated fibrosis or angiopathy.

Most small intestinal NETS occur in the ileum near the ileocecal valve. Small intestinal NETs may be multicentric in 30% of individuals and have a higher likelihood than NETs of arising from other portions of the gastrointestinal tract and metastasizing to regional lymph nodes and the liver. Because small intestinal NETs have the potential to metastasize, regardless of size, they should be removed surgically along with local lymph node resection. Patients with these tumors are most at risk for synchronous lesions (present in 30% of cases), so at surgery, the surgeon should thoroughly inspect the remaining small bowel. Resection may be required for palliation, even in patients with metastatic disease. The prognosis for patients with small intestinal NETs varies with the stage of disease. The 5-year survival rate ranges from 35% to 80%.

Appendix

Up to one-half of intestinal NETs are appendiceal tumors, and NETs are the most common neoplasms of the appendix. Patients are almost always asymptomatic, and typically these tumors are discovered incidentally at appendectomy. Incidental NETs are found in 0.5% of appendectomy specimens. Appendiceal NETs are often smaller than 1 cm and usually are solitary and benign. Although local invasion by appendiceal NETs is common, metastatic disease is rare.

If symptoms are present, they usually are associated with large tumors, tumors located at the base of the appendix, and tumors with associated metastatic disease. Approximately 10% of patients with appendiceal carcinoids have tumors at the base of the appendix, where the tumor can cause obstruction that may result in appendicitis. Patients with appendiceal NETs may present with carcinoid syndrome, but this occurs almost always with liver metastases.

Table 6.5.   Three Types of Gastric Neuroendocrine Tumors

Characteristic	Type 1	Type 2	Type 3
Tumor frequency, %	80	5	15
Tumor frequency by sex	Women more than men	Women same as men	Women less than men
Tumor features	<1 cm; multiple	1-2 cm; multiple	>2 cm; single
Gastric mucosa	Atrophic	Hyperplastic	Normal
Associated conditions	Gastric atrophy	MEN-1, ZES	None
Gastric pH	High	Low	Normal
Fasting serum gastrin	High	High	Normal
Treatment	<1 cm, EndoR; >2 cm, surgery	<1 cm, EndoR; >2 cm, surgery	Surgery

Abbreviations: EndoR, endoscopic resection; MEN, multiple endocrine neoplasia; ZES, Zollinger-Ellison syndrome.

The prognosis for patients with appendiceal NETs is determined by the size of the tumor. Tumors smaller than 2 cm (most tumors) are unlikely to have metastasized when diagnosed. Tumors larger than 2 cm are uncommon, but when they are present, up to 30% have metastasized at the time of diagnosis. Appendiceal tumors smaller than 2 cm can be treated with simple appendectomy. However, for larger tumors, right hemicolectomy should be performed.

The overall 5-year survival rate for patients with appendiceal NETs is 70% to 100%, but for patients with metastatic disease at the time of presentation, it ranges from 10% to 30%.

Colon

NET of the colon is rare. When it occurs, it is often located on the right side of the colon. Unlike patients with NETs in other locations, those with a NET of the colon may present with symptoms, and when they do, they often have locally advanced disease. Local resection of the tumor has been reported to be effective in the early stages of disease, but many patients require radical colectomy because of advanced disease at the time of diagnosis. Patients with colonic NETs rarely have carcinoid syndrome. The overall 5-year survival rate for patients with colonic NETs is 30% to 75%.

Rectum

Patients with rectal NETs are nearly always asymptomatic, and the tumors are found incidentally during screening colonoscopy. They are not associated with carcinoid syndrome. Tumors smaller than 1 cm can be treated with local excision. Radical excision is more appropriate for tumors larger than 2 cm or for smaller tumors that have invaded the muscularis propria. The overall 5-year survival rate for patients with rectal NETs ranges from 75% to 100%.

Diagnosis of NETs and Carcinoid Syndrome

Most NETs are found incidentally on endoscopy or cross-sectional imaging, such as CT performed for other indications. If symptoms of carcinoid syndrome are strongly suspected, the best initial evaluation is to measure urinary 5-hydroxyindoleacetic acid (5-HIAA), which is the end product of serotonin metabolism. This test has a sensitivity of more than 90% and a specificity of 90% for carcinoid syndrome. Sensitivity is less for patients who have NETs without symptoms of carcinoid syndrome. Measurement of urinary excretion of 5-HIAA is generally most useful in patients with primary tumors of the midgut (small bowel and right colon), which tend to produce the highest levels of serotonin. The normal rate of excretion of 5-HIAA over 24 hours is 2 to 8 mg daily. The rate of excretion may be up to 30 mg daily in patients with malabsorption syndromes, such as celiac disease and Whipple disease, as well as after the ingestion of large amounts of tryptophan- or serotonin-rich foods. Patients should avoid the ingestion of tryptophan- and serotonin-rich foods, such as bananas, tomatoes, avocados, and certain nuts at least 24 hours before and during the 24-hour urine collection.

Chromogranins are proteins that are stored and released with peptides and amines in various neuroendocrine tissues and are designated as chromogranin A (CgA), B, and C. Well-differentiated NETs are associated with high blood concentrations of chromogranins, which increase with a larger tumor burden.

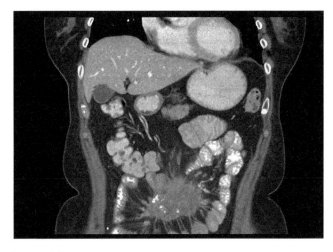

Figure 6.5.   Small-Bowel Carcinoid. Computed tomographic image, coronal view, shows classic spoke wheel sign in mesentery.

CgA is a more sensitive indicator of a NET than chromogranin B or C. Levels of CgA vary daily in healthy persons and in those with NETs. False-positive increases in CgA can be present in various other conditions, including inflammatory conditions and endocrine, gastrointestinal, and cardiovascular diseases, and as a result of medications, such as histamine-receptor antagonists and proton pump inhibitors. Because of its low specificity, measurement of CgA alone is not recommended as a screening test for the diagnosis of a NET or carcinoid syndrome. However, for patients with an established diagnosis, CgA can be used as an appropriate tumor marker to assess disease progression or response to therapy or after surgical resection.

✓ Gastroenteric NETs
  • Most patients are asymptomatic
  • Most patients have vague abdominal symptoms for years that mimic irritable bowel syndrome
✓ Carcinoid syndrome
  • To develop from gastroenteric NET, liver metastases must be present
  • Most common symptoms—diarrhea and facial flushing
✓ Small intestinal NETs
  • Propensity to metastasize even when small
  • Multicentric in 30% of cases
✓ Appendiceal NETs
  • Tumor size dictates management
  • Appendectomy if smaller than 2 cm
✓ Rectal NETs
  • Most often found incidentally at colonoscopy
  • Local excision—usual treatment if smaller than 1 cm
✓ Dotatate PET/CT—imaging test of choice to identify an occult primary NET

NETs are highly vascular, and those that originate in the small intestine often produce mesenteric masses with dense desmoplastic fibrosis. These features are usually well seen on CT or MRI scans of the abdomen and pelvis with the classic finding of the spoke wheel sign from mesenteric retraction (Figure 6.5). Both imaging modalities can show liver metastases, although MRI is probably more sensitive than contrast-enhanced CT. Most NETs express high levels of somatostatin receptors and can be detected with functional imaging assessing somatostatin receptor expression. Traditionally this imaging was done with somatostatin receptor scintigraphy (SRS) and a radiolabeled form of the

Table 6.6. WHO Histopathologic Classification of NETs

Classification and grade	Mitotic count[a]	Ki-67 index, %[b]
NET G1	<2	<3
NET G2	2-20	3-20
NET G3	>20	>20
NEC (G3), poorly differentiated, small or large cell	>20	>20

Abbreviations: G, grade; NEC, neuroendocrine carcinoma; NET, neuroendocrine tumor; WHO, World Health Organization.

[a] Mitotic count is determined from evaluation of mitoses in 50 high-power fields and indicated as number of mitoses per 2 mm².

[b] Ki-67 proliferation index is determined from more than 500 cells in the area of highest labeling (hot spot).

Data from Rindi G, Arnold R, Bosman FT, Capella C, Klimstra D, Kloppel G, et al. Nomenclature and classification of neuroendocrine neoplasms of the digestive system. In: Bosman FT, Carneiro F, Hruban RH, Theise ND, eds. WHO classification of tumours of the digestive system. 4th ed. International Agency for Research on Cancer; 2010:13.

somatostatin analogue octreotide (Octreoscan). However, PET with newer somatostatin-receptor–targeting radiotracers, such as gallium Ga 68 dotatate, is more sensitive than SRS, particularly for small tumors. Because of the greater sensitivity, gallium Ga 68 dotatate PET/CT is the imaging test of choice to identify an occult primary tumor. The World Health Organization histopathologic classification of NETs defines a grading system based on both mitotic index and Ki-67 index determined by immunohistochemistry (Table 6.6). This grading system along with staging is effective at defining risk groups of well-differentiated NETs across the entire gastroenteropancreatic spectrum.

Pancreatic Neuroendocrine Tumors

The most common pancreatic malignancy is adenocarcinoma, which arises from pancreatic exocrine cells. PNETs are less than 4% of all diagnosed pancreatic cancers. These malignancies may progress, and the tumor cells may spread to other sites such as lymph nodes, liver, lung, or bone. Advanced PNETs may be functional or nonfunctional. *Functional PNETs* produce hormones such as gastrin, insulin, and glucagon, which are released into the blood and cause symptoms. *Nonfunctional PNETs* are more difficult to diagnose, since they produce substances that often do not cause overt symptoms until the tumor has spread and continued to grow. PNETs include the following: gastrinoma, insulinoma, VIPoma, glucagonoma, and somatostatinoma. The functional NET syndromes are summarized in Table 6.7.

Gastrinoma

Gastrinomas produce the classic triad of symptoms called Zollinger-Ellison syndrome. This syndrome consists of peptic ulcer disease, gastric acid hypersecretion, and a gastrin-producing tumor. Gastrinomas are rare and occur in less than 1% of patients who have peptic ulcer disease. Gastrinomas are associated frequently with MEN-1 syndrome.

Etiology and Pathogenesis

The majority of gastrinomas occur in an anatomical area called the gastrinoma triangle (Figure 6.6) with 60% occurring in the duodenal wall; the pancreas is the second most common site.

Gastrinomas are slow growing, and it can be difficult to distinguish benign tumors from malignant ones. Approximately two-thirds of gastrinomas are malignant. The best indicator of malignancy is the presence of metastases, which most often affect the regional lymph nodes or the liver. It is important to determine whether liver metastases are present. If they are, the patient is not a candidate for surgical treatment.

Clinical Features

Peptic ulcer disease is the most common endoscopic sign of gastrinoma and occurs in more than 90% of patients. Traditionally, the ulcer disease associated with gastrinomas has been characterized by multiple duodenal ulcers (including postbulbar ulcers) and esophagitis refractory to medical treatment. However, the most common type of ulcer associated with gastrinoma is an ordinary duodenal bulb ulcer. Gastric folds in Zollinger-Ellison syndrome are characteristically enlarged from gastrin-stimulated hyperplasia of parietal cells (Figure 6.7).

As many as 70% of patients with a gastrinoma have symptoms or endoscopic findings of severe gastroesophageal reflux, which likely is caused by hypersecretion of gastric acid. Also, 50% of the patients have diarrhea due to the effect of acid hypersecretion on the small bowel. Increased acid exposure to the small bowel causes morphologic and inflammatory changes that can result in malabsorption. In addition, the low pH may inactivate pancreatic lipase and cause precipitation of bile salts, resulting in malabsorption of fat and steatorrhea, which is the most common mechanism of diarrhea in Zollinger-Ellison syndrome.

If a patient has a duodenal ulcer that is not caused by either *H pylori* infection or nonsteroidal anti-inflammatory drugs, or if a patient has duodenal ulcer disease and diarrhea, the concurrent presence of gastrinoma should be considered.

Table 6.7. Functional Neuroendocrine Tumor Syndromes

Tumor (syndrome)	Presentation	Location in pancreas, %	Malignant, %	MEN-1 associated, %
Gastrinoma (ZES)	Abdominal pain, diarrhea	30	70	25
Insulinoma	Hypoglycemic symptoms	100	10	10
VIPoma	Severe watery diarrhea, hypokalemia	90	80	5
Glucagonoma	4 D's[a]	100	60	5
Somatostatinoma	3 S's[b]	60	60	5

Abbreviations: MEN-1, multiple endocrine neoplasia type 1; ZES, Zollinger-Ellison syndrome.

[a] 4 D's is a mnemonic for dermatitis, diabetes, deep vein thrombosis, and diarrhea.

[b] 3 S's is a mnemonic for sugar (diabetes), stones (gallstones), and steatorrhea.

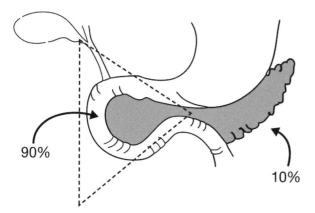

Figure 6.6. The Gastrinoma Triangle. Most gastrinomas (90%) occur inside this triangle.

Diagnostic Tests

For patients with the clinical manifestations of gastrinoma, the first screening test is measurement of the serum level of gastrin. This should be done after proton pump inhibitor therapy has been withheld for at least 7 days. A serum gastrin level of more than 1,000 pg/mL is suggestive of the presence of a gastrinoma but is not diagnostic. A level less than 1,000 pg/mL but more than 110 pg/mL may be consistent with several conditions that cause hypergastrinemia. The most common cause of hypergastrinemia generally is achlorhydria. The most common cause of achlorhydria, in turn, is atrophic gastritis. It is important to note that most patients with a gastrinoma have a serum gastrin level of approximately 600 pg/mL, and atrophic gastritis can cause serum gastrin levels greater than 1,000 pg/mL; therefore, no level of hypergastrinemia is diagnostic of Zollinger-Ellison syndrome. Other causes of hypergastrinemia associated with achlorhydria include gastric ulcer, gastric carcinoma, vagotomy, and current proton pump inhibitor therapy. Also, some disorders cause hypergastrinemia with normal or increased acid secretion; these are gastric outlet obstruction and retained gastric antrum in patients with previous gastric surgery.

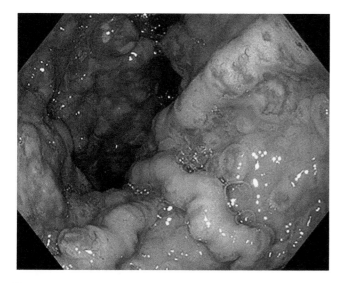

Figure 6.7. Zollinger-Ellison Syndrome. Endoscopic image shows enlarged gastric folds.

A gastric pH probe can be used to determine whether acid hypersecretion is present. For a patient who has not been receiving proton pump inhibitor therapy for at least 7 days, gastric pH less than 2 is consistent with a hypersecretory condition, and this, in combination with a markedly increased gastrin level, is nearly diagnostic of Zollinger-Ellison syndrome.

A secretin stimulation test is warranted for only a few clinical situations (Figure 6.8). If a patient has hypergastrinemia and acid hypersecretion, an intravenous secretin test is indicated. In patients with Zollinger-Ellison syndrome, the serum level of gastrin increases at least 120 pg/mL over the basal gastrin level. Patients with other causes of hypergastrinemic hyperchlorhydria have only a slight or no increase in the serum level of gastrin.

After there is biochemical evidence of gastrinoma, the tumor should be localized. Most gastrinomas have somatostatin receptors, and the test of choice for localizing these tumors is gallium Ga 68 dotatate PET/CT. Because most gastrinomas occur in the gastrinoma triangle, EUS is very sensitive for localizing the primary tumor but is less helpful for evaluating metastatic disease. CT of the abdomen detects approximately half the tumors and may be useful for directing biopsy of liver metastases, if present.

Treatment

Surgical resection is the treatment of choice for patients with resectable disease (ie, not metastatic or locally advanced). Patients with liver metastases or MEN-1 syndrome (with multifocal disease) may not be candidates for surgical treatment because they may have multiple tumors.

If resection is not possible, the objective in treating Zollinger-Ellison syndrome is to control gastric acid hypersecretion. Medical treatment to decrease gastric acid hypersecretion usually consists of high doses of proton pump inhibitors; often the dose can be gradually decreased. The administration of octreotide, which inhibits the secretion of gastrin, often produces an unpredictable clinical response and generally is not considered first-line therapy.

✓ Most common type of ulcer in Zollinger-Ellison syndrome—ordinary duodenal bulb ulcer
✓ Diagnostic threshold for a secretin stimulation test for gastrinoma is an increase in serum gastrin of at least 120 pg/mL
✓ Imaging modality of choice to localize a gastrinoma—gallium Ga 68 dotatate PET/CT

Insulinoma

Insulinomas are insulin-secreting islet cell tumors that originate in the pancreas and cause symptoms of hypoglycemia. They are usually solitary but, rarely, may be multiple.

Clinical Features

Most patients present with clinical manifestations of hypoglycemia: altered or loss of consciousness, confusion, dizziness, and visual disturbances. Symptoms may result also from catecholamine release caused by hypoglycemia. These symptoms are anxiety, weakness, fatigue, headache, palpitations, tremor, and sweating. Typically, symptoms occur with fasting, when a meal is delayed or missed, or during exercise. Patients may learn to avoid symptoms by eating frequently; as a result, 40% of patients have a history of weight gain from increased eating.

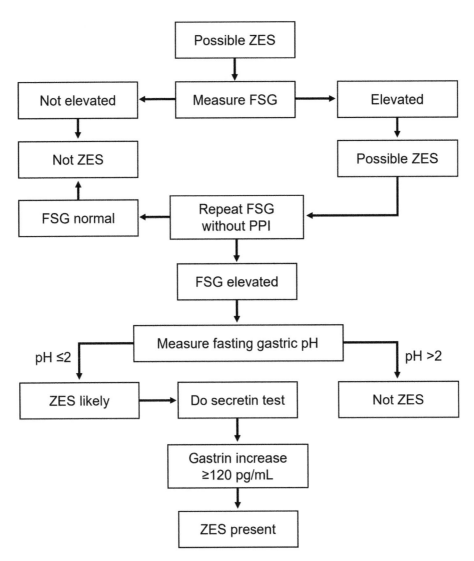

Figure 6.8. **Diagnostic Evaluation of Gastrinoma and Zollinger-Ellison Syndrome (ZES).** FSG indicates fasting serum gastrin; PPI, proton pump inhibitor.

Diagnosis

The presence of an insulinoma is determined by the combination of a low fasting blood glucose level and an inappropriately increased plasma level of insulin. This combination is identified in 65% of patients with insulinoma. For a definitive diagnosis, a 72-hour fast is required, with the serum levels of glucose and insulin determined at regular intervals and when the patient becomes symptomatic. With this fasting test, symptoms develop in 75% of patients with an insulinoma within 24 hours, in 95% by 48 hours, and in virtually 100% within 72 hours.

When there is biochemical evidence of an insulinoma, localization of the tumor can be difficult since most tumors are small. Because it is less common for insulinomas than for gastrinomas to have somatostatin receptors, functional imaging with somatostatin analogues can localize only 50% of the tumors. Also, CT of the abdomen shows only 50% of insulinomas because of their small size. These tumors are almost exclusively in the pancreas, and EUS, the imaging modality of choice, allows detection of nearly 90% of pancreatic insulinomas. Metastatic insulinoma is evaluated best with MRI.

Treatment

As for any GNET, definitive treatment is surgical removal of the tumor, and this is indicated for any patient in whom metastatic disease has not been identified. According to most reports, 70% to 95% of all patients are cured with surgical treatment.

For patients with metastatic disease and those with insulinomas that have not been removed by partial pancreatectomy, the disease can be managed with hyperglycemic agents such as diazoxide and octreotide. Also, patients with metastatic insulinoma may receive chemotherapy. The most effective combination chemotherapy is streptozocin and doxorubicin.

✓ Most insulinomas are small and located in the pancreas
✓ EUS—imaging modality of choice for detection of insulinomas

---

VIPoma

VIPoma is caused by a NET that produces vasoactive intestinal polypeptide (VIP). VIP induces intestinal water and chloride secretion and inhibits gastric acid secretion. This syndrome is characterized by severe watery diarrhea, hypokalemia, and achlorhydria and is known as the *WDHA* (watery diarrhea, hypokalemia, and achlorhydria) *syndrome*, Verner-Morrison syndrome, or pancreatic cholera.

Pathogenesis

Approximately 90% of VIPomas are in the pancreas. Although other tumors, including intestinal carcinoids, pheochromocytomas, and bronchogenic carcinomas, may produce VIP, they rarely cause VIPoma syndrome. VIPomas are usually solitary tumors, and more than 75% of them occur in the body or tail of the pancreas. Although these tumors are slow growing, they frequently become large before diagnosis; 75% of VIPomas are malignant, and 50% have metastasized at the time of diagnosis. VIPomas cannot be distinguished from other pancreatic endocrine tumors with conventional histologic or electron microscopic examination. However, the demonstration of immunoreactive VIP in the tumor and plasma establishes the diagnosis.

Clinical Features

As stated above, VIPomas cause secretory diarrhea, which results in hypokalemia and dehydration. Stool volume may exceed 3 L daily. The watery diarrhea resembles that of cholera, hence the term *pancreatic cholera* is sometimes used. Erythematous flushing of the head and trunk occurs in some patients. Also, hyperglycemia develops in some patients because of VIP- and hypokalemia-induced glycogenolysis in the liver.

Diagnosis

VIPoma should be suspected if patients present with high-volume watery diarrhea that persists despite fasting and is associated with hypokalemia and dehydration. The diagnosis is confirmed by the finding of an increased plasma concentration of VIP. Because these tumors are large, frequently malignant, and metastatic, the abdomen should be scanned with CT to localize and determine the extent of tumor involvement. MRI is also effective for localizing the tumor and identifying metastatic disease. Other imaging studies may not be necessary.

Treatment

The first priority of treatment is to correct the dehydration and electrolyte abnormalities. Patients may require at least 5 L of fluid daily with aggressive potassium replacement. Long-acting octreotide controls diarrhea in most patients with VIPoma, and this agent is considered the initial treatment of choice. For patients who do not have a response to somatostatin analogues, concomitant administration of glucocorticoids may be tried because the combination has had some success.

After imaging studies have been used to localize the tumor and determine the extent of tumor involvement, surgery should be considered for all patients who do not have evidence of metastatic disease. Surgical resection of a pancreatic VIPoma relieves all symptoms and is curative in approximately 30% of patients. Surgery also may be indicated to relieve local effects produced by the large size of the tumor.

For patients with metastatic disease, the best treatment option is chemotherapy. The most effective chemotherapy regimen is streptozocin in combination with either doxorubicin or fluorouracil, which achieves partial remission in up to 90% of patients.

✓ Large-volume secretory diarrhea with hypokalemia is the hallmark clinical presentation of VIPoma

✓ VIPomas are usually large pancreatic masses at presentation, and most are malignant

---

Glucagonoma

Glucagonomas produce a rare syndrome of dermatitis, glucose intolerance, weight loss, and anemia.

Pathogenesis

Glucagonomas usually are solitary, large tumors with an average size of 5 to 6 cm at the time of diagnosis; 65% are located in the head of the pancreas, and the other 35% occur equally in the body and tail. Most tumors are metastatic at the time of diagnosis.

Clinical Features

Glucagonomas occur in persons 45 to 70 years old. Typically, the patient presents with a distinct dermatitis called *necrolytic migratory erythema*, which usually develops a mean of 7 years before the onset of other symptoms. This rash starts as an erythematous area, typically in an intertriginous area such as the groin, buttocks, thighs, or perineum, or it may start in periorificial areas. The erythematous lesions spread laterally and then become raised, with superficial central blistering or bullous formation. When the bullae rupture, crusting occurs and the lesions begin to heal in the center. Healing is associated with hyperpigmentation. The entire sequence usually takes 1 to 2 weeks and consists of a mixed pattern of erythema, bullous formation, epidermal separation, crusting, and hyperpigmentation, which wax and wane. Glossitis, angular stomatitis, dystrophic nails, and hair thinning are other clinical findings. The majority of patients with glucagonoma also have hypoaminoacidemia, which may be responsible for the rash. The rash improves with treatment with amino acids and nutrition.

Glucagon stimulates glycogenolysis, gluconeogenesis, lipolysis, ketogenesis, and insulin secretion and inhibits pancreatic and gastric secretion and intestinal motility. Most patients have glucose intolerance, and some may have frank type 2 diabetes. Most patients with glucagonoma also have noticeable weight loss, even if the tumor is found incidentally and is small. It is believed that glucagon exerts a catabolic effect. Some patients also may have anorexia.

Diagnosis

If the clinical features of glucagonoma are present, the diagnosis can be confirmed by the finding of an increased plasma glucagon level of more than 1,000 pg/mL. Because glucagonomas occur in the pancreas and tend to be large and metastatic at the time of clinical presentation, CT of the abdomen usually localizes the tumor.

Treatment

The initial treatment objectives are to control the symptoms and hyperglycemia and to restore the nutritional status. The surgical risk for these patients usually is increased because of the catabolic effects of glucagon, glucose intolerance, and hypoaminoacidemia.

Patients should receive nutritional support, and the hyperglycemia should be corrected. The rash may improve with correction of the hypoaminoacidemia. If anemia is pronounced, transfusion may be needed. Octreotide is useful for controlling symptoms, and it improves the dermatitis, weight loss, diarrhea, and abdominal pain but not type 2 diabetes. Surgery is offered to all patients who are acceptable surgical risks and who do not have evidence of metastatic spread of the tumor, but it is curative in only 20% of them.

For patients with metastatic disease, it is important to remember that the tumors are slow growing and survival is good even for those who do not receive chemotherapy. There is no clear evidence that chemotherapy has any important effect on these tumors. The most commonly used chemotherapeutic agents are streptozocin in combination with either doxorubicin or fluorouracil.

✓ Necrolytic migratory erythema—the characteristic rash of glucagonoma
✓ Plasma glucagon level greater than 1,000 pg/mL is diagnostic of glucagonoma

---

Somatostatinoma

Somatostatinomas are the least common of the GNETs. They produce a distinct syndrome of type 2 diabetes, gallbladder disease, and steatorrhea.

Pathogenesis

Somatostatinomas are NETs that occur in the pancreas and intestine. Tumors that arise in the pancreas tend to have higher levels of somatostatin and are more likely to produce symptoms. Somatostatinomas are usually solitary and large, and the majority have metastasized at the time of diagnosis. Somatostatin inhibits insulin release, gallbladder motility, and secretion of pancreatic enzymes and bicarbonate. Somatostatinomas are associated with neurofibromatosis type 1.

Clinical Features

Type 2 diabetes occurs in half the patients with somatostatinoma. Gallbladder disease occurs in 65% of the patients and usually is manifested as cholelithiasis, acalculous cholecystitis, or obstructive jaundice from local tumor invasion. Steatorrhea occurs in one-third of the patients.

Diagnosis

Most somatostatinomas are found incidentally when laparotomy is performed for gallbladder disease. The diagnosis is established by the finding of somatostatin-containing D cells in the resected tumor and an increased plasma concentration of somatostatin-like immunoreactive material. Tumors are localized with CT, EUS, or ultrasonography of the abdomen.

Treatment

Diabetes usually is mild and responds to oral hypoglycemic agents or low doses of insulin. No specific medical treatment exists for treating somatostatinomas. Octreotide may be helpful in treatment. However, somatostatinomas are rare, and more reports are needed to determine the efficacy of octreotide.

Surgical excision is the treatment of choice, but most patients present with metastatic disease. Cytotoxic chemotherapy is offered to patients who have evidence of metastatic disease, but there is no clear evidence that this treatment is effective.

Management Principles for GNETs and PNETs

In general, the treatment of GNETs and PNETs is based on the following: localization of the tumor and identification of metastatic disease if present, resection of the primary tumor if appropriate, and control of symptoms, such as those associated with carcinoid syndrome.

The liver is the predominant site of metastatic disease. Liver resection is indicated for the treatment of metastatic liver disease in the absence of diffuse bilobar involvement, compromised liver function, or extensive extrahepatic metastases. Although surgery is not curative in the majority of cases, symptoms of hormone hypersecretion are effectively palliated and prolonged survival is often possible because these tumors are slow growing.

Other therapies can be directed at specific components of the syndrome. Patients who have carcinoid syndrome with flushing should avoid ingesting substances, such as alcohol, that can induce flushing. Also, physical therapy that could involve pressure or trauma to the right upper quadrant should be avoided. Certain drugs, such as codeine and cholestyramine, can help control flushing and diarrhea. Severe symptoms often require a somatostatin analogue such as octreotide.

Flushing and diarrhea can be ameliorated in up to 80% of patients treated with octreotide. The depot form of octreotide (Sandostatin LAR) allows for administration monthly, rather than 3 times daily. Typically, patients start a brief trial of the short-acting form of octreotide (to assess for symptomatic response and tolerance) and then start receiving a monthly dose of 20 mg intramuscularly, with a gradual increase in the dose as needed for control of symptoms. Patients also can be given short-acting, subcutaneous octreotide for breakthrough symptoms.

In addition to improving symptoms, octreotide may retard tumor growth. Because octreotide is not cytotoxic, the disease rarely regresses.

Patients who have progressive metastatic carcinoid tumors have few therapeutic options, and the best systemic therapy has not been defined. Several cytotoxic drugs (streptozocin in combination with either doxorubicin or fluorouracil) have been tried in various combinations and generally have had minimal effect on these tumors. The lack of effectiveness of any 1 agent or combination of agents has led to debate about whether chemotherapy is appropriate for these patients.

Metastatic Disease to the Stomach

When a patient presents with upper gastrointestinal tract symptoms and a history of a primary extragastric neoplasm, metastatic involvement of the stomach should be considered as a possible explanation of the symptoms.

Malignant melanoma is one of the most frequently encountered metastatic lesions to the stomach. At endoscopy, it usually appears as a slightly elevated black nodule or as a lesion with the appearance of a volcano (Figure 6.9). Cancer of the breast, lung, ovary, testis, liver, or colon or sarcoma can all involve the stomach.

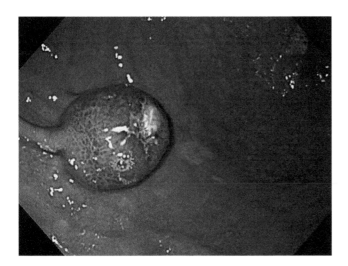

Figure 6.9. **Endoscopic Image of Metastatic Melanoma in Stomach.**
Lesion resembles a volcano.

Suggested Reading

Basuroy R, Srirajaskanthan R, Ramage JK. Neuroendocrine tumors. Gastroenterol Clin North Am. 2016 Sep;45(3):487–507.

Blair VR, McLeod M, Carneiro F, Coit DG, D'Addario JL, van Dieren JM, et al. Hereditary diffuse gastric cancer: updated clinical practice guidelines. Lancet Oncol. 2020 Aug;21(8):e386-e97.

Cives M, Strosberg J. Treatment strategies for metastatic neuroendocrine tumors of the gastrointestinal tract. Curr Treat Options Oncol. 2017 Mar;18(3):14.

Ito T, Jensen RT. Molecular imaging in neuroendocrine tumors: recent advances, controversies, unresolved issues, and roles in management. Curr Opin Endocrinol Diabetes Obes. 2017 Feb;24(1):15–24.

Singh S, Moody L, Chan DL, Metz DC, Strosberg J, Asmis T, et al. Follow-up recommendations for completely resected gastroenteropancreatic neuroendocrine tumors. JAMA Oncol. 2018 Nov 1;4(11):1597–604.

Trieu JA, Bilal M, Saraireh H, Wang AY. Update on the diagnosis and management of gastric intestinal metaplasia in the USA. Dig Dis Sci. 2019 May;64(5):1079–88.

Van Cutsem E, Sagaert X, Topal B, Haustermans K, Prenen H. Gastric cancer. Lancet. 2016 Nov 26;388(10060):2654–64.

7

Gastrointestinal Motility Disorders[a,b]

XIAO JING (IRIS) WANG, MD

Motility disorders result from impaired control of the neuromuscular apparatus of the gut. Symptoms vary according to which portion of the gastrointestinal tract is affected. Motility disorders specifically affecting the esophagus and colon are addressed in other chapters of this book and can lead to symptoms such as dysphagia (ineffective esophageal peristalsis, achalasia) or constipation (slow transit constipation). Gastroparesis, which affects the stomach, and intestinal pseudo-obstruction, which affects the small intestine and colon, are motility disorders that can cause symptoms of recurrent or chronic nausea, vomiting, bloating and abdominal discomfort, constipation, or diarrhea, all of which occur in the absence of a structural lesion. Occasionally, gastroparesis and intestinal pseudo-obstruction are associated with generalized disease and systemic or extraintestinal organ

dysfunction (eg, urinary bladder). For many people, the relation between motility and the generation of symptoms is unclear. Patients who have similar symptoms without structural or motility abnormalities are thought to have a disorder of gut-brain interaction (previously termed *functional gastrointestinal disorder*), specifically functional dyspepsia, which is discussed in this chapter.

Gastrointestinal Neuromuscular Function

Neuromuscular Control of the Gastrointestinal System

Motor function of the gastrointestinal tract depends on the contraction of smooth muscle cells, which is under the control of a complex neuronal network consisting of enteric and extrinsic nerves (via the central and autonomic nervous systems) and on the interstitial cells of Cajal, which serve as pacemaker cells in the wall of the gut. The central nervous system, autonomic nerves, and enteric nervous system all serve as neurogenic modulators of gastrointestinal motility. Extrinsic neural control of gastrointestinal motor function consists of the cranial and sacral parasympathetic outflow (excitatory to non-sphincteric muscle) and the thoracolumbar sympathetic supply (excitatory to sphincters and inhibitory to non-sphincteric muscle). The cranial outflow is predominantly through the vagus nerve, which innervates the gastrointestinal tract from the stomach to the right colon and consists of preganglionic cholinergic fibers that synapse with the enteric nervous system. The supply of sympathetic fibers to the stomach and small bowel arises from levels T5 to T10 of the intermediolateral column of the spinal cord. The prevertebral ganglia are important in the integration of afferent impulses between the gut and the central nervous system and reflex control of abdominal viscera.

[a] Portions of this chapter were adapted from Camilleri M. Disorders of gastrointestinal motility. In: Goldman L, Schafer AI, editors. Goldman's Cecil Medicine, 24th ed. Philadelphia (PA): WB Saunders; 2012. p. 862-8; used with permission. Camilleri M, Andresen V. Motility disorders. In: Waldman SA, Terzic A, eds. Pharmacology and therapeutics: Principles to practice. Saunders/Elsevier; 2009:475-86; used with permission. Locke GR, 3rd. Nonulcer dyspepsia: What it is and what it is not. Mayo Clin Proc. 1999 Oct;74(10):1011-4; used with permission. Ouyang A, Locke GR, 3rd. Overview of neurogastroenterology-gastrointestinal motility and functional GI disorders: Classification, prevalence, and epidemiology. Gastroenterol Clin North Am. 2007 Sep;36(3):485-98; used with permission.

[b] G. Richard Locke III, MD, Lawrence A. Szarka, MD, and Michael Camilleri, MD, are gratefully acknowledged as authors of this chapter in previous editions (parts of which appear in this edition).

Abbreviations: FDA, US Food and Drug Administration; 5-HT, serotonin; G-POEM, gastric peroral endoscopic myotomy; QTc, corrected QT interval; TPN, total parenteral nutrition

The enteric nervous system is an independent nervous system consisting of approximately 100 million neurons organized into ganglionated plexuses. The larger myenteric (or Auerbach) plexus is situated between the longitudinal and circular muscle layers of the muscularis externa and contains neurons responsible for gastrointestinal motility. The submucosal (or Meissner) plexus controls absorption, secretion, and mucosal blood flow. The enteric nervous system is also important in visceral afferent function.

The enteric nervous system develops in utero by migration of neural crest cells to the developing alimentary canal. This migration and the sequence of innervation of different levels of the gut are regulated by specific signaling molecules, which include transcription factors (eg, Mash1), neurotrophic factors (eg, glial-derived neurotrophic factor), and the neuregulin signaling system. These facilitate the growth, differentiation, and persistence of the migrating nerve cells after they arrive in the gut. The receptors for neuregulin proteins are tyrosine kinases, which are important in cell signaling.

Myogenic factors regulate the electrical activity generated by gastrointestinal smooth muscle cells. The interstitial cells of Cajal, located at the interface of the circular and longitudinal smooth muscle layers of the small intestine, form a nonneural pacemaker system and function as intermediaries between the neurogenic (enteric nervous system) and myogenic control systems. Electrical control activity generated by the interstitial cells of Cajal spreads through the contiguous segments of the gut through neurochemical activation by excitatory (eg, acetylcholine and substance P) and inhibitory (eg, nitric oxide, somatostatin, and vasoactive intestinal peptide) transmitters.

Gastric and Small-Bowel Motility

The motor functions of the stomach and small intestine are characterized by distinct manometric patterns of activity in the fasting and postprandial periods (Figure 7.1). The fasting (or interdigestive) period is characterized by a cyclic motor phenomenon called the *interdigestive migrating motor complex*. In healthy persons, 1 cycle of the interdigestive migrating motor complex is completed every 60 to 90 minutes, although it may occur much less frequently. The 3 phases of the interdigestive migrating motor complex are a period of quiescence (*phase I*), a period of intermittent pressure activity (*phase II*), and an activity front (*phase III*), during which the stomach and small intestine contract at a frequency that is maximal for each site: 3 per minute in the stomach and 12 per minute in the upper small intestine. The phase III activity front migrates for a variable distance through the small intestine; there is a gradient in the frequency of contractions from approximately 12 per minute in the duodenum to approximately 8 per minute in the ileum. Another characteristic interdigestive motor pattern in the distal small intestine is the *giant migrating complex*, or power contraction, which empties residue from the ileum into the colon in bolus transfers.

In the postprandial period, the interdigestive migrating motor complex is replaced by an irregular pressure response pattern of variable amplitude and frequency, which enables mixing and absorption. This pattern is observed in the regions in contact with food. The maximal frequency of contractions is lower than that noted during phase III of the interdigestive migrating motor complex. The duration of the postprandial motor activity is proportional to the number of calories consumed during the meal: approximately 1 hour for every 200 kcal ingested. Segments of the small intestine that are not in contact with food continue to display interdigestive motor patterns.

In the stomach, the response to stimuli indicating impending oral intake leads to gastric accommodation: a decrease in proximal stomach tone, which facilitates the ingestion of food without an increase in pressure. This reflex is mediated by the vagus nerve and involves an intrinsic neuronal network that inhibits contractions (eg, nitrergic neurons). The accommodation response, in conjunction with gastric emptying, allows for controlled transfer of gastric contents from the stomach to the small intestine.

Solids and liquids have different gastric emptying characteristics. Liquids empty from the stomach in an exponential

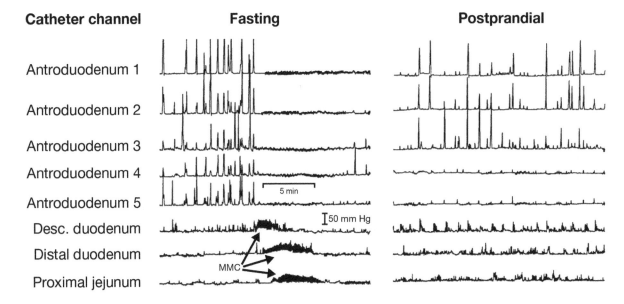

Figure 7.1. **Fasting and Postprandial Gastroduodenal Manometric Recordings From a Healthy Volunteer.** The volunteer ingested a 535-kcal meal during the study. The recordings show the cyclic interdigestive migrating motor complex (MMC) (left) and the sustained, high-amplitude but irregular pressure activity after the meal (right). Desc. indicates descending. (Adapted from Coulie B, Camilleri M. Intestinal pseudo-obstruction. Annu Rev Med. 1999;50:37-55; used with permission.)

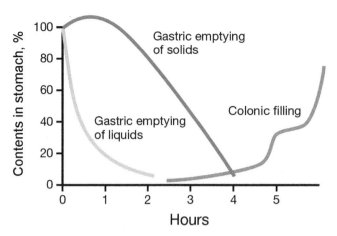

Figure 7.2. Schematic Representation of Typical Gastric Emptying and Colonic Filling Curves. Liquids are emptied at an exponential rate; solids are retained initially (lag phase) but then are emptied at a generally linear postlag rate. The colonic filling curve is characterized by intermittent bolus transfers.

manner (Figure 7.2). The gastric emptying half-time for non-nutrient liquids in healthy persons is usually less than 20 minutes. Solids are retained selectively in the stomach until particles have been triturated to less than 2 mm in diameter. Therefore, gastric emptying of solids is characterized by an initial lag period and then a linear postlag emptying phase. The small intestine transports solids and liquids at approximately the same rate. However, owing to the lag phase for the transport of solids from the stomach, liquids typically arrive in the colon before solids. Chyme moves from the ileum to the colon intermittently in boluses (Figure 7.2). The movement of gas in the intestines results from fluctuations in intestinal tone and capacitance that produce pressure gradients.

> ✓ Gastric accommodation, a vagally mediated response to food stimulus, leads to a decrease in proximal stomach tone
> ✓ Liquids empty from the stomach at an exponential rate, whereas solids empty in a sigmoidal fashion at a rate that has an initial lag phase and then a linear postlag phase

Gastroparesis and Intestinal Pseudo-obstruction

Definitions

Gastroparesis is a syndrome of objectively delayed gastric emptying of solids in the absence of mechanical obstruction; key symptoms are nausea, vomiting, postprandial fullness (early satiety), belching, bloating, and upper abdominal pain. *Intestinal pseudo-obstruction* is characterized by signs and symptoms of mechanical obstruction involving the small or large bowel in the absence of an anatomical lesion that obstructs the flow of contents.

> ✓ **Gastroparesis**—a syndrome of objectively delayed gastric emptying of solids in the absence of mechanical obstruction; key symptoms are nausea, vomiting, postprandial fullness (early satiety), belching, bloating, and upper abdominal pain
> ✓ **Intestinal pseudo-obstruction**—characterized by signs and symptoms of mechanical obstruction involving the small or large bowel in the absence of an anatomical lesion that obstructs the flow of contents

Table 7.1. Classification of Gastroparesis and Pseudo-obstruction

Type	Neuropathic	Myopathic
Infiltrative	Progressive systemic sclerosis	Progressive systemic sclerosis
	Amyloidosis	Amyloidosis
		Systemic lupus erythematosus
		Ehlers-Danlos syndrome
		Dermatomyositis
Familial	Familial visceral neuropathies	Familial visceral myopathies
		Metabolic myopathies
Idiopathic	Idiopathic intestinal pseudo-obstruction	Sporadic hollow visceral myopathy
Neurologic	Porphyria	Myotonia
	Heavy-metal poisoning	Other dystrophies
	Brainstem tumor	
	Parkinson disease	
	Multiple sclerosis	
	Spinal cord transection	
Infectious	Chagas disease	
	Cytomegalovirus	
	Norwalk virus	
	Epstein-Barr virus	
Drug-induced	Tricyclic antidepressants	
	Narcotic agents	
	Anticholinergic agents	
	Antihypertensive agents	
	Antipsychotics	
	Vincristine	
	Laxatives	
Paraneoplastic	Small cell lung carcinoma	
	Carcinoid syndrome	
Postoperative	Postvagotomy with or without pyloroplasty or gastric resection	
Endocrine	Type 2 diabetes	
	Hypothyroidism or hyperthyroidism	
	Hyperparathyroidism	

Adapted from Camilleri M. Disorders of gastrointestinal motility. In: Goldman L, Schafer AI, eds. Goldman's Cecil medicine. 24th ed. Elsevier Saunders; 2012:862-8; used with permission.

Pathogenesis

Gastrointestinal motility disturbances (Table 7.1) can result from disturbances at the level of the extrinsic nervous system, enteric nervous system, interstitial cells of Cajal (or intestinal pacemakers), or smooth muscle. In addition, some disorders affect both nerves and muscles (eg, systemic sclerosis, amyloidosis, and mitochondrial cytopathy) and can appear initially with neuropathic patterns that progress to myopathic characteristics during advanced disease. These disorders can be congenital (eg, disruption of the development of the motility apparatus) or acquired.

Congenital Disorders

Disruptions in the development of gut neuromuscular apparatus result from genetic defects in migration, differentiation, and survival of enteric neurons that have been identified in several causes of gut dysmotility. These genetic defects include abnormalities of *cRET* (OMIM 601496) (the gene that encodes for the tyrosine kinase receptor); the endothelin B system (which tends to retard development of neural elements, thereby facilitating colonization of the entire gut from the neural crest as primitive neural elements enter through the proximal and distal segments of the developing gut and migrate in oral and anal directions, respectively, and innervate the entire gut); Sox10 (a transcription factor that enhances the maturation of neural precursors); and c-kit (a marker for the interstitial cells of Cajal). Disturbances in these mechanisms result in syndromic motility disorders such as Hirschsprung disease, Waardenburg-Shah syndrome (pigmentary defects, piebaldism, neural deafness, and megacolon), and idiopathic hypertrophic pyloric stenosis.

Extrinsic Neuropathic Disorders

Extrinsic neuropathic processes that disrupt autonomic or central nervous system input include vagotomy, type 2 diabetes, trauma, Parkinson disease, amyloidosis, and a paraneoplastic syndrome usually associated with small cell carcinoma of the lung. Another common "neuropathic" problem encountered in clinical practice results from the effects of medications such as α_2-adrenergic agonists and anticholinergic agents on neural control.

Damage to the autonomic nerves from trauma, infection, neuropathy, or neurodegeneration may lead to motor, secretory, and sensory disturbances, most frequently resulting in constipation rather than upper gastrointestinal tract motility disorders. Parkinson disease and multiple sclerosis are 2 neurologic diseases involving the extrinsic nervous system that frequently are associated with constipation. A feature of Parkinson disease is a decrease in the number of dopamine-containing neurons and the presence of Lewy bodies in myenteric plexus neurons. Also, failure of the striated muscles of the pelvic floor to relax may be an extrapyramidal manifestation of Parkinson disease that aggravates the disturbance of colonic emptying and contributes to the common symptom of constipation, which often precedes other neurologic changes. Multiple sclerosis is associated with slow colonic transit and absence of the postprandial motor contractile response in the colon. Gastroparesis and pseudo-obstruction can occur but are less frequent than constipation in these diseases.

A broad spectrum of gastrointestinal motility disorders may be related to type 2 diabetes: gastroparesis, pylorospasm, intestinal pseudo-obstruction, diarrhea, constipation, and fecal incontinence. All these manifestations may be caused by autonomic dysfunction (Table 7.2), although evidence points to the importance of reversible changes in persons with acute hyperglycemia (blood glucose >250 mg/dL) and, more importantly, chronic persistent changes in the structure and function of the enteric nervous system or the interstitial cells of Cajal in persons with chronic hyperglycemia.

From a population perspective, constipation is the most important gastrointestinal symptom in patients with type 2 diabetes because it is the most prevalent symptom. In a large group that had screening tests for autonomic neuropathy, the prevalence of constipation was 22% among patients who had diabetes and neuropathy but only 9.2% among those without neuropathy, which was not significantly different from the percentage among persons in the healthy control group. In a questionnaire-based study of patients with diabetes in the community, constipation was more prevalent among patients who had type 1 diabetes than in patients who had type 2 diabetes and was associated with symptoms of dysautonomia and the use of constipating drugs (eg, calcium channel blockers). Gastroparesis frequently is encountered as a complication of diabetes in hospitalized patients. Apart from the added attention needed for metabolic control, management follows that of other causes of gastroparesis and pseudo-obstruction. Patients with diabetic gastroparesis (ie, symptoms and objective delay in gastric emptying) require more hospitalizations and physician visits and have higher morbidity and mortality than controls.

✓ Diabetes is associated with a wide spectrum of gastrointestinal motility disorders, including gastroparesis, pylorospasm, intestinal pseudo-obstruction, diarrhea, constipation, and fecal incontinence
✓ Diabetes-associated gastrointestinal motility disorders can be reversible if induced by acute hyperglycemia or irreversible if they result from chronic hyperglycemia-induced neuropathy

---

Enteric or Intrinsic Neuropathic Disorders

Enteric or intrinsic neuropathic disorders include disruptions to the enteric nervous system or to the interstitial cells of Cajal. Disorders of the enteric nervous system usually result from a degenerative, immune, or inflammatory process. Only rarely can the cause be ascertained in these disturbances. Infection may be an important predisposing factor, as suggested by virally induced gastroparesis (eg, *Rotavirus*, Norwalk virus, cytomegalovirus, or Epstein-Barr virus) and pseudo-obstruction as well as degenerative disorders associated with infiltration of the myenteric plexus by inflammatory cells. In idiopathic chronic intestinal pseudo-obstruction, there is no disturbance of extrinsic neural control and no identified cause for abnormality of the enteric nervous system.

A full-thickness biopsy specimen from the intestine may be required to evaluate the myenteric plexus and interstitial cells of Cajal. The decision to perform a biopsy needs to be weighed carefully against the risk of complications, including the subsequent formation of adhesions and, possibly, mechanical obstruction superimposed on episodes of pseudo-obstruction.

Smooth Muscle Disorders

Disturbances of smooth muscle may result in major disorders of gastric emptying and small-bowel and colonic transit. These disturbances include systemic sclerosis and amyloidosis. Dermatomyositis, myotonic dystrophy, and metabolic muscle disorders such as mitochondrial cytopathy are seen infrequently.

Table 7.2. Gastrointestinal Manifestations of Type 2 Diabetes

Manifestation	Associated disease	Clinical presentation
Decreased gallbladder motility		Gallstones
Antral hypomotility		Gastric stasis
Pylorospasm		Bezoars
Decreased α_2-adrenergic tone in enterocytes		Diarrhea, steatorrhea
SB dysmotility	SB bacterial overgrowth	Gastric or SB stasis or rapid SB transit
Colonic dysmotility	Bile acid malabsorption	Constipation or diarrhea
Anorectal dysfunction		Diarrhea or fecal incontinence
Sensory neuropathy		
IAS-sympathetic neuropathy		
EAS-pudendal neuropathy		

Abbreviations: EAS, external anal sphincter; IAS, internal anal sphincter; SB, small-bowel.

Adapted from Camilleri M. Gastrointestinal problems in diabetes. Endocrinol Metab Clin North Am. 1996 Jun;25(2):361-78; used with permission.

Abnormal facial and external ocular muscle functions may be useful clinical signs of these diseases. In rare instances, there is a positive family history (eg, hollow visceral myopathy may occur either sporadically or in families). Patients with more subtle motility disturbances often present with constipation from metabolic disorders such as hypothyroidism or hyperparathyroidism.

Scleroderma is a multisystemic disorder characterized by vascular dysfunction and progressive fibrosis with nearly 90% of patients showing some degree of gastrointestinal tract involvement, most frequently in the esophagus. Scleroderma in the gastrointestinal system initially presents with neuronal dysfunction and eventually progresses to muscle dysfunction and fibrosis. In the stomach and small bowel, it may result in focal or general dilatation, diverticula (often wide-mouthed, especially in the colon), and delayed transit at the levels affected. The amplitude of contractions is decreased (average <30 mm Hg in the distal esophagus, <40 mm Hg in the antrum, and <10 mm Hg in the small bowel) compared with that of controls, indicative of smooth muscle dysfunction. Bacterial overgrowth is common and may result in steatorrhea, and it is more likely to occur in myopathic disorders, often with concomitant dilation or diverticula of the small intestine.

A mitochondrial disorder that affects the gut is *mitochondrial neurogastrointestinal encephalomyopathy*. It is referred to also as *oculogastrointestinal muscular dystrophy* or *familial visceral myopathy type II* and is an example of a spectrum of diseases that affect oxidative phosphorylation. It is an autosomal recessive condition with gastrointestinal and liver manifestations that may occur at any age, typically with hepatomegaly or liver failure in the neonate, seizures or diarrhea in infants, and liver failure or chronic intestinal pseudo-obstruction in children and adults.

Mitochondrial neurogastrointestinal encephalomyopathy is characterized also by external ophthalmoplegia, ptosis, peripheral neuropathy, and leukoencephalopathy. The small intestine is dilated or has multiple diverticula, and the amplitude of contractions is low, typical of a myopathic disorder. Some patients have a combination of intestinal dysmotility or transfer dysphagia due to abnormal coordination and propagation of the swallow through the pharynx and the skeletal muscle portion of the esophagus. This becomes even more devastating when the smooth muscle portion of the esophagus is also affected by the cytopathy.

Presentation and Diagnosis of Gastroparesis and Intestinal Pseudo-obstruction

Evaluation of motility disorders should be considered in 4 categories:

1. Timing and chronicity: Are the symptoms acute or chronic?
2. Etiology: Is the disease due to neuropathy or myopathy? Is there an underlying systemic disorder?
3. Location: What regions of the digestive tract are affected?
4. Severity: What is the status of hydration and nutrition?

Clinical Features

The clinical features of gastroparesis and chronic intestinal pseudo-obstruction are similar and include nausea, vomiting, early satiety, abdominal discomfort, distention, bloating, and anorexia. Patients with severe stasis and vomiting may have considerable weight loss and depletion of mineral and vitamin stores. The severity of the motility problem often manifests itself most clearly in the degree of nutritional and electrolyte depletion. Disturbances of bowel movements, such as diarrhea and constipation, indicate that the motility disorder is more extensive than gastroparesis. Severe vomiting may be complicated by aspiration pneumonia or Mallory-Weiss tears that may result in gastrointestinal tract hemorrhage. When patients have a more generalized motility disorder, they also may have symptoms referable to abnormal swallowing or delayed colonic transit.

History and Risk Factors

A family history and medication history are essential for identifying underlying etiologic factors such as diabetes. Review of systems may be helpful to diagnose an underlying collagen vascular disease (eg, scleroderma) or disturbances of extrinsic neural control that also may be affecting the abdominal viscera. Such symptoms include orthostatic dizziness, difficulties with erection or ejaculation, recurrent urinary tract infections, difficulty with visual accommodation, absence of sweating, and dry mouth, eyes, or vagina.

Physical Examination

Physical examination findings are limited for diagnoses of a motility disorder but are helpful for evaluation of potential systemic causes. A succussion splash detected on physical examination usually indicates a region of stasis within the gastrointestinal tract, typically the stomach. The hands and mouth may show signs of Raynaud phenomenon or scleroderma. Testing pupillary responses to light and accommodation, testing external ocular movement, measuring blood pressure in the supine and standing positions, and noting the general features of peripheral neuropathy can be used to identify patients who have a neurologic disturbance or oculogastrointestinal dystrophy associated typically with mitochondrial cytopathy.

A motility disorder of the stomach or small bowel should be suspected whenever large volumes are aspirated from the stomach, particularly after an overnight fast or when undigested solid food or large volumes of liquids are observed during esophagogastroduodenoscopy.

Differential Diagnosis

In the evaluation of a suspected motility disorder, exclusion of mechanical obstruction (eg, from peptic stricture, obstructing masses in the stomach or intestines, or Crohn disease of the stomach or small bowel) is key as treatments to speed up bowel motility in pseudo-obstruction would be relatively contraindicated in patients with mechanical obstruction. Other considerations for patients who present with abdominal pain, nausea, and vomiting include disorders of gut-brain interaction such as functional dyspepsia, eating disorders such as anorexia nervosa, and rumination syndrome. The degree of impairment of gastric emptying in eating disorders is relatively minor compared with that of diabetic or postvagotomy gastric stasis.

Diagnostic Evaluation

The recommended sequence for diagnostic evaluation is as follows:

1. Rule out mechanical obstruction. The initial step in evaluation should be to exclude mechanical obstruction. This can be done with upper endoscopic and radiologic studies with an oral contrast agent,

including upper gastrointestinal series with small-bowel follow-through or computed tomographic enterography. Imaging findings that support pseudo-obstruction show dilated small-bowel loops with associated air-fluid levels but no transition points. Gross dilatation of the intestines, dilution of barium, and retained solid food within the stomach also provide support for a motility disorder but are rarely seen. Therefore, these studies are undertaken largely for exclusion of mechanical obstruction as opposed to positive diagnosis of a motility disorder. An exception is small-bowel systemic sclerosis, which is characterized by megaduodenum and packed valvulae conniventes in the small intestine resulting in the hidebound radiographic sign.

2. Diagnose dysmotility. For definitive assessment of a motility disorder, bowel transit studies should be performed to assess gastric and small-bowel function. For evaluating efficiency in the emptying of solids, scintigraphy offers the most sensitive measurement of upper gastrointestinal tract transit. Scans typically are performed at 0, 1, 2, 4, and 6 hours after ingestion of a radiolabeled meal and should be done after all medications that affect gastric emptying have been withheld for at least 48 hours. *Delayed gastric emptying* is defined as gastric retention of more than 10% at 4 hours or more than 60% at 2 hours (or both) after a standard low-fat, scrambled egg meal, although the 4-hour residual has higher sensitivity for diagnosis of delayed gastric emptying. Alternatives to measuring transit include use of the stable isotope breath test and the wireless motility capsule, but these tests are not as well validated as scintigraphic gastric emptying.

If the cause of the motility disturbance is obvious, such as gastroparesis in a patient with long-standing type 2 diabetes, further diagnostic testing usually is not needed. If the cause is unclear, gastroduodenal manometry, with the use of a multilumen tube with sensors in the distal stomach and proximal small intestine, can be used to distinguish between neuropathic and myopathic processes (Figure 7.3). Neuropathies are characterized by contractions with normal amplitude but with abnormal patterns of contractility. In contrast, the predominant disturbance in myopathic disorders is the low average amplitude of contractions in the segments affected (<40 mm Hg in the antrum; <10 mm Hg in the small intestine) (Figure 7.3).

Endoflip (Medtronic) is an endoscopically deployed device that has been used to measure the pyloric dimensions at rest and with distention as well as the distensibility of the pylorus to assess for hypertonicity at this junction.

3. Identify the pathogenesis. Causes of gastroparesis and intestinal pseudo-obstruction are outlined in Table 7.1. In the absence of a cause for a neuropathic pattern of motor activity in the small intestine, it is necessary to pursue additional investigations, including testing for autonomic dysfunction, antineuronal nuclear autoantibodies type 1 associated with paraneoplastic syndromes, and magnetic resonance imaging of the brain to exclude a brainstem lesion in patients with vomiting (Figure 7.4). Autonomic testing may include evaluation for orthostatic hypotension, assessment of supine and standing serum norepinephrine levels, measurement of the heart rate interval changes during deep breathing, and plasma pancreatic polypeptide response to modified sham feeding. This testing can identify sympathetic adrenergic or vagal neuropathy.

The identification of a myopathic disorder on initial testing should lead to a search for amyloidosis (immunoglobulin electrophoresis, fat aspirate, or rectal biopsy), systemic sclerosis (Scl-70), and a family history of gastrointestinal motility disorders.

Laboratory studies to consider include assessment of thyroid function and levels of antinuclear antibody, lactate, creatine phosphokinase, aldolase, and porphyrins and serologic study for Chagas disease. In certain cases, a laparoscopically obtained full-thickness biopsy specimen from the small intestine may be required. Special staining techniques may be needed to identify metabolic muscle disorders, including mitochondrial myopathy, for which genetic testing may be available.

4. Identify complications of the motility disorder. Morbidity in motility disorders is often due to complications that should be addressed to make the primary dysmotility more manageable. These complications include bacterial overgrowth, dehydration, and malnutrition. In patients with diarrhea, it is important to assess nutritional status (including essential mineral and vitamin levels) and to exclude bacterial overgrowth by culturing small-bowel aspirates or performing hydrogen breath testing. Bacterial overgrowth is relatively uncommon in neuropathic disorders but is more common in myopathic conditions, such as scleroderma, that are associated more often with bowel dilatation, low-amplitude contractions, or small-bowel diverticula that allow for bacterial proliferation. Bacterial overgrowth should be suspected in

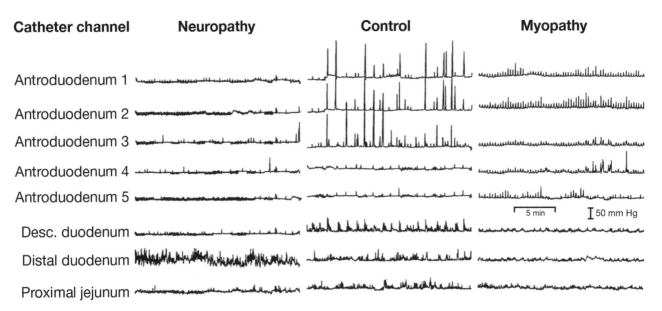

Figure 7.3. Gastroduodenal Manometric Profiles. Postprandial manometric profiles in small-bowel dysmotility due to neuropathy (left; type 2 diabetes) and myopathy (right; systemic sclerosis). In myopathy the profiles show simultaneous, prolonged contractions of low amplitude. Although the contraction amplitudes are normal in neuropathy, contractile activity is uncoordinated and contractile frequency is decreased. Desc. indicates descending. (Adapted from Coulie B, Camilleri M. Intestinal pseudo-obstruction. Annu Rev Med. 1999;50:37-55; used with permission.)

Abnormal gastric or small-bowel transit

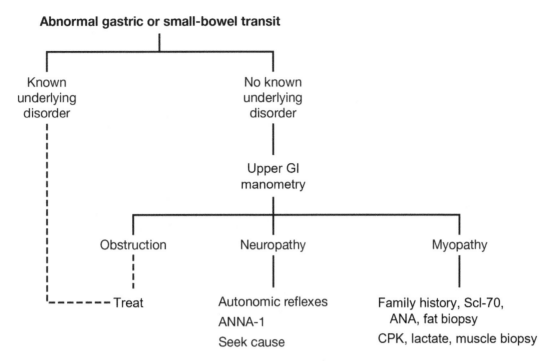

Figure 7.4. **Flow Diagram of Steps in Diagnosis of Gastroparesis and Intestinal Pseudo-obstruction.** ANA indicates antinuclear antibodies; ANNA-1, antineuronal nuclear antibodies type 1; CPK, creatine phosphokinase; GI, gastrointestinal. (Adapted from Camilleri M, Prather CM. Gastric motor physiology and motor disorders. In: Feldman M, Sleisenger MH, Scharschmidt BF, editors. Sleisenger & Fordtran's gastrointestinal and liver disease: pathophysiology, diagnosis, management. 6th ed. Philadelphia [PA]: Saunders; c1998. p. 572-86; used with permission.)

patients with an increased folate level but a deficiency of vitamin B_{12}. Bacterial overgrowth may be difficult to detect with culture of small-bowel aspirates; however, breath hydrogen after a glucose or lactulose load is a nonspecific test that should be interpreted with caution and in conjunction with small-bowel transit time because the early breath hydrogen peak may be due to bacterial metabolism of the substrate in the colon resulting from fast small-bowel transit. Often, an empirical trial of antibiotic therapy is used as a surrogate for formal testing.

Treatment of Gastroparesis and Intestinal Pseudo-obstruction

Treatment of gastroparesis and intestinal pseudo-obstruction should be tailored for each patient depending on complications present and the specific effects of the underlying motility disorder. In patients with a systemic disorder driving gastrointestinal motility, control of these disorders can occasionally improve motility but are of greater importance in preventing progression.

Management of Complications

Correction of Hydration and Nutritional Deficiencies

Rehydration, electrolyte repletion, and nutritional supplementation are particularly important during acute exacerbations of gastroparesis and chronic intestinal pseudo-obstruction. Restoration of nutrition can be achieved orally, enterally, or parenterally, depending on the severity of the clinical syndrome. Oral intake should be low in fiber and fat, both of which delay gastrointestinal transit, with the addition of iron, folate, calcium, and vitamins D, K, and B_{12}. Patients with more severe symptoms may require enteral or parenteral supplementation of nutrition. If enteral supplementation may be required for more

than 3 months, usually the best approach is to provide feedings through a jejunostomy tube. Gastrostomy tubes should be avoided in gastroparesis for delivery of nutrition, but combined gastrojejunal tubes can be considered so that gastric ports may be used for venting purposes. Many patients who require long-term parenteral nutrition continue to tolerate some oral feeding, which should be encouraged.

Management of Bacterial Overgrowth in the Small Intestine

Antibiotic therapy is indicated for patients who have documented symptomatic bacterial overgrowth (typically manifested as diarrhea and steatorrhea with bloating). Owing to persistent underlying motility disorder, patients with intestinal pseudo-obstruction typically have frequent recurrence of bacterial overgrowth and require cycling of various antibiotics for long-term suppression. Although formal clinical trials have not been conducted, common practice is to use different antibiotics for 7 to 10 days each month to avoid development of resistance. Common antibiotics include doxycycline (100 mg twice daily), metronidazole (500 mg 3 times daily), ciprofloxacin (500 mg twice daily), double-strength trimethoprim-sulfamethoxazole (2 tablets twice daily), and rifaximin (550 mg 3 times daily). Antibiotic therapy for patients with diarrhea and fat malabsorption due to bacterial overgrowth produces considerable symptomatic relief.

✓ Bacterial overgrowth in the small intestine
- High likelihood of recurrence if a patient has a motility disturbance
- Cycling of various antibiotics is often needed for long-term suppression

---

Management of Underlying Motility Disturbance

Medications

Medications may be used to treat neuromuscular motility disorders. However, there is little evidence that they are effective in primary myopathic disturbances, except for the rare case of myotonic dystrophy affecting the stomach and for small-bowel systemic sclerosis.

Erythromycin, a macrolide antibiotic that stimulates motilin receptors at higher doses (eg, 250-500 mg) and cholinergic mechanisms at lower doses (eg, 40-80 mg), results in the dumping of solids from the stomach. It has been shown to accelerate gastric emptying in gastroparesis; it also increases the amplitude of antral contractions and improves antroduodenal coordination. Erythromycin is most effective when it is given intravenously during acute exacerbations of gastroparesis or intestinal pseudo-obstruction. The usual dose of intravenous erythromycin lactobionate is 3 mg/kg infused over 45 minutes every 8 hours. The efficacy of oral erythromycin appears to be restricted by tolerance and gastrointestinal adverse effects, which often prevent treatment for longer than 1 month; sometimes a low dosage of liquid erythromycin (eg, 40-80 mg 3 times daily before meals) can be tolerated. The elixir formulation may improve absorption if the patient has dysmotility. Although studies demonstrated that 2 weeks of treatment was effective for patients with diabetic gastroparesis, there is little evidence that continued therapy produces long-term improvement in gastric emptying or associated symptoms. Similar benefit has been seen with other macrolides, including azithromycin and clarithromycin, but the use of these agents is similarly limited by concerns for tachyphylaxis, cardiac risks from potential drug interactions, and antibiotic resistance.

Metoclopramide is a dopamine antagonist that has both prokinetic and antiemetic properties. Antiemetic effects are due partly to its antiserotoninergic$_3$ antagonist actions. Long-term use of metoclopramide is limited by the adverse effects of tremor and Parkinson-like symptoms, a consequence of antidopaminergic activity in the central nervous system. Occasionally, tardive dyskinesia occurs. This led to a recommendation to limit use of metoclopramide to less than 3 months (the US Food and Drug Administration [FDA] ordered a boxed warning). It is available in tablet or elixir form and typically is taken 30 minutes before meals and at bedtime. Usual dosages range from 5 to 20 mg 4 times daily, but the drug is safest when the total daily dose is restricted to a maximum of 30 mg.

Domperidone, a dopamine D2 receptor antagonist that is not available in the US, has been made available for prescription through the FDA's Expanded Access to Investigational Drugs program. The efficacy of domperidone is generally like that of metoclopramide, but domperidone has fewer adverse effects on the central nervous system. The recommended starting dose of domperidone is 10 mg 3 times daily with the option to titrate the dose to 20 mg 4 times daily (before meals and at bedtime). Use of domperidone should be avoided in patients with a corrected QT interval (QTc) that is prolonged (>470 ms in men; >450 ms in women) because of the risk of cardiac dysrhythmias.

Serotonin (5-HT) receptor agonists may prove to be beneficial in the treatment of gastroparesis and intestinal pseudo-obstruction. The combined 5-HT$_4$ agonist and 5-HT$_3$ antagonist, cisapride, was previously the only medication for which there was evidence for medium- and long-term efficacy; however, the medication is no longer available for prescription because of the risks of cardiac dysrhythmias (torsades de pointes). Prucalopride, a selective 5-HT$_4$ receptor agonist, has been shown in trials to significantly decrease gastric emptying half-time compared to placebo and improve gastroparesis symptoms, but prucalopride has not received FDA approval for use in gastroparesis. Velusetrag, felcisetrag (TAK 954), and naronapride are other selective 5-HT$_4$ agonists with positive evidence in clinical trials for improving gastroparesis in various clinical settings with minimal cardiac adverse effects.

Neostigmine and pyridostigmine are acetylcholinesterase inhibitors that improve gastric and duodenal contractility and have been shown in trials to increase gastric and small bowel emptying. Neostigmine is limited to parenteral administration and must be administered under cardiac monitoring because of the potential for bradycardia and excess vagal tone. Pyridostigmine is available in enteral formulation as a liquid or a tablet and has been shown to improve chronic intestinal pseudo-obstruction, delayed small-bowel transit with gastroparesis, and chronic constipation in pediatric patients in open-label trials with dosing of 0.25 to 2.0 mg/kg daily. Neither medication has FDA approval for the indication of improving gastrointestinal motility.

Octreotide, a cyclized analogue of somatostatin, has been shown to induce activity fronts in the small intestine that mimic phase III activity of the interdigestive migrating motor complex. The clinical effects of octreotide include an initial acceleration of gastric emptying, a decrease in postprandial gastric motility, and inhibition of small-bowel transit. The therapeutic efficacy of octreotide in intestinal dysmotility associated with gastroparesis and pseudo-obstruction has not been demonstrated in clinical trials. Currently, octreotide administered before meals appears to be more useful in the treatment of dumping syndromes associated with accelerated transit. However, it may be useful just before bedtime to induce activity of the migrating motor complex and to propel residue toward the colon with the goal of avoiding bacterial overgrowth. If required during the daytime, octreotide is often given in combination with oral erythromycin to normalize the gastric emptying rate.

Antiemetics, including diphenhydramine, prochlorperazine, scopolamine, and metoclopramide, are important in the management of nausea and vomiting in patients with gastroparesis and intestinal pseudo-obstruction. The more expensive 5-HT$_3$ antagonists (eg, ondansetron) have not provided greater benefit than the less expensive alternatives. Ondansetron causes prolongation of the QTc and should be used with caution, particularly if patients are taking other medications that affect the QTc. Granisetron is a sustained-release transdermal patch that has shown improvement in gastroparesis symptoms in open-label trials.

Newer medications include neurokinin-1 antagonists such as aprepitant. Aprepitant, available parenterally and enterally, has FDA approval for the prevention of chemotherapy-induced or postoperative nausea and vomiting and has been shown in trials to improve overall symptoms, although it does not improve gastric emptying.

Several medications are currently undergoing investigation for the treatment of gastroparesis, including cannabidiol, a low-tetrahydrocannabinol extract from *Cannabis sativa*; tradipitant, a neurokinin-1 antagonist; relamorelin, a ghrelin receptor agonist; and trazpiroben, a dopamine D2/D3–receptor antagonist with limited effects on the central nervous system.

Decompression

Decompression is rarely necessary in patients with gastroparesis or chronic pseudo-obstruction. However, venting enterostomy (gastrostomy or jejunostomy) is effective in relieving abdominal distention and bloating. It has been shown to decrease the frequency of nasogastric intubations and hospitalizations for acute exacerbations of severe intestinal pseudo-obstruction in patients requiring central parenteral nutrition. Access to the small intestine by enterostomy also provides a way to deliver nutrients enterally and should be considered for patients with intermittent symptoms. The currently available enteral tubes allow for gastric aspiration and feeding by a single apparatus. However, because venting can lead to displacement, some patients need a feeding tube in the jejunum and a venting tube in the stomach.

Surgical and Endoscopic Interventions

Surgical treatment has a limited role in patients with gastroparesis and intestinal pseudo-obstruction. For patients who have had multiple abdominal operations, it becomes difficult to discern whether exacerbations of symptoms reflect an underlying disease or adhesions and mechanical obstruction. Recent advancements have focused more on therapy directed to the pylorus to address the pyloric dysfunction seen in a subset of patients who have gastroparesis with prolonged, intense tonic pyloric contractions (ie, pylorospasm).

Surgical Resection. Surgical treatment should be considered whenever the motility disorder is localized to a resectable portion of the gut. Three instances in which to consider this approach are 1) duodenojejunostomy or duodenoplasty for patients with megaduodenum or duodenal atresia in children; 2) near-total gastrectomy with Roux-en-Y reconstruction or completion gastrectomy for patients with postgastric surgical stasis syndrome; and 3) colectomy with ileorectostomy for intractable constipation associated with chronic colonic pseudo-obstruction.

Gastric Electrical Stimulation. Open-label treatment with externally provided gastric pacing improved gastric emptying and symptoms in patients with severe gastroparesis. Gastric pacing has not successfully entrained gastric slow waves to normalize gastric dysrhythmias or to accelerate gastric emptying, and placement of the device is associated with complications, including local infection and lead migration. Gastric electrical stimulation is an approved treatment (under the FDA's Humanitarian Device Exemption Program), but data on efficacy are inconclusive, and current guidelines do not provide consensus for which patients would benefit from this device.

Pylorus-Directed Interventions. Botulinum toxin injected into the pylorus has been shown to have short-term, dose-dependent efficacy for symptom improvement in a subset of patients with gastroparesis. Repeated injections, however, may induce pyloric fibrosis.

Surgical pyloroplasty that uses a longitudinal incision across the pylorus through the longitudinal and circular muscle layers (ie, Heineke-Mikulicz pyloroplasty) has improved gastric emptying and symptoms. Complication rates were high, however, and 10% of patients required subsequent surgical intervention.

Gastric peroral endoscopic myotomy (G-POEM) was developed to replicate the positive effects of surgical pyloroplasty in a minimally invasive manner to decrease morbidity. G-POEM is performed endoscopically and involves tunneling through the submucosa from the luminal stomach with the goal of severing the circular muscle layer without disrupting the longitudinal muscle layer. Early trial data are promising, but long-term results and large randomized trials to validate efficacy are necessary. In

the future, Endoflip may be used for guidance for the efficacy of G-POEM and as a predictor of response.

Small-Bowel Transplant. Small-bowel transplant is limited to patients with intestinal failure who have reversible total parenteral nutrition (TPN)-induced liver disease or life-threatening or recurrent catheter-related sepsis. Combined small-bowel and liver transplant is performed in patients with irreversible TPN-induced liver disease. Complications after small-bowel transplant include infection, rejection, and lymphoproliferative disorders due to long-term immunosuppression and Epstein-Barr virus infection. Studies have suggested that small-bowel transplant may improve quality of life and may be more cost-effective than long-term TPN. Improvements in immunosuppressive regimens, earlier detection of rejection, and treatment of cytomegalovirus infection have enhanced outcomes of small-bowel transplant for short bowel syndrome or severe pseudo-obstruction uncontrolled by TPN. In the meantime, parenteral nutrition is the treatment of choice for most patients.

Functional Dyspepsia

Functional dyspepsia is in the group of disorders now termed disorders of gut-brain interaction. The pathophysiology is not well understood, but some experts consider that functional dyspepsia exists along a continuum with gastroparesis because of the overlap of symptoms.

Symptoms of dyspepsia are encountered commonly in clinical practice. These include epigastric pain or discomfort, nausea, vomiting, early satiation, postprandial fullness, and upper abdominal bloating. The roles of gastroesophageal reflux, peptic ulcer disease, gastritis, and cancer in causing these symptoms are reviewed in other chapters in this book.

Several mechanisms have been postulated for functional dyspepsia (Table 7.3). Similarly, many different therapies have been tried. This multitude of diagnostic and therapeutic options underscores the fact that the cause of functional dyspepsia is not uniform; hence, treatment must be tailored to the identified disorder of function.

Definition

Dyspepsia is not a condition: It is a symptom complex. *Dyspepsia* can be defined as persistent or recurrent abdominal pain or abdominal discomfort centered in the upper abdomen. The term *discomfort* includes symptoms of nausea, vomiting, early satiety, postprandial fullness, and upper abdominal bloating. The Rome IV criteria (Box 7.1) define *functional dyspepsia* as 1 or more of the following: bothersome postprandial fullness, bothersome early satiation, bothersome epigastric pain, and bothersome epigastric burning in the absence of structural disease likely to explain the symptoms. The criteria must be fulfilled for the past 3 months with symptom onset at least 6 months before the diagnosis.

Functional dyspepsia is further categorized into postprandial distress syndrome and epigastric pain syndrome. *Postprandial*

Table 7.3. Proposed Causes of Functional Dyspepsia

Acid or Helicobacter pylori	*Motility or sensitivity*
H pylori infection	Gastroparesis
Gastritis, duodenitis	Abnormal relaxation
Missed peptic ulcer disease	Visceral hypersensitivity
Acid sensitivity	Brain-gut disorder
Occult gastroesophageal reflux disease	Psychologic disorder

distress syndrome necessitates bothersome postprandial fullness or bothersome early satiation (or both). *Epigastric pain syndrome* in contrast must include bothersome epigastric pain or bothersome epigastric burning (or both). These 2 conditions may coexist, but 1 generally is determined to be predominant.

Other symptoms that are often present in both disorders include epigastric bloating, excessive belching, and nausea. While the symptoms of heartburn and acid regurgitation frequently coexist, they are not considered dyspeptic symptoms and should prompt evaluation for gastroesophageal reflux disease. Patients with symptoms or signs typical for biliary tract or pancreatic disease should not be considered to have functional dyspepsia. Thus, right upper quadrant pain or epigastric pain that radiates to the back should not be included in the definition of *dyspepsia*. Presence of vomiting suggests another disorder.

Functional dyspepsia is diagnosed if the above symptom criteria are met for more than 3 months without an anatomical or biochemical abnormality. Typically, this means negative findings on blood tests and on evaluation of the upper gastrointestinal tract with endoscopy or barium radiography. However, describing endoscopic findings as negative for functional dyspepsia can be difficult. Does this include biopsy study of the esophagus for esophagitis or biopsy study of the stomach for gastritis or *H pylori* infection? Are erythema, erosions, and histologic inflammation meaningful findings? These issues are somewhat controversial.

Surveys have evaluated how many people in the community have symptoms of dyspepsia. The rates vary in large part because of the definitions used. Some surveys include the symptom of heartburn in the definition of *dyspepsia* and report a prevalence rate of 40%. Other surveys exclude persons with symptoms of heartburn or irritable bowel syndrome and report prevalence rates of less than 5%. Nonetheless, it is reasonable to state that 15% of the adult population (about 1 in 7) has dyspepsia. Not all these people with dyspepsia have functional dyspepsia. In 1 study, when a random sample of the population with dyspepsia underwent endoscopy, only 53% had normal endoscopic findings. The remarkable findings were esophagitis, peptic ulcer disease, duodenitis, and duodenogastric reflux. Furthermore, in this study only 66% of the asymptomatic controls had normal endoscopic findings. Peptic ulcer disease and duodenitis were more common in the persons with dyspepsia than in the controls. Other findings such as gastritis were found in a similar number of cases and controls.

Guidelines of the American Gastroenterological Association recommend that in the absence of visible lesions on endoscopy, esophageal and duodenal biopsies are not indicated. However, biopsies of the stomach can be performed to look for *H pylori* if the status of *H pylori* is unknown.

Pathophysiology

The most frequently mentioned etiologic possibilities for functional dyspepsia are listed in Table 7.3. The possible causes have been divided into 2 categories: acid or *H pylori* vs motility or sensitivity.

Whether *H pylori* infection causes symptoms in the absence of an ulcer is still debated. The prevalence of *H pylori* infection and gastritis is only slightly more common in patients with dyspepsia. Still, physicians, investigators, and patients have been interested in the idea that the histologic inflammation produces symptoms. In multicenter, placebo-controlled clinical trials, the effect of the eradication of *H pylori* on functional dyspepsia has been small.

Patients commonly take antacids for relief of dyspepsia, but gastric acid secretion is normal in patients with functional dyspepsia. One hypothesis is that patients with functional dyspepsia may have visceral hypersensitivity and be more sensitive to acid. Placebo-controlled trials have shown that acid suppression is modestly more effective than placebo in functional dyspepsia. The question has been whether this is due to occult gastroesophageal reflux that manifests as dyspepsia.

Although clinicians often focus on epigastric pain as the cardinal symptom of functional dyspepsia, most investigators include other symptoms, such as nausea, fullness, and early satiety. These symptoms suggest that motor abnormalities (delayed or paradoxically accelerated emptying or impaired accommodation) may be a factor in causing this condition. Of the patients with functional dyspepsia who are evaluated in gastrointestinal clinics of referral centers, one-third to one-half have delayed gastric emptying. Multiple studies, primarily in Europe, have evaluated the role of prokinetics in functional dyspepsia. Generally, prokinetics are 30% more effective than placebo, although the rates varied considerably among studies. Most of these studies were with cisapride or domperidone, neither of which is currently available in the US. They may be helpful in part because of their antiemetic effects. Treatment with metoclopramide for more than 3 months should be avoided because of the risk of tardive dyskinesia and other adverse effects.

More recently, attention has shifted from gastric emptying to gastric accommodation and gastric sensitivity. Like the heart, the stomach has both systolic and diastolic functions. Recent studies have shown that gastric accommodation (ie, the relaxation of the stomach in response to a meal) is abnormal in patients with functional dyspepsia. Medications such as the anxiolytic buspirone (a

---

Box 7.1. Rome IV Criteria for Selected Gastroduodenal Disorders

B1. Functional dyspepsia
≥1 of the following:
1. Bothersome postprandial fullness
2. Bothersome early satiation
3. Bothersome epigastric pain
4. Bothersome epigastric burning

and

No evidence of structural disease (including at upper endoscopy) that is likely to explain the symptoms

B1a. Postprandial distress syndrome
≥1 of the following ≥3 d/wk:
1. Bothersome postprandial fullness (ie, severe enough to affect usual activities)
2. Bothersome early satiation (ie, severe enough to prevent finishing a regular-size meal)

B1b. Epigastric pain syndrome
≥1 of the following symptoms ≥1 d/wk:
1. Bothersome epigastric pain (ie, severe enough to affect usual activities)
2. Bothersome epigastric burning (ie, severe enough to affect usual activities)

Adapted from Stanghellini V, Chan FKL, Hasler WL, Malagelada JR, Suzuki H, Tack J, et al. Gastroduodenal disorders. Gastroenterology. 2016 150(6):1380-92; used with permission.

5-HT$_{1A}$ receptor agonist) and the experimental anticholinesterase inhibitor acotiamide appear effective in clinical trials with patients who have functional dyspepsia.

The disorders of gut-brain interaction form a continuum of illnesses characterized by gastrointestinal symptoms and nondiagnostic findings on evaluations. The disorders have considerable overlap. Specifically, at least one-third of patients with functional dyspepsia also have symptoms of irritable bowel syndrome. Patients with irritable bowel syndrome have been shown to have a lower threshold for rectal distention. A similar phenomenon has been noted in functional dyspepsia for distention of the stomach. More recently, imaging of the central nervous system has highlighted the activation of different parts of the brain in persons with functional gastrointestinal disorders. Thus, the concept of visceral hypersensitivity remains a strong consideration in all the functional gastrointestinal disorders, including functional dyspepsia. Currently, however, no specific medication is available for visceral hypersensitivity, although new agents are being investigated. Clinically, low-dose antidepressants are being prescribed, but formal clinical trial data are not available.

Recommendations for Evaluation and Therapy

A test-and-treat approach for this *H pylori* infection is indicated and may be effective in relieving functional dyspepsia. Yet, many patients still have symptoms after testing and eradication of *H pylori*, and a trial of acid inhibition, usually with a proton pump inhibitor, is the next recommended treatment option. Because of the controversy from conflicting studies and inadequate data, practice guidelines recommend either a trial of acid inhibition or testing for *H pylori* infection before any diagnostic investigation for dyspepsia in the absence of alarm or high-risk symptoms (Figure 7.5). These include clinically significant weight loss (>5% body weight over 6-12 months), progressive dysphagia or odynophagia, unexplained iron deficiency anemia or covert gastrointestinal bleeding, persistent vomiting, family history of upper gastrointestinal cancer, palpable abdominal or epigastric mass or lymphadenopathy, and the patient being 60 years or older with new-onset symptoms. If 1 or more of these alarm symptoms is present, or if patients have no benefit from empirical dyspepsia treatment (Figure 7.5A), upper gastrointestinal endoscopy should be performed to exclude peptic ulcer disease, esophagitis, and

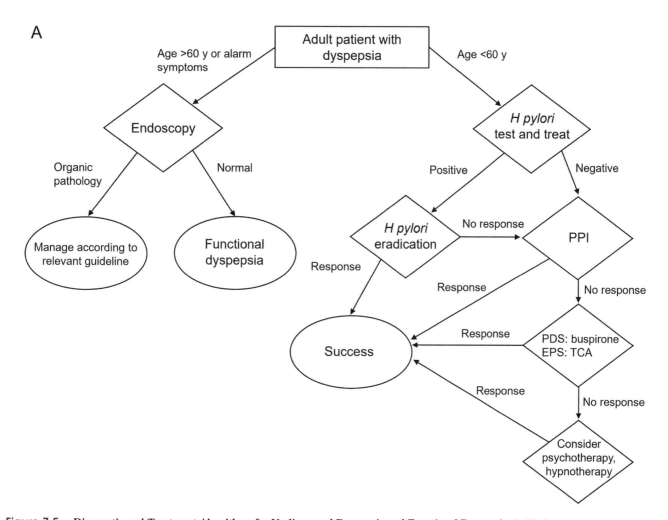

Figure 7.5. Diagnostic and Treatment Algorithms for Undiagnosed Dyspepsia and Functional Dyspepsia. A, Undiagnosed dyspepsia. Alarm symptoms are 1) clinically significant weight loss with progressive dysphagia or odynophagia; 2) unexplained iron deficiency anemia or overt gastrointestinal bleeding; 3) persistent vomiting; 4) family history of upper gastrointestinal cancer; 5) palpable abdominal or epigastric mass or lymphadenopathy; and 6) age older than 60 years with new-onset symptoms. B, Functional dyspepsia. EPS indicates epigastric pain syndrome; *H pylori*, *Helicobacter pylori*; PDS, postprandial distress syndrome; PPI, proton pump inhibitor; TCA, tricyclic antidepressant. (Adapted from Moayyedi P, Lacy BE, Andrews CN, Enns RA, Howden CW, Vakil N. ACG and CAG clinical guideline: management of dyspepsia. Am J Gastroenterol. 2017 Jul;112(7):988-1013; used with permission.)

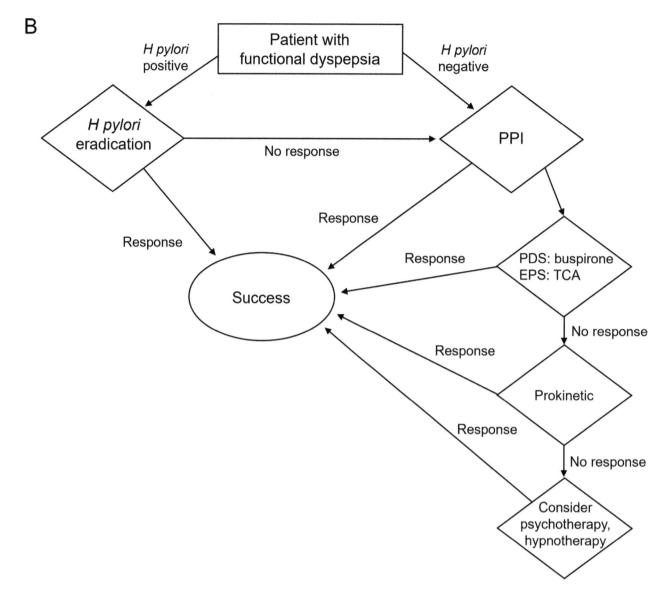

Figure 7.5. Continued

malignancy. After the diagnosis of functional dyspepsia has been made, the first step is to provide reassurance. Some patients with functional dyspepsia want only to be assured that they do not have cancer. They find their symptoms tolerable and require no further intervention. The more difficult decision is whether to perform additional diagnostic testing. The alternative is to proceed directly with empirical trials (Figure 7.5B). Often, the diagnostic tests can be interfaced with therapies that have shown benefit in functional dyspepsia, including *H pylori* eradication (if *H pylori* is present), proton pump inhibitors, intermittent use of prokinetics, buspirone for postprandial distress syndrome, or low-dose tricyclic antidepressants for epigastric pain syndrome.

An 8-week trial of a proton pump inhibitor should be started at once-daily dosing and discontinued if ineffective. If the therapy is effective, discontinuation of the therapy should be attempted every 6 to 12 months. Histamine blockers have modest effect, but antacids, bismuth, and sucralfate have not shown efficacy.

In postprandial distress syndrome, 4 weeks of buspirone administered at 10 mg 3 times daily has been shown to improve postprandial fullness, early satiation, and upper abdominal bloating with improvement in gastric accommodation and delay of gastric emptying of liquids. In epigastric pain syndrome, and in patients with postprandial distress who do not respond to buspirone, a tricyclic antidepressant can be tried. Tricyclic antidepressants are preferred over selective serotonin reuptake inhibitors and serotonin and norepinephrine reuptake inhibitors, although mirtazapine may be considered for patients with unintentional weight loss attributed to functional dyspepsia.

The use of prokinetic agents, including a short course of metoclopramide, can be considered at 5 to 10 mg 3 times daily if patients have not had a therapeutic response with a proton pump inhibitor, *H pylori* eradication, or a trial of an antidepressant. A second trial can be administered for recurrent symptoms. Psychological therapy with cognitive behavioral therapy, hypnotherapy, or psychotherapy can decrease visceral hypersensitivity and resulting symptoms and should be considered if patients have not had a response to medical therapies. Complementary medicines with data for functional dyspepsia include peppermint oil and caraway oil, which have been coformulated in various commercial products. In small trials, these products have been shown to improve symptoms in patients with functional dyspepsia, but current guidelines recommend against their routine use because of the low-quality evidence.

Summary

Disorders of gastric and small-bowel motility may result in either stasis or accelerated transit. Functional dyspepsia most likely resides on a continuum with disturbances in gastric sensation or function that are yet to be clinically defined. Understanding the mechanisms that control motility and the pathophysiologic mechanisms is the key to optimal management. Simple, quantitative measures of transit and an algorithmic approach to identifying the underlying cause may lead to correction of abnormal function. Correcting dehydration and nutritional abnormalities and providing symptomatic relief are important steps in the management of these disorders. More medications and interventions are in development to target the underlying neuromuscular disturbances in gastroparesis. Patient education is essential to avoid aggravation of symptoms caused by dietary indiscretions.

Suggested Reading

Camilleri M. Enteric nervous system disorders: genetic and molecular insights for the neurogastroenterologist. Neurogastroenterol Motil. 2001 Aug;13(4):277–95.

Camilleri M, Iturrino J, Bharucha AE, Burton D, Shin A, Jeong ID, et al. Performance characteristics of scintigraphic measurement of gastric emptying of solids in healthy participants. Neurogastroenterol Motil. 2012 Dec;24(12):1076–e562.

Camilleri M, Parkman HP, Shafi MA, Abell TL, Gerson L; American College of Gastroenterology. Clinical guideline: management of gastroparesis. Am J Gastroenterol. 2013 Jan;108(1):18–37.

Camilleri M, Sanders KM. Gastroparesis. Gastroenterology. 2022 Jan;162(1):68–87.

Camilleri M, Stanghellini V. Current management strategies and emerging treatments for functional dyspepsia. Nat Rev Gastroenterol Hepatol. 2013 Mar;10(3):187–94.

Moayyedi P, Lacy BE, Andrews CN, Enns RA, Howden CW, Vakil N. ACG and CAG clinical guideline: management of dyspepsia. Am J Gastroenterol. 2017 Jul;112(7):988–1013.

Moayyedi P, Soo S, Deeks J, Delaney B, Harris A, Innes M, et al. Eradication of helicobacter pylori for non-ulcer dyspepsia. Cochrane Database Syst Rev. 2006 Apr 19;(2):CD002096.

Parkman HP, Jones MP. Tests of gastric neuromuscular function. Gastroenterology. 2009 May;136(5):1526–43.

Tack J, Talley NJ, Camilleri M, Holtmann G, Hu P, Malagelada JR, et al. Functional gastroduodenal disorders. Gastroenterology. 2006 Apr;130(5):1466–79.

Questions and Answers

Questions

Abbreviations used:

CMV,   cytomegalovirus
CT,   computed tomography
EGD,   esophagogastroduodenoscopy
FDA,   US Food and Drug Administration
FSG,   fasting serum gastrin
GIST,   gastrointestinal stromal tumor
HDGC,   hereditary diffuse gastric cancer
NSAID,   nonsteroidal anti-inflammatory drug
PET,   positron emission tomography
PPI,   proton pump inhibitor
ZES,   Zollinger-Ellison syndrome

Multiple Choice (choose the best answer)

II.1. Peptic ulcers result from an imbalance between processes that damage the mucosa of the gastrointestinal tract and mechanisms that protect it. Which of the following is *not* a normal defense mechanism against gastric acid?

    a. Surface mucous layer
    b. Inhibition of prostaglandin synthesis
    c. Secretion of bicarbonate
    d. Epithelial cell restitution

II.2. A 75-year-old man is referred to your office for recurrent abdominal pain and bleeding from anastomotic and jejunal ulcers. He reports that he had surgery many years ago for peptic ulcer disease, but he is unsure about the type of surgery performed. Recent testing was negative for *Helicobacter pylori*. He does not take aspirin or other NSAIDs. He does not smoke, and he does not have

diarrhea. He says that he takes omeprazole 40 mg orally twice daily, but his symptoms have not improved. What is the most likely diagnosis?

    a. Gastrinoma
    b. Crohn disease
    c. Cryptogenic multifocal ulcerous stenosing enteritis
    d. Retained antrum syndrome

II.3. A 62-year-old woman presents with iron deficiency anemia. Results of a colonoscopy with terminal ileal examination were normal 1 month ago. She does not take aspirin or other NSAIDs. Her bowel movements have been normal. For the past 6 months, she has had mild epigastric discomfort and occasional reflux. What is the best next step in management?

    a. Stool test for *Helicobacter pylori*
    b. EGD with gastric biopsy
    c. Occult stool test
    d. Follow-up colonoscopy

II.4. A 35-year-old man with HIV presents with epigastric pain and melena. He does not take aspirin or other NSAIDs. Recently he declined antiretroviral therapy. EGD shows multiple ulcers in the antrum and lesser curvature of the stomach. Biopsy findings are negative for *Helicobacter pylori*. What is the most likely diagnosis?

    a. Epstein-Barr virus infection
    b. HIV ulcers
    c. CMV infection
    d. Gastric adenocarcinoma

II.5. A 45-year-old woman is referred to the gastroenterology clinic for epigastric pain, unintentional weight loss, and macroscopic anemia. Upper endoscopy shows decreased folds in the body and fundus of the stomach. Biopsy samples were collected, but results are not yet available. What laboratory findings would support the suspected diagnosis?

a. Autoantibodies to parietal cells and intrinsic factor, increased serum gastrin level, and low vitamin B_{12} level
b. Autoantibodies to parietal cells and intrinsic factor, decreased serum gastrin level, and low vitamin B_{12} level
c. Autoantibodies to chief cells and intrinsic factor, increased serum gastrin level, and low vitamin B_{12} level
d. Autoantibodies to G cells and D cells, decreased serum gastrin level, and low vitamin B_{12} level

II.6. A 60-year-old man underwent upper endoscopy for dyspepsia. The antrum appeared erythematous and was biopsied. Biopsy results were consistent with gastric intestinal metaplasia and *Helicobacter pylori* infection. What is the most important action to decrease his risk for gastric cancer?

a. Perform another upper endoscopy with gastric mapping biopsies
b. Recommend the use of proton pump inhibitor medication indefinitely
c. Treat the *H pylori* infection
d. Treat the *H pylori* infection and test for eradication

II.7. A 56-year-old woman presents with frank hematemesis with subsequent coffee-ground emesis. She was recently given a diagnosis of diffuse large B-cell lymphoma. She is hospitalized on the gastroenterology service and found to have a large gastric ulcer in the cardia of her stomach. Biopsy samples are obtained from the edge and center of the gastric ulceration. She does not use aspirin or other NSAIDs. The ulceration does not appear to be malignant. What is the most likely infectious cause of her gastric ulceration?

a. *Mycobacterium tuberculosis*
b. Herpes simplex virus
c. CMV
d. Mucormycosis

II.8. A 40-year-old woman presents for upper endoscopy because she has symptoms of nausea, vomiting, and heartburn that have progressively worsened over the past 3 months. Her primary care physician prescribed omeprazole 40 mg daily, but her symptoms have not improved. Upper endoscopy shows nodularity and erosions in the distal gastric body and antrum. You obtain biopsy samples to assess for *Helicobacter pylori*. The pathologist reports that staining for *H pylori* is negative. The biopsy samples show noncaseating granulomatous lesions with multinucleated giant cells. A subsequent chest radiograph shows bilateral hilar adenopathy. What is the most likely diagnosis?

a. NSAID-induced gastropathy
b. Sarcoidosis
c. Isolated granulomatous gastritis
d. Vasculitis-associated granulomas

II.9. A 24-year-old woman presents with postprandial nausea, vomiting, abdominal pain, and weight loss of 9.1 kg (20 lb). Symptoms have been present for 3 months and are progressive. Her father died of gastric cancer at age 39 years. On examination, she appears comfortable. Physical examination findings are remarkable for a nondistended abdomen with mild epigastric discomfort on palpation. Laboratory assessment shows a microcytic anemia with hemoglobin level of 7 g/dL. Upper endoscopy shows gastric luminal narrowing and poor distention of the stomach with air insufflation. The gastric mucosa appears normal. Gastric biopsy was performed, and the findings are shown below:

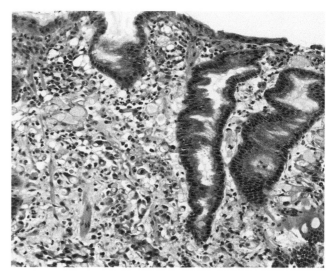

Adapted from Ravi K, Sweetser S. Gastroenterology. 2014;146(1):33; used with permission.

Which gene most likely has a sequence variation?

a. *APC*
b. *CDH1*
c. *MSH6*
d. *STK11*

II.10. A 33-year-old woman who has a history of gastroesophageal reflux disease treated with omeprazole presents with persistent substernal burning discomfort for 3 months. She appears well and physical examination findings are unremarkable. Upper endoscopy shows mild erosive esophagitis and a single superficial duodenal bulb ulcer without stigmata of recent hemorrhage. Laboratory study results are normal for a complete blood cell count and chemistry panel. The FSG level is 600 pg/mL (upper limit of the reference range, 100 pg/mL). What is the best next step?

a. Perform a secretin stimulation test
b. Perform a gallium Ga 68 PET/CT scan
c. Perform endoscopic ultrasonography
d. Recheck the FSG when she has not received PPI therapy for 1 week

II.11. A 56-year-old man presents with dyspepsia. He appears well, and abdominal examination findings are unremarkable. Upper endoscopy shows a 2-cm ulcerated lesion in the gastric body, which on biopsy shows monotonous sheets of small round cells with uniform nuclei consistent with a neuroendocrine tumor. The Ki-67 index is 10%. In addition, results from biopsies of the surrounding gastric mucosa are normal. Laboratory study results include a normal complete blood cell count and serum gastrin level. A gallium Ga 68 PET/CT scan shows no metastatic disease. Endoscopic ultrasonography shows that the lesion is confined to the submucosa. What is the best next step in management?

a. Surgical resection
b. Endoscopic submucosal resection
c. Ablation with argon plasma coagulation
d. Octreotide

I.12. A 25-year-old woman with no past medical history presents with a 1-week history of exertional dyspnea, melena, and abdominal discomfort. On physical examination she is a pale woman with a heart rate of 119 beats/min, respiratory rate of 26 breaths/min, and blood pressure of 87/51 mm Hg with orthostatic hypotension. Results of laboratory studies include hemoglobin, 5.6 g/dL; serum urea nitrogen, 35 mg/dL; and creatinine, 1.0 mg/dL. She receives volume resuscitation, transfused blood products, and a PPI. Upper endoscopy shows a gastric submucosal mass with central ulceration and visible vessel, as in the image below:

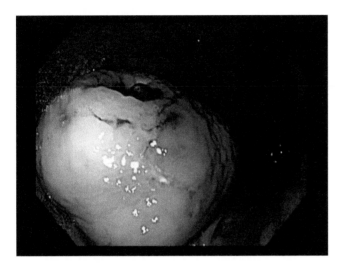

Subsequent CT imaging of the abdomen and pelvis with an intravenous contrast agent shows a 4.5-cm heterogeneously enhancing mass arising from the gastric fundus without adjacent lymphadenopathy, as shown in the image below:

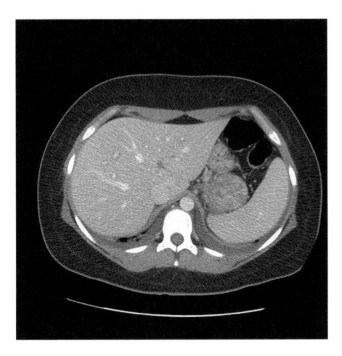

What is the most likely diagnosis?

a. GIST
b. Lymphoma
c. Adenocarcinoma
d. Carcinoid

II.13. A 38-year-old woman presents with a 12-month history of early satiation and postprandial pain occurring at least 5 times per week. She describes the pain as a vague sensation in the epigastrium that worsens 10 to 40 minutes after eating. She is eating only 50% of her previous meal sizes before feeling full. Eating more causes nausea, and rarely she has an episode of emesis. She has not had weight loss, dysphagia, blood in her emesis, or changes in her bowel habits. What is the best next step in management?

a. Perform upper endoscopy with small-bowel aspirates
b. Test for *Helicobacter pylori* stool antigen
c. Perform a gastric emptying study
d. Begin empirical treatment with omeprazole twice daily

II.14. A 67-year-old man presents with nausea, vomiting, epigastric abdominal pain, postprandial fullness, and decreased appetite. His past medical history is notable for hypertension, hyperlipidemia, and type 2 diabetes. His most recent hemoglobin A$_{1c}$ was 10%, and he recently received a diagnosis of peripheral neuropathy. EGD findings are unremarkable, and gastric biopsies do not show evidence of *Helicobacter pylori* infection. What is the best next step in diagnosis?

a. Gastric emptying study with radiolabeled high-fat liquid supplement for 4 hours
b. Gastric emptying study with radiolabeled oatmeal for 2 hours
c. Gastric emptying study with radiolabeled eggs and toast for 2 hours
d. Gastric emptying study with radiolabeled eggs and toast for 4 hours

II.15. A 43-year-old woman with a history of systemic sclerosis for the past 20 years presents for evaluation of abdominal discomfort, bloating, and diarrhea that started 3 months earlier and has been increasing in severity. She reports having increased abdominal distention about an hour after eating and mild fatigue. She has not had dysphagia or odynophagia, but she thinks her weight has decreased about 3 kg (6.6 lb) over the past 2 months. Her vital signs are unremarkable. Laboratory tests show the following: hemoglobin, 11.0 g/dL; MCV, 101 fL; iron studies, unremarkable; vitamin B$_{12}$, less than the lower limit of the reference range; and folate levels, greater than the upper limit of the reference range. What is the best next step in diagnosis?

a. Upper endoscopy with small-bowel aspirates
b. Abdominal fat pad aspirate
c. Esophageal manometry
d. Four-hour gastric emptying study

II.16. Which of the following patients is most likely to have adverse neurologic or extrapyramidal effects from use of metoclopramide for gastroparesis?

a. A 65-year-old man with idiopathic gastroparesis who has taken 10 mg metoclopramide 3 times daily for the past month
b. A 20-year-old man with diabetic gastroparesis who has taken 10 mg metoclopramide 4 times daily for the past 4 months
c. A 45-year-old woman with postviral gastroparesis who has taken 5 mg metoclopramide 3 times daily for the past 2 months
d. A 70-year-old woman with postsurgical gastroparesis who has taken 5 mg metoclopramide up to once daily as needed for the past 3 months

Answers

II.1. Answer b.

Several defense mechanisms protect against gastric acid, and many of these defense mechanisms are prostaglandin dependent. Therefore, inhibition of prostaglandin synthesis would lead to mucosal damage of the gastrointestinal tract.

II.2. Answer d.
The patient has a history of surgery for peptic ulcer disease. He most likely had a Billroth II operation, which is a partial gastrectomy. If removal of the distal antrum is inadequate, continued exposure to the alkaline fluid from the duodenum will cause it to secrete excessive acid and promote ulcer development. A secretin provocation test may help to differentiate retained antrum from a gastrinoma because the serum gastrin concentration will increase (>120 pg/mL) in Zollinger-Ellison syndrome and remain the same in retained antrum syndrome.

II.3. Answer b.
Iron deficiency anemia is an alarm sign for *Helicobacter pylori* infection. The patient also has had a new onset of dyspeptic symptoms at an age older than 60 years. An EGD with gastric biopsy is warranted to assess for *H pylori* and the cause of the iron deficiency anemia.

II.4. Answer c.
CMV infection is the most likely diagnosis since the biopsy findings were negative for *Helicobacter pylori*, and the patient is immunocompromised. CMV can infect various sites, including the gastrointestinal tract, lungs, liver, and central nervous system. Biopsy samples should be obtained from the center of the ulcers to increase the diagnostic yield.

II.5. Answer a.
This patient most likely has autoimmune atrophic gastritis (ie, pernicious anemia), which is the most common cause of vitamin B_{12} deficiency. Autoantibodies to the parietal cells and intrinsic factor are characteristic of autoimmune atrophic gastritis. The loss of parietal cells leads to an inability to secrete hydrochloric acid and a high gastric pH, which permits uninhibited gastrin release. Chief cells secrete pepsin and gastric lipase, G cells secrete gastrin, and D cells secrete somatostatin.

II.6. Answer d.
Helicobacter pylori is a gastric carcinogen and accounts for almost 90% of noncardia gastric cancers in the world. It is recommended that patients with gastric intestinal metaplasia be tested and treated for *H pylori*. Routine endoscopy surveillance is not recommended. Use of proton pump inhibitors alone without eradication of *H pylori* infection is not a recommended strategy.

II.7.Answer c.
CMV is the agent for the most recognized viral infection of the stomach. CMV gastrointestinal disease can occur in up to 5% of patients with advanced immunosuppression. The patient's new diagnosis of lymphoma has resulted in her being immunocompromised. Biopsy samples from the center of the ulceration aid in the diagnosis of CMV infection; samples from the edge of the ulceration aid in making the diagnosis of herpes simplex virus infection.

II.8. Answer b.
Sarcoidosis is a multisystemic disease characterized by the histologic presence of noncaseating granulomas. It most commonly affects the lungs. Gastrointestinal sarcoidosis is rare and usually asymptomatic. The most involved gastrointestinal organ is the stomach. The mainstay of treatment is glucocorticoids. NSAIDs are unlikely to cause noncaseating granulomatous inflammation, and isolated granulomatous gastritis and vasculitis are less likely causes of this clinical scenario given the radiographic finding of bilateral hilar adenopathy, which is highly suggestive of sarcoidosis.

II.9. Answer b.
This patient has diffuse gastric cancer, and gastric biopsy shows signet ring cell carcinoma. Given her young age, HDGC should be considered. HDGC is an autosomal dominant, inherited gastric cancer syndrome characterized by germline variation of the *CDH1* gene, which encodes for the cell-to-cell adhesion protein E-cadherin. HDGC is a relatively rare cancer syndrome but may account for approximately 1% of all cases of gastric carcinoma in populations with a low incidence of gastric cancer, such as in the US, Canada, and the UK. Diffuse-type gastric adenocarcinoma with signet ring cells is the most common cancer in carriers of germline *CDH1* variations. Genetic testing for *CDH1* variants is widely available. However, only 50% of families meeting diagnostic criteria carry a predisposing *CDH1* variant. Established diagnostic criteria for *CDH1* variant testing include any 1 of the following: 1) 2 persons with gastric cancer in a family, regardless of their ages, with at least 1 having a confirmed diffuse gastric cancer; 2) diffuse gastric cancer in a person younger than 40 years; and 3) personal or family history (first- or second-degree relative) of diffuse gastric cancer and lobular breast cancer, 1 of which was diagnosed when the patient was younger than 50 years. The other malignancy that occurs with an increased frequency in families with HDGC is lobular breast carcinoma. There is a high lifetime risk for advanced gastric cancer with HDGC (approximately 70%) by 80 years of age. The risk for advanced gastric cancer is age related and estimated to be less than 1% at 20 years and increasing to 4% at 30 years. Because most patients have advanced-stage gastric carcinoma at diagnosis, prophylactic gastrectomy is recommended in asymptomatic patients who carry the *CDH1* variant and are older than 20 years to prevent the development of this lethal cancer. If the patient declines prophylactic gastrectomy, intensive gastroscopic surveillance should be performed and the patient informed of the limitations with endoscopic detection of early lesions in HDGC. The *APC* gene (variants are involved in familial adenomatous polyposis), the *MSH6* gene (variants are involved in Lynch syndrome), and the *STK11* gene (variants are involved in Peutz-Jeghers syndrome) can all predispose a patient to gastric cancer; however, a diffuse signet ring cell carcinoma at a young age would be highly unusual with these gene variants.

II.10. Answer d.
This patient presents with acid peptic disease complications (erosive esophagitis and duodenal ulcer) while taking a PPI. The high FSG level increases concern for ZES. However, the use of a PPI can increase the FSG level. Therefore, the next step is to recheck the FSG when she has not received PPI therapy for 1 week. If that result is still high, the next step would be to measure a fasting gastric pH. If the gastric pH is greater than 2, ZES is unlikely. In contrast, if gastric pH is 2 or less, ZES is possible and a secretin stimulation test should be performed. Localization studies such as endoscopic ultrasonography or gallium Ga 68 PET/CT scan should be performed only after a gastrinoma has been confirmed biochemically.

II.11. Answer a.
This patient has a type 3 gastric carcinoid. Type 3 gastric carcinoids are more common in men and are typically 2 to 5 cm. With type 3 gastric carcinoids, the surrounding gastric mucosa is normal in contrast to type 1 gastric carcinoids (atrophic mucosa) and type 2 gastric carcinoids (hyperplastic mucosa). In addition, the fasting serum gastrin level in patients with type 3 gastric carcinoid is normal, whereas it is high in patients with types 1 or 2. The recommended treatment

of type 3 gastric carcinoid without evidence of distant metastases is surgical resection with removal of regional lymph nodes.

II.12. Answer a.

The morphologic features of the tumor and presentation with marked bleeding make GIST the most likely diagnosis. GISTs are the most common mesenchymal tumor of the gastrointestinal tract, with 60% of them occurring in the stomach. Patients with a GIST may present with gastrointestinal tract bleeding, abdominal pain or discomfort, and, rarely, signs of obstruction. More than 90% of patients with GISTs have sequence variants of the *c-KIT* proto-oncogene. Surgical resection would be the treatment of choice for this patient. A patient with gastric lymphoma would most likely present with adjacent lymphadenopathy and without a well-circumscribed lesion. In addition, adenocarcinoma is unlikely to occur as a well-circumscribed, submucosal lesion. Carcinoids arise in the submucosa but would not have this endoscopic appearance.

II.13. Answer b.

The Rome IV criteria define *functional dyspepsia* as 1 or more of the following symptoms: postprandial fullness, early satiation, epigastric pain, or epigastric burning over the past 3 months with onset of symptoms occurring at least 6 months before the diagnosis. *Helicobacter pylori* testing, either with stool antigen or urea breath testing, should be completed in the initial diagnostic evaluation for patients presenting with dyspepsia. Upper endoscopy is recommended for patients older than 60 years or those with alarm features, including dysphagia, weight loss, and treatment-resistant dyspepsia. A gastric emptying study is not recommended as part of the initial evaluation for dyspepsia but can be considered if symptoms of gastroparesis are present. An empirical trial with a PPI is reasonable after *H pylori* is ruled out but should be initiated at a standard daily dosage (not twice daily).

II.14. Answer d.

Gastroparesis, a known complication of poorly controlled diabetes, should be a strong consideration if a patient has consistent symptoms, concomitant neuropathic complications, and normal findings on endoscopic evaluation. The gastric emptying study should use a solid meal because it is the most sensitive means of detecting a delay in gastric emptying. Oatmeal-based meals are semiliquid and not validated to the same extent as meals of egg and toast, and gastric emptying should be measured for a full 4 hours.

II.15. Answer a.

Systemic sclerosis can be complicated by a motility disturbance leading to intestinal pseudo-obstruction. While this is generally neuropathic in early disease, progressive systemic sclerosis will lead to myopathic disease, which increases rates of small intestinal bacterial overgrowth. The best diagnostic step is to perform upper endoscopy and obtain duodenal aspirates to assess for the complication of small intestinal bacterial overgrowth. While amyloidosis can also cause myopathic motility disturbance and may be detected with an abdominal fat pad aspirate, this patient is known to have systemic sclerosis, which is probably a contributing risk factor for bacterial overgrowth in this case. Patients who have systemic sclerosis can have esophageal peristalsis disturbance and decreased lower esophageal sphincter tone. However, this patient does not have symptoms of esophageal dysfunction that would require esophageal manometric evaluation at this time. Gastroparesis can also be a complication of systemic sclerosis and can lead to symptoms such as bloating and abdominal discomfort. The patient may have gastroparesis; however, pursuing a gastric emptying study would be lower yield as small intestinal bacterial overgrowth is more likely the diagnosis because the patient has diarrhea, a low level of vitamin B_{12}, and a high level of folate.

II.16. Answer b.

The FDA has given metoclopramide a boxed warning for the development of tardive dyskinesia with a high dose or long-term use. The risk of tardive dyskinesia is directly related to duration of therapy, and the FDA recommendation is that the drug be used only if the duration is no longer than 12 weeks. In addition, tardive dyskinesia and other extrapyramidal signs are most likely to develop in pediatric patients, patients with diabetes, and elderly patients (especially women). When metoclopramide is used, the daily dose should not exceed 40 mg, and treatment duration should not exceed 3 months without an interruption in administration. A decreased dose should be considered for elderly patients and for patients with decreased kidney function. Answer choice *b* is correct because of the patient's young age, the cause of the gastroparesis, the high daily dose, and the long duration of drug use. The patients described in the other answer choices have lower risk because of 1 or more of the following: shorter duration of use, lower dose, and less frequent administration.

III

Small Bowel and Nutrition

8

Clinical Features of Malabsorptive Disorders, Small-Bowel Diseases, and Bacterial Overgrowth Syndromes

AMY S. OXENTENKO, MD

Malabsorptive Disorders and Diarrhea

Both *malabsorption* (a defect in the mucosal absorption of nutrients) and *maldigestion* (a defect in the hydrolysis of nutrients) imply disordered physiologic mechanisms in the gastrointestinal system. Malabsorption and maldigestion of nutritional substrates can occur in multiple phases: 1) the *luminal phase*, in which there is contact between ingested food and various digestive enzymes; 2) the *mucosal phase*, in which substances are assimilated and absorbed in the required constituent form; and 3) the *delivery phase*, in which nutrients are taken up into the cytoplasm and transported to the lymphatics or portal venous system (Table 8.1).

Carbohydrate Malabsorption

Starch, sucrose, and lactose account for nearly 85% of ingested carbohydrates, with starches alone comprising 50%. For starches to be absorbed, they first are digested by salivary α-amylase and pancreatic α-amylase—mainly the latter—into disaccharides and oligosaccharides of maltose, maltotriose, and α-dextrins, which are then hydrolyzed by brush border enzymes to form the monosaccharide glucose. Sucrose is hydrolyzed by sucrase to form glucose and fructose, whereas lactose is hydrolyzed by lactase to form glucose and galactose. After being cleaved by the brush border disaccharidases, these monosaccharides can be absorbed into the cytoplasm. Fructose is transported by facilitated diffusion, but glucose and galactose are transported by

Abbreviations: DGP, deamidated gliadin peptide; EATL, enteropathy-associated T-cell lymphoma; EMA, endomysial antibody; Ig, immunoglobulin; PAS, periodic acid–Schiff; PCR, polymerase chain reaction; SGLT-1, sodium–glucose-linked transporter 1; SIBO, small intestinal bacterial overgrowth; tTG, tissue transglutaminase

sodium–glucose-linked transporter 1 (SGLT-1); oral rehydration solutions are effective because of the inclusion of both sodium and glucose in concentrations that maximize use of this transport system (see below).

Carbohydrate malabsorption can be caused by either a decrease in mucosal surface area (absolute or relative) or a decrease in disaccharidases or transport proteins. Unabsorbed carbohydrates increase the osmolality within the intestinal lumen, resulting in more fluid being drawn into the lumen to maintain an isosmotic state, which can lead to diarrhea. Colonic bacterial fermentation of these malabsorbed substances increases intestinal gas. The most common clinical syndrome of carbohydrate malabsorption is from lactase deficiency. Congenital lactase deficiency is present at birth and is rare. Primary lactase deficiency has a delayed onset, with the highest prevalence among American Indians and people from sub-Saharan Africa and Asia. A secondary, or late-onset, acquired lactase deficiency may occur after intestinal resection, mucosal disease, or a postinfectious syndrome. Because lactase is present on the microvillous surface, it is often the first disaccharidase affected by small-bowel mucosal diseases. Less common conditions associated with disaccharidase deficiencies include sucrase-isomaltase deficiency (an inherited condition) and trehalase deficiency (trehalose is a sugar found in various mushrooms).

The clinical features of carbohydrate malabsorption include flatus, bloating, and osmotic diarrhea. Weight loss should not occur with isolated carbohydrate malabsorption; if weight loss has occurred, possible contributing conditions should be considered. A detailed dietary history can suggest the type of carbohydrate malabsorption that may be occurring. The diagnosis may be supported by the findings of an increased stool osmotic gap (>100 mOsm/kg) and stool pH less than 6 (the pH reflects the release of hydrogen and short-chain fatty acids from carbohydrate

Table 8.1.   Mechanisms of Malabsorption and Maldigestion

Defect	Cause	Examples
Luminal phase		
Defective fat hydrolysis	Decreased lipase	Pancreatic insufficiency
	Decreased duodenal pH	Zollinger-Ellison syndrome
	Impaired mixing	Postgastrectomy
Defective protein hydrolysis	Decreased proteases	Pancreatic insufficiency
	Absence of enterokinase	Congenital deficiency
Impaired solubilization	Decreased micelle formation	Liver disease
		Biliary obstruction
		Ileal resection or disease
		Drugs (cholestyramine)
	Deconjugation of bile salts	Bacterial overgrowth
Mucosal phase		
Diffuse mucosal damage	Diminished surface area, altered absorption or secretion	Celiac disease, tropical sprue, Crohn disease, Whipple disease, amyloidosis
Decreased brush border enzymes	Congenital or acquired deficiency	Lactase, trehalase, or sucrose deficiency
	Small-bowel damage	Postinfectious lactase deficiency
Transporter defects	Single enzyme defects	Hartnup disease, cystinuria
Delivery phase		
Lymphatic derangement	Ectasia of lymphatics	Lymphangiectasis
	Increased lymphatic pressure	Congestive heart failure, pericardial constriction, lymphoma, fibrosis

Data from Riley SA, Marsh MN. Maldigestion and malabsorption. In: Feldman M, Scharschmidt BF, Sleisenger MH, editors. Sleisenger & Fordtran's gastrointestinal and liver disease: pathophysiology, diagnosis, management. 6th ed. Vol 2. Philadelphia (PA): Saunders; c1998. p. 1501-22.

fermentation in the colon). The mucosal enzyme activity of the various disaccharidases can be quantified (rarely done for adult patients), but this practice is invasive and not widely available. Hydrogen breath tests have largely replaced oral tolerance tests; an increase in breath hydrogen of at least 20 ppm above baseline during the 3-hour study is indicative of colonic fermentation of the nonabsorbed carbohydrate by bacteria. False-positive results (small intestinal bacterial overgrowth [SIBO] or inadequate dietary instructions) and false-negative results (recent treatment with antibiotics or nonhydrogen producers) can occur with breath testing. Tolerance to lactose-containing products can be improved if they are ingested with other foods, especially in amounts less than 15 g (equivalent to about 300 mL of milk).

✓ Carbohydrates need to be broken down to monosaccharides to allow for absorption
✓ Lactase deficiency—the most common cause of carbohydrate malabsorption

---

Fat Malabsorption

Fat malabsorption is a complex process that requires adequate function of the pancreas, liver and biliary system, small-bowel mucosa, and lymphatic system. Triglycerides constitute the majority of dietary fat. Initial lipolytic activity begins in the stomach through the action of gastric lipase, although this contributes little to digestion in most people, whereas pancreatic lipase has a much larger role in hydrolyzing dietary triglycerides. Because the optimal activity of pancreatic lipase occurs at a pH of 8, it is inactivated in acid overproduction states (eg, Zollinger-Ellison syndrome and mastocytosis). Pancreatic lipase hydrolyzes dietary triglycerides into free fatty acids and β-monoglycerol. These constituents then combine with conjugated bile salts from the liver to form water-soluble micelles, which allow passage into enterocytes. At the level of the enterocyte, triglycerides are reesterified, synthesized into chylomicrons, and distributed systemically through the lymphatics. Although pancreatic function is required for fat digestion, a person may lose nearly 90% of lipase output from the pancreas before the efficiency of fat digestion and absorption is affected. Unlike long-chain triglycerides, which require bile salts and micelle production for absorption, medium-chain triglycerides do not require micelle formation for absorption and can be absorbed directly into the portal blood. This mechanism can be used to provide triglycerides in the diet without worsening fat malabsorption in patients with bile salt deficiency, such as patients who have had more than 100 cm of distal small bowel resected.

The clinical features of fat malabsorption include diarrhea, weight loss, and complications from deficiencies of fat-soluble vitamins (vitamins A, D, E, and K). Although the amount of fat in the stool can be assessed qualitatively with Sudan staining, this test has relatively low sensitivity and specificity. The test for fecal elastase is an indirect method for evaluation of pancreatic function; sensitivity increases according to the severity of the pancreatic insufficiency, and the specificity exceeds 90%. Quantification of fecal fat excretion is considered the gold standard for establishing the presence of fat malabsorption. The normal value for fecal fat excretion is less than 7 g daily, and levels of 7 to 14 g may be present when patients have chronic diarrhea without true fat malabsorption. A 72-hour stool collection is optimal; the patient should receive a diet containing 100 g of fat daily for several days before stool collection commences and continue to receive the high-fat diet throughout the stool collection process. The patient should be instructed to avoid antidiarrheal agents or pancreatic enzyme replacement immediately before and during the stool collection so that the stool volume and fat will be accurately reflected.

Once fat malabsorption has been confirmed, the cause should be determined. In some cases, the cause may be apparent clinically. The most common clinical conditions result from small-bowel diseases or pancreatic insufficiency. Evaluation for small-bowel abnormalities that can lead to fat malabsorption could include small-bowel biopsies (eg, celiac disease or amyloid), small-bowel cultures (eg, SIBO), and small-bowel imaging (eg, Crohn disease or radiation enteritis). To evaluate for pancreatic causes of fat malabsorption, imaging (computed tomography, magnetic resonance cholangiopancreatography, or endoscopic ultrasonography) can be used to examine for changes from chronic pancreatitis. Pancreatic calcifications seen on plain films can be helpful, but they are present infrequently. Tests of pancreatic function, which are not widely available, can be performed with secretin (to measure bicarbonate) and cholecystokinin (to measure lipase or trypsin). Alternatively, an empirical trial of pancreatic enzymes can be recommended, with fecal fat quantification before and after the trial to assess objectively for improvement.

✓ Up to 90% of lipase output from the pancreas (from resection or insufficiency) may be lost before fat digestion and absorption is affected
✓ Pancreatic lipase function is inhibited by acid hyperproduction states
✓ Long-chain triglycerides require bile salts and micelles for absorption; medium-chain triglycerides do not require micelles, so patients with bile salt deficiency can receive dietary triglycerides without worsening fat malabsorption

---

Protein Malabsorption

Protein digestion and absorption require adequate pancreatic function as well as integrity of the intestinal mucosa. Ingested proteins are cleaved initially by pepsin (an endopeptidase), which is produced from the precursor pepsinogen in response to a gastric pH of 1 to 3, with inactivation at a pH greater than 5. When gastric chyme reaches the small intestine, enterokinase from duodenal enterocytes activates trypsin. Trypsin then converts pancreatic proteases from inactive to active forms in a cascade fashion, subsequently cleaving proteins into various amino acids and small peptides. Additional mucosal brush border oligopeptidases further cleave small peptides, with free amino acids and oligopeptides crossing into the cytoplasm either freely or through carrier-mediated channels, some of which are sodium-mediated channels.

In addition to disorders that affect protein digestion and absorption, considerable amounts of protein can be lost from the intestinal tract; these conditions are referred to as *protein-losing enteropathies*. Although the liver can respond to protein loss by increasing the production of various proteins such as albumin, a protein-losing state develops when net loss exceeds net production. Three major categories of gastrointestinal-related disorders are associated with excess protein loss: 1) diseases with increased mucosal permeability without erosions, 2) diseases with mucosal erosions, and 3) diseases with increased lymphatic pressure. Examples of clinical conditions in each of these categories are listed in Box 8.1.

The clinical features of a protein-losing enteropathy may include diarrhea, edema, or ascites. Because isolated protein malabsorption or loss is infrequent, features of concomitant carbohydrate and fat malabsorption may also be apparent. Laboratory studies may show a low serum level of protein, albumin, and immunoglobulins, except for immunoglobulin (Ig) E, which has a short half-life and rapid synthesis. If the protein-losing state is from lymphangiectasia (primary or acquired), patients may also have lymphocytopenia. To diagnose

---

Box 8.1. Causes of Protein-Losing Enteropathies

Nonerosive disease
  Ménétrier disease
  Helicobacter pylori gastritis
  Eosinophilic gastroenteritis
  Celiac disease
  Small intestinal bacterial overgrowth
  Whipple disease
  Vasculitides

Erosive disease
  Amyloidosis
  Inflammatory bowel disease
  Graft-vs-host disease
  Clostridioides difficile colitis
  Ischemia

Increased lymphatic pressure
  Congestive heart failure
  Constrictive pericarditis
  Lymphangiectasia (primary vs acquired)
  Lymphatic obstruction (lymphoma)
  Mesenteric venous thrombosis
  Retroperitoneal fibrosis

Adapted from Greenwald DA. Protein-losing gastroenteropathy. In: Feldman M, Friedman LS, Brandt LJ, editors. Sleisenger & Fordtran's gastrointestinal and liver disease: pathophysiology, diagnosis, management. 9th ed. Vol 1. Philadelphia (PA): Saunders/Elsevier; c2010. p. 437-43; used with permission.

---

a protein-losing enteropathy, an α_1-antitrypsin clearance test should be performed. α_1-Antitrypsin is unique in that it is neither absorbed nor secreted from the intestinal mucosa, and unlike other proteins, it is resistant to proteolysis (with the exception of pepsin). Therefore, its clearance reflects a true protein-losing state. If a protein-losing gastropathy is suspected (eg, Ménétrier disease), the patient should receive acid-suppressive therapy before an α_1-antitrypsin clearance test is performed. This sequence avoids degradation of α_1-antitrypsin by pepsin, since the elevated pH from acid suppression will inactivate pepsin and hence allow adequate assessment of gastric loss.

✓ Protein malabsorption rarely occurs in isolation
✓ The α_1-antitrypsin clearance test is used to assess for protein-losing enteropathy

---

Diarrhea

The mechanism for diarrhea is often from a combination of decreased absorption (a villous function) and increased secretion (a crypt function). Diarrhea can be categorized as *inflammatory* or *noninflammatory* or as *secretory* or *osmotic*.

The clinical features of *inflammatory* diarrhea may include abdominal pain, fever, and tenesmus. Stools may be mucoid, bloody, smaller volume, and more frequent, unless the small bowel also is affected. Microscopically, the stools can contain blood and leukocytes. However, if the inflammation is microscopic, these clinical and stool features may be absent (eg, microscopic colitis). Common causes of inflammatory diarrhea include invasive infections, inflammatory bowel disease, radiation enteropathy, and ischemia.

Noninflammatory causes of diarrhea tend to produce watery diarrhea, without fever or gross blood, and the stool appears normal on microscopy. There are many causes, but infections, particularly by toxin-producing organisms, are a common cause of acute, self-limited diarrhea.

Distinguishing whether diarrhea is osmotic or secretory can be useful clinically in order to narrow the differential diagnosis. *Osmotic* diarrhea is due to the ingestion of poorly absorbed cations, anions, sugars, or sugar alcohols (such as sorbitol or xylitol). These ingested ions obligate retention of water in the intestinal lumen to maintain osmolality equal to that of other body fluids (290 mOsm/kg); this subsequently causes diarrhea. Osmotic diarrhea can occur also from maldigestion or malabsorption (pancreatic insufficiency or disaccharidase deficiency). The stool osmotic gap is calculated by adding the stool sodium and potassium concentrations, multiplying by 2, and subtracting this amount from 290 mOsm/kg. A gap greater than 100 mOsm/kg strongly supports an osmotic cause for the diarrhea, whereas a gap less than 50 mOsm/kg supports a secretory cause. Stool osmolality does not necessarily need to be measured because the value should be the same as that of the serum (290 mOsm/kg), with lower values indicating urine or water contamination and higher values indicating that the specimen was not processed readily. The utility of checking stool osmolality therefore lies in determining whether the stool specimen was processed properly. Stool volumes tend to be less with osmotic diarrhea than with secretory diarrhea, and diarrhea due to an osmotic cause tends to abate with fasting.

When *secretory* diarrhea occurs, the primary bowel function converts from net absorption to net secretion. Normally, up to 9 to 10 L of intestinal fluid crosses the ligament of Treitz each day, and all but 1.5 L crosses the ileocecal valve, demonstrating the tremendous absorptive capacity of the small bowel. The colon then absorbs all but 100 to 200 mL of the fluid, which is evacuated as stool. In secretory diarrhea, net absorption converts to net secretion, and the small bowel loses its normal capacity to absorb the large volume of fluid; thus, liters of fluid pass into the colon daily. Although the colon can adapt and absorb nearly 4 L of liquid from the stool each day, larger fluid loads cannot be absorbed, and this results in diarrhea (often liters per day). Secretory diarrhea does not abate with fasting. Dehydration can occur easily, and replacement fluids need to contain adequate concentrations of both sodium and glucose, as in oral rehydration solutions, to maximize small-bowel absorption of sodium and water. Consuming beverages that have low sodium concentrations (water, some sports drinks, or juices) may worsen the volume status of the patient because sodium will be secreted into the bowel lumen to maintain an isosmotic state, and the volume of water eliminated will increase because of the stool sodium loss. Sodium and glucose absorption from the small bowel occurs through the transporter SGLT-1. Characteristics, common causes, and testing strategies for secretory and osmotic diarrhea are listed in Table 8.2.

✓ Osmotic diarrhea—volume is usually smaller, stops with fasting, and leads to a stool osmotic gap greater than 100 mOsm/kg

✓ Secretory diarrhea—volume is usually larger, continues with fasting, and leads to a stool osmotic gap less than 50 mOsm/kg

---

Table 8.2. Comparison of Osmotic and Secretory Diarrhea

Osmotic diarrhea	*Secretory diarrhea*
Characteristics	
Daily stool volume <1 L	Daily stool volume >1 L
Stops with fasting	Continues with fasting
Stool osmotic gap >100 mOsm/kg	Stool osmotic gap <50 mOsm/kg
Common causes	
Disaccharidase deficiency	Infections and toxins
Lactase	Cholera
Trehalase	Bile acids
Sucrase-isomaltase	Microscopic colitis
Iatrogenic	Neuroendocrine tumors
Polyethylene glycol solution	Medullary carcinoma of thyroid
Lactulose	(calcitonin)
Magnesium antacids or	VIPoma
supplementation	Gastrin (not pure secretory)
Sweeteners and elixirs	Carcinoid syndrome
Sorbitol	Laxatives (nonosmotic)
Xylitol	Diabetic diarrhea
Fructose	Transporter defects or deficiencies
	Chloridorrhea
	Idiopathic
Testing strategies	
Dietary review	Stool cultures
Carbohydrate malabsorption	Structural or mucosal evaluation
Breath testing	Neuroendocrine hormone levels
Stool pH <6	Bile acid sequestrant trial
Avoidance	
Stool magnesium	

Intestinal Resections and Shortened Bowel

Diarrhea and malabsorption can result from any process that shortens the length of the functioning small bowel, whether from surgery or from relative shortening due to underlying disease. Whether diarrhea and malabsorption occur with a shortened small bowel depends on several factors: the length of the resected bowel, the location of the resected bowel, the integrity of the remaining bowel, and the presence of the colon.

The length and location of the resected small bowel affect the enterohepatic circulation of bile. Typically, bile salts are reabsorbed from the terminal ileum. If *less* than 100 cm of distal ileum is resected, the liver can compensate for the loss of absorptive capacity by producing an increased amount of bile salts, which enter the colon and cause a bile-irritant secretory diarrhea. This diarrhea is treated with a bile acid sequestrant, such as cholestyramine, which binds the excess bile salts and improves diarrhea. If *more* than 100 cm of distal small bowel is resected, including the terminal ileum, the liver can no longer compensate for the loss of absorptive capacity. The resulting bile salt deficiency leads to steatorrhea since micelle production is negatively affected and long-chain triglycerides cannot be effectively handled. This can be managed by prescribing a diet that consists of medium-chain triglycerides, which do not require bile salts or micelle formation for absorption because they are absorbed directly into the portal blood.

The location of the small-bowel resection is also important. The terminal ileum has the specialized function of absorbing and recirculating bile salts and binding the cobalamin-intrinsic factor complex. When the jejunum is resected, the ileum assumes all the functions of the jejunum. However, the opposite is not true; the jejunum cannot compensate for the loss of the specialized functions of the ileum.

Outcomes of ileal resection include diarrhea (from either an excess of bile salts or a deficiency of bile salts, depending on the length resected), vitamin B_{12} deficiency, SIBO (from resection of the ileocecal valve), gallstones (from disruption of the cholesterol pool), and calcium oxalate kidney stones. Normally, in the small bowel, calcium binds to oxalate, with this calcium oxalate complex passing into the colon and being excreted in stool. If the small bowel has been shortened and the colon is absent, calcium preferentially binds to fatty acids in the stool, leaving oxalate unbound. Unbound oxalate is incorporated into the stool and excreted through the ostomy. In the case of a shortened small bowel and intact colon, calcium again binds to the fatty acids, and the free or unbound oxalate is absorbed from the colon, leading to the formation of calcium oxalate kidney stones. Although the absolute length of resected small bowel is important, the integrity of the remaining bowel is crucial because diffuse pathologic processes such as Crohn disease or radiation enteritis can result in a functionally shortened bowel without surgical resection. Whether a patient has an intact colon is of considerable importance if there has been prior small-bowel resection. The colon can adapt by increasing water and sodium absorption, by acting as an intestinal "brake" to slow motility, and by salvaging nonabsorbed carbohydrates to provide additional calories for patients with short bowel syndrome. Patients who still have an intact colon may not need parenteral nutrition if they have 50 to 100 cm of small bowel remaining. However, patients who no longer have a colon may need parenteral nutrition when the length of the small bowel is less than 150 to 180 cm.

In short bowel syndrome, multiple mechanisms contribute to malabsorption. In the early postoperative stage, hypersecretion of gastric acid inactivates pancreatic enzymes, leading to diarrhea and steatorrhea. Until the remaining small bowel has time to adapt, intestinal transit is rapid because of the loss of surface area. As mentioned above, patients may be at risk for SIBO, and because of the disruption of the enterohepatic circulation of bile, bile acid excess (shorter resection) or deficiency associated with steatorrhea (longer resection) may develop. Early management of short bowel syndrome includes aggressive treatment with antidiarrheal agents, total parenteral nutrition, and gastric acid suppression. Later management includes the introduction of a low-fat enteral diet, with progressive increase in carbohydrates, medium-chain triglyceride supplementation as needed, lactose restriction, and treatment of SIBO if present or suspected.

✓ Small-bowel resection shorter than 100 cm tends to lead to bile acid–induced diarrhea, which can improve with a bile acid sequestrant
✓ Small-bowel resection longer than 100 cm leads to bile acid deficiency and steatorrhea, which can improve with an emphasis on the use of a medium-chain triglyceride diet

---

Small-Bowel Diseases

Celiac Disease

Celiac disease may occur in genetically susceptible persons (those with *HLA-DQ2* or *HLA-DQ8* positivity) as an immune response to gliadins in the diet. The prevalence is highest among persons of European descent, and the disease is being diagnosed with greater frequency in North America as clinicians become more familiar with the many manifestations of the disease. In the general population, the prevalence of celiac disease is nearing 1 in 100 (0.7%-1.0%). Celiac disease occurs in patients of all ages, but as many as 20% are older than 60 years at diagnosis.

The diagnosis of celiac disease can be facilitated with the following: 1) the presence of a clinical feature or features compatible with the disease, although they are not always present; 2) supportive, highly sensitive and specific serology; 3) characteristic small-bowel biopsy findings; and 4) a clinical response to a gluten-free diet. The diagnosis no longer requires rechallenging the patient with gluten to invoke symptoms because of the risk for highly sensitive patients. Before patients are tested for celiac disease, they need to be eating a gluten-containing diet. While diagnostic changes may be seen as early as 2 weeks after reintroducing gluten as part of a gluten challenge, a 6- to 8-week challenge, with the consumption of 3 to 5 g of gluten daily, may lead to definitive results. Patients with classic celiac disease have features of malabsorption, whereas those with nonclassical celiac disease tend to have extraintestinal manifestations. These nonclassical (previously referred to as "atypical") forms of celiac disease are now the most common clinical presentations of the disease. The gastrointestinal and extraintestinal manifestations of celiac disease are outlined in Table 8.3. The many diseases associated with celiac disease are listed in Table 8.4.

The available serologic tests for celiac disease measure levels of 1) antigliadin antibodies, 2) endomysial antibodies (EMAs), 3) tissue transglutaminase (tTG) antibodies, and 4) deamidated gliadin peptides (DGPs). The IgA-based tTG antibody test is considered the single best screening test for celiac disease in patients older than 2 years and has a sensitivity of about 95% and a specificity greater than 95%. The original antigliadin antibody test had less sensitivity and specificity than other serologic markers and should be avoided in practice. EMA testing may be more expensive and subjective than tTG antibody testing. A serum IgA level is often determined with the initial IgA tTG antibody testing because IgA deficiency affects 2% to 3% of patients with celiac disease. If patients are found to have or are known to have IgA deficiency, an IgG-based test (IgG tTG antibody or IgG DGP antibody) should be performed. In children younger than 2 years, EMA and tTG antibody testing may be less sensitive, so a combination of both tTG and DGP antibody testing is recommended in this age group. Panel testing (ie, checking >1 serology in adult patients) is not recommended to screen for celiac disease because it will increase the sensitivity but decrease the specificity.

Serologic tests for celiac disease should be considered for 1) patients with classic gastrointestinal manifestations of the disease, 2) patients with well-described nonclassic manifestations, 3) at-risk groups, and 4) patients who are being followed for their response to a gluten-free diet. For symptomatic patients, however, biopsies of the small bowel are needed regardless of the results of serologic testing. Also, any positive serologic results need to be confirmed with small-bowel biopsies. Recent guidelines support that the diagnosis of celiac disease can be made in children without small-bowel biopsies if the children have permissive celiac haplotyping and a tTG antibody level 10 times the upper limit of normal (confirmed with EMA testing); however, it is still recommended that all adults have histologic assessment to ensure baseline confirmation of the disease.

Endoscopic findings in celiac disease include loss of mucosal folds, a mosaic pattern, scalloping, and nodularity. The sensitivity of these endoscopic markers is quite poor; however, if the markers are seen, small-bowel biopsy specimens should be obtained regardless of the indication for upper endoscopy because of the high likelihood of demonstrating an enteropathy from celiac disease or a similar process. Small-bowel biopsies are required for the diagnosis of celiac disease and should be performed in all patients before treatment is initiated. The classic

Table 8.3.   Manifestations of Celiac Disease

Manifestation	Clinical features	Details
Gastrointestinal	Diarrhea, steatorrhea	
	Flatulence, distention	
	Weight loss, anorexia	
	Abdominal pain	
	Nausea, vomiting	
	Constipation	
	Aphthous stomatitis	
	Angular cheilosis	
Extraintestinal		
Laboratory findings	Anemia	Deficiencies of iron, vitamin B_{12}, folate (may be normocytic, dimorphic with >1 deficiency)
	Vitamin and mineral deficiencies	Examples: vitamin D, vitamin B_{12}, iron, zinc, copper
	Abnormal liver biochemistry values	Evaluate for AIH, PBC, PSC
Skin	Dermatitis herpetiformis	Pruritic, papulovesicular, on extensor surfaces
Hematologic	Splenic atrophy	Functional, predisposed to encapsulated organisms
Musculoskeletal	Osteopenia, osteoporosis	Calcium or vitamin D loss or lactose avoidance
	Osteomalacia	Vitamin D deficiency, increased bone alkaline phosphatase level
	Enamel defects	Similar to Sjögren syndrome
	Arthropathy	Nonerosive, polyarticular, symmetrical, large joint
	Muscle cramps, tetany	From low levels of calcium, vitamin D, or magnesium
Neurologic	Peripheral neuropathy	Symmetrical, distal, small-fiber most common
	Ataxia	Cerebellar
	Epilepsy	Bilateral parieto-occipital calcifications
Reproductive	Infertility	Female or male
	Recurrent miscarriage	
Psychiatric	Depression, anxiety	One-third of celiac patients

Abbreviations: AIH, autoimmune hepatitis; PBC, primary biliary cholangitis; PSC, primary sclerosing cholangitis.

Data from Farrell RJ, Kelly CP. Diagnosis of celiac sprue. Am J Gastroenterol. 2001 Dec;96(12):3237-46.

histologic findings include villous atrophy (total or partial), crypt hyperplasia, intraepithelial lymphocytosis (≥25 intraepithelial lymphocytes per 100 surface enterocytes), and chronic inflammatory cell infiltrate in the lamina propria (Figure 8.1). The spectrum of histologic findings in celiac disease is indicated by the modified Marsh (Oberhuber) classification (Figure 8.2). Early Marsh lesions are more likely to produce fewer or no symptoms than

Table 8.4.   Disorders Associated With Celiac Disease

Type of disorder	Disorder
Endocrine	Type 1 diabetes
	Autoimmune thyroiditis
	Adrenal insufficiency
Connective tissue disorders	Sjögren syndrome
	Rheumatoid arthritis
	Systemic lupus erythematosus
Immunologic	IgA deficiency
Inflammatory conditions	Inflammatory bowel disease
	Microscopic colitis
Hepatic	AIH, PSC, PBC
Neurologic	Epilepsy
Kidney	IgA mesangial nephropathy
Cardiopulmonary	Carditis
	Fibrosing alveolitis
	Pulmonary hemosiderosis
Other	Down syndrome, Turner syndrome

Abbreviations: AIH, autoimmune hepatitis; Ig, immunoglobulin; PBC, primary biliary cholangitis; PSC, primary sclerosing cholangitis.

Data from Farrell RJ, Kelly CP. Diagnosis of celiac sprue. Am J Gastroenterol. 2001 Dec;96(12):3237-46.

late Marsh lesions. An increase in the number of intraepithelial lymphocytes is the minimal histologic lesion needed for the diagnosis of celiac disease; villous atrophy alone is not sufficient for diagnosis because it is a nonspecific finding. Other conditions that may show either isolated intraepithelial lymphocytosis or villous flattening in small-bowel biopsy specimens are listed in Box 8.2. These should be considered, especially if the results of serologic studies are negative.

Approximately 95% of patients with celiac disease are positive for *HLA-DQ2*, and the other 5% are positive for *HLA-DQ8*. However, 30% to 40% of the general population is also positive for *HLA-DQ2* or *HLA-DQ8*. Therefore, the presence of 1 of these permissive genes is necessary but not sufficient for the diagnosis of celiac disease. HLA testing is not necessary for most patients being evaluated for celiac disease; however, the negative predictive value of nearly 100% can be useful in evaluating 1) patients who have early Marsh lesions, 2) patients who have negative serologic results but typical small-bowel histology, 3) patients who already have been prescribed a gluten-free diet and are unwilling to reintroduce gluten in the diet, or 4) at-risk patients (eg, patients with Down syndrome) for whom reporting symptoms may be difficult.

The only therapy for celiac disease is a lifelong gluten-free diet, which includes the avoidance of wheat, barley, and rye. Food items that contain oats can be tolerated by most patients with the disease, but cross-contamination or hypersensitivity may limit oat tolerability. Oats are generally avoided for the first year after diagnosis in severely symptomatic patients and then reintroduced if the patient is doing well clinically. Consultation with a skilled dietician is imperative for patients with celiac disease. Determining baseline vitamin and mineral levels and providing replacement therapy when needed is recommended.

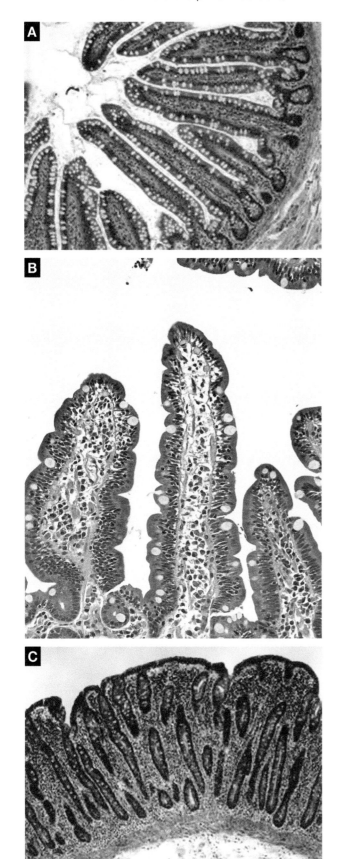

Figure 8.1. Small-Bowel Histopathologic Findings in Celiac Disease. A, Normal findings (hematoxylin-eosin). B, Intraepithelial lymphocytes alone as seen in an early Marsh lesion of celiac disease (hematoxylin-eosin). C, Classic histologic findings of celiac disease, with marked villous atrophy, crypt hyperplasia, and intraepithelial lymphocytosis, with a chronic inflammatory cell infiltrate in the lamina propria (hematoxylin-eosin).

In adults, consideration should be given for bone densitometry. Since patients are at risk for functional asplenia, vaccinations against the encapsulated organisms should be considered. First-degree relatives should be advised to be screened for celiac disease, often with an IgA tTG antibody test.

Dermatitis herpetiformis is an intensely pruritic papulo-vesicular rash, typically on the extensor surfaces, that represents an intestinal sensitivity to gliadins in the diet. Biopsy specimens from the skin adjacent to the affected area may show granular IgA deposits in the papillary dermis; these deposits are pathognomonic for dermatitis herpetiformis (Figure 8.3). Therapy for dermatitis herpetiformis, as for celiac disease, is a lifelong gluten-free diet. Dapsone may help with healing the skin, but it does not heal the intestinal abnormality.

For patients with celiac disease in whom initial therapy fails or symptoms recur after early clinical improvement, several questions should be answered. First, was the initial diagnosis of celiac disease correct? Results of the original small-bowel biopsies and serologic studies should be reviewed. Second, has there been inadvertent or surreptitious ingestion of gluten? The ingestion of gluten is the most likely cause of ongoing or recurring symptoms in a patient with celiac disease; thus, the patient's diet and medications should be reviewed. Also, patients with celiac disease are at risk for other conditions that can cause diarrhea, and these should be considered: microscopic colitis, SIBO, pancreatic insufficiency, lactase deficiency, fructose malabsorption, inflammatory bowel disease, and irritable bowel syndrome. Celiac-specific complications also need to be considered, including ulcerative jejunitis, refractory sprue, and malignancy. Patients with refractory celiac disease type 1 (without clonality) or type 2 (with clonality) can be initially treated with open-capsule budesonide with good clinical and histologic responses. Patients with celiac disease are at increased risk for a rare enteropathy-associated T-cell lymphoma (EATL), which may be manifested as a recurrence of symptoms. EATL is associated with poor survival. Compliance with a gluten-free diet can decrease the risk of EATL considerably. Patients with celiac disease are at increased risk for other malignancies, including other forms of non-Hodgkin lymphoma, small-bowel adenocarcinoma, and oropharyngeal and esophageal cancers.

✓ Iron deficiency anemia—the most common nonclassical feature of celiac disease
✓ Immunoglobulin A tissue transglutaminase antibody test—the serology of choice to screen for celiac disease
✓ The presence of either *HLA-DQ2* or *HLA-DQ8* is necessary for the diagnosis of celiac disease; their absence has nearly 100% negative predictive value in ruling out the disease
✓ Most common cause of nonresponsive celiac disease—gluten ingestion
✓ Several entities can mimic celiac disease, including medications such as olmesartan

---

Whipple Disease

Whipple disease is a multisystem disorder caused by the gram-positive bacillus *Tropheryma whipplei*. This disease usually occurs in White men in the fourth or fifth decade of life. The clinical features include diarrhea, weight loss, adenopathy, arthralgias, fevers, carditis, hyperpigmentation, pleural effusions, and ocular and neurologic symptoms. The diagnosis can be established with a combination of small-bowel biopsy studies and the polymerase chain reaction (PCR). Small-bowel biopsy specimens typically contain periodic acid–Schiff (PAS)-positive macrophages (Figure 8.4). *T whipplei* needs to be differentiated from *Mycobacterium*

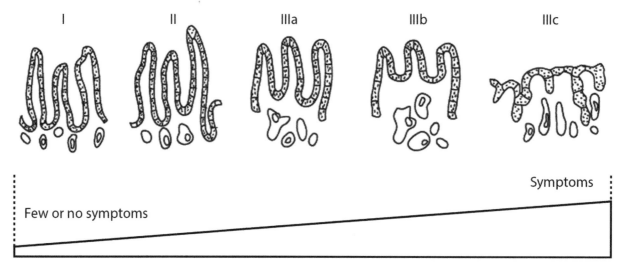

Figure 8.2.   Marsh Classification of the Spectrum of Histologic Findings in Celiac Disease. IEL indicates intraepithelial lymphocyte. (Adapted from Rostom A, Murray JA, Kagnoff MF. American Gastroenterological Association [AGA] Institute technical review on the diagnosis and management of celiac disease. Gastroenterology. 2006 Dec;131[6]:1981-2002; used with permission.)

avium-intracellulare complex, which, in addition to being PAS-positive, is also acid-fast–positive. Electron microscopy can be used to show sickle-shaped *T whipplei* bacteria with their trilaminar cell wall. If the biopsy specimens are PAS-positive and PCR is positive, the diagnosis is established. A testing algorithm is provided in Figure 8.5.

Treatment of Whipple disease includes long-term administration of antibiotics that penetrate the blood-brain barrier. In a randomized controlled study, 14 days of intravenous therapy with either ceftriaxone or meropenem, followed by 1 year of oral trimethoprim-sulfamethoxazole, was curative. Therapies that have had variable success include doxycycline, hydroxychloroquine, and interferon-based regimens.

Box 8.2.   Causes of Small-Bowel Biopsy Findings That May Mimic Celiac Disease

Small intestinal bacterial overgrowth
Nonsteroidal anti-inflammatory drugs
Helicobacter pylori infection
Giardiasis
Crohn disease
Viral gastroenteritis
Autoimmune enteropathy
Eosinophilic gastroenteritis
Combined variable immunodeficiency
Tropical sprue
Lymphoma
Zollinger-Ellison syndrome
Hypersensitivity to nongluten protein
Medications (olmesartan)

✓ Whipple disease is a multisystem disorder that typically occurs in White men in the fourth or fifth decade of life and can be diagnosed through polymerase chain reaction testing
✓ Treatment of Whipple disease includes intravenous antibiotics initially and then prolonged use of oral antibiotics

---

Tropical Sprue

Features of tropical sprue may be indistinguishable from those of classic celiac disease: diarrhea, weight loss, anorexia, and lactose intolerance. Tropical sprue needs to be considered if the patient has traveled to certain geographic areas, such as Asia, India, the Caribbean, and Central or South America. In patients with acute tropical sprue, the onset of clinical features is rapid and is independent of the length of stay in a tropical area. By comparison, in patients with chronic tropical sprue, clinical features occur gradually after several years of residence in a tropical area. Physical examination may show evidence of weight loss or cachexia, glossitis, and hyperactive bowel sounds. Laboratory features can indicate megaloblastic anemia with vitamin B_{12} and folate deficiencies and a protein-losing state. No specific test helps establish the diagnosis, and other infectious disorders need to be ruled out. Small-bowel biopsy specimens may show villous atrophy similar to what is found in celiac disease; therefore, for all patients with newly diagnosed celiac disease, the travel history must be documented, especially if the serologic test results are negative. Treatment with folate, 5 mg daily, and vitamin B_{12} replacement produces rapid improvement in the anemia, glossitis, and weight loss in many patients with tropical sprue. In addition, antibiotic therapy with tetracycline, 250 mg 4 times daily, may be needed in combination with folate for 3 to 6 months, especially to treat the chronic form of the disease.

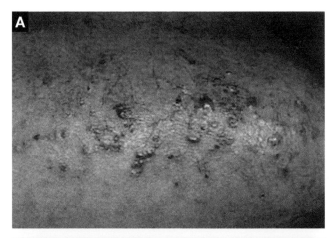

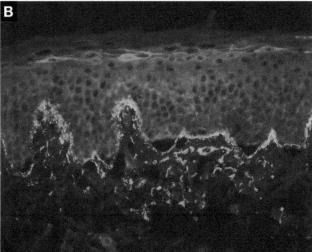

Figure 8.3. Dermatitis Herpetiformis. A, Pruritic papulovesicular rash on the extensor surface of the skin. (Adapted from Bennett ML, Jorizzo JL, Sherertz EF. Skin lesions associated with gastrointestinal and liver diseases. In: Yamada T, editor. Textbook of gastroenterology. 4th ed. Vol 1. Philadelphia [PA]: Lippincott Williams & Wilkins; c2003. p. 992-1009; used with permission.)

B, Immunofluorescence of biopsy specimen showing the characteristic immunoglobulin A deposits in the papillary dermis. (Courtesy of Dr Kristin M. Leiferman, Immunodermatology Laboratory, University of Utah; used with permission.)

✓ Tropical sprue may be indistinguishable from celiac disease clinically and histologically, but patients with tropical sprue are serologically negative
✓ Treatment of tropical sprue includes folate, vitamin B$_{12}$, and prolonged use of antibiotics

---

Eosinophilic Gastroenteritis

Eosinophilic gastroenteritis has various clinical manifestations depending on the location of bowel involvement. With mucosal disease, patients often have diarrhea, malabsorption, and evidence of a protein-losing enteropathy. Involvement of the muscularis layer may lead to features of bowel obstruction, whereas serosal involvement may lead to ascites and peritonitis.

Laboratory studies typically show an increased serum level of IgE and peripheral eosinophilia, with a greater increase in the

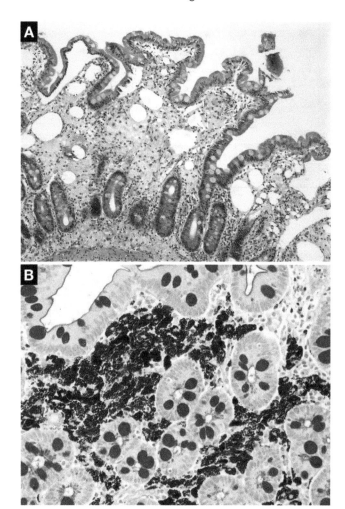

Figure 8.4. Histopathologic Features of Whipple Disease. A, The villi are widened (hematoxylin-eosin). B, The villi are filled with foamy macrophages that are periodic acid-Schiff–positive.

serum eosinophil count in patients with serosal disease. However, a normal serum eosinophil count does not exclude eosinophilic gastroenteritis. With the mucosal form of the disease, the diagnosis is established with intestinal biopsy specimens that show more than 20 to 25 eosinophils per high-power field. With muscular or serosal involvement, full-thickness biopsy may be required. Eosinophilia found on ascitic fluid analysis also can be suggestive. Parasitic infections need to be ruled out before eosinophilic gastroenteritis is diagnosed. Also, eosinophilic gastroenteritis needs to be differentiated from hypereosinophilic syndrome, which is characterized by a serum eosinophil count greater than 1.5×10^9/L for more than 6 months and multiorgan involvement.

An elimination diet may be incorporated in the treatment program for eosinophilic gastroenteritis, although it has a limited role. Prednisone, 20 to 40 mg orally daily, often produces a prompt clinical response, regardless of the layer of bowel involved. Treatment with mast cell stabilizers, such as sodium cromoglycate, and leukotriene receptor antagonists, such as montelukast, has had variable success. Open-capsule budesonide can be given in place of prednisone to patients who require ongoing maintenance therapy. The monoclonal antibody omalizumab has also been used.

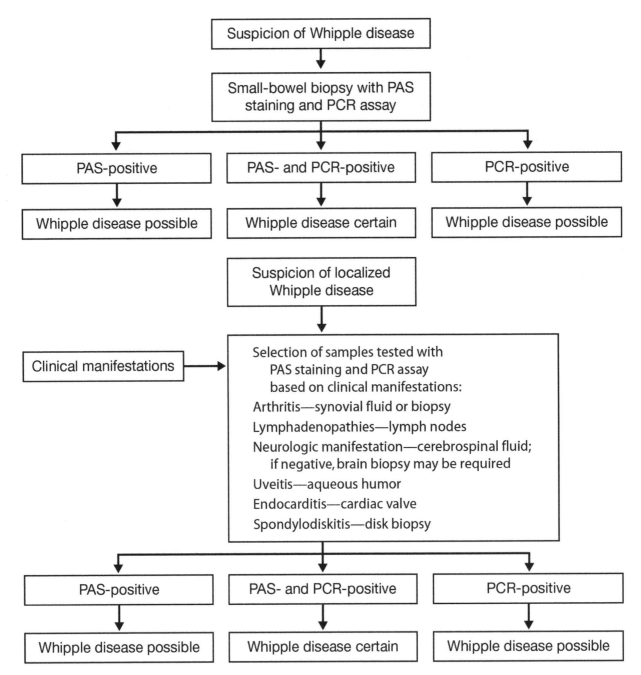

Figure 8.5   Strategy for Diagnosing Whipple Disease With Use of Periodic Acid-Schiff (PAS) Staining and Polymerase Chain Reaction (PCR) Assay. (Adapted from Fenollar F, Puechal X, Raoult D. Whipple's disease. N Engl J Med. 2007 Jan 4;356[1]:55-66; used with permission.)

✓ Eosinophilic gastroenteritis—clinical manifestations vary depending on whether involvement is mucosal, muscular, or serosal
✓ Eosinophilic gastroenteritis—parasitic infection must be ruled out

---

Intestinal Lymphangiectasia

Intestinal lymphangiectasia occurs as either a primary form or a secondary form. *Primary lymphangiectasia* is characterized by diffuse or localized ectasia of the enteric lymphatic system and often is diagnosed at a young age. *Secondary lymphangiectasia* occurs with conditions that produce impaired lymphatic flow; the causes are cardiac (congestive heart failure or constriction), neoplastic (lymphoma), or structural (retroperitoneal fibrosis).

Patients present with pronounced edema, diarrhea, nausea, and vomiting; also, chylothorax and chylous ascites may be present. Steatorrhea may be concurrent with a protein-losing enteropathy. Laboratory findings include a decrease in the plasma level of proteins and lymphocytopenia, which may affect cellular immunity. Endoscopically, punctate white dots may be seen on the bowel mucosa; histologic examination shows marked dilatation of the lacteals (Figure 8.6). Abnormalities of the lymphatics may also be assessed with contrast lymphangiography or nuclear scintigraphy after a high-fat load. The protein-losing state can be verified with an α_1-antitrypsin clearance test (described above).

Treatment of the primary form includes a low-fat, high-protein diet and supplementation with medium-chain triglycerides as needed. If the disease is localized, resection could be considered.

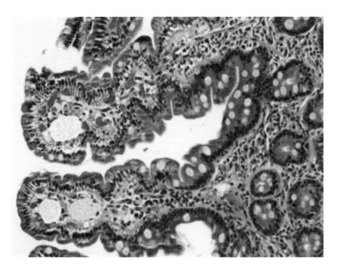

Figure 8.6.   Lymphangiectasia. Dilated lacteals are in several contiguous villi (hematoxylin-eosin).

Treatment of the secondary form should be directed at the underlying disease process.

Amyloidosis

Amyloidosis is a multisystem disease that frequently involves the gastrointestinal tract. Amyloid deposits can be found at various levels of the bowel wall, although they usually are detected in the submucosa. Amyloid also can be deposited in neuromuscular or perivascular sites. Patients with amyloidosis may have diarrhea for many reasons. Delayed transit related to autonomic neuropathy may lead to SIBO; accelerated transit related to autonomic neuropathy may lead to bile acid malabsorption. Also, the amyloid deposits may act as a barrier that prevents proper absorption; patients can have a combination of fat, protein, or carbohydrate malabsorption. They commonly have lactose malabsorption. Endoscopic findings in amyloidosis include granularity, friability, and erosions, but they are often normal. The yield of detecting amyloidosis involvement of the gastrointestinal tract depends on the site from which biopsy samples are obtained: esophagus, 70%; stomach, 75% to 95%; small intestine, 85% to 100%; and colorectum, 75% to 95%. A fat aspirate can be obtained for diagnostic purposes, but this may have a lower yield than intestinal biopsies if there is clinical suggestion of involvement of the gastrointestinal tract. Congo red staining can show apple-green birefringence, which is seen best in the walls of the vasculature if the biopsy specimens contain lamina propria. Treatment of amyloidosis involvement of the gastrointestinal tract includes treating the underlying disease, but treatment of SIBO and lactose avoidance should be considered.

✓ If a patient is suspected to have bowel involvement with amyloid, the greatest yields are from biopsies from the small bowel or colorectum

Other Conditions

Scleroderma

Patients with systemic scleroderma may have diarrhea and malabsorption from gastrointestinal disease. The diarrhea may be due to ineffectual motility, which may lead to SIBO. Patients

may also have small-bowel diverticulosis, another risk factor for SIBO. Also, chronic intestinal pseudo-obstruction may occur with systemic scleroderma. In addition, diarrhea may occur from decreased mucosal blood flow due to vasospasm, or diarrhea may result from lactose malabsorption. Treatment of diarrhea in patients with scleroderma includes antibiotics for SIBO and a lactose-restricted diet, as indicated. Treatment with low-dose octreotide, 50 µg at bedtime, could be considered because it can help stimulate intestinal motility and improve symptoms; however, octreotide can be prohibitively expensive.

Diabetes

Patients with diabetes may present with diarrhea or malabsorption (or both) for various reasons: 1) Several oral hypoglycemic agents, such as metformin and acarbose, are associated with diarrhea; the relation between the initiation of treatment with these medications and the onset of diarrhea needs to be determined. 2) Delayed intestinal transit in patients with diabetes puts them at risk for SIBO. 3) Because of the increased prevalence of celiac disease among patients with type 1 diabetes, celiac disease needs to be considered. 4) Pancreatic insufficiency needs to be considered because it may explain not only the diarrhea but also the hyperglycemia. 5) Patients with diabetes may ingest a considerable amount of sugar-free substances for better glycemic control; these substances often contain sorbitol, xylitol, or other sugar alcohols that may induce osmotic diarrhea. 6) In patients who have diabetes with end-organ involvement, an autonomic neuropathy may develop that will affect the gastrointestinal tract and lead to "diabetic diarrhea," for which clonidine therapy may be helpful if the patient does not have orthostatism.

Hospitalized Patients

New diarrhea or malabsorption in hospitalized patients has a broad differential diagnosis that includes the following causes: antibiotics, *Clostridium difficile* infection, tube feedings (based on the location of the tube in the bowel, concentration of the formula, and bolus effect of the nutrition), elixir medications (that contain sorbitol), magnesium (as in antacids and magnesium replacement or supplementation), intestinal ischemia (especially in critically ill patients), and fecal impaction with secondary overflow. Also, use of any new medication that was started during the hospitalization should be scrutinized as a cause of new-onset diarrhea. Diarrhea that is long-standing or was present before hospitalization requires diagnostic evaluation for chronic diarrhea (which can be done in the outpatient setting).

Miscellaneous

Many other conditions are associated with diarrhea, malabsorption, and mucosal disease of the small bowel but cannot be considered in detail here. Conditions to review include immunodeficiencies (IgA deficiency, combined variable immunodeficiency, and graft-vs-host disease), autoimmune enteropathy, collagen vascular diseases and vasculitides, radiation enteritis, ischemia, mastocytosis, abetalipoproteinemia, and endocrinopathies (thyroid and adrenal).

Bacterial Overgrowth Syndromes

Normally, the small-bowel flora contains a relatively small number of bacteria ($<10^3$ organisms/mL), with a predominance of gram-positive organisms. In contrast, the colonic flora has a

Table 8.5. Risk Factors for Small Intestinal Bacterial Overgrowth

Category	Risk factor
Structural	Small-bowel diverticula
	Intestinal strictures (Crohn disease, radiation, NSAIDs)
	Enterocolonic fistula
Surgical	Blind loops, afferent limbs
	Ileocecal valve resection
Dysmotility	Chronic intestinal pseudo-obstruction
	Scleroderma
	Gastroparesis
	Diabetic autonomic neuropathy
Diminished acid	Achlorhydria, gastric atrophy
	Gastric resection
	Acid suppression (PPI therapy)
Others	Cirrhosis
	Pancreatitis
	Immunodeficiencies
	Celiac disease
	Advanced age
	Idiopathic

Abbreviations: NSAID, nonsteroidal anti-inflammatory drug; PPI, proton pump inhibitor.

Adapted from Dukowicz AC, Lacy BE, Levine GM. Small intestinal bacterial overgrowth: a comprehensive review. Gastroenterol Hepatol (NY). 2007 Feb;3(2):112-22; used with permission.

significantly higher concentration of bacteria, which are largely gram-negative and anaerobic organisms. When there is stasis, altered motility, or loss of protective defenses in the proximal intestinal tract, bacteria that are more representative of colonic flora can overgrow in the small bowel and result in SIBO, a syndrome of diarrhea and nutritional deficiencies.

The many risk factors for SIBO are listed in Table 8.5; the principal causes are associated with stasis of small-bowel contents or loss of protective gastric acid. Structural or surgical changes in the bowel that produce relative stasis or reflux of colonic flora into the small bowel can be obtained from the history and radiographic imaging of the small bowel. Any motility disorder that affects the small bowel (scleroderma, diabetes, or pseudo-obstruction) can lead to stasis and overgrowth. Gastric acid is thought to be a protective barrier that keeps pathogenic bacteria out of the small intestine; when there is loss of gastric acid, SIBO may ensue. Advanced age alone may be a factor. In many patients, no discrete risk factor is identified.

Symptoms of SIBO include abdominal pain, bloating, flatulence, diarrhea, and weight loss. Malabsorption of fat, protein, or carbohydrates (or a combination of these) can occur with secondary diarrhea. Fat malabsorption results from bacterial deconjugation of bile salts and leads to steatorrhea. Carbohydrate malabsorption can occur because of early sugar breakdown and fermentation from bacteria as well as from decreased disaccharidase activity caused by mucosal damage and bacterial by-products. Mucosal damage is thought to have a role in protein malabsorption because of the effect on oligopeptidase levels.

A classic pattern of laboratory findings in SIBO includes a low serum level of vitamin B_{12} and an increased serum level of folate. The low level of vitamin B_{12} is the result of bacteria cleaving vitamin B_{12} prematurely from intrinsic factor and from the competitive binding and consumption of vitamin B_{12} by anaerobic bacteria. The increased serum level of folate is the result of folate synthesis by the intestinal bacteria. In addition to the

above laboratory findings, serum levels of iron, protein, albumin, and fat-soluble vitamins may be low, depending on the degree of malabsorption.

The reference standard for making the diagnosis of SIBO is small-bowel cultures from direct aspiration of the jejunum, with more than 10^5 organisms/mL of aerobes and anaerobes being diagnostic. Limitations of small-bowel cultures include availability,

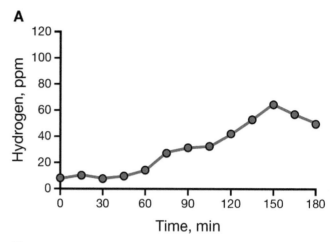

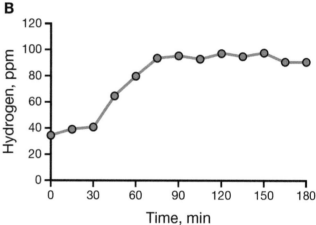

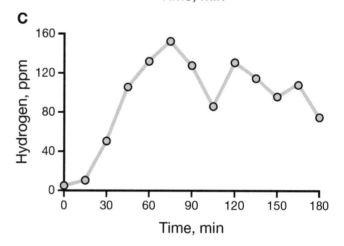

Figure 8.7. Breath Testing Patterns for Small Intestinal Bacterial Overgrowth. A, Lactulose breath test without bacterial overgrowth. B, Lactulose breath test with bacterial overgrowth. C, Lactulose breath test showing double-peak pattern. (Adapted from Dukowicz AC, Lacy BE, Levine GM. Small intestinal bacterial overgrowth: a comprehensive review. Gastroenterol Hepatol [NY]. 2007 Feb;3[2]:112-22; used with permission.)

lack of excess intestinal secretions for aspiration, recent antibiotic therapy, and decreased or no reimbursement for the test.

Breath testing can also be used to diagnose SIBO. The test involves giving an oral load of substrate (lactulose hydrogen, glucose hydrogen, or ^{14}C-xylose) and then measuring the breath hydrogen concentration every 15 to 30 minutes for 2 to 4 hours. Either glucose or lactulose hydrogen breath testing can be safely performed in children or pregnant women. A diagnosis of SIBO is supported by an increase of more than 12 ppm above baseline for glucose or 20 ppm above baseline for lactulose during the first 90 minutes. An increase is seen again as these substances reach the colon, thus producing a double-peak pattern that can also be used as a criterion for diagnosis (Figure 8.7). Breath testing for SIBO is not without challenges. False-positive results of breath testing can occur from rapid intestinal transit, in which the carbohydrate substance rapidly reaches the colon and produces an early but not double-peaked pattern. False-negative results of breath testing can occur from recent antibiotic therapy. Also, the results are falsely negative in 20% of the population who have methanogenic colonic bacteria; for those patients, breath methane levels rather than hydrogen levels can be checked. Breath testing results also can be affected by recent laxative use, high carbohydrate consumption, recent intense physical activity, and smoking.

Once SIBO is diagnosed on the basis of cultures or breath testing, evaluating for predisposing conditions could be considered. Also, an empirical trial of antibiotics could be considered for patients in whom testing for SIBO may not be available or may lead to inaccurate results.

Treatment of SIBO lies in managing the symptoms and replacing the deficiencies. Although modifying the underlying risk factor that predisposes to SIBO is feasible in only a small fraction of patients, it should be considered (tighter glycemic control in patients with diabetes, surgery for patients with stricturing disease, and possibly octreotide for patients with scleroderma). Vitamin and mineral levels should be measured and deficiencies corrected before irreversible sequelae ensue (eg, as with vitamin B$_{12}$ deficiency). The role of antibiotic therapy is not to sterilize the small bowel but rather to decrease and modify the bacterial makeup so that it more closely resembles the flora that should be present in the small intestine, with therapy targeting gram-negative and anaerobic organisms. Various antibiotics have been used, such as amoxicillin-clavulanate, fluoroquinolones, rifaximin, tetracycline derivatives, and metronidazole. Initial treatment may consist of 10 to 14 days of an antibiotic, with repeated shorter courses when symptoms recur. Some patients may need monthly rotation of antibiotic therapy, while others may not require retreatment for many months. Also, modified lactose intake should be considered in those with ongoing symptoms after antibiotic therapy, given the damaging effects that can be seen on the small-bowel microvilli due to SIBO.

✓ Among the many potential risk factors for small intestinal bacterial overgrowth (SIBO), the most common are stasis due to anatomical changes or altered motility
✓ SIBO may lead to low vitamin B$_{12}$ and high serum folate levels
✓ Breath testing for SIBO is fraught with the risk of both false-positive and false-negative results

---

Suggested Reading

Bushyhead D, Quigley EM. Small intestinal bacterial overgrowth. Gastroenterol Clin North Am. 2021 Jun;50(2):463–74.

Camilleri M, Nurko S. Bile acid diarrhea in adults and adolescents. Neurogastroenterol Motil. 2022 Apr;34(4):e14287.

Elli L, Topa M, Rimondi A. Protein-losing enteropathy. Curr Opin Gastroenterol. 2020 May;36(3):238–44.

Havlichek D, 3rd, Choung RS, Murray JA. Eosinophilic gastroenteritis: using presenting findings to predict disease course. Clin Transl Gastroenterol. 2021 Oct;12(10):e00394.

Kamboj AK, Oxentenko AS. Clinical and histologic mimickers of celiac disease. Clin Transl Gastroenterol. 2017 Aug;8(8):e114.

Marth T, Moos V, Muller C, Biagi F, Schneider T. Tropheryma whipplei infection and Whipple's disease. Lancet Infect Dis. 2016 Mar;16(3):e13–22.

Massironi S, Cavalcoli F, Rausa E, Invernizzi P, Braga M, Vecchi M. Understanding short bowel syndrome: Current status and future perspectives. Dig Liver Dis. 2020 Mar;52(3):253–61.

Oxentenko AS, Murray JA. Celiac disease: Ten things that every gastroenterologist should know. Clin Gastroenterol Hepatol. 2015 Aug;13(8):1396–404.

Sharma P, Baloda V, Gahlot GP, Singh A, Mehta R, Vishnubathla S, et al. Clinical, endoscopic, and histological differentiation between celiac disease and tropical sprue: A systematic review. J Gastroenterol Hepatol. 2019 Jan;34(1):74–83.

9

Nutritional Disorders: Vitamins and Minerals[a]
AMINDRA S. ARORA, MB, BCHIR

Vitamins and minerals are critical for normal health because they are essential in a vast assortment of metabolic functions. This chapter focuses on selected important vitamins and minerals and their relationships with gastrointestinal tract disorders.

Water-Soluble Vitamins

Vitamin B_{12}

Dietary intake of vitamin B_{12} (cobalamin) requires the ingestion of animal products (meat, dairy, fish, and shellfish). As cobalamin is bound to animal proteins, it is released in the stomach by a combination of gastric contractions, gastric acid, and pepsins. Free vitamin B_{12} then binds to salivary and gastric R proteins (also called haptocorrins), a process that is facilitated by the acidic gastric pH. The production and secretion of intrinsic factor by gastric parietal cells is critical for the binding of cobalamin from haptocorrins, which occurs in the duodenum and is facilitated by both the neutral pH and the pancreatic proteases. Finally, in the terminal ileum, the cobalamin–intrinsic factor complex is bound to specific receptors and vitamin B_{12} is absorbed into the circulation, where it binds to transcobalamin II. About half the circulating vitamin B_{12} in cobalamin–transcobalamin II is secreted into bile, of which half is recycled and the other half is excreted in stool. Cobalamin in bile is bound to a biliary haptocorrin, and this binding protein is then degraded by pancreatic proteases in the duodenum, once again liberating vitamin B_{12} for its binding to intrinsic factor. In healthy persons, overall about 70% of ingested cobalamin is absorbed.

Deficiency of vitamin B_{12}, like folic acid deficiency, results in megaloblastic anemia and hyperhomocysteinemia. However, in contrast to folic acid deficiency, vitamin B_{12} deficiency can cause neuropsychiatric abnormalities, including dementia, and disorders such as ataxia, paresthesia, chorea, dystonia, subacute combined degeneration of the posterior columns of the spinal cord (ie, loss of lower extremity vibratory and sometimes proprioceptive sensation), and loss of taste sensation. Both vitamin B_{12} deficiency and folate deficiency can cause glossitis, anorexia, and diarrhea.

Serum methylmalonic acid levels (which are normal in folic acid deficiency) may be abnormally increased before vitamin B_{12} levels are subnormal. Because large amounts of cobalamin (2.0-2.5 mg) are stored in the body, especially in the liver, the lack of adequate dietary vitamin B_{12} (eg, in a person who is a true vegan and does not take supplements) may take several years to cause cobalamin deficiency.

Achlorhydria is a common cause of vitamin B_{12} deficiency in elderly persons. Pernicious anemia causes vitamin B_{12} deficiency from the lack of intrinsic factor and gastric acid. In contrast to achlorhydria, hyperacidity (as in Zollinger-Ellison syndrome) can disrupt the duodenal phase of cobalamin absorption (by acidification of duodenal contents causing inactivation of pancreatic proteases) and result in cobalamin deficiency. Vitamin B_{12} deficiency rarely occurs with pancreatic insufficiency itself or with long-term treatment with acid-suppressive medications. Bacterial overgrowth, infestation with *Diphyllobothrium latum*, and ileal disease (Crohn disease and radiation enteritis) or resection also can result in vitamin B_{12} deficiency. Gastric bypass surgery is often complicated by subsequent cobalamin deficiency (lack of intrinsic factor, acid, and gastric grinding). Chronic use of the antidiabetic agents metformin and phenformin can decrease absorption of cobalamin, resulting in vitamin B_{12} deficiency.

[a] The author thanks Stephen C. Hauser, MD, who authored previous versions of this chapter.

Cobalamin deficiency, especially that due to pernicious anemia, gastrectomy, or ileal disease, generally is treated with parenteral cobalamin (1 mg daily for a week, then once weekly for a few weeks, and then once monthly). The use of high doses of oral cobalamin (1-2 mg daily) has a role in patients after cobalamin stores have been repleted or as initial therapy for persons who have a residual ability to absorb cobalamin and a mild cobalamin deficiency.

Folic Acid

Folic acid (vitamin B_9) has many dietary sources, including green leafy vegetables, grains, orange juice, and organ meats. Pregnant and lactating patients need higher daily doses than others. Unlike the body stores of vitamin B_{12}, those of folate are small, so deficiency can occur within a few months when intake is poor or absent. After brush border membrane hydrolysis of dietary folylpolyglutamates, active transport of folylmonoglutamates occurs, principally in the duodenum and upper jejunum.

Folic acid deficiency may lead to megaloblastic anemia, diarrhea (macrocytic enterocytes), glossitis, neural tube defects in newborns (maternal folic acid deficiency in the first 2 weeks of pregnancy), and increased risk of colorectal cancer and cardiovascular disease. The following increase a person's risk for folic acid deficiency: dietary deficiency of folic acid (body stores may last up to 4 months); gastric bypass surgery; small bowel malabsorption states; use of drugs such as sulfasalazine, phenytoin, methotrexate, and alcohol; pregnancy; lactation; chronic hemolytic anemia; and hemodialysis.

Folic acid by mouth, 1 to 5 mg daily, should be given for several weeks to persons with folic acid deficiency. Cobalamin deficiency needs to be ruled out or treated before folic acid therapy is begun.

Other Water-Soluble Vitamins

Vitamin C

Vitamin C deficiency results in scurvy due to decreased collagen synthesis. Clinical features may include perifollicular hyperkeratotic papules and petechiae; swollen, red, bleeding gums; or anemia. Severe malabsorptive disease and alcohol use disorder increase the risk of vitamin C deficiency, especially if the diet includes few fruits and vegetables. Vitamin C supplementation enhances iron absorption and can increase the risk of adverse cardiac arrhythmias in those with iron overload conditions. Supplementation with more than 250 mg daily of vitamin C also can produce false-negative results on fecal occult blood tests and increase the risk of oxalate kidney stones in persons with chronic kidney disease.

Thiamine (Vitamin B₁)

Thiamine (vitamin B_1) is involved in the decarboxylation of pyruvate, which is important in the citric acid cycle. It is found in yeast, cereals from whole grains, brown rice, and pork. Deficiency can result in wet beriberi with cardiac abnormalities (cardiomyopathy and high-output failure) or dry beriberi with neurologic disorders (peripheral neuropathy, cerebellar dysfunction, gaze pareses, or Wernicke-Korsakoff syndrome), which may be exacerbated by the administration of glucose to patients who are deficient in thiamine. Chronic alcohol use disorder, overuse of diuretics, long-term kidney dialysis, pregnancy, malabsorptive disorders (including gastric bypass surgery), and chronic malnutrition all are risk factors for thiamine deficiency. Thiamine has a relatively

short half-life, and storage in the body is limited, so deficiencies can occur quickly when oral intake is decreased.

Riboflavin (Vitamin B₂)

Riboflavin (vitamin B_2) deficiency can cause angular stomatitis, cheilosis, glossitis, seborrheic dermatitis, peripheral neuropathy, and impaired vision. Risk factors for deficiency include chronic alcohol use disorder and malabsorptive disorders. Riboflavin is found in many foods, including fortified cereals, milk, and eggs.

Niacin (Vitamin B₃)

Niacin (vitamin B_3) deficiency can occur as a result of malabsorptive syndromes, gastric bypass, chronic alcohol use disorder, carcinoid syndrome, or drug therapy (isoniazid, 6-mercaptopurine, or azathioprine). Persons with a niacin deficiency can have pellagra (diarrhea, dermatitis, and dementia occasionally resulting in death), glossitis, cheilosis, dyssebacia, and angular stomatitis. Excess niacin therapy for hyperlipidemia treatment (such as crystalline nicotinic acid) can cause flushing, nausea, diarrhea, and occasionally hepatocellular injury. Sources of niacin include tryptophan, fortified cereals, legumes, and fish.

Pyridoxine (Vitamin B₆)

Pyridoxine (vitamin B_6) deficiency is uncommon but can occur in patients receiving isoniazid, cycloserine, hydralazine, oral contraceptives, dopamine, or D-penicillamine, which directly interfere with vitamin B_6 metabolism. Malabsorptive syndromes and chronic alcohol use disorder also are risk factors. Manifestations include cheilosis, angular stomatitis, seborrheic dermatitis, sideroblastic anemia, seizures, and peripheral neuropathy. Vitamin B_6 deficiency may be responsible for both the limited increase in aminotransferase values and the increased ratio of aspartate aminotransferase to alanine aminotransferase in alcoholic hepatitis. Pyridoxine occurs in meat, fish, fortified cereals, and noncitrus fruit. Massive doses may cause sensory neuropathy.

Biotin

Although biotin deficiency is rare, it can occur in patients receiving total parenteral nutrition without biotin supplementation. They may have altered mental status, metabolic acidosis, and seborrheic dermatitis.

Fat-Soluble Vitamins

Vitamin A

As with other fat-soluble vitamins, the absorption of vitamin A requires luminal bile salts and pancreatic esterases, assembly into chylomicrons, and lymphatic transport. Lack of vitamin A can produce night blindness, xerophthalmia, a follicular hyperkeratotic rash, abnormalities of taste and smell, bone and muscle pain, and increased risk of infections. Deficiency of vitamin A can occur after bariatric surgery and in persons with chronic liver disease. Similar to other fat-soluble vitamins, excess vitamin A can cause toxicity (liver failure, increased cerebrospinal fluid pressure, desquamating rash, alopecia, or hypercalcemia).

Vitamin D

Adequate vitamin D levels are achieved mainly through exposure to sunlight. Few foods contain vitamin D, so they need to be fortified. Risk factors for vitamin D deficiency, in addition to lack of sunlight, are liver disease, kidney disease, and malabsorptive conditions. Hypercalcemia from excess vitamin D can result in anorexia, nausea, vomiting, constipation, confusion, and abdominal pain (from hypercalcemia). In addition, polyuria and kidney stones (from hypercalciuria) can occur. Vitamin D deficiency results in rickets and osteomalacia and may be associated with osteoporosis.

Vitamin E

Malabsorptive disorders and particularly chronic cholestasis in children are major risk factors for vitamin E deficiency. Manifestations of vitamin E deficiency include neurologic symptoms (posterior column disease, peripheral neuropathy, and brainstem and cranial nerve damage), retinal disease, and hemolysis. High doses of vitamin E may cause coagulation disorders.

Vitamin K

Vitamin K is acquired from exogenous dietary sources (green leafy vegetables) and endogenous sources (intestinal bacteria). Malabsorptive syndromes, dietary inadequacy, and antibiotic administration are risk factors for vitamin K deficiency. Factor VII usually is the rate-limiting factor for normal prothrombin time (or the international normalized ratio). Excessive doses of vitamin E can interfere with vitamin K–dependent metabolism, resulting in hemorrhage.

Minerals

Iron

Loss of endogenous iron from the gastrointestinal tract (usually 1.0-2.0 mg daily), urinary tract, and skin and menstrual loss in women needs to be matched by iron absorption from the duodenum and upper jejunum. Iron in the form of heme from meat is absorbed more readily (up to 25%) than inorganic ferric iron salts (3%-10%). Gastric grinding, gastric acid, and vitamin C help make ferric iron compounds more soluble. Ferric reductase (duodenal cytochrome B) on the brush border and ascorbate reduce inorganic iron from the ferric form (Fe^{3+}) to the ferrous form (Fe^{2+}). An iron transporter, divalent metal transporter 1, also on the brush border, facilitates the absorption of ferrous iron. This same transporter can also facilitate the absorption of divalent copper, zinc, lead, and manganese, each of which can compete with and inhibit the absorption of divalent iron.

Ferroportin 1 along with ferroxidase hephaestin (both located on the basolateral membrane) transports iron into the circulation, oxidizes it to the ferric form, and allows it to bind to apotransferrin, forming transferrin. The liver produces hepcidin, which regulates iron transport through its interactions with ferroportin 1, decreasing iron absorption. The basolateral membrane transferrin receptor, regulated by the hemochromatosis gene *HFE*, allows intestinal cell reuptake of iron from transferrin. Normally, with adequate total body iron stores, up to about 10% of dietary inorganic iron can be absorbed. With iron deficiency, this may increase to 30%.

Iron deficiency can result in microcytic hypochromic anemia, altered immune function, angular stomatitis, koilonychia, and atrophic lingual papillae. Causes of iron deficiency include lack of dietary iron, increased gastrointestinal loss of iron (bleeding), poor absorption of iron (celiac disease), surgical procedures that bypass the duodenum, achlorhydria, and *Helicobacter pylori*

infection. (Iron overload is discussed in Chapter 30, "Metabolic Liver Diseases.")

Zinc

Zinc is required as a cofactor for many enzymes (eg, alkaline phosphatase), and its deficiency impairs growth, development, and reproductive and immune functions. Meat and seafood are good sources. Risk factors for zinc deficiency are chronic diarrhea, short bowel syndrome, cystic fibrosis, pancreatic insufficiency, cirrhosis, alcohol use disorder, chronic kidney failure, anorexia nervosa, pregnancy, sickle cell anemia, and use of the drug D-penicillamine. A scaly red rash involving the face, groin, and hands may occur with zinc deficiency. Acrodermatitis enteropathica is an autosomal recessive condition with impaired zinc absorption. Other manifestations of zinc deficiency include alopecia, dysgeusia, growth retardation, poor wound healing, hypogonadism, diarrhea, and night blindness. Excess zinc intake (eg, supplements such as those used to treat Wilson disease) can cause copper deficiency.

Copper

Copper is present in meat, nuts, and grains. Copper deficiency can occur after gastrectomy or gastric bypass, celiac disease, and excessive zinc ingestion. Deficiency results in a microcytic hypochromic anemia, leukopenia, neutropenia, infections, diarrhea, neurologic disturbances mimicking vitamin B_{12} deficiency, hypopigmentation of the skin and hair, and bony changes. Toxicity from excess administration of oral copper includes acute hemorrhagic gastritis.

Phosphorus

Phosphorus deficiency is common in patients with malnutrition, malabsorptive disorders, and alcohol use disorder and in refeeding syndrome. Cardiac failure, hemolytic anemia, rhabdomyolysis, acidosis, and encephalopathy may develop with phosphorus deficiency.

Miscellaneous Minerals

Deficiencies of selenium (cardiomyopathy and myositis), chromium (hyperglycemia and neurologic symptoms), manganese (very rare, with nonspecific features), or molybdenum (neurologic symptoms) may develop in patients receiving long-term total parenteral nutrition or tube feeding without proper supplementation. Manganese excess may occur in patients who are oversupplemented with parenteral nutrition; they may present with headache, vomiting, and parkinsonian-like symptoms due to the effects on the basal ganglia.

Bariatric Surgery

Metabolic complications should be anticipated after bariatric surgery. Protein malnutrition or zinc deficiency can cause hair loss. Deficiencies of vitamins D, A, E, and B_{12} and thiamine, folate, iron, and copper may occur if supplementation and monitoring are deficient.

Suggested Reading

Buchman AL, Howard LJ, Guenter P, Nishikawa RA, Compher CW, Tappenden KA. Micronutrients in parenteral nutrition: too little or too much? The past, present, and recommendations for the future. Gastroenterology. 2009 Nov;137(5 Suppl):S1–6.

Khambatta S, Nguyen DL, Wittich CM. 38-Year-old woman with increasing fatigue and dyspnea. Mayo Clin Proc. 2010 Apr;85(4): 392–5.

Koch TR, Finelli FC. Postoperative metabolic and nutritional complications of bariatric surgery. Gastroenterol Clin North Am. 2010 Mar;39(1):109–24.

Merriman NA, Putt ME, Metz DC, Yang YX. Hip fracture risk in patients with a diagnosis of pernicious anemia. Gastroenterology. 2010 Apr;138(4):1330–7.

O'Donnell K. Severe micronutrient deficiencies in RYGB patients: rare but potentially devastating. Pract Gastroenterol. 2011;35(11):13–27.

Puig A, Mino-Kenudson M, Dighe AS. Case records of the Massachusetts General Hospital: case 13–2012: a 62-year-old man with paresthesias, weight loss, jaundice, and anemia. N Engl J Med. 2012 Apr;366(17):1626–33.

Stabler SP. Clinical practice: vitamin B12 deficiency. N Engl J Med. 2013 Jan;368(2):149–60.

Thacher TD, Clarke BL. Vitamin D insufficiency. Mayo Clin Proc. 2011 Jan;86(1):50–60.

Questions and Answers

Questions

Abbreviations used:

EATL,	enteropathy-associated T-cell lymphoma
EMA,	endomysial antibody
Ig,	immunoglobulin
MAC,	*Mycobacterium avium-intracellulare* complex
MCV,	mean corpuscular volume
PAS,	periodic acid–Schiff
PCR,	polymerase chain reaction
tTG,	tissue transglutaminase

Multiple Choice (choose the best answer)

III.1. A 27-year-old woman has a 1-year history of diarrhea and weight loss of 4.5 kg. She has not had fever, abdominal pain, or melena, and she has not traveled outside the US. She takes no medications. Laboratory results include the following: hemoglobin, 11.2 g/dL; MCV, 74 fL; and serum ferritin, 8 ng/mL. Which of the following antibody tests should be performed next?

a. IgA gliadin
b. IgA tTg
c. IgA and IgG deamidated gliadin peptide
d. IgA anti-EMA

III.2. A 32-year-old woman with celiac disease presents with recurrent diarrhea and weight loss. Celiac disease was diagnosed 4 years earlier when she had similar symptoms. At that time, testing showed an increased level of tTG, and biopsy findings were compatible with celiac disease. She initially had a good response to a gluten-free diet, and the tTG and biopsy results were normal. For the past several months, she has had recurrent symptoms. She says that her oral intake has not changed. Recently she moved and started a new job. When the tTG level is checked, it is high. Which of the following is the most likely?

a. Microscopic colitis
b. EATL
c. Gluten ingestion
d. Refractory celiac disease

III.3. A 72-year-old woman presents for evaluation of chronic diarrhea that has been present for 2 years. When she underwent a complete evaluation for diarrhea, results were negative for C-reactive protein and celiac serology, thyroid function results were normal, and findings were normal from random colonic biopsies. Small-bowel biopsy samples showed features consistent with celiac disease, but the patient has had no improvement while consuming a gluten-free diet. Her past medical history is notable for osteoporosis, hypertension, impaired fasting glucose, and mild depression; she has received therapy for all those. Which is the most likely to cause this presentation?

a. Metformin
b. Alendronate
c. Fluoxetine
d. Olmesartan

III.4. A 57-year-old farmer presents for evaluation of diarrhea and cognitive changes. Results for celiac serology are negative, and findings from colonoscopy with biopsies are unremarkable. Biopsy findings from the small intestine show broad villi with patchy atrophy. The biopsy samples stain positive with PAS and are acid-fast negative. Which of the following is the most likely diagnosis?

a. Whipple disease
b. Celiac disease
c. MAC infection
d. Tropical sprue

III.5. A 45-year-old woman is undergoing an evaluation for fatigue. Results of a 25-hydroxyvitamin D₂ and D₃ test were 11 ng/mL. She is interested in pursuing a "natural" way to supplement vitamin D. Which of the following would provide the most vitamin D?

a. Cheese
b. UV-A
c. UV-B
d. Carrots
e. Eggs

III.6. A 32-year-old professional body builder has been taking natural supplements daily for the past 12 years and presents with hematemesis and headache. He is hypotensive. Test results were hemoglobin, 7.1 g/dL, and platelet count, 88×10⁹/L. Varices were apparent on endoscopic examination. Which of the following supplements was the patient most likely taking in excess?

a. Selenium
b. Protein
c. Anabolic steroids
d. Vitamin A
e. Vitamin D

III.7. A 57-year-old woman is evaluated for confusion that has been progressively worsening over the past 6 months. Her only medication is thyroid replacement for a history of Hashimoto thyroiditis. On examination, she has vitiligo. On neurologic evaluation, her ankle and knee show hyperreflexia. Which of the following blood concentrations should be tested?

a. Ferritin
b. Vitamin A
c. Vitamin D
d. Vitamin B₁₂
e. Vitamin E

III.8. A 57-year-old woman presents with general fatigue. She has a history of atrophic gastritis and receives vitamin B₁₂ supplementation. On physical examination she has some conjunctival pallor, but findings are otherwise normal. What is the most likely cause of her symptoms?

a. Insufficient vitamin B₁₂ supplementation
b. Copper deficiency
c. Thiamine deficiency
d. Iron deficiency

Answers

III.1. Answer b.
The serologic test of choice to screen for celiac disease is IgA tTG antibody. This patient has a high probability of celiac disease given that she has diarrhea, weight loss, and iron deficiency anemia, all of which are characteristic of celiac disease. It would be prudent to start with celiac serology, but because the likelihood of disease is so strong for this patient, she would also need to have small-bowel biopsies even if the celiac serology were negative.

III.2. Answer c.
Ingestion of gluten, which may be inadvertent, is the most common reason a patient with celiac disease lacks a response to a gluten-free diet or has a recurrence of symptoms while eating a gluten-free diet. Abnormally high results for celiac serology also

indicate the presence of gluten in the diet. Microscopic colitis and refractory celiac disease can occur in patients with celiac disease, but gluten ingestion would be more likely given the high tTG results. Although patients with celiac disease are at increased risk for EATL, it is rare.

III.3. Answer d.
Olmesartan, an angiotensin-receptor blocker, has been reported to cause a small-bowel enteropathy that appears identical to celiac disease. The drug should be considered a possible factor if patients are receiving it and have a serologically negative enteropathy. Patients may receive the medication for years before they present with symptoms, but discontinuation of the drug results in marked improvement in symptoms and is often all that is needed. Other medications that can result in enteropathy include mycophenolate mofetil and checkpoint inhibitors. Metformin can cause diarrhea, and selective serotonin reuptake inhibitors (eg, fluoxetine) have been associated with microscopic colitis, but none of the answer choices besides olmesartan have been known to cause an enteropathy.

III.4. Answer a.
Both *Tropheryma whipplei* and MAC can infect the small bowel and cause macrophages to stain positive with PAS. However, acid-fast staining of biopsy samples will be positive if patients have MAC infection and negative if patients have Whipple disease. PCR for *T whipplei* is useful for confirmation of Whipple disease, which is rare but most often occurs in men in this age group who present with features of multisystem disease.

III.5. Answer c.
Sunshine is 95% UV-A and 5% UV-B. Only UV-B is required for vitamin D synthesis. In commercial tanning salons, UV-A is the major light source, and the exposure doses are considerably higher than those provided by the sun. Both UV-A and UV-B are implicated in skin damage and carcinogenesis. If a person eats normal portions of food sources of vitamin D, it is difficult to achieve the recommended daily allowance. However, vitamin D supplements are widely available and inexpensive. Vitamin D₃ is more potent than vitamin D₂.

III.6. Answer d.
Vitamin A toxicity is often associated with portal hypertension, rash, and headaches (pseudotumor cerebri).

III.7. Answer d.
Pernicious anemia is often associated with other autoimmune conditions (eg, Hashimoto thyroiditis and vitiligo). Deficiencies of vitamin B₁₂ take several years to develop as stores are quite high in the liver. In addition to a megaloblastic anemia, neurologic signs with spasticity and confusion can be present. Vitamin B₁₂ deficiency is easily treated with high doses of oral supplementation (1,000 μg daily) or subcutaneous injections monthly.

III.8. Answer d.
To be absorbed, iron must be in the reduced form (Fe²⁺), which requires gastric acid. Patients with atrophic gastritis have achlorhydria, and some of them may have iron deficiency. Younger patients with atrophic gastritis may present with iron deficiency before vitamin B₁₂ deficiency.

IV

Miscellaneous Disorders

10

Nonvariceal Gastrointestinal Tract Bleeding[a]

DAVID H. BRUINING, MD

JEFFREY A. ALEXANDER, MD

Upper Gastrointestinal Tract Bleeding

Introduction

Upper gastrointestinal (UGI) tract bleeding ("UGI bleeding") constitutes 75% to 80% of all cases of acute gastrointestinal tract bleeding. Although the incidence has decreased considerably, the mortality rate from acute UGI bleeding has decreased minimally in the past 50 years, ranging from 2.5% to 10%. This lack of change in the mortality rate likely is related to the older age of patients who present with UGI bleeding and the increase in associated comorbid conditions. Peptic ulcers (Box 10.1) are the most common source of UGI bleeding, accounting for about 40% to 50% of patients. Other major causes are gastric erosions (5%-25%), bleeding varices (5%-30%), and Mallory-Weiss tears (5%-15%). The use of aspirin or other nonsteroidal anti-inflammatory drugs (NSAIDs) is prevalent in 45% to 60% of all patients with acute bleeding. Moreover, the risk of UGI bleeding is increased in patients who take as few as 1 low-dose aspirin (81 mg) daily.

Initial Approach to Patients With UGI Bleeding

The initial evaluation of a patient with UGI bleeding should focus on assessment of 1) hemodynamic status and 2) comorbid conditions.

Melena can result when as little as 100 mL of blood is instilled into the UGI tract, and instillation of 1,000 mL or more initially leads to hematochezia. Hematochezia from UGI bleeding is a sign of significant bleeding and, if associated with a red nasogastric aspirate, the mortality rate is nearly 30%. Patients still

---

> **Box 10.1. Causes of Upper Gastrointestinal Tract Bleeding[a]**
>
> Peptic ulcer disease (40%-50%)
>
> Varices (5%-30%)
>
> Mallory-Weiss tear (5%-15%)
>
> Gastric erosions (5%-25%)
>
> Other
>
> > Tumor
> >
> > Dieulafoy lesion
> >
> > AVM, angioectasia
> >
> > GAVE
> >
> > Portal hypertensive gastropathy
>
> ---
>
> Abbreviations: AVM, arteriovenous malformation; GAVE, gastric antral vascular ectasia.
>
> [a] Percentages indicate percentage of patients.

---

[a] Portions previously published in Huprich J, Alexander J, Mullan B, Stanson A. Gastrointestinal Hemorrhage. In: Gore RM, Levine MS, eds. Textbook of gastrointestinal radiology. 4th ed. 2015:2271-81:chap 125; used with permission.

Abbreviations: CREST, calcinosis cutis, Raynaud phenomenon, esophageal dysfunction, sclerodactyly, and telangiectasia; CT, computed tomography; HHT, hereditary hemorrhagic telangiectasia; H$_2$, histamine; NSAID, nonsteroidal anti-inflammatory drug; PPI, proton pump inhibitor; UGI, upper gastrointestinal

bleed whole blood; therefore, the hematocrit may not decrease immediately with acute bleeding. Extravascular fluid will enter the vascular space and restore volume for up to 72 hours, thereby leading to a subsequent decrease in the hematocrit. Similarly, the hematocrit may continue to decrease for a few days after bleeding has stopped, and a decrease in hematocrit without clinical evidence of blood loss is not diagnostic of recurrent bleeding. Adequate intravenous access should be obtained. Volume resuscitation with stabilization of any comorbid active medical conditions should be achieved before endoscopy. Most guidelines support a restrictive transfusion threshold (<7 g/dL) in the absence of hemodynamic instability or cardiac comorbidities. Rarely, massive bleeding cannot be stabilized before endoscopy. Intubation for airway protection should be considered in patients with ongoing hematemesis or those with suspected active bleeding and decreased consciousness or loss of the gag reflex. Nasogastric tube aspiration should not be used routinely as it does not adequately differentiate UGI bleeding from lower gastrointestinal tract bleeding in patients presenting with melena, it does not allow for predicting the presence of high-risk lesions requiring endoscopic therapy, and it has not been shown to improve major clinical outcomes.

Prognostic Factors

Clinical

Age older than 70 years is a risk factor for death from UGI bleeding. Comorbid conditions that increase mortality include pulmonary disease (acute respiratory failure, pneumonia, and symptomatic chronic obstructive pulmonary disease), malignancy, liver disorders (cirrhosis and alcoholic hepatitis), neurologic disorders (delirium and recent stroke), sepsis, postoperative state, and possibly cardiac disease (congestive heart failure, ischemic heart disease, and dysrhythmia) and kidney disorders (acute kidney failure, creatinine >4 mg/dL, and dialysis). Signs of large-volume bleeding may include hematemesis or bright red nasogastric aspirate and shock, the 2 most predictive risk factors for death from UGI bleeding. Tachycardia (heart rate >100 beats/min), orthostasis, and hypotension (systolic blood pressure <100 mm Hg) are predictive of rebleeding. Vomitus that resembles coffee grounds ("coffee ground emesis") has no prognostic value. A transfusion requirement of 4 units of blood or more per resuscitative event is predictive of rebleeding and death from UGI bleeding. Laboratory findings of note include thrombocytopenia, leukocytosis, and abnormal coagulation profile, all of which increase mortality.

Endoscopic

Only the finding of varices or gastric cancer has been shown clearly to be a predictor of death from UGI bleeding. Active arterial spurting has been associated inconsistently with increased mortality. Endoscopic findings, however, have clear prognostic value in assessing rebleeding rates. For reliable prognostication of rebleeding, endoscopy should be performed within 24 hours after presentation. Nearly 94% of episodes of rebleeding occur within 72 hours and 98% within 96 hours. The 3 endoscopic observations that are independent predictors of rebleeding regardless of the type of lesion are arterial spurting (rebleeding in 70%-90% of cases), visible vessel or pigmented protuberance (40%-50%), and adherent clot resistant to washing (10%-35%). Ulcers larger than 2 cm and posterior duodenal bulb ulcers also are predictive of rebleeding.

Predictive Models

Multiple models are available for predicting survival and the need for endoscopic intervention. These models cannot unequivocally predict the need for intervention. However, a patient has a very small chance (<1%) of requiring intervention if the Blatchford score is 0 (serum urea nitrogen <18.2 mg/dL; hemoglobin ≥13.0 g/dL for men and ≥12.0 g/dL for women; systolic blood pressure ≥110 mm Hg; pulse rate <100/min; and an absence of melena, syncope, cardiac failure, and liver disease).

Specific Lesions

Peptic Ulcers

The approach to a patient who has bled from peptic ulcer disease is determined at endoscopy. There are many options for endoscopic therapy. Thermal-coaptive coagulation involves placement of the coagulating probe directly on the bleeding vessel. This is uniformly effective for vessels up to 2 mm in diameter with a bipolar hemostasis probe (14-16 W). Injection therapy results in short-term tamponade and vasospasm and can be induced with the liberal use of epinephrine (1:10,000). Vasodestruction is long-term and can be induced by sclerosants or alcohol (total injection volume ≤2 mL). Endoscopic clipping has not been shown to be any more effective than thermal therapy. However, it may have appeal for use in patients with coagulation disorders or when further coaptive coagulation may not be desirable. Hemostatic powder can be used when other treatment modalities have failed or are not reasonable options for temporizing tumor-related bleeding.

Endoscopic therapy is indicated for patients with active arterial bleeding and those with a nonbleeding visible vessel (pigmented protuberance). An adherent clot is a predictor of rebleeding and can be managed with endoscopic therapy or high-dose proton pump inhibitor (PPI) therapy (or both). All 3 endoscopic treatment options have been shown to have a relatively similar efficacy. However, the use of epinephrine injection with subsequent use of a more permanent form of treatment (coagulation, vasodestruction, or clipping) has been shown to be more effective than epinephrine therapy alone. Patients with a clean ulcer base (rebleeding rates <5%) and a flat pigmented spot (rebleeding rates, 5%-10%) do not require endoscopic therapy and likely could be discharged soon after endoscopy. Deep ulcers may expose larger vessels that may not be amenable to endoscopic coagulation. Deep ulcers in the stomach should not be treated, particularly if the ulcers are in the upper part of the body on the lesser curvature (left gastric artery) or posterior duodenal bulb (gastroduodenal artery) with nonbleeding visible vessels larger than 2 to 3 mm in diameter. Rebleeding after endoscopic therapy occurs 20% to 30% of the time. Re-treatment for recurrent bleeding achieves long-term hemostasis in more than 70% of patients. For patients with recurrent bleeding peptic ulcers, over-the-scope clips are more effective than standard endoscopic therapy for bleeding control.

If endoscopic therapy fails, angiographic embolization of the bleeding vessel is preferable to surgical intervention. No data support the use of histamine (H₂)-blockers or antacids in controlling peptic ulcer bleeding. High-dose PPI therapy is beneficial for patients with peptic ulcer bleeding and high-risk stigmata, both with and without endoscopic therapy. The presumed benefit is related to clot stabilization occurring in a nonacid environment. In vitro studies suggest that a pH greater than 6.0 is required for platelet aggregation and fibrin formation, whereas a pH less than 5.0 is associated with clot lysis. This pH increase is achieved best with PPI therapy administered as a continuous intravenous infusion. Because of its effects on decreasing splanchnic blood flow, octreotide can be considered for patients who have torrential bleeding and no response to intravenous PPI and endoscopic therapy.

Patients with UGI bleeding and *Helicobacter pylori* infection should be treated, and eradication of the *H pylori* infection should be confirmed. Patients taking NSAIDs should avoid them if possible. Patients without a reversible cause of peptic ulcer disease should receive long-term ulcer prophylaxis with a PPI. Without treatment, recurrent ulcer bleeding will occur in approximately one-third of these patients within 3 to 5 years. This rate can be decreased to less than 10% with full-dose H_2-blocker prophylaxis. Ulcer rebleeding is uncommon in patients with proven eradication of *H pylori* infection who avoid the use of NSAIDs. However, ulcer prophylaxis may be reasonable for patients in whom *H pylori* infection has been eradicated but who have a clinically important comorbid condition, especially if they take NSAIDs continuously or intermittently.

Mucosal Erosive Disease

Endoscopic esophagitis, gastritis, and duodenitis are defined by the endoscopic findings of hemorrhage, erythema, or erosions. These lesions rarely are associated with major UGI bleeding. Large hiatal hernias can be associated with chronic blood loss related to *Cameron lesions*, which are linear erosions along the crests of gastric folds at or near the diaphragmatic hiatus. Gastric erosive disease usually is related to NSAID use, alcohol intake, or stress gastritis. Bleeding generally is minor unless ulceration develops. Prophylaxis of NSAID injury with a PPI or treatment with cyclooxygenase-2–specific NSAIDs decreases the risk of ulcer development. Stress gastritis leads to clinically significant UGI bleeding in more than 3% of patients in intensive care units. Patients at higher risk are those receiving mechanical ventilation for more than 48 hours, patients with coagulopathy, and patients with head injury or extensive burn injuries. Prophylactic therapy should be reserved for these groups. Maintenance of gastric pH greater than 4, with enteral feedings and use of H_2-receptor antagonists or PPIs, is effective for preventing stress ulcer bleeding. PPI therapy appears more effective than H_2-blocker therapy for preventing bleeding. Sucralfate has been shown to be effective for prophylaxis of stress ulcer bleeding without affecting gastric pH; in some studies, it has been associated with less pneumonia and possibly less mortality than H_2 blockers.

Mallory-Weiss Tear

Mallory-Weiss tears occur at the gastroesophageal junction and often are present with a classic history of recurrent retching, frequently in a patient with alcohol use disorder, before the development of hematemesis. Most tears occur on the gastric side of the gastroesophageal junction, but 10% to 20% may involve the esophagus. Bleeding stops spontaneously in 80% to 90% of patients and rebleeding occurs in 2% to 5%. Endoscopic therapy with thermal coagulation, injection therapy, or banding is beneficial for active bleeding. Angiographic therapy with intraarterial vasopressin or embolization also can be effective, as can oversewing the lesion intraoperatively.

Portal Hypertensive Gastropathy

Portal hypertensive gastropathy is more frequent in the proximal portion of the stomach than the distal portion and gives the gastric mucosa a mosaic or snakeskin appearance, with or without red spots. Severe portal hypertensive gastropathy has a mosaic pattern and diffuse red spots and can be associated with both chronic and acute gastrointestinal tract bleeding. Bleeding usually is not massive, and therapy is directed at decreasing the portal pressure. Rebleeding can be decreased with nonselective β-blocker therapy.

Aortoenteric Fistula

Fistulas can occur between any major vascular structure and the gastrointestinal tract. Aortoesophageal fistulas are caused by thoracic aortic aneurysms, esophageal foreign bodies, or neoplasms. Up to 75% of aortoenteric fistulas communicate with the duodenum, usually in the distal third. These may develop from an aortic aneurysm but are related more commonly to abdominal aortic (graft) reconstructive surgery. Infection appears to have a major pathogenic role in the development of these fistulas, which usually develop off the origin of the graft, often with pseudoaneurysm formation. The classic "herald bleed," in which bleeding stops spontaneously hours to months before massive bleeding, occurs in about half of patients. The diagnostic test of choice is computed tomography (CT) with an intravenous contrast agent to show loss of the tissue plane between the graft and the bowel or to show air surrounding the graft near the duodenum. Extended upper endoscopy is often used next to exclude other causes of UGI bleeding; however, endoscopy has a low sensitivity for the diagnosis of an aortoenteric fistula. Explorative surgery is indicated for a patient with an aortic graft, severe bleeding, and no relevant radiologic and endoscopic findings. The correct diagnosis of an aortoenteric fistula is established preoperatively in as few as one-third of patients.

Hemobilia and Hemosuccus Pancreaticus

Hemobilia is manifested classically as UGI bleeding accompanied by biliary colic and jaundice. The diagnosis is suggested when blood is visualized coming from the ampulla at endoscopy. CT angiography is the diagnostic test of choice. The most common cause of hemobilia is trauma, including liver biopsy, to the liver or biliary tree. Extrahepatic or intrahepatic artery aneurysms often are caused by trauma and may communicate with the bile ducts. Bleeding can be caused also by gallstones, hepatic or bile duct tumors, and cholecystitis.

In hemosuccus pancreaticus, the bleeding is usually from peripancreatic blood vessels into the pancreatic duct. This commonly is due to rupture of true aneurysms or pseudoaneurysms often associated with necrotizing pancreatitis. CT angiography is the diagnostic test of choice; subsequent treatment is with transcatheter embolization. Surgery may be required for embolization failures.

Neoplasms

Bleeding can occur from primary UGI tumors (adenocarcinoma, stromal tumors, lymphomas, or neuroendocrine tumors) and, occasionally, metastatic UGI tumors (melanoma or breast cancer). Gastrointestinal stromal tumors often appear as a submucosal mass with central ulceration and may cause severe UGI bleeding. Effective therapy generally is surgical.

Vascular Anomalies

Anomalies With Skin Lesions. Vascular lesions can be seen throughout the gastrointestinal tract in several systemic diseases and syndromes such as Osler-Weber-Rendu disease (ie, hereditary hemorrhagic telangiectasia [HHT]), the elastic tissue disorders of pseudoxanthoma elasticum and Ehlers-Danlos syndrome, CREST (calcinosis cutis, Raynaud phenomenon, esophageal dysfunction, sclerodactyly, and telangiectasia) syndrome, and blue rubber bleb nevus syndrome. Endoscopic coagulation therapy is the treatment of choice. For patients who have HHT with acutely bleeding gastrointestinal telangiectasias, endoscopic coagulation treatment is indicated. Treatment of nonbleeding HHT-related telangiectasis is anti-angiogenic therapy with an agent such as bevacizumab. Endoscopic therapy of nonbleeding lesions is not recommended because thermal injury may incite further telangiectasia development.

Anomalies Without Skin Lesions. Vascular ectasias can occur anywhere in the UGI tract but are more common in the duodenum and stomach, particularly in older patients and those with chronic kidney failure or previous radiotherapy. These lesions are cherry red and often fernlike in appearance. Histologically, dilated, ectatic, or tortuous submucosal blood vessels (or a combination of these) are seen; the pathogenesis of these vessels is not known. These lesions may be diffuse or localized. Vascular ectasias are treated with endoscopic thermal coagulation.

Gastric antral vascular ectasia (also called watermelon stomach) is a specific type of localized ectasia often seen in elderly women who present with iron deficiency anemia and evidence of mild UGI tract blood loss. This lesion is associated with several other disease processes, most notably, connective tissue disorders, atrophic gastritis, pernicious anemia, and portal hypertension. Red streaks that traverse the gastric antrum and converge at the pylorus, resembling the stripes on a watermelon, are seen with endoscopy. Histologically, large blood vessels with intravascular fibrin thrombi and fibromuscular hyperplasia are seen, but the diagnosis usually is based on the classic endoscopic appearance. If iron replacement is inadequate to maintain a normal level of hemoglobin, endoscopic thermal therapy often is helpful. Argon plasma coagulation is the preferred thermal treatment for gastric antral vascular ectasia because of the large area usually requiring treatment. Rarely, antrectomy is necessary.

A Dieulafoy lesion (Figure 10.1) is an abnormally large submucosal artery that can rupture and bleed. The bleeding is arterial and is usually moderate to severe. Most of these lesions are within 6 cm of the esophageal junction, but they can occur in the duodenum and jejunum as well as in the esophagus, colon, rectum, and biliary tree. They can be difficult to diagnose when the bleeding has stopped, and endoscopy may need to be repeated several times to identify the lesion. When the lesion is identified, endoscopic tattooing of the lesion often is helpful, especially if surgical therapy is planned. A Dieulafoy lesion appears as a small protruding vessel surrounded by normal mucosa or as a minute mucosal defect. These lesions are amenable to conventional endoscopic therapy, band ligation, and endoscopic clipping. Rebleeding rates after endoscopic therapy are low. A nonbleeding visible vessel should be treated. Angiographic embolization can be effective in high-risk surgical patients.

Non-UGI Bleeding

Introduction

Gastrointestinal tract bleeding has been classified according to the level of the tract: 1) *upper*—proximal to the ampulla of

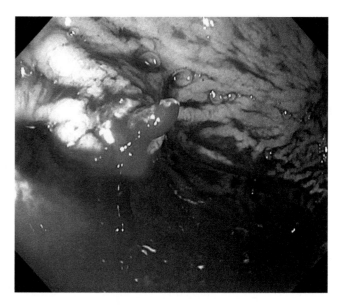

Figure 10.1. Dieulafoy Lesion. Endoscopic image shows active bleeding.

Vater; 2) *mid*—from the ampulla of Vater to the terminal ileum; and 3) *lower*—distal to the terminal ileum. Only 3% to 5% of episodes of gastrointestinal tract bleeding originate from a midbowel source.

Depending on the transit time, which in turn is determined by the volume of bleeding, patients with non-UGI bleeding may present with melena, hematochezia, or occult bleeding. An important point is that bacterial metabolism needs sufficient time for melena to be generated from fresh blood.

Hematochezia most commonly indicates bleeding from a colonic source. However, the source is more proximal in 5% to 10% of patients. It would be extremely uncommon for hematochezia to originate from a source in the proximal portion of the gastrointestinal tract without hemodynamic evidence of bleeding or clinical evidence of rapid gastrointestinal transit (eg, hyperperistalsis).

If blood is limited to the toilet paper or the surface of formed stool, a perianal source (eg, hemorrhoids or fissures) is likely. Tenesmus suggests a rectal origin (eg, proctitis). For all patients, the possibility of neoplasia must at least be considered and often excluded.

Specific Lesions

Diverticular Bleeding

Patients with diverticular bleeding typically present with acute blood loss, as manifested by maroon stools or hematochezia. Minor or occult bleeding is not characteristic of diverticular bleeding or diverticulosis. Diverticular bleeding and diverticulitis are distinct conditions that rarely occur together. Diverticular bleeding is painless except for the cramping that may occur with the cathartic effect of blood within the colon.

Diverticular bleeding is thought to originate more commonly from the right colon, where ostia tend to be wider and the colon wall thinner. Diverticular bleeding develops in an estimated 3% to 5% of patients with diverticulosis. Bleeding most commonly occurs during the sixth and seventh decades of life and stops spontaneously in more than 75% of patients. Generally, rebleeding occurs in about 15% to 20% of patients. After a second episode, the risk of rebleeding is approximately 25% to 50%.

For ongoing or recurrent bleeding, angiography often is performed with the intention of identifying an actively bleeding vessel. If the vessel is identified, transcatheter embolization can be attempted, although in some series colonic infarction has been as high as 20%. Transcatheter vasopressin can control bleeding in 90% of cases, but rebleeding rates are high. Endoscopic therapy is safe and effective, but locating the bleeding lesion is often difficult.

Vascular Ectasia

Vascular ectasias are typically smaller than 5 mm and are found in 3% to 6% of patients undergoing colonoscopy. Most commonly, they are in the right colon but may occur anywhere in the gastrointestinal tract. These lesions are usually angiodysplasias, which are often multiple and believed to be related to the aging process. Less than 10% of patients with angiodysplasia eventually have bleeding. Not uncommonly, these lesions become apparent because of a bleeding diathesis, such as anticoagulation or platelet dysfunction. The lesions may lead to acute overt as well as occult gastrointestinal tract bleeding.

For many patients, iron repletion therapy alone is sufficient. Endoscopic therapy is effective but is associated with a high rebleeding rate. Angiographic embolization can be used to control acute bleeding. Octreotide and thalidomide have been of benefit in small trials of patients with obscure gastrointestinal tract bleeding presumed to be related to vascular ectasias.

Neoplasm

Patients with neoplasm of the colon and small bowel may present with either acute or occult non-UGI bleeding. Tumors of the small intestine may be a relatively common cause of obscure non-UGI bleeding in patients younger than 50 years; two-thirds of the tumors are malignant. Carcinoids, adenocarcinomas, and gastrointestinal stromal tumors account for most of these lesions.

Colonic Ischemia

Patients with colonic ischemia often present with mild lower abdominal pain and bloody diarrhea or hematochezia. Colonic ischemia most often occurs in persons older than 60 years who have atherosclerotic cardiovascular risk factors, but it may occur in patients after abdominal vascular surgery, in patients who have vasculitis or clotting disorders, or in those who receive estrogen therapy. However, usually no etiologic factor is identified. It is the result of a low-flow, nonocclusive process in the colonic microvasculature. A large-vessel disease is rarely found, and angiography is not indicated for left-sided ischemic disease. There is no specific therapy, and recovery is usually complete in several days. Occasionally, however, a colonic stricture may develop.

Meckel Diverticulum

A Meckel diverticulum, a remnant of the vitelline duct, usually occurs 100 cm proximal to the ileocecal valve. Autopsy series suggest a prevalence rate of 2%. Approximately 50% of these diverticula contain gastric mucosa, and patients, typically a child or young adult, may present with bleeding from acid-induced ulceration of the ileum.

Inflammatory Bowel Disease

Patients with inflammatory bowel disease may present with bloody diarrhea or hematochezia, which is the classic presentation

for ulcerative colitis. Hemodynamically significant hemorrhage is uncommon.

Benign Rectoanal Disease

Patients with benign rectoanal disease often present with hematochezia. Painless hematochezia with blood on the toilet paper or the surface of formed stool is most suggestive of hemorrhoidal bleeding. Painful outlet bleeding is typical of a rectal fissure.

Stercoral ulcers are associated with constipation and occur most commonly in the rectosigmoid area or, occasionally, in the more proximal portion of the colon. They often become manifest after disimpaction. Solitary rectal ulcer syndrome often is associated with excessive straining. The ulcer usually occurs on the anterior wall, 6 to 10 cm above the anal verge. Both lesions may come to attention because of considerable bleeding.

Patients with radiation proctitis may present months to years after receiving radiotherapy to the prostate or pelvic organs. Sigmoidoscopy shows characteristic mucosal telangiectasias. The bleeding is rarely severe, and endoscopic argon plasma coagulation therapy is the treatment of choice.

Infection

Infections may be associated with non-UGI bleeding. Clues include a travel history or evidence of systemic toxicity such as fevers, rashes, arthralgias, eosinophilia, or diarrhea. In patients infected with HIV, common causes of non-UGI bleeding are cytomegalovirus colitis and lymphoma.

NSAID Enteropathy and Colonopathy

Increasingly, NSAID enteropathy and colonopathy are being recognized as explanations for non-UGI bleeding. Autopsy studies have documented small intestinal ulcers in 8% of patients who had taken NSAIDs within the preceding 6 months. Diaphragmatic strictures are strongly suggestive of NSAID-induced inflammation. NSAIDs may cause a flare of inflammatory bowel disease.

Approach

The evaluation and management of patients who present with non-UGI bleeding is determined largely by the clinical presentation and the differential diagnosis that has been generated. The following points are essential to keep in mind:

- Diagnostic colonoscopy is indicated for patients with positive findings on fecal occult blood testing. In addition, the presence of signs or symptoms of UGI tract disease or iron deficiency warrant upper endoscopy.
- Technetium Tc 99m–tagged red blood cell radionuclide scans can detect bleeding rates as low as 0.1 mL/min. The patient may undergo scanning repeatedly over a 12- to 24-hour period in an attempt to identify intermittent bleeding. Radionuclide scans generally are not useful for identifying a specific site of bleeding. They are more sensitive for bleeding, are less invasive than angiography, and often are used to determine the best timing for angiography. Tagged red blood cell scans are rarely used now with the availability of CT angiography.
- Mesenteric angiography is more accurate than radionuclide scans but requires a faster bleeding rate (>0.5 mL/min). Angiographic yields are much greater with active gastrointestinal tract bleeding (60%-70%) than when angiography is performed after bleeding has ceased (<20%). Angiographic therapy with transcatheter infusion

of vasopressin or embolization has been effective but carries a risk of bowel infarction.

- Capsule endoscopy is the method of choice for evaluating suspected small-bowel bleeding. It shows an abnormal finding about 70% of the time. Push enteroscopy has been reported to identify probable bleeding sites in 50% of patients with obscure gastrointestinal tract bleeding. This can be done with an adult or pediatric colonoscope. Approximately 25% of the diagnoses made with push enteroscopy are within the reach of a standard endoscope.
- Balloon-assisted endoscopy, with a single or double balloon, can be performed by the peroral or peranal route (or both), with a diagnostic yield greater than 60%. Endoscopic therapy can be administered. Double-balloon endoscopy appears to provide deeper small-bowel intubation than single-balloon or spiral endoscopy. Complete enteroscopy can be achieved with double-balloon endoscopy in over 40% of patients with the combined antegrade and retrograde approach.
- Intraoperative enteroscopy has been used to detect abnormalities in about 70% of patients. However, recurrent bleeding may occur, and only about 40% to 50% of these patients are free of bleeding at 2 years. Furthermore, it is rarely needed with the advent of capsule endoscopy and deep enteroscopy.
- CT enterography and CT angiography are having an increased role in the evaluation and localization of small-bowel blood loss. They are particularly useful in the evaluation of bleeding related to small-bowel mass lesions. CT angiography is preferred over red blood cell scintigraphy for hemodynamically unstable patients with lower gastrointestinal tract bleeding and allows transarterial embolization if CT angiography shows active extravasation.

✓ Resuscitation and risk stratification are critical for successful management of gastrointestinal tract bleeding
✓ Peptic ulcer disease—the most common cause of UGI bleeding
✓ Capsule endoscopy, CT enterography, or CT angiography (or >1 of these procedures) may be useful for suspected small-bowel bleeding

---

Suggested Reading

Alhazzani W, Alenezi F, Jaeschke RZ, Moayyedi P, Cook DJ. Proton pump inhibitors versus histamine 2 receptor antagonists for stress ulcer prophylaxis in critically ill patients: a systematic review and meta-analysis. Crit Care Med. 2013 Mar;41(3):693–705.

ASGE Standards of Practice Committee, Fisher L, Lee Krinsky M, Anderson MA, Appalaneni V, Banerjee S, et al. The role of endoscopy in the management of obscure GI bleeding. Gastrointest Endosc. 2010 Sep;72(3):471–9.

Barkun AN, Bardou M, Kuipers EJ, Sung J, Hunt RH, Martel M, et al. International consensus recommendations on the management of patients with nonvariceal upper gastrointestinal bleeding. Ann Intern Med. 2010 Jan;152(2):101–13.

Davila RE, Rajan E, Adler DG, Egan J, Hirota WK, Leighton JA, et al. ASGE Guideline: the role of endoscopy in the patient with lower-GI bleeding. Gastrointest Endosc. 2005 Nov;62(5):656–60.

Elmunzer BJ, Young SD, Inadomi JM, Schoenfeld P, Laine L. Systematic review of the predictors of recurrent hemorrhage after endoscopic hemostatic therapy for bleeding peptic ulcers. Am J Gastroenterol. 2008 Oct;103(10):2625–32.

Gerson LB, Fidler JL, Cave DR, Leighton JA. ACG Clinical Guideline: diagnosis and management of small bowel bleeding. Am J Gastroenterol. 2015 Sep;110(9):1265–87.

Gralnek IM, Barkun AN, Bardou M. Management of acute bleeding from a peptic ulcer. N Engl J Med. 2008 Aug;359(9):928–37.

Holster IL, van Beusekom HM, Kuipers EJ, Leebeek FW, de Maat MP, Tjwa ET. Effects of a hemostatic powder hemospray on coagulation and clot formation. Endoscopy. 2015 Jul;47(7):638–45.

Hwang JH, Fisher DA, Ben-Menachem T, Chandrasekhara V, Chathadi K, Decker GA, et al. The role of endoscopy in the management of acute non-variceal upper GI bleeding. Gastrointest Endosc. 2012 Jun;75(6):1132–8.

Laine L, Barkun AN, Saltzman JR, Martel M, Leontiadis GI. ACG Clinical Guideline: upper gastrointestinal and ulcer bleeding. Am J Gastroenterol. 2021 May;116(5):899–917.

Lanza FL, Chan FK, Quigley EM, Practice Parameters Committee of the American College of Gastroenterology. Guidelines for prevention of NSAID-related ulcer complications. Am J Gastroenterol. 2009 Mar;104(3):728–38.

Lau J, Sung JJ. From endoscopic hemostasis to bleeding peptic ulcers: strategies to prevent and treat recurrent bleeding. Gastroenterology. 2010 Apr;138(4):1252–4.

Rondonotti E, Sunada K, Yano T, Paggi S, Yamamoto H. Double-balloon endoscopy in clinical practice: where are we now? Dig Endosc. 2012 Jul;24(4):209–19.

Schmidt A, Golder S, Goetz M, Meining A, Lau J, von Delius S, et al. Over-the-scope clips are more effective than standard endoscopic therapy for patients with recurrent bleeding of peptic ulcers. Gastroenterology. 2018 Sep;155(3):674–86.

11

Vascular Disorders of the Gastrointestinal Tract

SETH R. SWEETSER, MD

Mesenteric Ischemia

Mesenteric ischemia (MI) is a broad term that includes several clinical conditions that occur when splanchnic blood flow is inadequate and thus fails to meet the metabolic demands of the intestines. The condition can result in symptomatic and life-threatening clinical presentations. The incidence of MI is increasing because of the aging population, increasing number of critically ill patients, and heightened clinical awareness. MI produces a spectrum of disorders that depend on many factors, including the acuity of the event, the vessel involved, and the length of bowel affected. In general, MI can be divided into 4 clinical syndromes: acute mesenteric ischemia (AMI), chronic mesenteric ischemia (CMI), colonic ischemia (CI), and focal segmental ischemia (FSI). These 4 syndromes account for most manifestations of ischemic injury to the gut (Table 11.1). This chapter reviews the epidemiology, pathophysiology, clinical presentation, and management of these conditions and discusses other vascular syndromes of the gastrointestinal tract.

> ✓ **Mesenteric ischemia**—a broad term that includes several clinical conditions that occur when splanchnic blood flow is inadequate and thus fails to meet the metabolic demands of the intestines

Abbreviations: AMI, acute mesenteric ischemia; ANCA, antineutrophil cytoplasmic antibody; CA, celiac artery; CI, colonic ischemia; CMI, chronic mesenteric ischemia; CTA, computed tomographic angiography; EDS, Ehlers-Danlos syndrome; FSI, focal segmental ischemia; IMA, inferior mesenteric artery; MALS, median arcuate ligament syndrome; MI, mesenteric ischemia; NOMI, nonocclusive mesenteric ischemia; RA, rheumatoid arthritis; SLE, systemic lupus erythematosus; SMA, superior mesenteric artery; SMAE, superior mesenteric artery embolus; SMAT, superior mesenteric artery thrombus; VAA, visceral artery aneurysm

Mesenteric Vascular Anatomy

The principal blood supply to the gut is from the celiac, superior mesenteric, and inferior mesenteric arteries, which arise directly from the aorta. The celiac artery (CA) has its origin from the anterior aorta and supplies blood to the stomach, the proximal duodenum, part of the pancreas, the liver, and the spleen. The superior mesenteric artery (SMA) arises from the anterior aorta at an acute angle (25°-60°) and supplies blood to the distal duodenum, jejunum, ileum, and proximal colon. The inferior mesenteric artery (IMA) arises just above the aortic bifurcation and supplies the large intestine from the distal transverse colon to the proximal rectum. The distal rectum is supplied by branches of the internal iliac artery.

The 3 major mesenteric vessels share an extensive collateral circulation that allows for redundant flow to mesenteric vascular territories in the event of arterial occlusion and protects the gut from episodes of arterial hypoperfusion. However, if the episodes of arterial hypoperfusion are abrupt, complete, or prolonged, the adaptive mechanisms are overwhelmed, and MI or mesenteric infarction (or both) occur. The major collateral pathways between the CA and SMA are the gastroduodenal and pancreaticoduodenal arteries and, less commonly, the *arc of Barkow* (an anastomosis between the left and right gastroepiploic arteries) and the *arc of Buhler* (a persistent communication between embryonic ventral

Table 11.1. Types and Frequencies of Mesenteric Ischemia

Type	Frequency, %
Colonic ischemia	70
Acute mesenteric ischemia	25
Chronic mesenteric ischemia	<5
Focal segmental ischemia	<5

segmental arteries). The SMA and IMA collateralize through the *arc of Riolan* (a connection between the middle and left colic arteries) and the *marginal artery of Drummond*, which consists of branches of the ileocolic and right, left, and middle colic arteries.

Acute Mesenteric Ischemia

Epidemiology and Pathogenesis

AMI is a rare condition that accounts for approximately 0.1% of hospital admissions and 25% of patients with MI. AMI is caused by an abrupt decrease in blood flow to the small bowel. Four distinct pathophysiologic processes can result in the clinical manifestations of AMI (Table 11.2): acute embolism, arterial thrombosis, mesenteric venous thrombosis, and nonocclusive mesenteric ischemia (NOMI). Intestinal infarction occurs with prolonged reduction in blood flow; therefore, AMI is an abdominal emergency with a high mortality rate.

Embolic disease most frequently affects the SMA because of its wide caliber and narrow takeoff angle from the abdominal aorta. SMA embolus (SMAE) is the most common cause of AMI (accounting for 50% of cases). The emboli usually originate from a left atrial or ventricular mural thrombus; an aortic origin (*atheromatous cholesterol embolism*) is less common. Emboli usually obstruct distally to the origin of the SMA, distal to the origin of the middle CA, and spare the proximal jejunum and the right colon. In contrast, embolic occlusion rarely occurs in the IMA because it has a small caliber, and embolism to the CA is uncommon because it arises from the aorta at a right angle. Major risk factors for SMAE are arrhythmias, cardioversion, cardiac catheterization, myocardial infarction or dyskinesia, congestive heart failure, valvular heart disease, atheromatous cholesterol embolism, previous embolism, and age older than 50 years.

SMA thrombus (SMAT) accounts for about 25% of cases of primary mesenteric small-bowel ischemia. Nonlaminar blood flow around vessel branch points makes the ostia of mesenteric vessels a common location for development of atherosclerotic disease; therefore, acute thrombosis often occurs at the origin of the SMA, which results in occlusion of blood flow at a level that is typically more proximal to that in embolic AMI. The result is a longer section of ischemic bowel and consequently a higher mortality rate. Risk factors for SMAT include old age; low-flow states (arrhythmia, hypotension, sepsis, dialysis, vasoconstrictive drugs, myocardial infarction, dyskinesia, and congestive heart failure); atherosclerosis (acute-on-chronic ischemia, hypertension, type 2 diabetes, hyperlipidemia, smoking history, and vasculopathy); hypercoagulable states; vasculitis; fibromuscular dysplasia; trauma; and aortic or mesenteric artery aneurysm. Up to one-third of patients with SMAT have a history of CMI (see below).

Mesenteric venous thrombosis, usually superior mesenteric vein thrombosis (up to 95% of cases), accounts for about 5% of

Table 11.2. Causes and Frequencies of Acute Mesenteric Ischemia

Cause	Frequency, %
SMA embolus	50
SMA thrombosis	25
Nonocclusive mesenteric ischemia	20
Mesenteric venous thrombosis	5

Abbreviation: SMA, superior mesenteric artery.

cases of AMI. Risk factors include a personal or family history of thrombophilia and a history of deep vein thrombosis. Causes include hypercoagulable states; hyperviscosity syndromes; intra-abdominal infections (pyelophlebitis, diverticulitis, and appendicitis) or inflammation (Crohn disease and pancreatitis); malignant obstruction; portal hypertension; vasculitis; and trauma.

NOMI, which accounts for 20% of cases of AMI, occurs when splanchnic vasoconstriction is precipitated by hypoperfusion in the context of decreased cardiac output (myocardial infarction or dyskinesia, arrhythmia, shock, sepsis, pancreatitis, burns, multiple organ failure, congestive heart failure, or hemorrhage); vasospasm (digoxin, α-adrenergic agonists, amphetamines, or cocaine); dialysis; and pre-existing atherosclerotic disease (hypertension, type 2 diabetes, hyperlipidemia, or vasculopathy).

Clinical Manifestations of AMI

Early diagnosis of AMI requires a high degree of clinical awareness. Patients most commonly present with abrupt onset of severe, unrelenting, periumbilical abdominal pain with a subsequent urge to defecate. The abdominal pain is constant, and the patient may subsequently have loose, nonbloody stools. Hematochezia, which occurs in a minority of patients with AMI (15%), signifies concomitant ischemia of the right colon. In the early course of AMI, findings from examination of the abdomen may be falsely reassuring without peritoneal signs or other abnormalities despite the patient's report of severe abdominal pain. This "pain out of proportion to physical examination findings" should immediately increase suspicion for early AMI. However, this classic descriptor is present in only 30% to 50% of patients, so its absence should not exclude the diagnosis. Compared to patients with AMI due to arterial embolus or thrombus, patients with NOMI have pain less often and more commonly present with nausea, abdominal distention, fever, diarrhea, and altered mental status. With a delayed or late presentation, intestinal ischemia progresses to infarction with peritoneal findings on abdominal examination.

Diagnosis of AMI

In the early course of AMI, before intestinal infarction develops, laboratory and abdominal imaging findings are nonspecific. The peripheral leukocyte count is usually high. A serum lactate concentration within the reference range should not be used to exclude the diagnosis.

Computed tomographic angiography (CTA), the recommended method of imaging for diagnosis of AMI, depicts the origins and lengths of vessels and characterizes the occlusion. CTA has a 95% sensitivity and specificity in the diagnosis of AMI. Given the potentially catastrophic consequences of a missed diagnosis of AMI, laboratory results that indicate a high creatinine value or kidney insufficiency should not preclude performance of CTA. Magnetic resonance angiography avoids the risks of radiation and contrast exposure but takes longer and is less sensitive for distal and nonocclusive disease. Duplex ultrasonography is an effective, low-cost method to assess the proximal mesenteric vessels, but adequate ultrasonography often cannot be performed in patients with AMI. The classic angiographic finding in obstructive AMI is an embolus or thrombus in the SMA (Figure 11.1). The diagnosis of NOMI is made by excluding an obstructive mesenteric process with the following angiographic features: 1) narrowing of the origins of the SMA branches, 2) irregularities of these branches, 3) spasm of the mesenteric arcades, and 4) impaired filling of intramural vessels. The most important factor in improving

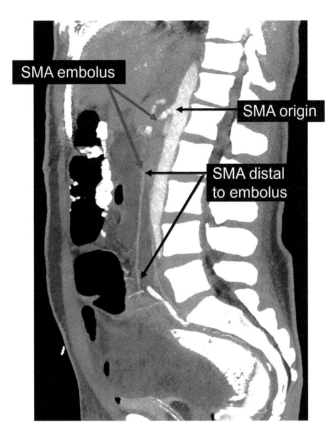

Figure 11.1. Embolic Occlusion of the Proximal Superior Mesenteric Artery (SMA). Computed tomographic angiography, sagittal view, shows the narrowed SMA distal to the embolus.

outcome in AMI is timely diagnosis before the occurrence of gut infarction. Once mesenteric infarction occurs, the mortality of patients with AMI exceeds 60% even with surgery.

Management of AMI

Management for patients with AMI can be remembered by the 3 *R*'s: resuscitation, rapid diagnosis, and revascularization.

After aggressive resuscitation and administration of intravenous heparin and broad-spectrum antibiotics, emergent surgery is indicated if mesenteric infarction is suggested from imaging findings such as gas within the intestinal wall (pneumatosis intestinalis) or in the portal vein (Figure 11.2). Otherwise, angiography with selective catheterization of the mesenteric vessels may be performed, along with endovascular intervention, if possible.

✓ **Acute mesenteric ischemia**—an abrupt decrease in blood flow to the small bowel

---

✓ Most common cause of acute mesenteric ischemia (AMI)—emboli to the superior mesenteric artery (SMA)
✓ Major risk factors for SMA embolus include arrhythmias, myocardial infarction, congestive heart failure, and valvular heart disease
✓ Early diagnosis of AMI requires a high degree of clinical awareness
✓ In the early course of AMI, findings from examination of the abdomen may be falsely reassuring with "pain out of proportion to physical examination findings"
✓ A serum lactate concentration within the reference range should not be used to exclude the diagnosis of AMI
✓ Computed tomographic angiography is the recommended method of imaging for diagnosis of AMI
✓ The 3 *R*'s for management of AMI: resuscitation, rapid diagnosis, and revascularization

Chronic Mesenteric Ischemia

Epidemiology and Pathogenesis

CMI is the least common ischemic gut syndrome (<5% of cases) and involves a gradual decrease in blood flow to the small intestine over months to years. It most commonly results from atherosclerosis involving the proximal segments of the mesenteric arteries (95% of cases), but it can also be a manifestation of nonatherosclerotic disorders such as median arcuate ligament syndrome, vasculitic syndromes, isolated dissection of the visceral arteries, radiation, and fibromuscular dysplasia. It

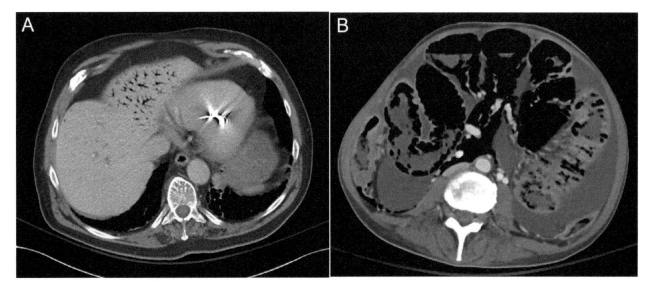

Figure 11.2. Mesenteric Infarction. Computed tomography of the abdomen, axial view, shows portal venous gas represented by linear branching lucencies in the liver (A) and pneumatosis intestinalis represented by linear lucencies in the bowel wall (B).

is thought that less than 1 in every 100,000 hospital admissions is due to CMI. A common history with atherosclerotic-related CMI includes previous vascular disease, hypertension, type 2 diabetes, kidney insufficiency, and smoking. CMI occurs with severe narrowing of 2 of the 3 adjacent mesenteric vessels (CA, SMA, and IMA).

> ✓ **Chronic mesenteric ischemia**—a gradual decrease in blood flow to the small intestine that most commonly results from atherosclerosis

Clinical Manifestations of CMI

Postprandial abdominal pain is the hallmark symptom of CMI. Occurrence of abdominal pain 30 to 60 minutes after eating is characteristic and is often self-treated with food restriction, which results in weight loss and often *sitophobia* (ie, fear of food). This classic symptom triad of postprandial abdominal pain, sitophobia, and weight loss is present in only 30% of patients with CMI, though, and CMI should be suspected in patients who have recurrent postprandial abdominal pain. The pain begins approximately 20 to 30 minutes after ingestion of food because the fixed narrowing of the mesenteric arteries prevents blood flow from increasing and meeting the increased functional demand of the stomach with resultant steal ischemia. If not treated, the condition in up to 50% of patients with CMI will progress to life-threatening AMI.

Diagnosis and Treatment of CMI

The diagnosis of CMI requires compatible ischemic symptoms, exclusion of alternative causes of postprandial abdominal pain and weight loss, and compatible angiographic findings (Box 11.1). A critical step is to rule out other intra-abdominal processes that cause postprandial pain and weight loss, such as peptic ulcer disease, pancreaticobiliary disease, and malignancy. CTA is the standard and preferred imaging modality for CMI. Most patients with ischemic symptoms have severe stenosis (>70%) in at least 2 of 3 mesenteric arteries because of the numerous collateral pathways that allow for redundant flow to the mesenteric vascular territories. However, patients may have ischemic symptoms even with single-vessel stenosis if they have poor collateral circulation, but this is uncommon (<5% of patients).

Traditionally, CMI was treated with either percutaneous endovascular stenting or surgical revascularization. The choice of therapy depended on operative risk and occlusive lesion characteristics. However, endovascular therapy with balloon expandable stents is now the preferred method for revascularization because of lower periprocedural morbidity and mortality when compared with surgical revascularization. Early diagnosis and treatment of CMI is important to prevent life-threatening acute-on-chronic MI.

> **Box 11.1. Criteria for Diagnosis of Chronic Mesenteric Ischemia**
> Consistent symptoms
> Exclusion of alternative causes
> Compatible angiographic findings

> ✓ Postprandial abdominal pain—the hallmark symptom of chronic mesenteric ischemia (CMI)
> ✓ Diagnosis of CMI requires compatible ischemic symptoms, exclusion of alternative causes of postprandial abdominal pain and weight loss, and compatible angiographic findings
> ✓ Most patients with ischemic symptoms have severe stenosis (>70%) in at least 2 of 3 mesenteric arteries
> ✓ CMI is treated with either percutaneous endovascular stenting or surgical revascularization

Colonic Ischemia
Epidemiology and Pathogenesis

CI is an acute event that is the most common form of ischemic bowel disease. The incidence of CI increased from 6 per 100,000 people in 1976-1980 to 23 per 100,000 in 2005-2009. This increase may have resulted from several factors, such as a longer life expectancy of patients who have many comorbid conditions and an increased recognition of CI. Most cases of CI are idiopathic and result from a nonocclusive low-flow state in microvessels, which occurs in the setting of hypovolemia or hypotension. Risk factors for CI include older age (>60 years), female sex, vasoconstrictive and antihypertension medications, irritable bowel syndrome, constipation, thrombophilia, and chronic obstructive pulmonary disease. The degree of ischemic injury is dependent on the duration of low-flow perfusion, the existence of collateral circulation, and the extent of the involved area.

> ✓ **Colonic ischemia**—an acute event that most often results from a nonocclusive low-flow state in microvessels

Anatomical Considerations

The SMA and the IMA supply most of the blood to the colon. Robust collateral vascular pathways (the marginal artery of Drummond and the arc of Riolan) protect the colon from ischemic injury. However, the right colon, splenic flexure, and rectosigmoid junction are regions of the colon that are more susceptible to ischemia. The right colon has less developed vasa recta (ie, end-arteries providing blood to the colonic wall), and the splenic flexure and rectosigmoid junction are watershed areas. These watershed regions are more susceptible to ischemia as they lie at the most distal reaches of the arterial blood supply (ie, the border zones between 2 arterial territories).

Clinical Manifestations of CI

CI manifests with a wide spectrum of injury that includes both reversible and irreversible ischemic disease. Reversible types of CI include colopathy (subepithelial hemorrhage and edema) and transient ulcerating colitis. Irreversible CI includes chronic segmental ulcerating colitis, fibrotic stricture, and gangrenous bowel. The initial presentation of CI is the same for both reversible and irreversible types.

Patients with CI most commonly present with an abrupt onset of lower abdominal discomfort that is mild to moderate and cramping; within 24 hours diarrhea and hematochezia occur. The onset of bleeding often prompts the patient to seek medical attention. On physical examination, a typical finding is mild lower abdominal tenderness over the involved bowel segment without peritoneal signs.

Diagnosis of CI

The diagnosis of CI is made clinically and supported by radiographic imaging and colonoscopic evaluation. Laboratory studies may show mild increases in the leukocyte count and the serum urea nitrogen level.

Plain radiographs of the abdomen may show evidence of submucosal edema and hemorrhage, so-called thumbprinting (Figure 11.3), or the findings may be normal. CT of the abdomen is indicated to assess the severity, phase, and distribution of CI. The phase of CI can be broadly described as *hemorrhagic* with marked thickening on CT or predominantly *ischemic* with wall thinning. CT findings in CI are nonspecific and include thickening of the bowel wall (Figure 11.4) and pericolonic *fat stranding* (ie, an increase in density within pericolonic fat secondary to inflammation), often in the distribution of the watershed areas of the colon (splenic flexure and rectosigmoid junction). CI is typically a segmental disease that can involve any region of the colon, but the left side is most affected. Pancolonic and rectal involvement are rare. Infections with agents such as the following can mimic CI and must be excluded: cytomegalovirus, *Clostridioides difficile*, and Shiga toxin–producing *Escherichia coli*. Colonoscopy with biopsy is the test of choice to confirm the diagnosis of CI. The findings vary in severity and include erythema, edema, friability, ulcerations, and blue-black nodules suggestive of gangrenous infarction (Figure 11.5). The colonic *single-stripe sign*, an erythematous band of ulceration along the longitudinal axis of the colon, is a highly specific endoscopic sign of CI and is a predictor of a good outcome (Figure 11.6). Biopsies should be performed unless there is evidence of infarction. Histopathology findings in CI are often nonspecific, showing

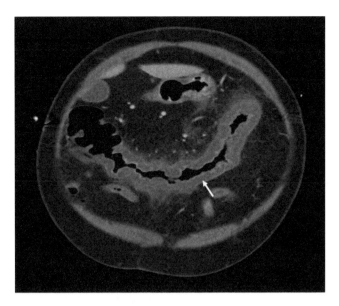

Figure 11.4. Bowel Wall Thickening in Colonic Ischemia. Computed tomography of the abdomen, axial view, shows segmental thickening of the transverse colon (arrow) in a patient with colonic ischemia.

epithelial necrosis, submucosal hemorrhage and edema, and neutrophilic infiltrate (Figure 11.7), but they are helpful in making the diagnosis when considered in clinical context.

Because CI is most often caused by a nonocclusive low-flow state of the microvasculature, dedicated imaging of the mesenteric arteries is of low yield and generally not indicated. The exception is right-sided CI, which can be a harbinger of AMI caused by a focal thrombus or embolus of the SMA. Therefore, patients with right-sided CI should undergo noninvasive imaging of the mesenteric vasculature to exclude an occlusive process of the SMA.

Treatment of CI

Most cases of CI are mild and transient, with a rapid spontaneous resolution. Patients who have more severe disease require hospitalization for supportive care with bowel rest, restoration of intravascular volume, antimicrobial therapy (in many cases), and close observation. Patients who have CI and several risk factors for poor outcome should receive broad-spectrum antibiotics. As an aid that can help guide antibiotic therapy, the American College of Gastroenterology has devised a risk stratification based on features associated with poor outcomes in patients with CI (Table 11.3). Antibiotics are predicted to improve outcomes by decreasing bacterial translocation from lack of mucosal integrity. Only a small percentage of patients with CI require operative intervention for necrotic bowel or irreversible complications, such as gangrene or fibrotic stricture.

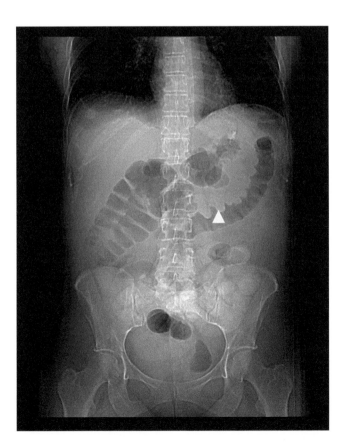

Figure 11.3. "Thumbprinting" in Colonic Ischemia. Abdominal radiograph shows thumbprinting (arrowhead), which indicates thickening of haustral folds from severe submucosal hemorrhage and edema.

✓ The splenic flexure and rectosigmoid junction are watershed areas that are more susceptible to ischemia
✓ Patients with CI usually present with an abrupt onset of cramping and mild to moderate discomfort in the lower abdomen; within 24 hours diarrhea and hematochezia occur
✓ Diagnosis of CI is made clinically and supported by radiographic and colonoscopic findings
✓ Colonoscopy with biopsy is the test of choice to confirm the diagnosis of CI
✓ Most cases of CI are mild and transient, with rapid spontaneous resolution

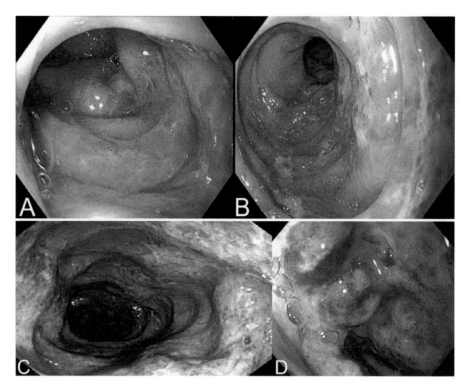

Figure 11.5. Spectrum of Endoscopic Findings in Colonic Ischemia. The range of findings includes mild edema and erythema (A); erythema, edema, and erosions (B); extensive ulceration (C); and hemorrhagic blue-black nodules (D).

Focal Segmental Ischemia

FSI is a condition characterized by vascular insults to short segments of the small intestine without the life-threatening consequences that characterize the other ischemic syndromes

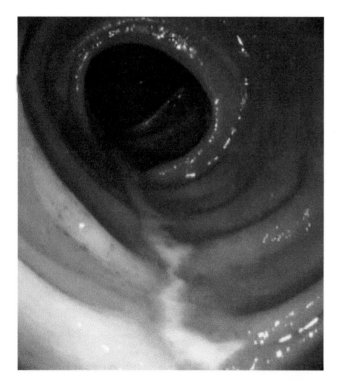

Figure 11.6. Colonic Single-Stripe Sign. The single-stripe sign is a highly specific endoscopic finding for colonic ischemia and indicates a favorable prognosis.

because the collateral blood flow is usually adequate to prevent transmural infarction. Among the many causes of FSI, the most frequent are atheromatous emboli, strangulated hernias, vasculitis, segmental venous thrombosis, and radiotherapy.

> ✓ **Focal segmental ischemia**—an ischemic syndrome characterized by vascular insults to short segments of the small intestine

FSI has a broad spectrum of clinical features but generally manifests in 1 of 3 ways: acute enteritis, chronic enteritis, or chronic small bowel obstruction. The acute enteritis form often mimics appendicitis with an acute abdomen. Patients with the chronic enteritis variety may appear to have Crohn disease with fever, intermittent cramping, abdominal pain, and diarrhea. The most common presentation of FSI is that of chronic small bowel obstruction from a stricture with intermittent abdominal pain. Radiologic evaluation of the acute and chronic enteritis forms usually shows segmental thickening of the small bowel (Figure 11.8). Imaging of chronic FSI typically shows a smooth, tapered stricture of variable length. Treatment of FSI is surgical resection of the involved bowel.

> ✓ FSI has a broad spectrum of clinical features but generally manifests in 1 of 3 ways: acute enteritis, chronic enteritis, or chronic small bowel obstruction
> ✓ Imaging of chronic FSI typically shows a smooth, tapered stricture of variable length
> ✓ Treatment of FSI—surgical resection of the involved bowel

Miscellaneous Syndromes

Median Arcuate Ligament Syndrome

Median arcuate ligament syndrome (MALS), also known as celiac artery compression syndrome, is a rare condition that results from

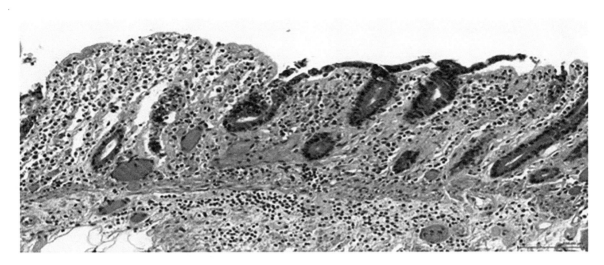

Figure 11.7. **Histologic Findings in Mild Colonic Ischemia.** The findings include surface and crypt epithelial necrosis with focal crypt preservation.

extrinsic compression of the celiac axis (celiac artery or celiac ganglion or both) by the MAL and diaphragmatic crura. Ischemia to the gut is unlikely to cause the pain (because only 1 vessel is affected, and collateral blood flow exists). Alternatively, the pain associated with MALS may be neuropathic resulting from compression and stimulation of the celiac ganglion. MALS most commonly occurs in women aged 30 to 50 years and in individuals who have a thin body habitus. Its hallmark characteristics include postprandial abdominal pain, nausea, vomiting, diarrhea, and weight loss. MALS is a diagnosis of exclusion; other possible causes of the symptoms must be excluded. On lateral mesenteric angiography, a typical concave defect is evident over the superior aspect of the celiac artery near its takeoff from the aorta (Figure 11.9) with respiratory variability. Treatment is laparoscopic surgical MAL release or celiac ganglionectomy (or both).

Vasculitis

Many types of vasculitis can involve the gastrointestinal tract, most commonly by FSI. Polyarteritis nodosa is a systemic necrotizing vasculitis involving small and medium-sized arteries and gastrointestinal manifestations due to mesenteric vasculitis and can occur in 60% of patients. Many patients have fever, abdominal pain, increased levels of inflammatory markers, hypertension, and multiple organ involvement. Some have gastrointestinal tract bleeding or perforation. Most cases of polyarteritis nodosa are idiopathic, although hepatitis B virus infection, hepatitis C virus infection, and hairy cell leukemia are important in the pathogenesis of some cases. The characteristic CTA finding is mesenteric arterial segmental microaneurysms. CTA can be used to detect aneurysms in vessels as small as 3 mm and is the recommended initial test in suspected cases. However, catheter-based angiography has superior spatial resolution and is preferred if suspicion is high despite negative CTA findings.

Immunoglobulin A vasculitis, formerly known as Henoch-Schönlein purpura, is an immune complex–mediated vasculitis affecting small blood vessels. Characteristic clinical features include palpable purpura, arthritis, kidney, and gastrointestinal tract involvement. A palpable purpuric skin rash occurs in all patients and predominates on the lower extremities. Gastrointestinal tract involvement occurs in 50% of patients; abdominal pain and

Table 11.3. CI Disease Severity and Use of Antibiotics

Disease severity	Features in a patient with typical signs and symptoms of CI	Antibiotics recommended?
Mild	No risk factors for poor outcome[a]	No
Moderate	≤3 Risk factors for poor outcome[a]	Yes
Severe	>3 Risk factors for poor outcome[a]	Yes
	or	
	Peritoneal signs, pneumatosis, portal venous gas, gangrene on colonic examination	

Abbreviation: CI, colonic ischemia.

[a] Risk factors for poor outcome: male gender; hypotension (systolic blood pressure <90 mm Hg); tachycardia (heart rate >100 beats/min); abdominal pain without rectal bleeding; colonic mucosal ulceration on colonic examination; increased serum urea nitrogen (>20 mg/dL), lactate dehydrogenase (>350 U/L), and white blood cell count (>15×10⁹/L); and decreased hemoglobin (<12 g/dL) and serum sodium (<136 mmol/L).

Adapted from Brandt LJ, Feuerstadt P, Longstreth GF, Boley SJ, American College of Gastroenterology. ACG clinical guideline: epidemiology, risk factors, patterns of presentation, diagnosis, and management of colon ischemia (CI). Am J Gastroenterol. 2015 Jan;110(1):18-44; used with permission.

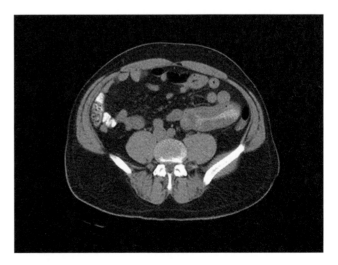

Figure 11.8. **Focal Segmental Ischemia.** Computed tomography of the abdomen, axial view, shows a region of jejunal thickening in a patient with immunoglobulin A vasculitis.

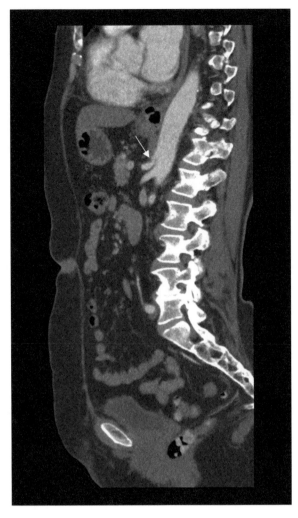

Figure 11.9. Median Arcuate Ligament Compression. Computed tomographic mesenteric angiogram, sagittal view, shows a concave defect in the celiac artery (arrow) related to compression of the median arcuate ligament.

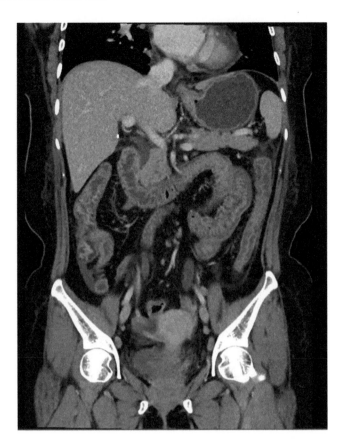

Figure 11.10. Lupus Enteritis. Computed tomography of the abdomen, coronal view, shows diffuse wall thickening and submucosal edema involving the entire small bowel and colon in a patient with lupus enteritis.

bleeding are frequent manifestations. In a subset of patients, gastrointestinal tract manifestations precede the onset of palpable purpura, which may confound the diagnosis.

Systemic lupus erythematosus (SLE) is a systemic autoimmune disease characterized by immune complex formation. SLE has the potential to affect virtually every organ system, including the gastrointestinal system. Mild gastrointestinal tract involvement is common and most commonly consists of nausea and vomiting, anorexia, and abdominal pain. A subset of SLE patients have mesenteric vasculitis (Figure 11.10), also termed *lupus enteritis*, and most commonly present with abdominal pain. Mesenteric vasculitis is usually associated with active disease involving other organs, and gastrointestinal tract activity arising in isolation without additional manifestations of active SLE is highly unusual. Mesenteric vasculitis leads to ischemia and infarctions of the bowel wall and perforation.

Antineutrophil cytoplasmic antibody (ANCA)-associated vasculitis includes 3 diseases: granulomatosis with polyangiitis (formerly Wegener granulomatosis), eosinophilic granulomatosis with polyangiitis (formerly Churg-Strauss syndrome), and microscopic polyangiitis. They are small-vessel necrotizing vasculitides that uncommonly affect the mesenteric circulation;

if gastrointestinal tract manifestations develop, they usually arise several months after other symptoms of ANCA-associated vasculitis. In a small percentage of patients with long-standing or uncontrolled rheumatoid arthritis (RA), small-vessel vasculitis may involve the gastrointestinal tract. Risk factors for development of RA-associated vasculitis include high titers of rheumatoid factor, subcutaneous nodules, and long-standing erosive arthritis. Patients with RA-associated mesenteric vasculitis present with abdominal pain and bleeding that results from ischemic ulceration of the gastrointestinal tract mucosa.

Behçet disease is a multisystem vasculitis characterized by oral and genital ulcers, skin lesions, and recurrent iritis. Gastrointestinal tract involvement most often affects the ileocecal region with large, deep ulcerations resulting in bleeding and perforation. This vasculitis often mimics Crohn disease in presentation.

Visceral Aneurysms

The most common location of visceral artery aneurysms (VAAs) is the splenic artery (70% of cases). Splenic artery aneurysms are more common in women and are associated with medial fibrodysplasia, multiple pregnancies, portal hypertension, and liver transplant. The second most common location of VAAs is the hepatic artery (20% of cases). They are usually extrahepatic and occur more frequently in men. Intrahepatic aneurysms typically develop from trauma or percutaneous interventions. Hemobilia may occur with hepatic artery aneurysms. Pseudoaneurysms of peripancreatic vessels, the most common being splenic artery, can complicate necrotizing pancreatitis and present with gastrointestinal tract or intraperitoneal hemorrhage. SMA aneurysms are rare and associated with endocarditis. Symptomatic aneurysms, sizable aneurysms (hepatic artery aneurysm ≥1 cm or splenic artery aneurysm ≥2 cm), and splenic artery aneurysms discovered during pregnancy should be treated, usually with interventional radiology.

Ehlers-Danlos syndrome (EDS) is a group of clinically and genetically heterogeneous, heritable connective tissue disorders affecting skin, bones, and other organs and systems. Life-threatening complications such as VAA formation and dissection and spontaneous organ rupture (most commonly colon and uterus) are limited to vascular EDS, previously known as EDS type 4. Vascular EDS is caused by alterations of the autosomal dominant gene *COL3A1* leading to defective type III collagen in the lungs, skin, intestines, and blood vessels. Vascular EDS is associated with characteristic facies, thin or translucent skin, and easy bruising.

✓ Diagnosis of median arcuate ligament syndrome requires exclusion of other possible causes of abdominal pain, nausea, vomiting, diarrhea, and weight loss
✓ Polyarteritis nodosa and immunoglobulin A vasculitis—systemic vasculitides that commonly have gastrointestinal tract involvement
✓ Behçet disease—gastrointestinal tract involvement most often affects the ileocecal region, where large, deep ulcerations result in bleeding and perforation

---

✓ Vascular EDS—life-threatening complications can occur (eg, VAA formation and dissection and spontaneous organ rupture)

Suggested Reading

Ahmed M. Ischemic bowel disease in 2021. World J Gastroenterol. 2021 Aug;27(29):4746–62.

Bala M, Kashuk J, Moore EE, Kluger Y, Biffl W, Gomes CA, et al. Acute mesenteric ischemia: guidelines of the World Society of Emergency Surgery. World J Emerg Surg. 2017;12:38.

Brandt LJ, Feuerstadt P, Longstreth GF, Boley SJ, American College of Gastroenterology. ACG clinical guideline: epidemiology, risk factors, patterns of presentation, diagnosis, and management of colon ischemia (CI). Am J Gastroenterol. 2015 Jan;110(1):18–44.

Clair DG, Beach JM. Mesenteric ischemia. N Engl J Med. 2016 Mar;374(10):959–68.

Cotter TG, Bledsoe AC, Sweetser S. Colon ischemia: an update for clinicians. Mayo Clin Proc. 2016 May;91(5):671–7.

Kim EN, Lamb K, Relles D, Moudgill N, DiMuzio PJ, Eisenberg JA. Median arcuate ligament syndrome: review of this rare disease. JAMA Surg. 2016 May;151(5):471–7.

Koster MJ, Warrington KJ. Vasculitis of the mesenteric circulation. Best Pract Res Clin Gastroenterol. 2017 Feb;31(1):85–96.

Luther B, Mamopoulos A, Lehmann C, Klar E. The ongoing challenge of acute mesenteric ischemia. Visc Med. 2018 Jul;34(3):217–23.

Sardar P, White CJ. Chronic mesenteric ischemia: diagnosis and management. Prog Cardiovasc Dis. 2021 Mar-Apr;65:71–5.

Singal AK, Kamath PS, Tefferi A. Mesenteric venous thrombosis. Mayo Clin Proc. 2013 Mar;88(3):285–94.

12

Gastrointestinal Manifestations of Systemic Disease[a]

SETH R. SWEETSER, MD

Many systemic diseases can have gastrointestinal (GI) manifestations. Both the gut and the liver may be the main targets of the disease process, or they may be affected indirectly; in either case, the GI symptoms or signs may be the initial reason for seeking medical attention. This chapter is an overview of the more common systemic disorders that have well-recognized GI and liver manifestations, with an emphasis on disorders not considered elsewhere in this book.

Cardiovascular Diseases

Aortic Stenosis

Aortic stenosis is associated with an increased incidence of GI bleeding (Heyde syndrome). The GI bleeding in patients with aortic stenosis is typically from small intestinal angiectasias. In patients with aortic stenosis, the aortic wall shear stress is high. As a result of high macrovascular shear stress, there is increased consumption of high-molecular-weight multimers of von Willebrand factor (vWF) from the increased activity of shear-dependent vWF-cleaving metalloprotease. This leads to a relative deficiency of high-molecular-weight multimers of vWF and an acquired type IIA von Willebrand disease that predisposes the patient to clinically manifest bleeding from angiectatic lesions in the GI tract. Support for this pathophysiologic mechanism comes from observations that the severity of GI bleeding from GI angiectasias decreases after aortic valve replacement, which is associated with a concomitant increase in the level of circulating high-molecular-weight vWF multimers. Similarly, hypertrophic obstructive cardiomyopathy has been associated with GI angiectasias.

Heart Failure

Impairment of myocardial filling or contraction results in inadequate perfusion of tissues and a resultant inability to maintain metabolic demands. Heart failure leads to congestion of the mesenteric venous system, which can manifest with anorexia, nausea, bloating, and abdominal pain. In extreme cases, mesenteric venous congestion results in diarrhea, malabsorption, protein-losing enteropathy, and the clinical picture of cardiac cachexia. Hepatic congestion from right-sided heart failure may cause hepatomegaly, jaundice, abnormal liver test results, and a high serum-ascites albumin gradient. In cases of prolonged hepatic congestion from heart failure, cardiac cirrhosis may develop.

> ✓ Aortic stenosis causing acquired von Willebrand disease that is associated with GI bleeding from small-intestinal angiectasias is known as Heyde syndrome

[a] Portions previously published in Sweetser S, Camilleri M. Gastrointestinal manifestations and management. In: Varga J, Denton CP, Wigley FM, eds. Scleroderma: from pathogenesis to comprehensive management. Springer; 2012:463-9 and Podboy A, Anderson BW, Sweetser S. 61-year-old man with chronic diarrhea. Mayo Clin Proc. 2016 Feb;91(2):e23-8; used with permission

Abbreviations: ALA, aminolevulinic acid; BD, Behçet disease; BRBNS, blue rubber bleb nevus syndrome; CF, cystic fibrosis; CVID, common variable immunodeficiency; DIOS, distal intestinal obstruction syndrome; DM, diabetes mellitus; EPS, encapsulating peritoneal sclerosis; GI, gastrointestinal; GVHD, graft-versus-host disease; HHT, hereditary hemorrhagic telangiectasia; HSP, Henoch-Schönlein purpura; KTW, Klippel-Trénaunay-Weber; PAN, polyarteritis nodosa; PCI, pneumatosis cystoides intestinalis; RA, rheumatoid arthritis; SCD, sickle cell disease; SIBO, small intestinal bacterial overgrowth; SLE, systemic lupus erythematosus; vWF, von Willebrand factor

✓ Heart failure may result in mesenteric venous congestion causing diarrhea, malabsorption, protein-losing enteropathy, and cardiac cachexia

Vascular Diseases

Hereditary Hemorrhagic Telangiectasia

Hereditary hemorrhagic telangiectasia (HHT) (Osler-Weber-Rendu syndrome) is an autosomal dominant disorder with high penetrance and an estimated prevalence of 1 per 10,000. It is characterized by the development of telangiectasias and arteriovenous malformations throughout the body, and it has a propensity to involve the small intestine. Mucocutaneous telangiectasias typically develop in the second decade of life, leading to recurrent, spontaneous epistaxis, which is the most common manifestation of HHT.

Clinical criteria for the diagnosis of HHT are the following:

1. *Epistaxis*—spontaneous, recurrent nosebleeds, usually present since adolescence
2. *Telangiectasias*—multiple lesions at characteristic sites (lips, oral cavity, fingers, nose)
3. *Visceral involvement*—pulmonary, liver, central nervous system, GI tract
4. *Family history*—a first-degree relative with definite HHT

If 3 of the 4 criteria are present, the clinical diagnosis of HHT is definite. If 2 criteria are present, the diagnosis of HHT is probable. If only 1 criterion is present, HHT is unlikely.

GI hemorrhage occurs in 30% of patients with HHT and does not usually start until the fourth or fifth decade of life. HHT is the most common cause of diffuse vascular malformations of the liver in adults. Although hepatic vascular malformations are present in most patients with HHT, symptoms occur in only 30%. With the dual blood supply to the liver, 3 types of vascular shunts may develop, which give rise to 3 distinct clinical presentations: high-output heart failure, portal hypertension, and biliary disease (Box 12.1).

After recurrent epistaxis, GI bleeding is the most common clinical manifestation of HHT. Telangiectasias are readily visible

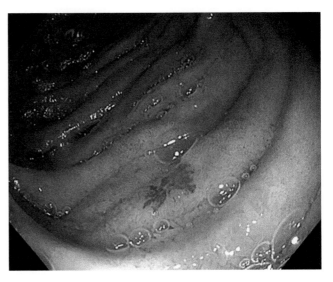

Figure 12.1. Endoscopic Finding of Jejunal Angiectasia in Hereditary Hemorrhagic Telangiectasia.

on endoscopy, occurring throughout the GI tract (Figure 12.1). Endoscopic ablation with argon plasma coagulation is commonly used for bleeding telangiectasias; antivascular endothelial growth factor therapy is the mainstay of treatment.

Blue Rubber Bleb Nevus Syndrome

Blue rubber bleb nevus syndrome (BRBNS) is a rare disorder characterized by the development of venous malformations in many organs; the skin and GI tract are the organs most involved (Figures 12.2 and 12.3). It is usually sporadic, but it may be inherited in an autosomal dominant fashion. The 2 most common manifestations of BRBNS are skin lesions alone or iron deficiency anemia from GI bleeding. Most patients with GI bleeding from BRBNS are asymptomatic and generally respond to blood transfusion and oral iron supplementation. Capsule endoscopy is a noninvasive way to exclude or confirm GI involvement (Figure 12.4), but the distribution of lesions is important to know only if bleeding cannot be controlled by conservative measures. Caution should be used when attempting endoscopic ablation of lesions, which may involve the full thickness of the bowel wall, so that perforation does not occur. The venous malformations can cause numerous extraintestinal complications, including orthopedic deformities, central nervous system involvement, spinal cord compression, hemothorax, and hemopericardium.

Klippel-Trénaunay-Weber Syndrome

Klippel-Trénaunay-Weber (KTW) syndrome is a rare congenital vascular anomaly characterized by the clinical triad of 1) soft tissue and bony hypertrophy of an extremity, 2) varicose veins limited to the affected side, and 3) vascular nevus of the hypertrophied extremity. The cause of this syndrome is unknown. KTW can be diagnosed by the presence of any 2 of these 3 clinical features, with 60% of KTW patients having the full triad. Visceral hemangiomas in KTW have been described involving organs such as the GI tract, liver, spleen, bladder, kidney, lung, and heart. GI hemorrhage is a potentially serious complication resulting from diffuse hemangiomatous involvement of the gut. Transfusion-dependent anemia and life-threatening bleeding may result from extensive cavernous hemangiomas involving the

---

Box 12.1. Three Distinct Clinical Manifestations of Liver Involvement in Hereditary Hemorrhagic Telangiectasia

1. *High-output heart failure* results from an arteriovenous shunt involving the hepatic artery and hepatic veins. This is the most common initial manifestation of liver involvement in hereditary hemorrhagic telangiectasia.

2. *Portal hypertension* results from a hepatic artery–portal vein fistula and occurs most commonly with ascites.

3. *Biliary disease* with bile duct abnormalities is similar to sclerosing cholangitis. Bile duct abnormalities result from ischemia of the biliary tree because the bile ducts obtain all their blood supply from the hepatic artery. Hepatic artery–hepatic vein or hepatic artery–portal vein fistulas may cause biliary ischemia. Clinical manifestations include right upper quadrant pain and cholestasis with or without cholangitis.

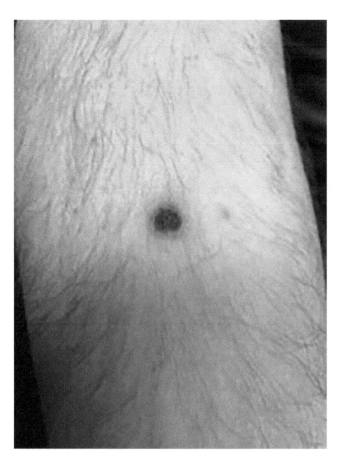

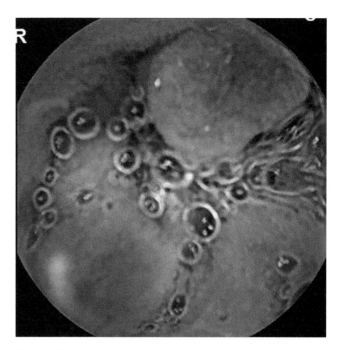

Figure 12.4. Capsule Endoscopic Finding of Characteristic Venous Lesions of Blue Rubber Bleb Nevus Syndrome in Jejunum.

Figure 12.2. Cutaneous Venous Bleb of Blue Rubber Bleb Nevus Syndrome.

rectum. Although diffuse cavernous hemangiomas of the distal colon and rectum are the most reported causes of GI bleeding in KTW, other potential causes of GI hemorrhage related to KTW include localized rectovaginal varices caused by an obstructed internal iliac system and portal hypertension–related bleeding from a hypoplastic portal venous system. GI bleeding in KTW

may be enhanced by consumption coagulopathy (Kasabach-Merritt syndrome) resulting from intravascular clotting within the venous sinusoids of the visceral hemangiomas. Endoscopic therapy has a limited role in the management of colorectal intestinal hemangiomas in KTW and is best reserved for management of localized lesions or ablation of postoperative residual disease. Resection of the involved bowel segment is usually necessary to adequately control bleeding.

Degos Disease

Degos disease (malignant atrophic papulosis) is a vasculopathy of unknown cause characterized by a predominantly non-inflammatory vascular occlusive process, mainly affecting arterioles. Progressive arteriolar occlusion results in tissue ischemia and infarction, which are responsible for the clinical manifestations of the disease. Age at onset of the disease ranges from the first months of life to the seventh decade. In the GI tract, the submucosal arteries are typically affected, causing infarction of the bowel. Endoscopic examination may show infarcts and ulcers throughout the GI tract. The most common cause of death in Degos disease is microvascular infarctions in the intestines, resulting in perforation and peritonitis. Cutaneous lesions typically precede visceral symptoms and have a characteristic appearance described as porcelain-white, atrophic, umbilicated papules with erythematous or telangiectatic borders. There is no known treatment for this disease, and it is usually fatal.

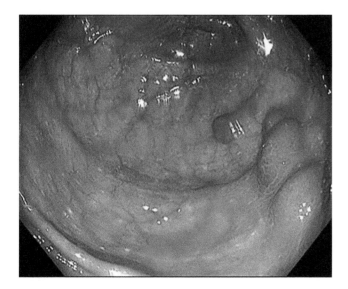

Figure 12.3. Colonoscopic Finding of Venous Lesions of Blue Rubber Bleb Nevus Syndrome.

✓ HHT is an autosomal dominant disorder characterized by telangiectasias and arteriovenous malformations involving the skin, GI tract, and other organs

✓ GI hemorrhage occurs in 30% of patients with HHT and typically begins in the fourth or fifth decade of life

✓ BRBNS is a rare disorder characterized by venous malformations involving mainly the skin and GI tract

✓ The clinical triad of KTW syndrome is soft tissue and bony hypertrophy of an extremity, varicose veins limited to the affected side,
and vascular nevus of the hypertrophied extremity
✓ GI bleeding in KTW syndrome is most commonly from a cavernous hemangioma of the distal colon or rectum

Dermatologic Diseases

The skin and the GI tract may be affected concurrently by the same
processes. Although many dermatologic diseases can manifest
with involvement of the GI tract, 3 with notable GI manifestations
are epidermolysis bullosa, lichen planus, and mastocytosis.
(Mastocytosis is discussed in the Hematologic Disorders section
of this chapter.)

Epidermolysis Bullosa

Epidermolysis bullosa is an inherited disorder characterized
by the development of trauma-induced blisters with resultant
scarring. It results from mutations of genes encoding for structural
proteins located at the dermal-epidermal junction. Disruption in
these structural proteins results in mechanical fragility of the skin
and other epithelialized organs. It is important for the gastroenterologist to be aware of this condition because it may lead to poor
dentition, dysphagia from esophageal strictures, malabsorption,
severe constipation, and anal fissures. Minor trauma from food
boluses leads to bullae, ulceration, and scarring of the esophageal
mucosa with formation of strictures, most commonly in the proximal esophagus. Supportive therapy is the mainstay of treatment
of epidermolysis bullosa. Minimizing trauma with a soft diet,
attention to wound care, and adequate nutritional support are
paramount. Antireflux measures and antisecretory medication
may help to minimize esophageal injury. It is important to be
aware of the risk of mucosal trauma from endoscopic procedures.
Esophageal strictures from epidermolysis bullosa are usually
dilated with balloons rather than bougies to avoid shearing forces
associated with bougies.

Lichen Planus

Lichen planus is a mucocutaneous, autoimmune, inflammatory
disease that most frequently involves the skin and oral mucosa.
Because lichen planus is a disease that affects squamous mucosa,
it can also involve the esophagus. Esophageal lichen planus is
predominantly a disease of middle-aged women. Up to 95% of
patients with esophageal lichen planus having preexisting oral
disease. Symptomatic esophageal involvement may be the initial
manifestation of the disease, and solid food dysphagia of variable severity is the predominant symptom of esophageal disease.
There is typically a long delay in diagnosis, often preceded by
multiple endoscopies, dilations, and treatment of reflux.

A proximal esophageal stricture is a common finding, although variations of esophageal disease include distal strictures,
multiple rings, and long esophageal strictures with a small-caliber
esophagus (Figure 12.5) that is radiologically identical to eosinophilic esophagitis. Common endoscopic findings include difficult passage of the endoscope through the proximal esophagus
on initial esophageal intubation, mucosal thickening with superficial ulceration, mucosal sloughing, and rings (Figure 12.6).
Mucosal sloughing is often evident on initial passage of the endoscope or on withdrawal. This shearing off of friable epidermis
from minor endoscopic trauma has been termed an endoscopic

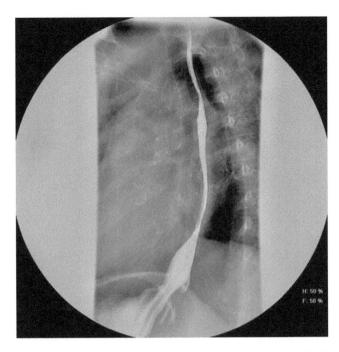

**Figure 12.5. Radiographic Findings in Lichen Planus of the
Esophagus.** Esophagogram shows diffuse esophageal narrowing and
areas of more focal narrowing.

Koebner phenomenon with a predilection for disease to flare in
sites of trauma. Therefore, although esophageal dilation is often a
necessary treatment to relieve dysphagia, unnecessary dilatations
actually might cause a disease flare, particularly if done without
concurrent therapies aimed at controlling the disease.

An increased risk of squamous cell carcinoma has been described
with lichen planus; however, there are no recommendations for
cancer screening of patients who have esophageal lichen planus,
although the co-occurrence should be entertained. The diagnosis
of esophageal lichen planus should be considered for patients with

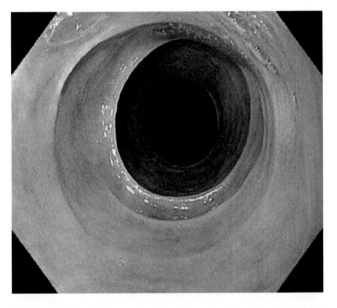

**Figure 12.6. Endoscopic Findings in Esophageal Lichen
Planus.** Endoscopic examination shows multiple, thin, membranous
webs and luminal narrowing.

refractory strictures, particularly middle-aged white women, with or without known lichen planus.

> ✓ Epidermolysis bullosa is an inherited blistering skin disease that can be complicated by esophageal strictures
> ✓ The typical profile of a patient with esophageal lichen planus is a middle-aged White woman with persistent dysphagia

Hematologic Disorders

Amyloidosis

Amyloidosis is characterized by the extracellular deposition of an abnormal fibrillar protein, which disrupts tissue structure and function. Amyloidosis can be acquired or hereditary, and systemic or localized to 1 or more organs, such as the liver or the GI tract. Amyloidosis is classified according to the type of precursor protein. The 2 major types of amyloidosis with clinically important GI involvement are primary and secondary amyloidosis. In primary (AL) amyloidosis, the protein fibrils are composed of fragments of monoclonal light chains; in reactive (secondary, AA) amyloidosis, the protein fibrils are composed of fragments of the circulating acute-phase reactant serum amyloid A protein.

GI disease in amyloidosis results from either mucosal infiltration or neuromuscular infiltration. Within the GI tract, the most common sites of infiltration are the descending duodenum (100%), the stomach and colorectum (>90%), and the esophagus (70%). Mucosal infiltration by amyloid causes polypoid protrusions, erosions, ulcerations (Figure 12.7), mucosal friability, and wall thickening.

Characteristic endoscopic findings in AL amyloidosis include submucosal hematomas and hemorrhagic bullous colitis. Neuromuscular infiltration initially affects the intrinsic enteric nervous system, resulting in a neuropathic process characterized by normal amplitude but uncoordinated contractions. In more advanced disease, tissue wall infiltration causes a myopathic process with low-amplitude contractions.

Symptomatic patients with GI amyloidosis have 4 major presentations: GI bleeding, chronic intestinal dysmotility, malabsorption, and protein-losing gastroenteropathy (Box 12.2).

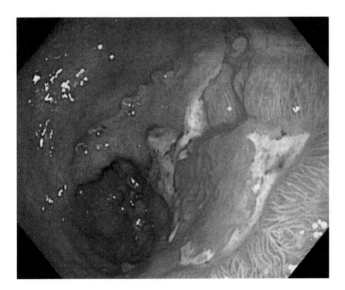

Figure 12.7. Amyloid Ulcer. This large amyloid ulcer with surrounding polypoid mucosa was in the gastric antrum.

> ### Box 12.2. Four Major Syndromic Presentations of Symptomatic Patients With Gastrointestinal Amyloidosis
> 1. *Gastrointestinal bleeding*—secondary to vascular fragility, mucosal lesions, or ischemia
> 2. *Intestinal dysmotility*—causing dysphagia, gastroparesis, chronic intestinal pseudo-obstruction, constipation, bacterial overgrowth, or bile acid malabsorption
> 3. *Malabsorption*—due to mucosal infiltration
> 4. *Protein-losing gastroenteropathy*—should be considered in patients with hypoalbuminemia and edema

Less common GI manifestations include intestinal obstruction from amyloid masses, called amyloidomas, and cholangitis from amyloid deposition around the ampulla of Vater, resulting in biliary obstruction. Liver involvement is common in both AL amyloidosis and AA amyloidosis. Common symptoms with hepatic amyloidosis include weight loss, fatigue, and abdominal pain. Most patients have hepatomegaly, with an elevated serum alkaline phosphatase level being the most frequent abnormal liver test result.

The diagnosis of GI amyloidosis can be challenging in patients without an established diagnosis of amyloidosis. It is important to maintain a high degree of awareness when patients have disorders known to be associated with amyloidosis, such as multiple myeloma and chronic inflammatory disorders. When AL amyloidosis is suspected, testing should be done to assess for the presence of serum or monoclonal proteins. However, diagnostic confirmation of GI involvement requires tissue biopsy of duodenal or colorectal mucosa, which is more sensitive than a subcutaneous fat biopsy. The diagnostic histologic finding is a red appearance of amyloid with Congo red stain under normal light microscopy and apple-green birefringence in polarized light (Figure 12.8). Treatment of amyloid-related GI complications is directed toward symptom control and the underlying cause of amyloidosis.

Porphyria

Porphyria results from a deficiency in 1 of the enzymes involved in the heme synthetic pathway. The porphyrias are commonly classified by clinical features into 2 main groups: acute porphyrias and cutaneous porphyrias. The *acute porphyrias* are characterized by dramatic and potentially life-threatening neurologic symptoms and usually present with severe abdominal pain, whereas the *cutaneous porphyrias* have no neurologic or abdominal symptoms but instead manifest with severe skin photosensitivity.

The 4 acute porphyrias are acute intermittent porphyria, variegate porphyria, hereditary coproporphyria, and aminolevulinic acid (ALA) dehydratase deficiency porphyria. Acute intermittent porphyria is the most common acute porphyria. Patients with any of the 4 acute porphyrias can present with acute neurovisceral attacks consisting of severe abdominal pain, nausea and vomiting, constipation, tachycardia, paresthesias, weakness, dark urine, and peripheral sensory deficits. The abdominal pain of acute attacks typically develops gradually over hours and lasts days. Factors that commonly precipitate an episode of acute porphyria include certain medications, alcohol ingestion, smoking, fasting or caloric restriction, infections, and pregnancy.

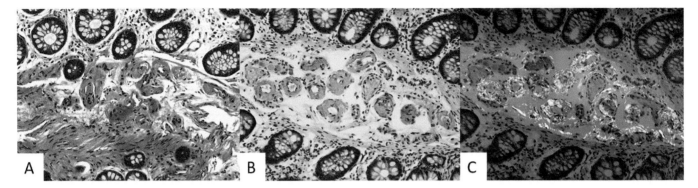

Figure 12.8. Histologic Appearance of Amyloid in Intestinal Biopsy Specimen. A, Subtle pink staining of thickened blood vessel walls in lamina propria suggestive of amyloid. B, Congo Red staining of amyloid. C, Characteristic apple-green birefringence of amyloid in blood vessel walls under polarized light.

Acute intermittent porphyria is inherited in an autosomal dominant manner with low penetrance. It is associated with increased levels of ALA and porphobilinogen; there are no skin findings. Variegate porphyria is characterized by increased levels of urine coproporphyrin and stool protoporphyrin and coproporphyrin; patients can have skin disease, with or without an abdominal attack. In hereditary coproporphyria, stool and urine coproporphyrin levels are increased; skin disease can be present, usually with an abdominal attack. In the very rare ALA dehydratase deficiency porphyria, only the ALA level is increased; there are no skin findings, and the condition is autosomal recessive. Urine ALA and porphobilinogen levels are always increased during an acute abdominal crisis (ALA accumulates in the absence of ALA dehydratase). In acute intermittent porphyria, urine ALA and porphobilinogen values usually are increased between attacks. The diagnostic test for acute intermittent porphyria is a spot urine sample for porphobilinogen.

The most common cutaneous porphyria is porphyria cutanea tarda, which affects only the skin and is associated with high alcohol intake, iron overload states such as hereditary hemochromatosis, hepatitis C virus infection, and systemic illnesses including systemic lupus erythematosus (SLE), diabetes mellitus (DM), and chronic kidney disease. Excess porphyrins, which are photoreactive, are deposited in the dermis, causing tissue damage that manifests as vesicles and bullae.

The second most common cutaneous porphyria is erythropoietic protoporphyria, with exquisite photosensitivity being its principal clinical manifestation. In addition, in 10% of patients, clinically evident liver disease (cirrhosis and liver failure) results from progressive hepatic accumulation of protoporphyrin (Figure 12.9). In patients with erythropoietic protoporphyria, liver disease typically occurs after age 30 years; the urine is notable in lacking porphyrin metabolites, which are detected only in the stool. The diagnosis of acute porphyria should be considered if patients have recurrent episodes of severe abdominal pain, constipation, dark urine, and neuropsychiatric disturbances, while the diagnosis of cutaneous porphyria should be considered if patients have typical dermatologic findings.

Management of an acute porphyric attack consists of quickly identifying and reversing the precipitating factors. Acetaminophen, meperidine, and morphine can be used safely for pain management. Ondansetron is the preferred antiemetic, and use of promethazine should be avoided. Intravenous glucose is beneficial. The definitive treatment of an acute porphyric attack is intravenous hemin, which replenishes the depleted heme pool and ameliorates signs and symptoms of the acute porphyric attack.

Givosiran is a small interfering RNA that neutralizes excess ALA synthase mRNA in hepatocytes, an effect that decreases the production of ALA and porphobilinogen. Givosiran is approved for treatment of acute intermittent porphyria and has been shown to

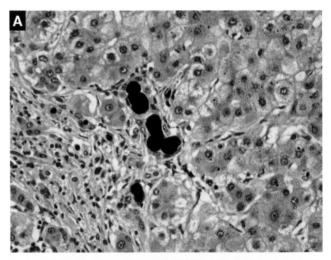

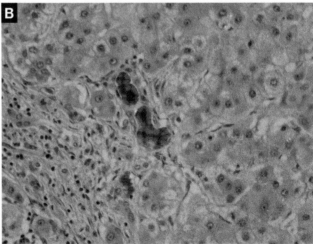

Figure 12.9. Erythropoietic Protoporphyria. A, Liver biopsy specimen shows distorted lobular architecture with red-brown protoporphyrin pigment in hepatocytes and lumen of bile canaliculi (hematoxylin-eosin, original magnification ×200). B, Polarizing microscopy shows characteristic bright red and centrally located Maltese cross appearance of globular protoporphyrin deposits (hematoxylin-eosin, original magnification ×200).

substantially decrease the rate of acute attacks. Liver transplant is the final treatment option for acute porphyrias.

Systemic Mastocytosis

Mastocytosis refers to the infiltration of mast cells in the skin or various other organs. Cutaneous mastocytosis is the most common form; however, the spectrum of disease includes symptoms related to the release of mast cell mediators (eg, histamine) and signs resulting from multiorgan mast cell infiltration, including infiltration of the liver and intestines. The characteristic dermatologic lesion is urticaria pigmentosa, which manifests as yellow-tan macules involving the extremities and trunk, with the classic finding of Darier sign (urticaria after scratching). GI manifestations of systemic mastocytosis are varied and include nausea, vomiting, diarrhea, and abdominal pain. Hyperhistaminemia can result in gastric acid hypersecretion and peptic ulcer disease. Infiltration of the liver causes hepatomegaly, liver test abnormalities, and portal hypertension. Mast cell infiltration of the small intestine and colon causes mast cell enterocolopathy. Systemic mastocytosis is a clonal disorder of mast cell progenitors and is associated with activating mutations of the *c-kit* gene. However, the tyrosine kinase inhibitors, such as imatinib mesylate, are rarely effective in systemic mastocytosis because the most common mutation interferes with drug binding.

Sickle Cell Disease

Sickle cell disease (SCD) is an autosomal recessive abnormality of the β-globin chain of hemoglobin that results in poorly deformable, sickled red blood cells that cause microvascular occlusion and hemolytic anemia. The spleen is nearly always involved in SCD, with hyposplenism or asplenism resulting from splenic infarction. Patients with splenic infarction present with left upper quadrant pain, nausea and vomiting, a friction rub over the splenic area, and leukocytosis. Splenic atrophy predisposes to infection with encapsulated bacteria. Liver and GI complications are common in SCD.

Several different acute and chronic processes can involve the liver in SCD. Hepatic injuries due to sickle cell anemia can be grouped as sickle cell hepatopathy. Acute hepatobiliary complications of SCD include acute hepatic crisis, sickle cell intrahepatic cholestasis, acute hepatic sequestration, and cholecystitis. Chronic liver disease in SCD may be due to hemosiderosis, chronic viral hepatitis, or nodular regenerative hyperplasia.

Patients with 1 of the 4 hepatobiliary complications of SCD most commonly present with right upper quadrant pain and acute painful hepatomegaly. High blood viscosity in SCD predisposes to liver ischemia and infarction despite the dual blood supply of the liver. Acute sickle hepatic crisis affects 10% of patients with a painful vasoocclusive crisis and simulates acute cholecystitis with fever, right upper quadrant pain, leukocytosis, and variable increases in liver enzymes. The liver is usually enlarged and tender in acute sickle hepatic crisis. Sickle cell intrahepatic cholestasis is a rare but potentially fatal complication. It is an unusually severe hepatic crisis caused by widespread sickling in the hepatic sinusoids, resulting in hepatic ischemia. It is characterized by profound conjugated hyperbilirubinemia (bilirubin level >50 g/dL) with renal failure, encephalopathy, and coagulopathy. Sickle cell intrahepatic cholestasis is treated with exchange transfusion, but affected patients often die of liver failure. Acute hepatic sequestration with jaundice is accompanied by a decrease in hemoglobin and is due to obstruction of sinusoidal blood flow by masses of sickled erythrocytes in the liver. The gallstones in SCD are typically of the black-pigment type as a result of increased bilirubin excretion. They are commonly seen on plain radiographs because the bilirubin is in the form of a calcium salt. There is an increased incidence of cholecystitis and choledocholithiasis in SCD. Cholecystectomy is the most frequent surgical procedure in patients with SCD, and some experts advocate early cholecystectomy in asymptomatic patients.

Liver abscesses are more common in SCD due to asplenism and an impaired reticuloendothelial system. Patients with SCD have a notable predisposition to liver abscesses due to *Yersinia enterocolitica* infection because of iron overload and deferoxamine therapy, which are 2 conditions that increase susceptibility to this organism.

Iron overload may cause chronic liver disease in SCD and is related to accumulation of transfused iron and continuous hemolysis. Chronic hepatitis C is more prevalent in patients with SCD who received transfusions before blood products were screened (June 1992).

Nodular regenerative hyperplasia may occur in SCD and is characterized by nodules of regenerative hepatocytes distributed diffusely throughout the liver, with atrophy of the intervening parenchyma (Figure 12.10). Lack of fibrosis and hepatic dysfunction differentiate it from cirrhosis. Nodular regenerative hyperplasia is believed to result from an obstructive portal venopathy and can be seen with hematologic disorders, rheumatologic conditions, and adverse effects of certain medications (eg, azathioprine).

GI complications of SCD include abdominal crisis, acute pancreatitis, peptic ulcer disease, and ischemic bowel. In an acute vasoocclusive crisis, small infarcts occur in the mesentery and abdominal viscera and cause severe abdominal pain and signs of peritoneal irritation with radiographic evidence of ileus. The crisis may mimic other acute abdominal processes but usually resolves with supportive care. Acute pancreatitis related to SCD may result from microvascular occlusion and ischemic injury. Peptic ulcer disease is more common in SCD and may be due to reduced mucosal resistance from ischemia. Ischemic bowel due to intravascular sickling, causing microvascular occlusion, is an uncommon complication of SCD.

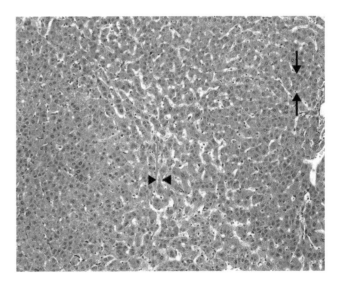

Figure 12.10. Nodular Regenerative Hyperplasia. Liver biopsy specimen shows atrophy of zone 3 hepatocytes (arrowheads) and hypertrophy of zone 1 hepatocytes (arrows) without fibrosis (hematoxylin-eosin, original magnification ×100).

✓ The 2 major types of amyloidosis involving the GI tract are AL and AA amyloidosis
✓ The most common segment of the GI tract to be involved by amyloid is the duodenum
✓ Submucosal hematomas are the characteristic endoscopic finding of AL amyloid
✓ The most common acute porphyria is acute intermittent porphyria
✓ Severe abdominal pain is the usual presentation of acute intermittent porphyria
✓ Laboratory analysis of a spot urine sample for porphobilinogen is the diagnostic test for acute intermittent porphyria
✓ GI manifestations of systemic mastocytosis are varied but include peptic ulcer disease and diarrhea
✓ The 4 acute hepatobiliary complications of SCD are acute hepatic crisis, sickle cell intrahepatic cholestasis, acute hepatic sequestration, and cholecystitis

Pulmonary Disorders

Cystic Fibrosis

Cystic fibrosis (CF) is an autosomal recessive disorder resulting from mutations in the CF transmembrane regulator (*CFTR*) gene. The *CFTR* gene encodes for a chloride channel protein in the apical surface of epithelial membranes. Dysfunction of *CFTR* results in altered electrolyte content in the environment external to the surface epithelial membranes, with desiccation and reduced clearance of secretions from tubular structures lined by affected epithelia. The pulmonary manifestations of CF are the most serious because they lead to respiratory failure. However, the CFTR protein is found throughout all GI tract epithelia, including the small intestine, pancreas, and hepatobiliary system. Therefore, *CFTR* dysfunction can result in many GI complications, including meconium ileus, pancreatic insufficiency, pancreatitis, gastroesophageal reflux disease, distal intestinal obstruction syndrome (DIOS), constipation, small intestinal bacterial overgrowth (SIBO), and liver disease. Because more than half of patients with CF in the US are adults, it is important to be able to recognize and manage the GI complications of CF.

The GI manifestations of CF begin in infancy. The earliest manifestation is meconium ileus, a neonatal bowel obstruction. It is the presenting symptom in 15% of infants with CF, and it classically manifests with signs of intestinal obstruction within 48 hours of birth. Characteristic radiographic findings show distended loops of bowel devoid of air-fluid levels. Acetylcysteine (Mucomyst), a mucolytic, is a safe and effective treatment to dissolve and dislodge meconium. Meconium-induced obstruction is also treated with diatrizoate (Gastrografin) enemas. Complicated meconium ileus requires surgical therapy.

Pancreatic insufficiency is the most common GI complication of CF. It often develops early in life with the more severe *CFTR* gene mutations. Pancreatic insufficiency leads to maldigestion and malabsorption of nutrients. Long-term sequelae of malnutrition include growth retardation, cognitive dysfunction related to vitamin E deficiency, and more rapid decline in pulmonary function. Measurement of fecal fat in a 72-hour stool collection can be done to screen for pancreatic insufficiency. Patients with pancreatic insufficiency require lifelong pancreatic enzyme replacement therapy. Fibrosing colonopathy is a severe intestinal fibrostenotic process that occurred in patients with CF who ingested large doses of pancreatic enzyme replacement therapy; because of this complication, the recommended upper limit is 2,500 lipase units per kg per meal.

Acute pancreatitis, which develops in 10% of patients with CF who have preserved pancreatic function, occurs when there is decreased ductal flow from inspissated secretions leading to premature activation of trypsinogen and local inflammation. Treatment of recurrent acute or chronic pancreatitis in patients with CF is like treatment in those without CF. Intravenous fluids are the cornerstone of management; however, use of narcotic analgesics should be minimized because they can precipitate constipation and DIOS (see below).

Gastroesophageal reflux disease occurs in approximately 30% of adults with CF. The basic mechanism, transient lower esophageal sphincter relaxation, is the same in patients with CF as in healthy controls. However, transient lower esophageal sphincter relaxations cause more frequent and more proximal reflux events in those with CF. Proton pump inhibitors are the first-line therapy for gastroesophageal reflux disease in CF. Lung function improves in patients who CF who have treatment with gastric acid suppression.

DIOS, a unique feature of CF, is characterized by partial or complete fecal obstruction of the ileocecal region. It occurs in patients with CF of all ages, including adults, and results from accumulation of viscous fecal material with adherence to the mucosa. Patients with DIOS present with acute or chronic intestinal obstruction with abdominal pain and distention. They may continue to have stool output. On physical examination, a right lower quadrant mass may be palpable. Radiographic imaging typically shows fecal loading in the right lower quadrant as evidenced by a bubbly-granular fecal mass (Figure 12.11). DIOS can be diagnosed from clinical symptoms, physical findings, and suggestive radiographic imaging. Management of DIOS includes surgical consultation, receiving nothing by mouth, nasogastric tube decompression, and intravenous fluids. In cases of complete obstruction, a hyperosmolar contrast enema such as diatrizoate should be administered to clear the impacted fecal mass. Hyperosmolar agents cause luminal hydration with resultant mobilization of the mucus-stool mass and relief of obstruction. With partial bowel obstructions, lavage with oral polyethylene glycol

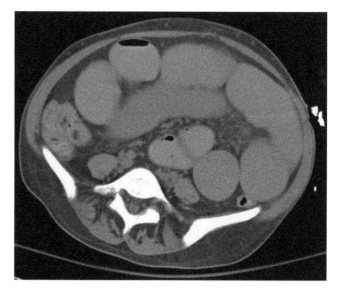

Figure 12.11. Distal Intestinal Obstruction Syndrome of Cystic Fibrosis. Computed tomographic image shows dilated loops of fluid-filled small bowel throughout the abdomen and pelvis with fecalization of bowel contents and gradual tapering of small-bowel caliber in the distal ileum.

solutions and oral laxatives can be effective. Surgical intervention remains the last resort when medical management fails or bowel ischemia develops. After recovery from an episode, prevention of recurrent episodes of DIOS with routine use of osmotic agents such as polyethylene glycol is critical.

Constipation is a frequent symptom in CF and, like DIOS, is related to decreased water secretion caused by the *CFTR* defect. In contrast to DIOS, which is an obstructive process that starts at the terminal ileum and extends distally, constipation in CF is an obstructive process that begins in the sigmoid colon and extends proximally. Osmotic laxatives are the first-line treatment of CF-related constipation.

SIBO occurs in up to 50% of patients with CF. Thick mucus secretions, intestinal dysmotility, and the use of acid-suppressing medications predispose patients to the development of SIBO. Diagnostic tests, such as culture of duodenal aspirates and breath hydrogen testing, have limitations. Empirical therapy with antibiotics is frequently performed for SIBO.

CF-related liver disease is becoming a more prevalent complication. There is a broad spectrum of hepatobiliary disease in CF, which includes microgallbladder, cholelithiasis, hepatic steatosis, nodular regenerative hyperplasia, and focal biliary cirrhosis with portal hypertension. Notably, asymptomatic increase in serum liver enzymes or hepatosplenomegaly may be the only clinical manifestations of CF-related liver disease.

The treatment of symptomatic liver disease in CF is a challenge and depends on the age of the patient and the extent of the liver disease. Cholestatic liver disease is best treated with ursodeoxycholic acid (15-20 mg/kg daily), and treatment should be initiated with early recognition of CF-related liver disease to improve the biochemical profile, facilitate biliary drainage, and delay progression of liver disease.

In addition to CF-related GI and liver complications, several GI diseases, including celiac disease and GI malignancies, are associated with CF. The prevalence of celiac disease is higher in patients with CF than in the general population. It is important to recognize that tissue transglutaminase IgA can be increased in CF even in the absence of histologic evidence of active celiac disease. Thus, the diagnosis of celiac disease should not be made solely because of positive IgA tissue transglutaminase serologic results and requires compatible small intestinal histologic changes and response to a gluten-free diet. Compared with the general population, patients with CF are at increased risk for esophageal, gastric, hepatobiliary, gallbladder, small intestinal, and colon cancers. The risk for colorectal cancer in these patients is markedly increased; most cases occur before 50 years of age. Therefore, the Cystic Fibrosis Foundation recommends that colorectal cancer screening begin at age 40 years in patients with CF and be continued every 5 years. In addition, patients with CF in whom adenomatous polyps have been found at colonoscopy should have surveillance in 3 years, unless a shorter interval is indicated by findings. Patients with CF who are older than 30 years and have recovered from solid-organ transplant should begin colorectal cancer screening within 2 years because of the additional risk for colorectal cancer in association with immunosuppression. Furthermore, the unique physiochemical characteristics of the stool and intestinal mucus in CF complicates bowel preparation for colonoscopy; therefore, increased intensity regimens are recommended to allow optimal examination.

Sarcoidosis

Sarcoidosis is a multisystem granulomatous disease that commonly involves the lungs and less frequently the liver and GI tract. Symptomatic liver involvement is infrequent. Most patients have only biochemical liver test abnormalities, most commonly an increased alkaline phosphatase level. However, in a small percentage of patients, progressive liver disease develops, including cholestasis, hepatitis, and nodular regenerative hyperplasia with resultant portal hypertension. In addition, portal vein thrombosis may occur because of stasis from obliteration of small portal veins by granulomatous phlebitis. Budd-Chiari syndrome may develop from extrinsic compression of hepatic veins by enlarged granulomatous lymph nodes.

In contrast to sarcoidosis involvement of the liver, sarcoidosis of the GI tract is rare, with the stomach being the most commonly involved portion of the GI tract. Patients with gastric sarcoidosis most commonly present with postprandial epigastric pain related either to peptic ulceration or to gastric luminal narrowing from granulomatous inflammation and fibrosis of the gastric wall. Patients may initially present with massive GI hemorrhage from ulceration. Endoscopic findings in gastric sarcoid include ulcerations, thickened gastric folds, mucosal polyps or nodules, and antral deformities. A characteristic finding on upper GI series is a resemblance to linitis plastica because of granulomatous involvement of the gastric wall. Involvement of other portions of the GI tract by sarcoidosis is much less common. Patients with esophageal involvement may present with dysphagia related to either dysmotility or mechanical obstruction. Patients with sarcoidosis of the small intestine may present with abdominal pain, diarrhea, malabsorption, or protein-losing enteropathy. Colonic involvement manifests with polypoid lesions, stenosis, and ulceration. Pancreatic sarcoidosis may simulate carcinoma with a mass in the head of the pancreas and associated obstructive jaundice and weight loss. Most patients with pancreatic sarcoidosis have bilateral hilar adenopathy.

The diagnosis of hepatic and luminal GI tract sarcoidosis is made from the presence of noncaseating granulomas on biopsy, extra-abdominal organ involvement, and exclusion of granulomatous infections. The differential diagnosis of GI sarcoidosis includes Crohn disease, foreign body reaction, tuberculosis, histoplasmosis, and syphilis. At times, sarcoidosis coexists with Crohn disease or ulcerative colitis. Treatment of GI sarcoidosis depends on the severity and extent of the disease, with asymptomatic patients requiring no treatment. Corticosteroids and other immunosuppressive agents are the treatment of choice for symptomatic patients.

✓ CF can result in many GI complications, including meconium ileus, pancreatic insufficiency, pancreatitis, gastroesophageal reflux disease, DIOS, constipation, SIBO, and liver disease

✓ Pancreatic insufficiency is the most common GI complication of CF

✓ DIOS is a unique complication of CF characterized by partial or complete fecal obstruction of the ileocecal region

✓ The spectrum of hepatobiliary disease in CF includes microgallbladder, cholelithiasis, hepatic steatosis, nodular regenerative hyperplasia, and focal biliary cirrhosis with portal hypertension

✓ Patients with CF are at increased risk of colorectal cancer when they are young; screening for this is recommended to begin at age 40 years with continued screening every 5 years

✓ Luminal GI tract involvement by sarcoidosis is uncommon; the stomach is the most commonly involved portion, presenting with a granulomatous gastritis

✓ A characteristic finding of the stomach on upper GI series in sarcoidosis is a linitis plastica appearance due to granulomatous involvement of the gastric wall

Immunologic Disorders

Angioedema

Angioedema affecting the intestinal tract causes severe abdominal pain with vomiting due to edematous bowel obstruction. Intestinal angioedema results from hereditary, acquired, or drug-induced causes. Hereditary angioedema is an autosomal dominant disorder characterized by quantitative or functional deficiency of C1 inhibitor protein, which inhibits complement proteases and coagulation system proteases. C1 inhibitor deficiency results in unregulated activation of the complement and coagulation systems and increased levels of bradykinin, which is responsible for angioedema. Hereditary angioedema is associated with localized swelling involving all layers of the skin or walls of hollow organs such as in the respiratory or GI tracts. GI manifestations include nausea, vomiting, abdominal pain, diarrhea, and ascites. Orthostatic symptoms may occur as a result of fluid shifts into the intestinal lumen or peritoneal cavity, which decrease the effective circulating volume. Symptoms are at maximum intensity for approximately 24 hours and can resolve spontaneously. Imaging may show edematous bowel (Figure 12.12) and ascites.

Measurement of a serum level of C4 is a cost-effective screening test to rule out hereditary angioedema because virtually all patients with hereditary angioedema have a persistently low C4 level. Subsequent measurement of quantitative and functional levels of C1 inhibitor confirms the diagnosis. On-demand treatment for acute attacks of hereditary angioedema includes administration of plasma or recombinant C1 inhibitor, blocking the bradykinin receptor with icatibant or inactivating plasma kallikrein with ecallantide.

Intestinal angioedema may be acquired, with C1 inhibitor deficiency related to collagen vascular diseases or lymphoproliferative disorders. Angiotensin-converting enzyme inhibitors can cause angioedema of the intestine, independently of diminished complement or C1 inhibitor levels. Angiotensin II receptor antagonists and renin inhibitors have also been implicated. Women taking medications containing estrogen may present with similar clinical manifestations.

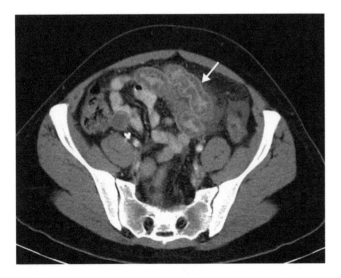

Figure 12.12. Mesenteric Angioedema. Computed tomographic image shows thickened small-bowel loop (arrow).

Common Variable Immunodeficiency

Common variable immunodeficiency (CVID) is a primary immunodeficiency disorder characterized by impaired B-lymphocyte maturation with hypogammaglobulinemia. T-lymphocyte dysfunction occurs variably in CVID. It is estimated to affect 1 in 25,000 individuals; age at onset is typically after puberty and before 30 years. Affected individuals have recurrent respiratory infections, autoimmune phenomena, and increased rates of malignancy. GI manifestations of CVID occur in up to 50% of individuals and include atrophic gastritis, chronic diarrhea, nodular lymphoid hyperplasia, and GI malignancies. Gastric manifestations of CVID include atrophic gastritis and achlorhydria, and the development of pernicious anemia is common. The risk of gastric carcinoma is markedly increased in patients with CVID, with concomitant *Helicobacter pylori* infection further increasing the risk. The most common GI manifestation of CVID is chronic diarrhea, which can be due to several conditions, including GI infections, a spruelike disorder, SIBO, inflammatory bowel disease, or small intestinal lymphoma.

Giardiasis is the most common GI infection in CVID and can be challenging to treat. It may cause refractory diarrhea, malabsorption, and weight loss. Other GI infections causing diarrhea in CVID include cytomegalovirus, cryptosporidiosis, and chronic norovirus infection.

A spruelike syndrome that occurs in CVID is distinct from celiac disease because it does not respond to a gluten-free diet. The absence of plasma cells in the lamina propria is a specific histologic feature that helps to distinguish CVID from other small intestinal enteropathies. Some patients with spruelike intestinal changes benefit from treatment with corticosteroids.

Liver disease with significant hepatic dysfunction occurs in approximately 10% of patients with CVID. The most common cause of liver dysfunction is nodular regenerative hyperplasia.

Initial evaluation of patients with CVID includes measurement of immunoglobulin levels and demonstration of an impaired response to vaccination. Referral to a clinical immunologist is indicated to determine the most appropriate therapies and to help monitor the patient for associated disorders.

Selective IgA Deficiency

Selective IgA deficiency is the most common primary immunodeficiency disorder, occurring in about 1 in 500 persons. It is characterized by selective loss of secretory and serum IgA. Individuals are susceptible to respiratory, urogenital, and GI infections (especially giardiasis). Celiac disease and pernicious anemia occur with increased frequency in patients with selective IgA deficiency.

✓ Intestinal angioedema can be hereditary or acquired and commonly manifests with abdominal pain and diarrhea
✓ Measurement of serum C4 levels is the screening test of choice to rule out hereditary angioedema
✓ GI manifestations of CVID are common and include diarrhea and spruelike disease, and the risk of gastric cancer and lymphoma is markedly increased in this disorder
✓ Giardiasis is the most common GI infection in CVID
✓ Patients with selective IgA deficiency have an increased frequency of celiac disease

Renal Diseases and Hemodialysis

Chronic Kidney Disease

Chronic kidney disease can be complicated by dysgeusia, anorexia, nausea, vomiting, esophagitis, gastritis, angiodysplasias of the GI tract, peptic ulcer disease, duodenitis, duodenal pseudomelanosis (asymptomatic), abdominal pain, constipation, pseudo-obstruction, perforated colonic diverticula, small-bowel and colonic ulceration, intussusception, GI tract bleeding, amyloidosis, diarrhea, fecal impaction, and SIBO.

Hemodialysis

In patients undergoing hemodialysis, a refractory exudative ascites of unclear pathogenesis can develop; this resolves with renal transplant. These patients also have a greater risk of colon ischemia. Infections and ulcerative complications of the GI tract, diverticulitis, and perforated colonic diverticula often develop in patients who have had renal transplant.

Peritoneal Dialysis

Patients undergoing continuous ambulatory peritoneal dialysis are at increased risk of bacterial peritonitis and a rare but serious complication, encapsulating peritoneal sclerosis (EPS). EPS is characterized by partial or intermittent bowel obstruction accompanied by marked sclerotic thickening of the peritoneal membrane. The bowel loops within the sclerotic membrane become adherent and encapsulated, leading to bowel obstruction. A typical computed tomographic feature of EPS is an enhancing thickened peritoneum, which may progress to peritoneal encapsulation of the involved bowel loops and is frequently described as "cocooning." Tamoxifen has been successful for decreasing EPS-related fibrosis and improving intestinal function.

Polycystic Kidney Disease

The adult form (autosomal dominant) of polycystic kidney disease is the most commonly inherited kidney disease; it affects between 1 in 400 to 1 in 1,000 people in the general population. It is a systemic disorder that is associated with numerous extrarenal manifestations, many of which occur in the GI tract. GI manifestations include hepatic cysts, diverticular disease, hernias, pancreatic cysts, choledochal cysts, common bile duct dilation, and splenic cysts. Liver cysts are common (Figure 12.13); their frequency increases with age, and they are more prevalent in women. Despite large cysts, liver function is preserved. Complications of hepatic cysts include infection and biliary obstruction, which requires antibiotic treatment and percutaneous drainage. Colonic diverticulosis is more common in adult polycystic kidney disease with end-stage renal disease. It may result from smooth muscle dysfunction leading to susceptibility for the development of diverticulosis. In addition, affected patients are more prone for the development of complicated diverticulitis. Hernias of the inguinal, incisional, and paraumbilical types are more common in adults with polycystic kidney disease. Hernias are suspected to be the result of abnormal extracellular matrix production and increased intra-abdominal pressure from cystic liver disease. Large bile duct abnormalities occur more frequently in polycystic kidney disease, including Caroli disease, which is multifocal cystic dilation of the intrahepatic bile ducts.

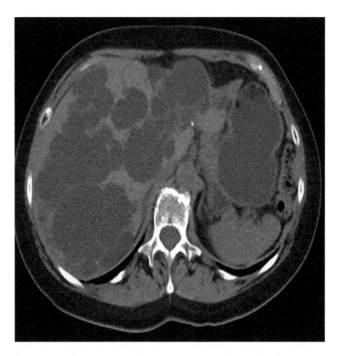

Figure 12.13. Computed Tomographic Finding of Multiple Liver Cysts in Adult Polycystic Kidney Disease.

✓ Angiodysplastic lesions of the GI tract occur more commonly in patients with chronic kidney disease
✓ Individuals undergoing hemodialysis have a greater risk of colon ischemia
✓ Bowel obstruction from EPS is a rare but serious complication of peritoneal dialysis
✓ Adult polycystic kidney disease has many GI manifestations, including hepatic cysts, diverticular disease, pancreatic cysts, and choledochal cysts

---

Endocrine Disorders

Diabetes Mellitus

GI symptoms are common in patients with DM. Autonomic neuropathy complicating DM can involve the entire GI tract. Dysphagia from esophageal dysmotility occurs as the result of vagal dysfunction. Esophageal stasis can predispose to *Candida* infection, and new-onset odynophagia in a patient with diabetes should suggest the presence of *Candida* esophagitis. Gastroparesis is a common complication of poorly controlled DM. Symptoms include early satiety, bloating, heartburn, nausea, and intermittent vomiting. A succussion splash may be appreciated on physical examination. Phase III of the migrating motor complex is frequently absent, which predisposes to the formation of gastric bezoars. Diarrhea and fecal incontinence are frequent complaints in DM. The diarrhea is often watery and nocturnal. Intestinal autonomic neuropathy may be the cause; however, other conditions to consider include celiac disease (more prevalent in type 1 DM), pancreatic exocrine insufficiency, and SIBO. Severe constipation associated with colonic dysmotility occurs in 20% of patients with diabetes who have neuropathy. Fecal incontinence is commonly due to anal sphincter dysfunction and decreased rectal sensation. Fatty liver disease is frequent.

Thyroid Disease

Hyperthyroidism may manifest as hyperphagia, weight loss, mild diarrhea, steatorrhea, abdominal pain, vomiting, concomitant atrophic gastritis, dysphagia, ascites, jaundice, and nonspecific mild abnormalities on liver function testing. Autoimmune hepatitis and primary biliary cholangitis also may be associated disorders. Hypothyroidism often results in anorexia, weight gain, constipation, dysphagia, heartburn, and, less often, intestinal pseudo-obstruction, achlorhydria, and ascites (high concentration of total protein and high serum-ascites albumin gradient). Associated GI diseases include pernicious anemia, ulcerative colitis, primary biliary cholangitis, autoimmune hepatitis, and celiac disease.

Parathyroid Disease

Hyperparathyroidism, with hypercalcemia, classically produces anorexia, nausea, vomiting, constipation, and abdominal pain; rarely, peptic ulcer disease and pancreatitis develop. Patients with hypoparathyroidism can present with diarrhea, steatorrhea, abdominal pain, pseudo-obstruction, protein-losing enteropathy, and lymphangiectasia; also, autoimmune hepatitis may develop.

✓ DM is associated with a spectrum of GI conditions, including gastroparesis, intestinal autonomic neuropathy, and colonic dysmotility
✓ Severe hypothyroidism can result in a high-protein and high serum-ascites albumin gradient

Oncologic Disorders

Leukemias and lymphomas commonly involve the GI tract and liver. Hodgkin disease can involve the liver, extrahepatic bile ducts, or lymph nodes, or it can manifest as intrahepatic cholestasis without hepatobiliary involvement. Unusual tumors affecting the gut include α chain disease (also called immunoproliferative small intestinal disease), which diffusely infiltrates the small intestine and adjacent lymph nodes (B cells and α heavy chains are produced in excess); mantle cell lymphomas, which mimic a multiple polyposis syndrome; multiple myeloma or amyloidosis, with focal plasmacytomas (mass, ulceration, bleeding, or obstruction), GI mucosal infiltration with malabsorption, or hyperviscosity syndrome (ischemia); Waldenström macroglobulinemia, with GI tract and hepatosplenic infiltration and malabsorption; and small cell lung carcinoma and other malignancies, with paraneoplastic pseudo-obstruction (patients may be positive for antineuronal nuclear antibody [anti-Hu], type 1 Purkinje cell antibody, or N-type calcium channel–binding antibody).

Allogenic bone marrow transplant often is complicated by graft-vs-host disease (GVHD). Usually occurring in the first 20 to 80 days after transplant, *acute GVHD* is characterized by erythematous maculopapular rashes, small and large intestinal mucosal involvement (diarrhea, protein-losing enteropathy, malabsorption, pain, bleeding, and crypt apoptotic bodies seen in biopsy specimens, even in areas that appear normal on endoscopy), and cholestatic liver disease. Usually occurring 80 to 400 days after transplant (and usually in persons with previous acute GVHD), *chronic GVHD* is characterized by cholestatic liver disease (vanishing bile ducts), esophageal disease (dysphagia, strictures, and webs), small-bowel disease (diarrhea or bacterial overgrowth), skin disease, and polyserositis. Sinusoidal obstruction syndrome of the liver, with bland, nonthrombotic obliteration of small hepatic veins and venules due to conditioning therapy (radiotherapy or chemotherapy), usually occurs 8 to 23 days after transplant.

✓ Mantle cell lymphoma may present as lymphomatous polyposis
✓ Small cell lung carcinoma is associated with a paraneoplastic pseudo-obstruction and positive anti-Hu antibodies
✓ The histologic hallmark of intestinal GVHD is crypt apoptotic bodies

Neuromuscular Disorders

Many neurologic and muscular disorders affect the GI tract. Acute head injury with intracranial hypertension, like many other serious illnesses, can result in stress gastritis. However, deep ulceration, sometimes with perforation, can occur with acute head injury, apparently as a result of vagal stimulation of gastrin and gastric acid production. Similar ulceration can occur after burns that cover a large surface area of the body. Abdominal pain, nausea, and vomiting rarely are attributed to migraine or temporal lobe epilepsy (temporal lobe epilepsy often includes central nervous system symptoms). Patients with cyclic vomiting may present with recurrent attacks of abdominal pain, nausea, and vomiting. Some persons with this disorder find relief with hot showers or baths and recover with cessation of the use of marijuana. Cerebrovascular disease and cerebral palsy commonly result in oropharyngeal dysphagia due to dysmotility.

Multiple sclerosis frequently affects the GI tract with oropharyngeal dysphagia, gastroparesis, constipation, or disorders of defecation or fecal incontinence. Patients with Parkinson disease often have oropharyngeal dysphagia, gastroesophageal reflux disease, esophageal dysphagia, constipation, and fecal incontinence. Both amyotrophic lateral sclerosis and myasthenia gravis can cause oropharyngeal dysphagia.

More diffuse GI tract dysmotility syndromes occur with poliomyelitis, Huntington chorea, dysautonomia syndromes, Shy-Drager syndrome, Chagas disease, and spinal cord injuries. Patients with dementia may be at risk for aspiration because of oropharyngeal dysphagia, and they may have weight loss because of decreased intake, poor diet, and pica.

Muscular dystrophies such as oculopharyngeal muscular dystrophy (third nerve palsy, often in persons who have French-Canadian ancestry) and Duchenne muscular dystrophy can be complicated by oropharyngeal dysphagia. Duchenne muscular dystrophy is associated with more widespread GI tract dysmotility.

✓ Multiple sclerosis frequently affects the GI tract from the mouth to anus
✓ Muscular dystrophies can be complicated by oropharyngeal dysphagia

Rheumatologic and Collagen Vascular Diseases

Scleroderma

Scleroderma is a chronic, connective tissue disease characterized by vascular damage and fibrosis of the skin and internal organs, including those in the GI tract. After skin involvement, the GI tract is the second most commonly involved organ system, with the esophagus being the most frequent segment involved. Involvement of the stomach, small intestine, colon, and anorectum is less common but may lead to severe complications and debility. The GI tract involvement is due to smooth muscle atrophy, fibrosis, small-vessel vasculitis, and neural damage. The esophagus is most frequently involved with smooth muscle atrophy and fibrosis of the distal two-thirds of the esophagus. Patients complain of dysphagia, heartburn, and regurgitation due to reflux and dysmotility. Most patients have Raynaud phenomena. Manometry classically shows an absence of peristaltic contractions and decreased lower esophageal sphincter pressure. Complications include strictures, Barrett esophagus, adenocarcinoma, and *Candida* esophagitis.

Replacement of the smooth muscle layers of the stomach by collagen leads to gastric hypomotility. In addition, a subset of scleroderma patients may have autonomic dysfunction affecting gastric emptying. Gastroparesis is reported to occur in up to 50% of patients and can result in significant morbidity and mortality. An additional gastric abnormality in scleroderma is gastric antral vascular ectasia.

The small intestine is frequently involved in scleroderma. Small intestinal complications include intestinal pseudo-obstruction, bacterial overgrowth, pneumatosis cystoides intestinalis, and perforation. Characteristic radiographic findings in cases of scleroderma pseudo-obstruction are dilatation of the small intestine and narrow valvulae conniventes, which remain tightly packed together despite the bowel dilatation and show the hidebound bowel sign (Figure 12.14). This characteristic mucosal fold pattern in scleroderma is caused by bowel shortening from fibrosis of the longitudinal muscle layer, with a relative decrease in the distance separating the valvulae conniventes for a given degree of small-bowel dilatation.

The intestinal stasis from pseudo-obstruction may cause abdominal distention and pain, with bacterial overgrowth resulting in diarrhea, steatorrhea, malabsorption, and weight loss. Treatment of episodes of pseudo-obstruction complicated by bacterial overgrowth involves cycled antibiotics and octreotide. When used at low doses (25-50 μg subcutaneously once nightly),

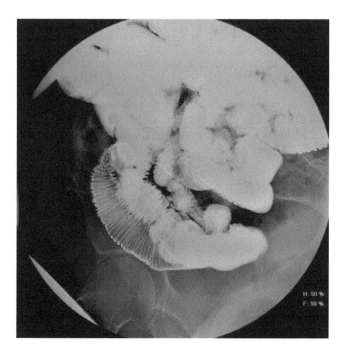

Figure 12.14. **Small-Bowel Radiographic Finding of "Hidebound" Bowel Sign of Scleroderma.**

octreotide stimulates small intestinal motility and is beneficial in patients with intestinal pseudo-obstruction and bacterial overgrowth. Despite these measures, many patients require home parenteral nutrition.

Pneumatosis cystoides intestinalis (PCI) is an uncommon condition characterized by multiple gas-filled cysts within the wall of the intestine. These cysts most commonly occur in the small bowel. PCI may be identified on plain radiographs or on computed tomographic scans. PCI is not a disease and can be classified as either primary (idiopathic) or secondary. Scleroderma is a secondary cause of PCI. The cysts of PCI may rupture, resulting in benign, chronic pneumoperitoneum. Patients with benign chronic pneumoperitoneum do not have signs of peritonitis, and no therapy is required for this condition.

Lower GI symptoms from anorectal dysfunction are not infrequent in scleroderma. Scleroderma patients with impaired anorectal function may complain of various symptoms including constipation, diarrhea, urgency, and fecal incontinence. The 2 main complications of anorectal involvement by scleroderma are fecal incontinence and rectal prolapse. Fecal incontinence associated with scleroderma is multifactorial and includes diarrhea, decreased rectal compliance, and weakening of the internal anal sphincter. Deposition of collagen in the rectal wall likely contributes to the development of rectal prolapse by weakening the rectal submucosa. Rectal prolapse may further exacerbate the already reduced capacity and compliance of the rectum in scleroderma. Therefore, rectal prolapse should be sought in all scleroderma patients with fecal incontinence, particularly because it is a potentially treatable cofactor of anorectal symptoms.

Rheumatoid Arthritis

GI manifestations of rheumatoid arthritis (RA) are varied and often catastrophic. The spectrum of GI involvement includes oropharyngeal dysphagia, esophageal dysphagia, mesenteric vasculitis, amyloidosis, and Felty syndrome.

Severe sicca manifestations from associated Sjögren syndrome may interfere with deglutition and cause oropharyngeal dysphagia in RA. Abnormal esophageal motility, with low-amplitude peristaltic contractions and reduced lower esophageal sphincter pressures, predisposes patients with RA to reflux, dysphagia, and esophagitis.

Rheumatoid vasculitis of the GI tract is rare but often catastrophic. Presentations vary with involvement of small arterioles causing ischemic ulcers and perforation, while large-vessel vasculitis results in extensive bowel infarction and intraperitoneal hemorrhage. Patients with rheumatoid mesenteric vasculitis may present with appendicitis, cholecystitis, or bowel obstruction from stricture formation.

RA is the most common disease that causes AA amyloidosis. Long-standing RA with poorly controlled inflammation is the major risk factor for development of AA amyloidosis. GI tract involvement is common with AA amyloidosis (see Amyloidosis subsection above). RA also is associated with liver disease, including mild liver function test abnormalities, autoimmune hepatitis, and primary biliary cholangitis. RA may be part of Felty syndrome (splenomegaly and neutropenia) with nodular regenerative hyperplasia and portal hypertension (variceal hemorrhage).

Systemic Lupus Erythematosus

SLE is a multisystem disease that predominantly affects women and can involve the entire GI tract and liver. Approximately 15%

of patients with SLE have skeletal myopathy that affects the upper one-third of the esophagus and results in hoarseness and dysphagia from involvement of laryngeal and pharyngeal muscles. Patients with esophageal dysmotility may have heartburn, regurgitation, and dysphagia. Mesenteric vasculitis can involve the stomach, small intestine, and colon. The presentation of patients with intestinal vasculitis ranges from nausea, vomiting, and abdominal pain to an acute abdomen. Mesenteric vasculitis is almost always accompanied by lupus involvement of other organ systems. Less common GI complications of SLE that may be the initial manifestation of lupus include intestinal pseudo-obstruction and protein-losing enteropathy. Primary lupus peritonitis is rare and sometimes occurs without ascites. Patients with primary lupus peritonitis present with abdominal pain simulating an acute abdomen, typically during a lupus flare. It responds to corticosteroids. Hepatic involvement in SLE includes mildly abnormal liver enzyme levels, fatty liver, nodular regenerative hyperplasia, autoimmune hepatitis, and primary biliary cholangitis.

✓ The GI tract is the second most commonly involved organ system in scleroderma

✓ Esophageal manometry in scleroderma classically shows absence of peristalsis and decreased lower esophageal sphincter pressure

✓ Small intestinal complications of scleroderma include intestinal pseudo-obstruction, bacterial overgrowth, pneumatosis cystoides intestinalis, and perforation

✓ The characteristic small-bowel radiographic finding in scleroderma is the hidebound bowel sign

✓ The 2 main complications of anorectal scleroderma involvement are fecal incontinence and rectal prolapse

✓ GI involvement by RA includes oropharyngeal dysphagia, esophageal dysphagia, mesenteric vasculitis, amyloidosis, and Felty syndrome

✓ RA is the most common disease that causes AA amyloidosis

✓ GI complications of SLE include mesenteric vasculitis, intestinal pseudo-obstruction, protein-losing enteropathy, and lupus peritonitis

---

Vasculitides

Systemic vasculitides involve the GI tract to a variable degree. Symptoms and signs of systemic vasculitis involving the GI tract result from mesenteric ischemia. The vasculitides with well-described and frequent GI involvement include Behçet disease (BD), polyarteritis nodosa (PAN), and IgA vasculitis (ie, Henoch-Schönlein purpura [HSP]).

Behçet Disease

BD is a vasculitis that may involve blood vessels of all sizes and both arterial and venous circulations. Recurrent oral ulceration is the sine qua non of BD. It typically affects individuals in the second through fourth decades of life. Its prevalence is similar in men and women, with more severe disease in men. GI involvement is variable. The small intestine and colon are the most frequently involved segments of the GI tract. Intestinal involvement may occur either from small-vessel disease with mucosal ulceration or from large-vessel disease resulting in ischemia and infarction. Intestinal lesions occur most frequently in the ileocecal region with the characteristic endoscopic finding of deep, punched-out ulcers. Complications include intestinal perforation from penetrating ulcers and type AA amyloidosis, with diarrhea and malabsorption.

BD with GI involvement may be difficult to distinguish from Crohn disease since oral and genital ulcers and rectal sparing

occur in both conditions. In addition, the 2 diseases share extraintestinal manifestations, such as uveitis, skin changes, and arthritis. However, a small-vessel vasculitis with deep ulcerations, no cobblestoning, and absence of granulomas characterizes BD. Large-vessel involvement may cause Budd-Chiari syndrome or portal vein thrombosis. BD has an unpredictable course, with immunosuppressive medications being the mainstay of treatment.

Polyarteritis Nodosa

PAN is a necrotizing vasculitis of medium-sized arteries that involves many different organ systems. It is associated with hepatitis B virus infection in about 7% of cases, but PAN develops in less than 1% of patients with hepatitis B. Patients with PAN have a variable clinical presentation; up to 65% of patients have GI involvement. The small intestine is the most commonly affected part of the GI tract, followed by the mesentery and colon. The most frequent symptom is postprandial abdominal pain from intestinal ischemia. Ischemia limited to the intestinal mucosa results in ulceration and GI bleeding. Bowel perforation may occur from transmural ischemic necrosis. Acalculous ischemic cholecystitis may develop from arteritis involving the wall of the gallbladder. Liver involvement may manifest as liver infarction, acute liver failure, nodular regenerative hyperplasia, and hemobilia from hepatic artery aneurysm rupture. Angiography, the main method of diagnosing PAN, typically shows saccular aneurysms. Tissue biopsy confirms the diagnosis—a common biopsy site is the sural nerve. Corticosteroids are the mainstay of treatment.

IgA Vasculitis (Henoch-Schönlein Purpura)

HSP is a systemic, small-vessel, leukocytoclastic vasculitis characterized by the tetrad of palpable purpura, arthralgias, renal disease, and GI involvement. It is the most common systemic vasculitis of children; however, it can occur in adults. The cutaneous hallmark of HSP is palpable purpura of dependent areas such as the legs and arms (Figure 12.15). In palpable purpura, blood leaks from injured vessels into the tissues. GI involvement in adult-onset HSP is common, with GI symptoms caused by immune complex deposition in vessel walls, which leads to impaired perfusion and ischemia. The most common GI features are abdominal pain and bleeding. The abdominal pain is characteristically located in the periumbilical area and, as in chronic mesenteric ischemia, the pain worsens after meals. The small intestine

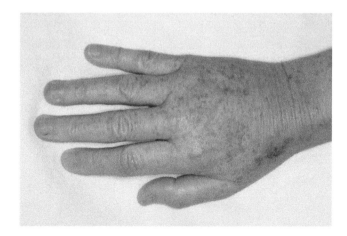

Figure 12.15.　IgA Vasculitis (Henoch-Schönlein Purpura). Discrete hemorrhagic papules on the hand of affected patient.

is the most frequently involved site in the GI tract. Computed to-mography characteristically shows small-bowel wall thickening involving mainly the jejunum and ileum. Complications include intussusception, perforation, and stricture.

The diagnosis is made from the presence of palpable purpura along with 1 of the following: abdominal pain, IgA deposition, arthritis, or renal involvement. HSP can be difficult to diagnose, especially if the GI symptoms develop before the characteristic cutaneous lesions, as in 15% of cases. In addition, when the ileum is involved, the presentation and findings mimic Crohn disease. GI manifestations of HSP typically resolve without treatment. The role of corticosteroids to prevent complications and relapses is controversial. Adults may have malignancies associated with HSP, with solid tumors being the most common (non–small cell lung carcinoma and prostate cancer). Appropriate cancer screening and surveillance among adults with a new diagnosis of HSP is important.

✓ Intestinal lesions of BD most frequently occur in the ileocecal region with the characteristic finding of deep, punched-out ulcers that can mimic Crohn disease
✓ PAN is a necrotizing vasculitis associated with hepatitis B virus infection; up to 65% of patients have GI involvement
✓ The clinical tetrad of HSP is palpable purpura, arthralgias, renal disease, and GI involvement
✓ In HSP, the small intestine is the most frequently involved site in the GI tract

---

Gynecologic Conditions

Endometriosis can affect the gut; most frequently, the sigmoid colon is involved. It can cause obstruction (adhesions), perforation, bleeding, diarrhea, and, more often, abdominal pain or constipation. These GI tract symptoms may or may not be cyclical. Associated gynecologic symptoms, such as pain with intercourse, are common. Estrogen administration after menopause may be associated with symptoms. Patients with Meigs syndrome present with ascites and, often, pleural effusion in association with benign ovarian neoplasms.

Miscellaneous Conditions

The vascular type (type IV) of Ehlers-Danlos syndrome, usually autosomal dominant, is associated often with bowel perforation, vascular aneurysms, arteriovenous fistulas, and rupture.

Paraneoplastic syndromes with diffuse GI tract motor dysfunction occur most often with small cell lung carcinoma, autonomic neuropathy, cerebellar degeneration, peripheral neuropathy, seizures, or syndrome of inappropriate secretion of antidiuretic hormone. Type 1 antineuronal nuclear (also known as anti-Hu) antibodies usually are detectable.

Suggested Reading

Bissell DM, Anderson KE, Bonkovsky HL. Porphyria. N Engl J Med. 2017 Aug 31;377(9):862–72.

Brito-Zeron P, Bari K, Baughman RP, Ramos-Casals M. Sarcoidosis involving the gastrointestinal tract: diagnostic and therapeutic management. Am J Gastroenterol. 2019 Aug;114(8):1238–47.

Busse PJ, Christiansen SC. Hereditary angioedema. N Engl J Med. 2020 Mar 19;382(12):1136–48.

Davila M, Bresalier RS. Gastrointestinal complications of oncologic therapy. Nat Clin Pract Gastroenterol Hepatol. 2008 Dec;5(12):682–96.

Ebert EC, Nagar M, Hagspiel KD. Gastrointestinal and hepatic complications of sickle cell disease. Clin Gastroenterol Hepatol. 2010 Jun;8(6):483–9.

Gelfond D, Borowitz D. Gastrointestinal complications of cystic fibrosis. Clin Gastroenterol Hepatol. 2013 Apr;11(4):333–42.

Iida T, Yamano H, Nakase H. Systemic amyloidosis with gastrointestinal involvement: diagnosis from endoscopic and histological views. J Gastroenterol Hepatol. 2018 Mar;33(3):583–90.

Jackson SB, Villano NP, Benhammou JN, Lewis M, Pisegna JR, Padua D. Gastrointestinal manifestations of hereditary hemorrhagic telangiectasia (HHT): a systematic review of the literature. Dig Dis Sci. 2017 Oct;62(10):2623–30.

Jacobs JW, Jr, Kukreja K, Camisa C, Richter JE. Demystifying esophageal lichen planus: a comprehensive review of a rare disease you will see in practice. Am J Gastroenterol. 2022 Jan 1;117(1):70–7.

Koster MJ, Warrington KJ. Vasculitis of the mesenteric circulation. Best Pract Res Clin Gastroenterol. 2017 Feb;31(1):85–96.

Kroner PT, Tolaymat OA, Bowman AW, Abril A, Lacy BE. Gastrointestinal manifestations of rheumatological diseases. Am J Gastroenterol. 2019 Sep;114(9):1441–54.

Loscalzo J. From clinical observation to mechanism: Heyde's syndrome. N Engl J Med. 2012 Nov 15;367(20):1954–6.

Mikolajczyk AE, Te HS, Chapman AB. Gastrointestinal manifestations of autosomal-dominant polycystic kidney disease. Clin Gastroenterol Hepatol. 2017 Jan;15(1):17–24.

Pikkarainen S, Martelius T, Ristimaki A, Siitonen S, Seppanen MRJ, Farkkila M. A high prevalence of gastrointestinal manifestations in common variable immunodeficiency. Am J Gastroenterol. 2019 Apr;114(4):648–55.

Shields HM, Shaffer K, O'Farrell R P, Travers R, Hayward JN, Becker LS, et al. Gastrointestinal manifestations of dermatologic disorders. Clin Gastroenterol Hepatol. 2007 Sep;5(9):1010–7.

Shreiner AB, Murray C, Denton C, Khanna D. Gastrointestinal manifestations of systemic sclerosis. J Scleroderma Relat Disord. 2016 1(3):247–56.

Stolzel U, Doss MO, Schuppan D. Clinical guide and update on porphyrias. Gastroenterology. 2019 Aug;157(2):365–81.

Thrash B, Patel M, Shah KR, Boland CR, Menter A. Cutaneous manifestations of gastrointestinal disease: Part II. J Am Acad Dermatol. 2013 Feb;68(2):211 e1–33.

13

Complications After Roux-en-Y Surgery

KHUSHBOO S. GALA, MBBS

ANDRES J. ACOSTA, MD, PHD

The incidence of obesity continues to increase at an alarming rate, the burden of disease having tripled since 1975. In the United States, nearly 50% of the population is obese. There has also been an associated increase in the incidence of obesity-related conditions, including heart disease, stroke, type 2 diabetes mellitus, and certain types of cancer. Bariatric surgery is the only effective treatment for severe obesity, resulting in sustained weight loss, improved obesity-associated comorbidities, and reduced mortality.

Roux-en-Y gastric bypass (RYGB) remains one of the most popular bariatric procedures. It is extremely effective for weight loss. Maximal weight loss is about 30% of total body weight within the 1 to 2 years after the procedure, and long-term data show that patients are able to maintain more than 25% of total weight loss even over 20 years. It is the bariatric procedure of choice in patients with insulin resistance (type 2 diabetes mellitus, nonalcoholic fatty liver disease, metabolic syndrome, and polycystic ovarian syndrome). It is also preferred for patients with Barrett esophagus, severe or complicated gastroesophageal reflux disease, or bile reflux. RYGB has a complication rate of approximately 15%, and most complications are minor. This chapter reviews the RYGB procedure and the related complications and their management.

Anatomy and Physiology of RYGB

To better understand complications associated with RYGB, it is necessary to understand the anatomy and physiology behind the procedure. It entails construction of a small gastric pouch that is divided and separated from the distal aspect of the stomach. The gastric pouch is generally 30 to 50 mL in volume, is composed primarily of the lesser curvature of the stomach, and is anastomosed to a limb of small bowel. The anastomosis is the gastrojejunal anastomosis. The limb is referred to as the Roux limb and is typically 75 to 150 cm in length. The other intestinal limb attached to the gastric remnant is known as the biliopancreatic limb; it helps to transport secretions from the gastric remnant, liver, and pancreas. The anastomosis of both limbs, known as the jejunojejunal anastomosis, is approximately 75 to 150 cm distally from the gastrojejunostomy (Figure 13.1).

The mechanism of weight loss in RYGB is multifactorial. The small gastric pouch and narrow anastomotic outlet serve as restrictive elements and limit caloric intake by inducing satiation. There is also a component of nutrients bypassing the biliopancreatic intestinal limb, which decreases the length of absorptive surface of the small intestine, and results in the food bolus reaching the distal intestine faster. Neurohormonal changes, including suppression of ghrelin and an increase in peptide YY, glucagon-like peptide-1, and plasma bile acids, contribute to an increase in satiation and reduction of food intake.

Abbreviations: ASL, anastomotic or staple leak; ASMBS, American Society for Metabolic and Bariatric Surgery; GGF, gastrogastric fistula; GI, gastrointestinal; PHH, postprandial hyperinsulinemic hypoglycemia; RYGB, Roux-en-Y gastric bypass; SBO, small-bowel obstruction; SIBO, small intestinal bacterial overgrowth

✓ **Roux-en-Y gastric bypass**—a bariatric surgery that involves creation of a small gastric pouch with anastomosis to a limb of jejunum that bypasses 75 to 150 cm of small bowel
✓ **Gastric pouch**—a small, divided pouch composed of the lesser curvature of the stomach that is created to restrict food intake

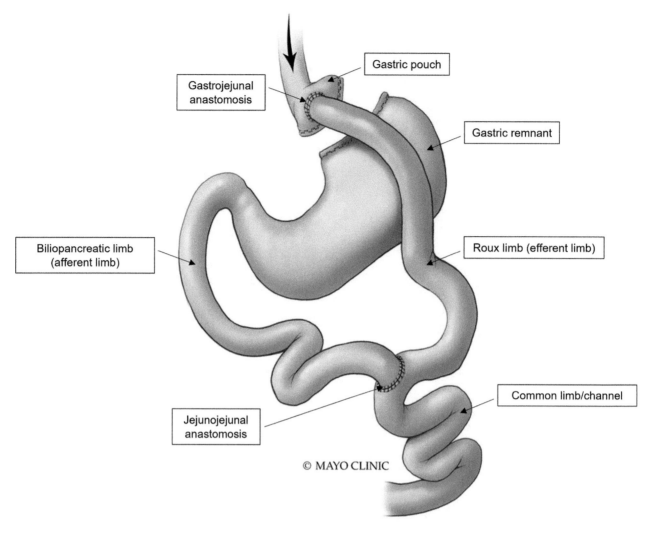

Figure 13.1.   **Anatomy of Roux-en-Y Gastric Bypass.** (Used with permission of Mayo Foundation for Medical Education and Research.)

✓ **Gastric remnant**—the portion of the stomach that is excluded during creation of the pouch; it includes the majority of the stomach, including fundus, greater curvature, and pylorus
✓ **Roux limb (efferent limb)**—the jejunal limb that is attached to the gastric pouch and serves as the primary recipient of food after the surgery
✓ **Biliopancreatic limb (afferent limb)**—the intestinal limb that is connected to the gastric remnant and serves as the recipient for biliary and pancreatic secretions
✓ **Common limb or channel**—the intestinal limb that is formed after anastomosis of the Roux and biliopancreatic limbs, 75 to 150 cm distally from the gastrojejunostomy

Endoscopic Anatomy of RYGB

Familiarity with postsurgical RYGB anatomy is important when performing endoscopy in patients who have had the procedure. The operative notes should be reviewed before performing an endoscopy to be aware of limb lengths, because these may vary by surgeons and centers. A patient with RYGB should have a normal esophagus and gastroesophageal junction. The endoscopically visualized stomach is the gastric pouch, which is typically 3 to 5 cm in length. This is anastomosed to the jejunum (the Roux limb). The gastrojejunal anastomosis is generally 10

to 12 mm in diameter and should permit passage of the standard adult gastroscope. The Roux limb is typically 100 to 150 cm in length; its anastomosis to the biliopancreatic limb forms the jejunojejunal anastomosis and common channel. The gastric remnant and biliopancreatic limb are not visualized during a routine endoscopy and require double balloon enteroscopy for examination.

Complications of RYGB

RYGB is associated with multiple surgical complications in both the early and the delayed postoperative periods. Complications in the immediate postoperative period (earlier than 1 month after the procedure) include anastomotic or staple line leak, postoperative hemorrhage, and bowel obstruction. Delayed complications (1 month or after) include anastomotic stricture, marginal ulceration, fistula formation, intestinal obstruction, and nutritional deficiencies.

Different surgical techniques have different rates of complications. In general, hand-sewn anastomoses have lower rates of postoperative bleeding, marginal ulcer, and strictures than stapled anastomoses. Specifically, circular stapling has a higher risk of postoperative hemorrhage, wound complications, anastomotic leaks, marginal ulcers, and anastomotic strictures.

Early Complications

Anastomotic or Staple Line Leaks

Anastomotic or staple line leaks (ASLs) are the most severe complication of RYGB and one of the major contributors to death. The frequency of ASL has been reported to be 0.5 to 5%; the lower rate is associated with more experienced surgeons. The frequency of ASL is higher in revisional RYGB. ASL generally occurs within the first week of hospitalization; in rare instances, it may occur up to 30 days postoperatively. ASLs occur most frequently at the gastrojejunal anastomosis. Many surgical techniques have been explored to decrease the risk of ASL, including appropriate staple sizing, staple-line reinforcement, hand-sewn otomy closures, placement of stay sutures, intraoperative leak testing, and placement of fibrin sealant.

Clinical Presentation and Diagnosis. ASL can have varied clinical presentations. The more obvious presentations include fever, abdominal pain, and purulent drain output. However, because clinical findings can frequently be subtle in patients with severe obesity, ASL can be challenging to diagnose. Sustained tachycardia (heart rate >120 beats per minute) postoperatively can be indicative of ASL.

The diagnosis of ASL requires a strong clinical suspicion. It can be confirmed radiographically with barium studies or contrast-enhanced computed tomography. Some centers routinely order postoperative upper gastrointestinal (GI) series on all patients with RYGB; however, there are no concrete data to support this practice. Use of intraoperative measures to evaluate for ASL, including methylene blue dye instillation with an orogastric tube or insufflation of air during intraoperative endoscopy, can help detect early leaks. If a leak is suspected clinically and the patient is unstable, surgical exploration should be prioritized to prevent progression to sepsis.

Management. Surgical exploration and management of leaks by repairing defects and draining the abdominal cavity are often feasible laparoscopically, especially at experienced centers. Minimally invasive endoscopic repair techniques, including use of glue, placement of covered stents, and placement of clips, can also be an option in clinically stable patients but should be considered adjuncts to surgical therapy.

Postoperative Hemorrhage

Hemorrhage after RYGB can be early (<30 days postoperatively) or late (≥30 days postoperatively). Early bleeding is likely due to bleeding from the anastomosis or staple line and is usually catastrophic. Late bleeding is generally caused by significant gastritis, marginal ulcers at the gastrojejunostomy, and ulcers in the pouch, gastric remnant stomach, or duodenum. A study of patients who had RYGB in the Metabolic and Bariatric Surgery Accreditation and Quality Improvement Program data set found an early postoperative hemorrhage rate of 1.5%. Postoperative bleeding leads to worse outcomes, including longer duration of stay, higher in-hospital mortality rate, higher 30-day mortality rate, discharge to an extended-care facility, and higher rates of major complications. Most patients are managed with reoperation or endoscopy. Endoscopy may be successful in minor bleeds with use of interventions such as clips, epinephrine injection, hemostatic powder, and thermal therapy.

Delayed Complications

Gastrojejunal Anastomotic Stricture

Anastomotic strictures (or stenosis) are a common complication of RYGB (approximate incidence is 15%). They generally occur within 2 to 3 months postoperatively. Risk factors for strictures include older age, circular stapled gastrojejunostomy, anastomotic leaks, and marginal ulceration. Strictures can have multiple causes, including ischemia, tension on the anastomosis, edema, or a foreign-body reaction.

Clinical Presentation and Diagnosis. Clinical manifestations of strictures include nausea, vomiting, dysphagia, gastroesophageal reflux, and eventually an inability to tolerate oral intake, including liquids. These generally present when the stricture narrows to less than 10 mm. Anastomotic strictures can be diagnosed from a thorough history and examination. The diagnosis can be confirmed with an upper GI series or upper endoscopy.

Management. Strictures can be managed either with endoscopic dilations or surgical revision. Endoscopic balloon dilation is a safe and effective treatment of anastomotic strictures. Strictures should generally be dilated to 12 to 16 mm; over-dilation should be avoided because it can reduce the restrictive effect of RYGB. Many centers schedule follow-up endoscopies because most patients require serial dilations every 2 to 3 weeks. Generally, strictures should not be dilated by more than 3 to 4 mm at a time to decrease the risk of perforation. There is a small risk of perforation after balloon dilation, reported to be less than 3%. Rarely, strictures can be refractory to multiple dilations and may require surgical revision of the gastrojejunostomy anastomosis.

Gastrojejunal Anastomosis (Marginal) Ulceration

Ulceration of any depth at the gastrojejunal junction is termed *marginal ulceration.* This is one of the most common complications after RYGB; the reported incidence is 15%. The pathophysiologic mechanism of marginal ulceration is multifactorial; the contributory factors differ for early and late ulceration. Local factors such as inflammation and the technical aspects of anastomosis creation contribute to early ulceration, whereas microvascular ischemia has a major role in late ulceration. A prominent risk factor for both early and late marginal ulceration is the use of nonsteroidal anti-inflammatory drugs. Other purported risk factors include diabetes mellitus, obstructive sleep apnea, female sex, smoking, and alcohol dependence. Preoperative *Helicobacter pylori* infection is associated with a risk for ulceration even after treatment, likely from persistent damage to the mucosal barrier that may precipitate marginal ulceration even when the organism has been eradicated. The technique used to perform the gastrojejunal anastomosis may also affect the rate of marginal ulcer formation.

Clinical Presentation and Diagnosis. Marginal ulceration can present with nausea, abdominal pain, and recurrent GI bleeding. Chronic marginal ulcers can lead to anastomotic stenosis. Gastrogastric fistulas have been known to develop from chronic marginal ulcers. In rare cases, perforation can be caused by marginal ulceration.

Marginal ulceration is usually diagnosed with endoscopic evaluation. It is located at the gastrojejunal anastomotic site, typically on the posterior aspect of the jejunum.

Management. Medical management is the first step in the treatment of marginal ulceration and is successful in most cases. It includes 6 to 8 weeks of antisecretory therapy with proton pump inhibitors alone or in combination with oral luminal coating agents, such as sucralfate. It is important to have the patient open the proton-pump-inhibitor capsules to allow better absorption within the RYGB anatomy. Testing and treating for *H pylori* infection are also strongly recommended. Avoidance of nonsteroidal anti-inflammatory drugs and smoking cessation are extremely important for preventing the progression of these ulcers.

A minority of patients (<10%) may have persistent symptoms, including intractable pain, despite medical management, and may have development of recurrent GI hemorrhage or perforation. In these cases, surgical or endoscopic revision is warranted. Generally, this includes revision of the gastrojejunostomy, with or without truncal vagotomy. Endoscopy and overstitch techniques have also been shown to be useful. In cases of perforation, a Graham patch and feeding tube can be placed for unstable patients, with formal revision after healing of the perforation.

Internal Hernias

Internal hernias are common after laparoscopic RYGB; the incidence varies from 0.5% to 10%. There are several types of internal hernias, including mesenteric, Petersen, and mesocolic.

- Mesenteric hernia: formed in the space adjacent to the jejunojejunal anastomosis, which is created by division of the jejunal mesentery
- Petersen hernia: formed in the space between the Roux limb and its mesentery anteriorly and the transverse colon and its mesentery posteriorly
- Mesocolic hernia: formed in a defect in the transverse colon mesentery. Only formed with retrocolic Roux limbs

Risk factors for formation of internal hernias include nonclosure or incomplete closure of mesenteric defects at the initial surgery, major weight loss, and pregnancy.

Clinical Presentation and Diagnosis.   Internal hernias most commonly present with intermittent abdominal pain that occurs because of transient incarceration that resolves spontaneously. This is more commonly found in antecolic constructions, which typically have wide internal defects that allow spontaneous reduction of the herniated intestines. Occasionally, internal hernias can present as small-bowel obstructions or incarcerations.

Diagnosis of internal hernias is challenging because they have a heterogeneous clinical presentation and, most commonly, present with vague intermittent symptoms. Imaging can confirm the presence of internal hernias; however, imaging findings must be strongly correlated to symptoms before confirming the diagnosis. The mesenteric swirl sign is the most sensitive radiographic sign for diagnosis of internal hernias; it is the swirled appearance of mesenteric vessels or fat at the root of the mesentery in hernia defects. If there is a clinical concern for internal herniation, computed tomographic scans should be carefully reviewed by an experienced radiologist and bariatric surgeon.

Management.   Management of internal hernias is primarily through surgical exploration and repair. A patient who has had RYGB and presents with acute severe pain, even in the absence of characteristic computed tomographic findings, should be evaluated by a surgical team and exploratory surgery considered. This approach is used because uncorrected bowel obstructions can lead to incarceration and bowel necrosis, which then require extensive bowel resection. Recommended measures to decrease the risk of formation of internal hernia are closure of all mesenteric defects, use of nonabsorbable running suture, and construction of an antecolic Roux limb.

Small-Bowel Obstruction

Small-bowel obstructions (SBOs) are common after RYGB; the lifetime incidence is 5%. The most common cause of SBO

after RYGB is internal hernias (described in detail above); other common causes are incisional hernias, jejunojejunostomy stenosis, and adhesions. Rare causes of SBO include intussusception (most commonly in the jejunojejunal anastomotic site) and bezoars. SBO is more common with laparoscopic RYGB (given the popularity of the procedure and predisposition for internal hernias, which are the most common cause of SBO); a retrocolic technique of laparoscopic RYGB is also a risk factor for SBO. In summary, causes for SBO among different types of surgery are as follows:

- Open RYGB: adhesive disease
- Laparoscopic RYGB: internal hernias
  - Retrocolic laparoscopic RYGB: internal hernias (mesocolic)
  - Anterocolic laparoscopic RYGB: jejunojejunostomy stenosis

Clinical Presentation, Diagnosis, and Management.   The symptoms of SBO are like those of internal hernias; there is a wide variety of presentations, from vague, intermittent abdominal pain to severe acute pain. A strong suspicion for and low threshold for surgical exploration are warranted in cases with SBO.

Nutritional Deficiencies

Clinical Presentation and Diagnosis.   Given the restrictive and malabsorptive state brought about by RYGB, both macronutrient and micronutrient deficiencies are common after the procedure. Also, preoperatively, the prevalence of micronutrient is high. The major macronutrient deficiency that occurs with RYGB is protein deficiency. Patients may have nausea and vomiting leading to electrolyte imbalances and thiamine deficiency. Fat malabsorption leads to deficiency of fat-soluble vitamins (vitamins A, D, E, and K) and zinc. Over time, patients are also at risk for vitamin B_{12}, calcium, iron, and copper deficiencies.

Postoperatively, protein deficiency occurs in patients with long Roux limbs (>150 cm), maladaptive eating behaviors, inadequate protein food sources, and protracted vomiting. Protein deficiency presents with generalized edema and low albumin level.

Preoperative screening for micronutrient deficiency is an important part of optimizing patients for bariatric surgery. Studies show that less than 25% of patients undergo preoperative screening for micronutrient deficiency. The American Society for Metabolic and Bariatric Surgery (ASMBS) guidelines for patients undergoing bariatric surgery suggest screening for most vitamins and minerals before RYGB. These include thiamine, folate, iron, calcium, zinc, copper, and vitamins A, B_{12}, and D. Screening recommendations are further summarized in Table 13.1.

Management.   All patients undergoing RYGB should have micronutrient supplementation postoperatively. In general, the ASMBS recommends multivitamin tablets daily. Generic multivitamins can be used after a careful review of the products' micronutrient contents; however, high-potency, bariatric surgery–specific multivitamins are also available. Multivitamins generally do not contain recommended doses of calcium, which must be supplemented separately. Detailed dosages are listed in Table 13.1.

In general, there should be a strong suspicion for micronutrient deficiencies postoperatively. Clinical signs and symptoms of various micronutrient deficiencies are listed in Table 13.2. Periodic screening for micronutrient deficiency can help with early detection of these deficiencies. ASMBS guidelines

Table 13.1. Micronutrient Screening[a] and Supplementation After Roux-en-Y Gastric Bypass

Micronutrient	Screening laboratory test	Standard postoperative supplementation dosage	Postoperative monitoring recommendations
Vitamin A	Vitamin A	5,000-10,000 IU/d	Optional (or based on signs and symptoms)
Vitamin B₁ (thiamine)	Thiamine	12 mg/d	Optional (or based on signs and symptoms)
Vitamin B₁₂ (cobalamin)	B₁₂; can also test for MMA	Oral or sublingual: 350-500 µg/d Intranasal: 1,000 µg/wk Intramuscular: 1,000 µg/mo	6, 12, 18, 24 mo and annually thereafter
Vitamin D	Vitamin D	Vitamin D₃ 3,000 IU/d	6, 12, 18, 24 mo and annually thereafter
Iron	Iron, TIBC, ferritin	45-60 mg/d	6, 12, 18, 24 mo and annually thereafter
Folate (folic acid)	Folate; can also test for RBC, folate, homocysteine, MMA	400-800 µg/d Women of childbearing age: 800-1,000 µg/d	6, 12, 18, 24 mo and annually thereafter
Calcium	Calcium	1,200-1,500 mg/d	6, 12, 18, 24 mo and annually thereafter
Zinc	Zinc	8-22 mg/d	Optional (or based on signs and symptoms)
Copper	Copper and ceruloplasmin	2 mg/d	Optional (or based on signs and symptoms)

Abbreviations: MMA, methylmalonic acid; RBC, red blood cell; TIBC, total iron-binding capacity.

[a] All patients should be screened for the listed nutrients.

recommend nutrient assessments every 3 to 6 months in the first year after bariatric surgery and annually thereafter with laboratory tests.

Dumping Syndrome

Clinical Presentation and Diagnosis. Dumping syndrome is a common complication of RYGB. It is classified as early or late, depending on timing of symptoms after meals. Early dumping happens within an hour of eating, whereas late dumping occurs 1 to 3 hours after meals. The pathogenesis and presentation of these 2 types differ.

Early dumping is primarily an osmotic process. Passage of undigested food into the small intestine triggers rapid fluid shifts into the intestinal lumen. These shifts result in a decrease in plasma volume and a consequent sympathetic nervous system response. The resulting symptoms occur within a few minutes to within an hour of eating and include hypotension and tachycardia, colicky abdominal pain, diarrhea, and nausea. Early dumping is common, occurring in 10% to 20% of patients after

Table 13.2. Clinical Signs and Symptoms of Micronutrient Deficiencies and Replacement Dosages After Roux-en-Y Gastric Bypass

Micronutrient	Clinical signs and symptoms of deficiency	Therapeutic replacement dose
Vitamin A	Xerophthalmia, loss of nocturnal vision, decreased immunity	Vitamin A deficiency without corneal changes: vitamin A 10,000-25,000 IU daily orally until clinical improvement is evident (1-2 wk) Vitamin A deficiency with corneal changes: vitamin A 50,000-100,000 IU IM for 3 d, followed by 50,000 IU daily IM for 2 wk Screen for concurrent iron or copper deficiencies because these can impair resolution of vitamin A deficiency
Thiamine	Neurologic symptoms (Wernicke-Korsakoff syndrome). Common in patients with rapid weight loss and alcohol use	Oral therapy: 100 mg 2-3 times daily until symptoms resolve IV therapy: 200 mg 3 times daily to 500 mg once or twice daily for 3-5 d, followed by 250 mg daily for 3-5 d or until symptoms resolve, then consider treatment with 100 mg daily orally, usually indefinitely or until risk factors have been resolved IM therapy: 250 mg once daily for 3-5 d or 100-250 mg monthly Simultaneous administration of magnesium, potassium, and phosphorus should be given to patients at risk for refeeding syndrome
Vitamin B₁₂ (cobalamin)	Pernicious anemia, tingling in fingers and toes, depression, dementia	1,000 mg daily
Vitamin D	Similar to those with calcium deficiency	Vitamin D₃ 3,000-6,000 IU daily Vitamin D₂ 50,000 IU 1-3 times weekly
Iron	Fatigue, koilonychia, pica, brittle hair, anemia	150-200 mg of elemental iron daily Consider IV supplementation in refractory cases
Folate (folic acid)	Macrocytic anemia, palpitations, fatigue, neural tube defects	1,000 mg daily
Calcium	Tetany, tingling, cramping, metabolic bone disease	1,200-1,500 mg daily
Zinc	Growth retardation, delayed sexual maturity, impotence, impaired immune function	60 mg elemental zinc orally twice a day
Copper	Microcytic anemia, neutropenia, ataxia	Mild to moderate deficiency (including low hematologic indices): 3-8 mg daily oral copper gluconate or sulfate until indices return to normal Severe deficiency: 2-4 mg daily IV copper can be initiated for 6 d or until serum levels return to normal and neurologic symptoms resolve

Abbreviations: IM, intramuscularly; IV, intravenously.

RYGB. Predictors of severe symptoms include younger age and a lower body mass index.

Late dumping is also known as postprandial hyperinsulinemic hypoglycemia (PHH). The pathophysiologic mechanism of PHH is complex and not completely understood but includes alterations in multiple hormonal and glycemic patterns. Incretin and insulin production increase, an effect that leads to hypoglycemia. Patients with PHH present with postprandial neuroglycopenic symptoms, including dizziness, diaphoresis, and weakness. These symptoms occur 1 to 3 hours after ingestion of a carbohydrate-rich meal. PHH generally presents at least 1 year after RYGB. It is a very uncommon phenomenon and occurs in less than 0.5% of cases.

Management. The initial management of early and late dumping syndrome is similar and revolves around dietary modifications. These include multiple small meals throughout the day and separating solid from liquid intake by 30 minutes. Meals should be high in fiber and protein and low in simple carbohydrates that can be rapidly absorbed. A multidisciplinary team including an experienced bariatric dietitian can be invaluable in the management of dumping syndrome. Early dumping is generally mild and resolves spontaneously over time. PHH may persist; in patients with refractory symptoms, pharmacotherapy or gastrostomy tube with feeding into the remnant stomach may be attempted. Drugs that have been shown to have some therapeutic benefit include nifedipine, acarbose, diazoxide, and octreotide. Partial pancreatectomy is not recommended. Surgical or endoscopic revision of RYGB is an option that can be explored in refractory cases.

Nephrolithiasis

The risk of nephrolithiasis is increased in patients who have had RYGB: a 2-fold increased risk in patients without a previous history of stones and a 4-fold increased risk in patients with a previous history of stones. RYGB is associated with several changes in the metabolic processing of calcium and oxalate in the urine, including an increase in urinary oxalate excretion, supersaturation of calcium oxalate, a low urine citrate level, and lower urine volume. All of these factors predispose patients to nephrolithiasis after RYGB. Most patients can be managed with dietary modifications (use of a low-fat, low-oxalate diet) and use of calcium as an oxalate binder. Rarely, chronic deposition of calcium oxalate in the renal parenchyma can result in oxalate nephropathy and chronic kidney disease after RYGB.

Small Intestinal Bacterial Overgrowth

RYGB is a common predisposing factor for small intestinal bacterial overgrowth (SIBO). This condition is thought to occur because of the intestinal bypass, with the pancreatobiliary limb acting as a relatively blind loop. This blind loop has abnormal motility and ineffective clearance of secretions, factors leading to bacterial stasis and overgrowth.

Clinical Presentation and Diagnosis. SIBO presents with vague and nonspecific symptoms, including abdominal pain, bloating, diarrhea, distention, and flatulence. It can be diagnosed with either noninvasive breath testing or culture of small-bowel aspirates obtained during endoscopy. Small-bowel cultures are considered more accurate in terms of testing; a threshold of more than 10^3 colony-forming units per milliliter is a positive test result

for SIBO. Breath testing involves ingestion of a carbohydrate substrate (glucose or lactulose); its metabolism when exposed to gut bacteria leads to the production of hydrogen and methane. However, postsurgical anatomy makes breath testing difficult to interpret.

Management. Management of SIBO involves use of antibiotics for bacterial eradication. The most studied and efficacious agent is rifaximin, which also has the advantage of being gut specific and nonsystemic. Other agents that have been proved efficacious include ciprofloxacin, norfloxacin, and metronidazole. Dietary approaches such as a low-FODMAP (fermentable oligosaccharides, disaccharides, monosaccharides, and polyols) diet and elemental diet have been tried with limited success and data. Many patients (up to 50%) may experience a recurrence in symptoms. Management for this group includes the following:

- Identification of offending organism with bacterial culture and use of targeted antibiotics
- Addressing any additional risk factors such as avoiding medications that delay gut transit, reducing proton pump inhibitor and opioid use, and improving glycemic control
- Cyclical monthly low-dose antibiotic therapy with 2 or 3 antibiotics
- Trial of prokinetic agents
- In rare instances, surgical or endoscopic revision of blind limb

Gastrogastric Fistula

A gastrogastric fistula (GGF) is an abnormal communication between the gastric pouch and the excluded stomach remnant, allowing ingested food to enter the bypassed foregut (stomach and duodenum). Historically, RYGB involved creation of a nondivided or partially divided gastric pouch, which resulted in GGF formation in close to 50% of patients. Contemporary techniques involve complete transection of the gastric segments, an approach that has led to a decrease in the incidence of GGF, now ranging from 1% to 3%.

There are multiple reasons for formation of GGF. As mentioned above, surgical technique or incomplete transection is a common iatrogenic reason for GGF formation. Anastomotic leaks from the gastrojejunal anastomosis or pouch staple-line disruption can also lead to GGF formation. Perforation of marginal ulcers and erosion of foreign bodies such as nonabsorbable suture material and preanastomotic rings may also cause GGF.

Clinical Presentation and Diagnosis. GGF most commonly presents with weight regain or intractable marginal ulceration leading to recurrent GI hemorrhage or pain. For differential diagnosis, GGF should be strongly considered in a patient with weight regain after a period of stable weight after RYGB. GGF can be diagnosed with upper GI series or computed tomography with oral contrast agent. It can also be visualized on upper endoscopy.

Management. Asymptomatic patients can be managed conservatively with proton pump inhibitor therapy and close follow-up. For symptomatic patients, GGF can be managed endoscopically or surgically. Endoscopic repair can be performed in multiple ways, including fibrin sealant, endoscopy clips, and endoscopic suturing systems. It is safe and feasible and can be used with good success for small fistulas or in the short term. Surgical repair in the form of laparoscopic fistula excision with or without revision of gastrojejunostomy anastomosis remains the definitive therapy.

Candy Cane Syndrome

This rare complication develops in patients with an abnormally long blind afferent Roux limb. The blind limb fills with food after meals and acts like an obstructed loop; the associated abdominal pain is relieved by vomiting or passage of food into the Roux limb. It occurs in patients with excessive length of the blind Roux limb just distal to the gastrojejunostomy; this length was reported to be 8 to 15 cm in one study. Other predisposing factors include GI dysmotility and progressive dilatation of the blind afferent limb.

Clinical Presentation and Diagnosis. Patients present with postprandial epigastric abdominal pain. This may occur either relatively early after surgery (as soon as 2-3 months postoperatively) or even years after surgery. Patients may also have nausea and symptoms of reflux or regurgitation. The pain is generally relieved after vomiting.

Candy cane syndrome should be suspected in patients with postprandial pain relieved by vomiting. It can be confirmed by upper GI contrast studies, which show contrast spillage into the blind afferent limb before passing into the Roux limb. Endoscopic visualization shows that the afferent limb is the direct outlet of the gastrojejunostomy, rather than the Roux limb.

Management. Surgical revision of the RYGB is the mainstay of treatment for candy cane syndrome. This generally includes laparoscopic resection of the afferent limb. Surgeons should attempt to minimize the length of the blind afferent limb and place the blind limb toward the right side to favor drainage by gravity as a means to prevent this complication.

Afferent Loop Syndrome

Afferent loop syndrome refers to a partial or complete obstruction of the biliopancreatic (afferent) limb along its course or at the anastomosis. It presents with symptoms of bowel obstruction but can also cause biliary dilatation or acute pancreatitis due to back pressure. It occurs after Billroth II or Roux-en-Y reconstruction; the reported incidence is 0.3% to 1%. Causes of afferent loop syndrome include entrapment and kinking of the afferent loop by postoperative adhesions, internal herniation, volvulus and intussusception of the afferent loop, and stenosis due to ulceration at the gastrojejunostomy site. Rarely, enteroliths, bezoars, and foreign bodies are responsible for the afferent loop.

Clinical Presentation and Diagnosis. Afferent loop syndrome may be acute or chronic. Acute cases generally occur early postoperatively and present with sudden onset of abdominal pain, nausea, and vomiting. In severe cases with ischemia and perforation, patients may have peritonitis and shock. Patients may also have jaundice due to biliary obstruction and features of acute pancreatitis.

Chronic afferent loop syndrome typically presents in the late postoperative period with postprandial abdominal pain and weight loss. The postprandial abdominal pain may lead to food aversion and malabsorption.

Afferent loop syndrome should be suspected in a patient with acute or chronic abdominal pain after RYGB. It can be diagnosed with abdominal computed tomography, which can show the bowel obstruction and complications including ischemia, perforation, pancreatitis, and biliary obstruction. A classic feature described on computed tomography is the C-loop sign (seen in the right upper quadrant, representing the dilated afferent limb). An upper GI series can also be used for the diagnosis of afferent loop syndrome and may show failure of contrast agent to enter the afferent limb; however, this finding is nonspecific.

Management. Most cases of acute afferent limb syndrome should be managed surgically. Nasojejunal decompression and intravenous fluids can be used as temporizing measures preoperatively. Endoscopic therapy is emerging as a safe and effective option for many patients. This includes stent placement, anastomotic stricture dilation, and endoscopic ultrasound-guided creation of a gastrojejunostomy.

Suggested Reading

Al Harakeh AB, Kallies KJ, Borgert AJ, Kothari SN. Bowel obstruction rates in antecolic/antegastric versus retrocolic/retrogastric Roux limb gastric bypass: a meta-analysis. Surg Obes Relat Dis. 2016 Jan;12(1):194–8.

Almby K, Edholm D. Anastomotic strictures after Roux-en-Y gastric bypass: a cohort study from the Scandinavian Obesity Surgery Registry. Obes Surg. 2019 Jan;29(1):172–7.

Aryaie AH, Fayezizadeh M, Wen Y, Alshehri M, Abbas M, Khaitan L. "Candy cane syndrome:" an underappreciated cause of abdominal pain and nausea after Roux-en-Y gastric bypass surgery. Surg Obes Relat Dis. 2017 Sep;13(9):1501–5.

Blouhos K, Boulas KA, Tsalis K, Hatzigeorgiadis A. Management of afferent loop obstruction: reoperation or endoscopic and percutaneous interventions? World J Gastrointest Surg. 2015 Sep 27;7(9):190–5.

Canales BK, Hatch M. Kidney stone incidence and metabolic urinary changes after modern bariatric surgery: review of clinical studies, experimental models, and prevention strategies. Surg Obes Relat Dis. 2014 Jul-Aug;10(4):734–42.

Chahine E, Kassir R, Dirani M, Joumaa S, Debs T, Chouillard E. Surgical management of gastrogastric fistula after Roux-en-Y gastric bypass: 10-year experience. Obes Surg. 2018 Apr;28(4):939–44.

Chowbey P, Baijal M, Kantharia NS, Khullar R, Sharma A, Soni V. Mesenteric defect closure decreases the incidence of internal hernias following laparoscopic Roux-en-Y gastric bypass: a retrospective cohort study. Obes Surg. 2016 Sep;26(9):2029–34.

Grotewiel RK, Cindass R. Afferent loop syndrome. Statpearls [internet]. StatPearls Publishing; 2022.

Parrott J, Frank L, Rabena R, Craggs-Dino L, Isom KA, Greiman L. American Society for Metabolic and Bariatric Surgery integrated health nutritional guidelines for the surgical weight loss patient 2016 update: micronutrients. Surg Obes Relat Dis. 2017 May;13(5):727–41.

Ramos-Andrade D, Andrade L, Ruivo C, Portilha MA, Caseiro-Alves F, Curvo-Semedo L. Imaging the postoperative patient: long-term complications of gastrointestinal surgery. Insights Imaging. 2016 Feb;7(1):7–20.

Termsinsuk P, Chantarojanasiri T, Pausawasdi N. Diagnosis and treatment of the afferent loop syndrome. Clin J Gastroenterol. 2020 Oct;13(5):660–8.

Vargas EJ, Abu Dayyeh BK, Storm AC, Bazerbachi F, Matar R, Vella A, et al. Endoscopic management of dumping syndrome after Roux-en-Y gastric bypass: a large international series and proposed management strategy. Gastrointest Endosc. 2020 Jul;92(1):91–6.

Zafar SN, Miller K, Felton J, Wise ES, Kligman M. Postoperative bleeding after laparoscopic Roux-en-Y gastric bypass: predictors and consequences. Surg Endosc. 2019 Jan;33(1):272–80.

14

Endoscopy for the Gastroenterology Board Examination

TAREK SAWAS, MD

DAVID H. BRUINING, MD

ANDREW C. STORM, MD

Quality Metrics for Colonoscopy

Colonoscopy is a widely used diagnostic and therapeutic tool. The goal of a screening colonoscopy is to detect and remove early neoplastic lesions to prevent the development of colorectal cancer in asymptomatic patients. Performing a high-quality colonoscopy with comprehensive mucosal visualization is essential. The following metrics have been proposed as indicators for high-quality examinations: colon preparation, cecal intubation rate, withdrawal time, and adenoma detection rate (ADR) (Table 14.1).

Colon Preparation

The yield of screening colonoscopy is dependent on the quality of the colon preparation. The American College of Gastroenterology and the American Society for Gastrointestinal Endoscopy Task Force on Quality in Endoscopy defined adequate examination as one that allows detection of lesions larger than 5 mm (Am J Gastroenterol. 2002 Jun;97[6]:1296-308). Inadequate colon preparation is the most common cause of incomplete colonoscopy and has been associated with missed neoplasia, prolonged procedure time, and a higher rate of adverse events. Preparation is inadequate in about 15% of colonoscopies. Multiple factors have been identified as predictors of poor colon cleansing. Patient factors

include advanced age, male sex, obesity, non-English speaking, enrolled in Medicaid insurance, inpatient, single, polypharmacy, and comorbidities such as diabetes mellitus, cerebrovascular accident, Parkinson disease, and dementia. An important nonpatient determinant of a poor preparation is a long interval between the end of preparation and the start of the procedure.

Patients should be carefully educated and instructed about the preparation process. Appropriate cleansing incorporates a combination of diet modification and a cathartic agent. Patients should be advised to follow a clear-liquid or low-residual diet the day before the procedure. Consuming the colon preparation in a split dose results in higher-quality examinations, higher adenoma detection rates, and improved patient tolerance. The quality of the colon preparation should be documented for each procedure. One of the proposed validated scoring tools is the Boston bowel preparation scale (Table 14.2). This scale has been shown to be positively associated with the ADR and procedural insertion and withdrawal times. Screening colonoscopy with inadequate preparation should be repeated in 1 year or less.

Table 14.1. Quality Metrics for Colonoscopy

Quality measure	Recommended target
Adequate colon preparation	≥90% of all colonoscopies
Cecal intubation rate	≥95% of screening colonoscopies
	≥90% of all colonoscopies
Adenoma detection rate	≥25%
	≥20% in women
	≥30% in men
Withdrawal time	≥6 minutes

Data from Rex DK, Schoenfeld PS, Cohen J, Pike IM, Adler DG, Fennerty MB, et al. Quality indicators for colonoscopy. Gastrointest Endosc. 2015 Jan;81(1):31-53.

Abbreviations: ADR, adenoma detection rate; CHA$_2$DS$_2$-VASc, cardiac failure or dysfunction, hypertension, age 65-74 years or older than 75 years, diabetes mellitus, and stroke, transient ischemic attack, or thromboembolism-vascular disease, and sex category (female); ERCP, endoscopic retrograde cholangiopancreatography; EUS, endoscopic ultrasonography; FNA, fine-needle aspiration; GI, gastrointestinal; INR, international normalized ratio; PEP, post-ERCP pancreatitis.

Table 14.2. Boston Bowel Preparation Scale

Score	Description
0	Unprepared colon segment with solid stool preventing mucosal visualization
1	Portion of the mucosal segment is not seen because of staining, solid stool, or opaque liquids
2	Minor amount of residual staining, residual stool, or opaque liquids but mucosa is well visualized
3	Entire mucosa is well visualized without residual staining, stool, or opaque liquid

Data from Lai EJ, Calderwood AH, Doros G, Fix OK, Jacobson BC. The Boston bowel preparation scale: a valid and reliable instrument for colonoscopy-oriented research. Gastrointest Endosc. 2009 Mar;69(3 Pt 2):620-5.

Cecal Intubation Rate

Cecal intubation is defined as advancement of the colonoscope tip proximal to the ileocecal valve to ensure adequate visualization of the cecal base. Low cecal intubation rates are associated with higher post-colonoscopy proximal colon cancer. The current quality guidelines recommend a cecal intubation rate of 95% for screening colonoscopies and 90% for all colonoscopies. Endoscopists are expected to photographically document anatomical landmarks (ileocecal valve and appendiceal orifice).

Withdrawal Time

The goal withdrawal time is an average of 6 or more minutes. Longer withdrawal time is associated with a higher ADR.

Adenoma Detection Rate

The ADR is the single most important quality measure for screening colonoscopy. It is defined as the percentage of patients aged 50 years or older undergoing screening colonoscopy who have 1 or more precancerous polyps detected. The ADR is inversely associated with the risk of colorectal cancer. The goal ADR is 25% or more (men ≥30% and women ≥20%). An ADR less than 20% is associated with a higher risk for post-colonoscopy colorectal cancer.

Management of Antithrombotic Agents

Antithrombotic medications can be categorized according to their mechanism of action into anticoagulants and antiplatelet agents. Anticoagulants prevent thrombosis by blocking the clotting cascade, whereas antiplatelet agents affect platelet function by preventing platelet aggregation. Management of antithrombotic agents in patients undergoing endoscopic procedures is challenging. Interrupting antithrombotic therapy increases the risk of thromboembolic events. Conversely, some endoscopic procedures are associated with a high risk of bleeding. Periprocedural management should consider 4 factors: 1) the risk of bleeding associated with the endoscopic procedure, 2) a patient's personal risk for thromboembolic events, 3) the urgency of the procedure, and 4) the pharmacokinetics of the antithrombotic agent.

Step 1: Determine the Risk of Bleeding (High vs Low)

The risk of bleeding is mainly driven by the need for therapeutic intervention (Box 14.1). Most diagnostic endoscopy is associated with a low risk of bleeding (<1%) and does not require interruption of anticoagulation or antiplatelet therapy. The most common low-risk procedures are upper endoscopy with biopsies, colonoscopy with biopsies, endoscopic retrograde cholangiopancreatography (ERCP) without sphincterotomy, and endoscopic ultrasonography (EUS) without fine-needle aspiration (FNA). High-risk

---

Box 14.1. Procedure Risk for Bleeding

High bleeding risk	Low bleeding risk
Varices treatment	Diagnostic EGD or colonoscopy with biopsy
Dilation	Enteral stent (controversial)
Polypectomy	Barrett esophagus ablation
ERCP with biliary or pancreatic sphincterotomy	ERCP with stent or papillary balloon dilation
Ampullectomy	Capsule endoscopy
EUS with FNA	EUS without FNA
Cystgastrostomy	EUS with FNA of solid masses and patient is receiving ASA or NSAIDs
PEG and PEJ tube placement	PEG placement and patient is receiving ASA or clopidogrel
Therapeutic BAE (except APC)	Diagnostic BAE
Endoscopic mucosal resection or endoscopic submucosal dissection	APC

Abbreviations: APC, argon plasma coagulation; ASA, aspirin; BAE, balloon-assisted enteroscopy; EGD, esophagogastroduodenoscopy; ERCP, endoscopic retrograde cholangiopancreatography; EUS, endoscopic ultrasound; FNA, fine-needle aspiration; NSAIDs, nonsteroidal anti-inflammatory drugs; PEG, percutaneous endoscopic gastrostomy; PEJ, percutaneous endoscopic jejunostomy.

Adapted from ASGE Standards of Practice Committee, Acosta RD, Abraham NS, Chandrasekhara V, Chathadi KV, Early DS, et al. The management of antithrombotic agents for patients undergoing GI endoscopy. Gastrointest Endosc. 2016 Jan;83(1):3-16; used with permission.

procedures require holding and possibly reversing the effect of antithrombotics to minimize the risk of bleeding. High-risk procedures include esophageal dilation, variceal banding, percutaneous feeding-tube placement, ERCP with sphincterotomy, EUS with FNA, and colonoscopy with removal of large polyps (>1 cm).

The risk of bleeding after polypectomy ranges from 0.3% to 10%. Factors associated with increased postpolypectomy bleeding include large polyp size (>10 mm), polyp location (higher risk in the right side), morphologic features (large sessile polyps and pedunculated thick-stalk polyps), resection technique (lower risk of delayed bleeding with cold snare polypectomy), and type of cautery used (higher risk with pure cutting mode of electrosurgical current).

Step 2: Determine the Risk of a Thromboembolic Event

If a procedure is deemed to be associated with a high risk of bleeding, the next step is to determine the risk for a thromboembolic event and thus the need for a bridging agent (Table 14.3). The risk depends on the underlying indication for anticoagulation or antiplatelet therapy. Patients receiving anticoagulation who have a low thromboembolic risk do not require bridging. Conversely, high-risk patients undergoing high-risk procedures require bridging with a short-acting anticoagulant before and after the procedure. Conditions that are associated with a low thromboembolic risk include nonvalvular atrial fibrillation with a CHA_2DS_2-VASc (cardiac failure or dysfunction, hypertension, age 65-74 years [1 point] or ≥75 years [2 points], diabetes mellitus, and stroke, transient ischemic attack, or thromboembolism [2 points]-vascular disease [2 points], and sex category [female]) risk score of 0 or 1, having a bileaflet aortic valve prosthesis without atrial fibrillation, and venous thromboembolism for more than 6 months before the procedure. High-risk conditions include having any prosthetic mitral valve or a caged-ball or tilting disk aortic valve prosthesis; cerebrovascular accident or transit ischemic attack within the past 6 months; venous thromboembolism in the past 3 months; and severe thrombophilia (protein C, protein S, and antithrombin deficiency and the antiphospholipid antibody syndrome). For patients receiving antiplatelet therapy,

high-risk conditions include placement of drug-eluting coronary stents in the past year or bare metal stents within the previous month. In these situations, endoscopic procedures should be delayed, if possible, until it is safe to withhold antiplatelet therapy. Patients with a history of an occluded coronary artery stent are at high risk for a second stent occlusion (20%) and cardiac death (28%) even after 1 year from stent placement.

Step 3: Determine the Urgency of the Procedure

Urgent situations include but are not limited to active gastrointestinal (GI) bleeding and acute cholangitis. Patients receiving warfarin who have life-threatening GI bleeding may require reversal of the effect of anticoagulation, whereas those with minor bleeding may be managed by withholding warfarin but not reversing its effect. For patients with active GI bleeding, some experts recommend a goal international normalized ratio (INR) of less than 2.5. One study suggested that the success rate of endoscopic hemostasis for patients with an INR between 1.3 and 2.7 is comparable to that of patients who are not receiving anticoagulants, and the study was not powered to determine the success rate for an INR of more than 2.7 (Am J Gastroenterol. 2007 Feb;102[2]:290-6). Accordingly, endoscopic therapy for serious GI bleeding should not be delayed in patients with an INR less than 2.5.

Step 4: Determine the Appropriate Duration to Withhold Medication

The risk of bleeding in patients taking a low-dose aspirin is low, and use of this medication does not need to be stopped even for patients undergoing a procedure associated with a high risk of bleeding. Other antiplatelet agents can be withheld on the basis of their elimination time: clopidogrel (5-7 days), prasugrel (5-7 days), ticagrelor (3-5 days), and ticlopidine (10-14 days). Warfarin should be withheld for 5 days before high-risk procedures. Because low-molecular-weight heparin has a short half-life, its use can be stopped 24 hours before the procedure. Novel oral anticoagulants include direct factor Xa inhibitors and

Table 14.3. Risk Stratification for Thromboembolic Event in Patients With Mechanical Valve or VTE

Valve or condition	Risk		
	High	Medium	Low
Mitral valve	Any mitral prosthesis	NA	NA
Aortic valve	Caged-ball or tilting disk aortic valve prosthesis	Bileaflet aortic valve prosthesis *and* 1 of the following: AF, prior CVA or TIA, hypertension, diabetes, CHF, age ≥75 y	Bileaflet aortic valve without risk factors
Cerebrovascular accident	TIA or CVA within past 6 months	NA	NA
VTE	VTE within 3 mo	VTE in past 3-12 mo Recurrent VTE Active cancer (treatment in the past 6 mo or palliative)	VTE >12 mo and no other risk factors
Thrombophilia	Severe thrombophilia (deficiency protein C/S/antithrombin, antiphospholipid antibodies)	Nonsevere thrombophilia (heterozygous factor V Leiden)	NA

Abbreviations: AF, atrial fibrillation; CHF, congestive heart failure; CVA, cerebrovascular accident; NA, not applicable; TIA, transient ischemic attack; VTE, venous thromboembolism.

Adapted from Douketis JD, Spyropoulos AC, Spencer FA, Mayr M, Jaffer AK, Eckman MH, et al. Perioperative management of antithrombotic therapy: antithrombotic therapy and prevention of thrombosis, 9th ed: American College of Chest Physicians evidence-based clinical practice guidelines. Chest. 2012 Feb;141(2 Suppl):e326S-e50S; used with permission.

Table 14.4.   Perioperative Management of Novel Oral Anticoagulant Agents[a]

Novel oral anticoagulant	Elective[b] (Cr clearance >90 mL/min)	Reversal agent	Hemodialysis (massive GI bleeding)
Direct thrombin inhibitor	NA	NA	NA
Dabigatran	Hold 2-3 d	Idarucizumab	Yes
Direct Xa inhibitors	NA	Recombinant factor Xa	NA
Rivaroxaban	Hold 1 d	NA	No
Apixaban	Hold 1-2 d	NA	No
Edoxaban	Hold 1 d	NA	No

Abbreviations: Cr, creatinine; GI, gastrointestinal; NA, not applicable.

[a] Based on procedural urgency and high-risk procedure.

[b] See guidelines for impaired renal function.

[c] Approved apixaban and rivaroxaban.

Data from ASGE Standards of Practice Committee, Acosta RD, Abraham NS, Chandrasekhara V, Chathadi KV, Early DS, et al. The management of antithrombotic agents for patients undergoing GI endoscopy. Gastrointest Endosc. 2016 Jan;83(1):3-16.

Table 14.5.   Antibiotic Prophylaxis in Cardiac Conditions

Cardiac condition	Indication for antibiotics
All cardiac conditions	No
Highest risk of IE	If established GI tract infection and for those who receive antibiotic therapy to prevent wound infection or sepsis associated with a GI procedure, use an antibiotic regimen with an agent active against enterococci
Prosthetic cardiac valve	NA
History of IE	
Cardiac transplant with valvulopathy	
CHD	
Unrepaired cyanotic CHD	
Repaired CHD (first 6 mo)	
Repaired CHD with residual defects	

Abbreviations: CHD, congenital heart disease; GI, gastrointestinal; IE, infective endocarditis; NA, not applicable.

Adapted from ASGE Standards of Practice Committee, Khashab MA, Chithadi KV, Acosta RD, Bruining DH, Chandrasekhara V, et al. Antibiotic prophylaxis for GI endoscopy. Gastrointest Endosc. 2015 Jan;81(1):81-9; used with permission.

direct thrombin inhibitor agents. The discontinuation duration varies according to kidney function. For most of these agents, an average of 1 to 2 days is appropriate in patients with normal creatinine clearance (Table 14.4). Patients with impaired renal function may require longer discontinuation times. Use of novel oral anticoagulants can be restarted once hemostasis is confirmed. Idarucizumab is a reversal agent for direct thrombin inhibitor (dabigatran), and recombinant factor Xa (Andexxa) is a reversal agent for apixaban and rivaroxaban.

Antibiotic Prophylaxis for Endoscopy

Although bacteremia is common after endoscopy, clinically significant infections are rare. Antibiotic prophylaxis to solely prevent infectious endocarditis is not recommended for most GI procedures, even in patients with high-risk cardiac conditions. Similarly, patients with synthetic vascular grafts or an orthopedic prosthesis who are undergoing GI endoscopic procedures do not require antibiotic prophylaxis. The only exceptions are patients with high-risk cardiac conditions (Table 14.5) and those with an established GI tract enterococcus infection such as cholangitis. Prophylactic antibiotics effective against gram-positive skin flora should be given before percutaneous endoscopic gastrostomy or jejunostomy tube placement. Patients who are having peritoneal dialysis and will undergo lower endoscopy should receive antibiotic prophylaxis with ampicillin and an aminoglycoside.

Antibiotic prophylaxis should be administered before ERCP in the following: 1) liver transplant recipients, 2) patients in whom biliary obstruction is suspected who have a possibility of incomplete biliary drainage, and 3) patients with primary sclerosing cholangitis (Table 14.6). The antibiotic chosen should be effective against biliary or enteric flora, including enteric gram-negative organisms and enterococci. Patients undergoing EUS or EUS with FNA of a solid lesion do not require prophylaxis. However, prophylactic antibiotics are suggested for EUS with FNA of mediastinal, pancreatic, and peripancreatic cystic lesions (Table 14.7).

Endoscopic Ultrasonography

EUS is both a diagnostic and a therapeutic tool. The diagnostic role includes evaluation and staging of GI mucosal and submucosal lesions and of pancreas and bile duct abnormalities and performance of EUS-guided FNA and biopsy. The wall of the GI tract is lined by 5 layers. Layers that contain muscle appear darker (hypoechoic) on EUS. The 5 layers from the inside out are as follows (Figure 14.1):

1.   Mucosa/epithelium (bright)
2.   Muscularis mucosa (dark)

Table 14.6.   Antibiotic Prophylaxis Before Endoscopic Procedures

Procedure	Indication for antibiotics
ERCP without cholangitis (complete drainage)	No
ERCP for obstruction without cholangitis (incomplete drainage)	Yes; continue after procedure
Liver transplant	Yes; continue after procedure
EUS-FNA of solid lesion (upper or lower GI tract)	No
EUS-FNA of mediastinal cysts	Suggested
EUS-FNA of pancreatic or peripancreatic cysts	Suggested
PEG or PEJ initial placement	Yes
Cirrhosis with GI bleeding	Yes
Synthetic vascular graft OR prosthetic joints	No
Lower endoscopy in patient undergoing peritoneal dialysis	Yes; ampicillin + aminoglycoside

Abbreviations: ERCP, endoscopic retrograde cholangiopancreatography; EUS, endoscopic ultrasound; FNA, fine-needle aspiration; GI, gastrointestinal; PEG, percutaneous endoscopic gastrostomy; PEJ, percutaneous endoscopic jejunostomy.

Adapted from ASGE Standards of Practice Committee, Khashab MA, Chithadi KV, Acosta RD, Bruining DH, Chandrasekhara V, et al. Antibiotic prophylaxis for GI endoscopy. Gastrointest Endosc. 2015 Jan;81(1):81-9; used with permission.

Table 14.7. Endoscopic Ultrasonography of Subepithelial Lesions

Lesion	Layer	Pattern	Stain	Miscellaneous
Carcinoid	2,3	Hypoechoic or isoechoic	NA	NA
Duplication cyst or varices	Cyst: 2,3,4,5 Varices: 3 (can course through all layers)	Anechoic	NA	Duplication cyst: Doppler negative Varices: Doppler positive
Pancreatic rest	2,3,4	Hypoechoic (usually)	NA	Central umbilication
Lipoma	3	Hyperechoic	NA	Pillow sign
Schwannoma	3,4	Hypoechoic	+S100	NA
Glomus tumor	3,4	Hypoechoic (usually)	+Vimentin	NA
Leiomyoma	4 (usually) 2,3 (rare)	Hypoechoic	+Desmin, +SMA, −CD117	NA
GIST	4 (usually) 2,3 (rare)	Hypoechoic	+CD117 (c-Kit) +PDGFRa	NA

Abbreviations: GIST, gastrointestinal stromal tumor; NA, not applicable; PDGFRa, platelet-derived growth factor receptor alpha; SMA, smooth muscle actin.

3. Submucosa (bright)
4. Muscularis propria (dark)
5. Serosa (bright)

Subepithelial tumors are identified in layers 2, 3, or 4. The appearance and location of the most commonly identified and important lesions are listed in Table 14.7.

Endoscopic Retrograde Cholangiopancreatography

ERCP is the cornerstone for management of pancreaticobiliary diseases. Familiarity with the following concepts is important for the board examination:

1. Adverse events associated with ERCP
2. High-yield cholangiograms
3. Biliary stents

ERCP-Associated Adverse Events

It is essential for gastroenterologists to understand the possible adverse events associated with ERCP. Post-ERCP pancreatitis (PEP) is the most common adverse event (5% of cases). Factors associated with a high risk for PEP include prior PEP, female sex,

recurrent pancreatitis, suspected sphincter of Oddi dysfunction, young age, absence of chronic pancreatitis, normal serum bilirubin value, difficult cannulation, repetitive pancreatic guidewire cannulation, pancreatic injection, pancreatic sphincterotomy, and papillary large-balloon dilation of an intact sphincter. Administration of rectal nonsteroidal anti-inflammatory drugs in high-risk patients substantially reduces the incidence and severity of PEP. Additional methods to reduce PEP involve placement of a prophylactic pancreatic plastic stent and periprocedural intravenous hydration.

Post-ERCP bleeding complicates less than 2% of procedures and most commonly is a result of sphincterotomy. Other less common causes of post-ERCP bleeding include stricture dilation, biopsy, and ablative therapy. Bleeding might be immediate or delayed up until several weeks after ERCP. Risk factors for post-ERCP bleeding include coagulopathy, active cholangitis, the use of anticoagulants within 3 days from the procedure, and the endoscopist's ERCP case volume. The length of sphincterotomy, periampullary diverticulum, and aspirin use have not been shown to increase the risk of bleeding.

Other possible adverse events associated with ERCP include cholangitis, cholecystitis, and perforation. Abdominal computed tomography with an oral contrast agent is the most reliable method to assess for perforation.

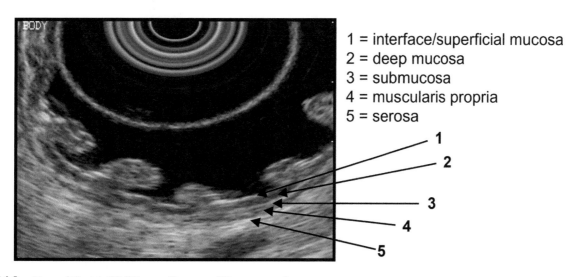

1 = interface/superficial mucosa
2 = deep mucosa
3 = submucosa
4 = muscularis propria
5 = serosa

Figure 14.1. **Normal Gastric Wall Layers Shown on Ultrasonography.**

High-Yield Cholangiograms or Pancreatograms

The following conditions are important to recognize on cholangiograms or pancreatograms:

1. Primary sclerosing cholangitis: the multifocal short biliary strictures and upstream dilatation result in the characteristic appearance of beads on a string.
2. Abnormal pancreaticobiliary junction: the junction of the biliary duct and pancreatic duct is outside the wall of the duodenum with a long common channel (Figure 14.2).
3. Post-cholecystectomy biliary leak: contrast extravasation from the cystic duct stump (most commonly) or within the gallbladder bed.
4. Pancreatic divisum (Figure 14.3): characterized by the presence of a short ventral duct at the major papilla and the dorsal pancreatic duct draining separately from the tail to the head at the minor papilla.
5. Annular pancreas (Figure 14.4): the ventral pancreatic duct encircles the duodenum.
6. Recurrent pyogenic cholangitis (Figure 14.5): the classic finding is the arrowhead sign. This sign results from multiple changes caused by periductal fibrosis, including dilated intrahepatic and extrahepatic ducts, straightened intrahepatic ducts with less acute angled branching, and decreased branching with acute tapering of the peripheral ducts.

Biliary Stents

Biliary stents can be either plastic or metal. All plastic stents are radiopaque. They have a small diameter and require exchange every 2 to 3 months. The 2 main adverse events associated with plastic stents are migration and occlusion. Metal stents have a larger diameter with longer patency time and a low risk for obstruction. Metal stents are either fully covered or uncovered. Uncovered metal stents are prone to tissue ingrowth, which makes stent extraction or manipulation extremely difficult after insertion. Covered metal stents prevent tissue ingrowth but are more likely to migrate. Self-expanding metal stents are preferred over plastic stents in selected patients with nonresectable malignant biliary obstruction given their longer patency and might be more cost effective in patients with a longer life expectancy and no metastasis and who have early occlusion of the plastic biliary stents.

✓ ADR is the single most important quality measure for screening colonoscopy and is inversely associated with the risk of post-colonoscopy colorectal cancer. The goal ADR is 25% or more.
✓ The goal withdrawal time for screening colonoscopy is an average of 6 minutes or more. Longer withdrawal times are associated with higher ADRs.

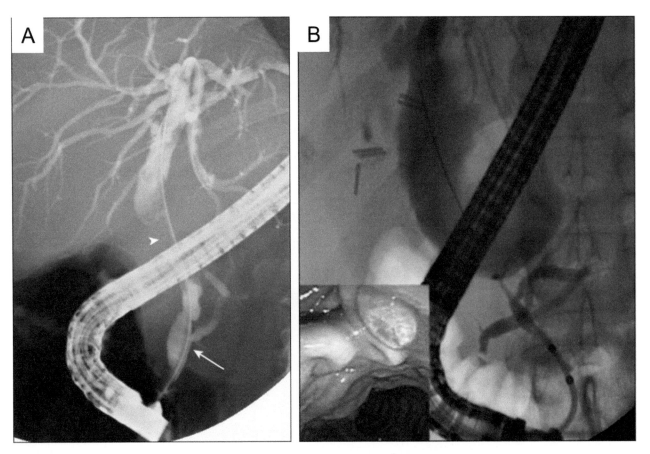

Figure 14.2.   Anomalous Pancreaticobiliary Junctions on Endoscopic Retrograde Cholangiopancreatography. A, Anomalous pancreaticobiliary junction (APBJ, arrow) with a bile duct stricture (arrowhead) caused by gallbladder cancer in a 32-year-old with obstructive jaundice. APBJ is a risk factor for development of gallbladder cancer. Note the absence of a bile duct cyst. B, Anomalous pancreaticobiliary junction with a cyst of the common bile duct. Bile drains to the duodenum via the minor papilla (inset). (Adapted from Topazian MD. Pancreas divisum, biliary cysts, and other congenital anomalies. In: Baron TH, Kozarek RA, Carr-Locke DL, eds. ERCP. 3rd ed. Elsevier; 2018:335-45; Figure 2B courtesy of Naoki Takahashi, MD, Diagnostic Radiology, Mayo Clinic; used with permission.)

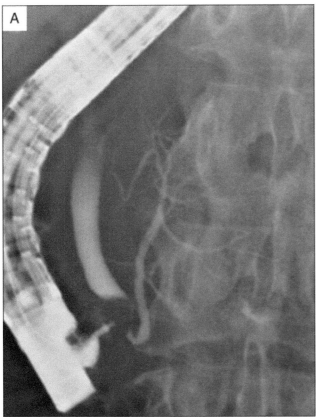

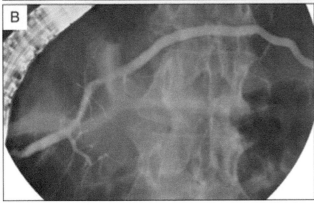

Figure 14.3. Pancreatic Divisum on Endoscopic Retrograde Cholangiopancreatography. A, Cannulation of the major papilla demonstrates an arborizing ventral pancreatic duct that does not cross the midline or give rise to an uncinate branch. B, Cannulation of the minor papilla demonstrates a dominant dorsal pancreatic duct, with no communication to the ventral pancreas. The uncinate branch arises from the dorsal pancreatic duct. (Adapted from Topazian MD. Pancreas divisum, biliary cysts, and other congenital anomalies. In: Baron TH, Kozarek RA, Carr-Locke DL, eds. ERCP. 3rd ed. Elsevier; 2018:335-45; used with permission.)

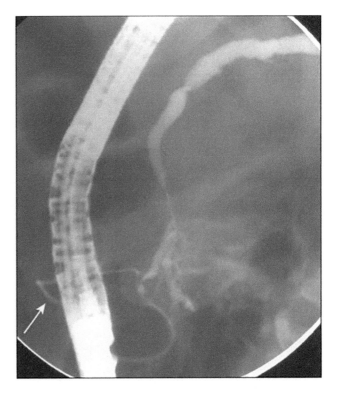

Figure 14.4. Annular Pancreas on Endoscopic Retrograde Cholangiopancreatography. The ventral pancreatic duct encircles the second duodenum (arrow). This patient also has a stricture of the main pancreatic duct, caused by pancreatic adenocarcinoma. (Adapted from Topazian MD. Pancreas divisum, biliary cysts, and other congenital anomalies. In: Baron TH, Kozarek RA, Carr-Locke DL, eds. ERCP. 3rd ed. Elsevier; 2018:335-45; used with permission.)

✓ Repeat colonoscopy within 1 year after a colonoscopy for which preparation was inadequate.

✓ Continue use of antithrombotics for procedures with a low bleeding risk. There is no need to interrupt the use of aspirin, even for procedures with a high bleeding risk.

✓ There is no need for prophylactic antibiotics for most GI procedures, even in the presence of high-risk cardiac conditions.

✓ Antibiotic prophylaxis should be used in the following cases: before ERCP in liver transplant recipients or patients with ongoing biliary obstruction, before EUS with FNA of a cystic lesion, before percutaneous endoscopic gastrostomy or jejunostomy tube placement, in patients who are having peritoneal dialysis and will undergo lower endoscopy, in patients with high-risk cardiac conditions, and in patients with established GI tract enterococcus infection.

✓ Administration of rectal nonsteroidal anti-inflammatory drugs in high-risk patients substantially reduces the incidence and severity of post-ERCP pancreatitis.

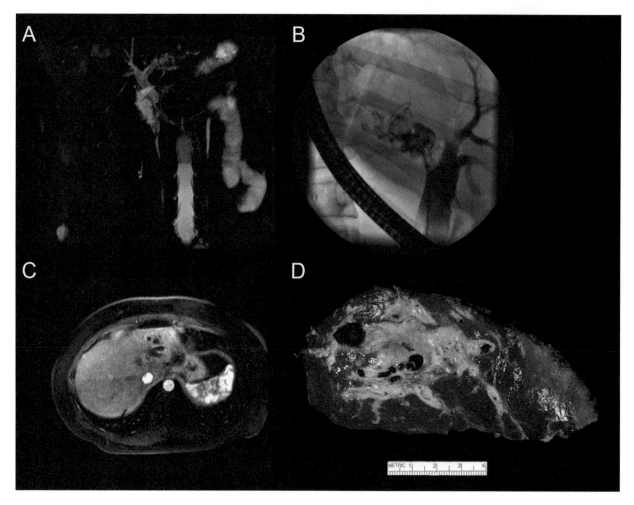

Figure 14.5. Recurrent Pyogenic Cholangitis. This condition is characterized by recurrent and progressively severe attacks of cholangitis with associated intrahepatic stones, secondary strictures, and upstream duct dilatation. These features often lead to segmental or lobar atrophy, as shown on magnetic resonance cholangiopancreatograpy (A), endoscopic retrograde cholangiography (B), computed tomography (C), and gross specimen (D). When disease is unilateral, isolated left lobe involvement is most common.

Suggested Reading

ASGE Standards of Practice Committee, Acosta RD, Abraham NS, Chandrasekhara V, Chathadi KV, Early DS, et al. The management of antithrombotic agents for patients undergoing GI endoscopy. Gastrointest Endosc. 2016 Jan;83(1):3–16.

ASGE Standards of Practice Committee, Chandrasekhara V, Khashab MA, Muthusamy VR, Acosta RD, Agrawal D, et al. Adverse events associated with ERCP. Gastrointest Endosc. 2017 Jan;85(1):32–47.

ASGE Standards of Practice Committee, Khashab MA, Chithadi KV, Acosta RD, Bruining DH, Chandrasekhara V, et al. Antibiotic prophylaxis for GI endoscopy. Gastrointest Endosc. 2015 Jan;81(1):81–9.

ASGE Standards of Practice Committee, Saltzman JR, Cash BD, Pasha SF, Early DS, Muthusamy VR, et al. Bowel preparation before colonoscopy. Gastrointest Endosc. 2015 Apr;81(4):781–94.

Rex DK, Boland CR, Dominitz JA, Giardiello FM, Johnson DA, Kaltenbach T, et al. Colorectal cancer screening: recommendations for physicians and patients from the US Multi-Society Task Force on Colorectal Cancer. Gastrointest Endosc. 2017 Jul;86(1):18–33.

Questions and Answers

Questions

Abbreviations used:

ALT,	alanine aminotransferase
ANCA,	antineutrophil cytoplasmic antibody
AST,	aspartate aminotransferase
BAE,	balloon-assisted endoscopy
CE,	capsule endoscopy
CI,	colonic ischemia
CT,	computed tomography
CTA,	computed tomographic angiography
CTE,	computed tomographic enterography
DBE,	double-balloon endoscopy
EGD,	esophagogastroduodenoscopy
ERCP,	endoscopic retrograde cholangiopancreatography
GAVE,	gastric antral vascular ectasia
GI,	gastrointestinal
HSP,	Henoch-Schönlein purpura
INR,	international normalized ratio
IRCI,	isolated right colonic ischemia
MRA,	magnetic resonance angiography
MRCP,	magnetic resonance cholangiopancreatography
NSAID,	nonsteroidal anti-inflammatory drug
PAN,	polyarteritis nodosa
PEG,	percutaneous gastrostomy
PEJ,	percutaneous jejunostomy
PUD,	peptic ulcer disease
RYGB,	Roux-en-Y gastric bypass
SSc,	systemic sclerosis

Multiple Choice (choose the best answer)

IV.1. **A 53-year-old man presents with a 7-day history of melena. Four years earlier, when EGD was performed for reflux, a 3-cm hiatal hernia was identified. Since then the patient has lost 6.8 kg with daily exercise, and he stopped taking omeprazole 1 year ago (he says that he does not have reflux symptoms now).**

He takes daily ibuprofen for tennis elbow. His medical history also includes a diagnosis of fatty liver disease and alcohol use disorder during his teenaged and college years. What is the most likely cause of the GI tract bleeding?

a. Diverticular bleeding
b. Cameron lesions
c. PUD
d. Small-bowel angiectasia
e. Esophageal varices

IV.2. **A 75-year-old man presents with a 3-month history of intermittent melena. His current hemoglobin level is 10.1 g/dL. He had an ileal carcinoid tumor resected 10 years earlier. He has daily bloating and intermittent distention when he eats high-fiber foods. EGD and colonoscopy are performed, but a bleeding source is not identified. He does not use NSAIDs or anticoagulants, and he has no history of kidney disease. What is the most appropriate next test for this patient?**

a. Antegrade BAE
b. Retrograde BAE
c. CE
d. CTA
e. CTE

IV.3. **A 44-year-old woman presents with a 3-day history of melena. Four years earlier, when EGD was performed for reflux, a 2-cm hiatal hernia was identified. The patient takes NSAIDs daily for chronic pain in her lower back. EGD for the present history of melena shows a large (1.5-cm diameter) ulcer with a 1-mm nonbleeding vessel in the lateral wall of the second portion of the duodenum. What is the most appropriate management plan?**

a. High doses of proton pump inhibitor and no endoscopic intervention
b. Epinephrine injection only
c. Hemostatic powder application

d. Epinephrine injection and bipolar probe therapy

e. Immediate referral to the interventional radiology service for embolization

IV.4. **A 24-year-old man presents with a 3-day history of melena. The hemoglobin concentration is 7.6 g/dL. The patient's past medical history is unremarkable, and he has not had any surgical procedures. He does not use NSAIDs, and he has not had diarrhea or abdominal pain. EGD and colonoscopy do not show evidence of the source of the bleeding. What is the most appropriate next test?**

a. Meckel scan

b. Antegrade DBE

c. Retrograde DBE

d. Follow-up EGD

e. Capsule endoscopy

IV.5. **A 70-year-old man is admitted to the hospital with sudden onset of cramping right lower quadrant abdominal pain of moderate severity. Several hours later, he has bloody bowel movements. He has hypertension and coronary artery disease; his medications are atorvastatin, metoprolol, and low-dose aspirin. On physical examination, he appears comfortable. Vital signs are normal. The abdomen is nondistended, and bowel sounds are normal. On deep palpation of the right lower quadrant, he has moderate tenderness with no rebound or guarding. CT without a contrast agent shows thickening of the ascending colon. Colonoscopy shows a segment with subepithelial hemorrhage, edema, and erythema from the cecum to the ascending colon. Which of the following is the most appropriate test to perform next?**

a. Selective catheter angiography

b. MRA

c. CTA

d. Duplex ultrasonography of mesenteric vessels

IV.6. **A 75-year-old woman is evaluated for early satiety, postprandial abdominal pain, and an unintentional 13.6-kg (30-lb) weight loss over the past 2 months. She also has coronary artery disease and hypertension and a 50 pack-year smoking history. Her medications are low-dose aspirin, metoprolol, lisinopril, hydrochlorothiazide, sublingual nitroglycerin, and rosuvastatin. On physical examination, her vital signs are normal, and body mass index is 20. The patient appears cachectic with temporal wasting. An abdominal bruit is heard, and mild epigastric tenderness is noted. Laboratory test results are as follows: hemoglobin, 11 g/dL; mean corpuscular volume, 90 fL; white blood cell count, 9.0×10⁹/L; and platelet count within the reference range. Ultrasonography of the mesenteric vessels shows increased velocity in the celiac and superior mesenteric arteries, which is consistent with high-grade stenosis of these vessels. Subsequent CTA shows severe stenosis of the celiac and superior mesenteric arteries and possible enlargement of pancreatic head. Which of the following is the most appropriate management?**

a. Catheter angiography with stenting of the celiac artery

b. Vascular surgery consultation for mesenteric arterial bypass

c. Four-hour solid meal gastric emptying study

d. Endoscopic ultrasonography of the pancreas with fine-needle aspiration

IV.7. **A 73-year-old man with hypertension presents with abrupt onset of mild, cramping abdominal pain in the left lower quadrant and subsequent bloody diarrhea several hours later. On physical examination, he is afebrile with normal hemodynamic status. On abdominal examination he has mild abdominal tenderness in the left lower quadrant without rebound or guarding. Laboratory study results include a white blood cell count of 12×10⁹/L and normal values for hemoglobin, lactate, serum urea nitrogen, and creatinine. CT of the abdomen and pelvis is performed (see image).**

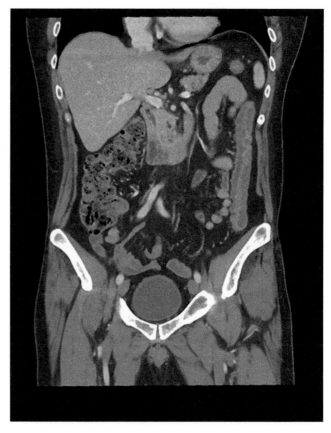

The patient is admitted to the hospital with a diagnosis of ischemic colitis. In addition to giving him nothing by mouth and providing intravenous fluids and narcotic analgesia, what else should be done?

a. Perform mesenteric CTA

b. Initiate therapy with intravenous broad-spectrum antibiotics

c. Start total parenteral nutrition

d. Perform flexible sigmoidoscopy

IV.8. **A 70-year-old woman with cerebrovascular and peripheral vascular disease presents to the emergency department for further evaluation of worsening abdominal pain and weight loss. She reports postprandial abdominal bloating and discomfort for the past 6 months associated with a 13.6-kg (30-lb) weight loss. She describes variable occurrence of abdominal distention and cramping with onset 20 to 40 minutes after eating. The postprandial pain gradually increases in severity and then slowly resolves over the next 1 to 3 hours. She does not use NSAIDs. Findings were unremarkable from previous laboratory testing, including Helicobacter pylori serology, liver biochemical tests, abdominal radiography, and carbohydrate antigen 19-9. Findings from upper endoscopy, colonoscopy, and capsule endoscopy have been unremarkable. What should be the next step in management?**

a. Duplex ultrasonography of the mesenteric vessels

b. Ultrasonography of the right upper quadrant

c. Mesenteric CTA

d. Gastric emptying study

IV.9. **A 25-year-old woman presents for evaluation of recurrent episodes of severe abdominal pain of prolonged duration that have required admissions to the hospital for intravenous fluids and narcotic analgesia. The pain episodes began 6 months previously after she underwent Roux-en-Y gastric bypass surgery for medically complicated obesity. During these episodes, she also has upper extremity pain, nausea, vomiting, and constipation. On review of the medical records, other presenting conditions were hypertension** and tachycardia. Laboratory studies done during pain found mild hyponatremia. Upper endoscopy and cross-sectional imaging of the abdomen performed during the pain crises had unremarkable findings. Between episodes, she is without symptoms. Currently, she feels well and is without symptoms. On physical examination, she is a well-appearing, slightly overweight woman with normal vital signs. Results of abdominal and anorectal examinations are normal. What is the most likely diagnosis?

a. Systemic mastocytosis
b. Adrenal insufficiency
c. Recurrent small-bowel obstruction
d. Acute intermittent porphyria

IV.10. A 60-year-old man presents with an 18-month history of progressively worsening, nonbloody diarrhea with multiple stools per day of varying volume. He reports a 16-kg weight loss since onset of the diarrhea and infrequent episodes of urge fecal incontinence. His medical history includes atrial fibrillation with onset at age 40 years and bilateral surgical release for carpal tunnel syndrome. On physical examination, he is a thin-appearing man with an unremarkable abdomen. Anorectal inspection shows intact perianal sensation and adequate resting and squeeze anal sphincter tones. A stool pathogen panel is negative. A 72-hour quantitative stool collection result is 55 g of fecal fat/24 hours.

Given the patient's history and the presence of chronic fatty diarrhea, which of the following is the most appropriate next step for evaluating this patient's diarrhea?

a. Small-bowel aspiration and culture
b. Empirical trial of pancreatic enzyme replacement
c. Upper endoscopy with duodenal biopsy
d. Colonoscopy with random biopsies

IV.11. A 26-year-old woman presents with 5 days of persistent abdominal pain associated with nausea, vomiting, and nonbloody stools that developed 2 weeks after an upper respiratory infection. Her only medication is ibuprofen for joint pain. Physical examination is notable for right lower quadrant tenderness and fullness. Laboratory examination indicates a mild leukocytosis. CT of the abdomen and pelvis shows circumferential wall thickening of the terminal ileum (arrow, image below). Stool studies are negative for infection. Colonoscopy shows normal colonic mucosa; however, in the ileum there is diffuse, circumferential ulceration and subepithelial hemorrhage that extends 15 cm. Ileal biopsies are interpreted as ulceration with ischemic-like changes. Three days after hospital admission, palpable purpura develops on the lower extremities, and a leukocytoclastic vasculitis with IgA deposits is detected with immunofluorescence of a skin biopsy specimen. Urinalysis results are mild proteinuria, leukocytes, and red cell casts.

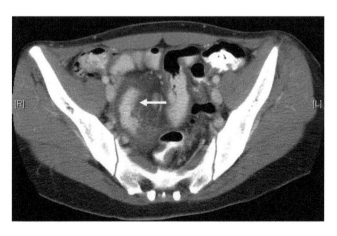

Which of the following diagnoses likely explains the patient's abdominal pain?

a. HSP
b. Granulomatosis with polyangiitis
c. PAN
d. Eosinophilic granulomatosis with polyangiitis

IV.12. A 78-year-old woman presents with a 1-year history of iron deficiency anemia with intermittent melena. She denies heartburn, regurgitation, dysphagia, and abdominal pain. Physical examination shows multiple facial telangiectasias, patchy vitiligo on the upper extremities, and hand sclerodactyly. Stool obtained on digital rectal examination is positive for occult blood. Which GI manifestation of systemic disease is the most likely cause of her iron deficiency anemia?

a. Gastroesophageal reflux
b. Wide-mouth colonic diverticula
c. GAVE
d. Mesenteric vasculitis

IV.13. A 56-year-old woman with a past medical history significant for type 2 diabetes mellitus and severe obesity (body mass index, 52) undergoes RYGB and is admitted for observation. On postoperative day 3, she is asymptomatic and appears well. On review of her medical record, you note that she has had mild tachycardia (heart rate 111 beats/min) during the past 24 hours and one recorded episode of a low-grade fever (37.2 °C). She requests dismissal from the hospital. What do you do next?

a. Order blood cultures and chest radiograph
b. Order CT of abdomen with oral contrast agent
c. Continue observation overnight
d. Dismiss with close follow-up

IV.14. A 45-year-old man underwent RYGB for severe obesity 2 months ago. He did very well postoperatively for the first month. During the past 1 month, he has noticed nausea and early satiety. On seeking medical attention, his bariatric team obtained an upper GI series, which confirmed an anastomotic stricture measuring 10 mm. What is the best next step in management?

a. Endoscopic balloon dilation to 15 mm
b. Endoscopic balloon dilation to 20 mm
c. Endoscopic stricturotomy with needle knife
d. Surgical revision of gastrojejunostomy

IV.15. A 47-year-old woman undergoes RYGB for obesity complicated by type 2 diabetes. She has an uneventful postoperative course. At her 6-month follow-up, she reports that she has had severe diarrhea since her surgery. This is most prominent about an hour after meals and associated with mild dizziness. She has not noticed any blood in her stools. She has lost 50 lb (22.68 kg) since her surgery. She has no other symptoms. What is the best next step?

a. Reassure the patient that this is an expected outcome after RYGB
b. Refer the patient to a dietitian
c. Obtain stool studies to rule out infection
d. Order EGD and colonoscopy with random biopsies

IV.16. A 54-year-old man undergoes RYGB for super-obesity (body mass index, 54). He has an uneventful postoperative course and loses 53% of his excess body weight in the first year after surgery. He presents for follow-up 3 years after surgery. He has now regained about 15% of his weight. On review of his medical record, he was noted to have increased his weight by 5% at his 2-year appointment. The patient reports that there have been no changes in his dietary habits and that he is adhering to his diet. What is the best next step in evaluation?

a. Continue to monitor closely because the weight gain is an expected stabilization of weight after initial weight loss

b. Refer him to a dietitian for further evaluation

c. Obtain a thyroid function test

d. Obtain an upper GI series

IV.17. A 58-year-old woman presented with severe right upper quadrant abdominal pain associated with fever, nausea, and vomiting that had been present for 1 day. Her medical history was clinically significant for coronary artery disease for which she was receiving aspirin and clopidogrel and for atrial fibrillation for which she was receiving warfarin. On presentation, her vital signs were as follows: temperature, 39.4 °C; blood pressure, 75/50 mm Hg; and heart rate, 120 beats per minute. Laboratory results were as follows: white blood cell count, 22 × 10⁹/L; ALT, 420 IU/L; AST, 250 IU/L; total bilirubin, 5.2 mg/dL; alkaline phosphatase, 350 IU/L; and INR, 3.5. On abdominal ultrasonography, cholelithiasis and a dilated common bile duct (16 mm) with an obstructing stone at the distal end were found. The patient was admitted to the intensive care unit and received fluid resuscitation and wide-spectrum antibiotics. What is the best next step in her management?

a. Perform ERCP with sphincterotomy for stone extraction

b. Perform MRCP

c. Refer to surgery for cholecystectomy

d. Perform ERCP for stent placement

e. Continue administration of fluid and antibiotics and delay ERCP until clopidogrel and warfarin have been discontinued for 1 week

IV.18. A 35-year-old woman with no clinically significant medical history presented to the emergency department with right upper quadrant abdominal pain associated with nausea and vomiting. Her vital signs were as follows: temperature, 36.1 °C; blood pressure, 120/80 mm Hg; and heart rate, 105 beats/min. Laboratory results were as follows: white blood cell count, 13 × 10⁹/L; ALT, 234 IU/L; AST, 178 IU/L; total bilirubin 4.2 mg/dL; and lipase, 60 IU/L. Ultrasonography showed cholelithiasis with a dilated common bile duct but no visual stone. The patient underwent ERCP with difficult biliary cannulation in which the wire accessed the pancreatic duct multiple times. A few hours after ERCP, severe epigastric pain radiating to her back developed. Her repeat lipase value was 980 IU/L. Which of the following could have decreased her risk of post-ERCP pancreatitis?

a. She should not have had ERCP because it was not indicated

b. Administration of indomethacin 100 mg rectally after the procedure

c. Performance of a sphincter balloon dilation instead of sphincterotomy

d. Placement of a biliary stent after sphincterotomy

e. Administration of ibuprofen 800 mg orally for 3 days

IV.19. A 73-year-old man with a history of right knee replacement surgery, aortic regurgitation, coronary artery disease, and ischemic cardiomyopathy is referred for an inpatient gastroenterology consultation regarding PEG placement. He experienced a cerebrovascular accident 10 days ago and had a recent failed swallow evaluation (oropharyngeal dysfunction with aspiration). Which of the following indications is the strongest for antibiotic prophylaxis with GI endoscopy?

a. Prosthetic joints

b. PEG placement

c. Cardiomyopathy

d. Aortic regurgitation

IV.20. An 84-year-old woman with a history of coronary artery disease (stent placement 6 months ago) and atrial fibrillation is referred for an inpatient gastroenterology consultation

regarding PEG placement. She experienced a cerebrovascular accident 7 days ago and failed a swallow evaluation (oropharyngeal dysfunction with aspiration). She is receiving clopidogrel 75 mg daily through a nasogastric tube. What is the correct recommendation regarding peri-procedural use of clopidogrel before PEG placement?

a. Continue administration of clopidogrel (low risk if not used as dual-antiplatelet therapy)

b. Withhold clopidogrel for 3 days before the procedure

c. Withhold clopidogrel for 5 days before the procedure

d. Withhold clopidogrel for 5 days before the procedure and start aspirin therapy now

e. Withhold clopidogrel for 5 days before the procedure and start heparin therapy as bridge

Answers

IV.1. Answer c.

A patient presentation with melena is most consistent with a bleeding source in the upper GI tract. Patients with diverticular bleeding are more likely to present with painless hematochezia. The history provided (no ascites or encephalopathy) does not suggest decompensated cirrhosis, so esophageal varices as a bleeding source are less likely. While patients with Cameron lesions (history of hiatal hernia) or small-bowel angioectasia can present with melena, the most likely cause of melena in this patient (who is taking NSAIDs) would be PUD.

IV.2. Answer e.

Small-bowel bleeding should be suspected in this patient who has melena without abnormalities apparent on EGD and colonoscopy. While BAE can be both diagnostic and therapeutic, it is typically performed after a target lesion has been identified with capsule endoscopy, CTE, or CTA. This patient, who had small-bowel surgery and who now has symptoms of possible obstruction, should undergo a patency capsule test before CE. CTA is typically done if active bleeding is present (this patient has had intermittent melena for several months). Therefore, CTE would be the most appropriate next test for this patient.

IV.3. Answer d.

In this patient, EGD showed an ulcer and a blood vessel with a high risk of bleeding. Endoscopic intervention would be appropriate. Because of the bleeding risk, the use of epinephrine alone would be inferior to the use of epinephrine in combination with either cautery (bipolar probe or heater probe) or hemoclip placement. Hemostatic powder is typically used for active bleeding that cannot be effectively managed with other modalities.

IV.4. Answer a.

The bleeding source is most likely in the small bowel since the findings from EGD and colonoscopy were unremarkable. Given the patient's young age and lack of comorbidities, a Meckel diverticulum would rank high in the differential diagnosis. BAE is typically performed after a lesion is identified on CE or CT.

IV.5. Answer c.

CTA is the best next test for this patient, whose clinical presentation with sudden onset of right-sided cramping abdominal pain and a subsequent bloody bowel movement is typical of IRCI. The CT findings of thickening of the ascending colon and the colonoscopy features are helpful in confirming this diagnosis. The most common cause of CI is a nonocclusive low-flow state in the colonic microvasculature. Most cases of CI involve the left colon, which is supplied by the inferior mesenteric artery. As with IRCI, the diagnosis is clinical and supported by CT and colonoscopy. Patients with left-sided CI tend to heal well with conservative therapy alone. However, IRCI can be the harbinger of acute mesenteric ischemia caused by a focal thrombus or embolus of the superior mesenteric artery. This artery supplies both the small intestine and the right colon, and the consequences of acute mesenteric ischemia involving the small bowel are severe, with mortality rates that can approach 60%. Therefore, patients with IRCI require urgent noninvasive imaging of the mesenteric vasculature to assess the extent of ischemia and nature of the intervention. CTA is the recommended method of imaging for the diagnosis of acute mesenteric ischemia because results can be obtained rapidly. CTA allows visualization of the origins and length of the vessels, characterizes the extent of occlusion, and aids in planning revascularization.

MRA provides information about mesenteric arterial flow and avoids the potential harms of radiation and use of contrast agents that are associated with CTA. However, MRA takes longer to perform than CTA, lacks the required resolution to identify arterial occlusion, and can lead to overestimation of the severity of stenosis. Selective catheter angiography was the standard method for diagnosing mesenteric ischemia. However, it is now used after a revascularization plan has been chosen, because CTA can be obtained rapidly and is noninvasive. Duplex ultrasonography is an effective, low-cost tool that can be used to assess the proximal visceral vessels but with limited ability to visualize distal vessels. It is best reserved for the evaluation of patients who have chronic mesenteric ischemia, which typically presents with postprandial abdominal pain, sitophobia, and weight loss.

IV.6. Answer d.

The patient has postprandial abdominal pain and weight loss, which can be the manifestation of chronic mesenteric arteriosclerotic disease. Mesenteric Doppler study and subsequent CTA showed severe stenosis of the celiac and superior mesenteric arteries, which in this clinical setting are suggestive of chronic mesenteric ischemia. However, the differential diagnosis for postprandial abdominal pain and weight loss include more common conditions such as peptic ulcer disease, intestinal obstruction, upper GI tract malignancy, chronic pancreatitis, and hepatobiliary pathology. CTA showed possible enlargement of the pancreatic head, which would be concerning for pancreatic adenocarcinoma causing malignant encasement and occlusion of the celiac and superior mesenteric arteries. Therefore, the most appropriate next step in management would be to perform endoscopic ultrasonography with fine-needle aspiration of the pancreatic head to exclude malignancy. Selective catheter angiography with stenting of the celiac artery and surgical mesenteric bypass would be potential treatment options if the cause of the arterial occlusion were atherosclerotic and not cancer. A 4-hour solid meal gastric emptying study would be helpful to assess for gastroparesis, which can be an atypical manifestation of chronic mesenteric ischemia, but this test would not be helpful in diagnosing the cause of mesenteric vascular occlusion.

IV.7. Answer d.

This patient most likely has CI, which is the most common form of intestinal ischemia. CI is often self-limiting and transient. The CT image shows thickening of the left colon without ominous features that suggest gangrenous bowel, such as pneumatosis linearis. When CI is suspected, endoscopy should be performed within 48 hours after presentation to confirm the diagnosis. For

this patient, limited colonoscopy (flexible sigmoidoscopy) would be appropriate to confirm the nature of the CT abnormality given the left-sided occurrence. The endoscopic procedure should be stopped at the most distal extent of disease, and biopsies of the colonic mucosa should be obtained unless gangrene is present. The pathophysiology of CI most often involves a nonocclusive, low-flow state in the colonic microvasculature, particularly when the left colon is involved. CTA would be appropriate if the CI were isolated to the right colon because IRCI can be the harbinger of acute mesenteric ischemia caused by a focal thrombus or embolus of the superior mesenteric artery. This artery supplies both the small intestine and the right colon, and the consequences of acute mesenteric ischemia involving the small bowel are severe, with mortality rates that can approach 60%. This patient has mild CI and initiation of therapy with intravenous antibiotics would not be indicated. In addition, starting total parenteral nutrition would not be indicated.

IV.8. Answer c.

The patient presents with postprandial abdominal pain and weight loss, which can be manifestations of chronic mesenteric ischemia. However, the differential diagnosis of postprandial abdominal pain and weight loss includes more common conditions such as peptic ulcer disease, intestinal obstruction, upper GI malignancy, chronic pancreatitis, and hepatobiliary disease. This patient, though, has undergone a multitude of laboratory and imaging studies, so these more common conditions are less likely. Demonstration of severe stenosis of the major mesenteric vessels is a requirement for a diagnosis of chronic mesenteric ischemia. For patients with suggestive symptoms, as in this patient, the American College of Radiology consensus opinion recommends CTA as the preferred initial imaging modality because it reliably identifies or excludes the presence of atherosclerotic vascular disease and can be used to rule out other abdominal disease as the source of symptoms. Duplex ultrasonography of the mesenteric vessels is a reasonable initial screening modality for the detection of high-grade celiac and superior mesenteric artery stenosis for patients examined in an office setting. When the results of duplex ultrasonography are assessed, technical considerations should be kept in mind because they can limit the accuracy of the findings; these include the expertise of the examiner, large body habitus, intestinal gas, and previous abdominal surgery. Ultrasonography of the right upper quadrant to assess for biliary pathology as a source of symptoms would be a low-yield procedure given the normal results of the liver biochemical tests. A gastric emptying study would be helpful to assess for gastroparesis, which can be an atypical manifestation of chronic mesenteric ischemia, but this test would not be helpful in assessing for mesenteric vascular occlusion.

IV.9. Answer d.

The differential diagnosis of abdominal pain after gastric bypass surgery for obesity is broad and includes complications of surgery such as small-bowel obstruction and ischemic or thrombotic disease of the gut. In this case, appropriate studies, including abdominal imaging and laboratory studies, ruled out many of these conditions. The possibility of acute porphyria should be considered in patients with recurrent, severe abdominal pain when clinical evaluation has not found a cause. Features that may occur in association with attacks of acute porphyria and that should increase suspicion for the diagnosis include systemic arterial hypertension, tachycardia, constipation, and hyponatremia (due to syndrome of inappropriate antidiuretic hormone secretion). Various factors can precipitate porphyria attacks, including fasting, poor intake of carbohydrates and energy, use of drugs or alcohol, smoking, infections, and other forms of stress. This patient's recurrent acute attacks were precipitated by the negative energy balance resulting from bariatric surgery. The diagnostic study of choice is measurement of 5-aminolevulinic acid and porphobilinogen in urine or serum. The absence of urticaria pigmentosa and intermittent symptoms makes systemic mastocytosis unlikely. Hyponatremia can occur with adrenal insufficiency, but the normal vital signs and intervening symptom-free periods makes this diagnosis unlikely.

IV.10. Answer c.

With the history of young-onset atrial fibrillation and bilateral carpal tunnel syndrome, clinical suspicion for an infiltrative disorder such as amyloidosis of the GI tract is high. The criterion standard for the diagnosis of GI involvement by amyloidosis is pathologic confirmation with biopsy. The highest degree of amyloid deposition in the GI tract is in the duodenum. Therefore, upper endoscopy with duodenal biopsy is the appropriate study to assess for GI involvement by amyloidosis. Small-bowel aspiration and culture is used for the evaluation of small intestinal bacterial overgrowth, which may complicate amyloidosis and other infiltrative diseases of the gut. Although bacterial overgrowth in the small intestine is associated with steatorrhea, small-bowel aspiration would be of little utility in evaluating for suspected amyloidosis. Pancreatic enzyme replacement may be useful for reducing the degree of steatorrhea in patients with steatorrhea due to pancreatic insufficiency. An empirical trial of pancreatic enzyme replacement has no role in the investigation of suspected GI involvement by amyloidosis. The colon can be involved by amyloidosis; however, because the presence of steatorrhea suggests intestinal malabsorption, colonoscopy with biopsy is a less correct choice.

IV.11. Answer a.

The clinical presentation and biopsy findings are diagnostic of HSP, a systemic vasculitis characterized by cutaneous involvement with tissue deposition of IgA-containing immune complexes. It occurs more often in children than adults and presents with the classic tetrad of rash, abdominal pain, arthralgias, and renal disease. The rash is typically the initial manifestation, is purpuric, and occurs in a symmetric distribution over the lower aspect of the legs. GI symptoms occur in most patients and are due to a local vasculitis causing intestinal ischemia. In the absence of the purpuric rash, the diagnosis of HSP may not be obvious. As in this patient, abdominal symptoms can precede the rash (15% of cases) and may initially obscure the diagnosis.

Granulomatosis with polyangiitis is a small-vessel vasculitis that rarely involves the gut. Histology-confirmed features of necrotizing granulomatous vasculitis facilitate a diagnosis of granulomatosis polyangiitis, which is frequently associated with c-ANCA and proteinase-3 antibodies. PAN is a non–ANCA-associated vasculitis that predominantly affects muscular medium-sized arteries of any organ system except the lungs. GI manifestations of PAN are variable but abdominal pain, often due to ischemia resulting from mesenteric arteritis, is the most common. Because PAN does not involve small vessels, a leukocytoclastic vasculitis rash does not occur. Eosinophilic granulomatosis with polyangiitis, or Churg-Strauss syndrome, although an important consideration in this case, is unlikely in the absence of concomitant asthma and peripheral eosinophilia.

IV.12. Answer c.

This patient has SSc, which commonly affects the GI tract. GI manifestations of SSc include gastroesophageal reflux, esophageal aperistalsis, GAVE, intestinal pseudo-obstruction, wide-mouth colonic diverticula, pneumatosis cystoides intestinalis, and anal incontinence. GAVE is associated with SSc and often presents with low-grade GI bleeding and iron deficiency anemia, as in this patient. SSc is the most common rheumatologic condition associated with GAVE. GAVE is also termed "watermelon stomach" because of the characteristic endoscopic appearance of longitudinal rows of red stripes radiating from the pylorus into the antrum that resemble the stripes on a watermelon. These red stripes represent ectatic mucosal vessels, which are prone to bleeding. Gastroesophageal reflux can cause erosive esophagitis, which can lead to iron deficiency anemia, but it is unlikely in the absence of heartburn, regurgitation, and dysphagia. Wide-mouth colonic diverticula are a characteristic feature of colon involvement by SSc but would not present with iron deficiency anemia. Mesenteric vasculitis can cause occult blood in the stool but would be associated with abdominal pain and is not a GI manifestation of SSc.

IV.13. Answer b.

Anastomotic leaks are one of the most severe complications after RYGB. Often, they can present subtly, especially in patients who have severe obesity. Postoperative tachycardia is a sensitive sign of a potential anastomotic leak. Clinicians should have a strong clinical suspicion for this complication and a low threshold for ordering contrast-enhanced imaging postoperatively.

IV.14. Answer a.

Anastomotic strictures are a common complication after RYGB and generally present within 2 to 3 months postoperatively. The first line of treatment should be endoscopic balloon dilation, which has proved to be a safe and effective therapy. Balloon dilation should be performed only up to 15 mm, because dilation to larger diameters may increase the risk of perforation and partly abolish the restrictive nature of the weight loss mechanism. Generally, serial dilations are needed to manage most strictures. Surgical revision of gastrojejunostomy should be reserved for refractory cases.

IV.15. Answer b.

Postprandial diarrhea in the setting of recent RYGB is concerning for early dumping syndrome. This occurs due to fluid shifts with hyperosmolar food entering the small intestinal lumen. Patients present with diarrhea, abdominal pain, dizziness, and hypotension a few minutes to an hour after eating. Most cases of early dumping syndrome are managed with dietary changes, including avoiding simple sugars and a diet consisting of high-fiber, complex carbohydrate, and protein-rich foods. A consultation with an experienced dietitian is most appropriate in this situation.

IV.16. Answer d.

Regaining weight after RYGB can occur in up to 20% of patients. One of the most common causes of weight regain is progressive noncompliant eating or behavioral change. In this patient, who reports adherence to diet, further evaluation for structural causes of weight regain is warranted. These include enlargement of the gastric pouch, dilation of the gastrojejunal anastomosis, or development of a gastrogastric fistula. All of these causes result in a decrease in the restrictive nature of the gastric bypass procedure.

An upper GI series will help in further evaluation of anatomical changes that may be promoting weight regain.

IV.17. Answer d.

At presentation, the patient had severe acute cholangitis and septic shock in the setting of an obstructing common bile duct stone. After fluid resuscitation and administration of antibiotics, she needs urgent biliary drainage. Ideally, this is achieved by performing ERCP with sphincterotomy for stone extraction. However, because she is receiving an antithrombotic, she is at high risk for post-sphincterotomy bleeding. Alternatively, ERCP with stent placement is the most appropriate next step and is not contraindicated in the setting of antithrombotic therapy. There is no role for MRCP because the diagnosis is already made based on the clinical picture and ultrasonographic findings. The patient is in septic shock, and delaying biliary drainage is inappropriate. Although the patient will need a cholecystectomy, she is currently unstable to undergo surgery. Once the patient is stable and not receiving an antithrombotic, she can undergo another ERCP for stone extraction followed by cholecystectomy.

IV.18. Answer b.

The patient presented with symptomatic choledocholithiasis, and ERCP is indicated for stone removal. She is at high risk for post ERCP-pancreatitis because of difficult cannulation and multiple accesses of the wire to the pancreatic duct. Rectal, not oral, NSAIDs have been shown to decrease the risk of post-ERCP pancreatitis in patients who are at high risk. Other methods to decrease post-ERCP pancreatitis include intravenous hydration and a pancreatic stent but not a biliary stent. Sphincter balloon dilation increases the risk for post-ERCP pancreatitis.

IV.19. Answer b.

Data support a reduction in peristomal infections when antibiotics are provided before the initial placement of PEG or PEJ tubes. The use of antibiotics solely to prevent endocarditis or septic arthritis is not recommended for patients undergoing GI endoscopy.

IV.20. Answer a.

Clopidogrel monotherapy (not when used as dual-antiplatelet therapy with aspirin) is considered a low bleeding risk for PEG placement. In this case, stopping treatment, changing to therapy with aspirin, or bridging with heparin therapy is not indicated.

V

Colon

15

Inflammatory Bowel Disease: Clinical Aspects

VICTOR G. CHEDID, MD, MS

NAYANTARA COELHO-PRABHU, MBBS

Inflammatory bowel disease (IBD) is a disease process characterized by chronic idiopathic intestinal inflammation along a spectrum that ranges from ulcerative colitis (UC) at one end to Crohn disease (CD) at the other. UC affects the colonic mucosa and extends proximally from the anal verge in an uninterrupted pattern that involves all or part of the colon. In contrast, CD is a transmural process that primarily affects the small bowel. However, CD can occur anywhere in the gastrointestinal tract from mouth to anus, manifesting as patchy inflammation with intervening areas of normal mucosa. *Indeterminate colitis*, now termed *IBD colitis, unclassified type*, in the middle of the spectrum, affects a small number of patients who have chronic colonic inflammation with features consistent with both UC and CD. All IBD, regardless of where it lies on the spectrum, can be associated with extraintestinal manifestations (EIMs).

✓ UC involves the colonic mucosa in a continuous distribution from the anal verge to all or part of the colon
✓ CD involves transmural patchy inflammation with intervening normal mucosa and can occur anywhere in the gastrointestinal tract from the mouth to the anus
✓ Indeterminate colitis has features of UC and CD
✓ EIMs can be present in all forms of IBD

Epidemiology

Onset of IBD is most frequent among adolescents, with a peak incidence between ages 15 and 25 years. A smaller second peak

occurs between the fifth and seventh decades. Men and women generally have a similar risk for IBD, but the overall incidence of CD is higher among women. IBD is more common among Ashkenazi Jews than among non-Jews. Historically, UC has been more common than CD.

The incidence of UC is 8.3 per 100,000 person-years in Olmsted County, Minnesota, and 14.2 per 100,000 person-years in Winnipeg, Manitoba. The prevalence in Olmsted County is 229 per 100,000 persons. The proportion of patients with ulcerative proctitis varies in different series from 17% to 49% of the totals.

The incidence of CD also varies among reporting centers. It is 6.9 per 100,000 person-years in Olmsted County and 14.6 per 100,000 person-years in Winnipeg. The prevalence in Olmsted County is 133 per 100,000 persons.

Mortality rates for persons with IBD may be slightly higher than those for the general population. In a study from Stockholm, Sweden, the standardized mortality ratio was 1.37 for UC and 1.51 for CD.

✓ **Proctitis**—inflammation isolated to the rectum

Genetics

The genetic influence on the development of IBD is a topic of considerable interest. From 10% to 15% of patients with UC have a relative with IBD, mainly UC and, less commonly, CD. Approximately 15% of patients with CD have a relative with IBD, mainly CD and, less commonly, UC. The phenotypic concordance appears to be higher for CD. Several genetic linkages have been identified, and specific genetic defects have been determined in IBD. The first to be characterized was the *CARD15/NOD2* gene, present in the homozygous form in up to 17% of patients with CD. This genetic defect is associated

Abbreviations: CD, Crohn disease; CT, computed tomographic; EIM, extraintestinal manifestation; IBD, inflammatory bowel disease; MR, magnetic resonance; PSC, primary sclerosing cholangitis; UC, ulcerative colitis

with fibrostenotic disease involving the distal ileum. Other associations are with the *IBD5* haplotype of chromosome 5 and the *IL23R* gene on chromosome 1p31. The *IL23R* gene encodes a proinflammatory cytokine, interleukin 23. Three genetic syndromes are associated with IBD: Turner syndrome; Hermansky-Pudlak syndrome (oculocutaneous albinism, a platelet aggregation defect, and a ceroid-like pigment deposition); and glycogen storage disease type IB.

Diet

Patients with IBD can often have food sensitivities, but only those with complications such as strictures need to follow restricted diets. Although lactose intolerance is more common among patients with CD than among the general population, lactose and other milk components do not seem to influence the inflammatory disease. Elemental diets and parenteral hyperalimentation are useful for correction of malnutrition and for growth failure in children with IBD. Parenteral nutrition has not been found to be superior to enteral nutrition for CD. The use of enteral nutrition or parenteral nutrition as primary therapy for CD is controversial; nutritional support is used primarily as an alternative to corticosteroids. There is no convincing evidence that elemental nutrition or parenteral nutrition is therapeutic for UC. Increased interest has led to the exploration of the use of anti-inflammatory diets for symptom management in patients with IBD, and large studies are underway to study the efficacy of these diets.

Pregnancy

Fertility is normal in patients with inactive IBD. Fertility is decreased in some women with active IBD, but most patients can conceive. Sulfasalazine causes reversible infertility in men as a result of abnormalities of spermatogenesis and decreased sperm motility. There is no clear evidence of birth defects in the offspring of a parent with IBD. Most studies do not show an increased risk in association with the disease or the treatments; however, methotrexate is contraindicated during pregnancy (its use should be discontinued ≥3 months before conception). The course of pregnancy is usually normal, although there is an increased chance of preterm delivery and decreased birth weight. Two-thirds of women with IBD in remission before pregnancy remain in remission through pregnancy and the postpartum period. Flares occur most commonly during the first trimester and the postpartum period. Previous colectomy with an end-ileostomy or with a continent ileal pouch does not preclude pregnancy, and for some women, vaginal delivery is still an option. Increased infertility has been reported in women after ileal pouch–anal anastomosis for UC. There is no definitive evidence to support the idea that breastfeeding is a protective factor against later development of IBD.

Environmental Influences

UC is primarily a disease of nonsmokers. Only 13% of patients with UC are current smokers, and the rest are nonsmokers or former smokers. Pouchitis after proctocolectomy with an ileal J-pouch–anal anastomosis for UC is less common among smokers. In contrast, patients with CD are more likely to be smokers than the general population, and smoking increases the risk of symptomatic recurrences. IBD is more common in colder climates than in warmer climates, and it is more common in developed countries than in developing countries.

✓ Among patients with CD and UC, 10% to 15% have a relative with CD or UC
✓ *CARD15/NOD2* gene—associated with fibrostenotic CD
✓ Patients with IBD—no specific dietary restrictions
✓ Women with active IBD—decreased fertility but able to conceive
✓ Sulfasalazine causes reversible azoospermia in men
✓ UC is a disease of nonsmokers, but smoking increases the risk of symptomatic recurrences in patients with CD

Diagnosis

The basis for suspicion of IBD is clinical presentation in combination with physical examination findings. The diagnosis is confirmed with findings from endoscopic, radiographic, serologic, and histopathology studies.

Clinical Presentations

Ulcerative Colitis

The onset of UC may be gradual or sudden, with an increase in bowel movements and bloody diarrhea, fecal urgency, cramping abdominal pain, and fever. The course is variable, with periods of exacerbation, improvement, and remission that may occur with or without specific medical therapy. About half the patients have disease involving the left colon to some extent, including proctitis, proctosigmoiditis, and disease extending from the splenic flexure distally. Constipation with rectal bleeding is a presenting symptom in about 25% of patients with disease limited to the rectum. Diarrhea, which is usually worse in the morning and immediately after meals, may vary from 1 to 20 or more loose or liquid stools daily; patients with moderate or severe symptoms often have nocturnal stools. Abdominal pain is usually cramping, which is worse after meals or bowel movements. Anorexia, weight loss, and nausea in the absence of bowel obstruction are common with severe and extensive disease but uncommon with mild to moderate disease or disease limited to the left colon. In children, urgency, incontinence, and upper gastrointestinal tract symptoms are more frequent and growth failure is common.

Crohn Disease

Symptoms of CD depend on the anatomical location of the disease. Typical symptoms with ileocecal disease are abdominal pain, diarrhea, and fever. With colonic disease, bloody bowel movements with diarrhea, weight loss, and low-grade fever are common. Patients with gastroduodenal CD often have burning epigastric pain and early satiety, and these symptoms usually overshadow the symptoms from coexisting ileal or colonic disease. The symptoms of oral or esophageal CD include dysphagia, odynophagia, and chest pain, even without eating. The findings in patients with perianal CD include perirectal abscesses, painful and edematous external hemorrhoids, and anal and perianal fistulas. Enterovesical fistulas can cause pneumaturia and recurrent polymicrobial urinary tract infections. Rectovaginal fistulas occur in up to 10% of women with rectal CD and may cause gas or stool to be passed from the vagina. In children, the onset of CD is often insidious; weight loss occurs in up to 87% before the diagnosis is made, and 30% of children have growth failure before the onset of intestinal symptoms.

Table 15.1. EIMs of IBD and Their Relationship With IBD Activity

EIM	Parallels IBD activity	Independent of IBD activity	May or may not parallel IBD activity
Axial arthropathy		✓	
Peripheral arthropathy			
Type 1 (pauciarticular)	✓		
Type 2 (polyarticular)		✓	
Erythema nodosum	✓		
Pyoderma gangrenosum			✓
Sweet syndrome	✓		
Oral aphthous ulcers	✓		
Episcleritis	✓		
Uveitis			✓
PSC			✓

Abbreviations: EIM, extraintestinal manifestation; IBD, inflammatory bowel disease; PSC, primary sclerosing cholangitis.

Extraintestinal Manifestations

Up to 36% of patients with IBD have EIMs. These may involve any organ system and can greatly affect the patient's function and quality of life. The most common EIM involves the joints as peripheral or axial arthropathy. Peripheral arthropathies are classified as *type 1*, with asymmetric involvement of fewer than 5 large joints (ie, *pauciarticular*), and *type 2*, with symmetric involvement of 5 or more small joints (ie, *polyarticular*). Skin manifestations include erythema nodosum, pyoderma gangrenosum, Sweet syndrome, and aphthous stomatitis. Eye involvement includes episcleritis and uveitis. Table 15.1 summarizes the EIMs and their relationship to the IBD activity.

Primary sclerosing cholangitis (PSC) is an EIM involving the hepatobiliary tract. Although PSC occurs in a relatively small percentage of patients with UC (2.4%-7.5%), a large percentage of patients with PSC (75%) typically have UC. When patients receive a diagnosis of PSC, they should undergo colonoscopy with colonic biopsy to evaluate for concomitant IBD. In addition, for patients with IBD, the presence of PSC is an independent risk factor for the development of colorectal dysplasia or cancer. Therefore, annual surveillance colonoscopies are recommended for patients who have IBD and PSC.

> ✓ Diagnostic testing for IBD—endoscopy, radiology, serology, and pathology
> ✓ Onset of UC—varies from mild and gradual to severe and sudden with bloody diarrhea, crampy abdominal pain, and fever
> ✓ Half the patients with UC have disease involving the left colon
> ✓ CD symptoms vary with anatomical location, severity of disease, and patient's phenotype

Physical Examination

When patients have mildly active UC, physical examination findings are often normal or the patients may have abdominal tenderness, particularly with palpation over the sigmoid colon. Patients with more severe disease may have pallor (from anemia), tachycardia (from dehydration), fever, diminished bowel sounds, and diffuse abdominal tenderness with rebound. Tenderness with rebound is ominous and suggests toxic dilatation or perforation.

When patients have CD, physical examination findings may be normal or may include 1 or more of the following: fever, weight loss, muscle wasting, abdominal tenderness (particularly in the lower abdomen), and a palpable mass, usually in the ileocecal region of the right lower quadrant of the abdomen. Rectal examination findings may include large, edematous, external hemorrhoidal tags; fistulas; anal canal fissures; and anal stenosis. Patients with CD may have ulcers on the lips, gingiva, or buccal mucosa.

Laboratory Findings

When patients have mild disease, laboratory test results may be normal. Iron deficiency anemia due to gastrointestinal tract blood loss may occur in UC and in CD, and anemia of chronic disease, presumably due to cytokine effects on the bone marrow, may occur with either disorder. Malabsorption of vitamin B_{12} or folate is another cause of anemia in patients with CD. Hypoalbuminemia, hypokalemia, and metabolic acidosis can occur with severe disease because of potassium and bicarbonate wasting with diarrhea. An increased leukocyte count may be a consequence of active IBD or a complicating abscess.

> ✓ **Toxic megacolon**—total or segmental nonobstructive dilatation of the colon with systemic toxicity in patients with IBD or infectious colitis

Laboratory values of acute phase reactants, including the erythrocyte sedimentation rate and C-reactive protein, can be increased but may also be normal in mildly active disease. Perinuclear antineutrophil cytoplasmic antibody test results are positive in about two-thirds of patients with UC and in about one-third of patients with CD. Anti–*Saccharomyces cerevisiae* antibody test results are positive in about two-thirds of patients with CD and in about one-third of patients with UC. These antibody tests may be used together to help distinguish between UC and CD. However, the positive predictive value of the 2 tests together is 63.6% for UC and 80% for CD; thus, distinguishing the 2 diseases with these serologic tests is less than ideal (Table 15.2). Several additional antimicrobial antibodies have been described, including those to *Escherichia coli* outer membrane protein C, *Bacteroides caccae* TonB-linked outer membrane protein W, CBir1 flagellin, and *Pseudomonas fluorescens*–related protein. The usefulness and role of these markers in IBD diagnostic and management algorithms is being assessed. With new-onset IBD or with relapse, infection should be ruled out with stool studies, including cultures for bacterial pathogens and examinations for ova and parasites and *Clostridioides difficile* toxin. For patients with systemic symptoms such as fever, malaise, and myalgias, cytomegalovirus infection should be ruled out with mucosal biopsy studies, particularly if the patient is receiving therapy with immunosuppressive agents.

Table 15.2. Positive Predictive Value of Serologic Markers in Patients With Indeterminate Colitis

Disease	Marker	Positive predictive value, %
Ulcerative colitis	pANCA+ ASCA−	63.6
Crohn disease	pANCA− ASCA+	80

Abbreviations: ASCA, anti–*Saccharomyces cerevisiae* antibody; pANCA, perinuclear antineutrophil cytoplasmic antibody.

✓ In a patient with UC, abdominal rebound tenderness is an ominous sign of possible toxic megacolon or perforation
✓ Thorough rectal examination in patients with CD may identify fistulas, fissures, anal stenosis, or perianal abscesses
✓ Iron deficiency anemia may occur with either UC or CD
✓ Vitamin B_{12} deficiency occurs more commonly with CD than with UC
✓ New-onset IBD or relapse—use stool studies to rule out infection, especially with *Clostridioides difficile*

Endoscopy

Flexible proctosigmoidoscopy or colonoscopy can be used to identify characteristic mucosal changes of UC, including loss of the normal vascular markings and the presence of mucosal granularity, friability, mucous exudate, and focal ulceration (Figure 15.1). With colonoscopy, the extent of disease can be determined and the terminal ileum can be examined for evidence of backwash ileitis in UC or ileal involvement in CD. Patients with left-sided UC may have inflammatory changes around the appendix, referred to as a *cecal patch*, as a manifestation of the disease; this finding should not be confused with segmental colitis due to CD. Only a limited examination of the rectosigmoid colon should be performed in patients with severely active colitis because of the risk of perforation. In CD, characteristic lesions at colonoscopy are deep linear ulcers (*rake ulcers*) with surrounding erythema and granularity and *skip areas* of normal-appearing mucosa between areas of involvement (Figure 15.2). Endoscopy of the upper gastrointestinal tract can be used to confirm the presence and distribution of disease in the upper gut and to define how severely the mucosa is affected.

Patients with IBD who have extensive, long-standing colonic inflammation have a risk for malignancy that is higher than that for the general population. For that reason, periodic colonoscopy with surveillance biopsies for dysplasia is indicated after 8 to 10 years of disease for patients who have extensive UC. The risk

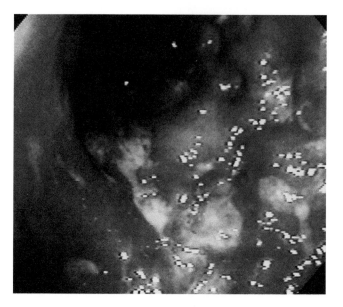

Figure 15.2.   Crohn Disease. Colonoscopy shows linear ulcers and surrounding mucosal erythema, edema, and granularity. These findings are typical of Crohn disease.

of malignancy for patients with less extensive UC (with involvement of the colon distal to the splenic flexure) also is increased, but the magnitude of the risk has not been defined. The risk of rectal cancer for patients with ulcerative proctitis without colitis above the rectum does not appear to be increased. Patients with either form of colitis that involves more than one-third of the colon should have periodic surveillance biopsies after 8 to 10 years of disease. The optimal interval between surveillance examinations has not been defined, and the examinations are usually performed at 1- to 2-year intervals.

Radiologic Features

If patients have severely active colitis, plain abdominal films with supine and upright views should be obtained to examine for complications, including perforation with free air or toxic dilatation. In CD, computed tomographic (CT) enterography (Figure 15.3), magnetic resonance (MR) enterography (Figure 15.4), or abdominal ultrasonography can be used to assess the location and extent of small-bowel disease and complications such as fistulas, strictures, or abscesses. CT enterography has been shown to have superior sensitivity and specificity compared with traditional small-bowel follow-through images for detecting active inflammation of the small intestine. MR enterography has the advantage of avoiding exposure to ionizing radiation and is safe in pregnancy (gadolinium should be avoided in the first trimester). Wireless capsule endoscopy may be useful for evaluation in some patients but should not be performed if obstructive or stricturing disease is suspected, because of the risk of capsule retention. A barium swallow may be useful for assessment of CD that involves the esophagus, stomach, and duodenum. MR imaging is the preferred imaging method for identifying pelvic and perianal abscesses.

Histology

Mucosal biopsy specimens from involved areas of the gastrointestinal tract are useful for excluding self-limited colitis and

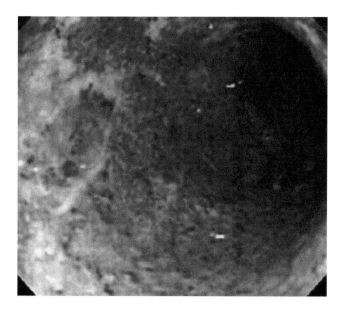

Figure 15.1.   Ulcerative Colitis. Colonoscopy shows diffuse changes of colitis with mucosal granularity, erythema, and exudate. These findings are typical of moderately active ulcerative colitis.

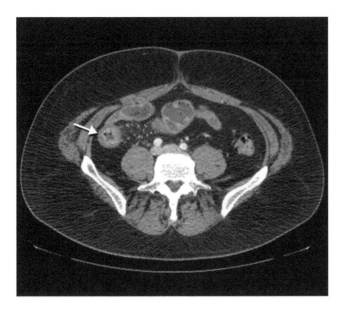

Figure 15.3. Computed Tomographic Enterography in Crohn Disease. This axial image shows wall thickening and mural enhancement (arrow) in the terminal ileum of a patient with active Crohn disease.

other infections and noninfectious causes of colitis, such as ischemia, drug effect, radiation injury, and solitary rectal ulcer syndrome. Noncaseating granulomas are a feature of CD and can be helpful in differentiating it from UC, but even when multiple specimens are taken, granulomas are identified in only 30% of specimens of resected CD. The presence of focal, patchy inflammation is characteristic of CD but not invariably identifiable.

✓ **Granuloma**—a structure formed during inflammation that is present in many diseases; it is a collection of cells known as macrophages

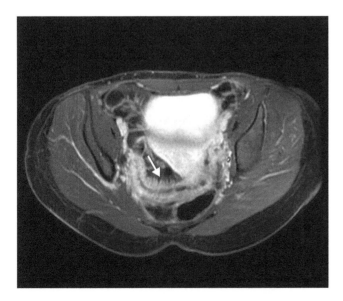

Figure 15.4. Magnetic Resonance Enterography in Crohn Disease. This axial image of a segment of ileum shows enhancement, thickening, and dilated vasa recta (arrow) (the comb sign) in a patient with Crohn disease.

Differential Diagnosis

UC and CD must be differentiated from infectious causes of colitis and also from noninfectious causes of inflammation in the colon and small intestine (Box 15.1). *Microscopic colitis* describes a syndrome of chronic watery diarrhea with characteristic histologic abnormalities but without specific endoscopic or radiographic features. Specific forms of microscopic colitis include *lymphocytic colitis*, in which intraepithelial lymphocytes and chronic inflammatory cells are present in the lamina propria, and *collagenous colitis*, which includes the features of lymphocytic colitis and also the presence of a subepithelial collagen band. Diverticular disease–associated chronic colitis is a segmental colitis in which there are chronic inflammatory changes of the mucosa limited to areas of the sigmoid colon where diverticula are present.

Nonsteroidal anti-inflammatory drugs can cause ulcerations throughout the gastrointestinal tract, including the colon and rectum, which can be confused with CD. Ischemia more commonly causes segmental colitis that may be confused with CD, but occasionally it causes a diffuse colitis that can resemble UC. Injury to the rectum from radiotherapy for prostate cancer or gynecologic malignancy may appear similar to ulcerative proctitis or CD with fistulas and strictures. Injury to the small intestine and more

---

Box 15.1. Differential Diagnosis of Inflammatory Bowel Disease

Acute self-limited colitis
  Bacteria
    Toxigenic *Escherichia coli*
    Salmonella
    Shigella
    Campylobacter
    Yersinia
    Mycobacterium
    Neisseria gonorrhoeae
    Clostridioides difficile
    Chlamydia
  Parasites
    Amebae
  Viruses
    Cytomegalovirus
    Herpes simplex virus
Collagenous colitis and lymphocytic colitis
Diverticular disease–associated colitis
Medication-induced colitis
    Nonsteroidal anti-inflammatory drugs
    Gold
Ischemic colitis
Radiation enterocolitis
Diverticulitis
Appendicitis
Neutropenic enterocolitis
Solitary rectal ulcer syndrome
Malignancy
    Carcinoma
    Lymphoma
    Leukemia

proximal colon from radiotherapy may cause chronic diarrhea, strictures, malabsorption, and other features that may mimic extensive CD. Solitary rectal ulcer syndrome may be confused with CD involving the rectum but can be differentiated on the basis of histologic features showing marked subepithelial fibrosis without inflammation. Diverticulitis may be confused with CD when patients present with fistulas, localized abscesses, and a segmental colitis.

✓ Endoscopic characteristics of UC—loss of normal vascular markings and the presence of mucosal granularity, friability, exudates, and focal ulcerations

✓ Left-sided UC can be associated with isolated inflammation around the appendix (known as a *cecal patch*)

✓ Endoscopic characteristics of CD—deep linear ulcers, erythema, granularity, and skip lesions

✓ Colonoscopy with surveillance biopsies for malignancy should be performed after 8 to 10 years from diagnosis with subsequent surveillance every 1 to 2 years

✓ CT or MR enterography can be used to assess the location and extent of small-bowel disease in CD

✓ MR imaging—the preferred method for evaluation of pelvic and perianal abscesses

---

Suggested Reading

Fletcher JG, Fidler JL, Bruining DH, Huprich JE. New concepts in intestinal imaging for inflammatory bowel diseases. Gastroenterology. 2011 May;140(6):1795–806.

Henckaerts L, Figueroa C, Vermeire S, Sans M. The role of genetics in inflammatory bowel disease. Curr Drug Targets. 2008 May;9(5):361–8.

Joossens S, Reinisch W, Vermeire S, Sendid B, Poulain D, Peeters M, et al. The value of serologic markers in indeterminate colitis: a prospective follow-up study. Gastroenterology. 2002 May;122(5):1242–7.

Loftus EV, Jr. Clinical epidemiology of inflammatory bowel disease: Incidence, prevalence, and environmental influences. Gastroenterology. 2004 May;126(6):1504–17.

Peyrin-Biroulet L, Loftus EV, Jr., Colombel JF, Sandborn WJ. The natural history of adult Crohn's disease in population-based cohorts. Am J Gastroenterol. 2010 Feb;105(2):289–97.

Podolsky DK. Inflammatory bowel disease. N Engl J Med. 2002 Aug 8;347(6):417–29.

Rubin DT, Ananthakrishnan AN, Siegel CA, Sauer BG, Long MD. ACG clinical guideline: ulcerative colitis in adults. Am J Gastroenterol. 2019 Mar;114(3):384–413.

16

Inflammatory Bowel Disease: Therapy

DARRELL S. PARDI, MD

VICTOR G. CHEDID, MD, MS

There are many therapies available for patients with inflammatory bowel disease (IBD). Medical therapies include aminosalicylate drugs such as sulfasalazine, olsalazine, balsalazide, and various formulations of mesalamine; antibiotics; corticosteroids; immunosuppressive medications such as azathioprine, 6-mercaptopurine (6-MP), methotrexate, and cyclosporine; and biotechnology medications such as anti–tumor necrosis factor (TNF) agents, anti-interleukins, anti-integrins, and other newer agents with different targets and mechanisms of action. This chapter reviews these various treatments and where they fit in the treatment algorithms for Crohn disease (CD) and ulcerative colitis (UC). Many surgical therapies also are used in patients with IBD, although a detailed review of these options is beyond the scope of this chapter.

Many of the treatments reviewed are used for both UC and CD, with some notable exceptions. Some of the treatments act systemically, but others are designed to deliver medication to specific areas of the bowel, so a thorough understanding of the anatomical distribution of inflammation is required in order to choose the optimal drug for a given patient.

UC is classified according to the extent of involvement as *ulcerative proctitis* (rectal involvement only), *ulcerative proctosigmoiditis* (involving the rectum and sigmoid colon),

left-sided UC (inflammation from the rectum to the splenic flexure), and *extensive colitis* or *pancolitis* (inflammation extends from the rectum to beyond the splenic flexure or involves the entire colon). CD, however, can involve any location in the gastrointestinal tract, from mouth to anus. Accordingly, it is divided into *ileitis*, *colitis*, and *ileocolitis*; involvement of the jejunum or the upper gastrointestinal tract is much less common. A subset of patients has perianal disease with fissures, fistulas, abscesses, and other findings.

Aminosalicylates

Sulfasalazine, oral mesalamine (Pentasa, Asacol, Delzicol, Lialda, and Apriso), rectal mesalamine (Rowasa and Canasa), olsalazine, and balsalazide (Colazal and Giazo) are drugs that deliver 5-aminosalicylate (5-ASA) to the bowel lumen (Table 16.1). With the exception of the Pentasa formulation of mesalamine, these medications primarily deliver drug to the colon.

Sulfasalazine, the first drug developed in this class, combines a 5-ASA molecule with sulfapyridine. This drug was originally developed to treat rheumatoid arthritis, and for that indication, the sulfapyridine moiety is thought to be the active component. Subsequently, sulfasalazine was discovered to be effective for UC, with the active ingredient being 5-ASA. This discovery led to the development of the newer generation of 5-ASA drugs that have fewer adverse effects than the sulfa-containing parent drug. In sulfasalazine, 5-ASA is linked to sulfapyridine by an azo bond, which keeps the 5-ASA inactivated until the azo bond is cleaved by bacterial enzymes. Therefore, active drug is delivered primarily to the colon.

Olsalazine and balsalazide are prodrugs with 5-ASA bound by an azo bond. In addition, 5-ASA is available covered with a pH-dependent polymer that dissolves in the terminal ileum and

Abbreviations: CD, Crohn disease; FDA, US Food and Drug Administration; 5-ASA, 5-aminosalicylate; IBD, inflammatory bowel disease; Ig, immunoglobulin; IL, interleukin; IPAA, ileal pouch–anal anastomosis; JAK, janus kinase; MAdCAM-1, mucosal addressin cell adhesion molecule 1; NUDT15, nudix hydrolase 15; 6-MP, 6-mercaptopurine; SONIC, Study of Biologic and Immunomodulator Naive Patients in Crohn's Disease; TNF, tumor necrosis factor; TPMT, thiopurine methyltransferase; UC, ulcerative colitis

Table 16.1. Preparations of 5-Aminosalicylate (5-ASA) for Treatment of Ulcerative Colitis

Generic name	Proprietary name	Formulation	Sites of delivery	Daily dose, g^a Active	Maintenance
Mesalamine	Rowasa	Enema suspension	From rectum to splenic flexure	4	4^b
	Canasa	Suppository	Rectum	1	1^b
	Pentasa	Ethylcellulose-coated granules (controlled-release)	Duodenum, jejunum, ileum, colon	2-4	1.5-4
	Asacol	Eudragit-S–coated tablets (dissolves at pH ≥7.0)	Terminal ileum, colon	2.4-4.8	1.6-4.8
	Delzicol	Eudragit-S–coated tablets (dissolves at pH ≥7.0)	Terminal ileum, colon	2.4-4.8	1.6-4.8
	Apriso	Enteric coating (dissolves at pH ≥6) around polymer matrix	Terminal ileum, colon	1.5	1.5
	Lialda	Enteric coating (dissolves at pH ≥7) around polymer matrix with lipophilic and hydrophilic matrices	Terminal ileum, colon	2.4-4.8	2.4
Olsalazine	Dipentum	5-ASA dimer linked by azo bond	Colon	2-3	1
Sulfasalazine	Azulfidine	5-ASA linked to sulfapyridine by azo bond	Colon	2-4	2-4
Balsalazide	Colazal	5-ASA linked to inert carrier by azo bond	Colon	6.75	4.5-6.75
	Giazo	5-ASA linked to inert carrier by azo bond	Colon	6.6	4.4-6.6

^{a} Dose ranges reflect those commonly used in clinical practice and are broader than those specifically studied in clinical trials.

^{b} When 5-ASA enemas or suppositories are used for maintenance therapy, the dose may be decreased to every second or third night.

cecum (Asacol and Delzicol), as ethylcellulose-coated granules that release drug throughout the gastrointestinal tract (Pentasa); or in more complex delivery systems that result in prolonged mesalamine release throughout the colon (Lialda and Apriso). Mesalamine can also be administered as an enema to treat left-sided colitis or proctosigmoiditis (Rowasa) or as a suppository to treat proctitis (Canasa).

All 5-ASA drugs are effective in inducing and maintaining remission in mildly to moderately active UC. The choice of drug therefore depends primarily on the distribution of inflammation. In contrast, the efficacy of 5-ASA drugs for CD is much less clear; the conclusion from a meta-analysis was that these drugs have little or no benefit over placebo. Drug-associated toxicity is common with sulfasalazine, including headache, epigastric pain, nausea and vomiting, and skin rash. Less common but severe adverse events include hepatitis, fever, autoimmune hemolysis, bone marrow toxicity, and others. Folate deficiency is induced by sulfasalazine, and therefore folate supplementation is required. Sulfasalazine can cause reversible azoospermia leading to male infertility. Sulfasalazine may be taken during pregnancy and breastfeeding.

Olsalazine, balsalazide, and mesalamine generally are better tolerated than sulfasalazine. Commonly occurring adverse events include headache, rash, and alopecia. Less common is a hypersensitivity reaction resulting in worsening diarrhea and abdominal pain that may be confused with a colitis flare. Rarely, patients have serious adverse events, including interstitial nephritis, pericarditis, pneumonitis, hepatitis, or pancreatitis. Periodic monitoring of kidney function is recommended with long-term treatment with any mesalamine formulation, although nephrotoxicity is rare. A secretory diarrhea can occur with olsalazine, which has limited its use. Olsalazine, balsalazide, and mesalamine may be taken during pregnancy and breastfeeding.

✓ Medical therapies for IBD include oral or rectal 5-ASA drugs, immunomodulators, biologicals, and other newer agents with different targets and mechanisms of action
✓ For patients with mild to moderate UC, 5-ASA drugs are effective for achieving remission and maintenance
✓ Rarely, patients have serious adverse events with 5-ASA drugs (eg, interstitial nephritis, pericarditis, pneumonitis, hepatitis, or pancreatitis)

Antibiotics

Controlled trials of various antibiotics have not demonstrated efficacy in treating UC. The data for use of antibiotics in CD are less clear-cut. Three small studies suggested efficacy of metronidazole and ciprofloxacin; however, a placebo-controlled trial of metronidazole did not demonstrate efficacy for inducing remission in patients with active CD. Similarly, another trial did not demonstrate an adjunctive role for antibiotics in patients receiving budesonide for active CD. Controlled trials of metronidazole and ornidazole after ileal resection showed that postoperative endoscopic recurrence of disease could be delayed after resection for CD, although adverse effects were common; in a small pilot study of ciprofloxacin after ileal resection, findings were negative. Because of these results, the use of antibiotic therapy for CD is debated, and in the absence of penetrating complications, such as a fistula or abscess, the role of antibiotics as primary therapy in CD is limited.

In contrast, uncontrolled studies and clinical experience indicate that antibiotics such as metronidazole and ciprofloxacin are effective for fistulizing CD, particularly perianal fistulas. No controlled trials have been performed, but antibiotic therapy is used widely for this treatment indication and is considered to be the first-line therapy in combination with immunosuppressive or biological therapies.

Small placebo-controlled and comparative trials have shown that metronidazole and ciprofloxacin are effective for inducing remission in patients with acute pouchitis after colectomy and ileoanal anastomosis for UC. Uncontrolled clinical observations have suggested that metronidazole and ciprofloxacin may be effective for maintaining remission in patients with chronic pouchitis.

Adverse effects with metronidazole include paresthesias, peripheral neuropathy, yeast infections, anorexia, dyspepsia, nausea, a metallic taste, and intolerance to alcohol. Adverse effects with ciprofloxacin are less common and include photosensitivity, nausea, rash, increased liver enzyme levels, and tendinopathy, rarely including tendon rupture. Ciprofloxacin should not be taken during pregnancy or breastfeeding. Metronidazole can be considered during pregnancy, but it is secreted in breast milk.

Corticosteroids

Corticosteroids are commonly used in patients with IBD. A dose-response study of patients with active UC showed that a prednisone dosage of 40 or 60 mg daily is more effective than 20 mg daily, and more adverse effects occur with 60 mg daily. Doses larger than 60 mg provide little if any additional efficacy with more adverse effects, so they should not be used. Similar data exist for corticosteroid therapy in patients with CD. Most clinicians initiate oral corticosteroid therapy with prednisone at a dosage of 40 to 60 mg daily. For patients with ileocolonic CD, controlled ileal-release budesonide is an alternative to prednisone, and for patients with UC, a colonic-release formulation of budesonide (multimatrix system budesonide) is available. Both formulations of budesonide offer effective therapy with fewer corticosteroid-related adverse effects (owing to high first-pass hepatic metabolism) but at a higher cost.

Placebo-controlled trials have shown that corticosteroid therapy is not effective for maintaining remission in patients with UC or CD; thus, for patients who respond to corticosteroid therapy, the dose is typically tapered over 2 to 4 months while use of another medication is begun for maintenance. Patients with severely active disease who do not have a response to oral corticosteroid therapy are often either hospitalized and given corticosteroids intravenously (eg, methylprednisolone, 40-60 mg daily) or treated with a biological agent.

Corticosteroid enemas are effective for inducing remission in left-sided UC or ulcerative proctosigmoiditis, and corticosteroid suppositories are effective for ulcerative proctitis. However, in clinical trials, topical mesalamine is superior to topical corticosteroids, and thus topical corticosteroids are typically reserved for patients who do not tolerate or have no response to mesalamine. Topical corticosteroids are not effective for maintaining remission.

Short- and long-term adverse events occur frequently in patients receiving corticosteroids. Short-term adverse events include weight gain, moon face, acne, ecchymoses, hypertension, hirsutism, petechial bleeding, striae, and psychosis. Long-term adverse events include type 2 diabetes, increased risk of infection, osteonecrosis, osteoporosis, myopathy, cataracts, and glaucoma among many others. Corticosteroids may be taken during pregnancy and breastfeeding.

Azathioprine and 6-MP

Azathioprine is a prodrug that is converted rapidly to 6-MP, which is then either inactivated (to 6-thiouric acid by xanthine oxidase or to 6-methylmercaptopurine by thiopurine methyltransferase) or activated through several enzyme steps to the active metabolite 6-thioguanine nucleotide. The enzyme activity of thiopurine methyltransferase (TPMT) is determined genetically: 1 in 300 patients (0.3%) have no enzyme activity and have a very high risk of serious toxicity, such that these drugs should not be used; 10% have intermediate enzyme activity, with an increased risk of toxicity that can be mitigated in most patients by dose reduction and careful follow-up; and 90% have normal enzyme activity.

The enzyme nudix hydrolase 15 (NUDT15) is directly involved in the metabolism of thiopurines by catalyzing the conversion of active metabolites to less toxic metabolites, thus preventing the incorporation of toxic metabolites into DNA. The frequency of the NUDT15 poor metabolizer phenotype is about 1 in every 50 patients of East Asian descent, so it is more common than the TPMT poor metabolizer phenotype in Europeans. NUDT15 deficiency is also more prevalent in individuals of Hispanic ethnicity, particularly those with a high degree of American Indian genetic ancestry.

Before these medications are prescribed, consideration should be given to checking for TPMT activity in all patients and for the NUDT15 genotype in certain populations (especially those with Asian, Latino, American Indian, or Finnish ancestry); patients with normal TPMT and NUDT15 activity may be treated with full-dose azathioprine or 6-MP. Trials have shown that azathioprine at dosages of 1.5 to 2.5 mg/kg daily is useful for its corticosteroid-sparing effects and for maintenance of remission in patients with UC. One study showed that azathioprine 2.0 mg/kg daily was more effective than oral mesalamine 3.2 g daily. Trials also have shown that azathioprine 2 to 3 mg/kg daily and 6-MP 1.5 mg/kg daily are effective for inducing remission, closing fistulas, corticosteroid sparing, and maintaining remission in patients with CD.

Adverse effects with azathioprine and 6-MP include fever, nausea, allergic reactions, pancreatitis, arthralgias, bone marrow suppression, hepatitis, infectious complications, and an increased risk of lymphoma and skin cancer. Although azathioprine and 6-MP are classified as pregnancy category D drugs, several recent publications indicated that these drugs can be administered safely during pregnancy. They are also probably safe for use during breastfeeding.

✓ Before azathioprine and 6-MP are administered, test all patients for TPMT and NUDT15 activity
✓ Patients with normal TPMT and NUDT15 activity may be treated with full-dose azathioprine or 6-MP

Methotrexate

Parenteral methotrexate at a dose of 25 mg weekly is effective for inducing and maintaining remission in patients with CD. Adverse events that may occur with methotrexate include rash, nausea, mucositis, diarrhea, bone marrow suppression, infections, pneumonitis, increased liver enzyme levels, and liver fibrosis or cirrhosis. Some toxicity can be mitigated by the concomitant administration of folic acid. Methotrexate is contraindicated for pregnant and lactating women.

Cyclosporine

Intravenous cyclosporine is effective for inducing remission in patients with severely active, corticosteroid-refractory UC. The efficacy of cyclosporine at a moderate dose (2 mg/kg) is similar to that at a higher dose (4 mg/kg). Many patients who have a response to cyclosporine undergo a colectomy within a few years; therefore, many clinicians do not feel that the risk is worth the long-term benefit. In placebo-controlled trials of oral cyclosporine, the drug was not efficacious for inducing or maintaining remission in patients with CD.

Adverse events that may occur with cyclosporine therapy include headache, tremor, paresthesias, seizures, hypertrichosis, gingival hyperplasia, kidney insufficiency, hypertension, infections, hepatotoxicity, and nausea and vomiting. Use of cyclosporine is generally avoided in pregnant women.

Anti-TNF Agents

Infliximab is a mouse-human chimeric, intravenously administered monoclonal antibody directed toward TNF-α. Adalimumab and golimumab are fully human monoclonal antibodies and certolizumab pegol is a pegylated humanized (mostly human)

Fab′ fragment; all 3 are administered by subcutaneous injection. Controlled trials have shown that infliximab is effective for inducing and maintaining remission and closing fistulas in CD and for inducing and maintaining remission in UC. Controlled trials have shown that adalimumab and certolizumab pegol are effective for inducing and maintaining remission in CD and UC. Data also indicate that use of adalimumab and certolizumab can result in fistula closure. Controlled trials have shown that golimumab is effective for inducing and maintaining remission in UC.

Adverse events that may occur with anti-TNF therapy include formation of antibodies against the therapy, infusion or injection site reactions, delayed hypersensitivity reactions, autoantibody formation, drug-induced lupus, infection (particularly tuberculosis and fungal infections such as histoplasmosis), psoriasis, and possibly lymphoma and skin cancers. Antibodies to infliximab lead to higher rates of infusion reactions and loss of efficacy in patients receiving infliximab. The frequency of formation of these antibodies is decreased when patients receive 3 induction doses of infliximab and then maintenance infusions every 8 weeks, with concomitant immunosuppressive therapy and pretreatment with corticosteroids before each dose. There are fewer studies and less experience with antibodies to adalimumab, certolizumab, or golimumab. Although data are limited, anti-TNF agents appear to be safe for use in pregnant women.

Vedolizumab

Vedolizumab is an immunoglobulin (Ig) G1 humanized monoclonal antibody that selectively inhibits the interaction between α4β7 integrin and mucosal addressin cell adhesion molecule 1 (MAdCAM-1). It prevents lymphocyte translocation from the blood into the inflamed gut tissue and thereby decreases local inflammation. Vedolizumab is effective for the induction and maintenance of remission in patients with UC and CD. It is approved for those with an inadequate response to either standard therapies or anti-TNFα.

With its gut-selective mechanism of action and no systemic effects, vedolizumab has a good safety profile with minimal immunogenicity. Progressive multifocal leukoencephalopathy has not been observed in patients treated with vedolizumab as compared to those treated with the non–gut selective anti-integrin, natalizumab. Vedolizumab is not associated with an increased risk of serious or opportunistic infections, does not increase the risk of malignancy, and is well tolerated by patients. There is no evidence for safety concerns regarding pregnancy outcomes associated with vedolizumab.

Ustekinumab

Ustekinumab is an IgG1 κ humanized monoclonal antibody that binds to interleukin (IL)-12 and IL-23. These cytokines modulate the function of lymphocytes, including T-helper-1 and T-helper-17 cell subsets. Ustekinumab is indicated for the treatment of adult patients with moderate to severely active CD and UC. Ustekinumab has been found to be safe with minimal long-term risks. It has also shown favorable outcomes in treating perianal disease in patients with CD. Safety data during pregnancy have been promising.

✓ Infliximab and adalimumab—anti-TNF antibodies
✓ Vedolizumab—an antibody against α4β7 integrin
✓ Ustekinumab targets IL-12 and IL-23

Risankizumab

Risankizumab is a humanized monoclonal antibody directed to the p19 subunit of IL-23. It has been recently approved for the treatment of adults who have moderate to severe CD. Risankizumab is also indicated for psoriasis and psoriatic arthritis. In clinical trials risankizumab was safe, and patients had few adverse reactions. Drug-induced liver injury has been reported, so pretreatment evaluation should include checking levels of liver enzymes and bilirubin in addition to the usual laboratory testing performed before administration of biologicals. Liver enzyme and bilirubin levels should be checked again 8 weeks after initiation of risankizumab therapy and every 3 to 6 months thereafter.

Janus Kinase Inhibitors

The inhibition of the janus kinase (JAK) family, which includes JAK1, JAK2, JAK3, and TYK2, can block several proinflammatory cytokines involved in immune function, such as IL-6, IL-12, and IL-23, which are important in the pathophysiology of UC and CD.

Tofacitinib is a pan-JAK inhibitor (blocking all JAK receptors) approved by the US Food and Drug Administration (FDA) for the treatment of UC. In the OCTAVE trials, tofacitinib was effective for induction and maintenance of remission in patients with UC. Results from studies in patients with CD were negative.

Nonselective JAK inhibitors may have more safety concerns related to the pan-JAK inhibition compared to selective JAK inhibitors. Hematopoietic or blood cell–related adverse effects such as anemia or neutropenia may occur with JAK2 inhibition. The biggest safety concern with tofacitinib thus far is venous thromboembolism, which occurred in a large study of patients older than 50 years who had 1 or more cardiac risk factors. This has led the FDA to add a black box warning to JAK inhibitors and restricted the use of tofacitinib to patients who have not had a therapeutic response to anti-TNFs or other biological therapies. However, increased rates of venous thromboembolisms have not been reported for patients with UC or CD who were treated with tofacitinib. Another concern with JAK inhibition is the reactivation of herpes zoster, which occurs in a dose-dependent manner with tofacitinib. Therefore, patients should be vaccinated with the recombinant shingles vaccine. In addition, patients beginning therapy with tofacitinib should be monitored with complete blood cell counts and lipid panels. There are no data on safety during pregnancy, so tofacitinib is not recommended during pregnancy.

Upadacitinib, a selective JAK1 inhibitor, has been recently approved by the FDA for UC (March 2022). It is only approved in patients that have failed anti-TNF therapy due to safety concerns with the class of JAK inhibitors. The U-ACHIEVE and U-ACCOMPLISH trials have shown excellent clinical remission and response for induction and maintenance in UC. The overall safety signals have been very favorable for upadacitinib, likely due to the selectivity of JAK1 inhibition. Similar to tofacitinib, it is recommended to monitor complete blood counts and lipid panels when starting upadacitinib and that patients be vaccinated with the recombinant shingles vaccine if they are to be treated with upadacitinib. There is no data on safety during pregnancy, and thus it is not recommended during pregnancy.

Ozanimod

Ozanimod is a selective sphingosine 1-phosphate receptor agonist, which was approved for UC by the FDA in 2021. It is effective in achieving clinical remission in induction and maintenance in UC. Ozanimod is contraindicated for patients who have had a myocardial infarction, unstable angina, stroke, transient ischemic attack, or decompensated heart failure in the previous 6 months. Other contraindications are Mobitz type II second or third degree atrioventricular block, sick sinus syndrome, or sinoatrial block unless the patient has a functioning pacemaker. Ozanimod is also not recommended for patients with severe untreated sleep apnea or for those receiving therapy with a monoamine oxidase inhibitor.

Patients should have a baseline complete blood cell count (to exclude lymphopenia) and liver enzyme testing, and they should be monitored for hypertension before and after initiation of therapy. Monitoring for signs and symptoms of macular edema is recommended. Pregnancy should be avoided during therapy with ozanimod and for 3 months after stopping therapy.

Surgery

The original operation for UC consisted of a total proctocolectomy with Brooke ileostomy (Figure 16.1). In the 1970s, the continent ileostomy, or Kock pouch, served as an alternative to the conventional ileostomy (Figure 16.1). However, dysfunction of the pouch, often requiring reoperation, was common. In the 1980s, the ileal pouch–anal anastomosis (IPAA) largely replaced the Kock pouch for patients with UC who required operation and is now the standard procedure for the majority of patients (Figure 16.1).

Colectomy is indicated for patients with UC who have colorectal cancer or dysplasia, patients who have disease refractory to medical therapy, and patients who have a complication (eg, toxic megacolon). Colectomy for low-grade dysplasia has been the subject of debate recently because of results from newer studies, and the procedure is dependent on other patient factors. Patients who elect not to proceed with colectomy should have more intensive surveillance colonoscopy and biopsies, ideally with chromoendoscopy, which increases the detection of dysplasia.

The most common complication after IPAA for UC is pouchitis, which is characterized by diarrhea, cramps, urgency, and often fecal incontinence. The cumulative frequency of acute pouchitis after IPAA for UC approaches 50% by 5 years. Most patients respond to a short course of antibiotics (often ciprofloxacin or metronidazole), although some patients have a prompt recurrence after discontinuation of antibiotic therapy (termed *antibiotic-dependent chronic pouchitis*). In these patients, long-term use of suppressive antibiotics can be helpful. A small subset of patients has antibiotic-refractory chronic pouchitis and requires treatment with corticosteroids (eg, budesonide), immunomodulatory medications, biologicals, or surgery (pouch excision or diversion). For these patients, the possibility of CD of the pouch must be considered.

The need for surgical resection in patients with CD increases with time. By 15 years after diagnosis, 70% of patients have had at least 1 operation, and half these patients have had 2 or more operations, but much of the data on the surgical natural history of CD are from the era before biologicals. Emerging data indicate that these highly effective medications are changing the natural history of this disease, resulting in fewer hospitalizations and operations. In patients with extensive stricturing or numerous previous operations (or both), bowel-sparing techniques such as stricturoplasty may be used (Figure 16.2). In patients with perianal fistulas, a fistulotomy or placement of setons or drains may be used to control symptoms, enhance the effectiveness of medical therapies, and ultimately avoid proctectomy.

Conventional ileostomy (Brooke)
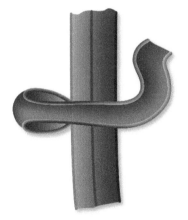

Continent ileostomy (Kock pouch)
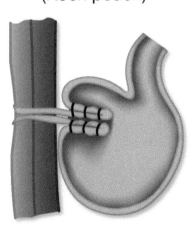

Ileoanal anastomosis with reservoir
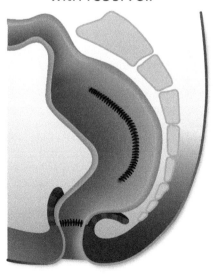

Figure 16.1. **Surgical Options for Ulcerative Colitis.**

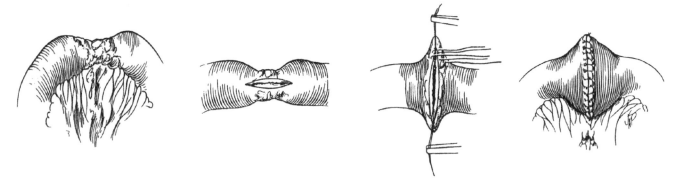

Figure 16.2. Stricturoplasty for Crohn Disease.

Treatment Strategies for UC

Induction of Remission

The aminosalicylates are effective for inducing remission in patients with mild to moderate UC. Patients with proctitis alone may be treated with mesalamine suppositories, and those with proctosigmoiditis or left-sided colitis may be treated with mesalamine enemas. Corticosteroid suppositories and enemas can also be used in these situations, although clinical trials and a meta-analysis have shown that mesalamine is superior to corticosteroids.

In patients who do not respond to topical therapy or who cannot administer or tolerate it and in those with pancolonic UC, oral 5-ASA drugs can be used, either alone or in combination with topical therapy. When the choice is between sulfasalazine and the other 5-ASA compounds, the trade-off between cost and adverse effects needs to be considered. In addition, for patients with arthralgias, sulfasalazine may be used to treat the joints and the colitis more effectively than other 5-ASA compounds. The pH is less than 7 in some patients with active UC who are treated with a 5-ASA formulation that is pH dependent (Table 16.1); thus, whole pills may pass in their stool. If this happens, an alternative formulation should be used.

For patients with more severe disease and those with moderate disease who do not respond to 5-ASA products, short-term therapy with corticosteroids is considered along with planning the corticosteroid-sparing agent of choice for induction and maintenance of remission. Patients with moderately severe disease can receive oral prednisone or an anti-TNF agent (eg, vedolizumab or ustekinumab) as an outpatient, while those with fulminant colitis (acute severe UC) are often hospitalized and treated with intravenous corticosteroids. Patients who respond to corticosteroid therapy require an alternative therapy for maintenance, as discussed below. In hospitalized patients who do not respond to intravenous corticosteroids, treatment with cyclosporine, an anti-TNF, or colectomy is indicated. Azathioprine or 6-MP can be considered, but usually neither is recommended for induction therapy because the data on efficacy are limited and the onset of action is slow. In patients with moderate to severe UC not requiring admission and with no response to anti-TNF therapy, a second agent should be considered such as vedolizumab, ustekinumab, ozanimod, or one of the new JAK inhibitors.

Maintenance of Remission

The 5-ASA drugs, including topical therapies in patients with proctitis and proctosigmoiditis, are effective for maintaining remission in UC. Prednisone is not effective for maintaining remission, and patients who respond to this therapy require a corticosteroid-sparing maintenance therapy such as azathioprine or 6-MP or biological therapy. Anti-TNFs, vedolizumab, and ustekinumab are effective for maintaining remission in patients who respond to these agents. In those with no response to anti-TNF therapy, a second agent should be considered such as vedolizumab, ustekinumab, ozanimod, or one of the new JAK inhibitors.

Treatment Strategies for CD

Induction of Remission

In 2 older studies, sulfasalazine was modestly effective for inducing remission in patients with active CD and colitis or ileocolitis, although a recent meta-analysis indicated that the effect size is small. Antibiotics and mesalamine are not consistently effective for inducing remission. Ileal-release budesonide is more effective than mesalamine and is as effective as prednisone (but with fewer adverse effects) in patients with ileocolonic disease. The colonic-release formulation of budesonide might be considered for induction of colonic CD.

For patients who have moderate to severe disease and for patients who had no response with budesonide or sulfasalazine, the next therapy to consider may be prednisone, an anti-TNF biological agent, ustekinumab, risankizumab, or vedolizumab. Data from meta-analyses and guidelines do not support the use of azathioprine and 6-MP as induction agents in patients with active CD. Methotrexate is sometimes considered as an induction agent in these patients.

Special Considerations

Combination Therapy

In the pivotal trials of anti-TNF therapy in CD, outcomes were no better for patients who were receiving an immunomodulator than for those who were not. However, these were all post hoc, uncontrolled observations and therefore not definitive conclusions. The Study of Biologic and Immunomodulator Naive Patients in Crohn's Disease (SONIC) compared azathioprine monotherapy, infliximab monotherapy, and combination therapy with both agents in patients with CD who were naive to both. The efficacy results showed that infliximab was superior to azathioprine and that combination therapy was superior to either treatment alone. In addition, the risk of serious adverse effects was not increased in the combination therapy group. Although the SONIC trial assessed infliximab, the same results would probably be found with the other anti-TNF agents. These data, together with several other lines of evidence showing benefits of combination therapy (eg, better efficacy and fewer antitherapeutic antibodies) has led to the recommendation to use combination therapy more often in patients with CD.

Top-Down Versus Step-Up

The use of biological therapy earlier in the course of CD has become standard of care. Several lines of evidence support this thinking, including the "top-down or step-up" study. Although the design of this study was not ideal with respect to current practice paradigms, it did support the notion that early use of anti-TNF therapy led to better outcomes than the traditional approach of using corticosteroids first, immunomodulators second, and then anti-TNF agents. Other evidence supporting the earlier use of anti-TNFs includes data from children and adults that show high response and remission rates when treatment is started earlier in the course of the disease. Similar data are emerging for other biologicals.

Maintenance of Medically Induced Remission

The 5-ASA drugs and prednisone are not effective for maintenance of medically induced remission. Budesonide prolongs the time to relapse, but a maintenance effect beyond 6 months has not been shown. Azathioprine, 6-MP, methotrexate, anti-TNF agents, ustekinumab, and vedolizumab are all effective for maintaining remission.

Postoperative Maintenance of Remission

The 5-ASA drugs provide minimal benefit for maintaining surgically induced remission. Metronidazole and ornidazole have had some efficacy in small studies, but adverse events are common. A pilot study of ciprofloxacin was negative. Azathioprine and 6-MP may be effective, but data are sparse and conflicting. A small study of infliximab has suggested a possible large benefit for postoperative maintenance of remission. A large randomized trial showed that infliximab is not superior to placebo in preventing clinical recurrence after CD-related resection; however, infliximab decreased endoscopically observed recurrence. The current approach to postoperative maintenance therapy is risk stratification of patients for the likelihood of postoperative recurrence. Those deemed to be at high risk are offered treatment with azathioprine, 6-MP, or preferably infliximab. Patients not considered to be at high risk, and those who opt not to receive medical therapy, are offered a colonoscopy 6 to 12 months after surgery. Patients who show evidence of endoscopic recurrence are then offered treatment.

Treatment of Perianal CD

Perianal fistulas can be divided into simple and complex fistulas. A *simple fistula* is below the sphincter complex, has a single external opening, and does not have an associated abscess, rectovaginal fistula, anorectal stricture, or macroscopically evident rectal inflammation. A *complex fistula* is high or has multiple external openings, a perianal abscess, rectovaginal fistula, anorectal stricture, or macroscopic evidence of rectal inflammation.

Antibiotics may be effective for fistula closure, especially for a simple fistula, but no placebo-controlled trial has been

performed, and the risk of recurrence is high after discontinuation if no other therapy is used. Similarly, azathioprine and 6-MP may be effective for perianal disease, but no controlled trials with fistula closure as the primary end point have been conducted. However, uncontrolled studies, post hoc analyses, and clinical experience have suggested that these treatments may be effective. Anti-TNF agents and ustekinumab appear to be effective for both inducing and maintaining fistula closure, although only infliximab has been assessed in randomized trials with fistula closure as the primary end point.

Conclusions

Several treatment options are available for CD and UC. Many of the drugs can be used for either condition, although some are used for only one or the other. Knowledge of the individual drugs and their characteristics with regard to whether the drug treats systemic disease or local disease, and where in the gastrointestinal tract it releases active drug, is critical for successful treatment of patients with IBD.

Suggested Reading

Colombel JF, Sandborn WJ, Reinisch W, Mantzaris GJ, Kornbluth A, Rachmilewitz D, et al. Infliximab, azathioprine, or combination therapy for Crohn's disease. N Engl J Med. 2010 Apr;362(15):1383–95.

D'Haens G, Baert F, van Assche G, Caenepeel P, Vergauwe P, Tuynman H, et al. Early combined immunosuppression or conventional management in patients with newly diagnosed Crohn's disease: an open randomised trial. Lancet. 2008 Feb;371(9613):660–7.

D'Haens G, Panaccione R, Baert F, Bossuyt P, Colombel JF, Danese S, et al. Risankizumab as induction therapy for Crohn's disease: results from the phase 3 ADVANCE and MOTIVATE induction trials. Lancet. 2022 May 28;399(10340):2015–30.

Engel T, Ungar B, Yung DE, Ben-Horin S, Eliakim R, Kopylov U. Vedolizumab in IBD-lessons from real-world experience; a systematic review and pooled analysis. J Crohns Colitis. 2018 Jan;12(2):245–57.

Feagan BG, Macdonald JK. Oral 5-aminosalicylic acid for induction of remission in ulcerative colitis. Cochrane Database Syst Rev. 2012 Oct;10:CD000543.

Feagan BG, Macdonald JK. Oral 5-aminosalicylic acid for maintenance of remission in ulcerative colitis. Cochrane Database Syst Rev. 2012 Oct;10:CD000544.

Ferrante M, Panaccione R, Baert F, Bossuyt P, Colombel JF, Danese S. Risankizumab as maintenance therapy for moderately to severely active Crohn's disease: results from the multicentre, randomised, double-blind, placebo-controlled, withdrawal phase 3 FORTIFY maintenance trial. Lancet. 2022 May 28;399(10340):2031–46.

Feuerstein JD, Ho EY, Shmidt E, Singh H, Falck-Ytter Y, Sultan S, et al. AGA clinical practice guidelines on the medical management of moderate to severe luminal and perianal fistulizing Crohn's disease. Gastroenterology. 2021 Jun;160(7):2496–508.

Ford AC, Bernstein CN, Khan KJ, Abreu MT, Marshall JK, Talley NJ, et al. Glucocorticosteroid therapy in inflammatory bowel disease: systematic review and meta-analysis. Am J Gastroenterol. 2011 Apr;106(4):590–9.

Ford AC, Kane SV, Khan KJ, Achkar JP, Talley NJ, Marshall JK, et al. Efficacy of 5-aminosalicylates in Crohn's disease: systematic review and meta-analysis. Am J Gastroenterol. 2011 Apr;106(4):617–29.

Hashash JG, Regueiro MD. The evolving management of postoperative Crohn's disease. Expert Rev Gastroenterol Hepatol. 2012 Sep;6(5):637–48.

Honap S, Meade S, Ibraheim H, Irving PM, Jones MP, Samaan MA. Effectiveness and safety of ustekinumab in inflammatory bowel disease: a systematic review and meta-analysis. Dig Dis Sci. 2022 Mar;67(3):1018–35.

Kornbluth A, Sachar DB; Practice Parameters Committee of the American College of Gastroenterology. Ulcerative colitis practice guidelines in adults: American College of Gastroenterology, Practice Parameters Committee. Am J Gastroenterol. 2010 Mar;105(3):501–23.

Lichtenstein GR, Feagan BG, Cohen RD, Salzberg BA, Diamond RH, Price S, et al. Serious infection and mortality in patients with Crohn's disease: more than 5 years of follow-up in the TREAT registry. Am J Gastroenterol. 2012 Sep;107(9):1409–22.

Lichtenstein GR, Hanauer SB, Sandborn WJ; Practice Parameters Committee of American College of Gastroenterology. Management of Crohn's disease in adults. Am J Gastroenterol. 2009 Feb;104(2):465–83.

Ng SW, Mahadevan U. Management of inflammatory bowel disease in pregnancy. Expert Rev Clin Immunol. 2013 Feb;9(2):161–73.

Pineton de Chambrun G, Peyrin-Biroulet L, Lemann M, Colombel JF. Clinical implications of mucosal healing for the management of IBD. Nat Rev Gastroenterol Hepatol. 2010 Jan;7(1):15–29.

Regueiro M, Feagan BG, Zou B, Johanns J, Blank MA, Chevrier M, et al. Infliximab reduces endoscopic, but not clinical, recurrence of Crohn's disease after ileocolonic resection. Gastroenterology. 2016 Jun;150(7):1568–78.

Sandborn WJ, Feagan BG, D'Haens G, Wolf DC, Jovanovic I, Hanauer SB, et al. Ozanimod as induction and maintenance therapy for ulcerative colitis. N Engl J Med. 2021 Sep;385(14):1280–91.

Sandborn WJ, Ghosh S, Panes J, Schreiber S, D'Haens G, Tanida S, et al. Efficacy of upadacitinib in a randomized trial of patients with active ulcerative colitis. Gastroenterology. 2020 Jun;158(8):2139–49.

Sandborn WJ, Su C, Sands BE, D'Haens GR, Vermeire S, Schreiber S, et al. Tofacitinib as induction and maintenance therapy for ulcerative colitis. N Engl J Med. 2017 May;376(18):1723–36.

Sands BE, Sandborn WJ, Panaccione R, O'Brien CD, Zhang H, Johanns J, et al. Ustekinumab as induction and maintenance therapy for ulcerative colitis. N Engl J Med. 2019 Sep;381(13):1201–14.

Shen B. Acute and chronic pouchitis: pathogenesis, diagnosis and treatment. Nat Rev Gastroenterol Hepatol. 2012 Apr;9(6):323–33.

Wiese DM, Schwartz DA. Managing perianal Crohn's disease. Curr Gastroenterol Rep. 2012 Apr;14(2):153–61.

17

Inflammatory Bowel Disease: Extraintestinal Manifestations and Colorectal Cancer

KEVIN P. QUINN, MD

LAURA E. RAFFALS, MD

Ulcerative colitis (UC) and Crohn disease (CD) are inflammatory disorders that affect the gastrointestinal tract. However, these diseases are systemic disorders that may involve other organ systems. Extraintestinal manifestations can affect any organ system, and while in many cases these symptoms are believed to be a result of the underlying intestinal inflammation, some extraintestinal manifestations are independent of the luminal disease course. Extraintestinal manifestations may precede the diagnosis of inflammatory bowel disease (IBD). Many patients who have extraintestinal manifestations have colonic disease, and in persons with 1 extraintestinal manifestation, another extraintestinal symptom is more likely to develop.

This chapter reviews the most common extraintestinal manifestations, their relation to luminal disease activity, and their treatment. Patients with IBD with colonic involvement (UC or CD involving the colon) are at increased risk for colorectal cancer (CRC). This chapter also reviews risk factors associated with CRC and provides guidelines for surveillance measures.

Musculoskeletal Manifestations

Musculoskeletal symptoms (pain) are the most common extraintestinal manifestations of IBD, affecting up to 53% of patients who have IBD (Box 17.1). Arthritis can affect the spine, the sacroiliac joints, or the peripheral joints. Peripheral and axial

arthritis can precede the diagnosis of IBD by many years. IBD arthropathies are seronegative (negative for rheumatoid factor). The prevalence of peripheral and axial arthritis is similar in CD and UC (5%-20%). However, inflammatory joint disease is more common in patients who have CD with colonic involvement than in patients who have other CD phenotypes. IBD arthropathy also appears to be less common in patients with ulcerative proctitis.

Peripheral Arthropathy

Patients with peripheral arthropathy have pain, increased local temperature, joint swelling, and stiffness. These patients generally have joint stiffness that improves with activity; this feature helps to differentiate IBD-associated arthropathy from osteoarthritis. Plain radiographs of involved joints typically do not show

---

> **Box 17.1. Bone and Joint Manifestations of Inflammatory Bowel Disease**
>
> Spondyloarthropathy
>
> > Axial skeleton
> > > Sacroiliitis
> > >
> > > Ankylosing spondylitis
> >
> > Peripheral
> > > Type 1 (oligoarticular)
> > >
> > > Type 2 (polyarticular) (rare)
>
> Metabolic bone diseases
>
> > Osteoporosis or osteopenia
> >
> > Osteomalacia (rare)
> >
> > Osteonecrosis (rare)

Abbreviations: CD, Crohn disease; COX-2, cyclooxygenase 2; CRC, colorectal cancer; DEXA, dual energy x-ray absorptiometry; EN, erythema nodosum; HLA, human leukocyte antigen; IBD, inflammatory bowel disease; NSAID, nonsteroidal anti-inflammatory drug; PG, pyoderma gangrenosum; PSC, primary sclerosing cholangitis; TNF, tumor necrosis factor; UC, ulcerative colitis; UDCA, ursodeoxycholic acid

destructive changes. Peripheral arthritis associated with IBD is divided into 2 subtypes.

Type 1 peripheral arthritis is pauciarticular, involving fewer than 5 joints. Larger joints are generally involved, and knees are the most commonly involved joints. This arthritis is associated with disease activity, generally in parallel with the severity of the luminal symptoms, and is also associated with other extraintestinal manifestations. Type 1 peripheral arthritis is self-limited and typically resolves within 1 to 2 months or as the bowel symptoms resolve.

Patients with *type 2 peripheral arthritis* have a polyarticular arthritis (affecting ≥5 joints) that is independent of IBD activity. The severity of type 2 peripheral arthritis is also independent of IBD severity. Smaller joints, such as metacarpophalangeal joints, are typically involved, and generally the distribution is symmetrical. This is a chronic arthritis that can last years. Type 2 peripheral arthritis may be associated with uveitis, but it is not associated with other extraintestinal manifestations.

Treatment of type 1 peripheral arthritis is generally aimed at treating the underlying bowel disease. Nonsteroidal anti-inflammatory drugs (NSAIDs) may provide symptomatic relief, although they are not commonly used because of the risk of flaring bowel inflammation. Alternatively, cyclooxygenase 2 (COX-2) inhibitors may provide symptomatic relief and are less likely to worsen underlying IBD. Sulfasalazine, with its antiarthritic sulfapyridine moiety, may provide some relief of arthritic symptoms. Methotrexate has also been used for the treatment of IBD-associated arthropathy. A short course of corticosteroids can be considered for more immediate relief. In refractory cases, tumor necrosis factor (TNF) antagonists may help relieve symptoms of peripheral arthritis. Tofacitinib and ustekinumab may also have some efficacy in relieving symptoms of type 1 peripheral arthritis. Conversely, vedolizumab, a gut-specific monoclonal antibody directed against α4β7 integrin, appears ineffective for treating peripheral arthritis.

Axial Arthropathy

Axial arthritis is also associated with IBD but is independent of IBD disease activity. Sacroiliitis, which is often asymptomatic, is more common than ankylosing spondylitis, which is present in only 1% to 6% of patients with IBD. Men tend to be affected more commonly than women, although less than previously believed. More recent studies show a 2:1 to 3:1 male to female ratio, compared with earlier studies that showed a 5:1 to 6:1 ratio.

Axial joint disease should be suspected if patients have inflammatory back pain. Inflammatory back pain is a clinical diagnosis based on a history of back pain of insidious onset before the age of 40 to 45 years, pain with stiffness that improves with exercise, pain that is not relieved with rest, and pain that has been present for at least 3 months. Axial arthritis is typically classified as sacroiliitis or ankylosing spondylitis. Sacroiliitis is more common and often remains undiagnosed. The majority of the patients are asymptomatic. Sacroiliitis is detected in 24% of asymptomatic IBD patients who undergo magnetic resonance imaging. In a subset of patients with sacroiliitis, the disease progresses and ankylosing spondylitis develops. Patients with sacroiliitis who test positive for human leukocyte antigen (HLA)-B27 have a greater risk for progression to ankylosing spondylitis. Sacroiliitis, spinal inflammation, and enthesitis are the characteristic features of ankylosing spondylitis. Progressive ankylosing spondylitis is measured by the presence of new bone formation (syndesmophytes) and ankylosis of the sacroiliac joints and vertebral column. Patients with ankylosing spondylitis may have limited spinal mobility and decreased chest expansion.

Treatment of sacroiliitis is guided by the patient's symptoms. Asymptomatic patients who have normal spinal mobility and who test negative for HLA-B27 do not need specific therapy. However, symptomatic patients should be referred to a physical therapist and monitored for disease progression. First-line therapy for ankylosing spondylitis is physical therapy and use of NSAIDs, which have been shown to prevent radiographic progression of disease. COX-2 inhibitors are the preferred NSAID because they carry a lower risk of exacerbating underlying IBD.

Treatment of ankylosing spondylitis has improved dramatically over recent years with the introduction of TNF antagonists. TNF antagonists have been shown to induce remission, particularly in the earlier stages of ankylosing spondylitis; therefore, TNF antagonists are preferred when NSAIDs have not helped. The opportunity to treat and prevent disease progression highlights the importance of early detection of ankylosing spondylitis. As with peripheral arthritis, the utility of vedolizumab for treating axial arthritis in IBD appears limited. Colectomy also has no effect on axial arthritis.

Osteoporosis

Osteoporosis is common in patients with IBD, with a prevalence rate of 22% to 70%. The overall fracture risk in IBD patients is 40% higher than in the general population. Common risk factors in this patient population include frequent use of corticosteroids, decreased physical activity, inflammation leading to increased cytokine release (interleukin 1, interleukin 6, and TNF-α) and thereby contributing to bone resorption, malabsorption of calcium and magnesium, vitamin D deficiency, and ileal resection. Patients who have been treated with corticosteroids for more than 3 months or who have had recurrent courses of corticosteroids should be evaluated for osteoporosis. The diagnostic standard for bone density measurement is dual energy x-ray absorptiometry (DEXA). Patients who have a low-trauma or fragility fracture, patients with hypogonadism, postmenopausal women, and men older than 50 years should also undergo DEXA. Despite the prevalence rate of osteoporosis in patients with IBD, only 23% of patients who have IBD and are at risk for osteoporosis undergo screening, which highlights the need for attention to this preventive measure.

✓ Two types of peripheral arthritis associated with IBD
  • Type 1—affects fewer than 5 joints, typically involves larger joints (knees are most common), and is associated with luminal disease activity
  • Type 2—affects 5 or more joints, typically involves smaller joints with symmetrical distribution (joints of hands commonly involved), and is independent of IBD activity
✓ Axial arthritis is independent of IBD activity
✓ Treatment of axial arthropathies, including ankylosing spondylitis
  • First-line therapy—physical therapy and NSAIDs (preferably COX-2 inhibitors)
  • If no response to initial therapy—TNF antagonists
✓ Indications for osteoporosis screening for patients with IBD—recurrent or persistent corticosteroid use (>3 months), low-trauma or fragility fracture, hypogonadism, postmenopausal woman, or man older than 50 years

---

Dermatologic Manifestations

Dermatologic manifestations are present in 10% of patients when IBD is diagnosed (Box 17.2). The incidence of skin conditions increases over time among patients with CD and UC.

Box 17.2. **Dermatologic Manifestations of Inflammatory Bowel Disease**

Common

> Pyoderma gangrenosum
>
> Erythema nodosum
>
> Cutaneous ("metastatic") Crohn disease
>
> Aphthous stomatitis

Less common

> Bowel-associated dermatosis-arthritis syndrome (bowel bypass syndrome)
>
> Sweet syndrome (acute neutrophilic dermatosis)
>
> Epidermolysis bullosa acquisita
>
> Mucosal cobblestoning of buccal mucosa and palate
>
> Pyostomatitis vegetans

The most common dermatologic manifestations of IBD are erythema nodosum (ED), pyoderma gangrenosum (PG), and oral ulcerations. Metastatic CD and Sweet syndrome are less commonly associated with IBD.

EN is the most common cutaneous lesion in patients with IBD. It occurs as deep, tender nodules on the extensor surfaces of the lower extremities, although these lesions can also occur on the arms and trunk. EN typically parallels bowel disease activity, and treatment is directed toward the underlying IBD. In patients with severe or refractory disease, corticosteroids can be helpful. EN is associated with conditions other than IBD, including Behçet syndrome and sarcoidosis. EN has also been described in patients with various infections, including *Yersinia* infection, tuberculosis, coccidioidomycosis, histoplasmosis, and blastomycosis.

PG is a painful, ulcerating skin disorder that typically manifests initially as a pustule, papule, or nodule that eventually breaks down into an ulcer with violaceous, undermined borders. These lesions are most commonly encountered on the lower extremities or peristomal region, but because this skin condition is pathergic (similar to Behçet syndrome), these lesions can occur in any area that is frequently traumatized (Figure 17.1). PG may or may not parallel disease activity. Because PG may be associated with active IBD, it is important to treat any underlying bowel inflammation when managing this condition. In addition to receiving therapy for active IBD, patients generally require therapy with corticosteroids at a high dose that is tapered. Topical tacrolimus can also be helpful in treating these lesions. Milder cases can be managed with dapsone. Despite these measures, PG can be extremely difficult to treat. Other treatments that can be considered for difficult-to-treat lesions include cyclosporine, tacrolimus, azathioprine, and anti–TNF-α agents. Vedolizumab appears to be less effective. Surgical measures should be avoided because of the risk of exacerbating the lesion or inducing new lesions from pathergy.

Oral lesions (aphthous stomatitis) are relatively common in patients with IBD, affecting 10% of patients with UC and 20% to 30% of patients with CD. Typical lesions are indistinguishable from canker sores, and often these lesions resolve when the underlying IBD is treated (Figure 17.2). Treatment is symptomatic. Topical anesthetics may be helpful. In some instances, a topical corticosteroid can be applied for more immediate relief.

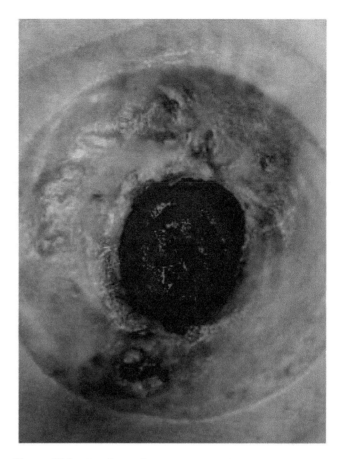

Figure 17.1. Pyoderma Gangrenosum Involving Peristomal Skin.

Metastatic CD is a rare skin manifestation of IBD that is characterized by ulcerating nodules typically present on the anterior abdominal wall, submammary area, arms, legs, or perianal region. Biopsy specimens from these lesions show noncaseating granulomas. The lesions may or may not parallel luminal activity. If luminal activity is present, treatment of the underlying IBD is generally helpful. Corticosteroids and immunosuppressives may also help alleviate these lesions. Case reports have described successful treatment of metastatic CD with metronidazole.

Sweet syndrome, also associated with IBD, occurs as raised, tender nodules on the face, arms, or trunk (Figure 17.3). Patients

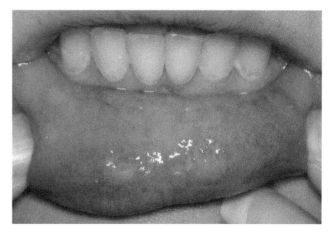

Figure 17.2. Aphthous Ulcers of the Lower Lip.

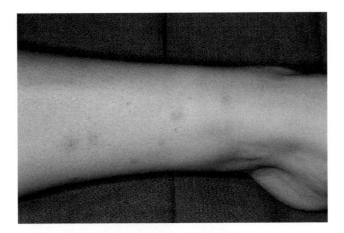

Figure 17.3. Sweet Syndrome Involving the Lower Extremity.

also have constitutional symptoms, including fever. Biopsy specimens from these lesions show intense neutrophilic infiltrates without underlying vasculitis. Treatment includes corticosteroids and treatment of the underlying IBD.

✓ Erythema nodosum
  • Most common skin lesion in IBD
  • Tender, subcutaneous nodules on extensor surfaces of lower extremities
  • Parallels IBD activity
✓ Pyoderma gangrenosum
  • Painful, violaceous skin ulcerations with irregular borders
  • Often preceded by trauma
  • May or may not parallel IBD disease activity

Ocular Manifestations

Ocular manifestations of IBD are present in up to 5% of patients (Box 17.3). Most patients with ocular symptoms have colonic involvement of IBD. Episcleritis is the most common ocular complication and parallels IBD activity. Patients with episcleritis present with acute redness in 1 or both eyes and a sensation of irritation or burning of the eye. No change in vision is associated with this ocular manifestation. Episcleritis generally resolves with treatment of the underlying bowel disease, although topical corticosteroids can be helpful.

Scleritis, a more severe ocular manifestation, may impair vision and warrants immediate evaluation by an ophthalmologist. The clinical presentation of scleritis is similar to episcleritis;

Box 17.3. Ocular Manifestations of Inflammatory Bowel Disease

Inflammatory
   Anterior uveitis (iritis)
   Scleritis
   Episcleritis
   Retinitis (rare)
Treatment-related (corticosteroids)
   Cataracts
   Glaucoma

---

therefore, it is reasonable to refer all patients who have IBD with ocular manifestations to an ophthalmologist for evaluation. Treatment is aimed at controlling the underlying bowel disease, but oral and topical corticosteroids are often required.

Anterior uveitis (iritis) is associated with other extraintestinal manifestations, including peripheral and axial arthritis and dermatologic manifestations (particularly EN). Test results are positive for HLA-B27 in approximately 50% of patients who have the acute form of uveitis. In these patients, uveitis does not always parallel disease activity. It is associated with eye pain, redness, visual blurring, photophobia, and headaches. This condition should also prompt a referral to an ophthalmologist since untreated uveitis can lead to complications such as cataracts or glaucoma. Characteristic findings on examination include a ciliary flush (intense redness in the center of the eye that lessens in intensity peripherally). Slit-lamp examination shows corneal clouding and conjunctival injection. Treatment consists of oral and topical corticosteroids. Anti–TNF-α agents have been used for refractory cases.

Ocular complications may also develop from medical therapy for IBD. Prolonged courses of corticosteroids can lead to the development of cataracts and glaucoma. Patients who have received long courses of corticosteroids should undergo regular examinations by an ophthalmologist.

✓ Episcleritis
  • Eye redness and irritation or burning without a change in vision
  • Parallels IBD activity and resolves with treatment of underlying bowel inflammation
✓ Eye redness or pain and a change in vision in a patient with IBD warrants immediate ophthalmologic evaluation for scleritis or anterior uveitis

---

Hepatobiliary and Pancreatic Manifestations

The most common hepatobiliary manifestation of IBD is primary sclerosing cholangitis (PSC) (Box 17.4). PSC is an idiopathic, chronic inflammatory disorder of the biliary tree. The inflammatory process can result in stricturing and fibrosis of the medium-sized and large intrahepatic and extrahepatic bile ducts, which leads to the classic "beads-on-a-string" finding on endoscopic or magnetic resonance cholangiography. A strong association exists between PSC and IBD. Although only 2% to 7% of patients with

---

Box 17.4. Hepatobiliary Manifestations of Inflammatory Bowel Disease

Biliary
   Primary sclerosing cholangitis (large duct)
   Small duct primary sclerosing cholangitis (formerly known as pericholangitis)
   Cholelithiasis or choledocholithiasis
   Cholangiocarcinoma (rare)
   Primary biliary cirrhosis (rare)
Hepatic
   Fatty liver or steatohepatitis
   Autoimmune hepatitis
   Drug-induced liver injury (thiopurines, methotrexate, 5-aminosalicylates)

UC have PSC, up to 80% of patients with PSC have IBD, most commonly UC. Patients often have mild pancolitis, although patients with PSC-associated colitis may also have rectal sparing or predominantly right-sided colitis with backwash ileitis. This pattern of inflammation is most likely a unique PSC phenotype of IBD. The majority of patients (approximately 80%) have positive test results for perinuclear antineutrophil cytoplasmic autoantibody.

PSC is often diagnosed after the onset of IBD, although PSC may develop years before the onset of bowel symptoms. The disease course of PSC is independent of IBD activity. PSC is typically a progressive disease leading to end-stage liver disease. The median survival time after diagnosis is 12 years. Patients with advanced disease may present with pruritus or jaundice. Earlier in the disease course, patients may be asymptomatic and present with findings of mildly abnormal levels of liver enzymes. Any patient with IBD and evidence of cholestasis (high alkaline phosphatase level) warrants further evaluation to exclude a diagnosis of PSC. Patients with PSC have an increased risk of cholangiocarcinoma, even in the absence of cirrhosis. The risk of CRC is also increased in this patient population, so annual surveillance colonoscopies are recommended.

No effective medical therapies are available for PSC. Therapeutic trials of ursodeoxycholic acid (UDCA) have yielded inconsistent results. High dosages of UDCA (25-30 mg/kg daily) may actually be harmful and should be avoided. Liver transplant is often an effective therapy for PSC, but PSC can recur after transplant.

Although rare, autoimmune hepatitis is associated with IBD. An overlap syndrome of autoimmune hepatitis and PSC is also recognized. The serologic findings are characteristic of autoimmune hepatitis (high levels of antinuclear antibodies, smooth muscle antibodies, and immunoglobulin G), and the cholangiographic findings are typical of PSC.

Cholelithiasis is more common in patients with IBD than in the general population. Patients with ileal CD (active inflammation of the terminal ileum or resection of the ileum) are at particular risk for cholelithiasis due to interruption of enterohepatic cycling of bile salts leading to disruption of the processing of cholesterol and phospholipids. Cholesterol stones may form in these patients.

Pancreatitis also occurs in patients with IBD. Pancreatitis is an adverse effect of thiopurine therapy and a less common adverse effect of 5-aminosalicylic acid or corticosteroid therapy. In patients with CD involving the duodenum, pancreatitis may develop if active disease disrupts the drainage of pancreatic juices into the bowel. In patients with CD, a granulomatous inflammatory process can involve the pancreas.

✓ Up to 80% of patients with PSC have IBD, most commonly UC
✓ Any patient with IBD and a high alkaline phosphatase level warrants evaluation for PSC, with magnetic resonance cholangiopancreatography being the test of choice
✓ Causes of pancreatitis in IBD
  • Medications (thiopurines more often than 5-aminosalicylates)
  • Active CD involving the duodenum
  • Autoimmune pancreatitis

Miscellaneous Complications

Patients with IBD may have various miscellaneous extraintestinal manifestations and complications (Box 17.5).

Box 17.5.   Miscellaneous Extraintestinal Manifestations and Complications of Inflammatory Bowel Disease

Renal
  Nephrolithiasis (oxalate, urate)
  Glomerulonephritis (rare)
  Right ureteral obstruction
  Urinary system fistulas (eg, enterovesical, colovesical, rectourethral)
  Tubulointerstitial nephritis (5-aminosalicylates)
  Secondary amyloidosis
Hematologic
  Anemia
    Iron deficiency
    Vitamin B_{12} deficiency
    Folic acid deficiency
    Anemia of chronic disease
    Autoimmune hemolytic anemia
  Neoplastic
    Myelodysplastic syndrome (rare)
    Promyelocytic leukemia (rare)
Cardiopulmonary
  Pericarditis (extraintestinal manifestation or drug-induced)
  Myocarditis
  Conduction abnormalities
  Pneumonitis
  Eosinophilic pneumonia
  Cryptogenic organizing pneumonia
  Bronchiectasis, bronchiolitis, bronchitis, and subglottic stenosis
Pancreatic
  Acute pancreatitis
    Drug-induced (purine analogues, 5-aminosalicylates)
    Duodenal Crohn disease
    Granulomatous involvement of pancreas (rare)
  Chronic pancreatitis
    Autoimmune pancreatitis
Thrombophilia
  Multifactorial

Nephrolithiasis is a recognized problem for patients with CD, particularly ileal CD. Disease or resection of the terminal ileum leads to bile salt malabsorption, and, in patients with extensive disease or resection, fat malabsorption. In patients with fat malabsorption, free calcium binds to fatty acids rather than oxalate within the intestinal lumen. The oxalate is then absorbed, leading to increased urinary oxalate excretion and a risk of calcium oxalate stone formation. In patients who have less extensive involvement of the terminal ileum and subsequent bile salt malabsorption, increased colonic permeability to small molecules develops from the exposure of the bile salts to the colonic epithelium. This increased permeability leads to absorption of oxalate and increased urinary oxalate excretion. In patients with IBD, uric acid stones may also develop as a result of hypovolemia and metabolic acidosis from diarrhea.

Secondary amyloidosis is a rare complication of many inflammatory diseases, including IBD. This complication more commonly affects patients with CD rather than UC. Patients may present with proteinuria or kidney failure. Treatment is aimed at the underlying bowel disease, but in some instances, kidney transplant may improve survival.

Patients receiving 5-aminosalicylate therapy should be monitored for interstitial nephritis, a rare idiosyncratic reaction to this class of medication. Kidney function should be monitored on a regular basis in these patients.

Thromboembolism is also a complication of IBD. Compared with the general population, patients with IBD have a 3-fold risk of deep vein thrombosis or pulmonary embolism. IBD is a risk factor for venous thromboembolism, whereas neither rheumatoid arthritis nor celiac disease increases the risk of thromboembolism. One-third of IBD patients with a venous thromboembolism have no risk factors for thromboembolism except a diagnosis of IBD. Thromboembolic events are most common in patients with active disease but can also occur in patients with disease in partial or full remission. Prevention is of utmost importance. All acquired risk factors for thrombosis should be addressed with any patient who has IBD. Effective treatment of luminal disease, maintenance of hydration, mobilization, treatment of vitamin deficiencies (folate, vitamins B_{12} and B_6), and prophylaxis for high-risk patients should be instituted. The American College of Chest Physicians recommends pharmacologic prophylaxis for any acutely ill hospitalized patient with IBD. Sequential compression devices should be used only if pharmacologic prophylaxis is contraindicated.

✓ All acutely ill hospitalized patients with IBD have an increased risk for thromboembolism and should receive pharmacologic prophylaxis

---

Colorectal Cancer

Patients with IBD involving the colon have an increased risk for CRC compared with the general population (Box 17.6). This risk increases as the duration of disease increases, with an estimated incidence rate of 18% after 30 years of disease in patients with UC. Methods to identify patients at greatest risk for CRC are imperfect. The current standard surveillance program includes multiple random biopsies obtained throughout the colon at regularly scheduled intervals. This approach has been the preferred method of surveillance for the past 30 years. Chromoendoscopy is also an effective surveillance tool in the IBD population, but it is tedious and time-consuming, and it is not performed by most endoscopists. Furthermore, the benefit of chromoendoscopy compared with targeted biopsies using high-definition colonoscopes has yet to be determined. As technology advances, strategies to detect neoplasia in patients with long-standing colitis will continue to evolve.

The risk of CRC increases with the extent of disease and disease duration. Generally, initiation of surveillance colonoscopies should begin 8 to 10 years after diagnosis. Patients with disease limited to the rectum do not have an increased risk for CRC and do not need to undergo surveillance colonoscopies. A minimum of 32 biopsies should be obtained throughout the colon, and many experts advocate 4-quadrant biopsies every 10 cm, with targeted biopsies of suspicious lesions.

The recommendations for interval surveillance colonoscopies vary among professional societies. There is agreement that patients with the highest risk for CRC (eg, patients with PSC

Box 17.6.   Risk Factors for Colorectal Cancer in Inflammatory Bowel Disease

Extent of colitis

Duration of disease

Family history of colorectal cancer

Primary sclerosing cholangitis

Medical nonadherence or lack of follow-up

No use or minimal use of sulfasalazine or 5-aminosalicylates

---

or prior dysplasia) should undergo annual colonoscopies. The American Gastroenterological Association recommends colonoscopy every 1 to 3 years, with more frequent colonoscopies for patients at higher risk.

Surveillance guidelines were developed with patients with UC in mind. However, patients with CD involving the colon also have an increased risk for neoplasia. Risk factors for neoplasia include younger age at diagnosis, longer disease course, and greater intervals between colonoscopies. For all practical purposes, patients with CD involving more than one-third of the colon are considered to have a CRC risk that is similar to the risk for patients with UC.

Patients who have flat, high-grade dysplasia have a high risk for synchronous cancer and a great risk for a CRC diagnosis at a subsequent examination. Given the high risk for CRC among these patients, colectomy is the standard of care. There is some debate on the most appropriate management when patients have flat, low-grade dysplasia. Colectomy is often offered to these patients as well, but in some situations, patients are monitored closely with surveillance colonoscopies every 3 to 6 months with or without chromoendoscopy. The management of polypoid dysplasia also varies among practicing physicians. In the absence of flat dysplasia in the mucosa surrounding the lesion, polypoid lesions may be removed endoscopically with close follow-up.

✓ Surveillance colonoscopies should begin 8 years after diagnosis for patients with either of the following:
  • UC extending beyond the rectum
  • CD involving more than one-third of the colon
✓ Patients with PSC should undergo screening colonoscopy yearly

---

Suggested Reading

Bennett AN, McGonagle D, O'Connor P, Hensor EM, Sivera F, Coates LC, et al. Severity of baseline magnetic resonance imaging-evident sacroiliitis and HLA-B27 status in early inflammatory back pain predict radiographically evident ankylosing spondylitis at eight years. Arthritis Rheum. 2008 Nov;58(11):3413–8.

Chedid VG, Kane SV. Bone health in patients with inflammatory bowel diseases. J Clin Densitom. 2020 Apr-Jun;23(2):182–9.

Dubinsky MC, Cross RK, Sandborn WJ, Long M, Song X, Shi N, et al. Extraintestinal manifestations in vedolizumab and anti-TNF-treated patients with inflammatory bowel disease. Inflamm Bowel Dis. 2018 Aug 16;24(9):1876–82.

Farraye FA, Melmed GY, Lichtenstein GR, Kane SV. ACG clinical guideline: preventive care in inflammatory bowel disease. Am J Gastroenterol. 2017 Feb;112(2):241–58.

Garber A, Regueiro M. Extraintestinal manifestations of inflammatory bowel disease: epidemiology, etiopathogenesis, and management. Curr Gastroenterol Rep. 2019 May 16;21(7):31.

Hagen JW, Swoger JM, Grandinetti LM. Cutaneous manifestations of Crohn disease. Dermatol Clin. 2015 Jul;33(3):417–31.

Hannuksela M. Human yersiniosis: a common cause of erythematous skin eruptions. Int J Dermatol. 1977 Oct;16(8):665–6.

Koutroumpakis EI, Tsiolakidou G, Koutroubakis IE. Risk of venous thromboembolism in patients with inflammatory bowel disease. Semin Thromb Hemost. 2013 Jul;39(5):461–8.

Lichtenstein GR, Loftus EV, Isaacs KL, Regueiro MD, Gerson LB, Sands BE. ACG clinical guideline: management of Crohn's disease in adults. Am J Gastroenterol. 2018 Apr;113(4):481–517.

Lofgren S. False positive seroreactions for syphilis in connection with erythema nodosum. Acta Derm Venereol. 1946 Jan;26:243–60.

Loftus EV, Jr., Harewood GC, Loftus CG, Tremaine WJ, Harmsen WS, Zinsmeister AR, et al. PSC-IBD: a unique form of inflammatory bowel disease associated with primary sclerosing cholangitis. Gut. 2005 Jan;54(1):91–6.

Mahadevan U, Loftus EV, Jr., Tremaine WJ, Sandborn WJ. Safety of selective cyclooxygenase-2 inhibitors in inflammatory bowel disease. Am J Gastroenterol. 2002 Apr;97(4):910–4.

Queiro R, Maiz O, Intxausti J, de Dios JR, Belzunegui J, Gonzalez C, et al. Subclinical sacroiliitis in inflammatory bowel disease: a clinical and follow-up study. Clin Rheumatol. 2000 19(6):445–9.

Rubin DT, Ananthakrishnan AN, Siegel CA, Sauer BG, Long MD. ACG clinical guideline: Ulcerative colitis in adults. Am J Gastroenterol. 2019 Mar;114(3):384–413.

Sandborn WJ, Stenson WF, Brynskov J, Lorenz RG, Steidle GM, Robbins JL, et al. Safety of celecoxib in patients with ulcerative colitis in remission: a randomized, placebo-controlled, pilot study. Clin Gastroenterol Hepatol. 2006 Feb;4(2):203–11.

Shah J, Shah A, Hassman L, Gutierrez A. Ocular manifestations of inflammatory bowel disease. Inflamm Bowel Dis. 2021 Oct 20;27(11):1832–8.

Tavarela Veloso F. Review article: Skin complications associated with inflammatory bowel disease. Aliment Pharmacol Ther. 2004 Oct;20 Suppl 4:50–3.

Umit H, Asil T, Celik Y, Tezel A, Dokmeci G, Tuncbilek N, et al. Cerebral sinus thrombosis in patients with inflammatory bowel disease: a case report. World J Gastroenterol. 2005 Sep 14;11(34):5404–7.

Vavricka SR, Brun L, Ballabeni P, Pittet V, Prinz Vavricka BM, Zeitz J, et al. Frequency and risk factors for extraintestinal manifestations in the Swiss inflammatory bowel disease cohort. Am J Gastroenterol. 2011 Jan;106(1):110–9.

Vavricka SR, Rogler G, Gantenbein C, Spoerri M, Prinz Vavricka M, Navarini AA, et al. Chronological order of appearance of extraintestinal manifestations relative to the time of IBD diagnosis in the Swiss inflammatory bowel disease cohort. Inflamm Bowel Dis. 2015 Aug;21(8):1794–800.

Weismuller TJ, Trivedi PJ, Bergquist A, Imam M, Lenzen H, Ponsioen CY, et al. Patient age, sex, and inflammatory bowel disease phenotype associate with course of primary sclerosing cholangitis. Gastroenterology. 2017 Jun;152(8):1975–84.

Wester AL, Vatn MH, Fausa O. Secondary amyloidosis in inflammatory bowel disease: a study of 18 patients admitted to Rikshospitalet University Hospital, Oslo, from 1962 to 1998. Inflamm Bowel Dis. 2001 Nov;7(4):295–300.

18

Intestinal Infections[a]

SAHIL KHANNA, MBBS, MS

Intestinal infections are common. An estimated 180 million illnesses occur annually in the US and over 1 billion cases of infectious diarrhea occur annually worldwide. Despite advances in diagnosis, supportive care, and antibiotic guidance, the mortality from these infections remains extremely high, especially in the pediatric age group. Some estimates indicate that enteric infectious diarrhea in children younger than 5 years leads to 1 death every 10 seconds. Infectious diarrhea from enteric pathogens is more common in children and in resource-limited countries than in adults in industrialized countries. The clinical features of infectious diarrhea vary, depending on whether the organism is invasive and whether the infection occurs in the small bowel or colon. Patients with small-bowel diarrhea have middle or diffuse abdominal pain and large-volume watery diarrhea. Patients with colonic infections typically have lower abdominal or rectal pain, and the stool is mucoid or bloody; the volume of stool is often small. Most pathogens are managed with supportive treatment, and antibiotics are indicated in a few instances. Infection from an anaerobic pathogen, *Clostridioides difficile*, is more common in industrialized countries than in resource-limited countries.

Another infection of the colon, acute diverticulitis, is common in adults older than 50 years.

This chapter discusses common viral, bacterial, and protozoal enteric infections; *C difficile* infections (CDIs) in particular; and diverticulitis.

Enteric Viral Infections

In the US, most cases of gastroenteritis are viral and are usually brief and self-limited. Viral gastroenteritis typically is characterized by diarrhea with a brief duration and is often associated with nausea and vomiting; affected persons do not have high fever, severe abdominal pain, or bloody diarrhea. Management is symptomatic with hydration, antiemetics, and antipyretics if needed.

Rotavirus

Rotavirus, an enteric adenovirus, is a common cause of diarrhea in young children worldwide; the incidence has been decreasing since the introduction of the rotavirus vaccine. Adult infections are often the result of contact with a sick child or as part of a local epidemic. Rotavirus infections occur year-round in tropical climates, whereas in temperate climates, the infections are more common in winter. Spread is by fecal-oral contamination, which is promoted by prolonged survival in the environment along with resistance to many disinfectants. Typically, symptoms (mild fever, diarrhea, vomiting) occur within 72 hours after exposure and can last up to 5 days. Most adults are mildly symptomatic or asymptomatic, but the disease can be severe if the person is immunocompromised or malnourished or has multiple comorbidities.

Diagnosis is made from a stool test (rather than a rectal swab) that uses an enzyme immunoassay or a polymerase chain reaction

[a] I acknowledge the contributions of Conor G. Loftus, MD, author of "Gastrointestinal Infections, *Clostridium difficile*–Associated Disease, and Diverticular Disease," in previous editions of this text.

Abbreviations: CDI, *Clostridioides difficile* infection; EAEC, enteroaggregative *Escherichia coli*; EHEC, enterohemorrhagic *Escherichia coli*; EIA, enzyme immunoassay; EIEC, enteroinvasive *Escherichia coli*; EPEC, enteropathogenic *Escherichia coli*; ETEC, enterotoxigenic *Escherichia coli*; FDA, US Food and Drug Administration; FMT, fecal microbiota transplant; GDH, glutamate dehydrogenase; HLA, human leukocyte antigen; HUS, hemolytic uremic syndrome; PCR, polymerase chain reaction; TMP-SMX, trimethoprim-sulfamethoxazole; TTP, thrombotic thrombocytopenic purpura

(PCR) test. Treatment focuses on rehydration, and oral rehydration is optimal because oral nutrition stimulates mucosal repair, shortens the duration, and lessens the severity of the illness. Use of antivirals is not recommended. Very young or elderly persons can die of dehydration and acidosis. Symptoms may be prolonged because of a transient disaccharidase deficiency caused by damage to small-bowel epithelial cells, with a resultant decrease in brush border enzymes.

Protective immunity may not develop after natural infections, although reinfection tends to be less severe. A rotavirus vaccine has been approved for use in infants. The vaccine should be administered to all infants who do not have a contraindication. Two orally administered rotavirus vaccines with a live, attenuated virus are available in the US: a pentavalent rotavirus vaccine (RotaTeq; Merck) given in a 3-dose schedule at ages 2, 4, and 6 months or a monovalent vaccine (Rotarix; GlaxoSmithKline Biologicals) given in a 2-dose schedule at ages 2 and 4 months. In the US, rotavirus vaccination is part of the recommended immunization schedule.

Norovirus

Norovirus (also known as Norwalk-like virus) is a calicivirus (small round-structured viruses) and is an important cause of viral gastroenteritis in young children and adults. Since the introduction of the rotavirus vaccine, norovirus is now the most common cause of viral enteritis. Outbreaks from norovirus are associated with contaminated food (eg, shellfish) or water or with person-to-person spread. Norovirus is highly contagious, as it has a very low infectious dose (about 20 viral particles), and the virus can withstand a wide range of temperatures and persists on environmental surfaces, in drinking water, and in various food items. Interestingly, viral shedding precedes the onset of illness and may continue long after symptoms have subsided. The incubation period is less than 48 hours; the illness lasts up to 3 days. Diagnosis is made with a stool PCR assay. The infection occurs in the proximal small bowel. Symptoms include vomiting and nonbloody diarrhea lasting up to 2 or 3 days. A low-grade fever is present during the first 24 hours in 40% of infections. Many strains exist, and cross-protection is lacking, so repeated infections are likely. Patients who are immunosuppressed, such as those who have received an organ transplant and are receiving immunosuppressive therapy or those who have common variable immunodeficiency, can have chronic and severe norovirus infection.

Astrovirus

Astrovirus is an important cause of diarrhea in infants and children, particularly in resource-limited countries because malnourishment is a risk factor. Nausea and vomiting are less commonly reported than with rotavirus infection, and diarrhea is the predominant symptom. The incubation period is 2 to 4 days. Illness is usually mild and lasts up to 5 days.

Enteric Adenovirus

Most adenoviruses cause respiratory infection, although some strains cause diarrhea. Respiratory symptoms may precede gastrointestinal manifestations. Diagnosis is made with an enzyme immunoassay or a PCR test. A long incubation period (up to 10 days) and diarrhea of long duration (1-2 weeks) are characteristic.

Coronavirus

The novel SARS-CoV-2 is a respiratory pathogen that also causes gastrointestinal symptoms because of the presence of angiotensin-converting enzyme 2 receptors in the intestines. The nucleocapsid protein of this virus is present in gastric, duodenal, and rectal glandular epithelial cells. The viral RNA is found in esophageal, gastric, duodenal, and rectal biopsies from patients who have severe disease. About 50% of patients have detectable viral RNA and live virus in the stool, but the infectious potential of the stool is unclear. Gastrointestinal symptoms include diarrhea, nausea and vomiting, and abdominal pain. These symptoms may appear earlier than respiratory symptoms and may delay the diagnosis.

✓ Acute infectious diarrhea
  • Detailed clinical and exposure history should be obtained to ascertain causes
  • Patient with fever or bloody diarrhea should be evaluated for enteric pathogens, especially if antimicrobial agents would be beneficial
✓ Traveler's diarrhea
  • If uncomplicated and unless treatment is indicated, diagnostic testing is not recommended
  • If diarrhea lasts 14 days or longer, stool testing should be performed (including testing for parasitic infections)
✓ Multiple-pathogen nucleic acid amplification test results should be interpreted with caution and within the appropriate clinical context—these assays detect DNA and not necessarily viable organisms
✓ Testing for fecal leukocytes or lactoferrin is typically not useful because of low sensitivity and specificity
✓ Postinfection and extraintestinal manifestations associated with enteric infections are common

---

Enteric Bacterial Infections

Compared to viral infections, enteric bacterial infections are relatively uncommon causes of acute diarrhea, and the indiscriminate culturing of stool from patients with acute diarrhea produces few positive findings, with an unacceptably high cost per culture with positive results. Stool should be tested for bacterial pathogens if patients have fever, bloody or mucoid stools, severe abdominal cramping or tenderness, or signs of sepsis. If patients who are immunocompromised are at high risk for disease but do not have fever or bloody stools, testing should be considered, especially during an outbreak. In most laboratories, routine stool cultures detect *Salmonella*, *Shigella*, and *Campylobacter*. Testing for *Escherichia coli* O157:H7, *Yersinia*, *Vibrio*, and others often requires a special request. Some PCR-based assays have the potential to detect multiple bacterial and viral pathogens with 1 test. These tests are typically known as pathogen panels and should be interpreted with caution because of a risk of false-positive results. Stool studies help guide antimicrobial use in certain instances (eg, *Salmonella*, *Shigella*, and some *Campylobacter* infections). Stool studies may also help prevent unnecessary additional testing and imaging and unnecessary use of antibiotics.

In healthy adults, many bacterial causes of diarrhea do not require antibiotic therapy. Empirical use of antimicrobials is not recommended for most patients who are immunocompetent, but it should be considered for 1) patients younger than 3 months who may have a bacterial infection, 2) patients who are immunocompromised, 3) patients who are immunocompetent and appear ill if *Shigella* infection is suspected, or 4) recent travelers who are febrile or have signs of sepsis. Empirical antimicrobial therapy in adults should be either a fluoroquinolone (eg, ciprofloxacin) or azithromycin, depending on the local susceptibility patterns and travel history. Antibiotics should be avoided for those with the Shiga toxin–producing *E coli* O157 strain because of evidence of harm. Antimicrobial treatment should be modified or discontinued when a clinically plausible organism is identified. Common exposures and conditions that lead to diarrhea are summarized in Table 18.1. Clinical presentations that suggest causes of infectious diarrhea are outlined in Table 18.2; recommended antimicrobial agents for pathogens, in Table 18.3; and common postinfection manifestations associated with enteric pathogens, in Table 18.4.

Campylobacter jejuni

Most enteric bacterial infections are due to *Campylobacter jejuni* and typically are acquired from contaminated poultry (up to 90% of chickens may be colonized) or unpasteurized milk in the summer or early fall. Infection is most common in very young children, teens, and young adults. Fever, myalgias, malaise, abdominal pain, and headache occur after an incubation period of 1 to 4 days. Diarrhea begins later, ranges from profuse and watery to bloody, and lasts up to 1 week. Prolonged carriage can occur for several months, and recurrent infection can occur in up to

25% of patients. A chronic carrier state is rare. Hemolytic uremic syndrome (HUS), reactive arthritis (human leukocyte antigen [HLA]-B27), and Guillain-Barré syndrome can occur.

In most healthy patients, symptoms are mild to moderate, and by the time the slow-growing *Campylobacter* is identified, the patient's condition has begun to improve. A PCR assay will provide a rapid result. For healthy patients, antibiotic therapy is unnecessary. Antibiotics are recommended for patients who have prolonged (>1 week) or worsening symptoms, dysentery, high fever, or bacteremia and for pregnant women and persons at risk for complications (extremes of age, immunocompromised state, or cirrhosis). The drug of choice is azithromycin because of increased resistance to quinolones, which are an alternative therapy for *Campylobacter* infection.

Salmonella

Infection with *Salmonella* leads to a spectrum of diseases ranging from acute gastroenteritis to typhoid fever (Table 18.5). The infection may get complicated by bacteremia resulting in disseminated infection. *Salmonella typhi* and *Salmonella paratyphi* cause typhoid fever. The other serotypes (about 2,000 have been described) cause nontyphoidal salmonellosis. *Salmonella enteritidis* and *Salmonella typhimurium* are the 2 serotypes most often isolated in the US.

Table 18.1. Exposures and Conditions Associated With Pathogens That Cause Diarrhea

Exposure or condition	Pathogen
Foodborne outbreaks at hotels, cruise ships, resorts, restaurants, or catered events	*Norovirus*, nontyphoidal *Salmonella*, *Clostridium perfringens*, *Bacillus cereus*, *Staphylococcus aureus*, *Campylobacter* species, ETEC, STEC, *Listeria*, *Shigella*, *Cyclospora cayetanensis*, *Cryptosporidium* species
Consumption of unpasteurized milk or dairy products	*Salmonella*, *Campylobacter*, *Yersinia enterocolitica*, *S aureus*, *Cryptosporidium*, STEC, *Listeria* (infrequently associated with diarrhea), *Brucella* (goat milk cheese), *Mycobacterium bovis*, *Coxiella burnetii*
Consumption of raw or undercooked meat or poultry	STEC (beef), *C perfringens* (beef, poultry), *Salmonella* (poultry), *Campylobacter* (poultry), *Yersinia* (pork, chitterlings), *S aureus* (poultry), *Trichinella* species (pork, wild game meat)
Consumption of fruits or unpasteurized fruit juices, vegetables, leafy greens, or sprouts	STEC, nontyphoidal *Salmonella*, *Cyclospora*, *Cryptosporidium*, *Norovirus*, hepatitis A virus, *Listeria monocytogenes*
Consumption of undercooked eggs	*Salmonella*, *Shigella* (egg salad)
Consumption of raw shellfish	*Vibrio* species, *Norovirus*, hepatitis A virus, *Plesiomonas*
Swimming in or drinking untreated fresh water	*Campylobacter*, *Cryptosporidium*, *Giardia*, *Shigella*, *Salmonella*, STEC, *Plesiomonas shigelloides*
Swimming in recreational water facility with treated water	*Cryptosporidium* and other potentially waterborne pathogens when disinfectant concentrations are inadequately maintained
Health care, long-term care, prison exposure, or employment	*Norovirus*, *Clostridioides difficile*, *Shigella*, *Cryptosporidium*, *Giardia*, STEC, *Rotavirus*
Child care center (attendance or employment)	*Rotavirus*, *Cryptosporidium*, *Giardia*, *Shigella*, STEC
Recent antimicrobial therapy	*C difficile*, multidrug-resistant *Salmonella*
Travel to resource-limited countries	*Escherichia coli* (enteroaggregative, enterotoxigenic, enteroinvasive), *Shigella*, *Salmonella typhi*, nontyphoidal *Salmonella*, *Campylobacter*, *Vibrio cholerae*, *Entamoeba histolytica*, *Giardia*, *Blastocystis*, *Cyclospora*, *Cystoisospora*, *Cryptosporidium*
Exposure to house pets with diarrhea	*Campylobacter*, *Yersinia*
Exposure to pig feces in certain parts of the world	*Balantidium coli*
Contact with young poultry or reptiles	Nontyphoidal *Salmonella*
Visit to a farm or petting zoo	STEC, *Cryptosporidium*, *Campylobacter*
Age	*Rotavirus* (6-18 mo), nontyphoidal *Salmonella* (birth to 3 mo; adults >50 y with a history of atherosclerosis), *Shigella* (1-7 y), *Campylobacter* (young adults)
Underlying immunocompromising condition	Nontyphoidal *Salmonella*, *Cryptosporidium*, *Campylobacter*, *Shigella*, *Yersinia*
Hemochromatosis or hemoglobinopathy	*Yersinia enterocolitica*, *Salmonella*
AIDS, immunosuppressive therapies	*Cryptosporidium*, *Cyclospora*, *Cystoisospora*, microsporidia, *Mycobacterium avium-intracellulare* complex, *Cytomegalovirus*
Anal-genital, oral-anal, or digital-anal contact	*Shigella*, *Salmonella*, *Campylobacter*, *E histolytica*, *Giardia lamblia*, *Cryptosporidium*, agents of sexually transmitted infections

Abbreviations: ETEC, enterotoxigenic *Escherichia coli*; STEC, Shiga toxin–producing *Escherichia coli*.

Adapted from Shane AL, Mody RK, Crump JA, Tarr PI, Steiner TS, Kotloff K, et al. 2017 Infectious Diseases Society of America clinical practice guidelines for the diagnosis and management of infectious diarrhea. Clin Infect Dis. 2017 Nov 29;65(12):e45-e80; used with permission.

Table 18.2. Clinical Presentations That Suggest Causes of Infectious Diarrhea

Finding	Likely pathogens and other comments
Persistent or chronic diarrhea	*Cryptosporidium* spp, *Giardia lamblia*, *Cyclospora cayetanensis*, *Cystoisospora belli*, *Entamoeba histolytica*
Visible blood in stool	STEC, *Shigella*, *Salmonella*, *Campylobacter*, *Entamoeba histolytica*, noncholera *Vibrio* species, *Yersinia*, *Balantidium coli*, *Plesiomonas*
Fever	Not highly discriminatory: viral, bacterial, and parasitic infections can cause fever
	In general, higher temperatures suggest bacterial agent or *E histolytica*
	Patients infected with STEC usually are not febrile at presentation
Abdominal pain	STEC, *Salmonella*, *Shigella*, *Campylobacter*, *Yersinia*, noncholera *Vibrio* species, *Clostridioides difficile*
Severe abdominal pain, often grossly bloody stools (occasionally nonbloody), and minimal or no fever	STEC, *Salmonella*, *Shigella*, *Campylobacter*, *Yersinia enterocolitica*
Persistent abdominal pain and fever	*Y enterocolitica* and *Y pseudotuberculosis* (findings may resemble those with appendicitis)
Nausea and vomiting lasting ≤24 h	Ingestion of *Staphylococcus aureus* enterotoxin or *Bacillus cereus* (short-incubation emetic syndrome)
Diarrhea and abdominal cramping lasting 1-2 d	Ingestion of *Clostridium perfringens* or *B cereus* (long-incubation emetic syndrome)
Vomiting and nonbloody diarrhea lasting ≤2-3 d	*Norovirus* (low-grade fever usually present during the first 24 h in 40% of infections)
Chronic watery diarrhea, often lasting ≥1 y	Brainerd diarrhea (etiologic agent has not been identified)
	Postinfectious irritable bowel syndrome

Abbreviation: STEC, Shiga toxin–producing *Escherichia coli*.

Adapted from Shane AL, Mody RK, Crump JA, Tarr PI, Steiner TS, Kotloff K, et al. 2017 Infectious Diseases Society of America clinical practice guidelines for the diagnosis and management of infectious diarrhea. Clin Infect Dis. 2017 Nov 29;65(12):e45-e80; used with permission.

Outbreaks typically occur in the summer or autumn and are associated with contaminated food (undercooked or raw poultry or eggs, meat, or dairy products), reflecting the high colonization rates of *Salmonella* in poultry and livestock. Pets, including turtles, reptiles, cats, and dogs, can carry and transmit the organism. Person-to-person spread is also important in outbreaks and in resource-limited countries. Because typhoidal *Salmonella* exists only in humans, a new case of typhoid fever indicates exposure to a carrier. Attack rates are highest among infants, elderly patients, and persons with decreased levels of stomach acid. Conditions that predispose to *Salmonella* infection, in addition to eating raw or undercooked eggs and poultry, are listed in Box 18.1.

Gastroenteritis occurs in 75% of infections and typically begins with nausea and vomiting within 48 hours after exposure with subsequent diarrhea and cramps. Diarrhea may range from mild to severe and from watery to bloody. Fever and abdominal pain are common. Localized tenderness can simulate an acute abdomen and is often localized to the right lower quadrant, reflecting the ileal location of most infections. Gastroenteritis usually lasts for no more than 7 days, although in unusual cases, primarily with colitis, symptoms can last for weeks. Bacteremia occurs in 5% to 10% of infections, often resulting in distant infections (eg, central nervous system infections, endocarditis, or osteomyelitis). Recurrent or persistent bacteremia can occur in immunocompromised patients such as those with HIV or AIDS.

Typhoid fever (enteric fever) is a systemic infection characterized by an incubation period of 1 to 2 weeks and subsequent systemic symptoms that include fever, malaise, arthralgia, myalgia, headache, and delirium. Gastrointestinal symptoms often have a delayed onset and include abdominal pain and constipation more frequently than diarrhea. Delayed bowel perforation and bleeding can occur. Physical examination findings include relative bradycardia (pulse-temperature dissociation), hepatosplenomegaly, lymphadenopathy, and a macular rash (rose spots). Typhoid fever is associated with recurrent or sustained bacteremia, which results in metastatic infections.

Symptoms typically last 4 weeks, although antibiotic therapy can hasten recovery. Recurrent infection, occurring 7 to 10 days after apparent recovery, is not uncommon. The incidence of typhoid fever is decreasing in the US.

Prolonged asymptomatic fecal shedding of *Salmonella* is common (average duration, about 5 weeks), although most patients clear the organism within 3 months. Chronic carriage (>1 year) occurs in less than 1% of patients with gastroenteritis and in up to 3% with typhoid fever. Risk factors include extremes of age and cholelithiasis (associated with chronic gallbladder infection).

Therapy for uncomplicated gastroenteritis includes rehydration and avoidance of antimotility agents. Antibiotics may prolong the carrier state and select for resistant organisms; they do not improve outcomes and are not indicated for healthy patients with uncomplicated gastroenteritis. Commonly used antibiotics include cephalosporins and quinolones; alternatives are amoxicillin and trimethoprim-sulfamethoxazole (TMP-SMX). Antibiotics are indicated for patients who have colitis, bacteremia or a risk for bacteremia (extremes of age, immunocompromised state [from HIV, medications, or malignancy], valvular heart disease, hemoglobinopathy, or orthopedic implants), or severe disease and for patients who are long-term carriers. Multidrug resistance is becoming a problem; therapy should be guided by sensitivity testing. Prolonged therapy is necessary for metastatic infections.

For typhoid fever, therapy is recommended. Typically, a third-generation cephalosporin or a quinolone is given as empirical therapy while sensitivity data are pending. In cases of fluoroquinolone resistance, azithromycin is the treatment of choice. Chloramphenicol, TMP-SMX, and ampicillin are inappropriate for empirical therapy because of resistance. Short-term use of corticosteroids may be beneficial for patients with severe disease (eg, known enteric fever and severe systemic illness with delirium, coma, or shock). For long-term carriers, therapy with a quinolone (eg, norfloxacin, 400 mg twice daily for 4 weeks) may lead to clearance. If not, cholecystectomy may be needed to remove the nidus of chronic infection.

Table 18.3. Recommended Antimicrobial Agents for Diarrhea

Pathogen	First choice	Alternative	Comments
Bacteria[a]			
Campylobacter	Azithromycin	Ciprofloxacin	
Nontyphoidal *Salmonella enterica*[b]	Usually not indicated for uncomplicated infection	NA	Antimicrobial therapy should be considered for groups at increased risk for invasive infection: neonates (≤3 mo old); persons older than 50 y with suspected atherosclerosis; persons with immunosuppression, cardiac disease (valvular or endovascular), or joint disease If susceptible, treatment with ceftriaxone, ciprofloxacin, TMP-SMX, or amoxicillin
Salmonella enterica Typhi or Paratyphi[b]	Ceftriaxone or ciprofloxacin	Ampicillin or TMP-SMX, or azithromycin	
Shigella[a]	Azithromycin[c] or ciprofloxacin[a], or ceftriaxone	TMP-SMX or ampicillin if susceptible	Clinicians treating people with shigellosis for whom antibiotic treatment is indicated should avoid prescribing fluoroquinolones if the ciprofloxacin MIC is ≥0.12 µg/mL even if the laboratory report identifies the isolate as susceptible[d]
Vibrio cholerae	Doxycycline[e]	Ciprofloxacin, azithromycin, or ceftriaxone	
Non–*Vibrio cholerae*[e]	For noninvasive disease: usually not indicated, but single-agent therapy if treated For invasive disease: ceftriaxone with doxycycline	For noninvasive disease: usually not indicated, but single-agent therapy if treated For invasive disease: TMP-SMX with an aminoglycoside	
Yersinia enterocolitica	TMP-SMX	Cefotaxime or ciprofloxacin	
Parasites			
Cryptosporidium spp	Nitazoxanide (HIV-uninfected, HIV-infected in combination with effective cART)	Effective cART: immune reconstitution may lead to microbiologic and clinical response	NA
Cyclospora cayetanensis	TMP-SMX	Nitazoxanide (limited data)	Patients with HIV infection may require higher doses or longer durations of TMP-SMX treatment
Giardia lamblia	Tinidazole (data from HIV-uninfected children) Nitazoxanide	Metronidazole (data from HIV-uninfected children)	Tinidazole—approved in US for children aged ≥3 y; available in tablets that can be crushed Metronidazole—high frequency of gastrointestinal adverse effects; pediatric suspension is not commercially available but can be compounded from tablets; not FDA approved for treatment of giardiasis
Cystoisospora belli	TMP-SMX	Pyrimethamine Potential second-line alternatives: ciprofloxacin, nitazoxanide	
Trichinella spp	Albendazole	Mebendazole	Therapy less effective in late stage of infection when larvae encapsulate in muscle

Abbreviations: cART, combination antiretroviral therapy; FDA, US Food and Drug Administration; MIC, minimum inhibitory concentration; NA, not applicable; TMP-SMX, trimethoprim-sulfamethoxazole.

[a] For information on susceptibility patterns in the US, see the National Antimicrobial Resistance Monitoring System for Enteric Bacteria (https://www.cdc.gov/narms/index.html). Susceptibility testing should be considered when a therapeutic agent is selected.

[b] If invasive disease is suspected or confirmed, ceftriaxone is preferred over ciprofloxacin because of increasing resistance to ciprofloxacin.

[c] Most clinical laboratories do not test for azithromycin susceptibility.

[d] For additional information, see https://emergency.cdc.gov/han/han00401.asp.

[e] Primary therapy is aggressive rehydration; antibiotics are adjunctive therapy.

Adapted from Shane AL, Mody RK, Crump JA, Tarr PI, Steiner TS, Kotloff K, et al. 2017 Infectious Diseases Society of America clinical practice guidelines for the diagnosis and management of infectious diarrhea. Clin Infect Dis. 2017 Nov 29;65(12):e45-e80; used with permission.

Shigella

Shigella has 40 serotypes in 4 species (*Shigella dysenteriae*, *Shigella flexneri*, *Shigella boydii*, and *Shigella sonnei*). Spread is typically person to person, facilitated by a low infective dose because of resistance to stomach acid. Outbreaks are related to contaminated food and water. *Shigella sonnei* produces the mildest disease and is the most common serotype in the US. Symptoms characteristically begin within 48 hours after ingestion and include fever, malaise, abdominal pain, and watery diarrhea. Rectal pain or burning can be a prominent symptom. Respiratory symptoms are common, and children may have

Table 18.4. Postinfectious Manifestations Associated With Enteric Pathogens

Manifestation	Organisms
Erythema nodosum	*Yersinia, Campylobacter, Salmonella, Shigella*
Glomerulonephritis	*Shigella, Campylobacter, Yersinia*
Guillain-Barré syndrome	*Campylobacter*
Hemolytic anemia	*Campylobacter, Yersinia*
Hemolytic uremic syndrome	STEC, *Shigella dysenteriae* serotype 1
Immunoglobulin A nephropathy	*Campylobacter*
Reactive arthritis[a]	*Salmonella, Shigella, Campylobacter, Yersinia, Giardia* (rarely), *Cyclospora cayetanensis*
Postinfectious irritable bowel syndrome	*Campylobacter, Salmonella, Shigella,* STEC, *Giardia*
Meningitis	*Listeria, Salmonella* (infants ≤3 mo old are at high risk)
Intestinal perforation	*Salmonella* (including *Salmonella* Typhi), *Shigella, Campylobacter, Yersinia, Entamoeba histolytica*
Ekiri syndrome (lethal, toxic encephalopathy) and/or seizure	*Shigella*
Aortitis, osteomyelitis, extravascular deep tissue focus	*Salmonella, Yersinia*

Abbreviation: STEC, Shiga toxin–producing *Escherichia coli.*

[a] Includes Reiter syndrome.

Adapted from Shane AL, Mody RK, Crump JA, Tarr PI, Steiner TS, Kotloff K, et al. 2017 Infectious Diseases Society of America clinical practice guidelines for the diagnosis and management of infectious diarrhea. Clin Infect Dis. 2017 Nov 29;65(12):e45-e80; used with permission.

Box 18.1. Conditions Predisposing to *Salmonella* Infection

Hemolytic anemia
  Sickle cell disease

Malignancy
  Lymphoma
  Leukemia
  Disseminated carcinoma

Immunosuppression
  AIDS
  Corticosteroids
  Chemotherapy, radiotherapy

Achlorhydria
  Gastric surgery
  Proton pump inhibitors
  Idiopathic

Ulcerative colitis

Schistosomiasis

Adapted from Giannella RA. Infectious enteritis and proctocolitis and bacterial food poisoning. In: Feldman M, Friedman L, Brandt LJ, eds. Sleisenger & Fordtran's gastrointestinal and liver disease. Saunders/Elsevier; 2010:1843-87; used with permission.

neurologic manifestations, including seizures. The diarrhea may decrease and become bloody with mucus and pus (ie, dysentery). The initial watery diarrhea is thought to be due to the Shiga toxin, whereas dysentery is due to mucosal invasion, which occurs primarily in the colon. This classic progression occurs in a small proportion of cases and is least common in *S sonnei* infections.

Predictors of severity include extremes of age, malnutrition, immunosuppression, and infection with *S dysenteriae*, which is most likely to cause complications such as HUS, dysentery, or toxic megacolon. Shigellosis typically lasts for 1 to 3 days in children and 5 to 7 days in adults. Although chronic carriage is unusual, prolonged infections can occur and may be difficult to differentiate from ulcerative colitis. A delayed, asymmetric large-joint arthritis can occur, usually in persons with HLA-B27.

Table 18.5. Clinical Syndromes of *Salmonella* Infection

Syndrome	Incidence, %
Gastroenteritis	75
Varies from mild to severe (dysentery)	
Bacteremia	5-10
With or without gastroenteritis	
Consider AIDS	
Typhoid (enteric) fever	5-10
With or without gastroenteritis	
Systemic infection	5
Osteomyelitis, arthritis, meningitis, cholecystitis, abscess	
Carrier state duration >1 y	<1

Adapted from Giannella RA. Infectious enteritis and proctocolitis and bacterial food poisoning. In: Feldman M, Friedman L, Brandt LJ, eds. Sleisenger & Fordtran's gastrointestinal and liver disease. Saunders/Elsevier; 2010:1843-87; used with permission.

Treatment focuses on rehydration and avoidance of antimotility agents. Antibiotics have been shown to decrease mortality and the duration of disease. Therefore, antibiotic therapy is indicated for most patients, particularly those with chronic illnesses (including malnutrition and HIV), elderly patients, day care or health care workers, and food handlers. Owing to increasing antimicrobial resistance, selection of therapy should be guided, if possible, by results of antimicrobial susceptibility testing. Treatment options include azithromycin, ciprofloxacin, or TMP-SMX. Before susceptibility testing results are available, fluroquinolone therapy can be initiated. Resistance to multiple antibiotics has been reported. Clinicians should avoid prescribing fluoroquinolones if the ciprofloxacin minimum inhibitory concentration is 0.12 µg/mL or higher even if the laboratory report identifies the isolate as susceptible.

Escherichia coli

The different types of *E coli* are summarized in Table 18.6.

Enterohemorrhagic *E coli*

Enterohemorrhagic *E coli* (EHEC) produces Shiga toxin and causes colitis after an incubation period of 3 to 5 days. *Escherichia coli* O157:H7 accounts for more than 90% of EHEC cases in the US; 100 other serotypes have been identified. Although several outbreaks have attracted considerable media attention, most cases of EHEC are sporadic. It has been estimated that 50% of cattle and 90% of hamburger lots are contaminated with EHEC. Thus, EHEC is associated with the ingestion of undercooked hamburger but also with the ingestion of salami, sprouts, and unpasteurized milk or juice. Although the infectious dose is low, EHEC is effectively killed at temperatures higher than 69 °C. A pink center in a hamburger is associated with lower temperatures and an

Table 18.6. Types of *Escherichia coli* Causing Infectious Diarrhea

Type of E coli	Patients affected	Pathophysiology	Clinical features
Enteropathogenic (EPEC)	Infants in resource-limited countries; some travelers	Attachment alters brush border	Watery diarrhea
Enterotoxigenic (ETEC)	Children in resource-limited countries; travelers	Enterotoxin-mediated secretion	Watery diarrhea
Enteroinvasive (EIEC)	All ages; rare; food and water outbreak	Direct invasion	Usually watery diarrhea; 10% have dysentery
Enterohemorrhagic (EHEC) (eg, E coli O157:H7)	All ages; food (hamburger); sporadic or outbreak	Shiga-like cytotoxins	Watery then bloody diarrhea; HUS or TTP
Enteroaggregative (EAEC)	Infants in resource-limited countries; HIV-positive adults	Adherence; toxins	Prolonged watery diarrhea

Abbreviations: HUS, hemolytic uremic syndrome; TTP, thrombotic thrombocytopenic purpura.

Adapted from Giannella RA. Infectious enteritis and proctocolitis and bacterial food poisoning. In: Feldman M, Friedman L, Brandt LJ, eds. Sleisenger & Fordtran's gastrointestinal and liver disease. Saunders/Elsevier; 2010:1843-87; used with permission.

increased risk of infection. Irradiation of hamburger also effectively kills EHEC, but whether the public will embrace irradiated foods is not known.

EHEC typically produces watery diarrhea that progresses to bloody diarrhea after a few hours to a few days. One study suggested that EHEC is the most common cause of bloody diarrhea in the US. Systemic symptoms (fatigue, myalgias, and headache), severe abdominal pain, nausea, and vomiting are common, but fever is not. Illness typically lasts 5 to 10 days. In the elderly, EHEC may be misdiagnosed as ischemic colitis.

EHEC can lead to HUS or thrombotic thrombocytopenic purpura (TTP) in 5% of patients, resulting in hemolytic anemia and kidney failure, with or without central nervous system symptoms. The pathophysiologic mechanism of EHEC appears to be vascular endothelial damage that leads to platelet aggregation and initiation of the coagulation cascade. This, in turn, leads to ischemia of the colon and results in hemorrhagic colitis. Some cases of "ischemic colitis" probably are misdiagnosed cases of EHEC. Similarly, thrombi and ischemia in the kidney may be the cause of kidney insufficiency in HUS. Morbidity and mortality rates are high among patients with HUS or TTP, particularly among those who are very young or very old.

In some laboratories, specific testing for *E coli* O157:H7 (with sorbitol-MacConkey agar or a newer stool toxin assay that may be more sensitive) must be requested; thus, the condition can be underdiagnosed. In several large series reported from North America, *E coli* O157:H7 was the second to fourth most identified bacterium in acute diarrheal illnesses. Antibiotics do not appear to be beneficial and may increase toxin production or release (or both). This, in turn, may increase the risk of HUS or TTP and, perhaps, death. Also, antimotility agents, including narcotics, may increase the risk of HUS. Thus, use of antibiotics and antimotility agents should be avoided if EHEC infection is suspected clinically (eg, absence of fever in a patient with bloody diarrhea of suspected infectious origin).

Contact isolation precautions are necessary for patients with EHEC, and any personal contacts who have gastrointestinal tract symptoms should be tested for EHEC. It has been recommended that children, food handlers, and health care workers delay their return to school or work until they are asymptomatic and have had several stool cultures negative for EHEC.

Enterotoxigenic *E coli*

Enterotoxigenic *E coli* (ETEC) is a common cause of diarrhea in travelers and in children in resource-limited countries. The organism attaches to the small bowel and causes diarrhea through enterotoxins. The disease ranges from mild to severe watery diarrhea and is often associated with mild upper gastrointestinal tract symptoms that last for 2 to 5 days. Rehydration is the mainstay of therapy. Routine antibiotic administration is not recommended because most cases are self-limiting and antibiotics would propagate the development of drug-resistant strains. Antibiotics may be considered for patients who have severe diarrhea, who need hospitalization because of dehydration, or who are immunocompromised. Azithromycin or a fluoroquinolone would be considered the drug of choice.

Enteropathogenic *E coli*

Enteropathogenic *E coli* (EPEC) is primarily a problem in infants. It caused several epidemics with high mortality in neonatal nurseries in the early 1970s. Currently, it occurs most often in resource-limited countries. EPEC attaches to the small-bowel mucosa and causes watery mucoid diarrhea by producing structural changes in the microvilli. Most people recover spontaneously and do not need antibiotic treatment. The importance of antibiotics even in severe or persistent disease is unknown. If antibiotics are chosen, fluoroquinolones such as ciprofloxacin, macrolides such as azithromycin, or rifaximin may be used.

Enteroinvasive *E coli*

Enteroinvasive *E coli* (EIEC) is a rare cause of diarrhea associated with fever and abdominal pain. The diarrhea is usually watery, but it can be accompanied by fever and leukocytes (ie, dysentery). EIEC is similar to *Shigella* in its ability to invade the colonic mucosa and produce a Shiga-like toxin. Data are limited on the benefit of antibiotic therapy because patients do recover spontaneously. If antibiotics are chosen, fluoroquinolones such as ciprofloxacin, macrolides such as azithromycin, or rifaximin may be used.

Enteroaggregative *E coli*

Enteroaggregative *E coli* (EAEC) is primarily a problem in infants in resource-limited countries and in adults infected with HIV, although it also can cause traveler's diarrhea. EAEC causes persistent diarrhea that can be watery or bloody. Testing for EAEC requires a tissue culture adherence assay or a PCR assay. Quinolones are an effective therapy, suggesting that empirical treatment with these agents may be reasonable for patients with HIV who have diarrhea and negative findings on evaluation.

Vibrio

Vibrio species are halophilic and associated with the consumption of raw or undercooked saltwater fish or shellfish (oysters, crabs, and mussels) or contamination of food with seawater.

Vibrio parahaemolyticus is a common cause of diarrhea in the coastal US and Japan, particularly during warm months. Several toxins can be produced, resulting in various clinical presentations. The incubation period is less than 1 to 2 days, and the primary symptom is watery diarrhea. Abdominal pain, vomiting, and headaches are also common. Uncommonly, *V parahaemolyticus* may cause frank dysentery and mucosal ulceration. The illness typically lasts 2 to 5 days, and antibiotics usually are not necessary. The importance of antibiotics is uncertain, even for patients with severe or prolonged symptoms. If antibiotics are administered, a reasonable choice is doxycycline.

Vibrio cholerae infection is not common in the US, although sporadic cases occur along the Gulf Coast and in travelers returning from endemic areas (Latin America, Africa, and Asia). The infectious dose is large, although hypochlorhydria decreases it. Cholera toxin can cause profound dehydration from profuse diarrhea (>1 L/h in some cases) and vomiting. However, milder cases (and asymptomatic carriage) are possible. In severe cases, stools are described as "rice water" because of the watery consistency with flecks of mucus. Hypotension, kidney failure, and hypokalemic acidosis occur in severe cases and, without aggressive rehydration, often lead to death. Oral rehydration solution can be lifesaving, but severe cases usually require intravenous fluids, with attention to potassium and bicarbonate replacement. Infection can be treated with various antibiotics, which most commonly include tetracycline or doxycycline. Azithromycin, erythromycin, or even a single dose of quinolone therapy can be effective, although resistance patterns are emerging.

Vibrio vulnificus also can cause diarrhea, and hemorrhagic bullae may appear. The organism can be acquired through wound contamination from contaminated seawater or by direct consumption, particularly in the summer months. In patients who are immunocompromised or those with chronic liver disease, systemic infection with sepsis is a risk, and the mortality rate is high. These patients should be instructed not to eat or handle raw seafood, particularly oysters.

Yersinia

Yersinia enterocolitica is less common in the US than in northern Europe. *Yersinia* typically is acquired in cold months from contaminated food, milk, or water and has an incubation period of 4 to 7 days. Many animals can harbor the organism and be a source of infection, which occurs primarily in the terminal ileum. Symptoms range from mild (fever, diarrhea, nausea, and cramps) to severe (reflecting invasion). Uncommonly, *Yersinia* causes bacteremia with sepsis or distant infection. Arthralgias and rash are more common in adults than in children. Postinfectious arthritis also can occur (HLA-B27).

In healthy patients, symptoms typically last 1 to 3 weeks. Antibiotic therapy has not been shown to be of benefit in uncomplicated disease. Patients at risk for sepsis (those with cirrhosis, iron overload, or an immunocompromised state) and those with severe or prolonged symptoms, bacteremia, or distant infections may benefit from antibiotic therapy (TMP-SMX, a cephalosporin, or a quinolone). Ileocolitis from *Yersinia* infection can simulate Crohn disease (including extraintestinal manifestations: aphthous ulcers, arthralgias, and erythema nodosum), and right lower quadrant tenderness with mesenteric lymphadenitis can simulate appendicitis.

Parasitic Intestinal Infections

Stool evaluation for ova and parasites is helpful when patients are immunocompromised or have an appropriate exposure or travel history. Most parasites are shed intermittently, and a single stool evaluation is relatively insensitive. To increase sensitivity, 3 or more separate stools should be analyzed. Newer antigen-based and molecular PCR-based assays have higher sensitivity than stool microscopic assays.

Giardia lamblia

Giardia lamblia (also known as *Giardia intestinalis* or *Giardia duodenalis*), the most common parasitic infection in the US, is acquired by the ingestion of water or food contaminated with cysts or by person-to-person spread (eg, day care centers and nursing homes). Cysts can survive for months in the environment and are resistant to chlorination. In the US, the peak incidence occurs in the summer and early autumn. Excystation occurs in the small bowel, where the trophozoites attach to and damage the mucosa. High-risk groups are travelers to endemic areas, children in day care, patients with immunoglobulin deficiencies, and men who have sex with men. Symptoms, including watery diarrhea, cramps, nausea, bloating, and flatulence, occur 1 to 2 weeks after ingestion. Patients initially may have acute disease, although diarrhea may be intermittent, leading to a delay in seeking medical attention. Chronic symptoms also may occur and can be associated with malabsorption. Some persons become asymptomatic carriers with long-term cyst passage.

Examination of multiple stools for trophozoites or cysts is insensitive. Preferred methods are fecal analysis for *Giardia* antigen, nucleic acid assay, or duodenal aspirate and biopsy (to confirm presence of organisms or lack of plasma cells). First-line therapy is with tinidazole (single 2-g dose) or nitazoxanide; use of metronidazole (250 mg 3 times daily for 5-7 days) is an alternative. Paromomycin is the treatment of choice if the patient is pregnant. Treatment of asymptomatic carriers provides no benefit for the patient but may help prevent outbreaks (eg, among day care or health care workers).

Cryptosporidium

Although *Cryptosporidium* increasingly has been recognized as a pathogen in patients with AIDS, it also can cause diarrhea in hosts who are immunocompetent. Infection commonly is acquired from contaminated water or person-to-person spread. The parasite can resist chlorination, resulting in outbreaks even in industrialized areas. Several US outbreaks have been attributed to contaminated water sources. *Cryptosporidium* invades the small-bowel mucosa and causes inflammation, villous blunting, and malabsorption. In most healthy patients, disease is mild and self-limited, with watery diarrhea, nausea, cramps, and flatulence developing 7 to 10 days after ingestion. Stools may be intermittent and mucoid but should not contain much blood or pus. Diarrhea can last 6 weeks or longer. Headaches, fevers, or myalgias are common. The diagnosis can be made by stool analysis (immunoassays are more sensitive than microscopy) or small-bowel biopsy. In healthy patients, treatment usually is not necessary.

Entamoeba histolytica

Amebiasis is the most common parasitic diarrhea in the world, although it is less common in the US. Most cases in the US occur in travelers or immigrants from endemic areas (Latin America, Africa, and India) and in men who have sex with men. Infection is acquired through the ingestion of contaminated food or water. Amebic cysts undergo excystation in the small bowel and infect the colon. Symptoms begin 7 to 21 days after ingestion and include bloody diarrhea, abdominal pain, fever, and tenesmus, consistent with invasive colitis. Amebic colitis can vary from mild to fulminant, with severe bleeding or perforation. Because the risk of perforation is increased by corticosteroid use, it is important to differentiate amebic colitis from ulcerative colitis. Amebic ulcers are caused by mucosal invasion by trophozoites. The ulcers vary from mild to severe, with the classic description being that of undermined edges leading to a flask-shaped ulcer. Amebae can penetrate the bowel wall, enter the portal circulation, and cause liver or splenic abscesses. Patients with liver abscesses tend to be male, and they may not have a discernible history of colitis. Distant infection (peritonitis, empyema, or central nervous system infection) also can occur. A localized infection surrounded by granulation tissue or a dense fibrous coat (ameboma) can resemble colon cancer.

Diagnosis is made by stool examination. Three or more samples may be needed to make the diagnosis with microscopy, although stool antigen testing and the PCR assay for E histolytica DNA are more sensitive. Metronidazole (750 mg 3 times daily for 7-10 days) is the drug of choice for treating colitis or liver abscesses. Cysts are relatively resistant to metronidazole and require a second agent such as diloxanide furoate, paromomycin, or iodoquinol. Drainage of liver abscesses is not recommended unless rupture is imminent or medical therapy is ineffective.

The human colon can be inhabited by numerous nonpathologic amebae, including Entamoeba coli, Entamoeba hartmanni, and Endolimax nana. Distinguishing between these organisms and E histolytica can be difficult with routine microscopy, even for experienced examiners, although serologic testing and stool PCR assay should help.

Blastocystis hominis

Blastocystis hominis is found occasionally on routine stool examinations for ova and parasites. Its pathogenicity is uncertain, particularly in hosts who are immunocompetent. However, if no other cause for a patient's symptoms is found, a trial of metronidazole or tinidazole can be considered.

Traveler's Diarrhea

Infectious diarrhea affects 40% to 60% of travelers to high-risk areas of Southeast Asia, the Middle East, India, Africa, and South America. The incidence of diarrhea varies depending on the specific area visited (eg, urban or rural), the traveler's age, time of year, and local conditions, such as flooding or a cholera outbreak. Bacteria cause 80% to 90% of cases of traveler's diarrhea, and the other 10% to 20% are due to parasites, viruses, or toxins. ETEC is a common cause. The unusual case of prolonged traveler's diarrhea is more likely to be caused by a parasite such as G intestinalis or Cyclospora cayetanensis. The risk of infection can be decreased by avoiding uncooked foods, local water (including ice), and unpasteurized drinks.

Symptoms typically begin several days after the person arrives in the area and last for 3 to 5 days. Watery diarrhea, bloating, fatigue, and cramps are common. Bloody diarrhea and high fever are uncommon; their presence suggests an invasive organism and should prompt an evaluation for a specific organism. For most travelers, antibiotic prophylaxis is not recommended. Bismuth subsalicylate (2 tablets 4 times daily) is a possible prophylaxis.

Mild cases of traveler's diarrhea can be treated with rehydration and antidiarrheals or bismuth (if no fever, severe pain, or bloody diarrhea) for 1 to 3 days. The recommendation for moderate to severe diarrhea is azithromycin, a quinolone, or rifaximin, often in combination with an antidiarrheal. Azithromycin has activity against fluoroquinolone-resistant Campylobacter, which may be encountered during travel in South and Southeast Asia.

Food Poisoning

Common symptoms of food poisoning and typical offending agents are listed in Table 18.7.

Staphylococcus aureus toxin causes 1 to 2 days of severe vomiting, cramps, and diarrhea that begin 2 to 6 hours after ingestion of contaminated food (eg, cream-filled pastries, meat, or potato or egg salad). Severe infection can cause dehydration.

Clostridium perfringens toxin produces 1 to 2 days of abdominal pain and watery diarrhea that usually begin 8 to 24 hours after ingestion of foods typically prepared in advance and left to sit unrefrigerated (eg, beef, poultry, or gravy). An uncommon strain of C perfringens produces the potentially fatal enteritis necroticans, or pigbel, a condition that occurs primarily in poor tropical regions.

Bacillus cereus toxin causes nausea and vomiting that usually occur within 2 to 6 hours after ingestion of contaminated food (eg, pork, creams or sauces, or fried rice) and last 6 to 10 hours. Diarrhea may occur later, probably from a toxin formed in vivo. In healthy hosts, antibiotic therapy is not necessary for these acute forms of food poisoning due to preformed enterotoxins.

Listeria monocytogenes can be found in many foods (eg, hot dogs, lunch meat, and cheeses), and its growth is not substantially inhibited by refrigeration. It can cause gastroenteritis, often with fever, that is typically mild and self-limited, lasting 1 to 2 days. However, in chronically ill or immunosuppressed patients and in patients who are very young, elderly, or pregnant, Listeria also can cause severe disease, with bacteremia and disseminated infection associated with a high mortality rate. Therapy, usually with ampicillin and gentamicin, is indicated.

Table 18.7. Food Poisoning Syndromes

Symptoms	Incubation period, h	Possible agents
Acute nausea, vomiting	6	Preformed toxins of Staphylococcus aureus, Bacillus cereus
Watery diarrhea	6-72	Clostridium perfringens, B cereus, ETEC, Vibrio cholerae, Giardia
Inflammatory ileocolitis ("dysentery")	16-72	Salmonella, Shigella, Campylobacter, EIEC, EHEC (O157:H7), Vibrio parahaemolyticus, Yersinia

Abbreviations: EHEC, enterohemorrhagic Escherichia coli; EIEC, enteroinvasive Escherichia coli; ETEC, enterotoxigenic Escherichia coli.

Data from Guerrant RL, Bobak DA. Bacterial and protozoal gastroenteritis. N Engl J Med. 1991 Aug 1;325(5):327-40.

C difficile Infection

Clostridium difficile, recently renamed and reclassified as *Clostridioides difficile*, is a spore-forming toxigenic bacterium that causes diarrhea and colitis, typically after antibiotic therapy. It is the most common health care infection in industrialized countries, and the number of cases of CDI in the community has increased sometimes in the absence of prior antibiotic exposure. Risk factors that predispose persons to CDI include age older than 65 years, antibiotic exposure, health care exposure, immunosuppression, chemotherapy, chronic kidney disease, surgery, malnutrition, proton pump inhibitor use, and critical illness.

These risk factors lead to disruption of the gut microbiome and predispose a person to colonization and active infection with *C difficile*. The acquisition and germination of spores, and an overgrowth of *C difficile* owing to a disrupted microbiome, leads to toxin production. Toxin A binds to mucosal receptors and causes cytotoxicity by disrupting cytoplasmic microfilaments and inducing apoptosis. Toxin B can then enter the damaged mucosa and cause further cytotoxicity, resulting in hemorrhage, inflammation, and cellular necrosis. The toxins also interfere with protein synthesis, stimulate granulocyte chemotaxis, increase capillary permeability, and promote peristalsis. In severe cases, inflammation and necrosis may involve deeper layers of the colon and result in toxic dilatation or perforation.

The spectrum of disease associated with CDI ranges from mild to moderate infection at 1 end to fulminant infection with sepsis or shock at the other. Colitis may range from minimal erythema or edema to ulceration, often with nodular exudates that may coalesce and form yellow pseudomembranes consisting of mucus and fibrin filled with dead leukocytes and mucosal cells (Figure 18.1).

Clinical Presentation

The time between the initiation of antibiotic therapy and the appearance of clinical symptoms varies from 1 day to 6 weeks and can be up to 12 weeks after antibiotic exposure. The clinical presentation ranges from only loose stools to toxic megacolon (nausea, vomiting, high-grade fever, and ileus) and colonic perforation. Typically, the disease manifests with watery or mucoid diarrhea, abdominal pain, and low-grade fever. Diarrhea may cause dehydration and electrolyte depletion. Rarely, disease is localized to the proximal colon; affected patients may present with an acute

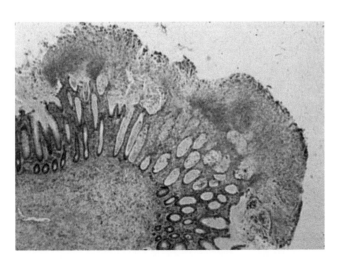

Figure 18.1. Pseudomembranous Colitis. Typical histologic appearance is shown (hematoxylin-eosin).

abdomen and localized rebound tenderness, no diarrhea, and normal findings on sigmoidoscopy. The overall mortality rate is low (2%-3%), although it is higher among elderly or debilitated patients (10%-20%) and patients with fulminant colitis or toxic megacolon (30%-80%).

Despite successful treatment, 20% to 30% of patients have a recurrence after a first infection; 40% to 50%, after a second infection; and more than 60%, after a third infection even after receiving guideline-based therapy.

Diagnostic Testing

An accurate diagnosis of CDI is based on a combination of risk factors, clinical findings, and stool testing. Endoscopy and biopsies have negligible value in the diagnosis of CDI owing to excellent sensitivity of available tests and a decreased incidence of pseudomembranes. Stool culture and cell cytotoxicity assays for *C difficile* are not used in clinical practice owing to the expense and the time required for the tests. An enzyme-linked immunosorbent assay for the detection of toxin A or B is limited by its lower sensitivity and is not used as an assay independently. Testing for fecal leukocytes lacks sensitivity and specificity.

Stool testing for CDI should not be performed in the absence of symptoms that suggest CDI, and a test of cure is not recommended after resolution of symptoms. Treatment of asymptomatic carriers is not recommended because it may prolong the carrier state and increase the risk of future CDI.

The most common test for CDI is a PCR assay, which has a sensitivity greater than 95% for a single stool sample. A PCR-based assay has limitations, including the inability to distinguish colonization from active infection because toxin production is not measured. Practice guidelines suggest that if PCR alone is used as an assay, it should be performed only when patients have otherwise unexplained diarrhea and CDI is a strong possibility. A test with negative results should not be repeated.

Most treatment guidelines now recommend a 2-step assay for an accurate diagnosis of CDI. The first step is to perform a glutamate dehydrogenase (GDH) assay and then an enzyme immunoassay (EIA) for toxins A and B. If results are positive for both GDH and EIA, the diagnosis is CDI. If results are negative for both GDH and EIA, CDI is ruled out. If the test results are discordant (ie, positive for GDH and negative for EIA), a PCR assay is performed. Interpretation of this testing algorithm is shown in Figure 18.2.

Treatment

Supportive therapy includes rehydration and, if possible, discontinuation of treatment with the offending antibiotic. Antidiarrheal agents and narcotics should be avoided because they may prolong exposure to toxins and result in more severe colitis. For severe disease, hospitalization for therapy and intravenous hydration may be necessary. If CDI is a strong possibility, empirical antibiotic therapy should be started after collecting a stool sample and before test results are known. Treatment options for CDI include therapy with antibiotics, a monoclonal antibody, and microbiome restoration. A management algorithm for CDI is included in Figure 18.3. Dosing regimens for CDI are included in Table 18.8.

Treatment of Primary Nonfulminant CDI

The preferred option for primary nonfulminant CDI is fidaxomicin 200 mg twice daily for 10 days. Fidaxomicin is as effective as vancomycin for clearing *C difficile* initially and is associated with

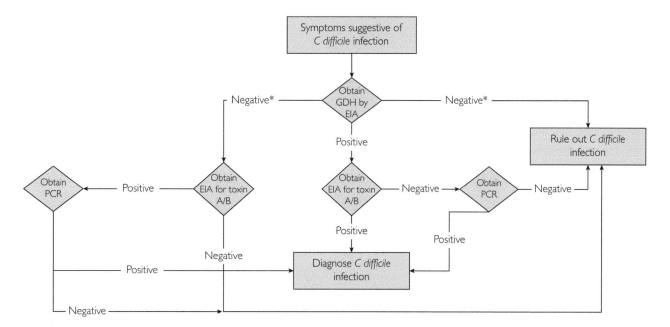

Figure 18.2. Algorithm for *Clostridioides difficile* Infection. Stepwise performance of 2-step testing algorithm for *C difficile* infection starts with glutamate dehydrogenase (GDH) assay, which is sensitive but not specific for *C difficile* infection, and subsequent enzyme immunoassay (EIA) for *C difficile* toxins. A polymerase chain reaction (PCR) test for *C difficile* is used to arbitrate discordant results. One asterisk (*) indicates that in most instances a negative result for GDH is not used to rule out *C difficile* infection; subsequent EIA for toxins A and B is performed (the diagnostic kits check for both GDH and the *C difficile* toxins). In some instances, a negative result for GDH may be used to rule out *C difficile* infection. (Adapted from Khanna S. My treatment approach to Clostridioides difficile infection. Mayo Clin Proc. 2021 Aug;96[8]:2192-204; used with permission.)

a lower likelihood of recurrent disease (recurrence rate, 25% with vancomycin and 15% with fidaxomicin). The use of fidaxomicin is limited by cost. An alternative to fidaxomicin is vancomycin at a dose of 125 mg 4 times daily for 10 days. Oral vancomycin is poorly absorbed, and a high concentration can be achieved in the stool without systemic adverse effects. If fidaxomicin and vancomycin are not available, metronidazole can be used (500 mg 3 times daily for 10 days).

Recurrences after CDI are common, and recurrent infection must be distinguished from developing postinfection irritable bowel syndrome. After resolution of CDI, postinfection irritable bowel syndrome develops in about 20% to 25% of patients, and symptoms may be overlapping. Patients with postinfection symptoms have fewer instances of diarrhea and may have intermittent constipation; their bowel habits are related to food, and their abdominal pain is relieved with defecation.

Treatment of First Recurrence of CDI

Most recurrences happen within 8 weeks of an initial infection. For a first recurrence, the general principle is to avoid repeating the course of antibiotics that was used for an initial infection. One option is a prolonged course of vancomycin therapy with a subsequent gradual tapering (eg, 125 mg 4 times daily for 2 weeks, 125 mg twice daily for 1 week, 125 mg daily for 1 week, 125 mg every other day for 1 week, and 125 mg every 3 days for 2 weeks). Other options include fidaxomicin, which can be given as a 10-day course or as an extended regimen (200 mg twice daily on days 1-5, none on day 6, and 200 mg once every other day on days 7-25).

Treatment of Multiply Recurrent CDI

Multiply recurrent CDI is managed with a course of antibiotics and subsequent microbiome restoration therapy, such as fecal

microbiota transplant (FMT) (which has been successful in more than 80%-90% of patients, as described below).

Treatment of Fulminant CDI

Fulminant CDI (such as in patients with sepsis, shock, or megacolon) is managed with a multidisciplinary approach, including a prompt surgical consultation. Vancomycin (500 mg 4 times daily) is administered orally or through a nasogastric tube supplemented with a vancomycin enema, especially in instances of paralytic ileus. In addition, intravenous metronidazole 500 mg 3 times daily is recommended. Diverting ileostomy or colectomy is performed for severe refractory disease or for complications such as perforation or megacolon. Because the risk of complications increases markedly after several days of ineffective therapy, some advocate surgery for patients with severe disease that does not respond after 2 to 7 days of treatment.

Antibody-Based Treatment

A 1-time dose of intravenous bezlotoxumab (10 mg/kg) can help with recurrent CDI. This treatment, approved by the US Food and Drug Administration (FDA), is not used as a sole treatment of CDI but as an adjunct to antibiotics during the antibiotic therapy. Bezlotoxumab is beneficial if at least 1 of the following risk factors is present: age older than 65 years, recent CDI (ie, in the past 6 months), immunosuppression, or presence of severe CDI (defined as a white blood cell count >15,000/μL or a creatinine value >1.5 mg/dL). A history of heart failure is a contraindication to the use of bezlotoxumab.

Microbiome-Based Therapies

Microbiome-based therapies, with FMT being the most common way to perform microbiome restoration, have shown promise in

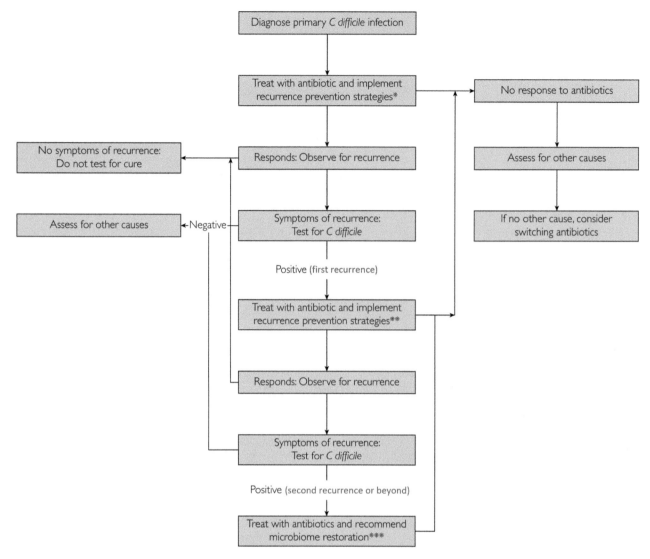

Figure 18.3. Management Algorithm for Nonfulminant *Clostridioides difficile* Infection. See Table 18.8 for dosing details. One asterisk (*) indicates use of oral vancomycin (standard) or fidaxomicin (standard or extended) and consideration of intravenous bezlotoxumab in patients at high risk for recurrence. Two asterisks (**) indicate use of oral vancomycin (taper and pulse) or fidaxomicin (standard or extended) while avoiding use of the same regimen as for the first episode and considering use of intravenous bezlotoxumab. Three asterisks (***) indicate use of a standard course of antibiotics with subsequent use of microbiota restoration therapies such as fecal microbiota transplant; alternatively, vancomycin (taper and pulse) or rifaximin chaser or fidaxomicin (extend) may be used. (Adapted from Khanna S. My treatment approach to Clostridioides difficile infection. Mayo Clin Proc. 2021 Aug;96[8]:2192-204; used with permission.)

Table 18.8. Dosing Regimens for *Clostridioides difficile* Infection

Regimen	Dosage
Vancomycin standard regimen	Vancomycin 125 mg orally 4 times daily for 10 d
Fidaxomicin standard regimen	Fidaxomicin 200 mg orally 2 times daily for 10 d
Fidaxomicin extended regimen	Fidaxomicin 200 mg orally 2 times daily for 5 d; then 200 mg once every other day on days 7-25 (20 doses)
Vancomycin taper and pulse	Vancomycin 125 mg orally 4 times daily for 14 d; then 2 times daily for 7 d, once daily for 7 d, once every other day for 8 d, and once every 3 d for 15 d (86 doses)
Rifaximin chaser regimen	Vancomycin 125 mg orally 4 times daily for 10-14 d; then rifaximin 550 mg orally twice daily for 10-14 d
Fulminant *C difficile* regimen	Vancomycin 500 mg orally 4 times daily in combination with IV metronidazole 500 mg 3 times daily (vancomycin 500 mg can be added rectally for ileus or suboptimal response)
Bezlotoxumab	One-time IV dose (10 mg/kg body weight) administered during an antibiotic course

Abbreviation: IV, intravenous.

Adapted from Khanna S. My treatment approach to Clostridioides difficile infection. Mayo Clin Proc. 2021 Aug;96(8):2192-204; used with permission.

the treatment of multiply recurrent CDI. Even though it is not an FDA-approved therapy, FMT is used commonly in this situation after completion of antibiotic therapy for an acute episode. FMT is dependent on the availability of stool from donors who have undergone screening for overall health and infectious diseases. Donors are excluded if they are very young or very old or if they have a disease associated with microbiome alterations. FMT is a heterogeneous practice, and recent FDA alerts warn of possible transmission of diarrheagenic and multidrug-resistant *E coli* and SARS-CoV-2.

- ✓ CDI—increased number of cases in the community with and without antibiotic exposure
- ✓ CDI diagnosis—2-step algorithm (glutamate dehydrogenase assay; then enzyme immunoassay for toxins A and B) with subsequent PCR if results are discordant
- ✓ CDI treatment
  - Fidaxomicin—first-line treatment; fewer recurrences compared to vancomycin
  - For first recurrence—vancomycin with a tapering dose; then pulse therapy
  - Metronidazole—not recommended in most instances
  - Intravenous bezlotoxumab—helps prevent recurrences in patients with high risk for recurrence
- ✓ Microbiome restoration by fecal microbiota transplant—experimental therapy with high efficacy for multiply recurrent CDI

Diverticulitis

In Western societies, colonic diverticulosis affects 5% to 10% of the population older than 45 years and 80% of those older than 80 years. Diverticulosis affects predominantly the sigmoid colon but may involve the entire colon. There is an association between diverticulosis and a Western diet high in refined carbohydrates and low in dietary fiber; whether this is a causal association is unproved. Patients with uninflamed and nonbleeding diverticula are usually asymptomatic. Diverticulitis is one of the most common gastrointestinal diagnoses in hospitals in the US.

Approximately 20% of patients with diverticula have an episode of symptomatic diverticulitis. If the neck of a diverticulum is obstructed, it may distend and lead to bacterial overgrowth and invasion, sometimes perforation, which is generally walled off by the adjacent mesocolon or appendices epiploicae. Stage I diverticulitis is characterized by small confined pericolonic abscesses, and stage II disease includes larger confined pericolonic collections. Stage III involves generalized suppurative peritonitis (perforated diverticulitis); because the diverticular neck is generally obstructed by a fecalith, peritoneal contamination by feces may not occur. Stage IV indicates fecal peritonitis.

Clinical Features

Symptoms of diverticulitis include lower abdominal pain, fever, and altered bowel habits (typically, diarrhea). Dysuria, urinary frequency, and urinary urgency reflect bladder irritation, whereas pneumaturia, fecaluria, and recurrent polymicrobial urinary tract infection suggest a colovesical fistula. Physical findings include fever, tenderness in the left lower quadrant of the abdomen, or a mass.

Rupture of a peridiverticular abscess or uninflamed diverticulum causes peritonitis, occurs more commonly in elderly and immunosuppressed persons, and is associated with a high mortality rate. Repeated episodes of acute diverticulitis may lead

to colonic obstruction. Jaundice or hepatic abscesses suggest pylephlebitis. A massively dilated (>10 cm) cecum, signs of cecal necrosis (ie, air in the bowel wall), or marked tenderness mandate immediate surgical consultation. Colovesical and, less frequently, colovaginal and colocutaneous fistulas may occur.

Diagnosis

The initial evaluation when diverticulitis is suspected should include a clinical evaluation and appropriate laboratory evaluation including a complete blood cell count. Computed tomography, the standard test for a diagnosis of diverticulitis, is used to assess disease severity and the risk of complications. If the clinical features are highly suggestive of mild uncomplicated diverticulitis, imaging studies may not be needed if patients have a history of diverticulitis.

Treatment

Treatment is influenced by severity, ability to tolerate oral intake, previous history of diverticulitis or bleeding, and complications. Mild diverticulitis can be treated without antibiotics and with bowel rest. Moderate or severe infections (including those with abscesses smaller than 3 cm) are managed with antibiotic courses. Percutaneous drainage is usually recommended for patients in stable condition who have an abscess larger than 3 cm. After an episode of acute complicated diverticulitis has resolved, a colonoscopy should be performed at around 6 to 8 weeks to exclude neoplasm.

If surgical treatment can be deferred until the acute inflammation heals, a single-stage primary resection and reanastomosis, perhaps laparoscopically, can be accomplished with minimal morbidity and mortality. Indications for elective surgery include recent diverticulitis with abscess or diverticulitis complicated by fistula, obstruction, or stricture. Elective surgical resection on the basis of a patient's young age at presentation is no longer recommended, and elective sigmoid colectomy after recovery from uncomplicated acute diverticulitis should be an individualized decision.

Indications for emergency surgery include diffuse peritonitis and failure of nonoperative management of acute diverticulitis. For emergency indications, the first stage of a 2-stage procedure involves resection of the diseased segment and creation of an end colostomy with oversewing of the distal colonic or rectal stump (Hartmann procedure). Colonic continuity may be reestablished in a second operation.

Prevention

A high-fiber diet, decreased intake of red meat, adequate water intake, and measures to avoid constipation may help prevent diverticulitis. The avoidance of nuts and popcorn does not prevent diverticulitis. Smoking cessation, physical activity, and weight loss are recommended to possibly decrease the risk of diverticulitis. The use of mesalamine, rifaximin, or probiotics does not decrease the risk of diverticulitis.

- ✓ Diverticular disease
  - Common, and incidence increases with age
  - Diverticulitis—most common complication
- ✓ Computed tomography of the abdomen and pelvis—most appropriate initial imaging when diverticulitis is suspected
- ✓ Treatment of diverticulitis
  - No antibiotics for mild uncomplicated diverticulitis
  - Percutaneous drainage for abscesses larger than 3 cm

- Most cases do not need surgical intervention
- Decisions related to surgery should be individualized on the basis of recurrent episodes and immunosuppression
- Elective colectomy is recommended for diverticulitis complicated by fistula, obstruction, or stricture
- Urgent partial colectomy is recommended for diffuse peritonitis or for failure of nonoperative management

✓ After resolution of acute diverticulitis, a colonoscopy should be performed 6 to 8 weeks later if one has not been performed recently

✓ Prevention—high-fiber diet; nuts and popcorn do not need to be limited

Suggested Reading

Hall J, Hardiman K, Lee S, Lightner A, Stocchi L, Paquette IM, et al. The American Society of Colon and Rectal Surgeons clinical practice guidelines for the treatment of left-sided colonic diverticulitis. Dis Colon Rectum. 2020 Jun;63(6):728–47.

Johnson S, Lavergne V, Skinner AM, Gonzales-Luna AJ, Garey KW, Kelly CP, et al. Clinical practice guideline by the Infectious Diseases Society of America (IDSA) and Society for Healthcare Epidemiology of America (SHEA): 2021 focused update guidelines on management of *Clostridioides* difficile infection in adults. Clin Infect Dis. 2021 Sep 7;73(5):755–7.

Khanna S. My treatment approach to *Clostridioides difficile* infection. Mayo Clin Proc. 2021 Aug;96(8):2192–204.

McDonald LC, Gerding DN, Johnson S, Bakken JS, Carroll KC, Coffin SE, et al. Clinical practice guidelines for *Clostridium difficile* infection in adults and children: 2017 update by the Infectious Diseases Society of America (IDSA) and Society for Healthcare Epidemiology of America (SHEA). Clin Infect Dis. 2018 Mar 19;66(7):e1–e48.

Shane AL, Mody RK, Crump JA, Tarr PI, Steiner TS, Kotloff K, et al. 2017 Infectious Diseases Society of America clinical practice guidelines for the diagnosis and management of infectious diarrhea. Clin Infect Dis. 2017 Nov 29;65(12):e45–e80.

19

Colorectal Neoplasms[a]

DEREK W. EBNER, MD

JOHN B. KISIEL, MD

Colorectal cancer (CRC) is primarily a disease of urban, industrialized societies. In the US, the lifetime risk of CRC is similar for men (4.4%) and women (4.1%). Recent data have suggested that the incidence rates of CRC may be decreasing gradually in some subgroups of the population but increasing in adults younger than 50 years. However, the mechanisms underlying these trends have not been defined completely. Several national organizations have endorsed screening and surveillance guidelines, which undoubtedly have contributed to more effective prevention of CRC.

Clinical Features

Definitions

Most cases (>95%) of CRC are adenocarcinomas. Less common cancer subtypes include lymphoma, neuroendocrine, and leiomyosarcoma. Metastatic lesions to the colorectum can include lymphoma, leiomyosarcoma, malignant melanoma, and adenocarcinomas of the breast, ovary, prostate, lung, and stomach. Because of the relative rarity of the other primary malignancies, the term *CRC* is used throughout the rest of this chapter to refer to *primary colon adenocarcinoma*. The term *colorectal neoplasia* is used to refer to either *malignant adenocarcinomas* or *premalignant precursor lesions*, as described in more detail below.

✓ **Colorectal cancer**—primary adenocarcinoma; can also include neuroendocrine, sarcomatous, and lymphomatous malignancies primary to the colon, but excludes metastasis
✓ **Colorectal neoplasia**—malignant adenocarcinoma or premalignant precursor lesions
✓ **Advanced colorectal neoplasia**—cancers and premalignant lesions with advanced features
✓ **Advanced features**—high-grade dysplasia, 1 cm or larger, and villous features
✓ **High-risk features**—advanced features or 3 or more premalignant precursors (or both); predictive of future advanced colorectal neoplasia

[a] Portions previously published in Limburg PJ, Ahlquist DA. Colorectal adenocarcinoma. In: Johnson LR, ed. Encyclopedia of gastroenterology. Academic Press; 2004:457-66 and Hawk ET, Limburg PJ, Viner JL. Epidemiology and prevention of colorectal cancer. Surg Clin North Am. 2002 Oct;82(5):905-41; used with permission.

Abbreviations: CMS, consensus molecular subtype; COX-2, cyclooxygenase 2; CRC, colorectal cancer; CT, computed tomography; EGFR, epidermal growth factor receptor; FAP, familial adenomatous polyposis; FOLFIRI, 5-fluorouricil, leucovorin, and irinotecan; FOLFOX, 5-fluorouracil, leucovorin, and oxaliplatin; HNPCC, hereditary nonpolyposis colorectal cancer; MAP, *MUTYH*-associated polyposis; MMR, mismatch repair; MSI, microsatellite instability; NCCN, National Comprehensive Cancer Network; SEER, Surveillance, Epidemiology, and End Results; SSL, sessile serrated lesion

Presentation

Clinical manifestations of CRC are often related to tumor size and location. Common signs and symptoms with proximal neoplasms (cecum to splenic flexure) include ill-defined abdominal pain, weight loss, and occult bleeding. Patients with distal neoplasms (descending colon to rectum) may present with altered bowel habits, decreased stool caliber, hematochezia, or a combination of these features. Colonoscopy is the test of choice for the diagnostic evaluation of any signs or symptoms suggestive of CRC because tissue specimens can be obtained at the time of visual inspection. Up to 7% of patients with CRC may have additional, synchronous malignancies in the colon or rectum at the time of the index cancer diagnosis. At the initial diagnosis of CRC, 37% of patients have localized disease, 35% have regional metastases, and 21% have distant metastases. Distant metastases typically occur in the liver, peritoneal cavity, and lungs. Less common sites of metastases are the adrenal glands, ovaries, and bones. Central nervous system metastases are rare.

Adenoma-Carcinoma Sequence

Most CRCs are thought to develop through an ordered series of events: Normal colonic mucosa develops into mucosa at risk, which develops into an adenoma, which develops into adenocarcinoma. Indirect evidence to support this adenoma-carcinoma sequence includes the following: 1) prevalence rates cosegregate within populations, 2) subsite distribution patterns within the colorectum are similar, 3) benign adenomatous tissue is often juxtaposed with invasive cancer in early-stage malignancies, and 4) incidence rates of CRC are decreased by endoscopic polypectomy.

A diverse group of molecular alterations has been associated with the adenoma-carcinoma sequence (Figure 19.1). Rather than a sequential progression through all these molecular alterations, several aberrancies commonly cluster together. The consensus molecular subtype (CMS) classification was developed to account for this molecular heterogeneity. CMS1 (immune) tumors show sequence variations or instability in normally repetitive regions

called microsatellites. In addition to microsatellite instability (MSI), CMS1 CRCs have aberrant hypermethylation in CpG islands, *BRAF* (OMIM 164757) sequence variants, and immune cell infiltration. CMS2 (canonical) tumors are characterized by chromosomal instability and activation of Wnt by *APC* (OMIM 611731) variation or other mechanisms. CMS3 (metabolic) CRCs harbor *KRAS* (OMIM 190070) variants and are typically low in DNA methylation. CMS4 (mesenchymal) cancers show stromal infiltration and transforming growth factor β activation. These features are useful for prognosis and selection of specific therapies (discussed below).

Polyp Subtypes

Adenomatous polyps are considered to have malignant potential, whereas hyperplastic, inflammatory, and hamartomatous (juvenile) polyps generally do not. Sessile serrated lesions (SSLs) confer an increased risk of future CRC and are implicated in being precursor lesions for microsatellite-unstable CRC (Figure 19.2). Adenomas can be classified further as tubular (70%-85%), villous (<5%), or tubulovillous (10%-25%) on the basis of their glandular histologic features and as low-grade or high-grade on the basis of their degree of dysplasia. "Advanced" adenomas are associated with an increased risk of CRC and usually are defined by 1) large size (≥1 cm), 2) any villous histologic features, or 3) high-grade dysplasia. Multiple (≥3) synchronous adenomas also are associated with an increased risk of CRC.

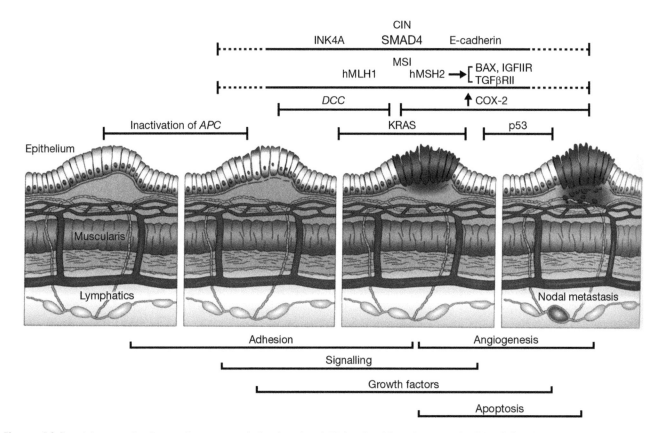

Figure 19.1.   Adenoma-Carcinoma Sequence and the Associated Molecular Alterations Involved in Colon Cancer Development. *APC* indicates adenomatous polyposis coli tumor suppressor gene; CIN, chromosomal instability; COX-2, cyclooxygenase 2; *DCC*, deleted in colorectal cancer gene; MSI, microsatellite instability. (Adapted from Van Schaeybroeck S, Lawler M, Johnston B, Salto-Tellez M, Lee J, Loughlin P, et al. Colorectal cancer. In: Niederhuber JE, Armitage JO, Doroshow JH, Kastan MB, Tepper JE, editors. Abeloff's clinical oncology. 5th ed. Philadelphia [PA]: Elsevier Churchill Livingstone; c2014. p. 1278-335.e14; used with permission.)

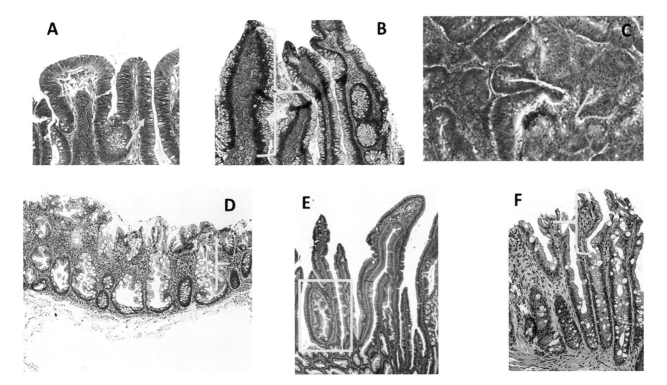

Figure 19.2. **Colon Polyp Architecture.** A, Tubular adenoma resembles normal colonic architecture but has irregular, crowded, and hyperchromatic nuclei (arrow). B, Villous adenoma has epithelial fingerlike projections (bracket) formed by fibrovascular cores and lined with dysplastic epithelium. C, High-grade dysplasia has architectural complexity, loss of nuclear polarity, and prominent nucleoli (arrow). D, Sessile serrated lesions (SSLs) often occur in the right colon. They have serrations that extend the length of the crypt (bracket) and boot-shaped deformity at the crypt base (arrow). E, Traditional serrated adenomas have "ectopic" crypts, which appear to be free-floating rather than anchored to the muscularis mucosae (frame). These lesions have malignant potential, are often in the left colon, and are much less common than SSLs. F, A hyperplastic polyp has serrations in only the upper half of the crypt (bracket). These are typically rectosigmoid in location and have no malignant potential. (Photos A, B, and C courtesy of Rondell P. Graham, MBBS, Anatomic Pathology, Mayo Clinic. Photos D, E, and F adapted from Sweetser S, Smyrk TC, Sinicrope FA. Serrated colon polyps as precursors to colorectal cancer. Clin Gastroenterol Hepatol. 2013 Jul;11[7]:760-7; used with permission.)

Staging and Prognosis

The American Joint Commission on Cancer system is commonly used to stage colon and rectal cancers (Table 19.1). It subcategorizes the pathologic stage of the tumor to correlate with prognosis. This classification system subdivides pathologic stages further to account for worse prognosis on the basis of the depth of tumor invasion, number of metastatic regional nodes, and number of metastatic sites. For colon cancers, the preoperative, or clinical, stage typically is determined by physical examination, computed tomography (CT), and chest radiography. For rectal cancer, endoscopic ultrasonography or pelvic magnetic resonance imaging can provide additional information about the depth of tumor invasion and regional lymph node status. The final CRC stage incorporates pathology review (lowercase letter *p*) of the resected tumor (T) tissue, lymph nodes (N), and biopsy of distant metastatic (M) disease. Before neoadjuvant radiochemotherapy, rectal cancers may be given a clinical stage according to imaging findings and designated by a lowercase letter *c,* or a lowercase *u* for endorectal ultrasonography, noted before the TNM scores; pathologic staging determined after neoadjuvant radiotherapy is designated by the lowercase letter *y.* Pathologic stage is the best predictor of survival. The overall 5-year survival rates for colon cancer and rectal cancer are generally similar (64%). By stage, 5-year survival rates are as follows: localized, 90%; regional (invaded nearby tissue or spread to nearby lymph nodes), 71%; and distant metastatic, 14%.

✓ Presenting symptoms of CRC
  • Proximal colon: ill-defined abdominal pain, weight loss, and occult bleeding
  • Distal colon: altered bowel habits and decreased stool caliber with or without hematochezia
  • Diagnostic colonoscopy is required for evaluation
✓ Adenoma carcinoma sequence
  • Up to 10 years for malignant transformation from early precursor to invasive cancer
  • Accumulation of molecular events that promote tumorigenesis
  • Molecular events aggregate into subtypes that have therapeutic and prognostic implications
✓ Precursor polyp lesions have different levels of risk for future advanced neoplasia
  • Removal of premalignant polyps results in lower population incidence of CRC
✓ Staging and prognosis
  • Pathologic stage is best predictor of survival
  • Five-year survival rate: 64% (localized, 90%; regional, 71%; and distant, 14%)

Epidemiologic Factors

General Distribution

Worldwide, CRC ranks third in cancer incidence for men and second for women. However, the incidence rates vary by global

Table 19.1. Colorectal Cancer Staging

Stage	TNM Classification[a,b]
0	Tis N0 M0
I	T1 or T2 N0 M0
IIA	T3 N0 M0
IIB	T4a N0 M0
IIC	T4b N0 M0
IIIA	T1-T2 N1/N1c M0
	T1 N2a M0
IIIB	T3-T4a N1/N1c M0
	T2-T3 N2a M0
	T1-T2 N2b M0
IIIC	T4a N2a M0
	T3-T4a N2b M0
	T4b N1-N2 M0
IVA	Any T any N M1a
IVB	Any T any N M1b
IVC	Any T any N M1c

[a] T category (primary tumor): Tis, tumor confined to mucosa; T1, tumor invades the submucosa; T2, tumor invades through the submucosa and into the muscularis propria; T3, tumor invades through the muscularis propria and into pericolorectal tissues; T4, tumor invades through the entire colorectal wall and into nearby tissues and organs.

[b] Prognosis varies with the following: 1) *Depth of tumor penetration*: T4a penetrates the surface of the visceral peritoneum and T4b invades into or adheres to other organs. 2) *Number of nodes*: N0 (no nodal metastases); N1a (metastasis in 1 regional node); N1b (metastasis in 2-3 regional nodes); N1c (no regional nodes but tumor in subserosa, mesentery, or nonperitonealized pericolic, or perirectal or mesorectal tissue); N2a (metastasis in 4-6 nodes); and N2b (metastasis in ≥7 nodes). 3) *Metastatic sites*: M0 (no distant metastasis); M1a (single metastatic site); M1b (multiple metastatic sites); and M1c (peritoneal carcinomatosis).

Adapted from Jessup J, Goldberg R, Asare E, Benson A, Brierly J, Chang G, et al. Colon and rectum. In: Amin MB, Edge SB, Greene FL, American Joint Committee on Cancer, eds. AJCC cancer staging manual. 8th ed. 2017:251-74; used with permission.

region (10-fold difference); most cases occur in industrialized regions. Areas with the highest reported incidence rates of CRC include North America, Australia and New Zealand, Western Europe, and Japan. Conversely, most parts of Africa and Asia report low incidence rates. In the US, both the incidence and the mortality for CRC decreased approximately 2% annually from 2007 to 2016. However, the incidence has increased among persons younger than 50 years. In the US, CRC is projected to account for 8% of new cancer diagnoses and for 9% of cancer-associated deaths among men and 8% among women in 2023.

Race and Ethnicity

Of the 5 major racial-ethnic population subgroups monitored by the Surveillance, Epidemiology, and End Results (SEER) program, Blacks in the US have the highest incidence and mortality rates for CRC. Although this likely is explained, at least partly, by differences in the stage of disease at the time of diagnosis, the survival gap persists when within-stage comparisons are made. Racial disparities in CRC burden are likely exacerbated by limited access to screening and lack of access to high-quality treatment.

Anatomical Subsite

Anatomical subsites of the colorectum differ in their embryologic origin, physiologic function, and vascular supply. Differences in the morphology, histology, and genetics of CRC have been observed across regions within the large bowel. Subsite-specific

incidence rates also differ, and the proportion of cases of CRC located in the proximal colon appears to be increasing compared with the proportion of cases in the distal colon and rectum.

Age

As with most malignancies, the incidence rates of CRC increase with advancing age. Less than 7% of cases occur among persons younger than 45 years. SEER data suggest that age-specific incidence rates of CRC begin to increase more rapidly during the fifth decade. The prevalence of adenomatous polyps also increases with age, with estimates of 30% at 50 years, 40% to 50% at 60 years, and 50% to 65% at 70 years. Also, several important clinical features of adenomas may be age-related. In the National Polyp Study, the risk of having a polyp with high-grade dysplasia was 80% higher among participants 60 years or older than among younger participants.

Personal History of Colorectal Neoplasia

Persons with a personal history of colorectal adenomas or adenocarcinomas are at increased risk (up to 6-fold) for additional, or metachronous, neoplasms. Adenoma characteristics associated with future tumor development include large size (≥1 cm), villous histology, and 3 or more lifetime colonic adenomas. Neither rectosigmoid hyperplastic polyps nor small, solitary tubular adenomas are strong risk factors for metachronous neoplasms. After resection of CRC, the annual incidence rate of a second primary colon or rectal cancer has been estimated at 0.35%.

Family History of Colorectal Neoplasia

Familial clustering occurs in approximately 20% of all cases of CRC, including patients with heritable cancer syndromes (see below). In the absence of an identifiable syndrome, a strong family history of colorectal neoplasia (typically defined as having 1 first-degree relative with colorectal neoplasia diagnosed before age 60 years or ≥2 first-degree relatives with colorectal neoplasia diagnosed at any age) appears to confer an approximately 1.5- to 2-fold increase in the risk of CRC.

Inflammatory Bowel Disease

Chronic ulcerative colitis and Crohn colitis are associated with an increased risk of CRC. In the US and Europe, the incidence of colitis-associated cancers appears to have decreased in recent decades but remains strongly correlated to the duration of chronic colitis. The extent of colitis has been positively associated with CRC risk (ie, the risk with pancolitis is greater than the risk with distal colitis, which is greater than the risk with proctitis), but the effects of disease activity have not been defined completely. Primary sclerosing cholangitis and a family history of CRC are additional risk factors. However, the effects of disease activity on the risk of CRC are not conclusively known. Screening for dysplasia is encouraged at 8 to 10 years after diagnosis of colonic inflammatory bowel disease and repeated every 1 to 5 years. Fewer data are available on the association between Crohn disease and CRC, but the risk appears to be comparable to that of chronic ulcerative colitis when more than one-third of the colon has been involved after a similar duration. Current data do not support an increased CRC risk for patients with lymphocytic or collagenous colitis.

Dietary Components

Excess body weight has been associated with a 1.5- to 2-fold increase in the risk of CRC, although not all observational studies have had consistent results. Red meat, particularly when consumed with a heavily browned surface, has been proposed as a risk factor for both benign and malignant colorectal neoplasia. Meats processed by salting, curing, fermentation, or smoking are listed by the World Health Organization as carcinogenic to humans.

Vegetables and fruits contain a wide array of potentially anticarcinogenic substances that may function through 1 or several independent or codependent mechanisms. Generally, vegetable consumption has been 1 of the most consistent predictors of reduced risk of CRC, but fruit consumption appears to be associated less strongly with reductions in large-bowel tumorigenesis.

Fiber enhances stool bulk, decreases the concentration of procarcinogenic secondary bile acids, and increases the concentration of anticarcinogenic short-chain fatty acids. Although multiple case-control studies initially suggested a protective effect from increased intake of dietary fiber, subsequent intervention trials have not shown appreciable reductions in the risk of CRC.

Calcium binds to intraluminal toxins and also influences mucosal proliferation within the colorectum. In 1 clinical trial, calcium supplementation was associated with a statistically significant 19% decrease in the recurrence of adenoma in postpolypectomy patients after 4 years. However, in another large, randomized, controlled trial of postmenopausal women, calcium and vitamin D supplementation for 7 years had no appreciable effect on incident CRC.

Antioxidants (including retinoids, carotenoids, ascorbic acid, α-tocopherol, and selenium) have been hypothesized to prevent carcinogen formation by neutralizing free radical compounds. So far, observational and experimental data have been unimpressive, with the exception that selenium decreased the risk of CRC by 58% when measured as a secondary end point in a skin cancer prevention study.

Folate and methionine supply methyl groups necessary for critical cellular functions such as nucleotide synthesis and gene regulation. Particularly in the context of excess alcohol consumption, dietary deficiencies of these compounds may be a risk factor for CRC. Nonetheless, in a recent multicenter clinical trial of participants with a previous history of benign colorectal neoplasia, folic acid 1 mg daily was associated with an increased risk of both recurrent advanced adenomas and noncolorectal cancers.

Lifestyle

Alcohol induces cellular proliferation, blocks methyl group donation, and inhibits DNA repair. Many observational studies have suggested a 2- to 3-fold increase in the risk of CRC with excess alcohol consumption, although a meta-analysis of 27 case-control and cohort studies found only a 10% increase in risk among daily alcohol users.

Tobacco smoke contains numerous putative carcinogens, including polycyclic aromatic hydrocarbons, nitrosamines, and aromatic amines. On the basis of data from several large cohort studies, smoking appears to be a risk factor for CRC after a prolonged latency of 20 or more years.

Physical activity has been associated consistently with a 40% to 50% decrease in the risk for CRC, particularly in the distal colon, through the stimulation of intestinal transit, decreased prostaglandin E_2 levels, or other undefined mechanisms.

Other

In a meta-analysis of data from 15 observational studies, patients with type 2 diabetes had a 30% increase in the risk for CRC compared with those without diabetes. Insulin resistance has been proposed as the underlying mechanism of tumorigenesis.

Persons with acromegaly may be predisposed metabolically or anatomically to higher risks for CRC. Because of the relative rarity of this condition, most observational studies have lacked adequate statistical power, but the preponderance of evidence supports a positive risk association.

Cholecystectomy results in an altered fecal bile acid composition. Two meta-analyses have reported moderately increased risks of 11% to 34% for CRC (mainly in the proximal colon) after gallbladder surgery.

✓ CRC epidemiology
- Third most common and fatal cancer in men (after lung and prostate cancers), third most common and fatal cancer in women (after lung and breast cancers), second most common and fatal cancer in men and women combined
- Incidence and mortality are increasing among persons younger than 50 years
- Blacks in the US have the highest incidence and mortality
- Incidence increases with age and male sex
- Personal history of advanced or high-risk colorectal neoplasia is the strongest risk factor for subsequent (metachronous) advanced neoplasia, including cancer
- Family history of CRC is identified in about 20% of all cases
- Inflammatory bowel disease involving the colon is a strong risk factor that increases the lifetime incidence by 2- to 3-fold
- Weaker risk factors: sedentary lifestyle, obesity, type 2 diabetes, alcohol, tobacco, and processed meat consumption

---

Heritable Syndromes

Well-defined hereditary CRC genetic syndromes account for approximately 2% to 5% of all large-bowel malignancies. An important point is that patients with gene variations are also at increased risk for target organ cancers outside the colorectum.

Familial Adenomatous Polyposis

Germline mutations in the *APC* gene form the basic molecular foundation for familial adenomatous polyposis (FAP) (an autosomal dominant condition). As many as 1 in 5 cases may result from new-onset spontaneous mutations. The estimated prevalence is 1 per 5,000 to 7,500 persons. Additional but unidentified genetic and environmental factors seem likely to influence the clinical manifestations of FAP because phenotypic features vary widely despite similar inherited *APC* alterations. The hallmark lesion of FAP is diffuse colorectal polyposis, and, typically, hundreds to thousands of adenomas develop during adolescence. Other findings include duodenal adenomas, gastric (fundic) gland hyperplasia, mandibular osteomas, and supernumerary teeth. In the absence of prophylactic colectomy, CRC inevitably is diagnosed in patients with FAP at a mean age of approximately 40 years. Even after colectomy, patients have an increased risk for cancer, particularly in the periampullary region of the duodenum and in the retained rectal remnant (if partial colectomy was performed).

Gardner syndrome is a variant of FAP in which patients with *APC* alterations have the same phenotypic features as in classic FAP, but they also can have osteomas of the skull and long bones, congenital hypertrophy of the retinal pigmented epithelium, desmoid tumors, epidermoid cysts, fibromas, and lipomas.

Attenuated FAP

Compared with classic FAP, attenuated FAP is associated with relatively fewer adenomas (<100) and a later onset of CRC (approximate age at onset, 55 years). About 40% of these cases are associated with germline *APC* alterations. Because both the adenomas and the cancers appear to arise in the proximal colon, at-risk family members should have screening with full colonoscopy rather than with flexible sigmoidoscopy, as recommended for screening in classic FAP kindreds.

Lynch Syndrome

Hereditary nonpolyposis CRC (HNPCC) is a clinical phenotype, and family history suggests that it is an autosomal dominant syndrome; features include early-onset CRC, usually located in the proximal colon, and increased risk of extracolonic malignancies (in the uterus, ovaries, stomach, urinary tract, small bowel, and bile duct). The clinical criteria for considering a person to be at risk for HNPCC are the Amsterdam criteria (Box 19.1). Lynch syndrome is a common cause of HNPCC. Lynch syndrome is genetically defined by the presence of a germline alteration in the DNA mismatch repair (MMR) genes or *EPCAM* gene (OMIM 185535). Because the Amsterdam criteria are not sufficiently sensitive to identify all cases of Lynch syndrome, and because MMR expression has therapeutic value, the National Comprehensive Cancer Network (NCCN) recommends that all colorectal primary tumors should be tested for phenotypes MMR deficiency (either MSI testing or MMR expression testing) (see the Universal Molecular Testing of Colon Cancer section below). If results are positive, germline variations should be sought in the DNA MMR genes (*MLH1* [OMIM 120436], *MSH2* [OMIM 609309], *MSH6* [OMIM 600678], and *PMS2* [OMIM 600259]) and *EPCAM*,

which maintain nucleic acid sequence integrity during replication. According to the NCCN, the specific germline variant can be used to further individualize the frequency of endoscopic screening and surveillance. Adenomas are believed to precede carcinomas in most instances, and CRC develops in 75% to 80% of patients with Lynch syndrome, at a median age of 46 years. It has been reported that for persons with Lynch syndrome, regularly performed colonoscopy with polypectomy can decrease the risk of large-bowel adenocarcinoma by approximately 60%. Patients who receive a diagnosis of CRC with Lynch syndrome are often treated with subtotal colectomy rather than segmental surgical resection. Women with Lynch syndrome have a very high risk for endometrial cancer and should be offered total hysterectomy or endometrial biopsy every 1 to 2 years. Not all patients with HNPCC have Lynch syndrome. Patients who meet the Amsterdam criteria for HNPCC and have MMR-proficient tumors are considered to have familial CRC type X, and those who have MMR-deficient tumors but no somatic or germline MMR gene variations are considered to have Lynch-like syndrome.

Turcot Syndrome

Turcot syndrome is a familial predisposition for both colonic polyposis and central nervous system tumors. It likely is a constellation of molecular features that can be variants of either FAP or Lynch syndrome. Patients with early-onset colonic polyposis associated with *APC* variations tend to have medulloblastomas (an FAP variant), whereas those with DNA mismatch repair gene variations are prone to the development of glioblastoma multiforme (a Lynch syndrome variant). Of interest, glioblastoma multiforme that arises in Turcot syndrome tends to occur at an earlier age and carry a better prognosis than the sporadic form of the tumor.

Muir-Torre Syndrome

Patients with Muir-Torre syndrome have sebaceous neoplasms, urogenital malignancies, and gastrointestinal tract adenocarcinomas in association with defective DNA mismatch repair. The ratio of affected men to women is 2:1.

Box 19.1.   Amsterdam Clinical Criteria for Hereditary Nonpolyposis Colorectal Cancer Syndrome

At least 3 relatives have had Lynch syndrome–related cancers[a]

At least 1 relative is a first-degree relative of 2 other affected persons

At least 2 successive generations have been affected

At least 1 relative received diagnosis before age 50 y

Familial adenomatous polyposis should be excluded in the colorectal cancer case(s) if any

Tumors should be verified by pathologic examination

---

[a] Including cancer of the colorectum, endometrium, small bowel, ureter, or renal pelvis.

Adapted from Vasen HF, Watson P, Mecklin JP, Lynch HT. New clinical criteria for hereditary nonpolyposis colorectal cancer (HNPCC, Lynch syndrome) proposed by the International Collaborative Group on HNPCC. Gastroenterology. 1999 Jun;116(6):1453-6; used with permission.

✓ **Hereditary nonpolyposis colorectal cancer (HNPCC)**—clinical phenotype of young-onset colon cancer, familial cancers associated with Lynch syndrome, and family history suggesting an autosomal dominant syndrome (Amsterdam criteria describe the clinical criteria)

✓ **Lynch syndrome**—1 of several diseases causing HNPCC; defined by germline variations in 1 of 4 DNA mismatch repair (MMR) genes (*MLH1, MSH2, MSH6, PMS2*) or *EPCAM*

✓ **Deficient MMR**—phenotypic feature of Lynch syndrome and other forms of HNPCC, which is measured by immunohistochemistry for MMR proteins or by microsatellite instability polymerase chain reaction testing and can be due to somatic (nonhereditary) events

✓ **Lynch-like syndrome**—deficient MMR phenotype but negative results with genetic testing for germline Lynch mutations and somatic (primary tumor) mutations in MMR genes

✓ **Familial CRC type X**—meets pedigree phenotype of HNPCC but has MMR-proficient tumors

✓ **Turcot syndrome**—familial predisposition for CRC and brain tumors and is likely a variant of FAP (medulloblastomas) or Lynch syndrome (glioblastomas)

✓ **Muir-Torre syndrome**—sebaceous neoplasms, urogenital malignancies, and gastrointestinal tract adenocarcinomas in association with deficient MMR

MUTYH-Associated Polyposis

MYH is a DNA base excision repair enzyme coded for by the gene *MUTYH* (OMIM 604933). *MUTYH*-associated polyposis (MAP) is an autosomal recessive syndrome with a wide-ranging phenotype. The colorectal adenoma burden in MAP can be similar to that in attenuated FAP, but there are reports of patients with MAP who have more than 100 adenomas. Also, duodenal and periampullary adenomas can be found in patients with MAP, although the true incidence of upper gastrointestinal tract neoplasia is not known. Biallelic carriers, or persons with variations in both *MUTYH* alleles, have an 80% cumulative risk of CRC by age 70 years, but monoallelic carriers do not appear to have an increased risk for CRC.

Hamartomatous Polyposis Syndromes

Peutz-Jeghers Syndrome

Peutz-Jeghers syndrome is an autosomal dominant condition characterized by multiple hamartomatous polyps scattered throughout the gastrointestinal tract. Up to 60% of cases of the syndrome are related to germline variations in the *LKB1* (*STK11*) gene (OMIM 602216). Melanin deposits usually can be seen around the lips, buccal mucosa, face, genitalia, hands, and feet, although occasionally the skin and intestinal lesions are inherited separately. Foci of adenomatous epithelium can develop within Peutz-Jeghers polyps and may be associated directly with an increased risk of CRC. Extracolonic malignancies include other gastrointestinal tract cancers (in the duodenum, jejunum, ileum, pancreas, biliary tree, and gallbladder), ovarian sex cord tumors, Sertoli cell testicular tumors, and breast cancer.

Tuberous Sclerosis

Tuberous sclerosis (an autosomal dominant condition) is associated with hamartomas, intellectual disability, epilepsy, and adenoma sebaceum. Adenomatous polyps may occur, particularly in the distal colon.

Juvenile Polyposis Syndrome

Juvenile polyposis syndrome is an autosomal dominant condition in which juvenile mucous retention polyps (misnamed hamartomata) can arise in the colon, stomach, or elsewhere in the gastrointestinal tract. Variations of genes in the transforming growth factor β pathway (*SMAD4* [OMIM 600993], *BMPR1A* [OMIM 601299], and *ENG* [OMIM 131195]) have been implicated as genetic causes of the syndrome. Symptoms of bleeding or obstruction may arise during childhood and may warrant surgery on the affected intestinal segments for treatment of anemia or obstruction or for cancer prevention. The risk of CRC is increased when synchronous adenomas or mixed juvenile-adenomatous polyps are present. If prophylactic or therapeutic colonic resection is performed, ileorectostomy or total proctocolectomy should be considered because of an increased risk of recurrent juvenile polyps within the retained colorectal segment. Of note, the presence of fewer than 5 juvenile polyps (including solitary polyps) in a person with no family history of juvenile polyposis syndrome does not indicate a heritable syndrome and, on the basis of current knowledge, does not warrant further diagnostic testing or aggressive cancer surveillance.

Cowden Disease

Cowden disease is an autosomal dominant condition in which persons with variations in the *PTEN* gene (OMIM 158350) may have trichilemmomas, other skin lesions, and alimentary tract polyps that are histologically similar to the polyps of juvenile polyposis syndrome. Patients with Cowden disease are at increased risk for breast cancer (often bilateral) and papillary thyroid cancer. The risk of CRC is not well-defined in this syndrome, but colonoscopy should be included in the original diagnostic evaluation.

Cronkhite-Canada Syndrome

Cronkhite-Canada syndrome is a noninherited condition manifested by signs and symptoms of malnutrition or malabsorption. Characteristic clinical features include alopecia and hyperkeratosis of the fingernails and toenails. In the US and Europe, Cronkhite-Canada syndrome typically develops in men, whereas in Asian countries, women appear to be affected more often. The neoplastic potential of gastrointestinal tract hamartomas in Cronkhite-Canada is uncertain; case reports of CRC in these patients suggest involvement of both typical adenomatous and serrated lesion pathways.

Prevention

Screening and Surveillance

For patients with average risk (defined as asymptomatic adults who are 45-75 years old [screening is individualized for patients 76-85 years old] and who do not have other known CRC risk factors), the US Multi-Society Task Force on Colorectal Cancer has endorsed the following screening options:

- Colonoscopy every 10 years
- Fecal immunochemical test annually
- Stool DNA test every 3 years
- Flexible sigmoidoscopy every 5-10 years
- CT colonography every 5 years
- Capsule colonoscopy every 5 years

Diagnostic colonoscopy should be performed in follow-up of any noninvasive screening test with positive findings.

For patients with a strong family history of colorectal neoplasia (excluding FAP, Lynch syndrome, and other identifiable syndromes), colonoscopy is advised every 5 years beginning at age 40 years (or 10 years before the youngest age at diagnosis in the family, whichever is earlier). *Strong family history* refers to patients with 1 first-degree relative who received a diagnosis of CRC or advanced adenoma when younger than 60 years or 2 second-degree relatives with CRC or advanced adenomas diagnosed at any age.

Recommendations for patients with high risk are shown in Table 19.2.

History of Colorectal Neoplasia in Persons Without High-Risk Diseases

After a complete clearing colonoscopy (ie, the bowel preparation was adequate and all colonic polyps were removed), subsequent examinations are determined according to polyp histology, size, and number.

✓ Risk-stratified intervals for follow-up colonoscopy
- Lowest risk (10 years): normal colonoscopy or no more than 20 hyperplastic polyps smaller than 10 mm

Table 19.2.   Screening and Surveillance Recommendations for Patients With High Risk for Colorectal Cancer

Condition	Gene(s)	Clinical features	Cancer risk reduction strategy
Lynch syndrome	MLH1 MSH2 and EPCAM MSH6 PMS2	Accelerated adenoma-carcinoma sequence Microsatellite instability (MSI) Risk of extracolonic cancers	Colonoscopy: baseline as early as age 20-25 y; follow-up varies with germline mutation (may be as short as every 1-2 y) EGD: starting at age 30-40 y; repeated every 2-4 y Consider prophylactic hysterectomy and bilateral salpingo-oophorectomy after childbearing Skin examination (annually) Consider pancreatic cancer evaluation (except for PMS2 carriers)
Familial adenomatous polyposis (FAP)	APC	≥100 Cumulative adenomas (10-99 in attenuated form and right-side predilection) Risk of gastric, duodenal, and ampullary carcinoma	Baseline colonoscopy at puberty; individualized time to colectomy; then ileorectal evaluation, pouchoscopy, or ileoscopy every 6-12 mo EGD: baseline at age 20-25 y with follow-up pending findings Thyroid evaluation (every 2-5 y)
MUTYH-associated polyposis (MAP)	MUTYH	Similar to attenuated FAP	Colonoscopy: baseline at age 25-30 y; repeat every 1-2 y EGD: baseline at age 30-35 y with follow-up pending findings
Peutz-Jeghers syndrome (PJS)	STK11	Clinical diagnosis if ≥2 of the following: ≥2 PJS polyps in GI tract Mucocutaneous pigmentation Family history	Colonoscopy and EGD: baseline at age 8-10 y; repeat every 2-3 y pending findings Small bowel: video capsule or enterography every 2-3 y Pancreatic cancer evaluation (annually) Additional extraintestinal screening
Juvenile polyposis syndrome (JPS)	SMAD4 BMPR1A	Clinical diagnosis if ≥5 juvenile polyps of the colon or multiple juvenile polyps throughout GI tract or any in patient with family history of JPS HHT with SMAD4	Colonoscopy and EGD: baseline at age 12-15 y; repeat every 2-3 y pending findings Screen for features associated with HHT among those with SMAD4 at first diagnosis
Serrated polyposis syndrome (SPS)	Unknown	≥5 Serrated lesions proximal to rectum, all ≥5 mm in size (≥2 being ≥10 mm in size) or >20 serrated lesions of any size throughout the colon with ≥5 proximal to rectum Polyp count is cumulative over lifetime	Surveillance colonoscopy every 1-3 y
Cowden syndrome	PTEN	Macrocephaly Trichilemmomas Marked esophageal glycogenic acanthosis	Colonoscopy: baseline at age 35 y; repeat every 5 y EGD: no screening recommendation Clinical breast examination and annual mammography Endometrial cancer screening with discussion of prophylactic hysterectomy Evaluation of skin (annually), thyroid (annually), and kidneys (every 1-2 y)
Inflammatory bowel disease (IBD)	NA	Ulcerative colitis and Crohn disease involving ≥33% of colon	Colonoscopy: baseline screening for flat dysplasia 8-10 y after symptom onset Random 4-quadrant biopsies every 10 cm Targeted biopsies should be handled separately Colonoscopy annually for patients with primary sclerosing cholangitis; otherwise, every 1-5 y according to cumulative risk factors (extent and duration of inflammation, family history, personal history of colorectal dysplasia) Pouch surveillance annually for patients with primary sclerosing cholangitis and personal history of colorectal cancer

Abbreviations: EGD, esophagogastroduodenoscopy; GI, gastrointestinal; HHT, hereditary hemorrhagic telangiectasia; NA, not applicable.

- Low-risk adenomas (7-10 years): 1 or 2 adenomas smaller than 10 mm
- Low-risk sessile serrated lesions (SSLs) (5-10 years): 1 or 2 SSLs smaller than 10 mm
- Moderate increased risk (3-5 years): 3 or 4 adenomas or SSLs smaller than 10 mm; large (≥10 mm) hyperplastic polyps (may be a misdiagnosed SSL)
- High-risk (3 years): 5 to 10 adenomas or SSLs (even if small); adenoma or SSL 10 mm or larger; villous architecture or high-grade dysplasia; traditional serrated adenoma
- Highest risk (1 year): more than 10 adenomas; serrated polyposis syndrome

Malignant polyps, defined as neoplasms with dysplastic cells invading through the muscularis mucosa into the submucosa, can be treated endoscopically, particularly for pedunculated polyps. However, for sessile polyps with endoscopic features suggesting submucosal invasion (depression, disrupted vessels, or amorphous pattern) there is greater risk for nodal metastases; biopsy, tattooing, and referral to surgery should be pursued preferentially in an otherwise surgically fit patient. The success of endoscopic management depends on 1) complete excision of the lesion and thorough examination (ideally en bloc) by a pathologist; 2) the depth of invasion and grade of differentiation; 3) the absence of high-risk features (poor differentiation, vascular invasion, and lymphatic involvement); and 4) the margin of excision being free of cancer cells by at least 1 mm. Follow-up colonoscopy should be performed at 3 months for malignant polyps that meet these favorable prognostic criteria.

Patients with potentially curable colon or rectal cancer should have a clearing colonoscopy preoperatively or within 3 to

6 months postoperatively if obstructive lesions prevented preoperative colonoscopy. After clearing colonoscopy, subsequent surveillance examinations can be performed at 1 year, 3 years, and 5 years if no additional colorectal neoplasia is found. In addition, histologically favorable tumor stage 1 rectal cancers treated endoscopically or by transanal excision (without complete surgical staging to obtain lymph nodes) should be assessed with endoscopic ultrasonography or magnetic resonance imaging of the pelvis every 6 months for 5 years.

Chemoprevention

Chemoprevention is the use of chemical compounds to prevent, inhibit, or reverse carcinogenesis before the invasion of dysplastic epithelial cells across the basement membrane. In its broadest sense, chemoprevention includes both nutritional and pharmaceutical interventions. With regard to pharmaceutical agents, nonsteroidal anti-inflammatory drugs are structurally diverse, yet they appear to share abilities to decrease proliferation, slow cell cycle progression, and stimulate apoptosis. Extensive epidemiologic data uphold a negative risk (40%-60%) association between the regular use of nonsteroidal anti-inflammatory drugs and colorectal tumors. The chemopreventive effects of these drugs are thought to be derived through cyclooxygenase 2 (COX-2) inhibition. In several large clinical trials, agents that selectively block this enzyme isoform (celecoxib and rofecoxib) have been shown to decrease the recurrence rates of adenoma. However, selective COX-2 inhibitors have been associated also with increased cardiovascular toxicity, which has limited their chemopreventive applications to high-risk clinical settings. Emerging research suggests that combining COX-2 inhibitors with targeted epidermal growth factor receptor (EGFR) inhibitors (eg, erlotinib) may greatly decrease the duodenal polyp burden in patients with FAP.

Universal Molecular Testing of Colon Cancer

At the time of CRC diagnosis, testing of the primary tumor for deficiency of MMR enzymes is recommended by the US Preventive Services Task Force and the NCCN. The phenotypes of MMR deficiency include MSI marker polymerase chain reaction and deficient expression by immunohistochemistry. Either test may be ordered depending on local expertise. Positive results require confirmation with germline sequencing of Lynch syndrome causative variations; if those results are negative, other causes of MMR deficiency, *MLH1* hypermethylation and *BRAF* alteration, should be investigated. Testing for these are advised to confirm that these sporadic events (not requiring genetic testing of relatives) caused the MMR deficiency phenotype. Universal testing is used 1) to diagnose Lynch syndrome and refer family members for genetic testing and 2) to select therapy for patients with metastatic disease.

Treatment of CRC

Treatment of tumors above the peritoneal reflection differ from treatment of those in the rectum. The approaches are therefore described separately.

For most patients who have colon cancer proximal to the rectum, in the absence of known distant metastases or prohibitive comorbid conditions, surgical excision is the initial treatment. Chemotherapy with or without radiotherapy is not provided before surgical resection; it may be considered for selected patients who have advanced disease or if local cancer is inoperable. Extended segmental resection is performed to ensure sufficient sampling of a minimum of 12 lymph nodes for accurate staging. The procedure, if feasible, is preferentially performed laparoscopically as opposed to an open incision because of faster recovery and otherwise comparable morbidity and mortality. Subtotal colectomy or total proctocolectomy may be performed in patients who have colorectal neoplasia in multiple colonic segments or in patients who have familial cancer syndromes. Operative intervention also may be considered for selected patients who have isolated liver or lung metastases. For surgically incurable patients, resection of the primary cancer is usually indicated only if there is bleeding, obstruction, or impending obstruction. Postoperative, or adjuvant, cytotoxic chemotherapy is recommended for patients with stage III (lymph node involvement) colon cancer. It should be considered also for patients with stage II colon cancer who have poor prognostic factors (poor differentiation, lymphovascular or perineural invasion, T4 primary cancer, perforation, indeterminate or positive margins, or tumor budding) according to pathology review. The preferred regimen is FOLFOX (5-fluorouracil, leucovorin, and oxaliplatin) for 6 months.

Rectal adenocarcinoma should be managed through a multidisciplinary surgical, radiation, and medical oncology team. Adenocarcinomas in the middle and upper rectum usually are removed by a sphincter-sparing endoscopic resection or surgery. Cancers in the lower rectum (0-5 cm above the anal verge) often require abdominoperineal resection, with a permanent colostomy. However, sphincter-sparing procedures may be offered if complete resection is possible, if small rectal tumors are present, or while waiting for the response of large or invasive tumors to preoperative chemoradiotherapy or radiotherapy. Preoperative, or neoadjuvant, treatment with 5-fluorouracil–based chemotherapy in combination with radiotherapy generally is indicated for patients with tumors that are staged as T3 and higher or N1 and higher by CT of the chest abdomen and pelvis, retrograde endoscopic ultrasonography, or magnetic resonance imaging of the pelvis. Adjuvant chemotherapy with 5-fluorouracil and leucovorin (with or without oxaliplatin) is recommended for patients with stage II or stage III rectal cancer. For palliation of metastatic disease, both FOLFOX and FOLFIRI (a regimen containing irinotecan in place of oxaliplatin) are accepted as first-line cytotoxic regimens. Molecularly targeted therapies have shown benefits for subsets of patients with metastatic or advanced CRC; emerging data show benefit for those with early-stage rectal cancer. Bevacizumab is a humanized monoclonal antibody that targets vascular endothelial growth factor, impairing the proliferation of endothelial cells and formation of new blood vessels. Cetuximab and panitumumab are monoclonal antibodies that target EGFR. Pembrolizumab and nivolumab are monoclonal antibodies that act as immune checkpoint inhibitors, which bind to programmed cell death 1 on T cells and promote immune-mediating destruction of cancer cells. Ipilimumab is also a monoclonal antibody checkpoint inhibitor that binds to cytotoxic T-lymphocyte antigen-4, activating antitumor immunity. Checkpoint inhibitors are most likely beneficial in those with MSI high/MMR-deficient CRC. *KRAS* tumor testing is used to select which patients will respond best to an EGFR inhibitor, which may improve outcomes for patients with advanced tumors with wild-type *KRAS*. In contrast, mutant *KRAS* constitutively activates the RAS-RAF-ERK pathway downstream from EGFR, resulting in resistance to anti-EGFR therapy.

Suggested Reading

American Cancer Society. Colorectal cancer facts & figures. American Cancer Society; 2023.

Cooper K, Squires H, Carroll C, Papaioannou D, Booth A, Logan RF, et al. Chemoprevention of colorectal cancer: systematic review and economic evaluation. Health Technol Assess. 2010 Jun;14(32):1–206.

Gbolahan O, O'Neil B. Update on systemic therapy for colorectal cancer: biologics take sides. Transl Gastroenterol Hepatol. 2019 4:9.

Giardiello FM, Allen JI, Axilbund JE, Boland CR, Burke CA, Burt RW, et al. Guidelines on genetic evaluation and management of Lynch syndrome: a consensus statement by the us multi-society task force on colorectal cancer. Am J Gastroenterol. 2014 Aug;109(8):1159–79.

Guinney J, Dienstmann R, Wang X, de Reynies A, Schlicker A, Soneson C, et al. The consensus molecular subtypes of colorectal cancer. Nat Med. 2015 Nov;21(11):1350–6.

Gupta S, Lieberman D, Anderson JC, Burke CA, Dominitz JA, Kaltenbach T, et al. Recommendations for follow-up after colonoscopy and polypectomy: a consensus update by the US Multi-Society Task Force on Colorectal Cancer. Gastrointest Endosc. 2020 Mar;91(3):463–85.

Ma H, Brosens LAA, Offerhaus GJA, Giardiello FM, de Leng WWJ, Montgomery EA. Pathology and genetics of hereditary colorectal cancer. Pathology. 2018 Jan;50(1):49–59.

Murthy SK, Feuerstein JD, Nguyen GC, Velayos FS. AGA clinical practice update on endoscopic surveillance and management of colorectal dysplasia in inflammatory bowel diseases: expert review. Gastroenterology. 2021 Sep;161(3):1043–51.

National Cancer Institute. Cancer stat facts: colorectal cancer. https://seer.cancer.gov/statfacts/html/colorect.html

Rex DK, Boland CR, Dominitz JA, Giardiello FM, Johnson DA, Kaltenbach T, et al. Colorectal cancer screening: recommendations for physicians and patients from the US Multi-Society Task Force on Colorectal Cancer. Am J Gastroenterol. 2017 Jul;112(7):1016–30.

Syngal S, Brand RE, Church JM, Giardiello FM, Hampel HL, Burt RW, et al. ACG clinical guideline: genetic testing and management of hereditary gastrointestinal cancer syndromes. Am J Gastroenterol. 2015 Feb;110(2):223–62.

US Preventive Services Task Force, Davidson KW, Barry MJ, Mangione CM, Cabana M, Caughey AB, et al. Screening for colorectal cancer: US Preventive Services Task Force recommendation statement. JAMA. 2021 May 18;325(19):1965–77.

Wolpin BM, Mayer RJ. Systemic treatment of colorectal cancer. Gastroenterology. 2008 May;134(5):1296–310.

20

Irritable Bowel Syndrome

PRIYA VIJAYVARGIYA, MD

DAVID O. PRICHARD, MB, BCH, PHD

Irritable bowel syndrome (IBS) is characterized by abdominal pain and altered bowel habits in the absence of detectable biochemical or structural abnormalities. The goal of therapy is to improve the patient's symptoms, prevent suffering, and improve quality of life. Altered bowel habits and abdominal pain may need to be treated independently. The bidirectional relationship between gastrointestinal symptoms and psychological issues is well established, and behavioral therapies are effective.

Definition

The current symptom criteria for the diagnosis of IBS, based on the Rome IV criteria, are presented in Box 20.1. The Rome criteria were developed in conjunction with the World Congress of Gastroenterology held in Rome, Italy, in 1988 and were revised in 1999 (Rome II), 2006 (Rome III), and 2016 (Rome IV). The Rome criteria are similar to the criteria established by Manning and colleagues in 1978. However, the Rome criteria incorporate constipation-type symptoms into the definition. The dominant bowel pattern of patients is used to classify IBS into 4 categories: diarrhea-predominant IBS (IBS-D), constipation-predominant IBS (IBS-C), mixed-type IBS (IBS-M), and unclassified IBS (IBS-U) (Figure 20.1).

As with any set of criteria, there is a trade-off between sensitivity and specificity, depending on the threshold used. In clinical practice, this can be helpful. The more criteria a patient meets, the more likely the patient is to have IBS.

Epidemiology

IBS is a common condition, affecting 10% to 20% of the population in industrialized countries. Not everyone with IBS seeks medical care, so incidence data are difficult to obtain. One estimate of the incidence of clinically diagnosed IBS is 196 per 100,000 person-years. However, about 10% of the general population reports the onset of IBS symptoms over a 1-year period. The difference between the clinical incidence and onset figures likely reflects the limited use of health care by some persons with IBS and the fluctuating pattern of IBS symptoms. Still, this is much higher than the incidence of colon cancer (50 per 100,000

Box 20.1. Diagnostic Criteria for Irritable Bowel Syndrome[a]

Recurrent abdominal pain on an average of ≥1 d/wk with ≥2 of the following:

   a. Pain related to defecation

   b. Associated with a change in frequency of stool

   c. Associated with a change in form (appearance) of stool

---

[a] Criteria fulfilled for the past 3 months, with symptom onset at least 6 months before diagnosis.

Adapted from Lacy BE, Mearin F, Chang L, Chey WD, Lembo AJ, Simren M, et al. Bowel disorders. Gastroenterology. 2016;150(6):1393-407; used with permission.

Abbreviations: FDA, US Food and Drug Administration; FODMAP, fermentable oligosaccharides, disaccharides, monosaccharides, and polyols; HLA, human leukocyte antigen; IBS, irritable bowel syndrome; IBS-C, constipation-predominant irritable bowel syndrome; IBS-D, diarrhea-predominant irritable bowel syndrome; IBS-M, mixed-type irritable bowel syndrome; IBS-U, unclassified irritable bowel syndrome.

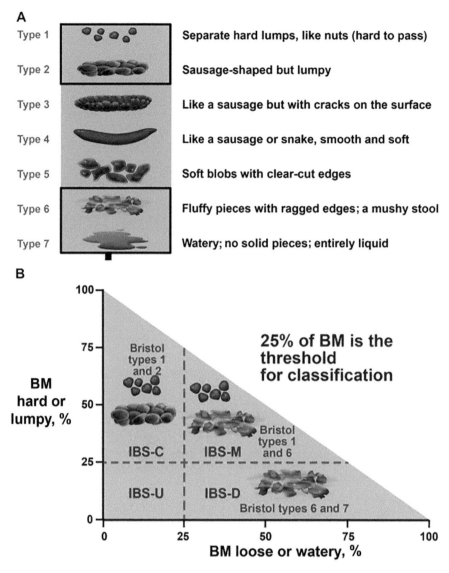

Figure 20.1. **Relationship Between Predominant Bowel Habit and Subtypes of Irritable Bowel Syndrome (IBS).** A, The Bristol Stool Form Scale recognizes 7 types of stool consistency. B, The stool type in the bowel movement (BM) is used to classify IBS subtypes as constipation-predominant IBS (IBS-C), diarrhea-predominant IBS (IBS-D), mixed-type IBS (IBS-M), or unclassified IBS (IBS-U). (Adapted from Lacy BE, Mearin F, Chang L, Chey WD, Lembo AJ, Simren M, et al. Bowel disorders. Gastroenterology. 2016;150[6]:1393-407; used with permission.)

person-years) and inflammatory bowel disease (10 per 100,000 person-years).

Risk Factors

Multiple risk factors have been proposed for IBS. In clinic-based studies, there is a strong association with sex. However, the female to male ratio in the community is approximately 2:1. Thus, sex may have a role not only in the onset of IBS but also in health care–seeking behavior. Even though the prevalence of IBS decreases slightly with age, new symptoms may occur in the elderly. Prevalence estimates are available from around the world, but no consistent racial or ethnic differences have been identified.

Multiple studies have assessed the role of personality characteristics, psychiatric illness, and physical and sexual abuse in the development of IBS. These associated characteristics are seen more frequently in patients with IBS evaluated in academic medical centers, likely reflecting the severity of IBS or personality traits (or both).

Many patients with IBS report that a family member also has the condition. Familial aggregation of IBS exists, and twin studies have suggested a genetic component. Other studies have shown that health care for gastrointestinal problems is sought more frequently among children of parents who have gastrointestinal symptoms. Additional study is needed to characterize the influence of nature and nurture in the development of IBS.

Postinfectious IBS is a well-recognized subtype of IBS that develops de novo after bacterial or viral gastroenteritis. The propensity for postinfectious IBS to develop is associated with female sex, duration of illness, and the psychological state (anxiety and depression) of the person at the time of infection. It usually develops into a diarrhea-predominant phenotype.

Food sensitivities also may have a role in the development of IBS. Patients with IBS symptoms report more sensitivity to food than people without symptoms. This could potentially be secondary to increased colonic contractions after eating associated with the gastrocolic reflex, alteration in the microbiome, insoluble foods that may result in increased gas production and water secretion, or changes in intestinal epithelial barrier function. To date, the data on exclusion diets have not convincingly shown that food is a cause of the symptoms. Moreover, only 25% of patients who completed a double-blind reintroduction of known symptomatic foods experienced a return of abdominal symptoms.

Pathogenesis

The cause of IBS is unknown. In the past, the predominant pathophysiologic mechanisms in IBS were perceived to be abnormalities intrinsic to the smooth muscle of the gut, visceral hypersensitivity, and psychological stress. Current models of pathophysiology suggest a role for altered motility, intraluminal intestinal irritants such as maldigested carbohydrates or fats, excess bile acids, gluten intolerance, visceral hypersensitivity, autonomic dysfunction, immune activation, and alterations in gut microbiome and epithelial permeability. A bidirectional association between the brain and gut has been established. Where conditions involving both are present, the psychiatric and psychological conditions preceded gastrointestinal symptoms in 50% of patients, and gastrointestinal symptoms preceded psychiatric and psychological conditions in the other 50%.

Slow colonic transit occurs in 25% of patients with IBS-C. Disorders of rectal evacuation, such as functional defecatory disorders and descending perineum syndrome, may mimic symptoms of IBS-C and are important to consider in the differential diagnosis.

Rapid colon transit occurs in up to 45% of patients with IBS-D. Disorders that mimic IBS-D include disaccharidase deficiencies, celiac disease, microscopic colitis, gluten intolerance without celiac disease, and idiopathic bile acid malabsorption. In selected studies, approximately 25% of patients with IBS-D had high concentrations of fecal bile acids; whether this is the cause or the consequence of accelerated colonic transit is unclear.

There is an association between ingestion of food and the induction of gastrointestinal symptoms in IBS. The fat content of the meal appears to have a key role in provoking gastrointestinal symptoms in IBS by inducing high-amplitude colonic contractions. In addition, ingestion of poorly absorbed, fermentable oligosaccharides, disaccharides, monosaccharides, and polyols (FODMAP) may induce symptoms of IBS. Studies have demonstrated that patients with human leukocyte antigen (HLA)-DQ2 or HLA-DQ8 genotypes without celiac disease are more likely to respond to gluten withdrawal than patients without these genotypes.

Alterations in the intestinal microbiome may be a relevant pathophysiologic mechanism in IBS. Small intestinal bacterial overgrowth may be the cause of IBS-like symptoms.

Diagnosis

The diagnosis of IBS is symptom based (Box 20.1). IBS can be categorized according to the patient's predominant bowel habits or most bothersome symptom (Figure 20.1). IBS-D is strictly defined as type 6 or 7 on the Bristol Stool Form Scale. IBS-C is characterized by stools described as type 1 or 2. The presence of other functional gastrointestinal disorders (eg, functional dyspepsia), nongastrointestinal disorders (eg, fibromyalgia or chronic fatigue), or psychological comorbidities (eg, depression or anxiety) support the diagnosis of IBS.

A symptom-based diagnosis is recommended when patients fulfill the diagnostic criteria, clinical examination findings are normal, and the patient does not have warning symptoms (no overt blood within the stool, weight loss, recent change in bowel habits, nocturnal pain or passage of stools, family history of colorectal cancer or inflammatory bowel disease, palpable abdominal mass or lymphadenopathy, or iron deficiency anemia). Only limited investigation should be performed. A complete blood cell count, celiac serology, and C-reactive protein can be evaluated for all patients. Thyrotropin test, fecal calprotectin test, and stool culture and microscopy can be considered. Colonoscopy should be offered to patients older than 50 years who are not current with high-quality colon cancer screening.

Some patients who have pronounced symptoms despite empirical therapy (discussed below) will seek further care. For these patients, an approach that considers the patient's predominant symptom is recommended (Figure 20.2). For patients with IBS-C, a detailed rectal examination should be performed to exclude a functional defecatory disorder or other anorectal pathology. Tests to consider for patients with IBS-D include measurement of fecal bile acids, duodenal aspirate or hydrogen breath testing for bacterial overgrowth, and colonic biopsies for microscopic colitis. The yield of these tests is low, but they are useful for evaluating patients who have chronic diarrhea with increased stool volume. Rarely, stool chemistry tests for surreptitious laxative abuse may be considered. If pain is predominant, a plain radiograph of the abdomen when the patient is having severe pain may help to exclude obstruction.

✓ IBS—symptom-based diagnosis defined by recurrent abdominal pain associated with 2 or more of the following:
- Pain associated with defecation
- Change in stool frequency
- Change in stool consistency

✓ IBS—in the absence of alarm features, only limited investigations should be performed

---

Prognosis

The natural history of IBS is becoming better understood. In approximately 30% of patients, the symptoms resolve within a year. This contributes to the placebo response rate, which has made evaluation of investigative agents difficult. Although IBS symptoms may resolve, symptoms of another functional gastrointestinal disorder develop in almost half the patients. Thus, the degree to which the gastrointestinal symptoms resolve completely is not clear. A pattern of the condition coming, going, and changing over time is quite common. Ten years after diagnosis, 50% to 70% of patients continue to have symptoms.

Management

Management of IBS requires an integrative approach based on an understanding of the patient's desired outcomes (ie, what symptoms are most bothersome). Patients must be educated about IBS and reassured about the low probability of organic disease. Simple investigations, as described above, should be performed. Abnormal bowel habits and abdominal pain should be treated with the simplest and safest agents. However, physicians must be aware that altering stool frequency or consistency may not reduce abdominal pain; each may require independent treatment. Coexisting psychological factors must be addressed with appropriate pharmacologic and nonpharmacologic means. Until an initial therapeutic trial is complete (ie, 3-6 weeks), further investigations should be

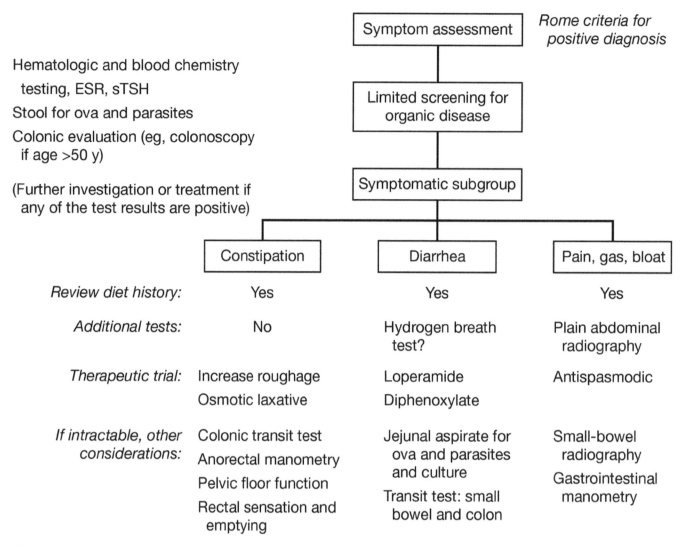

Figure 20.2. **Management of Irritable Bowel Syndrome.** ESR indicates erythrocyte sedimentation rate; sTSH, sensitive thyrotropin. (Adapted from Drossman DA, Whitehead WE, Camilleri M. Irritable bowel syndrome: a technical review for practice guideline development. Gastroenterology. 1997 Jun;112[6]:2120-37; used with permission.)

deferred. The hope is that the patient will be reassured about the diagnosis and will have a response to the initial therapy.

Exercise

Moderate to vigorous exercise (eg, walking, aerobics, and cycling) can decrease the severity of IBS symptoms. Patients who continue to exercise frequently can also experience long-term improvement in sleep, energy, and physical functioning. Different exercises may offer different benefits. For example, yoga and walking both decrease gastrointestinal symptoms. However, yoga may be more beneficial for reducing somatic symptoms (eg, nausea, dizziness, and fatigue), while walking may be more beneficial for depression and anxiety. It is not known whether exercise benefits 1 type of IBS more than others. A small proportion of people have worse symptoms with exercise.

Dietary Management

For every patient, a dietary history is important to ensure that the patient is not consuming products that may inadvertently cause

diarrhea, constipation, or bloating. Based on the observation that food can trigger or exacerbate symptoms, 4 specific dietary interventions can be offered to patients with IBS: general dietary advice, soluble fiber, low-FODMAP, and a gluten-free diet.

General dietary recommendations are to consume small meals, regularly spaced throughout the day, and avoid insoluble fiber, fatty foods, and caffeine. Soluble fiber (eg, psyllium) but not insoluble fiber (eg, wheat bran) reduces global symptoms in both IBS-D and IBS-C. Greater response rates are seen in patients with IBS-C. When only a limited number of food triggers are present, specific avoidance is the simplest restriction diet. When dietary triggers are numerous or unclear, a low-FODMAP or gluten-free diet, undertaken with the help of a dietician, may be beneficial. A low-FODMAP diet has been found to decrease abdominal bloating and gas production. Correctly undertaking this diet requires the complete elimination of all FODMAPs to determine symptomatic response, with subsequent stepwise reintroduction of FODMAP groups to identify those that provoke symptoms. Only FODMAPs associated with symptoms should be excluded thereafter. Notably, the low-FODMAP diet has not been shown to be superior to conventional, less restrictive diets. A gluten-free diet may offer similar benefit but is predominantly beneficial for patients with HLA-DQ2 and HLA-DQ8 haplotypes. The long-term consequences for patients with IBS continuing to eat a low-FODMAP or gluten-free diet are unknown.

Alterations of the Microbiome

In randomized controlled trials, the minimally absorbed antibiotic rifaximin relieved bloating, abdominal pain, and watery stools in patients with IBS-D. The mechanism underlying the beneficial effect is unclear. Symptoms recur in a high proportion of patients, and retreatment may be required. Rifaximin is approved by the US Food and Drug Administration (FDA) for the treatment of IBS-D. There are insufficient data from patients with IBS to support the use of prebiotics or probiotics.

Medications for Abdominal Pain

Several medications can be used to treat IBS-associated abdominal pain. No randomized controlled trials have directly compared their clinical efficacy.

The antispasmodics hyoscyamine and dicyclomine promote smooth muscle relaxation by antagonism of acetylcholine at the muscarinic receptor. The data supporting the efficacy of these medications is low to moderate, but both demonstrate a good safety profile. These medications can be given to treat existent pain (eg, hyoscyamine sublingually) or prophylactically (eg, 20 minutes before eating) to decrease postprandial symptoms. These medications inhibit intraluminal fluid secretion and may offer greater benefit to patients with IBS-D. Peppermint oil, which inhibits smooth muscle contraction through calcium channel blockade, has shown more efficacy than placebo in reducing the symptom burden in patients who have IBS-D or IBS-M.

Neuromodulators can provide considerable pain relief to patients with IBS. The choice of antidepressant should consider the underlying subtype of IBS and other psychological and physical factors. Tricyclic antidepressants (eg, amitriptyline, nortriptyline, and desipramine) are associated with a reduction in IBS symptom severity, particularly pain, discrete from alterations in mood. They prolong intestinal transit and are preferentially used in patients with IBS-D. They may also improve sleep and anxiety. A serotonin norepinephrine reuptake inhibitor such as duloxetine may reduce visceral pain in patients with fibromyalgia and depression. Pooled data suggest that selective serotonin reuptake inhibitors (eg, citalopram, paroxetine, and fluoxetine) do not improve global symptoms. However, where anxiety or stress are exacerbating symptoms, these medications may be of benefit. Selective serotonin reuptake inhibitors can shorten intestinal transit time and may be more appropriate for patients with IBS-C. These medications do not have FDA approval for the treatment of IBS, so care should be taken when counseling patients on potential benefits and adverse effects.

Pregabalin, a structural derivative of the neurotransmitter γ-aminobutyric acid, showed more efficacy than placebo in a double-blind placebo-controlled trial for reducing abdominal pain and overall symptom severity in patients with IBS-D, IBS-C, or IBS-M. In addition, subscores were lower for diarrhea and bloating but not constipation. Similar to the situation with antidepressants, pregabalin is not approved by the FDA for the treatment of IBS.

Medications for Diarrhea

Loperamide and eluxadoline are approved by the FDA for the treatment of IBS. Loperamide, a μ-opioid receptor agonist with anticholinergic effects, decreased bowel motion frequency, increased stool consistency, and decreased abdominal pain in small clinical trials involving patients with IBS-U. It worsened symptoms in patients with constipation. Eluxadoline, a novel μ- and κ-opioid receptor agonist and δ-opioid receptor antagonist, showed efficacy for decreasing abdominal pain and improving stool consistency on the same day for at least 50% of the days. The effects on stool frequency and form were greater than the effect on abdominal pain. Owing to an increased risk of pancreatitis, eluxadoline should be prescribed only to patients who have an intact gallbladder and minimal alcohol intake. The use of diphenoxylate (a μ- and δ-opioid receptor agonist) in combination with atropine (an antimuscarinic) is approved by the FDA only for the treatment of diarrhea.

In patients with IBS-D, the type 3 serotonin receptor antagonists ondansetron and alosetron decreased symptom severity, urgency, and frequency to a greater extent than placebo. In addition, ondansetron reduced the severity of bloating. Alosetron, but not ondansetron, is approved by the FDA for the treatment of IBS. In approximately 0.3% of patients receiving alosetron, ischemic colitis develops, so patients must be counseled about this risk.

Bile acid sequestrants can be used to treat diarrhea. Use of cholestyramine, available only in a powder formulation, carries the highest rates of nausea, but the drug is most readily covered by insurance companies. Colesevelam and colestipol are available in pill formulation. In patients with IBS-D, colesevelam increased stool consistency but had no effect on stool frequency. In general, bile acid sequestrants have few serious adverse effects. Constipation and bloating can be avoided by starting at a low dose and increasing it slowly to the lowest dose that relieves symptoms. Patients should be advised that bile acid sequestrants will also bind other medications and therefore should be taken 2 hours before or 4 hours after other medications. None has FDA approval for the treatment of bile acid diarrhea or IBS.

In truly refractory cases, treatment with clonidine, verapamil, or octreotide may be considered. However, use of these treatments is off-label.

Medications for Constipation

Simple laxatives (ie, osmotic or stimulant) are first-line therapy for the treatment of IBS-C, although they do not have FDA approval for this indication. Osmotic laxatives (eg, polyethylene glycol, magnesium, sodium phosphate, and nonabsorbable carbohydrates such as lactulose or sorbitol) retain fluid in the intestinal lumen and accelerate colonic transit. Use of lactulose and sorbitol should be avoided in patients with IBS because of the bloating associated with these medications. Stimulant laxatives (eg, Senokot [Avrio Health LP], bisacodyl, and glycerin) induce high-amplitude propagated colonic contractions. There is little evidence to suggest that patients become dependent on these medications with long-term use. Stimulant laxatives are best used as rescue agents when the patient has not had a bowel movement for several days.

Three secretagogues have FDA approval for IBS-C. By stimulating a net efflux of ions and water into the intestinal lumen, these secretagogues accelerate transit and facilitate defecation. Lubiprostone, a bicyclic fatty acid derivative of prostaglandin E_1, works mainly by activating apical type 2 chloride channels. Nausea, a common adverse effect of lubiprostone, may be lessened by ingestion with food. Linaclotide and plecanatide are guanylate cyclase-C agonists that induce opening of cystic fibrosis transmembrane regulator chloride channels on intestinal mucosa cells. At high doses (290 µg daily), linaclotide reduces abdominal pain; the effect is greater in patients with more severe pain.

The type 4 serotonin receptor agonist prucalopride, recently approved for the treatment of chronic idiopathic constipation, has not been approved by the FDA for the treatment of IBS.

Alternative Therapies

The bidirectional association between psychological distress and IBS is well established. When formal psychiatric disorders are present, appropriate therapy is mandatory. Even when a psychiatric disorder has not been diagnosed, the use of psychological intervention is helpful in the management of IBS. Cognitive behavioral therapy, dynamic psychotherapy, and hypnotherapy are effective psychological therapies in the management of IBS. These may be particularly beneficial when established precipitants of anxiety or stress worsen gastrointestinal symptoms. Overall, the number needed to treat for psychological therapies is 4 (95% CI, 3-5). Psychology-based self-aid (ie, education) has been shown to be beneficial for treating all subtypes of IBS. In addition, patients with IBS may benefit from formal pain management approaches.

✓ Patient education about the underlying disease process of IBS (eg, visceral hypersensitivity or central sensitization) increases acceptance of the diagnosis and decreases the use of health care
✓ Initial treatment of IBS—lifestyle and dietary modifications with symptomatic remedies
✓ Pain and bowel symptoms in IBS may require independent treatment
✓ A bidirectional association exists between psychological distress and IBS
  • Cognitive behavioral therapy and hypnotherapy are effective psychological therapies
  • Formal psychiatric disorders (eg, depression) should be treated concurrently by an appropriately trained physician
✓ Patients with persistent gastrointestinal symptoms despite empirical therapies may require tests to identify causative factors

---

Health Care Use

Older data suggest that IBS accounts for 3.5 million physician visits, 2.2 million prescriptions, and 35,000 hospitalizations annually. Primary care physicians provide most care for patients with IBS, although a survey of gastroenterologists indicated that 28% of their patient population had IBS. Expenditures accountable to IBS are difficult to determine. Recent estimates suggest that the additional costs of health care for patients with IBS, when compared with control groups, are approximately $2,250 for patients with IBS-D and $3,850 for patients with IBS-C. For both, 78% was from medical costs and 22% was from prescription costs. Additionally, IBS is associated with higher absenteeism, which is 75% higher among patients with IBS-D compared with control groups. These direct and indirect costs make the total cost of IBS considerable.

Summary

The diagnosis of IBS is symptom based. Routine serologic screening for celiac disease in patients with IBS is recommended. Initial treatment involves lifestyle and dietary modifications with symptomatic remedies. Patients with persistent gastrointestinal symptoms despite these initial measures should undergo tests to identify causative factors.

Suggested Reading

Camilleri M. Peripheral mechanisms in irritable bowel syndrome. N Engl J Med. 2012 Oct 25;367(17):1626–35.
Canavan C, West J, Card T. The epidemiology of irritable bowel syndrome. Clin Epidemiol. 2014 6:71–80.
Dionne J, Ford AC, Yuan Y, Chey WD, Lacy BE, Saito YA, et al. A systematic review and meta-analysis evaluating the efficacy of a gluten-free diet and a low FODMAPs diet in treating symptoms of irritable bowel syndrome. Am J Gastroenterol. 2018 Sep;113(9):1290–300.
Enck P, Aziz Q, Barbara G, Farmer AD, Fukudo S, Mayer EA, et al. Irritable bowel syndrome. Nat Rev Dis Primers. 2016 Mar 24;2:16014.
Ford AC, Lacy BE, Talley NJ. Irritable bowel syndrome. N Engl J Med. 2017 Jun 29;376(26):2566–78.
Ford AC, Quigley EM, Lacy BE, Lembo AJ, Saito YA, Schiller LR, et al. Effect of antidepressants and psychological therapies, including hypnotherapy, in irritable bowel syndrome: systematic review and meta-analysis. Am J Gastroenterol. 2014 Sep;109(9):1350–65.
Lacy BE, Mearin F, Chang L, Chey WD, Lembo AJ, Simren M, et al. Bowel disorders. Gastroenterology. 2016;150(6):1393–407.
Locke GR, 3rd. Natural history of irritable bowel syndrome and durability of the diagnosis. Rev Gastroenterol Disord. 2003 3 Suppl 3:S12–7.
Saito YA, Mitra N, Mayer EA. Genetic approaches to functional gastrointestinal disorders. Gastroenterology. 2010 Apr;138(4):1276–85.

21

Constipation and Fecal Incontinence[a]
ADIL E. BHARUCHA, MBBS, MD

Constipation

Colonic Motor Physiology and Pathophysiology: Salient Aspects

Function

Colonic functions include the absorption of water and electrolytes, storage of intraluminal contents until elimination is socially convenient, and nutrient salvage from bacterial metabolism of carbohydrates that are not absorbed in the small intestine. The colon absorbs all but 100 mL of fluid and 1 mEq of sodium and chloride from approximately 1,500 mL of chyme received over 24 hours. Absorptive capacity can increase to 5 to 6 L of fluid and 800 to 1,000 mEq of sodium and chloride daily. In a healthy person, the average mouth-to-cecum transit time is approximately 6 hours, and average regional transit times through the right, left, and sigmoid colon are about 12 hours each, with an average total colonic transit time of 36 hours. (The physiology of defecation is discussed in the "Disorders of Pelvic Floor Function" section below.)

Regional Differences in Colonic Motor Function

The right colon is a reservoir that mixes and stores contents and absorbs fluid and electrolytes. The left colon is primarily a conduit, whereas the rectum and anal canal are responsible for continence and defecation. The ileocolic sphincter regulates the intermittent transfer of ileal contents into the colon, a process that normalizes in response to augmented storage capacity in the residual transverse and descending colon within 6 months after right hemicolectomy.

Motor Patterns

Colonic motor activity is extremely irregular, ranging from quiescence (particularly at night) to isolated contractions, bursts of contractions, or propagated contractions. This activity is in contrast to that of the small intestine, where rhythmic migrating motor complexes occur. Colonic contractions are *tonic* or sustained, lasting several minutes to hours, and shorter or *phasic*. *Propagated phasic contractions* propel colonic contents over longer distances than nonpropagated phasic contractions. *High-amplitude propagated contractions* are more than 75 mm Hg in amplitude, occur about 6 times daily (frequently after awakening and after meals), are responsible for mass movement of colonic contents, and frequently precede defecation. Stimulant laxatives such as bisacodyl (Dulcolax; Sanofi Consumer Health Inc) and glycerol induce high-amplitude propagated contractions.

Colonic Contractile Response to a Meal

Neurohormonal mechanisms are responsible for increased colonic motor activity beginning within a few minutes after ingestion of a meal of 500 kcal or more. The term *gastrocolic reflex* is a misnomer because this response, induced by gastric distention and chemical stimulation by nutrients, is observed even after gastrectomy. This response may explain postprandial urgency and abdominal discomfort in patients with irritable bowel syndrome (IBS).

[a] Portions of this chapter have been adapted from Bharucha AE. Treatment of severe and intractable constipation. Curr Treat Options Gastroenterol. 2004 Aug;7(4):291-8; used with permission and Bharucha AE, Knowles CH, Mack I, Malcolm A, Oblizajek N, Rao S, et al. Faecal incontinence in adults. Nat Rev Dis Primers. 2022 Aug 10;8(1):53.

Abbreviations: DD, defecatory disorder; 5-HT, 5-hydroxytryptamine (serotonin); IBS, irritable bowel syndrome; MR, magnetic resonance; MRI, magnetic resonance imaging; NASHA/Dx, nonanimal stabilized hyaluronic acid/dextranomer; PNTML, pudendal nerve terminal motor latency

Colonic Relaxation

Colonic relaxation resulting from sympathetic stimulation or opiates may cause acute colonic pseudo-obstruction, or Ogilvie syndrome. Stimulation of α_2-adrenergic receptors decreases the release of acetylcholine from excitatory cholinergic terminals in the myenteric plexus, thereby inhibiting gastrointestinal motility. Conversely, reduced tonic inhibition of the sympathetic system impairs the net absorption of water and electrolytes and accelerates transit in patients who have diabetic neuropathy, thus explaining their diarrhea. Clonidine restores the sympathetic brake, reducing diarrhea.

Colocolonic Inhibitory Reflexes

Peristalsis is a local reflex mediated by intrinsic nerve pathways and characterized by contraction proximal to the distended segment and relaxation distal to the distended segment. In addition, rectal or colonic distention can inhibit motor activity in the stomach, small intestine, or colon. These inhibitory reflexes are mediated by extrinsic reflex pathways with synapses in the prevertebral ganglia, independent of the central nervous system. They may account for delayed left colonic transit or small intestinal transit (or both) in patients with obstructive defecation.

Serotonin and the Gut

About 95% of the body's serotonin (5-hydroxytryptamine [5-HT]), a monoamine neurotransmitter, is in the gut: 90% in enterochromaffin cells and 10% in enteric neurons. The effects of 5-HT are mediated by receptors located on gut neurons, smooth muscle, and enterochromaffin cells. There are 7 families of 5-HT receptors. The 5-HT$_3$ and 5-HT$_4$ receptors and, to a lesser degree, the 5-HT$_{1p}$, 5-HT$_{1a}$, and 5-HT$_2$ receptors are important targets of pharmacologic modulation in the gut. Cisapride, prucalopride, and tegaserod maleate (Zelnorm; Alfasigma USA, Inc) are 5-HT$_4$ receptor agonists. Alosetron is a more potent 5-HT$_3$ receptor antagonist than ondansetron.

The effects of 5-HT are motor and sensory. Motor effects involve stimulation of serotoninergic 5-HT$_4$ receptors, which facilitate both components of the peristaltic reflex: proximal excitation coordinated with distal inhibition. Thus, stimulation of 5-HT$_4$ receptors located on cholinergic enteric neurons induces the

release of acetylcholine and enhances contractility, whereas 5-HT$_4$ receptor–mediated stimulation of inhibitory neurons releases inhibitory neurotransmitters (eg, nitric oxide or vasoactive intestinal polypeptide), which relax smooth muscle.

Sensory effects involve the 5-HT$_3$ and 5-HT$_4$ receptors located on intrinsic primary afferent neurons, which initiate peristaltic and secretory reflexes. The 5-HT$_3$ receptors are located also on extrinsic sensory afferents and vagal afferents, which partly explains why 5-HT$_3$ antagonists reduce nausea.

Assessment of Colonic Transit

Colonic transit can be measured with commercially available radiopaque markers (Sitzmarks; CMX Medical Imaging), scintigraphy, or a wireless pH and pressure-sensing capsule. These techniques entail counting the number of orally ingested markers that remain in the colon as seen on plain radiographs of the abdomen. One approach is to administer a capsule containing 20 markers on day 1. Delayed colonic transit is indicated if 8 or more markers are seen on plain films on day 3 or if 5 or more markers are seen on day 5. With scintigraphy, the isotope (generally technetium Tc 99m or indium In 111) is delivered into the colon by orocecal intubation or within a delayed-release capsule. The delayed-release capsule contains radiolabeled activated charcoal covered with a pH-sensitive polymer (methacrylate) designed to dissolve in the alkaline pH of the distal ileum. This releases the radioisotope within the ascending colon. Gamma camera scans taken 4, 24, and, if necessary, 48 hours after ingestion of the isotope show the colonic distribution of isotope. Regions of interest are drawn around the ascending, transverse, descending, and sigmoid colon and the rectum; counts in these areas are weighted by factors 1 through 4, respectively, and stool counts are weighted by a factor of 5. Thus, colonic transit may be summarized as an overall geometric center (Figure 21.1). The 4-hour scan identifies rapid colonic transit, and the 24-hour and 48-hour scans show slow colonic transit. Assessments of colonic transit made with radiopaque markers, scintigraphy, and the pH and pressure capsule are comparable. The radiopaque marker technique is simpler and more widely available. However, with scintigraphy, colonic transit can be assessed in 48 hours, compared with 5 to 7 days for radiopaque markers. Moreover, gastric, small intestinal, and

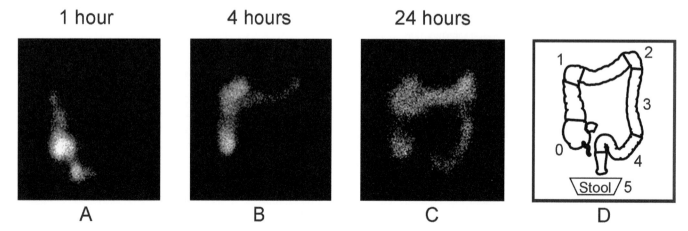

1 hour   **4 hours**   **24 hours**

A   B   C   D

Figure 21.1. Scintigraphic Assessment of Colonic Transit. Images show progression of isotope through cecum and ascending colon at 1 hour (A), ascending and transverse colon at 4 hours (B), and ascending, transverse, descending, and rectosigmoid colon at 24 hours (C). D, Numbers represent average isotope distribution corresponding to a geometric center of 1 to 5. In this patient, the geometric center at 24 hours was 2.2 (normal, 1.6-3.8). (Adapted from Bharucha AE, Klingele CJ. Autonomic and somatic systems to the anorectum and pelvic floor. In: Dyck PJ, Thomas PK, eds. Peripheral neuropathy. 4th ed. Philadelphia [PA]: Elsevier; 2005: 279-98; used with permission.)

colonic transit can be assessed simultaneously with scintigraphy and the wireless pH and pressure capsule.

Constipation

Definition and Classification

Chronic constipation may be classified on the basis of symptoms or according to colonic transit and anorectal functions. The symptom-based criteria (ie, the Rome criteria), which were developed by a committee of experts, are essential for clinical trials and research studies but are also useful in clinical practice. By convention, these symptom criteria need to be present for at least 3 months, with a total symptom duration of at least 6 months.

Functional constipation is defined by 2 or more of the following symptoms: 1) fewer than 3 defecations per week, 2) straining, 3) lumpy or hard stools, 4) sensation of incomplete evacuations, 5) sensation of anorectal obstruction or blockage, and 6) manual maneuvers to facilitate defecation. For symptoms 2 through 6 (as listed above) to be considered present, they should occur with one-fourth of defecations.

Constipation-predominant IBS is defined by abdominal discomfort and at least 2 of the following 3 symptoms: 1) abdominal discomfort associated with change in stool form (ie, hard stools), 2) abdominal discomfort associated with change in stool frequency (ie, less frequent stools), and 3) abdominal discomfort relieved by defecation.

However, many patients satisfy criteria for functional constipation and constipation-predominant IBS. Hence, a more practical approach is to characterize constipation as *painful* or *painless*. Patients with painful constipation report more abdominal pain, disability, somatic symptoms, and urinary urgency than those with painless constipation. (*Diarrhea-predominant syndrome* is defined by loose and less frequent stools instead of hard and more frequent stools.) Table 21.1 summarizes the salient differences between functional constipation and constipation-predominant IBS.

Clinical Assessment

Clinical assessment of constipation should focus on identifying 1) secondary causes (Table 21.2 and Box 21.1); 2) inadequate

dietary intake of calories and fiber; 3) a history of physical, emotional, or sexual abuse; and 4) obstructive defecation. Bowel diaries are more accurate than self-reporting for characterizing bowel habits, particularly stool frequency. As characterized by the Bristol Stool Form Scale, stools that are hard, small pebbles correlate with delayed colonic transit, and stools that are watery (at the other extreme) correlate strongly with accelerated colonic transit. In contrast to stool frequency recorded in diaries, frequency reported from recall alone does not correlate with colonic transit. Certain symptoms (prolonged straining, sense of anorectal blockage, tendency to facilitate defecation by assuming different positions, difficult evacuation of soft stool, and digital maneuvers to facilitate defecation) are suggestive but not diagnostic of functional defecatory disorders (DDs). The examination may identify anismus, inadequate perineal descent, or, conversely, ballooning of the perineum with excessive descent.

Practical Classification of Constipation

A practical approach to classifying and managing chronic constipation is shown in Figure 21.2. After secondary causes of constipation have been excluded, anorectal functions should be assessed in patients who have constipation that does not respond to dietary fiber supplementation or over-the-counter laxatives (or both in combination). Anorectal tests are necessary because symptoms alone cannot be used to distinguish among constipation resulting from DDs, normal transit, and slow transit. DDs, which are characterized by symptoms of constipation and anorectal test results indicative of disordered defecation, should be primarily managed with pelvic floor retraining (biofeedback therapy). When anorectal test results are normal, colonic transit should be assessed to distinguish normal from slow transit constipation. When anorectal test results are abnormal (ie, they indicate a DD), it is not essential to evaluate colonic transit before biofeedback therapy because the management is the same, regardless of whether colonic transit is normal or slow; 50% of patients with DD have slow colonic transit. However, colonic transit should be evaluated in patients with DD who do not respond to biofeedback therapy.

Table 21.1. Differences Between Functional Constipation and Constipation-Predominant IBS

Variable	Functional constipation	Constipation-predominant IBS
Symptom criteria	Symptoms for ≥6 mo and for >25% of defecations during preceding 3 mo: • Straining • Lumpy or hard stools • Sensation of incomplete evacuation • Sensation of anorectal obstruction/blockage • Manual maneuvers to facilitate defecations <3 defecations/wk • Loose stools not present and insufficient criteria for IBS	Recurrent abdominal pain or discomfort ≥3 d/mo in the preceding 3 mo associated with ≥2 of the following: • Improvement with defecation • Onset associated with change in frequency of stool • Onset associated with change in form (appearance) of stool • <25% of bowel movement were loose stools
Upper gastrointestinal tract symptoms (eg, heartburn, dyspepsia), anxiety and depression, urinary symptoms	Less common[a]	More common[a]
Prevalence of defecatory disorder	About 50% of patients	About 50% of patients
Prevalence of increased rectal sensation	Less common[b]	More common[b]

Abbreviation: IBS, irritable bowel syndrome.
[a] The prevalence of these symptoms varies by individual symptom; hence, specific figures are not provided.
[b] The prevalence of increased rectal sensation varies among studies.

Adapted from Bharucha AE, Wald A. Chronic constipation. Mayo Clin Proc. 2019 Nov;94(11):2340-57; used with permission.

Table 21.2.   Medications Associated With Constipation

Class	Examples
5-HT$_3$ receptor antagonists	Ondansetron
Analgesics	
Opiates[a]	Morphine
NSAIDs[a]	Ibuprofen
Anticholinergic agents	Librax, belladonna
Tricyclic antidepressants[a]	Amitriptyline > nortriptyline
Antiparkinsonian drugs	Benzatropine
Antipsychotics	Chlorpromazine
Antispasmodics[a]	Dicyclomine
Antihistamines[a]	Diphenhydramine
Anticonvulsants[a]	Carbamazepine
Antihypertensives	
Calcium channel blockers	Verapamil, nifedipine
Diuretics[a,b]	Furosemide
Centrally acting	Clonidine
Antiarrhythmics	Amiodarone
β-Adrenoceptor antagonist	Atenolol
Bile acid sequestrants	Cholestyramine, colestipol
Cation-containing agents	
Aluminum[a]	Antacids, sucralfate
Calcium	Antacids, supplements
Bismuth	
Iron supplements	Ferrous sulfate
Lithium	
Chemotherapy agents	
Vinca alkaloids	Vincristine
Alkylating agents	Cyclophosphamide
Miscellaneous compounds	Barium sulfate, oral contraceptives, polystyrene resins
Endocrine medications	Pamidronate and alendronic acid
Other antidepressants	Monoamine oxidase inhibitors
Other antipsychotics	Clozapine, haloperidol, risperidone
Other antiparkinsonian drugs	Dopamine agonists
Other antispasmodics	Mebeverine, peppermint oil
Sympathomimetics	Ephedrine, terbutaline

Abbreviations: 5-HT, 5-hydroxytryptamine (serotonin); NSAID, nonsteroidal anti-inflammatory drug.
[a] Drugs associated with constipation in community-based studies.
[b] Perhaps related to electrolyte disturbances.

Adapted from Branch RL, Butt TF. Drug-induced constipation. Adverse Drug React Bull. 2009 (257):987-90; used with permission.

Box 21.1.   Medical Conditions Associated With Constipation

Drug effects
Mechanical obstruction
  Colon cancer
  External compression from malignant lesion
  Strictures: diverticular or postischemic
  Rectocele (some)
Metabolic conditions
  Type 2 diabetes
  Hypothyroidism (severe)
  Hypercalcemia (severe)
  Hypokalemia
  Hypomagnesemia
  Heavy metal poisoning
Myopathies
  Amyloidosis
  Scleroderma
Neuropathies
  Parkinson disease[a]
  Spinal cord injury or tumor[a]
  Cerebrovascular disease
  Multiple sclerosis[a]
Other conditions
  Depression
  Autonomic neuropathy
  Cognitive impairment
  Immobility[a]

[a] Condition frequently encountered in clinical practice and associated with constipation.

Adapted from Bharucha AE, Wald A. Chronic constipation. Mayo Clin Proc. 2019 Nov;94(11):2340-57; used with permission.

Normal transit constipation includes IBS and functional constipation. In IBS, abdominal pain is associated with defecation or a change in bowel habits (ie, harder or less frequent stools). Patients with functional constipation also may have abdominal pain, but by definition the pain is not relieved by defecation or associated temporally with harder or less frequent stools. Most patients with DD also have delayed colonic transit. Consequently, delayed colonic transit does not imply slow transit constipation.

Colonic inertia refers to severe colonic motor dysfunction that is identified by reduced colonic contractile responses to a meal and stimulants such as bisacodyl or neostigmine, as assessed with intraluminal measurements of pressure activity or tone.

Management of Constipation

Principles. Reassurance and education about normal bowel habits, the need for adequate caloric intake and dietary fiber supplementation, and the absence of a "serious disorder" are vital. Deficient caloric intake can cause or exacerbate constipation, whereas refeeding may restore colonic transit.

Medical Therapy. A stepwise approach that begins with dietary fiber supplementation and osmotic or stimulant laxatives should be used to manage constipation. These agents are relatively safe, inexpensive, and widely used, and, in many cases, efficacy has been proved in controlled trials. Further testing to identify the pathogenesis of constipation is warranted if patients do not have a response to these agents (Table 21.3). This evaluation should be considered earlier if DDs are strongly suspected clinically. For normal transit and slow transit constipation, treatment with laxatives or a secretagogue (ie, lubiprostone), or both, should be considered.

Increasing dietary fiber either with food or a fiber supplement increases stool weight and accelerates colonic transit. Fiber intake should be increased gradually to 12 to 15 g daily with products such as the following: 1) psyllium (Konsyl, Konsyl Pharmaceuticals, Inc; Metamucil, Procter & Gamble), daily with fluid, or methylcellulose (Citrucel, Haleon Group), 1 teaspoon up to 3 times daily; 2) calcium polycarbophil (FiberCon, Foundation Consumer Brands), 2 to 4 tablets daily; or 3) bran, 1 cup daily. Fiber supplements are more effective in normal transit or "fiber-deficiency" constipation than in slow transit constipation or

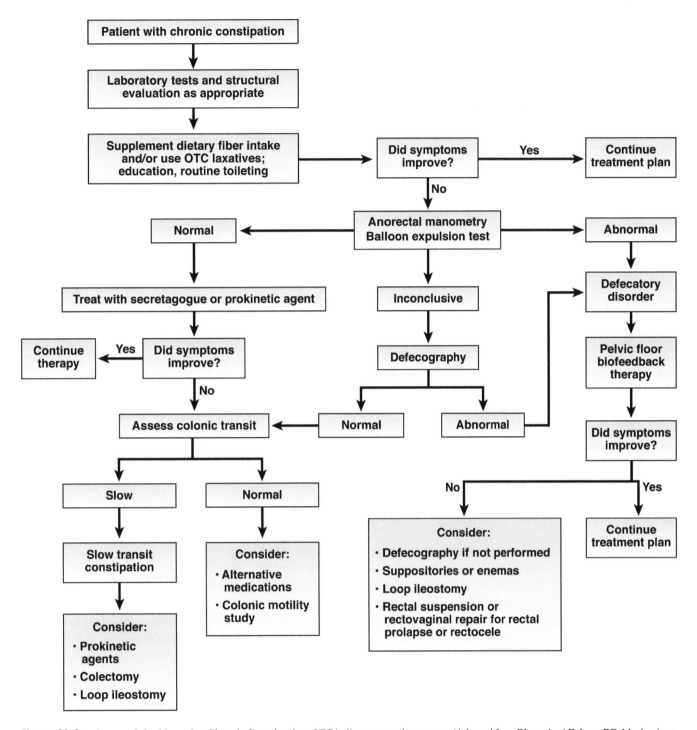

Figure 21.2.   Approach for Managing Chronic Constipation. OTC indicates over-the-counter. (Adapted from Bharucha AE, Lacy BE. Mechanisms, evaluation, and management of chronic constipation. Gastroenterology. 2020; 158[5]:1232-49; used with permission.)

Table 21.3.   Classification of Chronic Constipation

	Category		
Feature	Normal transit constipation	Slow transit constipation	Defecatory disorder
Colon transit	Normal	Slow	Normal or slow
Anorectal function	Normal	Normal	Abnormal
Management	Fiber supplementation	Fiber supplementation	Anorectal biofeedback
	Laxatives	Laxatives	therapy
		Surgery	

pelvic floor dysfunction. Fiber supplementation should start at a small dose administered twice daily (morning and evening) with fluids or meals, increasing the dose gradually after 7 to 10 days. Patients should be reassured that although fiber supplements may increase gaseousness, this often subsides with time. A response to fiber supplements is evident over several weeks, not days as with a laxative. Bloating may be reduced by gradually titrating the dose of dietary fiber to the recommended dose or by switching to a synthetic fiber preparation such as methylcellulose. Bran impairs absorption of iron and calcium. Fiber supplements are contraindicated for patients with intestinal obstruction, fecal impaction, or severe vomiting.

✓ Dietary fiber content should be increased gradually to 12 to 15 g daily for patients with constipation
✓ In normal transit constipation, 80% of patients have a symptomatic response to dietary fiber supplementation

---

Hyperosmolar agents, such as sorbitol or lactulose (15-30 mL once or twice daily), are nonabsorbable disaccharides metabolized by colonic bacteria into acetic and other short-chain fatty acids. Sorbitol and lactulose accelerate proximal colonic transit in healthy patients. Both agents may cause transient abdominal cramps and flatulence. They are equally effective for treating constipation in elderly patients. However, lactulose is extremely sweet and generally more expensive than sorbitol. A controlled study showed that polyethylene glycol (MiraLAX; Bayer Consumer Health), 17 g daily for 6 months, is superior to placebo for improving symptoms in chronic constipation. Oral sodium phosphate solution is used for bowel cleansing, occasionally by patients with severe constipation. However, acute phosphate nephropathy (acute nephrocalcinosis), a type of acute kidney failure, which rarely progresses to chronic kidney impairment and long-term dialysis, has occurred in patients who took oral sodium phosphate. Kidney tubular injury occurs from the deposition of calcium phosphate crystals in the distal tubules and collecting ducts, as shown histologically. Crystals form because of an abnormally high concentration of calcium phosphate from oral sodium phosphate–induced dehydration, decreased intravascular volume, and hyperphosphatemia, which is compounded further by reabsorption of water from kidney tubules. Risk factors for acute phosphate nephropathy include older age (greater severity for patients 57 years or older), decreased intravascular volume (eg, congestive heart failure, cirrhosis, or nephrotic syndrome), acute or chronic kidney disease, and concomitant use of drugs that affect kidney perfusion or function (diuretics, angiotensin-converting enzyme inhibitors, angiotensin receptor blockers, and possibly nonsteroidal anti-inflammatory drugs).

A saline laxative, milk of magnesia (15-30 mL once or twice daily), draws fluid osmotically into the lumen, stimulates the release of cholecystokinin, and accelerates colonic transit. It may cause hypermagnesemia, particularly in patients with kidney insufficiency.

✓ Patients with slow transit constipation can take saline laxatives or hyperosmolar agents daily and stimulant laxatives on an as-needed basis
✓ Sorbitol is as effective as lactulose but less expensive and less sweet
✓ Oral sodium phosphate solution should be used with care because rarely it can cause acute phosphate nephropathy and kidney failure

---

Stimulant laxatives affect mucosal transport and motility and include surface-active agents (docusate sodium [Colace, Avrio Health LP], 100 mg orally twice daily), diphenylmethane derivatives, ricinoleic acid, anthraquinones, glycerin (suppository), and bisacodyl (10-mg tablet or suppository). Stool softeners such as docusate sodium have limited efficacy. Glycerin and bisacodyl, taken up to once every other day, work by inducing colonic high-amplitude propagated contractions. Bisacodyl tablets take effect in 6 to 8 hours, and suppositories should be administered 30 minutes after eating to maximize synergism with the gastrocolic reflex. Of the diphenylmethane derivatives, phenolphthalein was withdrawn from the US market after animal studies suggested that it may be carcinogenic; however, no epidemiologic evidence supports this claim. The anthraquinone compounds may cause allergic reactions, electrolyte depletion, melanosis coli, and cathartic colon. *Melanosis coli* refers to brownish black colorectal pigmentation of unknown composition associated with apoptosis of colonic epithelial cells. *Cathartic colon* refers to altered colonic structure observed on barium enema studies and associated with long-term use of stimulant laxatives. The altered structure includes colonic dilatation, loss of haustral folds, strictures, colonic redundancy, and wide gaping of the ileocecal valve. Early reports implicating laxative-induced destruction of myenteric plexus neurons in cathartic colon have been disputed. Although anthraquinones may induce colorectal tumors in animal models, several cohorts and a recent case-control study did not find an association between anthraquinones and colon cancer.

✓ Bisacodyl and glycerin facilitate defecation by inducing colonic high-amplitude propagated contractions
✓ Melanosis coli indicates recent laxative use, but the evidence linking anthraquinones to colon cancer and destruction of the myenteric plexus is inconclusive

---

The secretagogues lubiprostone, linaclotide, and plecanatide increase the intestinal secretion of chloride; tenapanor, which is a locally acting, selective small-molecule inhibitor of the intestinal sodium-hydrogen exchanger 3 increases luminal sodium. As a result, all these drugs promote the efflux of fluid into the gut lumen and maintain osmotic balance. The US Food and Drug Administration has approved these 4 drugs for treating constipation-predominant IBS in adults; lubiprostone and linaclotide are also approved for treating chronic idiopathic constipation, and lubiprostone is also approved for treating opioid-induced constipation in adult patients who have chronic, noncancer pain.

✓ Lubiprostone stimulates intestinal secretion by activating chloride channels; it also improves stool consistency and relieves constipation

---

Lubiprostone is a bicyclic fatty acid derivative that promotes intestinal secretion by activating intestinal chloride channels. Lubiprostone accelerates colonic transit in healthy patients but not in those with chronic constipation. The effects of lubiprostone are more pronounced on stool consistency and frequency than on abdominal bloating, discomfort, and straining. Lubiprostone is well tolerated; nausea and headache are the most common adverse effects. In clinical trials, 33% of patients reported nausea, which generally was mild and could be reduced by taking the medication with meals.

Similar to the natriuretic peptides uroguanylin and guanylin and the heat-stable enterotoxins of *Escherichia coli* that cause traveler's diarrhea, linaclotide and plecanatide are peptide-based guanylate cyclase-C receptor agonists that increase the synthesis of cyclic guanosine monophosphate. In turn, these effects stimulate chloride and bicarbonate secretion through cystic fibrosis transmembrane conductance regulator channel–dependent and, to a lesser extent, channel-independent mechanisms. Linaclotide also acts on a sodium proton exchanger and thereby inhibits the absorption of sodium from the lumen. Linaclotide and plecanatide are comparably effective; there are minor differences between these drugs. The activation of guanylate cyclase-C is pH independent, and the activation of linaclotide and plecanatide is pH dependent, but the consequences of these differences on the beneficial and adverse effects is unclear. Evidence that the drugs decrease nociception during colonic distention in animal models and in humans is stronger for linaclotide than for plecanatide and is absent for tenapanor. In contrast to lubiprostone, linaclotide accelerates colonic transit in constipation-predominant IBS. Diarrhea is the most common adverse effect of all drugs in this class. In constipation-predominant IBS trials, 10% of patients discontinued use of linaclotide because of troublesome diarrhea.

Newer serotoninergic 5-HT$_4$ agonists are more specific for 5-HT$_4$ receptors and have fewer cardiovascular effects than older 5-HT$_4$ agonists (eg, cisapride). Prucalopride and tegaserod accelerate colonic transit in patients with constipation; prucalopride also accelerates gastric emptying. In the US, prucalopride is approved for treating chronic idiopathic constipation; tegaserod is approved for treating constipation-predominant IBS in women younger than 65 years.

Other pharmacologic approaches that have been used to manage constipation include colchicine and misoprostol (Cytotec, Pfizer Inc). Colchicine, 0.6 mg orally 3 times daily, and misoprostol, 1,200 mg daily, cause diarrhea. Colchicine should be used cautiously, if at all, for treating constipation, because long-term use may be associated with neuromyopathy. Other adverse effects include hypersensitivity reactions, bone marrow suppression, and kidney damage. Misoprostol should not be used to treat constipation because it is expensive, may cause miscarriage in pregnant women, and may exacerbate abdominal bloating. Moreover, its beneficial effects appear to decrease with time.

✓ Colchicine and misoprostol are unproven, potentially deleterious agents for treating slow transit constipation

---

Enemas, which are especially useful in patients with fecal impaction in the rectosigmoid colon, as may occur in obstructive defecation, include mineral oil retention enema, 100 to 250 mL daily per rectum; phosphate enema (Fleet; C B Fleet Co, Inc), 1 unit per rectum; tap water enema, 500 mL per rectum; and soapsuds enema, 1,500 mL per rectum. All the preparations are contraindicated for patients with rectal inflammation, and phosphate enemas are contraindicated for patients with hyperphosphatemia or hypernatremia. Mineral oil taken orally is associated with lipid pneumonia, malabsorption of fat-soluble vitamins, dehydration, and fecal incontinence.

✓ Enemas may be used judiciously on an as-needed basis for constipation

---

In summary, management should initially include dietary fiber supplements and osmotic laxatives, supplemented on an as-needed basis (eg, if a patient does not have a bowel movement for 2 days) with stimulant laxatives administered orally or as suppositories. In patients with chronic functional (ie, painless) constipation, these simple laxatives are as effective and much less expensive than newer agents (eg, secretagogues or prokinetic agents). When patients do not have a response to simple laxatives, secretagogues, which may also have antinociceptive effects, should be considered, especially in patients with marked abdominal bloating or pain (ie, painful constipation or constipation-predominant IBS), and anorectal testing should be considered, especially when the clinical features suggest a DD.

Surgical Therapy. Subtotal colectomy with ileorectal anastomosis is effective and occasionally indicated for patients with medically refractory, severe slow transit constipation, provided that pelvic floor dysfunction has been excluded or treated. In patients with megarectum, the rectum is also resected. Postoperative ileus and delayed mechanical small-bowel obstruction each occur in approximately 10% of patients. Diarrhea is common shortly after the operation but tends to resolve with time. It is extremely important to identify and treat pelvic floor dysfunction with biofeedback therapy preoperatively in patients with slow transit constipation.

✓ Subtotal colectomy is necessary and beneficial for patients with slow transit constipation who do not have a response to medical management

---

Disorders of Pelvic Floor Function

Disorders of pelvic floor function include functional DDs and fecal incontinence. Fecal incontinence, or involuntary leakage of stool from the anus, is a common symptom, particularly in the elderly. In community-based surveys, the prevalence of fecal incontinence among women 50 years or older is nearly 15%. The prevalence among nursing home residents is as high as 40%. At Mayo Clinic, 50% of patients who had chronic constipation also had a component of pelvic floor dysfunction.

Physiology of Defecation

Rectal distention evokes the desire to defecate and induces relaxation of the internal anal sphincter by an involuntary reflex (Figure 21.3). Defecation is completed by adoption of a suitable posture, contraction of the diaphragm and abdominal muscles to increase intra-abdominal pressure, and relaxation of the puborectalis muscle and external anal sphincter, both striated muscles. Relaxation of the puborectalis muscle allows widening and lowering of the anorectal angle, with perineal descent (Figure 21.4). The coordination between abdominal contraction and pelvic floor relaxation is crucial to the process. Although colonic high-amplitude propagated contractions may precede defecation, the contribution of rectal contraction to defecation is unclear.

Functional DDs

Functional DDs (also called *obstructive defecation, pelvic floor dyssynergia,* and *pelvic floor dysfunction*) are characterized by disordered defecation caused by functional obstruction that results from impaired relaxation of the external anal sphincter, impaired relaxation of the puborectalis muscle, or inadequate propulsive forces (ie, intrarectal pressure), or a combination of

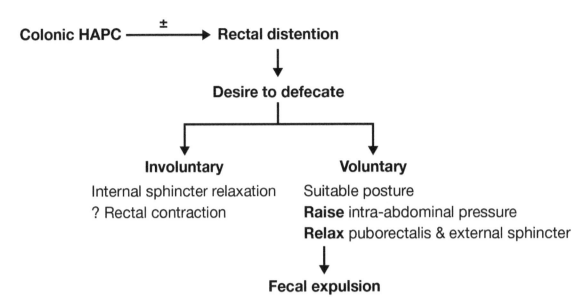

Figure 21.3. Physiology of Defecation. HAPC indicates high-amplitude propagated contraction. (Adapted from Bharucha AE, Camilleri M. Physiology of the colon. In: Zuidema GD, Yeo CJ, eds. Shackelford's surgery of the alimentary tract. 5th ed. Philadelphia [PA]: WB Saunders Company; 2002: 29-39; used with permission.)

these. Although certain symptoms are considered suggestive of DDs (eg, frequent straining, a sensation of incomplete evacuation, dyschezia, and digital evacuation of feces), symptoms alone are not sufficiently specific for distinguishing between functional DDs and other causes of constipation (ie, normal transit and slow transit constipation). A thorough digital rectal examination with assessment of anal resting tone and anorectal motion when patients contract their muscles (ie, squeeze) and simulate evacuation is useful for identifying DDs. Anal resting pressure is gauged by the resistance to the insertion of a finger in the anal canal. When patients squeeze, the anal sphincter and puborectalis muscles contract; the latter lifts the palpating finger toward the umbilicus. Conversely, simulated evacuation should be accompanied

by perineal descent (2-4 cm) and relaxation of the puborectalis muscle. In patients with functional DDs, digital rectal examination may show 1) increased resting pressure or 2) increased or decreased perineal descent or 3) both. When rectal prolapse is suspected, patients should be examined in the seated position on a commode.

Tests

Anorectal tests are necessary because DDs cannot be identified from clinical features alone. Anorectal manometry and rectal balloon expulsion tests usually are sufficient to confirm or exclude functional DDs. Defecography with barium or magnetic

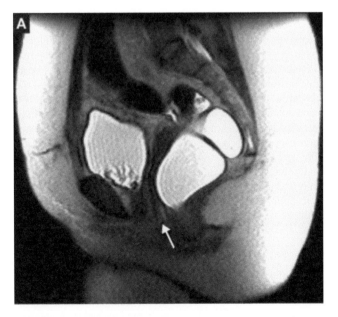
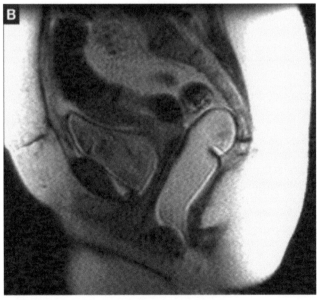

Figure 21.4. Magnetic Resonance Fluoroscopic Images of the Pelvis. A, At rest. B, During simulated defecation. Defecation is accompanied by opening of the anorectal junction (arrow), pelvic descent, and widening of the anorectal angle from 101° at rest to 124° during defecation. The rectum was filled with ultrasound gel.

resonance (MR) imaging (MRI) may be necessary in selected patients (eg, when findings from manometry and the balloon expulsion test are discrepant or these test results differ from the clinical impression, or when a rectocele is suspected). Because false-positive and false-negative results may occur, anorectal function tests need to be interpreted in the context of the clinical features.

Anorectal Manometry. Anorectal manometry can be conducted with traditional (ie, water- or air-perfused or solid-state) or high-resolution manometric catheters. The advantage of high-resolution manometric catheters is that sensors are evenly distributed along the catheter. Hence, when the catheter is positioned appropriately, the sensors straddle the entire anal canal, allowing pressures to be assessed without a pull-through maneuver, in contrast to traditional manometry.

Patients with DD may have 1 or more of several abnormalities. Arguably, the most useful parameter is a smaller rectoanal pressure gradient (ie, rectal pressure minus anal pressure), which may result from a low rectal pressure or a high anal pressure (or both), during simulated defecation. Other disturbances include high resting anal sphincter pressure and reduced rectal sensation (Figure 21.5). Normal values for anal pressures measured with manometry are technique-dependent and influenced by age, sex, and perhaps parity. Anal pressures are lower in women than in men and decrease with age, even in asymptomatic persons. Hence, the pressures must be compared against appropriate normal values.

Rectal Balloon Expulsion Test. Rectal expulsion can be evaluated by asking patients to expel from the rectum a balloon filled with water. While the patient is seated on a commode chair behind a privacy screen, the time required to expel a rectal balloon is measured. Depending on the technique, patients with normal pelvic floor functions can expel a rectal balloon within 1 to 2 minutes. The rectal balloon expulsion test is highly sensitive and specific (>85%) for identifying functional DDs. In 1 study, for the diagnosis of a DD, the positive predictive value was 64% and the negative predictive value was 97%. However, in this study the rectal balloon was not inflated to a fixed volume, which is the typical approach; instead, it was inflated until patients felt the desire to defecate (average volume, 183 mL), which may compensate for reduced rectal sensation of some patients with DD. Moreover, an abnormal result on the rectal balloon expulsion test predicts the response to pelvic floor retraining by biofeedback therapy.

Barium or MR Proctography. During dynamic (ie, barium or MR) proctography, anorectal anatomy and pelvic floor motion are recorded with the patient at rest and while coughing, squeezing, and straining to expel barium from the rectum. The anorectal angle and position of the anorectal junction are tracked during these maneuvers, as are the retention and evacuation of contrast material. Dynamic imaging can identify inadequate or excessive perineal descent, internal rectal intussusception, rectoceles, sigmoidoceles, and enteroceles. Also, puborectalis muscle dysfunction can be characterized during squeeze and evacuation. MR proctography is preferred to barium proctography because 1) it does not entail radiation exposure, 2) it is easier to visualize the bladder and uterus together with the anorectum, and 3) the bony landmarks (pubis and sacrococcygeal junction) necessary to measure anorectal descent are visualized more distinctly during MRI. Therefore, measurements of anorectal motion are more reproducible with MR proctography than with barium proctography. However, proctography findings need to be interpreted in the overall clinical context. For example, rectoceles are particularly common in multiparous persons. Clinically important rectoceles are generally large (>3 cm) or do not empty completely during defecation. Moreover, women with clinically important rectoceles often apply posterior vaginal pressure to facilitate defecation. Rectoceles usually are due to inadequate pelvic floor relaxation rather than to the primary abnormality.

Colonic Transit. Delayed colonic transit is common in DD. Hence, the finding of slow colonic transit does not exclude the diagnosis of DD.

✓ Anorectal manometry and the rectal balloon expulsion test generally are sufficient for diagnosing functional DDs; proctography is necessary in selected cases only
✓ Rectal balloon expulsion test
   • Highly sensitive and specific for diagnosis of functional DDs
   • Abnormal test result predicts the response to biofeedback therapy

---

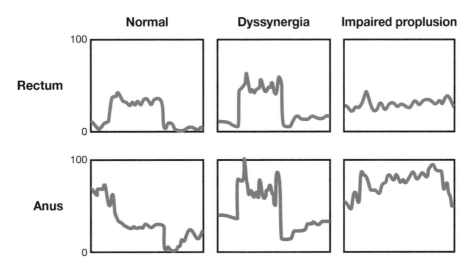

Figure 21.5. Rectoanal Pressure Profiles During Defecation in Health and Functional Defecatory Disorders (Dyssynergia and Impaired Propulsion). In contrast to patients with a normal pattern (left) (ie, increased rectal pressure and anal relaxation) during simulated evacuation, patients with defecatory disorders may either paradoxically contract the anal sphincters (center) or generate inadequate rectal propulsive forces (right).

- Some patients with a DD may have normal results on balloon expulsion test, so defecography should be performed when clinically indicated
✓ Colonic transit is delayed in the majority of patients who have functional DDs
✓ Anorectal function tests
  - False-positive and false-negative results may occur, so results must be interpreted in the context of the clinical features
  - In up to 20% of healthy persons, the anal sphincter paradoxically contracts instead of relaxes during evacuation

Treatment

Pelvic floor retraining with biofeedback therapy improves symptoms in 70% of patients who have a functional DD. Biofeedback therapy is conducted with sensors that measure surface electromyographic activity or pressures in the anorectum. By providing auditory or visual feedback of this activity, patients are taught to relax the pelvic floor and improve coordination between abdominal wall and diaphragmatic contraction and pelvic relaxation during defecation. Measures to contract the pelvic floor muscle (eg, Kegel exercises) are not appropriate for obstructive defecation. Strong rapport between patients and therapists is critical for biofeedback therapy. Controlled trials have shown that pelvic floor retraining is superior to laxatives for relieving constipation in patients with obstructive defecation. This symptomatic improvement has been sustained for 2 years. Biofeedback therapy also normalizes colonic transit and anal relaxation during defecation.

Fecal Incontinence

Fecal continence is maintained by anatomical factors and complex sensory and motor interactions among the sphincters, the anorectum, central and peripheral awareness, and the physical ability to get to a toilet. *Fecal incontinence* is defined as the involuntary leakage of liquid or solid stool from the anus; anal incontinence also includes leakage of gas. Up to 40% of nursing home residents have fecal incontinence, which is also common in the community. Up to 1 in 10 of all women and 1 in 5 women 40 years or older in the community have fecal incontinence. Patients with chronic fecal incontinence lead a restricted lifestyle, are afraid of having an embarrassing episode, and often miss work. The symptom frequently coexists with urinary incontinence and contributes to institutionalization. People with fecal incontinence are embarrassed to admit to their family and physician that they have this condition, even though their symptoms may affect their quality of life. Therefore, it is essential to ask patients with diarrhea or type 2 diabetes whether they have incontinence.

Etiology

In most patients, fecal incontinence is attributable to disordered anorectal continence mechanisms compounded by bowel disturbances, generally diarrhea. Several important diseases contribute to fecal incontinence.

Sphincter Damage. Sphincter damage includes obstetric and surgical (eg, hemorrhoidectomy) damage. Known obstetric risk factors for sphincter damage include forceps delivery, median episiotomy, and high birth weight.

Pudendal Neuropathy. Pudendal neuropathy may be attributable to obstetric trauma or type 2 diabetes. Also, patients with constipation may strain excessively during defecation and cause stretch injury to the pudendal nerve, soft tissue laxity, and excessive perineal descent. Eventually, sphincter weakness develops, predisposing to fecal incontinence.

Neurologic Causes. Neurologic causes include multiple sclerosis, Parkinson disease, Alzheimer disease, stroke, diabetic neuropathy, and cauda equina or conus medullaris lesions. Cauda equina lesions that cause fecal incontinence usually are accompanied by other neurologic symptoms and signs.

Other Local Causes. Examples of other local causes are perianal sepsis, radiation proctitis, and systemic sclerosis. In radiation proctitis, the entry of stool into a noncompliant (stiff) rectum may overwhelm continence mechanisms and cause incontinence. Scleroderma is associated with fibrosis of the internal anal sphincter and weak resting pressures.

Diarrhea. Fecal incontinence is a common complication of IBS, cholecystectomy, and inflammatory bowel disease.

Assessment

Patients with diarrhea must be asked specifically about fecal incontinence because they may not volunteer the information. The severity, risk factors, and circumstances of fecal incontinence and its effect on lifestyle should be assessed. Patients with urge incontinence generally are incontinent only for liquid or semiformed stools, have a brief warning time, and cannot reach the toilet in time. In contrast, patients with passive incontinence are aware of stool leakage only after the episode. Patients with urge incontinence have a decreased anal squeeze pressure or squeeze duration (or both), whereas those with passive incontinence have a reduced anal resting pressure. Some patients with urge fecal incontinence also may have rectal hypersensitivity, perhaps from a stiffer rectum. Nocturnal fecal incontinence occurs in patients with type 2 diabetes or scleroderma and is suggestive of weakness of the internal anal sphincter. A complete physical examination should include perianal assessment to identify common causes of perianal soiling, such as hemorrhoidal prolapse, perianal fistula, rectal mucosal prolapse, fecal impaction, anal stricture, and rectal mass. The perianal area must be inspected closely with the patient in the left lateral decubitus position and with the patient seated on the toilet. A thorough digital examination, as described above, should be performed. Flexible sigmoidoscopy, with or without anoscopy, is the final component in this phase of evaluation.

Tests

A combination of tests is necessary to evaluate the various components of anorectal anatomy and function. For each patient, the intensity of investigation depends on the patient's age, severity of fecal incontinence, clinical assessment of risk factors and anal sphincter pressures, and response to previous therapy (Figure 21.6).

Anorectal Manometry. Frequently, anal resting and squeeze pressures are decreased in fecal incontinence. Anal pressures should be compared with normal values obtained with the same technique in age- and sex-matched asymptomatic persons. Among patients with weak or normal anal pressures, other factors (eg, diarrhea or disturbances of rectal compliance or sensation) also may contribute to fecal incontinence.

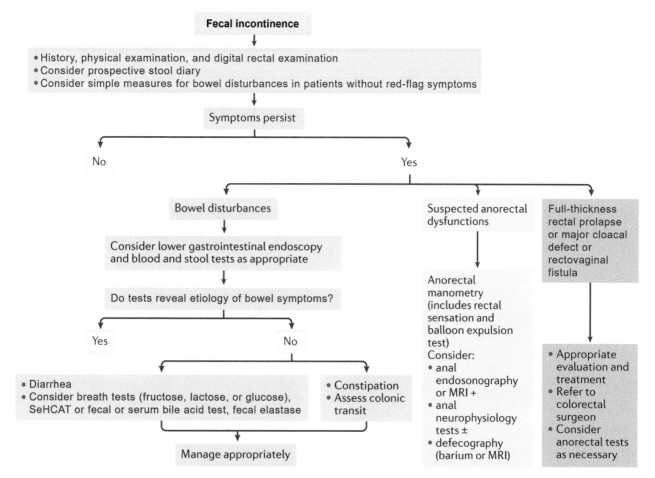

Figure 21.6. **Diagnostic Approach for Fecal Incontinence.** MRI indicates magnetic resonance imaging; SeHCAT, selenium homocholic acid taurine test. (Adapted from Bharucha AE, Knowles CH, Mack I, Malcolm A, Oblizajek N, Rao S, et al. Faecal incontinence in adults. Nat Rev Dis Primers. 2022 Aug 10;8[1]:53.)

Anal Ultrasonography. Anal ultrasonography reliably identifies anatomical defects or thinning of the internal anal sphincter and defects of the external anal sphincter that often are unrecognized clinically or are amenable to surgical repair (or both). However, compared with the interpretation of images of the internal sphincter, the interpretation of images of the external anal sphincter is more subjective, operator-dependent, and confounded by normal anatomical variations of the external anal sphincter. Even asymptomatic women may have an external anal sphincter defect after a vaginal delivery. Therefore, it can be challenging to interpret the clinical significance of anal sphincter defects (ie, the extent to which a sphincter defect explains anal weakness). Among women with obstetric injury, isolated injury of the external sphincter is more common; internal anal sphincter injury, in addition to external sphincter injury, increases the risk for fecal incontinence.

Evacuation Proctography. Dynamic proctography is indicated for fecal incontinence when clinical features suggest excessive perineal descent, a clinically significant rectocele (eg, in patients who splint the vagina to facilitate rectal emptying), an enterocele, or internal rectal intussusception.

Sphincter Denervation Measurements. The pudendal nerve may be injured (with or without damage to the sphincter) during vaginal delivery or by repetitive straining in patients with

chronic constipation. Pudendal nerve terminal motor latency (PNTML) can be measured by placing the examining finger, covered by a glove containing stimulating and recording electrodes, as close as possible to the pudendal nerve as it courses around the pelvic brim. PNTML measures the function of the fastest conducting fibers. Initial studies showed prolonged PNTML in fecal incontinence. However, PNTML measurements are operator-dependent and lack adequate sensitivity and specificity for identifying pudendal nerve damage. Patients with prolonged PNTML may have normal anal canal squeeze pressures. In contrast to data from earlier studies, recent data have suggested that prolonged PNTML does not predict success after surgical repair of sphincter defects. According to a position statement from the American Gastroenterological Association, PNTML should not be used to evaluate fecal incontinence. Needle electromyographic examination of the external anal sphincter provides a sensitive measure of denervation and usually can identify myopathic, neurogenic, or mixed injury.

Rectal Compliance and Sensation. Sensation is assessed by asking patients to report when they perceive the first detectable sensation, the desire to defecate (or urgency), and maximal tolerable discomfort during rectal balloon distention, generally with a handheld syringe. Alternatively, a balloon can be inflated at a controlled rate with a barostat, which is a continuous-infusion pump. During distention with a barostat, rectal pressures and volumes and, thus, rectal compliance (pressure-volume relationships) and capacity also can be assessed. Rectal sensation may be normal, decreased, or increased in fecal incontinence. When rectal sensation is decreased, stool may leak before the external anal sphincter contracts. By improving rectal sensation, sensory retraining can restore the coordinated contraction of the external anal sphincter and improve fecal continence. Conversely, some patients with fecal incontinence have exaggerated rectal sensation, perhaps because of a stiffer or smaller rectum.

Pelvic MRI. MRI is a relatively new method for imaging anal sphincter anatomy and pelvic floor motion during defecation and squeeze without radiation exposure. The anal sphincters also can be visualized, preferably with an endoanal MRI coil. MRI is superior to ultrasonography for visualizing morphologic features, particularly atrophy, of the external anal sphincter. In contrast to evacuation proctography, dynamic MRI does not entail radiation exposure and it provides direct visualization of the pelvic floor, including the anterior (bladder) and middle (uterus) compartments.

Treatment

Much can be accomplished by regulating bowel habits in patients who have diarrhea or constipation (Figure 21.7). The use of dietary fiber supplementation (eg, psyllium 15 g daily) has been shown to decrease episodes of loose or liquid fecal incontinence compared to placebo or other dietary fibers. In a crossover study,

therapy with a low dose of psyllium and loperamide reduced the frequency of fecal incontinence compared with use of placebo, but differences were not statistically significant. However, a recommendation to increase fiber intake in patients with diarrhea may be counterintuitive since increased fiber intake is commonly advised for treating constipation. Further study is necessary.

It is sensible to recommend limiting intake of caffeine, alcohol, fatty foods, fructose, and lactose, which predispose to loose stools and fecal incontinence. Weight loss may be attempted for patients who are overweight or who have obesity. Scheduled toileting may also be helpful, particularly for patients who have limited mobility.

Diarrhea should be managed by treatment of the underlying condition (eg, antibiotics for small intestinal bacterial overgrowth and dietary restriction for carbohydrate malabsorption) or with antidiarrheal agents, which must be prescribed in adequate doses. Loperamide hydrochloride (2 mg; maximal dose, 16 mg daily), diphenoxylate hydrochloride with atropine sulfate (5 mg), or codeine sulfate (30-60 mg) may need to be taken regularly, preferably 30 minutes before meals, perhaps up to several times daily. Loperamide not only delays gastrointestinal transit but also improves anal resting tone. Similarly, amitriptyline improves fecal continence by restoring stool consistency and reducing rectal irritability. The bile acid–binding resins cholestyramine and colesevelam are useful for patients with postcholecystectomy diarrhea. Scheduled rectal emptying with suppositories or enemas is often useful for fecal impaction and overflow incontinence.

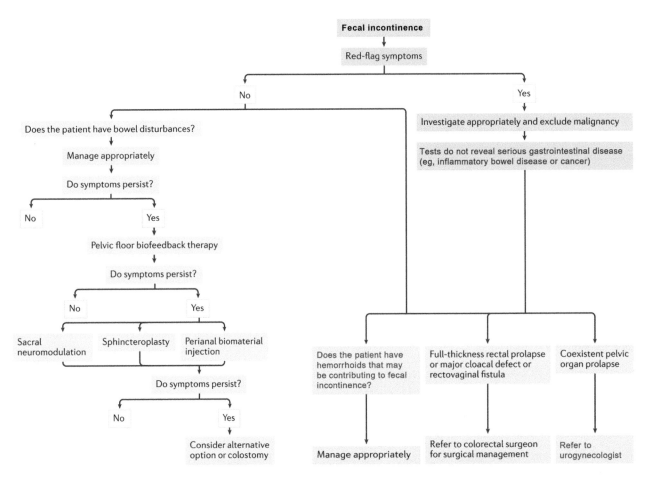

Figure 21.7. Treatment of Fecal Incontinence. (Adapted from Bharucha AE, Knowles CH, Mack I, Malcolm A, Oblizajek N, Rao S, et al. Faecal incontinence in adults. Nat Rev Dis Primers. 2022 Aug 10;8[1]:53.)

When individualized to the underlying anorectal dysfunction, pelvic floor rehabilitation may improve anal sphincter contractions, sensory dysfunction, and coordination, and rehabilitation may be supplemented with biofeedback to augment training through visual or auditory electronically amplified feedback. Among patients who did not respond to education and medical management, biofeedback-assisted pelvic floor rehabilitation provided additional benefit beyond pelvic floor exercises alone. By contrast, results with biofeedback were not different from results with education among 300 women who had fecal incontinence. In another randomized controlled trial, biofeedback improved fecal incontinence symptoms more than attention-control therapy. Together, these data justify biofeedback therapy when the response to dietary modifications and bowel management is insufficient. In patients with coexisting rectal evacuation disorders, biofeedback may provide the added benefit of teaching pelvic floor relaxation.

If initial therapies are unsuccessful, transanal irrigation or barrier devices may be considered. Patients with neurogenic bowel disorders or chronic constipation and fecal retention may benefit from transanal irrigation to facilitate rectal cleansing and prevent unwanted stool leakage. Barrier devices (eg, Renew anal insert [Renew Medical Inc] and Eclipse vaginal bowel-control system [Laborie Medical Technologies Corp]) are well tolerated and have improved symptoms in open-label trials. In 1 open-label trial, 62% of patients treated with Renew inserts completed therapy and had a decrease in the frequency of fecal incontinence of at least 50%. In an open-label trial of the Eclipse vaginal insert, of the 55% of patients who were successfully fitted, 79% had a decrease in the frequency of fecal incontinence episodes of at least 50%.

In patients whose symptoms are refractory to rigorously implemented conservative therapy, the key surgical options are sacral neuromodulation, sphincteroplasty, some implantable biomaterials and, as a final resort, colonic stoma. Artificial anal sphincter and dynamic graciloplasty are associated with considerable morbidity, particularly wound infections, and are not used in the US. In large observational cohorts and national registries, success rates after sacral neuromodulation have been about 50% at 5 to 10 years. Serious harm is very unlikely to occur. However, the process is a 2-stage procedure that entails a lifelong commitment to use the device, potentially a battery charge or change, and other troubleshooting interventions, which are not uncommon.

Especially for patients with an internal sphincter defect and reduced anal resting tone who often have predominantly passive incontinence, injectable biomaterials may be considered (ie, nonanimal stabilized hyaluronic acid/dextranomer [NASHA/Dx], which is the only approved submucosal agent). In 1 study, NASHA/Dx was superior to placebo but not to pelvic floor biofeedback therapy. The potential adverse effects with NASHA/Dx include proctalgia, bleeding, and infection.

Continence improves in 80% to 90% of patients shortly after repair of anal sphincter defects but then worsens over time; less than 20% of patients are continent at 5 years after the operation. Hence, sphincteroplasty is typically reserved for younger women (eg, younger than 45 years) who often have a sphincter defect shortly after obstetric injury. The risks include a high risk of minor wound infection (>50%), a moderate risk (about 20%) of wound breakdown, and a small risk (about 5%) of complete breakdown with iatrogenic fistulation or cloacal defect, which may necessitate a diverting stoma.

A colostomy is often the last resort for patients with medically refractory fecal incontinence. Conservative measures, including management of bowel disturbances, often can improve fecal continence.

✓ Patients who do not benefit from conservative measures alone may benefit from pelvic floor retraining
✓ After surgical repair of anal sphincter defects, fecal continence initially improves but then worsens

---

Suggested Reading

Bharucha AE. Pelvic floor: Anatomy and function. Neurogastroenterol Motil. 2006 Jul;18(7):507–19.

Bharucha AE, Basilisco G, Malcolm A, Lee TH, Hoy MB, Scott SM, et al. Review of the indications, methods, and clinical utility of anorectal manometry and the rectal balloon expulsion test. Neurogastroenterol Motil. 2022 Sep;34(9):e14335.

Bharucha AE, Dunivan G, Goode PS, Lukacz ES, Markland AD, Matthews CA, et al. Epidemiology, pathophysiology, and classification of fecal incontinence: state of the science summary for the National Institute of Diabetes and Digestive and Kidney Diseases (NIDDK) workshop. Am J Gastroenterol. 2015 Jan;110(1):127–36.

Bharucha AE, Knowles CH, Mack I, Malcolm A, Oblizajek N, Rao S, et al. Faecal incontinence in adults. Nat Rev Dis Primers. 2022 Aug 10;8(1):53.

Bharucha AE, Lacy BE. Mechanisms, evaluation, and management of chronic constipation. Gastroenterology. 2020 Apr;158(5):1232–49.

Bharucha AE, Sharma M. Painful and painless constipation: all roads lead to (a change in) Rome. Dig Dis Sci. 2018 Jul;63(7):1671–4.

Oblizajek NR, Gandhi S, Sharma M, Chakraborty S, Muthyala A, Prichard D, et al. Anorectal pressures measured with high-resolution manometry in healthy people-normal values and asymptomatic pelvic floor dysfunction. Neurogastroenterol Motil. 2019 Jul;31(7):e13597.

Rao SSC, Bharucha AE, Chiarioni G, Felt-Bersma R, Knowles C, Malcolm A, et al. Anorectal disorders. Gastroenterology. 2016;150(6):1430–42.

Wald A, Bharucha AE, Limketkai B, Malcolm A, Remes-Troche JM, Whitehead WE, et al. ACG clinical guidelines: management of benign anorectal disorders. Am J Gastroenterol. 2021 Oct;116(10):1987–2008.

Whitehead WE, Rao SS, Lowry A, Nagle D, Varma M, Bitar KN, et al. Treatment of fecal incontinence: state of the science summary for the National Institute of Diabetes and Digestive and Kidney Diseases workshop. Am J Gastroenterol. 2015 Jan;110(1):138–46.

22

Gastrointestinal Disease and Pregnancy[a]

SUNANDA V. KANE, MD

Pharmacotherapy for the management of common gastrointestinal illnesses continues to evolve. Women with chronic illnesses who would have been unwilling or unable to conceive in the past are now healthy enough to consider pregnancy. In addition, many women are deferring childbearing until later in life, when polypharmacy and illness may be more common. This chapter discusses the use of medications during pregnancy according to the best available evidence. Because the amount of high-quality controlled data in pregnancy is limited, absolute safety is not guaranteed with any medication. Instead, the risk of the underlying condition and the safety of the medications used to treat it should be balanced against the overall health of the mother and the fetus in each case. All conversations about medications, along with possible consequences of not treating the disease during pregnancy, should be documented carefully. Communication with the patient's obstetrician during this time is also paramount. The US Food and Drug Administration (FDA) has moved away from its safety rating system and now expects manufacturers to include paragraphs in the prescribing information related to fertility, pregnancy, and lactation. Any animal and human data

are presented, and the clinician must decide which information should be discussed with each particular patient. However, the rating system is still cited and thus is included here.

This chapter covers the treatment of common gastrointestinal and liver diseases, the management of common gastrointestinal symptoms, and the use of medications during endoscopy. The majority of medications can be categorized on the basis of existing reports; the categories are summarized in Table 22.1.

Table 22.1. US Food and Drug Administration (FDA) Categories for the Use of Medications in Pregnancy[a]

FDA category	Definition
A	Controlled studies in animals and women have shown no risk in the first trimester, and possible fetal harm is remote
B	Either animal studies have not demonstrated a fetal risk, but there are no controlled studies in pregnant women, or animal studies have shown an adverse effect that was not confirmed in controlled studies in women in the first trimester
C	No controlled studies in humans have been performed, and animal studies have shown adverse events, or studies in humans and animals are not available; give the medication if the potential benefit outweighs the risk
D	Positive evidence of fetal risk is available, but the benefits may outweigh the risk if the disease is life-threatening or serious
X	Studies in animals or humans show fetal abnormalities; the drug is contraindicated

[a] The categories are now considered historical.

Adapted from Mahadevan U, Kane S. American Gastroenterological Association Institute technical review on the use of gastrointestinal medications in pregnancy. Gastroenterology. 2006 Jul;131(1):283-311; used with permission.

---

[a] Portions of this chapter were adapted from Mahadevan U, Kane S. American Gastroenterological Association Institute technical review on the use of gastrointestinal medications in pregnancy. Gastroenterology. 2006 Jul;131(1):283-311 and Mahadevan U. Gastrointestinal medications in pregnancy. Best Pract Res Clin Gastroenterol. 2007;21(5):849-77; used with permission.

Abbreviations: ERCP, endoscopic retrograde cholangiopancreatography; FDA, US Food and Drug Administration; HBV, hepatitis B virus; H$_2$, histamine; IBD, inflammatory bowel disease; IBS, irritable bowel syndrome; Ig, immunoglobulin; OR, odds ratio; SSRI, selective serotonin reuptake inhibitor; TREAT, Crohn's Therapy, Resource, Evaluation, and Assessment Tool; UDCA, ursodeoxycholic acid

✓ The FDA no longer uses a rating system for safety of medications and expects all prescribing information to include sections on fertility, pregnancy, and lactation

Endoscopy

Endoscopy constitutes a large portion of the gastroenterologist's role in patient care. Although many pregnant women have appropriate indications for endoscopy, fetal drug safety is a major consideration in the choice and dosage of endoscopic medications. For particularly high-risk endoscopy, such as therapeutic endoscopic retrograde cholangiopancreatography (ERCP), an anesthesiologist may be helpful in titration of medications and patient monitoring. For patients who present with gastrointestinal tract hemorrhage, in which diagnosis and therapeutic intervention are necessary, therapeutic scopes should be used. The use of medications for endoscopy is summarized in Table 22.2.

Meperidine

Meperidine is transferred rapidly across the placenta. Physicians have extensive experience prescribing meperidine during pregnancy, particularly during labor. Two large studies did not show teratogenicity from the administration of meperidine during the first trimester. The Collaborative Perinatal Project, a national study with the primary aim of documenting the teratogenicity of drugs taken during the first 4 months of pregnancy, followed more than 50,000 women in 12 US centers between 1959 and 1965 and reported no teratogenicity from meperidine use in 268 mothers with first-trimester exposure. Meperidine is preferred to morphine for obstetric pain because meperidine crosses the fetal blood-brain barrier more slowly. Meperidine can cause diminished fetal beat-to-beat cardiac variability that lasts for approximately 1 hour after being administered intravenously to the mother and is a common cause of decreased fetal cardiac variability during endoscopy.

The labeling approved by the FDA for meperidine carries the following warning: "Meperidine should not be used in pregnant women prior to the labor period, unless in the judgment of the physician the potential benefits outweigh the possible risks, because safe use in pregnancy prior to labor has not been established relative to possible effects on fetal development." Meperidine is preferred to diazepam or midazolam as an endoscopic premedication during pregnancy. The meperidine dosage should be titrated to produce calmness, restfulness, and mild analgesia without somnolence.

Fentanyl

Fentanyl is rated a category C drug during pregnancy, and accumulated anecdotal experience suggests that it may be used in low doses for endoscopy. Fentanyl is sometimes used as an alternative to meperidine during endoscopy because of its more rapid onset of action. In several human studies, administration of fentanyl to the mother during labor produced no neonatal toxicity.

Propofol

Propofol is a category B drug and is now a preferred agent for sedation in some endoscopy centers. However, it has not been studied extensively in women in the first and second trimesters and, thus, is not recommended for use during this time because of the dearth of studies in the obstetric literature. Propofol rapidly transfers across the placenta near term. In 1 study, 20 infants exposed to propofol during parturition had depressed Apgar scores at birth compared with unexposed controls, but the neurodepression rapidly reversed. Numerous other studies have not demonstrated any neonatal toxicity when propofol was administered during parturition; however, the safety of exposure in the first trimester has not been studied adequately.

Naloxone

The FDA classifies naloxone as a category B drug during pregnancy. In opiate-dependent patients, small doses of naloxone precipitate a syndrome resembling that produced by opiate withdrawal. Symptoms include restlessness, anxiety, insomnia,

Table 22.2.   Medications Used for Endoscopy

Drug	FDA category	Recommendations for pregnancy	Recommendations for breastfeeding
Ampicillin	B	Safe to use when required	Compatible
Benzocaine	C	Avoid unless benefit outweighs risk	No human data: potential toxicity
Diatrizoate	D	Minimal use for therapeutic ERCP	Limited human data: probably compatible
Diazepam	D	Midazolam is the preferred benzodiazepine	Limited human data: potential toxicity
Electricity	None	Use for therapeutic ERCP	No human data: potential toxicity
Epinephrine	C	Avoid unless for hemostasis	No human data: potential toxicity
Fentanyl	C	Use in low doses	Compatible
Flumazenil	C	Only for severe benzodiazepine overdose	No human data: probably compatible
Glucagon	B	Avoid except for ERCP	No human data
Lidocaine	B	Gargle and spit (oral form)	Limited human data: probably compatible
Meperidine	B	Use in low doses	Compatible
Midazolam	D	Use in low doses	Limited human data: potential toxicity
Naloxone	B	Only for severe narcotic overdoses	No human data: probably compatible
Piperacillin-tazobactam	B	Useful in cholangitis or biliary sepsis	Safe
Polyethylene glycol electrolyte	C	No human studies available	Probably safe
Propofol	B	Avoid in first and second trimesters	Limited human data: probably compatible
Simethicone	C	Can be avoided but low risk	No human data: probably compatible
Sodium glycol electrolyte	C	Low risk with 1-time use	No human data

Abbreviations: ERCP, endoscopic retrograde cholangiopancreatography; FDA, US Food and Drug Administration.

Adapted from Mahadevan U, Kane S. American Gastroenterological Association Institute technical review on the use of gastrointestinal medications in pregnancy. Gastroenterology. 2006 Jul;131(1):283-311; used with permission.

irritability, hyperalgesia, nausea, and muscle cramps. Because opiates cross the placenta, the administration of naloxone is dangerous and contraindicated in a pregnant patient who is specifically opiate dependent. The FDA-approved labeling for naloxone has the following precaution about use during pregnancy: "Naloxone should be used in pregnancy only if clearly needed." The administration of naloxone is appropriate, however, for pregnant patients who have serious signs of potential meperidine toxicity, such as respiratory depression, systemic hypotension, or unresponsiveness.

Benzodiazepines

Diazepam and midazolam, category D drugs, should have restricted use during endoscopy, particularly during the first trimester. Benzodiazepines, including diazepam and midazolam, are commonly administered before gastrointestinal endoscopy to reduce anxiety, induce brief amnesia, and produce muscle relaxation. Diazepam freely and rapidly crosses the placenta and accumulates in the fetal circulation at levels equal to or higher than those of maternal serum. The FDA-approved labeling for diazepam carries the following warning about use in pregnancy: "An increased risk of congenital malformations associated with the use of minor tranquilizers . . . during the first trimester of pregnancy has been suggested in several studies. Because use of these drugs is rarely a matter of urgency, their use during this period should almost always be avoided." Diazepam is not recommended by the American Academy of Pediatrics because it, along with its metabolite N-demethyldiazepam, can accumulate in breastfed infants.

Many endoscopists prefer midazolam to diazepam for endoscopic premedication because of faster onset and recovery time, more intense transient antegrade amnesia, and lower risk of thrombophlebitis. Midazolam crosses the human placenta, but fetal serum levels increase to only about one-third to two-thirds of those of maternal serum after oral, intramuscular, or intravenous administration in the mother. Midazolam appears to be preferable to diazepam for endoscopy during pregnancy because of the potential association between diazepam and oral clefts and neonatal neurobehavioral abnormalities. Because the mechanism of action is similar to that of diazepam, midazolam should be used cautiously and in low doses during pregnancy, particularly during the first trimester. Dosages should be titrated carefully to an end point of relaxation and calmness but not somnolence.

Flumazenil

Flumazenil, a category C drug, is a benzodiazepine antagonist that rapidly reverses the central effects of benzodiazepines. Little is known about the safety of flumazenil during pregnancy or in infants; thus, it should be used during pregnancy only if the potential benefit clearly outweighs the risks. The need for flumazenil can be prevented by carefully and slowly titrating the benzodiazepine dosage and by using the minimal benzodiazepine dosage required for endoscopic examination.

Simethicone

The FDA has classified simethicone as a category C drug. Many endoscopists use simethicone to reduce gastric foam before upper endoscopy. A surveillance study of Michigan Medicaid patients did not show a statistically significant difference between pregnant women exposed to the drug and those not exposed to it.

Simethicone use carries a low risk during endoscopy because it is not absorbed systemically.

Glucagon

The FDA classifies glucagon as a category B drug during pregnancy. However, no adequate and well-controlled studies have involved pregnant women. Thus, this drug should be used during pregnancy only if clearly needed. Although fetal risk has not been characterized completely, the administration of glucagon appears to be justified to decrease intestinal motility to help reduce procedure time and to aid in cannulation of the bile duct and sphincterotomy during therapeutic ERCP, which is performed because of the high risk of untreated maternal cholangitis. If electrocautery is used, the grounding pad should be positioned so that the uterus is not directly between the electrical catheter and the grounding pad.

Antibiotics

Ampicillin

The FDA classifies ampicillin as a category B drug during pregnancy. This penicillin antibiotic may be used when *Enterococcus* infection is a concern. Ampicillin rapidly crosses the placenta, and fetal serum levels equilibrate with those of the maternal serum within 3 hours after the drug is administered to the mother.

Piperacillin-Tazobactam

Piperacillin-tazobactam, in FDA category B, is a good choice for pregnant patients who present with features of cholangitis or biliary sepsis. It may also be used before ERCP as prophylaxis against biliary sepsis when an obstructed biliary tree is suspected. Piperacillin-tazobactam covers most biliary and enteric pathogens (eg, *Escherichia* and *Klebsiella*) and also covers *Enterococcus* species. The drug does cross the placenta but is deemed safe in all trimeters of pregnancy. This antibiotic may also be used in women who breastfeed.

Colonic Lavage Preparations

Polyethylene glycol electrolyte solution has not been studied extensively in pregnancy, and it is not known whether it can cause fetal harm. A study of 225 patients showed that the agent was safe when used to treat constipation. Because full colonoscopy rarely is indicated during pregnancy, tap water enemas are recommended as bowel preparation for lower endoscopy.

Topical Anesthetics

Lidocaine

Lidocaine, an FDA category B drug, can be applied topically to the oropharynx before upper endoscopy and ERCP, although it is rarely needed. Additionally, lidocaine gel can be used topically around the perianal area before lower endoscopy in patients with painful hemorrhoids and fissures. No fetal harm was noted during parturition in the Collaborative Perinatal Project, in which 293 infants were exposed in the first trimester. The pregnant patient who is administered topical lidocaine should be instructed to gargle and spit out the preparation, rather than swallow it, to minimize systemic absorption.

Table 22.3.   Medications Used for Nausea and Vomiting During Pregnancy

Drug	FDA category	Recommendations for pregnancy	Recommendations for breastfeeding
Dolasetron	B	No human studies	No human data: probably compatible
Domperidone	C	Safety unknown	Limited human data: probably compatible
Granisetron	B	No human studies	No human data: probably compatible
Metoclopramide	B	No teratogenicity; low risk (population-based study)	Limited human data: potential toxicity
Ondansetron	B	No teratogenicity; low risk (controlled trial)	No human data: probably compatible
Prochlorperazine	C	No teratogenicity; low risk (large database study)	No human data: potential toxicity
Promethazine	C	No teratogenicity; low risk (large database study)	No human data: probably compatible
Pyridoxine	A	Considered safest therapy for nausea and vomiting; available without prescription	Compatible
Trimethobenzamide	C	No teratogenicity; low risk (case series)	No human data: probably compatible

Abbreviation: FDA, US Food and Drug Administration.

Adapted from Mahadevan U, Kane S. American Gastroenterological Association Institute technical review on the use of gastrointestinal medications in pregnancy. Gastroenterology. 2006 Jul;131(1):283-311; used with permission.

Benzocaine

Benzocaine aerosols, gels, and solutions are used to anesthetize the oropharynx before upper endoscopic procedures. However, benzocaine is an FDA category C drug and should be considered only if the benefit of the medication outweighs the risk to the fetus.

Therapeutic Agents for Hemostasis

Epinephrine is injected during endoscopy to achieve hemostasis of actively bleeding lesions. During therapeutic endoscopy, epinephrine is used to stop active bleeding; in this clinical scenario, the benefit outweighs the potential risk of its use.

Electricity is transferred readily across the uterus because amniotic fluid is an excellent conductor. Fetal risk depends on the voltage and on the current amplitude, duration, and frequency time as well as on the location on the body. Fetal mortality is rare from electroconvulsive therapy or direct current cardioversion during pregnancy. During endoscopy, bipolar electrocautery should be used because no grounding pad is necessary.

Contrast Dye

Diatrizoate, a contrast agent injected into the biliary tree, has been used in diagnostic and therapeutic amniography without harming the fetus. Although it has been documented to impair fetal thyroid function and is an FDA category D medication, the risk of its use for cholangiography is less than for amniography because of the doses used. In the appropriate clinical setting, the risk of maternal cholangitis likely outweighs the theoretical risk of transient fetal hypothyroidism.

- ✓ Indications for endoscopy in pregnant women are the same as those in women who are not pregnant
- ✓ Propofol—the preferred agent for sedation (if sedation is to be used)

Nausea and Vomiting

Nausea and vomiting are extremely common during pregnancy and have multiple causes. Most women can be supported through episodes without the use of antiemetics. However, for women who have a protracted course or underlying conditions that may predispose to nausea and vomiting, medical therapy is warranted to prevent complications from volume depletion. The use of antiemetic medications during pregnancy is summarized in Table 22.3.

Ginger

Ginger extract, which comes in many forms, is popular for homeopathic treatment of nausea and vomiting during pregnancy. At least 4 randomized controlled trials have compared ginger with placebo, and another 4 have compared ginger with pyridoxine. All these trials have shown that ginger is beneficial for symptoms without raising clinically significant safety concerns.

Pyridoxine

First-line therapy for nausea and vomiting during pregnancy is pyridoxine (vitamin B$_6$). Several randomized controlled trials have demonstrated its effectiveness at 10 to 25 mg every 8 hours in the treatment of nausea and vomiting during pregnancy. Pyridoxine in combination with doxylamine has also been shown to be effective and safe and is classified in FDA category A.

Metoclopramide

The use of metoclopramide as an antiemetic usually is confined to the first trimester, but it also is used to enhance gastric emptying throughout pregnancy. A Danish study compared, over a 5-year period, 309 women who had singleton pregnancies and prescriptions for metoclopramide with 13,327 controls. The study reported no major differences in the risk of malformations (odds ratio [OR], 1.11; 95% CI, 0.6-2.1); low birth weight (OR, 1.79; 95% CI, 0.8-3.9); or preterm delivery (OR, 1.02; 95% CI, 0.6-1.7). While metoclopramide is an FDA category B medication, the risk of metoclopramide-induced movement disorders with long-term use needs to be considered.

Prochlorperazine

Prochlorperazine, a category C drug, readily crosses the placenta. However, most studies have not found an increased risk of adverse outcomes in pregnancy.

Promethazine

Promethazine is another category C drug. It is an antihistamine that is used occasionally as an antiemetic during pregnancy and also as adjunctive therapy for narcotics during labor.

Table 22.4. Medications Used for Gastroesophageal Reflux and Peptic Ulcer Disease

Drug	FDA category	Recommendations for pregnancy	Recommendations for breastfeeding
Antacids			
Aluminum-containing antacids	None	Most safe: minimal absorption	Low risk
Calcium-containing antacids	None	Most safe: minimal absorption	Low risk
Magnesium-containing antacids	None	Most safe: minimal absorption	Low risk
Magnesium trisilicates	None	Avoid long-term use or high doses	Low risk
Sodium bicarbonate	None	Not safe: alkalosis	Low risk
Mucosal protectants			
Sucralfate	B	Safe	No human data: probably compatible
Histamine receptor antagonists			
Cimetidine	B	Controlled data: low risk	Compatible
Famotidine	B	Paucity of safety data	Limited human data: probably compatible
Nizatidine	B	Limited human data (low risk in animals)	Limited human data: probably compatible
Ranitidine	B	Low risk	Limited human data: probably compatible
Proton pump inhibitors			
Dexlansoprazole	B	Limited data: low risk	No human data: potential toxicity
Esomeprazole	B	Limited data: low risk	No human data: potential toxicity
Lansoprazole	B	Limited data: low risk	No human data: potential toxicity
Omeprazole	C	Embryonic and fetal toxicity	Limited human data: potential toxicity
Pantoprazole	B	Limited data: low risk	No human data: potential toxicity
Rabeprazole	B	Limited data: low risk	No human data: potential toxicity
Promotility agents			
Cisapride	C	Controlled study: low risk, limited availability	Limited human data: probably compatible
Metoclopromide	B	Low risk	Limited human data: potential toxicity
Treatment of *Helicobacter pylori* infection			
Amoxicillin	B	Safe	Compatible
Bismuth	C	Not safe: teratogenicity	No human data: potential toxicity
Clarithromycin	C	Avoid in first trimester	No human data: probably compatible
Metronidazole	B	Low risk: avoid in first trimester	Limited human data: potential toxicity
Tetracycline	D	Not safe: teratogenicity	Compatible

Abbreviation: FDA, US Food and Drug Administration.

Adapted from Mahadevan U, Kane S. American Gastroenterological Association Institute technical review on the use of gastrointestinal medications in pregnancy. Gastroenterology. 2006 Jul;131(1):283-311; used with permission.

Trimethobenzamide

Trimethobenzamide is a category C drug. Three studies have followed outcomes among women who took trimethobenzamide during the first trimester for nausea and vomiting. In all 3 studies, there was no increase in the incidence of malformations with the use of trimethobenzamide.

Ondansetron

Ondansetron, a category B drug, is used for the prevention and treatment of chemotherapy-induced nausea and vomiting and for hyperemesis gravidarum. A randomized, double-blind study compared intravenous ondansetron with promethazine for hyperemesis. Ondansetron was well tolerated and efficacious with no adverse effects; however, outcomes among infants were not reported. Results from teratogen information services databases do not show an increase in major malformations in comparison with exposure to other antiemetics or healthy controls.

Granisetron and Dolasetron

Both granisetron and dolasetron are category B drugs. There have not been any studies on pregnant women exposed to these agents. However, studies of pregnant rats and rabbits that were given up to 146 times the human dose did not show any adverse outcomes.

Domperidone

Domperidone, a category C drug, is a dopamine antagonist used for short-term treatment of nausea and vomiting and for its prokinetic properties. Currently, it is not available in the US by prescription. Whether it crosses the placenta is not known, but its bioavailability after oral ingestion is low.

✓ Nausea and vomiting—extremely common during pregnancy
✓ Natural entities such as ginger and pyridoxine are effective first-line therapy for mild symptoms related to nausea and vomiting

Gastroesophageal Reflux Disease

Heartburn is estimated to occur in 30% to 50% of pregnancies. For mild symptoms, only lifestyle and dietary modifications may be required. Medications for treating gastroesophageal reflux disease have not been tested routinely in randomized controlled trials with pregnant women. The medications used to treat gastroesophageal reflux disease and peptic ulcer disease are summarized in Table 22.4.

Antacids

Antacids that contain magnesium, aluminum, or calcium are not teratogenic in animal studies. Although 1 case-control study reported a significant increase in major and minor congenital abnormalities in infants exposed to antacids during the first trimester of pregnancy, no analysis of individual agents was done and, currently, most antacids at normal therapeutic doses are considered acceptable during pregnancy. Magnesium trisilicate, found in alginic acid, can lead to fetal nephrolithiasis, hypotonia, and respiratory distress if used long term and in high doses. Antacids containing sodium bicarbonate should not be used because they can cause maternal or fetal metabolic alkalosis and fluid overload. Excessive intake of calcium carbonate can result in milk-alkali syndrome, characterized by hypercalcemia, kidney impairment, and metabolic alkalosis. None of the antacids have been shown to concentrate in breast milk, so they are acceptable when breastfeeding.

Sucralfate

Sucralfate, a category B drug, is a nonabsorbable drug that exerts a local rather than systemic effect and has been tested in a prospective randomized controlled trial. Women with gastroesophageal reflux disease treated with sucralfate had a higher frequency of symptomatic remission than controls (90% vs 43%, P<.05).

Cimetidine

Cimetidine is a category B drug. Multiple large cohort studies have shown that the rate of major birth defects among pregnant women taking cimetidine is the same as that for healthy controls.

Ranitidine

Ranitidine, like the other histamine (H$_2$) blockers, is a category B drug. In the most recently published study of ranitidine use during pregnancy, data were collected prospectively from a large network database for teratology information. The study reported on 335 pregnant women exposed to ranitidine, 113 to cimetidine, 75 to famotidine, and 15 to nizatidine. The incidence of premature deliveries was higher in the exposed group than in the control group, but there was no increase in the incidence of major malformations. The authors concluded that there was no indication of an increased risk of major malformations after the use of H$_2$ blockers during pregnancy.

Famotidine and Nizatidine

Although both famotidine and nizatidine are category B drugs, the relatively smaller amount of data available from animal and human studies compared with that for other H$_2$ blockers makes the choice of another agent prudent. Studies of animals treated with nizatidine, at 300 times the recommended human dose, reported more abortions, lower fetal weight, and fewer live fetuses among the treated animals than among the controls. Another study showed a higher rate of abortions in rabbits treated with large doses of the drug.

Promotility Agents

Metoclopramide

Metoclopramide is a category B drug. No congenital malformations or other neonatal toxicities in humans have been reported with the use of metoclopramide. Reproductive studies of mice, rats, and rabbits that received up to 250 times the recommended human dose have not demonstrated any increase in fetal toxicity. Metoclopramide has been used as a lactation stimulant, and the total daily dose that would be consumed by a nursing infant if the mother took 30 mg daily is much less than the maximum daily dose of 500 µg/kg recommend for infants.

Therefore, maternal doses of 45 mg or less daily should not have adverse effects on a breastfeeding infant.

Cisapride

Cisapride is a category C drug. A prospective, multicenter study compared the outcomes of 129 Canadian women who took cisapride between November 1996 and November 1998 with those of matched controls. No differences in the rates of major or minor congenital malformations were reported for the 2 groups. In July 2000, Janssen Pharmaceuticals, Inc, removed cisapride from the market because of concern about cardiovascular effects, and it is available only through a limited-access program.

Omeprazole

Omeprazole, the first proton pump inhibitor, is a category C drug. This drug has been shown to produce dose-related embryonic and fetal mortality in pregnant rats and rabbits administered doses similar to those for humans. However, several prospective database studies have shown the safety of omeprazole. The incidence of major abnormalities in pregnant women exposed to omeprazole was 5.1%, compared with 3.1% for those taking H$_2$ blockers and 3.0% for the untreated group. Because of the paucity of data about their effects, proton pump inhibitors are not recommended for mothers who are breastfeeding.

Lansoprazole

Lansoprazole is a category B drug. In 1 nonobservational cohort study, 6 pregnant patients exposed to lansoprazole during the first trimester delivered 7 healthy newborns. The relative risk for a congenital malformation was 1.6 (95% CI, 0.1-5.2); for low birth weight, 1.8 (95% CI, 0.2-13.1).

Pantoprazole

Pantoprazole is also a category B drug. In a European cohort study, 53 pregnant women were exposed to pantoprazole, and the rate observed for congenital anomalies was 2.1%. Although the newer proton pump inhibitors rabeprazole and esomeprazole are also category B drugs, no controlled data are available about them; thus, their use is not recommended during pregnancy.

Esomeprazole

Esomeprazole is a category B drug. Most of its safety data come from studies done with its isomer, omeprazole. The single study that used esomeprazole showed a nonsignificant increase in the incidence of birth defects when the drug was used 4 weeks before pregnancy or in the first trimester.

Dexlansoprazole

Dexlansoprazole is a category B drug as well. To date, no controlled studies have been performed with humans. In reproductive studies with rodents given up to 40 times the recommended human dose, there was no evidence of adverse events.

Rabeprazole

Compared with studies of other proton pump inhibitors, rabeprazole studies have the least amount of human data. Studies with rodents given doses considered supratherapeutic for humans did not show any increase in adverse events. Thus, rabeprazole is a category B drug.

> ✓ Heartburn—extremely common during pregnancy, particularly during later stages
> ✓ Omeprazole—the only proton pump inhibitor that is discouraged as treatment according to early animal data
> ✓ Avoid use of heartburn remedies that contain sodium bicarbonate, calcium carbonate, or trisilicates

Peptic Ulcer Disease

Treatment of peptic ulcer disease involves the use of proton pump inhibitors or H₂ blockers, which are discussed above in the Gastroesophageal Reflux Disease section. If peptic ulcer disease is related to *Helicobacter pylori* infection, treatment of the infection can be deferred until after pregnancy. The most common regimen involves triple therapy with a proton pump inhibitor, amoxicillin, and clarithromycin. Alternatively, metronidazole, bismuth, and tetracycline may be used if needed. In the unusual case when treatment is warranted during the gravid period, tetracycline and bismuth should not be used.

Amoxicillin

Amoxicillin is a category B drug. A population-based study of 401 women treated with amoxicillin did not show any increased risk of congenital malformation or any other adverse event compared with pregnant women not treated with amoxicillin.

Clarithromycin

Clarithromycin, a category C drug, has a higher rate of placental passage than other macrolide antibiotics. In a prospective study of clarithromycin in pregnancy, no increased risk of congenital malformations was reported; however, the rate of spontaneous abortions was higher than in the unexposed group. A retrospective surveillance study of clarithromycin exposure within 270 days of delivery showed no increase in congenital malformations compared with that of the general population of pregnant women.

Tetracycline

Tetracycline, a category D drug, is possibly unsafe to use during lactation. It is discussed below in the Infectious Diarrhea section.

Metronidazole

Metronidazole is a category B drug and carries a low risk during lactation. It is discussed below in the Infectious Diarrhea section.

Bismuth

Bismuth, a category C drug, is one of the most commonly used over-the-counter antacids. Fetotoxicity from bismuth has been described for animals. Exposure to bismuth subsalicylate during late pregnancy may increase the risk of closure or constriction of the fetal ductus arteriosus, resulting in pulmonary hypertension. Bismuth is considered as possibly unsafe during lactation.

> ✓ Unless *H pylori* infection has been diagnosed in a patient with acute bleeding in the gastrointestinal tract, it is reasonable to defer treatment until after delivery

Acute and Chronic Pancreatitis

Acute pancreatitis often resolves with supportive care. If analgesia is required, meperidine and fentanyl are the preferred medications (discussed above in the Endoscopy section). If the patient cannot tolerate nutrition by mouth because of ongoing pain or ileus, early enteral feedings are recommended.

Chronic pancreatitis is managed with alcohol cessation, small low-fat meals, analgesia, and pancreatic enzyme supplements. Pancreatic enzymes are a category C drug because animal reproduction studies have not been performed. The data on safety during pregnancy and lactation are limited. Generally, unless these medications are essential, their use should be avoided. However, in patients with cystic fibrosis and pancreatic insufficiency, maintenance of nutritional status is a critical factor in pregnancy outcome. In a study of 23 women with 33 pregnancies, 91% of the women received pancreatic supplementation during pregnancy. The severity of lung disease predicted preterm delivery, and no congenital malformations were noted.

Biliary Tract Disease

Cholecystitis and Choledocholithiasis

Laparoscopic cholecystectomy has become the standard of care for the management of cholecystitis and symptomatic choledocholithiasis. Surgical intervention during pregnancy does not appear to be associated with an increase in complications, and if cholecystectomy is indicated during pregnancy, the second trimester is the best time. Nonsurgical approaches, such as oral chenodeoxycholic acid, oral ursodiol (ursodeoxycholic acid [UDCA]), and extracorporeal shock wave lithotripsy, have not been used in pregnancy and are not recommended. Chenodeoxycholic acid and UDCA have been used with limited success in the treatment of cholesterol gallstones in the general population. No data are available about chenodeoxycholic acid in pregnancy (UDCA is discussed below with primary sclerosing cholangitis).

Primary Sclerosing Cholangitis

There is no effective medical therapy for primary sclerosing cholangitis. The medication that has been used most commonly is UDCA, a category B drug. Its safety during lactation is not known. Human fetotoxicity from UDCA has not been reported; however, the data are not sufficient to determine risk in the first trimester. Therapeutic trials with UDCA have yielded inconsistent results, and high doses (25-30 mg/kg daily) may actually be harmful and should be avoided. UDCA can be administered during pregnancy, especially after the first trimester, to reduce cholestasis and accompanying sequelae such as pruritus.

Diseases of the Liver

The use of medications for diseases of the liver, including liver transplant, is summarized in Table 22.5.

Viral Hepatitis

Hepatitis A is a self-limited condition, and the treatment of pregnant women is similar to that of nonpregnant women. Both the inactivated vaccine against hepatitis A and postexposure immune globulin prophylaxis are safe to administer during pregnancy.

Table 22.5.   Medications Used in the Treatment of Diseases of the Liver

Drug	FDA category	Recommendations for pregnancy	Recommendations for breastfeeding
Adefovir dipivoxil	C	Minimal data: no teratogenicity	No human data: probably compatible (hepatitis B)
Antithymocyte globulin	C	Human-specific agent	Safety unknown
Cyclosporine	C	Safest of immunosuppressants	Limited human data: potential toxicity
Entecavir	B	Not recommended: alternatives available	No human data
Interferon	C	Not recommended: defer treatment until after delivery	Limited human data: probably compatible
Lamivudine	C	Low risk	Contraindicated
Muromonab-CD3 (Orthoclone OKT3[a])	C	No pregnancy data but probably low risk	Contraindicated
Mycophenolate mofetil	D	Not recommended	Contraindicated
Nadolol	C: First trimester	Prolonged half-life, so use alternative	Limited human data: potential toxicity
	D: Second and third trimesters	Risk of IUGR in second or third trimester	
Obeticholic acid	No rating	Acceptable to use if appropriate	Likely compatible
Penicillamine	D	Severe embryopathy	No human data: potential toxicity
		If required, decrease dose to 250 mg daily 6 wk before delivery	
Propranolol	C: First trimester	Fetal bradycardia	Limited human data: potential toxicity
	D: Second and third trimesters	IUGR in second and third trimesters	
Ribavirin	X	Contraindicated	No human data: potential toxicity
		Severe fetal neurotoxicity	
Sirolimus	C	Not recommended	No human data: potential toxicity
Tacrolimus	C	Use if mother's health mandates	Limited human data: potential toxicity
Tenofovir	B	Safe for use during pregnancy	Probably compatible (hepatitis B)
Trientine	C	Limited human data: alternative to penicillamine	No human data: potential toxicity
Ursodiol	B	Low risk	No human data: probably compatible
		Used for intrahepatic cholestasis of pregnancy	

Abbreviations: FDA, US Food and Drug Administration; IUGR, intrauterine growth retardation.

[a] Janssen-Cilag.

Adapted from Mahadevan U, Kane S. American Gastroenterological Association Institute technical review on the use of gastrointestinal medications in pregnancy. Gastroenterology. 2006 Jul;131(1):283-311; used with permission.

Hepatitis B infection carries a high rate of vertical transmission, and the indications to treat are much greater during pregnancy. The vaccine is safe to use. Passive and active immunization, given together, are very effective in preventing neonatal transmission, reducing the carrier state of infants born to women who test positive for hepatitis B e antigen and hepatitis B surface antigen (carrier state decreases from 70% to 90% to almost zero).

Lamivudine

The FDA has classified lamivudine as a category C drug. For women with chronic hepatitis B, studies have documented the safety of lamivudine for continued treatment during pregnancy. Standard doses of lamivudine have been continued through pregnancy with a hepatitis B virus (HBV)-DNA seroconversion rate of 92%, with no reported complications or congenital abnormalities. In an earlier study, investigators treated 8 highly viremic women with 150 mg lamivudine in the third trimester of pregnancy in an attempt to prevent perinatal transmission of HBV infection. One child was delivered early because of intrauterine growth retardation. All but 1 woman had a marked decrease in HBV DNA levels before delivery, and vertical transmission occurred in only 1 child.

In the medical literature on HIV, the Antiretroviral Pregnancy Registry contains 526 live births that were exposed to lamivudine during the first trimester, with a congenital defect rate of 1.7%. Of 1,256 live births, 25 had a history of exposure during pregnancy and showed a slightly higher rate, 2.5% (95% CI, 1.3%-3.0%),

but this was not statistically higher than expected. Lamivudine is contraindicated during breastfeeding because it is excreted into milk in high concentrations.

Adefovir Dipivoxil

Adefovir dipivoxil is a category C drug. No adequate well-controlled studies have been conducted on the use of adefovir dipivoxil in pregnant women. This drug is indicated for the treatment of chronic hepatitis B in adults who have evidence of active viral replication and evidence of either persistent increase in the serum levels of aminotransferases or histologically active disease. During clinical trials with this agent, 16 pregnancies with known outcomes were reported. Ten women had a therapeutic abortion, 2 had a spontaneous abortion, 3 delivered healthy babies, and 1 delivered a live infant at 25 weeks' gestation who died 4 days later. Studies conducted with adefovir dipivoxil administered orally in doses up to 23 times that achieved in humans have not shown any embryotoxicity or teratogenicity in laboratory animals. No human studies have been performed on the use of this drug during lactation, and its use during lactation is not recommended.

Tenofovir

Tenofovir is a nucleotide reverse transcriptase inhibitor. In a recent review, tenofovir was determined to provide more benefit than harm during pregnancy, and it is a reasonable choice when the viral load is greater than 200,000 U/mL at 26 to 28 weeks' gestation.

Telbivudine

Telbivudine is a nucleoside reverse transcriptase inhibitor that is not available in the US. It can be used if the viral load is greater than 200,000 U/mL at 26 to 28 weeks' gestation, but, as with other drugs in this class, lactic acidosis and kidney insufficiency can occur.

Entecavir

Entecavir is a cyclopentyl guanosine analogue used to treat active hepatitis B. It is not recommended for use during pregnancy because animal data have shown a teratogenic effect.

Interferon

Interferon, a category C drug, is contraindicated during pregnancy because of its antiproliferative activity. When interferon was administered to pregnant rhesus monkeys, they had a statistically significant increase in the number of spontaneous abortions. No teratogenic effects were observed in this species when doses of 1 million to 25 million IU/kg daily were administered during the early-fetal to mid-fetal period. To date, only 27 pregnancies have been reported after exposure to interferon. The majority of these women were being treated for essential thrombocythemia and not hepatitis B. Premature delivery occurred in 15% and intrauterine growth retardation in 22% of the patients (6 of 27). A total of 8 children have been born to mothers receiving interferon who were thought to be at high risk for chronic hepatitis infection. With the advent of effective direct-acting antiviral therapy, interferon is no longer used for the treatment of hepatitis C. Interferon is rarely indicated for treatment of chronic hepatitis B and should not be given during pregnancy because of the risk of teratogenicity.

Ribavirin

Ribavirin is indicated in some situations along with direct-acting antiviral therapy for treatment of hepatitis C. However, ribavirin is known to cause dose-related teratogenic effects and embryolethality in all animal species tested. It is a category X drug and is contraindicated in pregnancy. Furthermore, the risk of teratogenicity persists for up to 6 months after drug cessation in women taking ribavirin and in female partners of men taking ribavirin.

✓ Hepatitis B infection during pregnancy—use of passive and active immune therapy at birth is recommended
✓ Agents for treatment of hepatitis B that pose a low risk during pregnancy—lamivudine, tenofovir, and telbivudine
✓ Treatment of hepatitis B should be provided when the viral load exceeds 200,000 U/mL
✓ Interferon, adefovir, and entecavir are not recommended for use during pregnancy

---

While there are several FDA-approved regimens for hepatitis C with sustained viral response, the indications for treatment during pregnancy are individualized. Very small studies have demonstrated safety. However, there are not enough safety data to recommend use of direct-acting antiviral therapy during

pregnancy. For women who are pregnant and have hepatitis C virus infection, the guidance from the American Association for the Study of Liver Diseases and the Infectious Diseases Society of America is that "treatment can be considered during pregnancy on an individual basis after a patient-physician discussion about the potential risks and benefits."

✓ Generally, there is no need to use drug therapy for hepatitis C during pregnancy because the risks outweigh the benefits

---

Wilson Disease
Penicillamine

Penicillamine, a category D drug, is a chelating agent that is first-line therapy for Wilson disease. Only a few reports are available about the outcome of pregnancies in women with Wilson disease. The largest recent case series is from India, where 59 pregnancies in 16 women were studied retrospectively. This group included 24 spontaneous abortions, 3 stillbirths, 2 terminations, and 30 successful pregnancies. The majority of the spontaneous abortions were in women who were not receiving therapy. Other case reports have documented severe embryopathy characterized by micrognathia, diffuse cutis laxa, and agenesis of the corpus callosum in addition to transient fetal myelosuppression. It is debated whether penicillamine therapy should be continued during pregnancy; various authors have disagreed on whether to use the agent and, if so, how much to administer.

Trientine

Trientine is a category C drug and is used if no other alternatives are appropriate to treat the mother's liver disease. This chelating agent is an alternative to penicillamine and is available only as an orphan drug for use in Wilson disease. Because there are few other options, the benefit is thought to outweigh the risk.

Primary Biliary Cirrhosis
Ursodeoxycholic Acid

UDCA is a category B drug. Because of the paucity of data about its safety in the first trimester, its use during this time is not recommended unless essential. It has been administered to women during the second and third trimesters without apparent deterioration of liver function. No fetal loss or unfavorable outcomes were reported among 10 women receiving the drug. In a randomized controlled trial of UDCA in women with intrahepatic cholestasis of pregnancy, UDCA improved pruritus and liver enzyme levels, and it allowed for delivery closer to term. A second randomized controlled trial, which compared UDCA with cholestyramine, reported similar results: Among the patients treated with UDCA, symptoms were alleviated and babies were delivered much closer to term.

Obeticholic Acid

The FDA recently approved obeticholic acid to treat primary biliary cirrhosis. The drug is used when the response to ursodiol is inadequate or as monotherapy for patients unable to tolerate ursodiol. Animal data did not demonstrate a risk of adverse outcomes, so obeticholic acid can be used during pregnancy if the maternal benefit outweighs the risk of fetal harm.

Portal Hypertension

Propranolol

Propranolol, a category C drug, is a nonselective β-adrenergic blocking agent used for prophylaxis against variceal bleeding in patients with cirrhosis. It has been administered during pregnancy to treat maternal thyrotoxicosis, arrhythmias, and hypertension. It readily crosses the placenta and, thus, is used also to treat fetal arrhythmias. Adverse outcomes have not been clearly linked to its use, but daily doses greater than 160 mg appear to produce more serious fetal cardiac complications. No data have been reported for outcomes among women who took this drug for variceal prophylaxis. Propranolol is not a teratogen, but fetal and neonatal toxicity may occur. Maternal use after the second trimester can result in marked weight reductions in the infant. Therefore, it is not recommended for use after the first trimester unless the underlying condition of the mother requires continued β-blockade.

Nadolol

Nadolol, a category C drug, is another nonselective β-adrenergic blocker. It is an alternative to propranolol. Nadolol is used predominantly as an antihypertensive, and no data are available for its use for variceal prophylaxis. Because the characteristics of nadolol include a long half-life, low protein binding, and lack of metabolism, the use of alternative agents in this class is recommended if treatment is strongly indicated.

Liver Transplant

The best data available about medications for transplant recipients are from the National Transplantation Pregnancy Registry. Every year, an updated report is presented with the results from a prospective database of all transplant recipients. In a recent report, the rate of live births was 77% for women receiving cyclosporine, 82% for those receiving cyclosporine as Neoral (Novartis), and 72% for those receiving tacrolimus. Two patients were receiving mycophenolate mofetil therapy and delivered healthy infants. The mean gestational age was 37 weeks, and the rate of low birth weight was 29% to 42%. The conclusion of the advisory board was that "the majority of pregnancy outcomes reported to the Registry appear favorable for parent and newborn."

Cyclosporine

Cyclosporine is a category C drug. A meta-analysis of 15 studies of pregnancy outcomes after cyclosporine therapy reported on 410 patients. For major malformations, the calculated OR (3.83; 95% CI, 0.75-19.6) was not statistically significant, and the rate of malformations (4.1%) was not different from that of the general population. The conclusion from the study was that cyclosporine did not appear to be a major human teratogen. The American Academy of Pediatrics considers cyclosporine contraindicated during breastfeeding because of the potential for immunosuppression and neutropenia.

Tacrolimus

Tacrolimus is another category C drug. The earliest experience with this medication was in 1997, with a report of 27 pregnancies with exposure to tacrolimus. Another study from Germany reported on 100 pregnancies in transplant recipients followed from 1992 to 1998. The live birth rate was 68%, the spontaneous abortion rate was 12%, the stillbirth rate was 3%, and 59% of the infants were premature. Malformations occurred in 4 neonates, with no consistent defects. More recent data from the National Transplantation Pregnancy Registry showed a birth defect rate of 4.2% among live births with exposure to tacrolimus, which was not different from the background rate of birth defects in the US (3%-5%). Tacrolimus is the most commonly used immunosuppressive drug after liver transplant and is generally used at the lowest acceptable dose during pregnancy to prevent rejection. Tacrolimus is contraindicated during lactation because of the high concentrations found in breast milk.

Sirolimus

Sirolimus is a category C drug. Little is known about its effect in humans. Sirolimus is another agent used for immunosuppression in transplant recipients. Three patients in the National Transplantation Pregnancy Registry were treated with sirolimus, but they were kidney recipients. Because of the relative paucity of information, and the reasonable alternatives for immunosuppression, this agent is not recommended during pregnancy.

Mycophenolate Mofetil

Mycophenolate mofetil, a category D drug, has been shown to have teratogenic properties in laboratory animals. In a single case report in the obstetric literature, a kidney transplant recipient was treated with mycophenolate mofetil before conception and during the first trimester of pregnancy. The fetus had facial dysmorphology and multiple midline anomalies. The molecular weight of this agent is low enough that it most likely crosses the placenta. Its use is contraindicated in pregnancy. The manufacturer recommends that women use effective contraception before and during therapy and for 6 weeks after therapy has stopped.

Irritable Bowel Syndrome

Irritable bowel syndrome (IBS) is a heterogeneous disorder without a standardized therapeutic regimen. No large epidemiologic studies have been conducted with pregnant women who have preexisting IBS. If possible, medications should be avoided and dietary alterations and fiber supplementation should be the first step for symptoms of constipation. The following summarizes available safety data about drugs for IBS if medication is required. However, most drug therapies for the treatment of this syndrome have not demonstrated efficacy over placebo. The use of medications for IBS during pregnancy is summarized in Table 22.6.

> ✓ For any symptom in a patient with IBS, dietary modification should always be tried before medications

Constipation

For a pregnant woman with constipation, first-line therapy should be fiber supplements, introduced gradually to avoid excessive gas and bloating, and adequate water intake. New-onset constipation during early pregnancy is often due to iron therapy, and symptomatic relief can be achieved with docusate, now a component of some prenatal vitamins. When these methods are inadequate, an osmotic laxative should be considered, particularly a polyethylene glycol solution. Osmotic laxatives include saline osmotics (magnesium and sodium salts), saccharated osmotics

Table 22.6. Medications Used in the Treatment of Irritable Bowel Syndrome

Drug	FDA category	Recommendations for pregnancy	Recommendations for breastfeeding
Alosetron	B	Avoid: restricted access	No human data: potential toxicity
Amitriptyline	C	Avoid: no malformations, but worse outcomes	Limited human data: potential toxicity
Bisacodyl	C	Safe with short-term use	Safety unknown
Bismuth subsalicylate	C	Not safe: teratogenicity	No human data: potential toxicity
Castor oil	X	Uterine contraction and rupture	Possibly unsafe
Cholestyramine	C	Low risk, but can lead to infant coagulopathy	Compatible
Desipramine	C	Avoid: no malformations, but worse outcome	Limited human data: potential toxicity
Dicyclomine	B	Avoid: possible congenital anomalies	Limited human data: potential toxicity
Diphenoxylate-atropine	C	Teratogenic in animals; no human data	Limited human data: potential toxicity
Docusate	C	Safe	Compatible
Hyoscyamine	C	No available data	No human data: probably compatible
Imipramine	D	Avoid: no malformations, but worse outcomes	Limited human data: potential toxicity
Kaopectate (bismuth subsalicylate)[a]	C	Unsafe; now contains bismuth subsalicylate	No human data: probably compatible
Lactulose	B	No human studies	No human data: probably compatible
Linaclotide	B	Low risk if appropriate	Limited human data: probably compatible
Loperamide	B	Low risk: possibly increased cardiovascular defects	Limited human data: probably compatible
Lubiprostone	C	Limited human data: use when benefit outweighs risk	No human data: not recommended
Magnesium citrate	B	Avoid long-term use: hypermagnesemia, hyperphosphatemia, dehydration	Compatible
Mineral oil	C	Avoid: neonatal coagulopathy and hemorrhage	Possibly unsafe
Nortriptyline	D	Avoid: no malformations, but worse outcomes	Limited human data: potential toxicity
Paroxetine	D	Avoid: twice as many birth defects as other antidepressants	Potential toxicity
Plecanatide	B	Low risk if indicated	Low risk
Polyethylene glycol	C	First-choice laxative in pregnancy	Low risk
Senna	C	Safe with short-term use	Compatible
Selective serotonin reuptake inhibitors (except paroxetine)	C	Avoid: no malformations, but increased adverse fetal events	Limited human data: potential toxicity
Simethicone	C	No available data Low risk	No human data: probably compatible
Sodium phosphate	None	Avoid long-term use: hypermagnesemia, hyperphosphatemia, dehydration	Safety unknown
Tegaserod	B	Low risk: human data negative for malformations	Safety unknown

Abbreviation: FDA, US Food and Drug Administration.

[a] Kramer Laboratories.

Adapted from Mahadevan U, Kane S. American Gastroenterological Association Institute technical review on the use of gastrointestinal medications in pregnancy. Gastroenterology. 2006 Jul;131(1):283-311; used with permission.

(lactulose and sorbitol), and polyethylene glycol. Saline osmotic laxatives such as magnesium citrate (category B) and sodium phosphate have rapid onset of action but are intended for short-term intermittent relief. Long-term use can result in hypermagnesemia, hyperphosphatemia, and dehydration. No human studies are available on the use of lactulose (category B) during pregnancy. Polyethylene glycol (category C) is negligibly absorbed and metabolized in humans, making it unlikely to cause malformations. Also, it is effective and well tolerated compared with lactulose. The results of animal teratogenesis studies have been negative. A consensus meeting on the management of constipation in pregnancy considered polyethylene glycol to meet the criteria for an ideal laxative in pregnancy: effective, not absorbed (nonteratogenic), well tolerated, and safe. However, the consensus members thought that current data were insufficient to demonstrate conclusively whether absorption of polyethylene glycol affects the fetus.

Stimulant laxatives such as senna (category C) and bisacodyl (category C) are considered safe for short-term use, but long-term use is not recommended. Because senna is excreted in breast milk, it should be used with caution during lactation. Docusate (category C), a stool softener, is generally considered safe. Castor oil (category X) should be avoided because it is associated with uterine contraction and rupture. Mineral oil also should be avoided because it can impair maternal fat-soluble

vitamin absorption and lead to neonatal coagulopathy and hemorrhage.

Tegaserod (category B), a type 4 serotonin receptor agonist, was approved by the FDA for the treatment of constipation-predominant IBS and chronic constipation. It was withdrawn from the market in 2007 because of concern about an increased risk of cardiac events with its use, but it has been reintroduced and is available. Current guidelines suggest that it not be used in patients who have risk factors for cardiac disease.

Lubiprostone is a chloride channel activator that is approved by the FDA to treat chronic constipation and constipation-predominant IBS. It is a category C drug with limited human data, and animal studies have shown adverse events with exposure. It is not recommended for use when breastfeeding.

Linaclotide and plecanatide are both guanylate cyclase-C receptor agonists approved for treatment of chronic constipation. However, these are relatively new therapies, and few data are available from studies of pregnant women, so agents with other mechanisms of action should be used.

- ✓ Fiber should be the first-line therapy for constipation during pregnancy
- ✓ Short-term use of stimulant laxatives is acceptable
- ✓ Castor oil is absolutely contraindicated because of the risk of uterine rupture

Diarrhea

In a trial of 105 women exposed to loperamide (category B) during pregnancy, loperamide was not associated with an increased risk of congenital malformations, although 20% of the infants were 200 g smaller than infants in the control group. At least 187 cases of first-trimester exposure have been reported, with no evidence of developmental toxicity. Cholestyramine (category C), an anion exchange resin, is often used to treat cholestasis of pregnancy and can be used to manage diarrhea resulting from ileal resection or cholecystectomy. However, fat-soluble vitamin deficiency, including coagulopathy, can occur, so it should be used with caution. Kaolin in combination with pectin (Kaopectate; Kramer Laboratories) (category B) was an antidiarrheal of choice because it was not absorbed and did not cross the placenta, but concern arose over the potential for kaolin-induced iron deficiency anemia. In 2003, Kaopectate was reformulated to contain bismuth subsalicylate (category C). Bismuth subsalicylate, alone or in Kaopectate, should be avoided in pregnancy because the salicylates can be absorbed and lead to increased perinatal mortality, premature closure of the ductus arteriosus, neonatal hemorrhage, decreased birth weight, prolonged gestation and labor, and possible teratogenicity. Alosetron (category B) has restricted access because of concern about ischemic colitis. Its use generally should be avoided during pregnancy.

Eluxadoline is approved to treat diarrhea associated with IBS. Although data from studies with pregnant women are limited, eluxadoline is considered low risk for use during pregnancy and breastfeeding.

For pregnant women with diarrhea, dietary modification, with reduction of fats and dairy, can improve symptoms. Although human data are limited, both loperamide and diphenoxylate are considered "low risk" and can be used with discretion.

Tricyclic antidepressants (amitriptyline and desipramine, both category C drugs, and nortriptyline and imipramine, both category D drugs) and selective serotonin reuptake inhibitors (SSRIs) (generally category C drugs) are frequently used in the management of IBS. Overall, the newer antidepressants (citalopram, escitalopram, fluoxetine, fluvoxamine, sertraline, reboxetine, venlafaxine, nefazodone, trazodone, mirtazapine, and bupropion) are not associated with an increased rate of major malformations compared with that of the general population. Recently, however, an unpublished GlaxoSmithKline study of 3,500 pregnant women noted twice as many birth defects with paroxetine than with other antidepressants (Table 22.6). In the first trimester, for paroxetine users the absolute rate of major congenital malformations was 4% and the absolute rate of cardiovascular malformations was 2%. Infants exposed to antidepressants are also at higher risk for other adverse events. In a large Swedish study of 997 infants exposed to antidepressants during pregnancy, the infants had an increased risk of preterm birth, low birth weight, low Apgar score, respiratory distress, neonatal convulsions, and hypoglycemia. The data suggested that outcomes were worse with tricyclic antidepressants compared with SSRIs. Multiple studies with SSRIs have confirmed that the rate of congenital malformations for infants exposed to these drugs is similar to that for the general population; however, the studies also have noted a higher rate of premature delivery, respiratory difficulty, cyanosis on feeding, and jitteriness as well as low birth weight and neonatal convulsions among infants exposed to SSRIs. The effect of SSRI exposure through the placenta on neonatal adaptation and long-term neurocognitive development is debated. If the antidepressant is being administered

solely to treat symptoms of IBS and not an associated major depression, strong consideration should be given to stopping the drug therapy during the gravid period.

Antispasmodics are prescribed frequently for the management of abdominal pain in IBS. Dicyclomine (category B), in combination with pyridoxine and doxylamine (Bendectin; Merrell Dow Pharmaceuticals, Inc), has been associated with multiple congenital anomalies, but the studies have not been conclusive. Hyoscyamine (category C) has not been studied in pregnancy.

✓ During pregnancy, antidiarrheal agents containing salicylates should be avoided
✓ Loperamide, eluxadoline, and tricyclic antidepressants are acceptable to use for diarrhea caused by IBS

Infectious Diarrhea

Diarrhea can be described as acute (<14 days), persistent (>14 days), or chronic (>30 days). Although most episodes of diarrhea are self-limited and treatment is not required, certain pathogens require treatment. The common medications used to treat infectious diarrhea are summarized in Table 22.7.

Albendazole

Albendazole, a category C drug, is used in the treatment of microsporidial infection, cysticercosis, helminth infection, and hydatid disease. The drug is embryotoxic and teratogenic (skeletal malformations) in rats and rabbits. Human data are limited. Albendazole therapy for the eradication of helminths during pregnancy is associated with significantly less maternal anemia and no increase in adverse pregnancy outcomes, prompting the World Health Organization to recommend antihelminthic therapy in pregnancy.

Ampicillin

Ampicillin, a category B drug, is not considered teratogenic. It is second-line treatment of *Shigella* infection. Ampicillin passes through the placenta by simple diffusion and is excreted into breast milk in low concentrations.

Azithromycin

Azithromycin, a macrolide antibiotic, is in pregnancy category B and is a second-line treatment of *Cryptosporidium* and *Entamoeba histolytica* infections. In pregnant women with traveler's diarrhea, azithromycin or a third-generation cephalosporin is considered the treatment of choice. A study of 20 women who received the drug for *Chlamydia trachomatis* infection noted that 40% reported moderate to severe gastrointestinal adverse effects. A trial of 94 pregnant women with *Trichomonas vaginalis* treated with a combination of azithromycin, cefixime, and metronidazole demonstrated increased rates of infant low birth weight, preterm birth, and 2-year mortality compared with rates for the children of 112 infected mothers who were not treated for the same infection.

Doxycycline and Tetracycline

Doxycycline and tetracycline are both category D drugs. Doxycycline is used as second-line treatment of infections with *Vibrio cholerae*, *Campylobacter*, and enterotoxigenic *Escherichia*

Table 22.7. Medications Used for the Treatment of Infectious Diarrhea

Drug	FDA category	Recommendations for pregnancy	Recommendations for breastfeeding
Albendazole	C	Embryotoxic in animals Avoid in first trimester Human data support improved pregnancy outcomes with helminth eradication	No human data: probably compatible
Ampicillin	B	Safe	Compatible
Azithromycin	B	Low risk	Limited human data: probably compatible
Ciprofloxacin (all quinolones)	C	Potential toxicity to cartilage: avoid	Limited human data: probably compatible
Doxycycline	D	Contraindicated: teratogenic	Compatible
Fidaxomicin	B	Low risk but expensive	No human data: potential toxicity
Furazolidone	C	Low risk Limited data	No human data: potential toxicity
Metronidazole	B	Low risk: question of increased risk of cleft lip with or without cleft palate	Limited human data: potential toxicity
Rifaximin	C	Animal teratogen No human data	No human data: probably compatible
Tetracycline	D	Not safe: teratogenicity	Compatible
Tinidazole	C	Low risk Limited data	Unsafe
Trimethoprim-sulfamethoxazole	C	Teratogenic	Compatible
Vancomycin	C	Low risk	Limited human data: probably compatible

Abbreviation: FDA, US Food and Drug Administration.

Adapted from Mahadevan U, Kane S. American Gastroenterological Association Institute technical review on the use of gastrointestinal medications in pregnancy. Gastroenterology. 2006 Jul;131(1):283-311; used with permission.

coli. Similar to tetracycline, this class of medications crosses the placenta and is bound by chelating with calcium in developing bone and teeth. This results in discoloration of the teeth, hypoplasia of enamel, and inhibition of skeletal growth. A population-based study found a higher rate of congenital anomalies in the infants of mothers who used doxycycline during pregnancy; however, the case-control pair analysis did not show a significantly higher rate of doxycycline treatment in the second and third months of gestation in any group of congenital abnormalities.

Fidaxomicin

Fidaxomicin, a category B drug, recently received FDA approval for treatment of *Clostridioides difficile* infection. Its use is limited by its cost, and it has not been studied in large numbers of pregnancies to date.

Furazolidone

Furazolidone, a category C drug, is second-line treatment of giardiasis. Few data are available on the safety of furazolidone in pregnancy, but the Collaborative Perinatal Project monitored 50,282 mother-child pairs, and 132 had exposure to furazolidone in the first trimester with no association with congenital malformations.

Metronidazole

Metronidazole, a category B drug, is used to treat *C difficile* infection, amebiasis, and giardiasis. Multiple studies have suggested that exposure to metronidazole prenatally is not associated with birth defects. These studies include 2 meta-analyses, 2 retrospective cohort studies, and a prospective controlled study of 228 women exposed to metronidazole during pregnancy. A population-based case-control study found that overall teratogenic risk was low, but infants of women exposed to metronidazole in the second to third months of pregnancy had higher rates

of cleft lip, with or without cleft palate. This increase was slight and not thought to be clinically significant.

Quinolones

Quinolones (eg, ciprofloxacin, levofloxacin, and norfloxacin), category C drugs, are used to treat infections with *Shigella*, *Campylobacter*, *Yersinia*, enterotoxigenic and enteroinvasive *E coli*, and *V cholerae*. Quinolones have a high affinity for bone tissue and cartilage and may cause arthropathies in children. The manufacturer reports damage to cartilage in weight-bearing joints after quinolone exposure in immature rats and dogs. However, a prospective controlled study of 200 women exposed to quinolones and a population-based cohort study of 57 women exposed to quinolones did not find an increased risk of congenital malformations. Overall, the risk is thought to be minimal, but because safer alternatives are available, quinolones should be avoided in pregnancy.

Rifaximin

Rifaximin, a category C drug, can be used to treat traveler's diarrhea, although azithromycin is the antibiotic of choice for pregnant patients with traveler's diarrhea. Little information exists about the safety of rifaximin in pregnancy. Rifaximin has not been found to affect fertility or pregnancy outcome in rats or, in 1 study, to cause teratogenic complications in rats and rabbits. However, other studies have noted teratogenicity in rats and rabbits, including cleft palate and incomplete ossification.

Tinidazole

Tinidazole, a category C drug, is a second-line treatment of giardiasis and amebiasis. Placental transfer of tinidazole occurs early in pregnancy, raising concern about its use in the first trimester.

A population-based study from Hungary did not note an increased rate of congenital malformations when the drug was administered during pregnancy; however, the number of women treated with tinidazole was small.

Trimethoprim-Sulfamethoxazole

Trimethoprim-sulfamethoxazole, a category C drug, is first-line treatment of infections with *Cystoisospora* (previously known as *Isospora*) or *Cyclospora* and second-line treatment of infections with *Shigella*, *Yersinia*, or enterotoxigenic *E coli*. Trimethoprim has antifolate effects, increasing the potential for congenital anomalies. A study of 2,296 Michigan Medicaid recipients with first-trimester exposure to trimethoprim noted an increased risk of birth defects, particularly cardiovascular defects. A population-based case-control study in Hungary noted a higher rate of multiple congenital anomalies and cardiovascular malformations. On the basis of these data, use of trimethoprim-sulfamethoxazole should be avoided in pregnancy.

Vancomycin

Vancomycin, a category C drug, is used in the treatment of severe *C difficile* colitis, or *C difficile* infection that is refractory to treatment with metronidazole. Studies in rats and rabbits have not demonstrated teratogenic effects. No cases of congenital defects attributable to vancomycin have been located, and the drug is considered low risk in pregnancy.

> ✓ Quinolones should be avoided as alternatives are available for treating infectious diarrhea

Inflammatory Bowel Disease

For patients with Crohn disease and ulcerative colitis, disease activity at the time of conception can be associated with a higher risk of spontaneous abortion, and disease activity during the course of pregnancy can be associated with higher rates of low birth weight and premature infants. It is advisable that the disease be in remission when patients are considering pregnancy, and for the majority, this requires continued use of the medications. Medications used to treat inflammatory bowel disease (IBD) are summarized in Table 22.8.

Aminosalicylates

All aminosalicylates (sulfasalazine, mesalamine, and balsalazide) are category B drugs except olsalazine, and the mesalamine products Asacol and Asacol HD (AbbVie), which are in category C. A population-based study using the Hungarian Case-Control Surveillance of Congenital Abnormalities database did not show a significant increase in the prevalence of congenital abnormalities in the children of women treated with sulfasalazine. Because of concern about potential antifolate effects of sulfasalazine, it is recommended that women take folic acid 1 mg twice daily in the

Table 22.8. Medications Used in the Treatment of Inflammatory Bowel Disease (IBD)

Drug	FDA category	Recommendations for pregnancy	Recommendations for breastfeeding
Adalimumab	B	Limited human data: low risk	No human data: probably compatible
Amoxicillin-clavulinic acid	B	Low risk	Probably compatible
Azathioprine and 6-mercaptopurine	D	Data in IBD and transplant literature suggest low risk	No human data: potential toxicity
Balsalazide	B	Low risk	No human data: potential diarrhea
Certolizumab pegol	B	Low risk	No human data
Ciprofloxacin	C	Avoid: potential toxicity to cartilage	Limited human data: probably compatible
Corticosteroids	C	Low risk: possibly increased risk of cleft palate, adrenal insufficiency, premature rupture of membranes	Compatible
Cyclosporine	C	Low risk	Limited human data: potential toxicity
Fish oil supplements	None	Safe / Possible benefit	No human data
Golimumab	B	Low risk	Human data: probably compatible
Infliximab	B	Low risk	No human data: probably compatible
Mesalamine	B	Low risk	Limited human data: potential diarrhea
Methotrexate	X	Contraindicated: teratogenic	Contraindicated
Metronidazole	B	Avoid: limited efficacy in IBD and risk of cleft palate	Limited human data: potential toxicity
Natalizumab	B	Low risk	No human data
Olsalazine	C	Low risk	Limited human data: potential diarrhea
Ozanimod	No rating	Animal risk; no human data	No human data: possible toxicity
Rifaximin	C	Animal teratogen / No human data	No human data: probably compatible
Sulfasalazine	B	Considered safe / Give folate 2 mg daily	Limited human data: potential diarrhea
Tacrolimus	C	Use if mother's health mandates	Limited human data: potential toxicity
Thalidomide	X	Contraindicated: teratogenic	No human data: potential toxicity
Upadacitinib	No rating	Possible teratogen	Limited human data: probably compatible
Ustekinumab	No rating	Human data: low risk	Limited human data: probably compatible
Vedolizumab	No rating	Human data: low risk	Limited human data: probably compatible

Abbreviation: FDA, US Food and Drug Administration.

Adapted from Mahadevan U, Kane S. American Gastroenterological Association Institute technical review on the use of gastrointestinal medications in pregnancy. Gastroenterology. 2006 Jul;131(1):283-311; used with permission.

prenatal period and throughout pregnancy. Unlike with other sulfonamides, bilirubin displacement and, thus, kernicterus do not occur in the infant. Sulfasalazine has been clearly associated with infertility in men. Abnormalities in sperm number, motility, and morphology have been noted. This effect appears to be reversible: When mesalamine was substituted for sulfasalazine, semen quality returned to normal. An association has been described between sulfasalazine use in the parent and congenital malformations in the progeny. Because the lifespan of sperm is 120 days, men considering conception should either stop taking sulfasalazine or switch to mesalamine at least 3 months before attempting conception.

Case series of mesalamine use in pregnancy do not suggest an increased risk to the fetus. This has been supported by a prospective controlled trial of 165 women exposed to mesalamine who were compared with matched controls with no exposure and by a population-based cohort study from Denmark. The formulations of Asacol and Asacol HD have been changed, so dibutyl phthalate is no longer present in any mesalamine products.

Antibiotics

Metronidazole, the quinolones, and rifaximin are covered in the Infectious Diarrhea section above. Because of the limited evidence of the effectiveness of these agents in treating IBD and the extended duration of use in the treatment of Crohn disease and ulcerative colitis, use of these drugs should be avoided during pregnancy. Short courses for the treatment of pouchitis can be considered on the basis of the safety data presented above. An alternative antibiotic for pouchitis is amoxicillin-clavulanic acid, a category B drug.

Corticosteroids

Corticosteroids are category C drugs. A case-control study of corticosteroid use during the first trimester of pregnancy noted an increased risk of oral clefts in newborns. This was confirmed by a large case-control study and a meta-analysis, which reported a summary OR for case-control studies examining the risk of oral clefts (OR, 3.35; 95% CI, 1.97-5.69). However, the population was treated for various conditions, and the overall risk of major malformations was low (OR, 1.45; 95% CI, 0.80-2.60). A prospective controlled study of 311 women who received corticosteroids during the first trimester did not note an increased rate of major anomalies, and cases of oral cleft were not noted. The study was powered to find a 2.5-fold increase in the overall rate of major anomalies. An increased risk of premature rupture of membranes and adrenal insufficiency in the newborn has been reported for transplant patients. Overall, the use of corticosteroids poses a small risk to the developing infant, and the benefit of treating active disease outweighs the fetal risk. Systemic corticosteroids should be used at the lowest effective dose because prolonged exposure leads to increased risk of gestational diabetes and premature lung maturity in the fetus. A small retrospective review of patients with IBD treated with budesonide during pregnancy did not document congenital malformations or an increase in adverse outcomes.

Immunomodulators

The immunomodulators are the most controversial agents used to treat IBD in pregnant women.

Methotrexate

Methotrexate, a category X drug, is clearly teratogenic and should not be administered to women or men who are considering conception. Methotrexate is a folic acid antagonist, and its use during the critical period of organogenesis (6-8 weeks postconception) is associated with multiple congenital anomalies collectively called *methotrexate embryopathy* or *fetal aminopterin-methotrexate syndrome*. This syndrome is characterized by intrauterine growth retardation; decreased ossification of the calvarium; hypoplastic supraorbital ridges; small, low-set ears; micrognathia; limb abnormalities; and, occasionally, intellectual disability. Exposure in the second and third trimesters may be associated with fetal toxicity and death. Methotrexate may cause reversible oligospermia in men. No case reports have been published on congenital anomalies occurring in the offspring of men receiving methotrexate therapy. Methotrexate may persist in tissues for long periods, and it has been suggested that patients wait at least 3 to 6 months after discontinuation of treatment with the drug before attempting conception.

Azathioprine and 6-Mercaptopurine

The drug 6-mercaptopurine and its prodrug azathioprine are in category D. Animal studies have demonstrated teratogenicity, with increased frequencies of cleft palate and open-eye and skeletal anomalies in mice exposed to azathioprine and cleft palate and skeletal and urogenital anomalies in rats. Transplacental and transamniotic transmission of azathioprine and its metabolites from the mother to the fetus can occur. The oral bioavailability of azathioprine (47%) and 6-mercaptopurine (16%) is low, and the early fetal liver lacks the enzyme inosinate pyrophosphorylase, which is needed to convert azathioprine to 6-mercaptopurine. Both features may protect the fetus from toxic drug exposure during the crucial period of organogenesis. The largest evidence on safety comes from transplant studies, in which rates of anomalies ranged from zero to 11.8%, and no evidence emerged for recurrent patterns of congenital anomalies. Multiple case series of IBD have not noted an increase in congenital anomalies. On the basis of the large experience with transplant patients and the body of evidence in IBD, use of the drugs is often continued during pregnancy to maintain remission in the mother. A flare of disease during pregnancy may be more deleterious to neonatal outcome than any potential risk from the medication.

Cyclosporine and Tacrolimus

These agents are considered in the Liver Transplant section. For severe corticosteroid-refractory ulcerative colitis, cyclosporine may be a better treatment option than colectomy, which is associated with a considerable morbidity rate for mother and fetus.

Thalidomide

Thalidomide, a category X drug, has some anti–tumor necrosis factor effects and has been used successfully for the treatment of Crohn disease. However, its teratogenicity has been documented extensively and includes limb defects, central nervous system effects, and abnormalities of the respiratory, cardiovascular, gastrointestinal, and genitourinary systems. Thalidomide is contraindicated during pregnancy and for women of childbearing age who are not using 2 reliable methods of contraception for 1 month before starting therapy, during therapy, and for 1 month after stopping therapy.

✓ Immunomodulators safe to use in pregnancy include thiopurines and calcineurin inhibitors
✓ Methotrexate and thalidomide—contraindicated in pregnancy

Biological Therapy

Infliximab

Infliximab, a category B drug, is used in the management of Crohn disease and ulcerative colitis. A growing body of evidence suggests that infliximab is low risk in pregnancy. The 2 largest studies are from the Crohn's Therapy, Resource, Evaluation, and Assessment Tool (TREAT) Registry and the infliximab safety database maintained by Janssen Biotech, Inc. The TREAT Registry is a prospective registry of patients with Crohn disease, and the patients may or may not be treated with infliximab. Among the 5,807 patients enrolled, 66 pregnancies were reported, and 36 of the 66 had prior exposure to infliximab. Fetal malformations have not occurred in any of the pregnancies. The rates of miscarriage (11.1% vs 7.1%, P=.53) and neonatal complications (8.3% vs 7.1%, P=.78) were higher for infliximab-treated patients than for infliximab-naïve patients, but the differences were not statistically significant.

In the infliximab safety database, a retrospective data collection, pregnancy outcome data are available for 96 women who had direct exposure to infliximab. The 96 pregnancies resulted in 100 births. The expected outcomes and the observed outcomes for women exposed to infliximab were not different from those of the general population. In a series of 10 women who received maintenance therapy with infliximab throughout pregnancy, all 10 pregnancies ended in live births and no congenital malformations were reported.

Infliximab probably crosses the placenta, beginning at approximately week 20. Currently, if maternal health warrants infliximab therapy, it is continued through pregnancy.

Adalimumab

Adalimumab, a category B drug, is approved for induction and maintenance therapy for both Crohn disease and ulcerative colitis. It is an immunoglobulin (Ig)G1 molecule that crosses the placenta, but retrospective and prospective data show its safety during pregnancy.

Certolizumab Pegol

Certolizumab is a pegylated Fab′ fragment of IgG1 antibody against tumor necrosis factor α and is approved to treat Crohn disease. Studies have shown the lack of placental transfer of certolizumab, and it may thus have an advantage for use in pregnancy. Certolizumab pegol therapy is warranted during pregnancy for active IBD or maintenance of remission.

Golimumab

Golimumab is an IgG1 monoclonal antibody approved for ulcerative colitis. Like the other anti–tumor necrosis factor molecules, it crosses the placenta but is not associated with any adverse outcomes in pregnancy and should be continued before conception and during pregnancy.

Natalizumab

Natalizumab is a monoclonal antibody of the IgG4 class directed against α integrins and approved for the treatment of Crohn disease. On the basis of animal and trial data, it is listed as an FDA

category B drug. Few postmarketing data are available about its use in pregnancy. Currently, there are no firm recommendations about its use in treating IBD in pregnant women, but given the availability of more targeted anti-integrins, this agent is not commonly used for Crohn disease.

Vedolizumab

Vedolizumab is a more targeted IgG1 monoclonal antibody to α integrins. It is approved for the treatment of both Crohn disease and ulcerative colitis. While it does cross the placenta, it is thought to present only low risk during pregnancy, so therapy should not be discontinued before conception or during pregnancy.

Ustekinumab

Ustekinumab is an IgG1 monoclonal antibody targeted toward interleukins 12 and 23. It is approved for the treatment of both Crohn disease and ulcerative colitis. It also crosses the placenta, but in retrospective studies and registries, it is considered safe to use before and during pregnancy, so therapy should not be stopped.

✓ All biologicals except certolizumab cross the placenta but are not associated with an increase in adverse outcomes
✓ All biologicals should be continued before and during pregnancy to maintain maternal health

Small Molecules

Tofacitinib

Tofacitinib is a nonselective Janus kinase inhibitor that is approved to treat ulcerative colitis. Because of its potential effect on the placenta and the relative lack of safety data, it is not recommended for use in women actively interested in starting a family. For women receiving tofacitinib whose disease is in remission and who are pregnant, the recommendation is that they continue therapy but be monitored closely.

Upadacitinib

Upadacitinib is a selective Janus kinase 1 inhibitor that is approved to treat ulcerative colitis. As with tofacitinib, because of its potential effect on the placenta and the relative lack of safety data, it is not recommended for use in women actively interested in starting a family. For women receiving upadacitinib whose disease is in remission and who are pregnant, the recommendation is that they continue therapy but be monitored closely.

Ozanimod

Ozanimod is a sphingosine-1-phosphate receptor modulator recently approved to treat ulcerative colitis. Animal data suggest that fetal harm can occur with exposure, so it is not recommended for women interested in childbearing.

✓ The effect of small molecules in pregnancy is unclear, so therapy that uses other mechanisms of action should be used

Fish Oil Supplements

Many patients who have IBD take fish oil supplements as an adjunct to standard medical therapy. Because fish oil is a supplement and not a drug, it is not rated by the FDA. A randomized controlled trial of fish oil supplementation showed a prolongation of pregnancy without detrimental effects on the growth of the fetus or the course of labor. Fish oil supplementation may help prevent miscarriage associated with the antiphospholipid antibody syndrome. In women with IBD who may be at increased risk for preterm birth and miscarriage, fish oil supplementation is not harmful and may provide some benefit.

Suggested Reading

Akbari M, Shah S, Velayos FS, Mahadevan U, Cheifetz AS. Systematic review and meta-analysis on the effects of thiopurines on birth outcomes from female and male patients with inflammatory bowel disease. Inflamm Bowel Dis. 2013 Jan;19(1):15–22.

American Academy of Pediatrics Committee on Drugs. Transfer of drugs and other chemicals into human milk. Pediatrics. 2001 Sep;108(3):776–89.

Antiretroviral Pregnancy Registry Steering Committee. Antiretroviral pregnancy registry interim report for 1 January 1989 through 31 July 2022. Registry Coordinating Center.www.APRegistry.com.

Armenti VT, Radomski JS, Moritz MJ, Gaughan WJ, McGrory CH, Coscia LA. Report from the National Transplantation Pregnancy Registry (NTPR): outcomes of pregnancy after transplantation. Clin Transpl. 2003:131–41.

ASGE Standard of Practice Committee, Shergill AK, Ben-Menachem T, Chandrasekhara V, Chathadi K, Decker GA, et al. Guidelines for endoscopy in pregnant and lactating women. Gastrointest Endosc. 2012 Jul;76(1):18–24.

Bradley CS, Kennedy CM, Turcea AM, Rao SS, Nygaard IE. Constipation in pregnancy: prevalence, symptoms, and risk factors. Obstet Gynecol. 2007 Dec;110(6):1351–7.

Briggs GG, Freeman RK, Yaffe SJ. Drugs in pregnancy and lactation: a reference guide to fetal and neonatal risk. 7th ed. Lippincott Williams & Wilkins; 2005: 1,858 pages.

Brown RS, Jr., Verna EC, Pereira MR, Tilson HH, Aguilar C, Leu CS, et al. Hepatitis B virus and human immunodeficiency virus drugs in pregnancy: findings from the antiretroviral pregnancy registry. J Hepatol. 2012 Nov;57(5):953–9.

Deshpande NA, James NT, Kucirka LM, Boyarsky BJ, Garonzik-Wang JM, Cameron AM, et al. Pregnancy outcomes of liver transplant recipients: a systematic review and meta-analysis. Liver Transpl. 2012 Jun;18(6):621–9.

Diav-Citrin O, Shechtman S, Gotteiner T, Arnon J, Ornoy A. Pregnancy outcome after gestational exposure to metronidazole: a prospective controlled cohort study. Teratology. 2001 May;63(5):186–92.

Garbis H, Elefant E, Diav-Citrin O, Mastroiacovo P, Schaefer C, Vial T, et al. Pregnancy outcome after exposure to ranitidine and other H2-blockers: a collaborative study of the European Network of Teratology Information Services. Reprod Toxicol. 2005 Mar-Apr;19(4):453–8.

Hasler WL. The irritable bowel syndrome during pregnancy. Gastroenterol Clin North Am. 2003 Mar;32(1):385–406.

Lu EJ, Curet MJ, El-Sayed YY, Kirkwood KS. Medical versus surgical management of biliary tract disease in pregnancy. Am J Surg. 2004 Dec;188(6):755–9.

Mahadevan U, Kane S. American Gastroenterological Association Institute technical review on the use of gastrointestinal medications in pregnancy. Gastroenterology. 2006 Jul;131(1):283–311.

Mahadevan U, Robinson C, Bernasko N, Boland B, Chambers C, Dubinsky M, et al. Inflammatory bowel disease in pregnancy clinical care pathway: a report from the American Gastroenterological Association IBD Parenthood Project Working Group. Gastroenterology. 2019 Apr;156(5):1508–24.

Majithia R, Johnson DA. Are proton pump inhibitors safe during pregnancy and lactation? Evidence to date. Drugs. 2012 Jan;72(2):171–9.

Niebyl JR. Clinical practice: nausea and vomiting in pregnancy. N Engl J Med. 2010 Oct;363(16):1544–50.

Papadakis EP, Sarigianni M, Mikhailidis DP, Mamopoulos A, Karagiannis V. Acute pancreatitis in pregnancy: an overview. Eur J Obstet Gynecol Reprod Biol. 2011 Dec;159(2):261–6.

Ramin KD, Ramsey PS. Disease of the gallbladder and pancreas in pregnancy. Obstet Gynecol Clin North Am. 2001 Sep;28(3):571–80.

Su GG, Pan KH, Zhao NF, Fang SH, Yang DH, Zhou Y. Efficacy and safety of lamivudine treatment for chronic hepatitis B in pregnancy. World J Gastroenterol. 2004 Mar 15;10(6):910–2.

Questions and Answers

Questions

Abbreviations used:

ALT,	alanine aminotransferase
CD,	Crohn disease
CRC,	colorectal cancer
CT,	computed tomographic
DD,	defecatory disorder
ERCP,	endoscopic retrograde cholangiopancreatography
HBV,	hepatitis B virus
HLA,	human leukocyte antigen
IBD,	inflammatory bowel disease
IBS,	irritable bowel syndrome
MRCP,	magnetic resonance cholangiopancreatography
MRI,	magnetic resonance imaging
PCR,	polymerase chain reaction
PSC,	primary sclerosing cholangitis
UC,	ulcerative colitis

Multiple Choice (choose the best answer)

V.1.   A 44-year-old woman who received a diagnosis of UC 20 years ago is receiving therapy with a fourth biological after having a lack of response to previous agents because of antibody formation. She has been having 6 to 8 nonbloody bowel movements (Bristol type 4-6) daily for 6 months. Her weight has been stable. On surveillance colonoscopy, she has evidence of severe inflammation characterized by erosions, erythema, friability, granularity, and loss of vascularity in all the examined colon (Mayo score 3). Surveillance biopsies from the cecum and the ascending, transverse, descending, and rectosigmoid areas show moderate, active chronic colitis with ulcerations and no granulomas. Additionally, low-grade dysplasia is identified in random biopsy samples from the cecum and the ascending and rectosigmoid areas, and high-grade dysplasia is identified in

random biopsy samples of the transverse colon. What is the best next step in management?

a. Change the therapy to a different biological
b. Perform chromoendoscopy now
c. Refer her to a colorectal surgeon now
d. Perform follow-up colonoscopy in 6 months
e. Do nothing since she is asymptomatic

V.2.   A 34-year-old man who was previously healthy presents with a 2-month history of recurrent fevers, abdominal pain in the right lower quadrant, and weight loss. He also reports having intermittent, nonbloody diarrhea for the past 6 months. He has not traveled outside the US. He is not taking any medications. He has no family history of colorectal cancer or IBD. On physical examination he has tachycardia, a cachectic appearance, and a scaphoid abdomen with tenderness in the right lower quadrant but no guarding or rebound tenderness. Laboratory test results are notable for the following: leukocytes, 19×10^9/L; hemoglobin, 8.6 g/dL; mean corpuscular volume, 73 fL; and C-reactive protein, 95 mg/L. CT enterography with an intravenous contrast agent shows severe inflammation in the terminal ileum connecting to a 3-cm abscess in the right iliopsoas muscle. No areas of inflammation are apparent in the small bowel. What is the most likely diagnosis?

a. UC with backwash ileitis
b. *Mycobacterium tuberculosis* infection
c. CD
d. Acute appendicitis

V.3.   A 62-year-old man has a 30-year history of UC. His disease has been well controlled for the past 5 years with infliximab every 8 weeks. Previous chromoendoscopy for dysplasia surveillance showed a large number of pseudopolyps extending throughout the descending and sigmoid colon. Random biopsies were negative for dysplasia. A 15-mm lesion (Paris classification type Is) was removed en bloc with endoscopic mucosal resection from the transverse colon; the lesion was a tubular adenoma with low-grade dysplasia. There was no active inflammation. What is the most appropriate recommendation?

a. Perform high-definition white-light colonoscopy in 5 years
b. Refer to the surgery service for colectomy
c. Increase the dose of infliximab
d. Perform high-definition colonoscopy in 1 year
e. Perform chromoendoscopy now

V.4.   A 45-year-old woman presents to the IBD clinic for her annual follow-up. She has a 30-year history of mild, uncomplicated UC involving the left colon. She has been receiving mesalamine, and the disease has been in histologic remission for over 10 years. Findings from her most recent colonoscopy 1 year ago were normal. For several years, she has also had pain bilaterally in her metacarpophalangeal and metatarsophalangeal joints and in her ankles. She has not had back or hip pain. What is the most likely cause of the arthritis?

a. Parvovirus
b. Fibromyalgia
c. Type 1 IBD–related arthritis
d. Osteoarthritis
e. Type 2 IBD–related arthritis

V.5.   A 25-year-old man with a history of stricturing ileocolonic CD underwent an ileocecal resection for a stricture at the ileocecal valve. Before surgery, he was treated with azathioprine as a single agent. What would be the best approach for treatment after surgery?

a. Monitor symptoms for recurrence of disease, and treat if symptomatic
b. Initiate infliximab therapy now for prevention of postoperative CD
c. Offer colonoscopy at 12 months after surgery to assess for postoperative recurrence
d. Initiate budesonide treatment now for prevention of postoperative CD

V.6.   A 30-year-old man with a diagnosis of mild to moderate UC achieved and maintained remission with sulfasalazine about 4 years ago. He has been doing well with no recurrence of disease and continues to take sulfasalazine daily. He and his partner have been trying to get pregnant for over a year and have not been successful. How would you counsel him about fertility?

a. UC is associated with higher rates of infertility in men
b. The partner might have infertility issues, and they should seek care from an infertility specialist
c. His medication should be switched to mesalamine
d. His medication should be switched to vedolizumab

V.7.   A 28-year-old woman is admitted to the hospital with acute severe UC. *Clostridioides difficile* infection has been ruled out, and therapy was started with intravenous methylprednisolone. On the third day after admission, she continues to have 10 bloody bowel movements daily and abdominal pain, and her C-reactive protein level is still high. She is otherwise hemodynamically stable with no involuntary guarding on abdominal examination. What would be the best next step in management?

a. Initiate infliximab therapy
b. Refer her for a total proctocolectomy
c. Initiate azathioprine treatment
d. Increase the dose of intravenous methylprednisolone

V.8.   A 35-year-old woman received a diagnosis of moderate to severe UC, but she has not responded to treatment with infliximab and vedolizumab. You plan to begin therapy with tofacitinib. What are important considerations related to tofacitinib?

a. She should be evaluated for sleep apnea
b. She should be evaluated by an ophthalmologist
c. She should undergo electrocardiography before she begins therapy
d. She should receive the recombinant shingles vaccine

V.9.   A 36-year-old man returns for follow-up after he received a diagnosis of extensive UC 6 months ago. He is receiving adalimumab monotherapy. He feels well with 1 or 2 nonbloody bowel movements daily. However, follow-up colonoscopy shows mild inflammation from the sigmoid colon to the cecum with relative sparing of the rectum. The terminal ileum appears normal. Laboratory test results are notable for an alkaline phosphatase value of 176 U/L (reference range, 40-129 U/L); other liver enzyme results are normal. What is the best next step?

a. Perform MRCP
b. Perform liver biopsy
c. Repeat liver enzyme testing in 6 months
d. Perform ERCP

V.10. A 52-year-old woman with CD and ileocolitis for the past 4 years returns for her annual follow-up. She has been treated with vedolizumab every 8 weeks for the past 12 months. When she previously used adalimumab, antibodies developed. Her current symptoms include 3 or 4 loose stools daily with abdominal cramping. Within the past several months, she has also had pain, swelling, and stiffness in her left knee and right ankle. Those symptoms improve with activity. Laboratory test results are normal. Colonoscopy shows mild inflammation with scattered aphthous ulcerations in the terminal ileum and mild, patchy inflammation throughout the transverse colon. What is the best next step in management?

a. Increase the frequency of vedolizumab to every 4 weeks
b. Perform MRI of the affected joints
c. Discontinue the use of vedolizumab and prescribe infliximab
d. Continue the use of vedolizumab at the current dosage

V.11. A 60-year-old man with UC and PSC returns for his annual examination. The UC is currently in remission with his use of oral mesalamine. Surveillance colonoscopy shows a normal-appearing terminal ileum and colon without inflammation or polyps. Biopsies are obtained in 4 quadrants every 10 cm for surveillance. Histopathology shows high-grade dysplasia in the cecum and descending colon. What is the best next step in management?

a. Repeat the colonoscopy in 6 months with chromoendoscopy
b. Repeat the surveillance colonoscopy in 1 year
c. Repeat the colonoscopy in 3 months with chromoendoscopy
d. Perform a colectomy

V.12. Which of the following is associated with IBD activity and is likely to respond to treatment of the underlying bowel inflammation?

a. Peripheral arthritis involving joints of the hands bilaterally
b. Erythema nodosum
c. Ankylosing spondylitis
d. Scleritis

V.13. A 28-year-old man, a second-year resident in internal medicine, presents in the emergency department with nausea, vomiting, and diarrhea along with crampy abdominal pain that started 2 days ago during a flight. He had traveled to Cancun, Mexico, to present research findings. He is otherwise healthy, has a normal body mass index, and exercises 5 times per week. Before the trip, he missed an appointment in the travel medicine clinic because of his clinical schedule. He appears dehydrated and has blood in his stool. He says that he ate "quite a bit" of street food on the trip. On physical examination he has tachycardia (other vital signs are normal), and his abdomen is tender. What is the next step in his management?

a. Initiate loperamide for traveler's diarrhea
b. Perform a stool multiplex PCR panel for enteric pathogens
c. Perform a stool PCR assay for *Clostridioides difficile*
d. Admit him to the hospital for intravenous antibiotics
e. Begin empirical therapy with an oral outpatient antibiotic for traveler's diarrhea

V.14. **A 60-year-old woman with a history of hypertension and reflux disease (treated with atenolol and omeprazole) presents to the outpatient clinic with diarrhea for the past 9 days. Previously she had not had consistent diarrhea that required evaluation. She has daytime and nighttime stools and abdominal pain but no blood in the stool. She has lost 1.8 kg (4 lb) since the onset. About 3 weeks before the diarrhea began, she had received amoxicillin for routine dental cleaning. On physical examination, she has normal vital signs and mild tenderness on deep palpation of the abdomen. On laboratory evaluation, results are normal for hemoglobin, white blood cell count (8,500 cells/µL), electrolytes, and serum creatinine. PCR test results are positive for *Clostridioides difficile*. What treatment would you recommend for clinical cure with a low chance of recurrence?**

a. Metronidazole 500 mg 3 times daily for 10 days
b. Vancomycin 125 mg 4 times daily for 10 days
c. Fidaxomicin 200 mg 2 times daily for 10 days
d. Vancomycin 125 mg 4 times daily for 10 days in combination with intravenous bezlotoxumab 10 mg/kg

V.15. **A 60-year-old woman with a history of hypertension and reflux disease (treated with atenolol and omeprazole) received a diagnosis of a first episode of mild *Clostridioides difficile* infection after receiving amoxicillin for routine dental cleaning. When she was treated with a course of fidaxomicin, her diarrhea symptoms resolved on day 5, and she completed the 10-day course. She returns to the clinic 2 weeks after finishing treatment because she has gastrointestinal distress with occasional loose stools. She has regained the 1.8 kg (4 lb) that she had lost, but she thinks that the infection has not resolved. On physical examination in the office, she has normal vital signs and minimal abdominal tenderness. A resident physician orders a *C difficile* stool PCR test, and the results are positive. What is the next step in her management?**

a. Repeat the course of fidaxomicin because the infection has not completely resolved
b. Prescribe vancomycin 125 mg 4 times daily for 10 days
c. Perform a 2-step toxin-based assay for *C difficile* infection
d. Obtain a detailed symptom history to evaluate for a postinfection state

V.16. **A 41-year-old man with obesity (body mass index, 27) is receiving therapy for hyperlipidemia and reflux disease and presents to the emergency department with abdominal pain in the left lower quadrant that has worsened in the past 3 days. He has felt feverish but has not had diarrhea or blood in the stool. On examination, he has mild tenderness in the left lower quadrant of the abdomen but no peritoneal signs. The white blood cell count is 8,500/µL. CT with oral and intravenous contrast agents shows inflammation and stranding around diverticula in the sigmoid region and changes consistent with diverticulitis. No abscess or perforation is seen. What is the best next step in management?**

a. Outpatient management with a liquid diet, no antibiotics, and colonoscopy in 6 weeks
b. Outpatient management with antibiotics and colonoscopy in 6 weeks

c. Outpatient management with antibiotics, colonoscopy in 6 weeks, and surgical referral for sigmoid colectomy
d. Hospital admission, bowel rest, intravenous antibiotics, and colonoscopy in 3 days

V.17. **Which of the following statements correctly describes the epidemiology of CRC?**

a. The incidence of CRC is increasing for adults of all ages in the US
b. In the US, the mortality of CRC is higher for Blacks than Whites, even when adjusted for stage
c. The incidence of CRC is decreasing in resource-limited countries
d. Cigarette smoking decreases the risk for CRC

V.18. **A 62-year-old woman is found to have colon cancer during routine screening colonoscopy. Mismatch repair enzyme expression testing by immunohistochemistry shows an absence of *MLH1* and *PMS2*. Staging CT scans of the chest, abdomen, and pelvis do not show obvious lymph node involvement or metastatic disease. Her mother had endometrial cancer at age 48 years and her brother had a cancer of the upper urothelial tract. What is the best next step in management?**

a. Refer for prophylactic hysterectomy
b. Initiate annual colonoscopy for all first-degree relatives older than 20 years
c. Refer for germline genetic testing
d. Order PCR testing for microsatellite instability

V.19. **A 48-year-old man says that he has had hematochezia every 1 to 3 days for the past 6 weeks. At colonoscopy, a 2.5-cm pedunculated polyp is found in the rectum 10 cm from the anal verge; the polyp is removed with a snare with electrocautery. Pathology examination of the polyp shows a poorly differentiated adenocarcinoma with a focus of invasion into the submucosa. Although the margins are clear by at least 2 mm, lymphovascular invasion is present. Staging CT scans do not show distant metastasis. Which of the following is the best next step in management?**

a. Refer for transanal excision of the polyp at the base
b. Refer for low anterior resection and lymph node staging
c. Do not refer for surgery now, but repeat the colonoscopy in 1 year
d. Do not refer for surgery now, but perform endoscopic ultrasonography in 6 months

V.20. **During colonoscopy for a 53-year-old man, you find 4 sessile serrated polyps in the right colon; the diameters are 6 to 9 mm. At the patient's first screening colonoscopy 3 years ago, 2 sessile serrated lesions (12-15 mm in diameter) were removed from the ascending colon; no residual polyp tissue is seen near the well-healed scars from the previous polypectomy. When should he return for his next surveillance examination?**

a. In 1 year
b. In 3 to 5 years
c. In 7 years
d. In 10 years

V.21. **A 17-year-old adolescent girl presents with abdominal pain associated with defecation. She describes having 1 bowel movement every 4 days that is Bristol type 1 or 2. She says that she does not have any warning symptoms. She has received a diagnosis of constipation-predominant IBS and now wants to try further management options. Which of the following tests should be completed before further empirical treatment options are offered?**

a. Celiac disease testing
b. Colonoscopy
c. CT of the abdomen and pelvis
d. Colonic transit study

V.22. A 45-year-old man presents with abdominal pain and diarrhea. He has a past surgical history of cholecystectomy. He says that he does not have any warning symptoms. He has tried to increase his fiber intake, and he has received loperamide and antispasmodic therapy without any improvement in the diarrhea or the abdominal pain. What treatment option should *not* be offered to this patient?

   a. Tricyclic antidepressants
   b. Diphenoxylate-atropine
   c. Eluxadoline
   d. A serotonin-norepinephrine reuptake inhibitor

V.23. A 23-year-old woman with constipation presents with diarrhea and abdominal pain associated with defecation. The diarrhea is characterized by 3 bowel movements daily, which are Bristol type 6 and contain some blood. The symptoms have been present for the past 12 months. Her abdominal pain gets worse after bowel movements and is associated with eating. Blood test results were normal for hemoglobin, iron, C-reactive protein, fecal calprotectin, and a celiac panel, and a fecal sample was negative for *Clostridioides difficile*. Celiac genotype testing identified HLA-DQ1 and HLA-DQ4 haplotypes. What is the best next step in management?

   a. Trial treatment with dietary fiber supplementation
   b. Colonoscopy
   c. No further testing or treatment because the symptoms will resolve on their own
   d. Trial treatment with a gluten-free diet

V.24. A 24-year-old woman returns to your clinic. At her initial visit 6 months ago, she described a 6-month history of weekly abdominal pain and bloating associated with harder, less frequent stool. The pain was reportedly relieved by satisfactory defecation. A symptom-based diagnosis of constipation-predominant IBS was made. In the past 6 months her symptoms have not improved with increased aerobic exercise, increased consumption of soluble fiber, and use of osmotic and stimulant laxatives. She describes feeling frustration because of her symptoms and her doubts about the diagnosis. What is the next step in management?

   a. Digital rectal examination
   b. Colonoscopy
   c. Therapy with rifaximin
   d. Therapy with prucalopride

V.25. A 40-year-old woman presents to your office with chronic constipation for the past 20 years. She describes having hard stools, straining excessively to defecate, and having a sense of anal blockage during defecation and a sense of incomplete evacuation thereafter. Her symptoms have not responded to several laxatives or linaclotide. She does not have alarm symptoms or a family history of colon cancer. What is the best response at this point?

   a. Perform defecography
   b. Prescribe a cyclic guanosine monophosphate agonist (eg, lubiprostone or plecanatide)
   c. Perform a careful digital rectal examination, anorectal manometry, and rectal balloon expulsion test
   d. Perform a colonoscopy

V.26. A 45-year-old woman presents to your office with fecal incontinence for the past 15 years. She describes having accidental bowel leakage of a moderate amount of semiformed stool preceded by marked urgency once weekly. The symptom is embarrassing and has prompted her to withdraw from social activities. She describes having postprandial abdominal discomfort and rectal urgency that are relieved by passing 3 semiformed to loose stools daily. Her past medical history is notable for diarrhea-predominant IBS and a complicated

vaginal delivery with anal sphincter tear 20 years ago. She does not take any medications. Dietary fiber supplementation aggravated her diarrhea. On digital rectal examination she has normal anal resting tone, a weak squeeze response, and normal anorectal descent during evacuation. Results were normal from a complete blood cell count, serologic tests for celiac disease, and flexible sigmoidoscopy. What is the best next step?

   a. Perform endoanal ultrasonography and refer her to a colorectal surgeon for anal sphincteroplasty
   b. Recommend that she limit her intake of caffeine and foods containing artificial sugars, and if diarrhea persists, try loperamide (2 mg) beginning with 1 tablet 30 minutes before breakfast and lunch and titrated thereafter to a maximum of 16 mg daily
   c. Perform anal manometry
   d. Recommend anorectal biofeedback therapy

V.27. Which of the following statements about isolated slow transit constipation is most accurate?

   a. Every patient who has constipation with slow transit has slow transit constipation
   b. Opioids do not delay colon transit
   c. Patients with DDs may also have slow colon transit
   d. All patients with slow transit constipation need a colectomy

V.28. Which statement correctly describes anorectal tests for chronic constipation?

   a. A rectal balloon expulsion test is the preferred initial test for diagnosing DDs
   b. In healthy people, the rectoanal gradient during evacuation measured with high-resolution manometry is positive
   c. A negative rectoanal gradient is not associated with an abnormal result on the rectal balloon expulsion test
   d. Anorectal high-resolution manometry is the gold standard test for the diagnosis of DDs

V.29. A 24-year-old woman presents to your office at 13 weeks' gestation. She is having a little heartburn, particularly after she eats spicy foods. She does not have dysphagia, nausea, or vomiting. She is otherwise healthy and does not have a history of heartburn or gastroesophageal reflux disease before this pregnancy. Which of the following should you recommend for her heartburn symptoms?

   a. Calcium carbonate 4 times daily
   b. Sodium bicarbonate 3 times daily
   c. Magnesium trisilicate twice daily
   d. Famotidine once daily

V.30. A 28-year-old female immigrant from Southeast Asia presents to your clinic at 16 weeks' gestation and tells you that she has hepatitis B. Results for hepatitis B serology are positive for hepatitis B surface antigen and hepatitis B e antigen and negative for anti-hepatitis B e antigen. Her viral load, checked by her obstetrician last week, was 190,000 IU/mL; the ALT level was 110 U/L. She does not have cirrhosis. You counsel her about the use of hepatitis B immune globulin at the time of delivery. Which drug should be used now to treat her hepatitis B?

   a. Tenofovir
   b. Adefovir
   c. Interferon
   d. Entecavir

V.31. A 30-year-old woman at 26 weeks' gestation comes to your office because of constipation. She did not have constipation before her pregnancy. She is gaining weight appropriately, she works full-time, and she exercises 4 times weekly. Every other day she has a bowel movement that is type 1 or 2 on the Bristol Stool Form Scale, but she feels uncomfortable on the days when she does not have a bowel movement. She says that she does not have bleeding, excessive straining, or abdominal pain. What should you recommend that she try first?

a. Daily senna
b. Fiber supplementation
c. Castor oil
d. Eluxadoline

V.32. A 24-year-old woman with a history of UC who had a hypersensitivity reaction to mesalamine is currently taking delayed-release budesonide. She is contemplating pregnancy and wants your advice about a safe therapy for UC if she were to stop taking budesonide. She is currently asymptomatic with once-daily budesonide. What should you recommend for therapy?

a. Continue budesonide indefinitely until she is pregnant
b. Use a biological as a steroid-sparing agent
c. Use tofacitinib as it is another oral agent that is convenient
d. Stop the use of budesonide and evaluate the response

Answers

V.1. Answer c.
This patient should be referred to a colorectal surgeon now for a total proctocolectomy since she has evidence of multifocal dysplasia of the colon in addition to UC. The patient would also be a candidate for total proctocolectomy instead of a segmental colectomy since dysplasia is involving the rectum as well. While therapy with a different biological would be appropriate to help achieve remission, the presence of multifocal dysplasia poses a high risk of progression to colorectal cancer. Also, since therapy with other agents has already failed, the likelihood of endoscopic remission is much lower. The performance of chromoendoscopy to detect dysplastic lesions is limited by the presence of severe inflammation and hence would not be helpful in this patient. Although follow-up colonoscopy in 6 months might be appropriate, it would carry a high risk that the disease would progress to colorectal cancer or that high-grade dysplasia or carcinoma in situ would be missed. Doing nothing would not be an appropriate option as this time.

V.2. Answer c.
The history and imaging findings are most consistent with CD, and the patient most likely has severe fistulizing CD that involves the terminal ileum with abscess formation. He does not have UC because there is no evidence of colonic inflammation, and UC does not typically result in fistulas or abscesses. He does not have risk factors for *Mycobacterium tuberculosis* infection. Tuberculosis can involve the terminal ileum and mimic CD but does not commonly cause a communicating abscess. Acute appendicitis does not involve the terminal ileum, so that is not the diagnosis.

V.3. Answer d.
The patient has colonic pseudopolyposis with UC. Patients who have a long history of UC should undergo colonoscopy with high-definition white-light endoscopy or chromoendoscopy for dysplasia surveillance. This should be performed every 1 to 3 years (not every 5 years) when adenomatous dysplasia has been identified. Pseudopolyps are irregularly shaped islands of residual colonic mucosa that are the result of the mucosal ulceration and regeneration that occur in IBD. These lesions are not precancerous by themselves. Surgery should be discussed with patients, but it would not be performed because pseudopolyps are not precancerous and because the adenomatous lesions

were completely removed. The yield of chromoendoscopy is decreased when inflammation or pseudopolyposis is prominent. The most appropriate approach would be surveillance with high-definition white-light endoscopy with random and targeted biopsies of lesions of interest.

V.4. Answer e.
The most likely cause is type 2 IBD–related arthritis, which is polyarticular, involves smaller joints, is symmetrical, and does not parallel the IBD activity. Parvovirus is unlikely because the patient has no other symptoms that would suggest that infection. While fibromyalgia is possible, her symptoms suggest an inflammatory cause and are known extraintestinal manifestations. Type 1 IBD–related arthritis typically is pauciarticular and not symmetrical and usually parallels the IBD activity. She is too young for the development of osteoarthritis.

V.5. Answer b.
This patient should begin infliximab therapy now. The current approach to postoperative maintenance therapy is risk stratification of patients for the likelihood of postoperative recurrence. Those deemed to be at high risk are offered treatment with azathioprine, 6-mercaptopurine, or preferably infliximab. The patient in this vignette is a young man with a history of stricturing CD, which are high risk features. Patients not considered to have a high risk and those who opt not to receive medical therapy are offered colonoscopy 6 to 12 months after surgery. Patients who show evidence of endoscopic recurrence are then offered treatment.

V.6. Answer c.
Sulfasalazine is associated with reversible azoospermia and thus is the cause of infertility in this patient. Since he has been in deep remission with sulfasalazine, it would be reasonable to switch him to mesalamine at this point to maintain remission. Mesalamine therapy does not pose the reversible azoospermia risk. A switch to vedolizumab would not be necessary since he is in remission with an aminosalicylate. UC is not associated with higher rates of male infertility, and seeking care from an infertility specialist would not be necessary at this point.

V.7. Answer a.
This patient was admitted to the hospital for management of acute severe UC. If patients have not responded to intravenous methylprednisolone by the third day after admission, it is reasonable to try infliximab therapy before referring them for surgery. A surgical consultation is also indicated at this point, but a trial of infliximab should be considered first since the patient is hemodynamically stable with no signs of toxic megacolon. Initiation of azathioprine at this point would not be indicated because it has a slow onset of action. Use of a higher dose of methylprednisolone now would not have an added benefit and would increase the risk of infections and possible surgical complications.

V.8. Answer d.
Janus kinase inhibition is associated with reactivation of herpes zoster, which occurs with dose-dependent increases of tofacitinib. Patients should receive the recombinant shingles vaccine if they will be treated with tofacitinib. Sleep apnea and heart blocks are contraindications for ozanimod but not tofacitinib. Also, macular edema is associated with ozanimod but not tofacitinib.

V.9. Answer a.
In a patient with IBD and an increased alkaline phosphatase level, further evaluation for possible PSC is warranted. MRCP

is the diagnostic test of choice for PSC because it is sensitive for detecting characteristic bile duct changes and is noninvasive. Liver biopsy findings may support a diagnosis of PSC, but they are often nondiagnostic, and liver biopsy is rarely necessary if a patient has characteristic findings with cholangiography. However, a liver biopsy may be necessary if there is a strong possibility of small duct PSC or an overlap condition with autoimmune hepatitis. Repeating liver enzyme testing in 6 months would be inappropriate without further evaluation because it could delay the diagnosis of PSC. While ERCP is also sensitive for detection of PSC, it is invasive and typically not used as the initial diagnostic test.

V.10.　Answer c.

This patient has type 1 peripheral arthritis, which tends to affect fewer than 5 joints and often involves larger joints such as the knees. Type 1 peripheral arthritis tends to parallel IBD activity. In this patient with evidence of active CD, starting infliximab therapy would help to treat underlying IBD and arthritis. Vedolizumab, a gut-specific monoclonal antibody directed against α4β7 integrin, is thought to have less benefit in treating extraintestinal manifestations of IBD. Therefore, increasing the frequency of vedolizumab to every 4 weeks would be unlikely to provide effective treatment of her arthritis. Her symptoms, which improve with activity, are most consistent with inflammatory arthritis. MRI is unlikely to aid in diagnosis. Since she is symptomatic and has evidence of active inflammation on colonoscopy, a change in management is warranted rather than continuing therapy with vedolizumab at the current dosage.

V.11.　Answer d.

This patient, who has UC and PSC and an increased risk for colorectal cancer, appropriately underwent surveillance colonoscopy. The presence of multifocal, high-grade dysplasia suggests a high risk for synchronous cancer or development of colorectal cancer, especially with PSC. Therefore, colectomy is the most appropriate next step in management. Further surveillance with or without chromoendoscopy would not be appropriate for this patient who has multiple high-risk features.

V.12.　Answer b.

Patients with erythema nodosum, the most common cutaneous manifestation of IBD, have tender subcutaneous nodules on the anterior extensor surfaces of the lower extremities. The status of erythema nodosum tends to parallel IBD luminal activity and improves with treatment of the underlying disease. Type 2 peripheral arthritis typically involves more than 5 small joints (polyarticular) and is independent of IBD activity. Similarly, axial arthropathies associated with IBD, including ankylosing spondylitis and sacroiliitis, are independent of IBD activity. However, therapy with anti–tumor necrosis factor may induce remission in patients with ankylosing spondylitis, especially in the early stages. Among the extraintestinal manifestations involving the eye, scleritis and anterior uveitis are independent of IBD activity, while episcleritis may parallel luminal disease.

V.13.　Answer b.

The correct response is to perform stool testing when acute infectious diarrhea is suspected and the patient has fever, bloody or mucoid stools, severe abdominal tenderness, or signs of sepsis. Positive stool study results would help determine antimicrobial use (eg, for *Salmonella*, *Shigella*, or *Campylobacter*, in certain cases) and may prevent unnecessary additional testing and imaging. Loperamide would not be indicated because the patient has

blood in the stool. He does not have risk factors for *Clostridioides difficile*, and testing for *C difficile* alone would not be sufficient. A decision to admit to the hospital would be based on the overall clinical picture, and in most instances intravenous antibiotics are not needed. If there is no access to a stool test, empirical therapy with an antibiotic for traveler's diarrhea may be considered.

V.14.　Answer c.

This patient is having a first episode of mild *Clostridioides difficile* infection. The use of fidaxomicin has high rates of clinical cure (similar to those with vancomycin) but lower rates of recurrence compared to vancomycin. Metronidazole is no longer recommended, even in mild cases, owing to high rates of treatment failure and adverse effects. Use of vancomycin has a higher rate of recurrence compared to fidaxomicin. The addition of intravenous bezlotoxumab to vancomycin therapy would not improve cure rates in this situation because of the absence of risk factors (which include age >65 years), *C difficile* infection in the past 6 months, immunosuppression, and the presence of severe *C difficile* infection.

V.15.　Answer d.

This patient has had 1 episode of *Clostridioides difficile* infection and is at a risk for recurrent infection. She is also at risk for postinfection symptoms, which include occasional loose stools, sometimes with alternating constipation, and symptoms related to meals. A detailed symptom history is important. A stool PCR assay can have false-positive results in up to 30% to 50% of infections after successful treatment. Treatment with antibiotics is not indicated, and treatment with vancomycin may increase the risk for future C *difficile* infection. While performing a 2-step toxin-based assay would be reasonable, it should be done only if a patient has clinical signs and symptoms of *C difficile* infection.

V.16.　Answer a.

This patient presents with a first episode of acute uncomplicated diverticulitis. Since he is tolerating oral intake without difficulty, outpatient management would be recommended. Recent guidelines suggest that patients with uncomplicated acute diverticulitis be managed without antibiotics as outcomes are similar to those for patients treated with antibiotics in this situation. Hospital admission for bowel rest and intravenous antibiotics should be reserved for patients who have evidence of a complication (abscess) or for patients who cannot tolerate oral intake. Colonoscopy is contraindicated during an episode of acute diverticulitis and is not recommended until 6 to 8 weeks after the acute episode has resolved. Surgical referral for colectomy because a patient is young at onset is no longer recommended.

V.17.　Answer b.

In the US, Blacks have a disproportionately high mortality rate from CRC, which persists when adjusted for stage at diagnosis. Owing largely to population-level screening, the incidence of CRC in the US is decreasing for most age groups. However, CRC incidence and mortality are progressively increasing for persons younger than 50 years. While decreasing in industrialized nations, the incidence of CRC is increasing in many resource-limited countries. This is thought to be due to lifestyle factors that increase risk; these factors include cigarette smoking, obesity, and diets high in saturated fat or red (especially processed) meat.

V.18.　Answer c.

Lynch syndrome should be suspected in patients with an autosomal dominant pedigree of familial cancers. While mismatch repair deficiency is a hallmark of Lynch syndrome, there are other somatic events that can result in this phenotype. Therefore, genetic testing to confirm a germline mutation in 1 of the genes coding for mismatch repair enzymes is required for a diagnosis of Lynch syndrome. Additionally, the patient's primary tumor should be tested for *BRAF* variation and hypermethylation of *MLH1*. The Amsterdam criteria are useful for identifying patients with hereditary nonpolyposis CRC who should be tested for mismatch-repair deficiency to direct genetic testing for a diagnosis of Lynch syndrome. This diagnosis may lead to a subtotal colectomy rather than segmental resection. Women who have Lynch syndrome and have completed childbearing can consider hysterectomy, but this patient's diagnosis is not yet confirmed. When Lynch syndrome is diagnosed, cascade genetic testing should be offered to first-degree relatives to rule out the disease and offer surveillance to confirmed mutation carriers. Since the patient's tumor shows deficient mismatch repair phenotype by immunohistochemistry for mismatch repair enzymes, microsatellite instability testing does not offer any additional information. Use of immunohistochemistry or microsatellite instability testing depends on local availability and laboratory expertise.

V.19. Answer b.

The patient has a malignant rectal polyp. Although the histologic margin is clear, the poor tumor differentiation and lymphovascular invasion are both strong predictors of lymph node involvement and are associated with distant metastatic recurrent disease. In this situation, complete surgical staging by low anterior resection with pathologic lymph node staging is recommended by National Comprehensive Cancer Network guidelines. Transanal excision may be offered to patients with low-risk T1 rectal cancers. After transanal excision, surveillance by endoscopic ultrasonography and MRI should be performed every 6 months with colonoscopic surveillance at 1-, 3-, and 5-year intervals. Colonoscopy or endoscopic ultrasonography alone is not advised because the patient requires surgical staging.

V.20. Answer a.

The patient has a lifetime history of 5 or more sessile serrated lesions (2 were confirmed at a previous colonoscopy, and 4 are presumed according to the endoscopic features and polyp location), and all are 5 mm or larger in diameter with at least 2 lesions 10 mm or larger in diameter; he therefore meets 1 of 2 World Health Organization phenotypes for serrated polyposis syndrome (the second phenotype is >20 serrated lesions or polyps of any size distributed throughout the large bowel, with ≥5 being proximal to the rectum). Although surveillance may be personalized to include longer intervals, most guidelines recommend annual surveillance. A surveillance interval of 3 to 5 years is appropriate for patients with 3 or 4 serrated lesions that do not meet the criteria for serrated polyposis syndrome. An interval of 7 to 10 years is recommended for patients with 1 or 2 small adenomas. A 10-year interval is recommended if colonoscopy findings are normal or if only small hyperplastic lesions are found.

V.21. Answer a.

Up to 30% of patients with celiac disease present with constipation. All patients with IBS should be evaluated for celiac disease. This patient does not have warning symptoms, so she does not require further evaluation with colonoscopy or CT of the abdomen and pelvis. A colonic transit study could be considered if conservative therapy does not help the patient. Additionally,

colonic transit testing should be completed after a functional defecatory disorder has been ruled out because patients with defecatory disorders can have slow colonic transit, which will normalize after the pelvic floor is rehabilitated.

V.22. Answer c.

Eluxadoline increases the risk of pancreatitis in patients who have liver disease, who consume more than 3 alcoholic drinks daily, or who have had a cholecystectomy. The mechanism of action is believed to be related to a dysfunction of the sphincter of Oddi due to partial delta opioid antagonism. The other medications listed are appropriate for both abdominal pain and diarrhea.

V.23. Answer b.

The patient describes having blood in her stool, which is a concerning warning symptom, and requires a more thorough evaluation, including a colonoscopy to rule out IBD. If she did not have warning symptoms, trying supplementation with dietary fiber or foregoing further testing or treatment would be reasonable. A trial with a gluten-free diet has helped patients who have genes permissive for celiac disease (ie, *HLA-DQ2* or *HLA-DQ8*) but would not be appropriate in this situation.

V.24. Answer a.

This patient has persistent, bothersome symptoms despite an appropriate symptom-based diagnosis and appropriate therapy. Further investigation can be considered at this time. Functional defecatory disorders can mimic constipation-predominant IBS. A digital rectal examination should be performed to exclude organic anal pathology and to evaluate for a functional defecatory disorder. Anorectal manometry can be considered thereafter. A colonoscopy is not indicated in the absence of alarm symptoms. Rifaximin is approved for the treatment of only diarrhea-predominant IBS. Prucalopride is not approved by the US Food and Drug Administration for the diagnosis of IBS and may not affect her abdominal pain.

V.25. Answer c.

Defecatory disorders are managed with pelvic floor biofeedback therapy rather than with laxatives. Although symptoms and digital rectal examination findings may prompt a suspicion of DDs, anorectal tests are necessary because a clinical assessment alone does not suffice for identifying a DD. In patients with a DD, anal inspection may disclose an anal fissure or hemorrhoids; digital rectal examination may disclose anismus (ie, high anal resting pressure), reduced or excessive perineal descent, or rectal prolapse. The puborectalis muscle may not relax normally, or paradoxically it may contract during simulated evacuation. Initially, anal manometry and a rectal balloon expulsion test are preferred to barium defecography, which entails radiation exposure, or magnetic resonance defecography, which is more expensive. If a patient with long-standing constipation does not have alarm symptoms or a family history of colon cancer, a colonoscopy is not warranted. Since symptoms have not responded to lubiprostone, which is a secretagogue, anorectal tests rather than a trial with lubiprostone or plecanatide is the appropriate next step.

V.26. Answer b.

If patients do not have organic disease (eg, UC), the use of symptomatic measures to manage bowel disturbances is the preferred initial step and is often effective for managing fecal incontinence. If fecal incontinence persists despite the use of adequate measures to manage the bowel disturbances, anal manometry and then anorectal biofeedback therapy should be considered. Less than 20% of patients are continent at 5 years after anal sphincteroplasty. Hence, sphincteroplasty is typically reserved for younger women who often have a sphincter defect identified shortly after obstetric injury.

V.27. Answer c.
Many patients with DDs also have slow colon transit. Hence, the diagnosis of slow transit constipation applies to patients who do not have impaired rectal evacuation. Because opioids delay colonic transit, their use should be discontinued when feasible in patients with constipation. Colectomy is reserved for a small fraction of patients with slow transit constipation whose symptoms are most likely explained by slow colon transit and do not respond to laxatives.

V.28. Answer a.
The rectal balloon expulsion test is the preferred initial test for diagnosing DDs. Failure to expel a rectal balloon in 60 seconds is considered to be abnormal. Measured with manometry, the rectoanal gradient (ie, rectal pressure minus anal pressure) during evacuation is typically negative even in healthy women and men. Hence, this gradient is abnormal only if it is more negative than the lower limit of normal. A more negative rectoanal gradient is associated with an abnormal balloon expulsion test.

V.29. Answer d.
Heartburn is a common symptom during pregnancy and can get worse as the pregnancy progresses. Over-the-counter calcium supplements are appropriate for mild heartburn during pregnancy, but they should not be taken more than 3 times daily because higher amounts of carbonate can cause metabolic derangement. Similarly, sodium bicarbonate should not be used because it can cause milk-alkali syndrome. Trisilicates also can cause metabolic derangement and should not be used for extended periods. Histamine blockers are appropriate therapy for mild heartburn and can be used for the duration of the pregnancy if needed.

V.30. Answer a.
Treatment of hepatitis B depends on the viral load and ALT level. This patient should be treated. She has chronic hepatitis B in the immune-active phase and meets treatment thresholds (independent of pregnancy) with high levels of HBV DNA (>20,000 IU/mL) and ALT (≥2 times the upper limit of the reference range). Women who have an undetectable viral load can defer treatment and be monitored. To reduce the risk of maternal-fetal transmission, HBV DNA should be checked at 26 to 28 weeks' gestation, and antiviral therapy should be initiated if the viral load exceeds 200,000 IU/mL. Of the drugs listed in the answer choices, tenofovir has the most evidence for safety during pregnancy. Adefovir and entecavir are considered less safe, and interferon is contraindicated.

V.31. Answer b.
Constipation is common during pregnancy, particularly in advanced stages. First-line therapy is fiber supplementation because it is safe and effective for most patients. Senna can be used for a short duration, but as a stimulant laxative, it can cause cramps. Castor oil is contraindicated as it is associated with uterine rupture. Eluxadoline is safe during pregnancy but should be used only after other modalities, such as fiber and osmotic laxatives, have been tried.

V.32. Answer b.
Prolonged use of corticosteroids, including budesonide, is not an optimum strategy for conception or during pregnancy. All the biologicals currently approved for UC carry a low risk and would be appropriate to use to control the disease and to spare continued use of the corticosteroid. Tofacitinib is currently not suggested as first-line therapy for use in a patient contemplating pregnancy because data from animal studies suggest a teratogenic effect.

VI

Liver

23

Approach to the Patient With Abnormal Liver Test Results and Acute Liver Failure[a]

JOHN J. POTERUCHA, MD

Abnormal Liver Test Results

Definitions and Prevalence

Abnormal liver test results are defined as abnormal results for aminotransferases (aspartate aminotransferase [AST] or alanine aminotransferase [ALT]) or hepatic alkaline phosphatase (ALP). Determination of currently used "normal" values most likely included patients who had clinically unrecognized liver disease such as nonalcoholic fatty liver disease. It has been suggested that the upper limit of the normal value for ALT should be 33 U/L for men and 25 U/L for women. Population-based studies suggest that 25% of the population has an abnormal ALT value and 33% an abnormal ALP value. Abnormal liver test results are generally defined as *acute* if the duration is less than 3 months or *chronic* if the duration is more than 3 months.

✓ Hepatocellular disease—predominant elevation of ALT
✓ Cholestatic liver disease—predominant elevation of ALP
✓ Acute liver disease—elevation of liver enzymes for less than 3 months

---

[a] Portions previously published in Poterucha JJ. Fulminant hepatic failure. In: Johnson LR, editor. Encyclopedia of gastroenterology. Vol 2. Elsevier Academic Press; 2004: 70-4; Poterucha JJ. Hepatitis. In: Bland KI, Sarr MG, Buchler MW, Csendes A, Garden OJ, Wong J, editors. General surgery: principles and international practice. 2nd ed. Springer; 2009: 921-32; and Poterucha JJ, Gunneson TJ. Liver biopsy and paracentesis. In: Talley NJ, Lindor KD, Vargas HE, editors. Practical gastroenterology and hepatology: liver and biliary disease. Wiley-Blackwell; 2010: 80-6; used with permission.

Abbreviations: ALP, alkaline phosphatase; ALT, alanine aminotransferase; AST, aspartate aminotransferase; INR, international normalized ratio; MELD, Model for End-stage Liver Disease; MELD-Na, Model for End-stage Liver Disease with determination of sodium; PBC, primary biliary cholangitis; PSC, primary sclerosing cholangitis

✓ Chronic liver disease—elevation of liver enzymes for more than 3 months

Aminotransferases (ALT and AST)

ALT and AST are in hepatocytes, and elevated serum levels are an indication of hepatocellular disease. Injury of the hepatocyte membrane allows these enzymes to "leak" out of hepatocytes, and within a few hours after liver injury, the serum levels of the enzymes increase. ALT elevation is more specific for liver injury than is AST elevation, although severe muscle injury may result in serum elevations of both enzymes. ALT has a longer half-life than AST; thus, improvements in ALT levels lag those of AST.

Alkaline Phosphatase

ALP is an enzyme located on the hepatocyte membrane bordering the bile canaliculus. Because ALP is found also in bone and placenta, an increase in its level without other indication of liver disease should prompt further testing to discover whether the increase is from liver or from other tissues. One way of doing this is to determine the concentration of ALP isoenzymes. Another way is to determine the level of γ-glutamyltransferase, an enzyme of intrahepatic biliary canaliculi.

Bilirubin

Bilirubin is the water-insoluble product of heme metabolism that is taken up by hepatocytes and conjugated with glucuronic acid to form monoglucuronides and diglucuronides through the activity of the enzyme uridine diphosphate glucuronosyltransferase. Conjugation makes bilirubin water-soluble, allowing it to be excreted into the bile canaliculus. The serum concentration of bilirubin is measured in direct (conjugated) and indirect (unconjugated) fractions. Diseases characterized by overproduction of bilirubin, such as hemolysis or resorption of a hematoma, are characterized by hyperbilirubinemia that is 20% or less conjugated bilirubin. Hepatocyte dysfunction or impaired bile flow produces hyperbilirubinemia that is usually 20% to 80% conjugated bilirubin. Patients with an inherited disorder of bilirubin excretion into the canaliculus, such as Dubin-Johnson syndrome or Rotor syndrome, have hyperbilirubinemia that is more than 80% conjugated. Because conjugated bilirubin is water-soluble and may be excreted in urine, patients with conjugated hyperbilirubinemia may note dark urine. In these patients, the stools are lighter in color because of the absence of pigments that result from the presence of bilirubin in the intestine.

Prothrombin Time and Albumin

Abnormalities of prothrombin time and albumin occur with liver dysfunction and should prompt immediate evaluation. Prothrombin time is a measure of the activity of coagulation factors II, V, VII, and X, all of which are synthesized in the liver. These factors are dependent also on vitamin K for synthesis. Vitamin K deficiency may be caused by antibiotics, prolonged fasting, small-bowel mucosal disorders such as celiac disease, or severe cholestasis with an inability to absorb fat-soluble vitamins. Liver dysfunction is characterized by an inability to synthesize clotting factors despite adequate stores of vitamin K. Administration of vitamin K improves prothrombin time within 48 hours in a patient with vitamin K deficiency but has little effect if the prolonged prothrombin time is due to liver disease with poor hepatocellular function.

Because albumin has a half-life of 21 days, decreases due to liver dysfunction do not occur suddenly; however, the serum level of albumin can decrease relatively quickly in a patient who has an acute inflammatory illness such as bacteremia. This rapid decrease likely is caused by the release of cytokines, which accelerate the metabolism of albumin. Other causes of hypoalbuminemia include urinary or gastrointestinal tract losses, and these should be considered in a patient who has hypoalbuminemia in the absence of liver disease.

Platelet Count and Other Tests

Although most patients with significant liver injury have abnormal levels of liver enzymes, occasionally patients with cirrhosis may have normal liver enzyme levels and preserved liver function. A decreased platelet count due to hypersplenism may be a clue to the presence of significant liver injury, and the presence of thrombocytopenia requires exclusion of portal hypertension even when the results of other liver tests are normal. Most patients with thrombocytopenia due to portal hypertension have splenomegaly and, often, other features of portal hypertension such as esophageal varices.

Scoring Systems to Assess Liver Disease Severity

The Child-Turcotte-Pugh score (Table 23.1) uses encephalopathy, ascites, bilirubin, albumin, and prothrombin time (or international normalized ratio [INR]). The measurement of ascites and encephalopathy is subjective, leading to interobserver variation.

The Model for End-stage Liver Disease (MELD) with determination of sodium (MELD-Na) is based on measurements of INR, bilirubin, creatinine, and sodium and is used to predict survival of patients with chronic liver disease, to prioritize patients

Table 23.1. Child-Turcotte-Pugh Score

| Measure | Number of points[a] | | |
	1	2	3
Encephalopathy	None	Stage 1 or 2	Stage 3 or 4
Ascites	None	Mild or moderate	Severe
Bilirubin, mg/dL	<2	2-3	>3
Albumin, g/dL	>3.5	2.8-3.5	<2.8
INR	<1.7	1.7-2.3	>2.3

Abbreviation: INR, international normalized ratio.

[a] Interpretation: class A (compensated disease), 5 or 6 points; class B (functional compromise), 7-9 points; class C (decompensated disease), 10-15 points.

for deceased donor liver transplant, and to assess surgical risk for patients with cirrhosis. Online tools are available to calculate scores for MELD and MELD-Na to help stratify outcome for patients with chronic liver disease.

Hepatocellular Disorders

Acute Hepatitis

Symptoms of acute hepatitis include malaise, anorexia, abdominal pain, and jaundice. Common causes of acute hepatitis are listed in Table 23.2.

Acute hepatitis caused by viruses or drugs usually produces a marked increase in aminotransferase levels (often >1,000 U/L). Aminotransferase levels of more than 5,000 U/L usually are due to acetaminophen hepatotoxicity, ischemic hepatitis (shock liver), or, rarely, hepatitis caused by unusual viruses, such as herpesvirus. Ischemic liver injury occurs after an episode of hypotension and is seen most often in patients with preexisting cardiac dysfunction. Lactate dehydrogenase is also often markedly elevated. In patients with ischemic liver injury, aminotransferase levels increase quickly and improve within a few days. Acute and transient increases in aminotransferase levels (as high as 1,000 U/L) may also be caused by a sudden increase in intrabiliary pressure, usually from a common bile duct stone. In patients with pancreatitis, a transient increase in ALT is suggestive of gallstone pancreatitis. Alcoholic hepatitis is characterized by more modest increases in aminotransferase levels, nearly always less than 400 U/L, with an AST:ALT ratio greater than 2:1. If muscle injury has been excluded, the higher the AST:ALT ratio, the more likely a patient is to have alcoholic liver disease. Patients with alcoholic

Table 23.2. Common Causes of Acute Hepatitis

Disease	Clinical clue	Diagnostic test
Hepatitis A	Exposure history	IgM anti-HAV
Hepatitis B	Risk factors	HBsAg, IgM anti-HBc
Hepatitis C	Risk factors	HCV RNA more reliable than anti-HCV
Drug-induced	Compatible medication	Improvement after agent is withdrawn
Alcoholic hepatitis	History of alcohol excess, AST:ALT >2:1, AST <400 U/L	Liver biopsy, improvement with abstinence
Ischemic hepatitis	History of severe hypotension	Rapid improvement of aminotransferase levels

Abbreviations: ALT, alanine aminotransferase; AST, aspartate aminotransferase; HAV, hepatitis A virus; HBc, hepatitis B core; HBsAg, hepatitis B surface antigen; HCV, hepatitis C virus.

hepatitis frequently have an increase in bilirubin level that is out of proportion to the increase in aminotransferase levels.

When common causes of acute hepatitis have been excluded, considerations should include cytomegalovirus or Epstein-Barr virus, hepatitis E, severe cardiovascular disease, seronegative autoimmune hepatitis, and a previously unrecognized drug or toxin.

Chronic Hepatitis

In chronic hepatitis, the increase in the ALT level is generally more modest (1.5-5 times the upper limit of the reference range) than that in acute hepatitis. Usually the ALT is higher than the AST, although as the disease progresses to advanced fibrosis, the AST may be higher than the ALT. The most important and common disorders that cause chronic hepatitis are listed in Table 23.3.

Patients with nonalcoholic fatty liver disease usually have obesity and type 2 diabetes or hyperlipidemia. Risk factors for hepatitis C include a history of intravenous drug use or exposure to blood products. Most patients with hepatitis B are from an area where the disease is endemic, such as parts of Asia or Africa, or they have a history of illegal drug use or multiple sexual contacts. A complete history is needed to help diagnose drug-induced or alcohol-induced liver disease. Autoimmune hepatitis may manifest as acute or chronic hepatitis. Patients usually have an ALT serum level of 200 to 800 U/L, higher than that in other disorders that cause chronic hepatitis. Autoantibodies, hypergammaglobulinemia, and other autoimmune disorders are helpful clues to the diagnosis of autoimmune hepatitis.

When the most common causes of liver disease have been excluded, other diseases that should be considered are chronic drug-induced liver injury, celiac disease, and nonalcoholic fatty liver disease that is not apparent on imaging. About 30% to 50% of patients with celiac disease have elevated aminotransferase levels, and these abnormalities often improve with a gluten-free diet. Celiac disease may also accompany immune-mediated liver diseases such as autoimmune hepatitis, primary biliary cirrhosis, and primary sclerosing cholangitis. Chronic liver disease due to drug-induced liver injury is uncommon, although it should be considered if a patient has a history of severe cholestatic drug-induced liver injury.

Cholestatic Disorders

Diseases that affect predominantly the biliary system are termed *cholestatic diseases*. These can affect the microscopic ducts (eg,

primary biliary cholangitis [PBC]), large bile ducts (eg, pancreatic cancer obstructing the common bile duct), or both (eg, primary sclerosing cholangitis [PSC]). In these disorders, the predominant abnormality is the level of ALP rather than ALT. A markedly increased ALP level (>1,000 U/L) suggests an intrahepatic rather than obstructive problem. Some causes of cholestasis are listed in Table 23.4.

PBC usually occurs in women and can cause fatigue or pruritus. Of the patients with PSC, 70% to 80% also have ulcerative colitis. Patients with PBC or PSC often are asymptomatic but may have jaundice, fatigue, or pruritus. Large bile duct obstruction often is due to stones or to benign or malignant strictures. Acute bile duct obstruction from a stone is accompanied by abdominal pain and often fever and, as noted above, may produce marked increases in the ALT level. Because ALP must be synthesized before excretion, acute biliary obstruction may not cause an elevated ALP level. Gradual onset of biliary obstruction, such as that caused by a malignant stricture, is initially painless and not accompanied by fever. Infiltrative disorders such as amyloidosis, sarcoidosis, or lymphoma may produce a markedly increased ALP level with a normal bilirubin concentration. Any systemic inflammatory process such as infection or immune disorder may produce nonspecific liver test result abnormalities. The abnormalities usually show a mixed cholestatic (ALP) and hepatocellular (ALT or AST) pattern, and patients often have jaundice.

Hyperbilirubinemia

Jaundice may be the initial manifestation of hepatobiliary disease and occurs when the bilirubin concentration is more than 2.5 mg/dL. A common disorder that produces unconjugated hyperbilirubinemia (but not usually jaundice) is Gilbert syndrome due to an inherited deficiency of uridine diphosphate glucuronosyltransferase. In Gilbert syndrome, total bilirubin is generally less than 3.0 mg/dL, whereas direct bilirubin is 0.5 mg/dL or less. The bilirubin level usually is highest when a patient is ill or fasting. A presumptive diagnosis of Gilbert syndrome can be made in an otherwise well patient who has unconjugated hyperbilirubinemia, normal liver enzyme values, and a normal concentration of hemoglobin (to exclude hemolysis). Genetic testing for Gilbert syndrome is available but usually unnecessary for diagnosis.

Direct hyperbilirubinemia can result from a nonobstructive condition or from an obstructive condition. Obstruction is suggested by abdominal pain, fever, or a palpable gallbladder (or a combination of these). Jaundice due to hepatocellular dysfunction is suggested by risk factors for viral hepatitis, recent ingestion of a potentially hepatotoxic drug, a bilirubin concentration of more than 15 mg/dL, and persistently high aminotransferase levels. In patients with resolving acute hepatitis, improvement in bilirubin concentration occurs more slowly than improvement in ALT level. In diseases resulting in large bile duct obstruction, extrahepatic and intrahepatic biliary dilatation can be identified on imaging studies, especially if the bilirubin concentration is more than 10 mg/dL and the patient has had jaundice for more than 2 weeks. Acute large bile duct obstruction, usually from a stone, may not cause dilatation of the bile ducts, and if the clinical suspicion is strong for bile duct obstruction even though ultrasonography or computed tomography shows normal-sized bile ducts, the biliary tree should be imaged with magnetic resonance cholangiopancreatography,

Table 23.3. Common Causes of Chronic Hepatitis

Disease	Clinical clue	Diagnostic test
Hepatitis C	Risk factors	Anti-HCV, HCV RNA
Hepatitis B	Risk factors	HBsAg
Nonalcoholic fatty liver disease	Obesity, type 2 diabetes, hyperlipidemia	Ultrasonography, liver biopsy
Alcoholic liver disease	History, AST:ALT >2:1	Liver biopsy, improvement with abstinence
Autoimmune hepatitis	ALT 200-1,500 U/L, usually female, other autoimmune disease	Antinuclear or anti–smooth muscle antibody, biopsy

Abbreviations: ALT, alanine aminotransferase; AST, aspartate aminotransferase; HBsAg, hepatitis B surface antigen; HCV, hepatitis C virus.

Table 23.4. Common Causes of Cholestasis

Disease	Clinical clue	Diagnostic test
Primary biliary cholangitis	Woman	Antimitochondrial antibody
Primary sclerosing cholangitis	Association with ulcerative colitis	MRCP
Large bile duct obstruction	Jaundice and pain are common	Ultrasonography, CT, MRCP, ERCP
Drug-induced	Compatible medication or timing	Improvement after agent is withdrawn
Infiltrative disorder	History of malignancy, amyloidosis, sarcoidosis	Ultrasonography, CT, MRI
Inflammation-associated	Symptoms of underlying inflammatory disorder	Blood cultures, appropriate antibody tests

Abbreviations: CT, computed tomography; ERCP, endoscopic retrograde cholangiopancreatography; MRCP, magnetic resonance cholangiopancreatography; MRI, magnetic resonance imaging.

endoscopic retrograde cholangiopancreatography, or endoscopic ultrasonography.

General Approach to Abnormal Liver Test Results

Disease in a patient with abnormal liver test results can usually be categorized into 1 of the clinical syndromes in Box 23.1, although overlap among these categories is considerable. The approach to patients with acute hepatitis, chronic hepatitis, cholestasis, and jaundice is outlined above. Patients with a "first-time," often incidental, increase in liver enzyme levels are usually asymptomatic. Observation is reasonable, with the test repeated in a few months, if 1) the patient is asymptomatic, 2) risk factors for liver disease are not identified, 3) liver enzyme levels are less than 3 times normal, and 4) liver function is preserved. About 30% of patients with incidental elevations of liver test results have normal values on subsequent testing. If the subsequent test results are still abnormal, the patient's condition fits the category of chronic hepatitis or cholestasis, and appropriate evaluation should be initiated. A similar approach can be taken with incidentally discovered abnormal results from patients who are taking medications that only rarely cause liver disease.

Patients also may present with cirrhosis or portal hypertension. Most patients with portal hypertension have cirrhosis, although occasionally patients present with noncirrhotic portal hypertension that is idiopathic or due to portal vein thrombosis. The evaluation of a patient who has cirrhosis is like that of a patient who has chronic hepatitis and cholestasis (as discussed above). In patients with α_1-antitrypsin deficiency, genetic hemochromatosis, alcoholic liver disease, or nonalcoholic fatty liver disease, cirrhosis is frequently the first manifestation of liver disease.

- ✓ Upper limit of normal ALT value: for men, 33 U/L; for women, 25 U/L
- ✓ ALT has a longer half-life than AST; therefore, improvements in ALT lag behind those of AST

Box 23.1. Abnormal Liver Test Results: Clinical Syndromes

"First-time" increase in liver enzymes

Acute hepatitis

Chronic hepatitis

Cholestasis without hepatitis or jaundice

Jaundice

Cirrhosis or portal hypertension

- ✓ Thrombocytopenia—often the first manifestation of cirrhosis with portal hypertension
- ✓ ALT level greater than 5,000 U/L—usually due to hepatic ischemia, acetaminophen drug-induced liver disease, or herpes hepatitis
- ✓ Acute biliary obstruction from a common duct stone may increase ALT up to 1,000 U/L
- ✓ An AST:ALT ratio greater than 2 suggests liver disease associated with alcohol; an AST:ALT ratio greater than 1 in patients with hepatitis C or NASH suggests advanced hepatic fibrosis
- ✓ Infiltrative disorders such as amyloidosis or sarcoidosis cause an elevated ALP with a normal bilirubin level
- ✓ Patients with acute hepatitis without a common cause identified often have an unrecognized drug- or toxin-induced liver injury, infection, or cardiovascular disease
- ✓ Patients with a chronic liver injury without a readily identifiable cause often have nonalcoholic fatty liver disease
- ✓ Acute severe drug-induced liver injury may lead to a long-term increase in the ALP level
- ✓ Ultrasound- and MRI-based elastography have largely replaced liver biopsy for assessment of hepatic fibrosis

Liver Biopsy

Technique and Safety

Most liver biopsies are performed percutaneously and guided by imaging, usually ultrasonography. In patients with ascites or coagulopathy, specimens may also be obtained with transvenous access from the jugular vein. Transvenous approaches also allow for measurement of the wedged hepatic vein pressure gradient to assess for sinusoidal portal hypertension. If open or laparoscopic abdominal surgery is necessary for another indication, biopsy specimens may also be obtained under direct visualization. Finally, an increasing number of biopsies are done at the time of endoscopic ultrasonography. The most common complication of liver biopsy is pain, which can usually be controlled with simple analgesics. The most serious risk is bleeding, which occurs in 0.1% to 0.3% of all liver biopsies. Bleeding usually subsides without the need for transfusion or other intervention. Persistent bleeding may require transarterial embolization. Immediate severe pain after liver biopsy is suggestive of a bile leak.

General Utility

Liver histopathologic findings are often nonspecific. A common report might include a lymphoplasmacytic portal infiltrate consistent with viral, drug, or autoimmune hepatitis. Clinical information is then required to help differentiate a cause. When the liver biopsy is done for diagnostic reasons, the pathologist and clinician should communicate, when possible, to allow an exchange of relevant information. This kind of dialogue is much more effective than if the clinician merely relies on the biopsy report or the pathologist relies on printed clinical information, much of which may be incomplete. In patients with acute liver disease, a diagnosis is usually forthcoming with the help of the clinical history and blood tests for infections and inherited and metabolic disorders; therefore, biopsy is generally not performed. Occasionally, liver biopsy is needed to help in the diagnosis of a sudden onset of autoimmune hepatitis, drug-induced liver injury, diffuse intrahepatic malignancy not identified on imaging, Wilson disease, alcoholic liver disease when clinical history is uncertain, and unusual infections such as herpes or Q fever. Liver biopsy may detect clinically unsuspected chronic liver disease in a patient presenting with acute hepatitis.

Patients with long-term liver enzyme elevations and negative or normal results on blood tests are frequently referred to hepatology clinics for evaluation for causes of chronic liver disease. Studies incorporating liver biopsy show that most of these patients have nonalcoholic fatty liver disease with mild histologic changes. About 19% of patients have normal liver histology or minimal abnormalities. Predictors of minimal changes are female sex and body mass index (calculated as weight in kilograms divided by height in meters squared) less than 25. Predictors of significant fibrosis are tobacco use, body mass index less than 25, and presence of type 2 diabetes.

The availability of noninvasive tests for fibrosis (eg, blood test panels and scoring systems, transient elastography, shear-wave elastography, and magnetic resonance elastography) have decreased the need for liver biopsy to assess degree of fibrosis.

Acute Liver Failure

Definition and Etiology

Acute liver failure is the development of severe acute liver injury, including INR greater than 1.5 and encephalopathy, developing within 26 weeks after the onset of symptoms in a patient without a previous history of chronic liver disease. Patients with an acute presentation of Wilson disease or a flare of hepatitis B may be still characterized as having acute liver failure even if they have histologic features of chronic liver injury. About 2,000 cases of acute liver failure occur annually in the US. Because many of the patients are young and previously healthy, a poor outcome of this relatively unusual condition is particularly tragic.

Determining the cause of acute liver failure is important for 2 reasons: 1) specific therapy may be available, as for acetaminophen hepatotoxicity or herpes hepatitis, and 2) the prognosis differs depending on the cause. For instance, the spontaneous recovery rate for patients with acute liver failure due to acetaminophen or hepatitis A is more than 50%; consequently, a more cautious approach would be advised before proceeding with liver transplant. In comparison, spontaneous recovery from acute liver failure due to Wilson disease is unusual and early liver transplant would be recommended. In the US, the most common identifiable causes are acetaminophen hepatotoxicity, idiosyncratic drug reactions, Wilson disease, hepatitis B, and ischemia. Acetaminophen-protein adducts have also been identified in about 20% of patients with idiopathic acute liver failure, suggesting that acetaminophen hepatotoxicity may have a role in this patient subset. History should be obtained promptly, before mental status declines and a reliable history cannot be obtained. A history of prescription and nonprescription drugs, use of illicit substances, and alcohol use is important in making a decision about the patient's candidacy for liver transplant. If the cause of acute liver failure cannot be determined from the history and blood tests, biopsy can be considered to exclude malignancy and autoimmune hepatitis.

✓ Acute liver failure—severe liver injury, including international normalized ratio greater than 1.5 and hepatic encephalopathy, developing within 26 weeks after onset of symptoms without evidence of preexisting liver disease

Presentation

The presenting symptoms of patients with acute liver failure are usually those of acute hepatitis, including malaise, nausea, and jaundice. Hepatic encephalopathy is a required feature of the syndrome, and manifestations may range from subtle mental status changes, such as difficulty with concentration, to coma (Table 23.5). Because encephalopathy in a patient with acute liver disease is an ominous sign, the mental status of patients with acute hepatitis should be assessed frequently. Laboratory features are consistent with severe liver dysfunction. Aminotransferase levels are variably increased, although they usually are more than 1,000 U/L. Acetaminophen hepatotoxicity usually causes ALT to be more than 3,500 U/L. Fulminant Wilson disease is characterized by only modest increases in aminotransferase levels and a low or normal ALP level despite clinical evidence of liver failure, such as a prolonged prothrombin time and high bilirubin concentration. An ALP to total bilirubin ratio less than 4 is suggestive of Wilson disease.

The encephalopathy associated with acute liver failure, unlike that of chronic liver disease, has a propensity to progress to cerebral edema. The mechanisms for the development of cerebral edema have not been clarified but may involve disruption of the blood-brain barrier and interference with mechanisms of cellular osmolarity. Clinically, the encephalopathy often is associated with a marked increase in the serum level of ammonia, although alterations in unidentified neurotransmitters likely are involved in causing mental status changes. Ammonia levels of more than 150 μmol/L have been associated with intracranial hypertension and a poor outcome.

Cerebral edema and superimposed infection are the more common causes of death when patients have acute liver failure. Cerebral edema leads to death by causing brain ischemia and cerebral herniation. Patients with acute liver failure are predisposed to infections likely due to severe illness and the need for numerous interventions and monitoring. The clinical features typical of infection, such as fever and leukocytosis, may not occur in patients with acute liver failure, so a high level of awareness for infection needs to be maintained. Any clinical deterioration should mandate a search for infection, and the threshold for antimicrobial therapy should be low.

Hypoglycemia occurs frequently and is a poor prognostic sign. It is likely due to both inadequate degradation of insulin and diminished production of glucose by the diseased liver.

A hyperdynamic circulation and a decrease in systemic vascular resistance are seen in patients with acute liver failure. These features may be well tolerated by patients, but occasionally hemodynamic compromise can develop. Monitored parameters

Table 23.5. Stages of Hepatic Encephalopathy

Stage	Features
I	Changes in behavior, with minimal change in level of consciousness
II	Gross disorientation, gross slowness of mentation, drowsiness, asterixis, inappropriate behavior, maintenance of sphincter tone
III	Sleeping most of the time, arousable to vocal stimuli, marked confusion, incoherent speech
IV	Comatose, unresponsive to pain, decorticate or decerebrate posturing

may mimic sepsis. Fluid resuscitation usually is necessary, although caution is advised because the administration of excessive fluid may worsen intracranial pressure.

Kidney and electrolyte abnormalities occur because of underlying disease such as Wilson disease, functional kidney failure due to sepsis or hepatorenal syndrome, or acute tubular necrosis. Kidney dysfunction is particularly common in acetaminophen-induced acute liver failure. Monitoring of electrolytes, including sodium, potassium, bicarbonate, magnesium, and phosphorus, is important, and the presence of acidosis is a risk factor for poor outcome in acute liver failure and has been incorporated into some prognostic models.

Management

The appearance of encephalopathy precedes cerebral edema; therefore, patients with acute hepatitis and evidence of liver failure need to be monitored carefully for mental status changes. Lactulose is less effective in encephalopathy associated with acute liver failure compared with encephalopathy associated with chronic liver disease and may not prevent cerebral edema from developing later; nevertheless, it is often given with monitoring for gaseous distention of the intestines. Rifaximin may also be used, although its benefit has not been proved. Patients with stage II encephalopathy usually are admitted to an intensive care unit for close monitoring of mental status and vital signs. Sedatives should be avoided initially to allow close monitoring of mental status. Computed tomography or magnetic resonance imaging of the head is performed to exclude an alternative cause of mental status changes.

Patients who reach stage III encephalopathy are at considerable risk for progression to cerebral edema. Because clinical signs and computed tomography are insensitive for detecting increased intracranial pressure, many centers institute intracranial pressure monitoring when patients reach stage III encephalopathy. Endotracheal intubation and mechanical ventilation usually precede placement of the intracranial pressure monitor. Various monitors are used, but infection and bleeding can complicate any monitoring. The goal of intracranial pressure monitoring is to allow treatment of high pressure and to identify which patients are too ill for liver transplant because of a prolonged period of excessively high intracranial pressure. Generally, the goal is to maintain intracranial pressure less than 40 mm Hg and cerebral perfusion pressure (the difference between mean arterial pressure and intracranial pressure) between 60 and 100 mm Hg. Excessively high cerebral perfusion pressures (>120 mm Hg) can increase cerebral edema.

Maneuvers that cause straining, including endotracheal suctioning, should be avoided or limited. Paralyzing agents and sedatives may be necessary, although they may limit further assessment of neurologic status. Administration of hypertonic saline until the serum sodium level is 145 to 155 mmol/L decreases the risk of intracranial hypertension. If intracranial pressure is more than 20 mm Hg or cerebral perfusion pressure less than 60 mm Hg, the following steps are advised: elevation of the head to 20°, hyperventilation to a $Paco_2$ of 25 mm Hg, and administration of mannitol (if kidney function is intact). Barbiturate-induced coma can be used for refractory cases. Glucocorticoids are ineffective. A prolonged increase in intracranial pressure above mean arterial pressure may signify brain death and generally is a contraindication to liver transplant. A sudden decrease in intracranial pressure may indicate brain herniation.

Box 23.2.   King's College Criteria for Liver Transplant in Fulminant Liver Failure[a]

1. Fulminant liver failure due to Wilson disease or Budd-Chari syndrome
2. Acetaminophen-induced if either of the following are met:
   a. pH <7.3 at 24 h after overdose
   b. Creatinine >3.4 mg/dL, prothrombin time >100 s, and stage III or IV encephalopathy
3. Non-acetaminophen-induced if either of the following are met:
   a. INR >6.5 or
   b. Any 3 of the following: INR >3.5, >7 d from jaundice to encephalopathy, indeterminate or drug-induced cause, age <10 y, age >40 y, bilirubin >17.5 mg/dL

Abbreviation: INR, international normalized ratio.

[a] Any 1 of the 3 criteria.

In patients with acute liver failure, the prothrombin time is a simple noninvasive measure to follow, and coagulopathy is not corrected unless there is bleeding or an intervention is planned (eg, placement of a monitoring device). If bleeding occurs or an invasive procedure is necessary, fresh frozen plasma usually is administered first, although platelets, fibrinogen, and even recombinant activated factor VII may be necessary. Continuous infusion of 5% or 10% dextrose is used to keep the plasma glucose level between 100 and 200 mg/dL. The plasma glucose level should be monitored at least twice daily. Both bacteremia and fungemia are sufficiently frequent that periodic blood cultures are advised and prophylaxis with antimicrobials may be initiated, although this practice has not been shown to affect survival.

One randomized trial suggested that administration of *N*-acetylcysteine may be beneficial in some patients who have acute liver failure even when acetaminophen hepatotoxicity has been excluded. Patients with early-stage encephalopathy treated with *N*-acetylcysteine had better transplant-free survival than untreated patients.

Models to predict the outcome of acute liver failure have been developed to facilitate the optimal timing of liver transplant before the patient becomes so ill that transplant is contraindicated yet still allow time for spontaneous recovery. The most well-known and widely used model is the King's College criteria (Box 23.2). A MELD score higher than 32 is also associated with a poor liver transplant-free survival. Acute liver failure is the indication for 6% of liver transplants in the US. Even though 1-year survival with transplant for acute liver failure is lower than that for transplant for other indications, outcomes are an improvement over the dismal survival rates for patients with acute liver failure who meet poor prognostic markers such as the King's College criteria, and long-term survival after transplant is excellent.

✓ Patients with acute hepatic failure who are potential transplant candidates should be promptly referred to a liver transplant center
✓ Clues to the diagnosis of acute liver failure due to Wilson disease include a low ALP and evidence of hemolysis
✓ Encephalopathy associated with acute liver failure predisposes to cerebral edema and responds less well to lactulose than that associated with chronic liver disease

✓ Cerebral edema and infections are common causes of death in patients with acute liver failure
✓ The prognosis with acute liver failure due to acetaminophen hepatotoxicity and hepatitis A is better than that from other causes; the prognosis with acute liver failure associated with Wilson disease and drugs other than acetaminophen is particularly poor

Suggested Reading

Biggins SW, Kim WR, Terrault NA, Saab S, Balan V, Schiano T, et al. Evidence-based incorporation of serum sodium concentration into meld. Gastroenterology. 2006 May;130(6):1652–60.

Chalasani N, Bonkovsky HL, Fontana R, Lee W, Stolz A, Talwalkar J, et al. Features and outcomes of 899 patients with drug-induced liver injury: the DILIN prospective study. Gastroenterology. 2015 Jun;148(7):1340–52.

de Ledinghen V, Ratziu V, Causse X, Le Bail B, Capron D, Renou C, et al. Diagnostic and predictive factors of significant liver fibrosis and minimal lesions in patients with persistent unexplained elevated transaminases: a prospective multicenter study. J Hepatol. 2006 Oct;45(4):592–9.

Flamm SL, Yang YX, Singh S, Falck-Ytter YT, AGA Institute Clinical Guidelines Committee. American Gastroenterological Association Institute guidelines for the diagnosis and management of acute liver failure. Gastroenterology. 2017 Feb;152(3):644–7.

Kwo PY, Cohen SM, Lim JK. ACG clinical guideline: evaluation of abnormal liver chemistries. Am J Gastroenterol. 2017 Jan;112(1):18–35.

Lee WM, Hynan LS, Rossaro L, Fontana RJ, Stravitz RT, Larson AM, et al. Intravenous n-acetylcysteine improves transplant-free survival in early stage non-acetaminophen acute liver failure. Gastroenterology. 2009 Sep;137(3):856–64.

O'Grady JG, Alexander GJ, Hayllar KM, Williams R. Early indicators of prognosis in fulminant hepatic failure. Gastroenterology. 1989 Aug;97(2):439–45.

Stravitz RT, Lee WM. Acute liver failure. Lancet. 2019 Sep 7;394(10201): 869–81.

Tapper EB, Lok AS. Use of liver imaging and biopsy in clinical practice. N Engl J Med. 2017 Aug 24;377(8):756–68.

24

Viral Hepatitis[a,b]

MICHAEL D. LEISE, MD

Viral infections are important causes of liver disease worldwide. The 5 primary hepatitis viruses that have been identified are A, B, C, D (or delta), and E. Other viruses, such as cytomegalovirus and Epstein-Barr virus, also can result in hepatitis as part of a systemic infection. In addition, medications, toxins, autoimmune hepatitis, or Wilson disease may cause acute or chronic hepatitis.

It is useful to divide hepatitis syndromes into acute and chronic forms. *Acute hepatitis* can last from a few weeks to 6 months and is often accompanied by jaundice. Symptoms of acute hepatitis tend to be similar regardless of cause and include anorexia, malaise, dark urine, fever, and mild abdominal pain. In *chronic hepatitis*, patients are often asymptomatic but may complain of fatigue. Occasionally, they have manifestations of advanced liver disease (ascites, variceal bleeding, or encephalopathy) at the initial presentation with chronic hepatitis. Each hepatitis virus

causes acute hepatitis, but only hepatitis B, C, and D viruses cause chronic hepatitis, although chronic hepatitis E can develop in the context of immunosuppression.

The purpose of this chapter is to review the primary hepatitis viruses. More comprehensive discussions of acute hepatitis are found in other chapters. The 4 common hepatitis viruses are compared in Table 24.1, and the disease burden of the 3 most important viruses in the US is summarized in Table 24.2.

Hepatitis A

Epidemiology

The incidence of acute hepatitis A virus (HAV) infection is decreasing in the US owing to the recommendation for universal childhood vaccination. However, outbreaks resulting in 37,000 new cases from 2016 through 2021 were identified primarily among persons experiencing homelessness and those with a history of injection or noninjection drug use. Common routes of transmission of HAV are ingestion of contaminated food or water and contact with an infected person. Groups at particularly high risk include people living in or traveling to resource-limited countries, children in day care centers, men who have sex with men, and perhaps persons who ingest raw shellfish. The incubation period for HAV is 2 to 6 weeks.

Clinical Presentation and Natural History

The most important determinant of the severity of acute hepatitis A is the age at which infection occurs. Persons infected when younger than 6 years have nonspecific symptoms that rarely include jaundice. Adolescents or adults who acquire HAV infection usually have jaundice. Hepatitis A is almost always a self-limited infection. There may be a prolonged cholestatic phase

[a] Portions previously published in Poterucha JJ. Hepatitis. In: Bland KI, Sarr MG, Buchler MW, Csendes A, Garden OJ, Wong J, eds. General surgery: principles and international practice. 2nd Ed. London (England): Springer-Verlag; 2009: 921-32; used with permission.

[b] I acknowledge John J. Poterucha, MD, for his contributions to this chapter in previous editions of this text.

Abbreviations: AASLD, American Association for the Study of Liver Diseases; ALT, alanine aminotransferase; anti-HAV, antibody to hepatitis A virus; anti-HBc, antibody to hepatitis B core antigen; anti-HBs, antibody to hepatitis B surface antigen; anti-HCV, antibody to hepatitis C virus; APRI, aspartate aminotransferase to platelet ratio index; DAA, direct-acting antiviral; HAV, hepatitis A virus; HBeAg, hepatitis B e antigen; HBsAg, hepatitis B surface antigen; HBV, hepatitis B virus; HCC, hepatocellular carcinoma; HCV, hepatitis C virus; HDV, hepatitis D virus; IDSA, Infectious Diseases Society of America; Ig, immunoglobulin; MELD, Model for End-stage Liver Disease; MR, magnetic resonance; RAS, resistance-associated substitution; SVR, sustained virologic response; ULRR, upper limit of the reference range

Table 24.1.   Comparison of the 4 Primary Hepatitis Viruses

Feature	HAV	HBV	HDV	HCV
Incubation, d	15-50	30-160	Unknown	14-160
Jaundice	Common	30% of patients	Common	Uncommon
Course	Acute	Acute or chronic	Acute or chronic	Acute or chronic
Transmission	Fecal-oral	Parenteral	Parenteral	Parenteral
Test for diagnosis	IgM anti-HAV	HBsAg	Anti-HDV	HCV RNA

Abbreviations: anti-HAV, antibody to hepatitis A virus; anti-HDV, antibody to hepatitis D virus; HAV, hepatitis A virus; HBsAg, hepatitis B surface antigen; HBV, hepatitis B virus; HCV, hepatitis C virus; HDV, hepatitis D virus; Ig, immunoglobulin.

characterized by persistence of jaundice for up to 6 months. Rarely, acute hepatitis A manifests as acute liver failure that may require liver transplant. HAV does not cause chronic infection and should not be in the differential diagnosis of chronic hepatitis.

Diagnostic Tests

The diagnosis of acute hepatitis A is established by the presence of immunoglobulin (Ig)M antibody to hepatitis A virus (anti-HAV), which appears at the onset of the acute phase of the illness and becomes undetectable in 3 to 6 months. During the acute phase, IgG anti-HAV is also present, but it persists for decades and is a marker of immunity from further infection. A patient with IgG anti-HAV, but not IgM anti-HAV, has had an infection in the remote past or has been vaccinated.

Treatment

The treatment of acute hepatitis A is supportive. For those exposed to an infected person or contaminated food, postexposure prophylaxis with hepatitis A vaccine or immune serum globulin (or both) is advised, depending on the patient's age and overall health status.

Prevention

Immunization with hepatitis A vaccine is recommended for all children at 12 months of age. Hepatitis A vaccine should be offered also to travelers to areas with an intermediate or high prevalence of hepatitis A, to men who have sex with men, to intravenous drug users, to recipients of clotting factor concentrates, and to patients with chronic liver disease.

✓ Atypical presentation of hepatitis A—a relapsing -remitting cholestatic course lasting up to 6 months
---

Table 24.2.   Clinical Effects of Hepatitis Viruses in the US[a]

Feature	HAV	HBV	HCV
Acute hepatitis, No. of clinical cases annually	11,000	12,000	2,900
Fulminant hepatitis, No. of deaths annually	50	100	Rare
Chronic hepatitis, No. of clinical cases annually	0	800,000-1.4 million	2.7-3.9 million
Chronic liver disease, No. of deaths annually	0	3,000	12,000

Abbreviations: HAV, hepatitis A virus; HBV, hepatitis B virus; HCV, hepatitis C virus.

[a] Data from the Centers for Disease Control and Prevention (2008 data).

Hepatitis B

Epidemiology

Hepatitis B virus (HBV) is a DNA virus that causes about 30% of the cases of acute viral hepatitis and 15% of the cases of chronic viral hepatitis in the US. Most persons with chronic infection in the US are immigrants from Asia and Africa, where infection is acquired at birth or in early childhood. Major risk factors for adult disease acquisition in the US are sexual contact with an infected person and intravenous drug use.

Clinical Presentation and Natural History

The incubation period after HBV infection ranges from 60 to 150 days. About 30% of adolescents or adults with acute hepatitis B have icterus. Complete recovery with subsequent lifelong immunity occurs in 95% of infected adults. *Chronic infection*, defined as persistence of hepatitis B surface antigen (HBsAg) for more than 6 months, develops in about 5% of infected adults. Immunosuppressed persons with acute HBV infection are more likely to become chronically infected, presumably because of an insufficient immune response against the virus.

Patients with chronic hepatitis B infection present in 1 of 4 phases (Figure 24.1). An *immune tolerant phase* is recognized in many Asian patients who are infected perinatally. This phase, usually encountered in patients younger than 35 years, is characterized by the presence of hepatitis B e antigen (HBeAg) and very high HBV DNA levels yet normal levels of alanine aminotransferase (ALT). Generally, liver biopsy specimens from these patients show minimal changes except for ground-glass hepatocytes. The immune tolerant phase evolves under immune pressure into the *HBeAg-positive chronic hepatitis B phase*, characterized by increased ALT levels, persistence of HBeAg, and more than 10^4 IU/mL of HBV DNA. Active inflammation and often fibrosis, seen in liver biopsy specimens, lead to progressive liver injury. At a rate of about 10% per year, patients mount enough of an immune response to achieve a decrease in ALT levels, clearance of HBeAg and development of antibody to HBeAg (seroconversion), and a decrease in HBV DNA to less than 10^4 IU/mL. The resulting *inactive carrier phase* usually is not accompanied by progressive liver damage. In cross-sectional studies, about 60% of patients with chronic hepatitis B are in the inactive carrier phase. Many patients remain in this phase for many years and have a better prognosis than those with active liver inflammation and HBV DNA levels of more than 10^4 IU/mL.

About one-third of inactive carriers have a reactivation of active hepatitis characterized by abnormal ALT levels and HBV DNA levels of more than 10^4 IU/mL. This may be associated with a reversion to the HBeAg-positive state, but more commonly it is due to a precore or core promoter variant. This *HBeAg-negative chronic hepatitis B phase* is associated with progression of liver

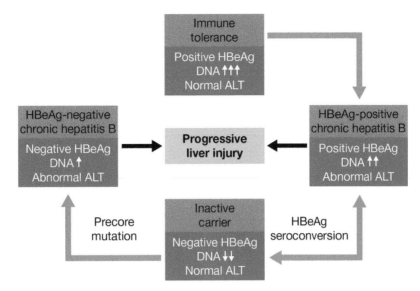

Figure 24.1. **Phases of Chronic Hepatitis B Virus Infection.** Black arrows indicate histopathologic changes; gray arrows, changes in serologic markers between phases. White arrows indicate increase or decrease of DNA level (↑, low increase;↑↑, moderate increase;↓↓, moderate decrease;↑↑↑, high increase). ALT indicates alanine aminotransferase; HBeAg, hepatitis B e antigen. (Adapted from Pungpapong S, Kim WR, Poterucha JJ. Natural history of hepatitis B virus infection: an update for clinicians. Mayo Clin Proc. 2007 Aug;82[8]:967-75; used with permission of Mayo Foundation for Medical Education and Research.)

damage. Patients with HBeAg-negative chronic hepatitis B are more likely to have a fluctuating course than patients with HBeAg-positive chronic hepatitis B. Also, the patients generally are older and have more advanced fibrosis because HBeAg-negative chronic hepatitis B tends to occur later in the course of infection.

Patients with chronic hepatitis B may experience spontaneous flares of disease characterized by markedly abnormal ALT levels, deterioration in liver function, and often seroconversion of HBeAg. The differential diagnosis for acute hepatitis in patients with chronic hepatitis B is listed in Table 24.3. Because disease activity changes in patients with chronic hepatitis B, even after years in the inactive carrier state, periodic monitoring with liver tests and hepatitis B markers is necessary. Each year HBsAg clears spontaneously in about 1% of patients who have chronic infection.

In about 15% to 40% of patients with chronic HBV infection, serious sequelae develop—either decompensated liver disease or hepatocellular carcinoma (HCC). Factors associated with the development of cirrhosis are older age; coinfection with hepatitis C

virus (HCV), HIV, or hepatitis D virus (HDV); hepatitis B genotype C; longer duration of infection; high HBV DNA levels; and alcohol use. Many of these factors, including HBV DNA level, are associated also with an increased risk of HCC.

Patients with chronic hepatitis B and cirrhosis are at high risk for the development of HCC, and surveillance every 6 to 12 months is advised. Surveillance also is advised for patients without cirrhosis who meet 1 of the following criteria: family history of HCC, Asian man older than 40 years, Asian woman older than 50 years, Black African older than 20 years, and persistent increase in ALT level together with an HBV DNA value of more than 10^4 IU/mL. The method of surveillance varies among centers, but many use ultrasonography at 6-month intervals with or without monitoring serum alpha fetoprotein levels.

Eight hepatitis B genotypes, labeled A through H, have been identified, and the genotype for a patient is determined largely by the country in which infection is acquired. All genotypes have been identified in the US. Asian patients who have genotype B have a better prognosis than those with genotype C, including a higher rate of clearance of HBeAg, a slower rate of progression to cirrhosis, and a lower likelihood of the development of hepatocellular cancer.

Diagnostic Tests

A brief guide to serologic markers for hepatitis B is provided in Table 24.4. The interpretation of serologic patterns is shown in Table 24.5. Rarely, a patient with acute hepatitis B (usually with a severe presentation such as acute liver failure) lacks HBsAg and has only IgM antibody to hepatitis B core antigen (anti-HBc) as the marker for recent infection. Patients with an acute flare of chronic hepatitis B may redevelop IgM anti-HBc. Most patients with HBsAg have detectable serum levels of HBV DNA. HBV DNA levels greater than 10^4 IU/mL are associated with an increased risk of cirrhosis and HCC.

Occasionally, patients have IgG anti-HBc as the only positive hepatitis B serologic marker. A common explanation for a

Table 24.3. Causes of Acute Hepatitis in Patients With Chronic Hepatitis B

Cause	Clinical clues
Spontaneous "reactivation" of hepatitis B	Seroconversion of HBeAg, reappearance of IgM anti-HBc
Flare due to immunosuppression	Chemotherapy, antirejection therapy, corticosteroids, anti–tumor necrosis factor agents
Induced by antiviral therapy	Interferon (common), oral agents (rare)
Superimposed infection with other viruses, especially HDV	Exposure to HDV (usually due to illicit drug use), HAV, or HCV
Other causes of acute hepatitis	History of excessive use of alcohol, medications, or illegal drugs

Abbreviations: anti-HBc, antibody to hepatitis B core antigen; HAV, hepatitis A virus; HBeAg, hepatitis B e antigen; HCV, hepatitis C virus; HDV, hepatitis D virus; Ig, immunoglobulin.

Table 24.4. Hepatitis B Serologic Markers

Test	Interpretation of positive result
Hepatitis B surface antigen (HBsAg)	Current infection
Antibody to hepatitis B surface antigen (anti-HBs)	Immunity (immunization or resolved infection)
IgM antibody to hepatitis B core antigen (IgM anti-HBc)	Recent infection or "reactivation" of chronic infection
IgG antibody to hepatitis B core antigen (IgG anti-HBc)	Remote infection
Hepatitis B e antigen (HBeAg) or hepatitis B virus DNA >10⁴ IU/mL (or both)	Active viral replication (high infectivity)

Abbreviation: Ig, immunoglobulin.

population without risk factors for disease acquisition is a false-positive test result (the results are often repeatedly positive). Another explanation is a previous, resolved HBV infection in which the level of antibody to hepatitis B surface antigen (anti-HBs) has decreased below the limit of detection. This can be supported by demonstrating an anamnestic type of response to hepatitis B vaccine. Rarely, patients with hepatitis B may have HBsAg levels that are below the level of detection, so that IgG anti-HBc is the only marker of infection. Although the importance of this low-level infection is unclear, these patients can be identified by the presence of HBV DNA in serum or liver.

The accuracy of serologic and nucleic acid tests obviates the need for liver biopsy in the diagnosis of hepatitis B; however, liver biopsy is useful for grading inflammatory activity and determining the stage of fibrosis. Histologic features of hepatitis B are inflammation that is usually around the portal tract, variable fibrosis that initially is also portocentric, and the presence of ground-glass hepatocytes. *Ground-glass hepatocytes* are hepatocytes with cytoplasm that has a hazy, eosinophilic appearance. With immunostaining, these cells are positive for HBsAg (Figure 24.2). Even though liver biopsy is the gold standard for diagnosing cirrhosis, it usually is not necessary for patients who have other features of cirrhosis, such as portal hypertension.

Treatment

Generally, hepatitis B is treated if the patient is at risk for disease progression. This includes patients who have HBeAg-positive chronic hepatitis B with ALT at least twice the upper limit of the reference range (ULRR) and HBV DNA greater than 20,000 IU/mL and patients who have HBeAg-negative chronic hepatitis B with ALT at least twice the ULRR and HBV DNA greater than

2,000 IU/mL. All patients with cirrhosis should be treated with an oral antiviral regardless of the phase of the disease or the HBV DNA level. Acute liver failure due to acute hepatitis B should be treated with an oral agent. In some patients, oral antiviral therapy can reverse liver failure.

Patients with hepatitis B generally do not require liver biopsy before a decision about the need for treatment. Liver biopsy is helpful for patients who otherwise do not meet clear criteria for treatment. In those who do not meet treatment criteria, treatment should still be initiated if they have a fibrosis stage of F2 or higher on liver biopsy or considerable inflammation. Liver biopsy also can be used to diagnose advanced fibrosis, which could mandate a change in management, such as evaluation for esophageal varices or surveillance for HCC. Noninvasive testing such as transient or magnetic resonance (MR) elastography can also be used instead of liver biopsy.

Hepatitis B can be treated with peginterferon or an oral agent (preferably entecavir or tenofovir). Peginterferon has replaced standard interferon because of its once-weekly dosing and perhaps better efficacy, and 1 year of treatment is advised. Seroconversion may occur months or even years after completion of treatment. Predictors of a greater likelihood of response to peginterferon include higher ALT level, lower HBV DNA level, shorter duration of disease, genotype A or B, and female sex. Patients treated with peginterferon may experience a flare of hepatitis (likely due to immune system activation) about 4 to 8 weeks after beginning treatment. Treatment should be continued despite this flare unless there is clinical or biochemical evidence of decompensation. Patients with Child-Turcotte-Pugh class B or C cirrhosis should not be treated with interferons because of the risk of precipitating decompensation with this flare. Adverse effects of peginterferon are common and are considered below (in the Hepatitis C section). Peginterferon is not used often.

The oral agents are prescribed more frequently than peginterferon for chronic hepatitis B. They are compared in Table 24.6. These oral agents are well tolerated, and they are useful particularly in patients with decompensated cirrhosis because these drugs may improve liver function. The flare of hepatitis that may occur during interferon therapy is unusual with the oral agents. Because of their high barrier to resistance, tenofovir and entecavir are the agents most commonly prescribed for hepatitis B. About 15% to 20% of patients with HBeAg-positive disease who are treated with oral agents have seroconversion and are positive for antibody to HBeAg after 1 to 2 years of therapy; treatment should be continued for 12 months after seroconversion. Patients without seroconversion of HBeAg need to continue treatment indefinitely. Seroconversion of HBsAg with the oral agents is unusual;

Table 24.5. Interpretation of Hepatitis B Serologic Patterns

HBsAg	Anti-HBs	IgM anti-HBc	IgG anti-HBc	HBeAg	Anti-HBe	HBV DNA, IU/mL	Interpretation
+	−	+	−	+	−	+	Acute infection or, less commonly, acute flare of chronic hepatitis B
−	+	−	+	−	±	−	Previous infection with immunity
−	+	−	+	−	−	−	Vaccination with immunity
+	−	−	+	−	+	<10⁴	Hepatitis B inactive carrier state
+	−	−	+	+	−	>10⁴	Chronic hepatitis B
+	−	−	+	−	+	>10⁴	HBeAg-negative chronic hepatitis B (often "precore" or "core promoter" variants)

Abbreviations: anti-HBc, antibody to hepatitis B core antigen; anti-HBe, antibody to hepatitis B e antigen; anti-HBs, antibody to hepatitis B surface antigen; HBeAg, hepatitis B e antigen; HBsAg, hepatitis B surface antigen; HBV, hepatitis B virus; Ig, immunoglobulin.

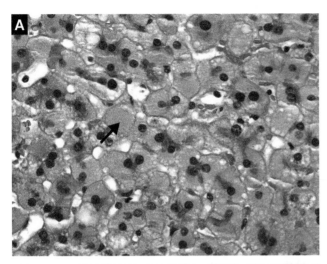

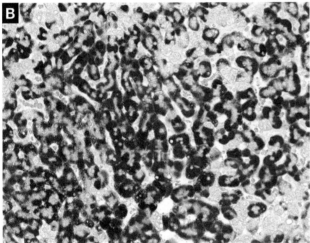

Figure 24.2. Liver Biopsy Specimen From Patient With Hepatitis B. A, Ground-glass hepatocyte (arrow) (hematoxylin-eosin). B, Immunostain for hepatitis B surface antigen shows positive staining of hepatocyte cytoplasm.

therefore, most patients with HBeAg-negative chronic hepatitis will require prolonged or even indefinite therapy.

The choice of therapeutic agent for hepatitis B depends on several factors. Peginterferon is reasonable for patients without cirrhosis who have an ALT level greater than 200 U/L and who can tolerate the numerous adverse effects of the drug. Peginterferon is most effective against hepatitis B genotypes A and B; thus, genotyping is advised for patients for whom peginterferon therapy is being considered. Entecavir or tenofovir is preferred

for patients who have cirrhosis. Tenofovir alafenamide is associated with lower risk of bone and kidney complications as compared to tenofovir disoproxil fumarate. Oral agents are preferred also for patients who are undergoing immunosuppression, for example, after organ transplant or infection with HIV.

Patients who test positive for HBsAg and need chemotherapy or immunosuppression are at risk for disease flare, and treatment with an oral agent is advised during therapy and for at least 6 months after therapy has been completed. Patients with isolated anti-HBc positivity are also at risk, although the risk is much smaller than for those with HBsAg positivity. Patients with isolated anti-HBc positivity who are treated with rituximab or hematologic stem cell transplant are at high enough risk for disease activation to warrant prophylactic HBV treatment, which should be continued for 12 months after the last dose of rituximab or other B-cell–depleting agents. For others with isolated anti-HBc positivity, monitoring of ALT and HBV DNA levels during immunosuppression therapy is advised, and treatment with oral agents should be given if HBV DNA becomes detectable.

For patients with end-stage liver disease or HCC due to hepatitis B, liver transplant results in excellent outcomes. Patients with hepatitis B who have HBeAg or high HBV DNA levels (or both) before liver transplant are at particularly high risk for recurrence after transplant. For these patients, oral agents are recommended before transplant, and a combination of hepatitis B immune globulin and an oral agent after transplant. Even among patients without detectable HBV DNA, recurrence rates are sufficiently high that most transplant groups still give an oral agent for both preoperative therapy and postoperative therapy.

Prevention

Hepatitis B immune globulin should be given to nonimmune household and sexual contacts of patients who have acute hepatitis B. All infants should receive hepatitis B vaccine. Neonates often acquire hepatitis B perinatally if the mother is infected; therefore, all pregnant women should undergo HBsAg testing. Infants born to women who have HBsAg positivity should receive both hepatitis B immune globulin and hepatitis B vaccine. In addition, oral agents can be administered during the third trimester to pregnant women who have HBV DNA levels higher than 200,000 IU/mL. Tenofovir is a category B drug for pregnant women and is a safe choice for treatment during pregnancy.

✓ HCC can develop without cirrhosis in patients with hepatitis B
✓ Surveillance is advised for patients without cirrhosis who meet 1 of the following criteria:
  • Family history of HCC
  • Asian man older than 40 years
  • Asian woman older than 50 years

Table 24.6. Oral Agents for Treatment of Hepatitis B

Feature	Lamivudine	Adefovir	Entecavir	Telbivudine	Tenofovir
Monthly charge, $[a]	150	1,086	970	890	860
HBeAg seroconversion, % of patients	20	12	21	22	20
Loss of HBV DNA, % of patients	40	21	67	60	90
Resistance, % of patients	20 at 1 y	0 at 1 y	Naive: <1 at 2 y	4 at 1 y	None
	70 at 5 y	29 at 5 y	Lamivudine resistance: 7 at 1 y	21 at 2 y	
Durability of response, % of responding patients	50-80	90	69	80	Unknown

Abbreviations: HBeAg, hepatitis B e antigen; HBV, hepatitis B virus.

[a] Data from http://cashcard.lc.healthtrans.com (2012).

- Black African older than 20 years
- Persistent increase in ALT level and HBV DNA value greater than 10^4 IU/mL
✓ A simplified approach to determine who requires hepatitis B treatment
  - ALT values at least twice the ULRR
  - Presence of cirrhosis, acute liver failure, fibrosis stage of F2 or higher, or significant inflammation on liver biopsy
✓ Treatment of hepatitis B in most patients—entecavir or tenofovir
✓ Tenofovir alafenamide—associated with fewer adverse events affecting kidneys or bones compared to other tenofovir formulations
✓ Use tenofovir to treat pregnant women at gestational weeks 26 through 28 who have HBV DNA levels greater than 200,000 IU/mL

Hepatitis D

HDV requires the presence of HBsAg to replicate. HDV infection can occur simultaneously with HBV (coinfection) or as a superinfection in persons with established hepatitis B. Hepatitis D is diagnosed with antibodies to HDV and should be suspected if a patient has acute hepatitis B or an acute exacerbation of chronic hepatitis B. In the US, intravenous drug users are the group of HBV patients at highest risk for acquiring HDV. Although HDV does not commonly require treatment (indication for treatment is elevated ALT and HDV RNA levels), peginterferon for 12 months can be used with sustained virologic clearance in about 30% of treated patients.

Hepatitis C

Epidemiology

As of 2016, HCV infection was estimated to affect 3.5 million Americans; estimates included 41,200 acute cases per year and 20,000 deaths per year. In 2013, the annual age-adjusted mortality from hepatitis C surpassed that of a combination of 60 other reportable infectious diseases, which included hepatitis B and HIV

infection. Historically, HCV: infection was the most common chronic bloodborne infection in the US, with about 70% of infected patients having abnormal ALT levels. With the advent of direct-acting antiviral (DAA) therapy, the prevalence of chronic hepatitis C is decreasing owing to the effectiveness of these therapies. While hepatitis C was once the most common indication for liver transplant, it is now the third leading indication behind alcohol-associated liver disease and nonalcoholic fatty liver disease.

Clinical Presentation and Natural History

The incubation period of HCV ranges from 2 to 23 weeks (mean, 7.5 weeks). Patients infected with HCV rarely present clinically with acute hepatitis, although retrospective studies have suggested that 10% to 20% of patients have an icteric illness with acute infection. Of those who acquire hepatitis C, chronic infection develops in 60% to 85% (Figure 24.3). Once chronic infection has been established, subsequent spontaneous loss of the virus is rare. Consequently, most patients with hepatitis C present with chronic hepatitis, with a mild to moderate increase in ALT levels. For patients with abnormal ALT levels, the degree of increase does not correlate with the histologic severity of disease.

Up to 30% of patients with chronic HCV infection have a persistently normal level of ALT. As a group, these patients generally have less aggressive histologic features and a lower risk for disease progression than patients with hepatitis C and abnormal ALT levels, but it is recommended that patients with normal ALT levels and patients with abnormal ALT levels be managed similarly and undergo biopsy when necessary to help make management decisions.

Cirrhosis accounts for nearly all mortality and most morbidity associated with hepatitis C. In about 20% to 30% of patients with chronic hepatitis C, cirrhosis develops over a 20-year period (Figure 24.3). Factors that lead to a higher risk for advanced fibrosis are duration of infection, alcohol intake of more than 50 g daily, steatosis, coinfection with HIV or HBV, and male sex. Patients with cirrhosis due to HCV generally have had the disease longer than 20 years.

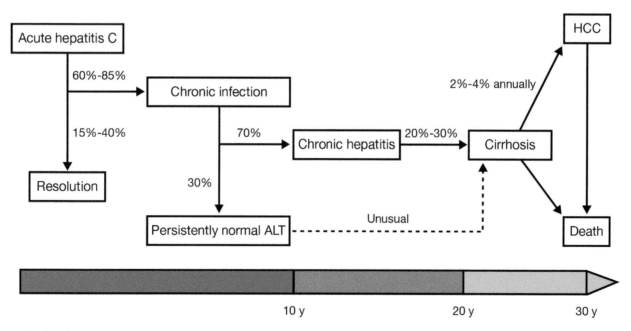

Figure 24.3. **Natural History of Hepatitis C.** Percentage values refer to patients. ALT indicates alanine aminotransferase; HCC, hepatocellular carcinoma.

An important predictive factor for the development of cirrhosis is the severity of the histologic features of the liver at presentation. Liver biopsy specimens need to be interpreted with knowledge of the duration of infection (if known). Patients who have only mild portal hepatitis without fibrosis, despite many years of infection, have a significantly lower risk of progression to cirrhosis than those who have more advanced disease with a similar duration of infection. Histologic markers of more advanced disease include moderate degrees of inflammation and necrosis and septal fibrosis. Biopsy is not necessary before hepatitis C treatment but may be helpful for decisions about the timing of treatment and surveillance for varices and HCC.

Screening

Risk factors that require testing for hepatitis C are shown in Box 24.1. Initial screening recommendations were applied to patients born between 1945 and 1965, as this population was projected to have a 5-fold increase in risk for hepatitis C as compared to other populations. However, the most recent screening recommendation from the American Association for the Study of Liver Diseases (AASLD) and the Infectious Diseases Society of America (IDSA) is for universal screening for all persons 18 to 79 years old. This is particularly important for persons 20 to 39 years old because of the increase in acute hepatitis C infections due to the opioid epidemic in this age group. Furthermore, a 1-time screening is recommended for persons younger than 18 years who have behaviors, exposures, or circumstances that increase their risk for hepatitis C infection. Periodic follow-up hepatitis C testing should be offered to all persons who have ongoing behaviors, exposures, or circumstances that increase their risk for hepatitis C infection. Annual hepatitis C testing is recommended for all persons who inject drugs and for men with HIV infection who have unprotected sex with men.

Box 24.1. Risk Factors That Require Testing for Hepatitis C

Use of injection drugs or illicit intranasal drugs (at any time in life)

Long-term treatment with hemodialysis (at any time in life)

Percutaneous or parenteral exposure to HCV in an unregulated setting

Needlesticks, sharps, or mucosal exposures to HCV-infected blood

Child of an HCV-infected mother

Receipt of blood or blood components, transfusion, or organ transplant before July 1992

Receipt of clotting factor concentrates produced before 1987

History of incarceration

HIV infection

Sexually active person who will begin preexposure prophylaxis for HIV

Person with undiagnosed chronic liver disease

Abnormally high level of ALT

Living organ donor or deceased liver donor

Abbreviation: ALT, alanine aminotransferase; HCV, hepatitis C virus.

Diagnostic Tests

Antibody to HCV (anti-HCV) indicates either current infection or a previous infection with subsequent clearance. Even after clearance of the infection, anti-HCV is no longer detectable in only about 10% of patients. The diagnosis of hepatitis C infection is confirmed by the presence of HCV RNA in serum. Levels of HCV RNA do not correlate with either disease severity or prognosis; the main use of HCV RNA quantitation is to help stratify response to therapy. Patients with viral levels higher than 800,000 IU/mL are less likely to have a response to treatment than those with lower HCV RNA levels.

Identification of the HCV genotype is necessary to help determine the optimal treatment regimen. Liver biopsy is not necessary for the diagnosis of hepatitis C but may be helpful in assessing the severity of disease for making decisions about treatment and screening. Typical biopsy findings include a mononuclear (predominantly lymphocytic) portal hepatitis with lymphoid follicles and mild steatosis (Figure 24.4). Patients with risk factors for nonalcoholic fatty liver disease and those with HCV genotype 3 have more prominent steatosis than other patients with HCV. Staging of fibrosis is often done with a 5-point scale, from 0 (no fibrosis) to 4 (cirrhosis).

Treatment

The treatment of hepatitis C has improved dramatically since 2013 but continues to evolve. Nomenclature used to define outcomes of hepatitis C treatment is shown in Table 24.7. Patients who respond to treatment and remain HCV RNA negative 24 weeks after completion of therapy (ie, they have a sustained virologic response [SVR]) are cured of hepatitis C infection and have improved outcomes compared with those who do not clear the virus. However, patients with cirrhosis remain at risk for HCC despite having an SVR, and continued monitoring is advised.

The treatment of hepatitis C has become more straightforward with the advent of DAA therapies. According to the AASLD-IDSA guidelines, treatment is recommended for all patients who have chronic hepatitis C infection except those who have a short life expectancy that cannot be improved by treatment of hepatitis C with transplant or other directed therapy. The care of

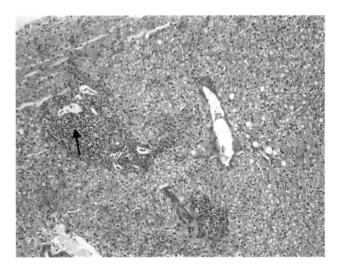

Figure 24.4. Biopsy Specimen From Patient With Hepatitis C. Specimen shows portal infiltrate, lymphoid follicle (arrow), and mild steatosis.

Table 24.7. Hepatitis C Treatment Response Definitions

Virologic response	Definition
End-of-treatment response	HCV RNA negative at end of treatment
Sustained virologic response	HCV RNA negative 24 wk after end of treatment
Breakthrough	Reappearance of HCV RNA during treatment
Relapse	End-of-treatment response without sustained response
Nonresponder	Failure to clear HCV RNA during treatment
Null responder	Usually used for peginterferon-ribavirin dual therapy; failure to decrease HCV RNA by week 12 of therapy
Partial responder	Usually used for peginterferon-ribavirin dual therapy; 2 $\log_{10}$ decrease in HCV RNA by week 12 of therapy, but still HCV RNA positive at 24 wk

Abbreviation: HCV, hepatitis C virus.

Adapted from Ghany MG, Strader DB, Thomas DL, Seeff LB; American Association for the Study of Liver Diseases. Diagnosis, management, and treatment of hepatitis C: an update. Hepatology. 2009 Apr;49(4):1335-74; used with permission.

patients with a short life expectancy should be managed by an expert specialist. After candidacy for hepatitis C treatment is determined, requisite pretreatment testing should include a complete blood cell count; liver tests; creatinine level; HBsAg, anti-HBs, and anti-HBc testing; and HIV screening. Hepatitis B testing is important because hepatitis B reactivation can occur during DAA therapy, particularly in patients with HBsAg positivity and detectable but not quantifiable hepatitis B DNA levels or low levels of hepatitis B DNA. The HCV RNA level and genotype should be checked. Additionally, fibrosis should be assessed and, if available, transient elastography or MR elastography should be performed. If transient or MR elastography is not available, non-invasive blood-based assessments of fibrosis can be used. These include the aspartate aminotransferase to platelet ratio index (APRI), Fibrosis-4 index, FibroTest (BioPredictive SAS), and Enhanced Liver Fibrosis (ELF) test (Siemens Medical Solutions USA, Inc).

The 3 main classes of DAA therapies for hepatitis C are shown in Figure 24.5, and Table 24.8 shows how these classes of DAA therapies are used together. Although several regimens are available, a streamlined approached has been published.

For patients who are treatment naïve and have genotype 1 hepatitis with or without cirrhosis, the preferred regimen (in no particular order) is glecaprevir-pibrentasvir for 8 weeks or sofosbuvir-velpatasvir for 12 weeks. For patients with genotype 2 or 3 with or without compensated cirrhosis, the preferred treatment (in no particular order) is glecaprevir-pibrentasvir for 8 weeks or sofosbuvir-velpatasvir for 12 weeks.

The recommendation for patients with genotype 3 is to undergo resistance-associated substitution testing for the *Y93H* variant before treatment with sofosbuvir-velpatasvir. If the patient tests positive for the *Y93H* variant, the recommendation is to add ribavirin to the regimen or use sofosbuvir-velpatasvir-voxilaprevir for 12 weeks.

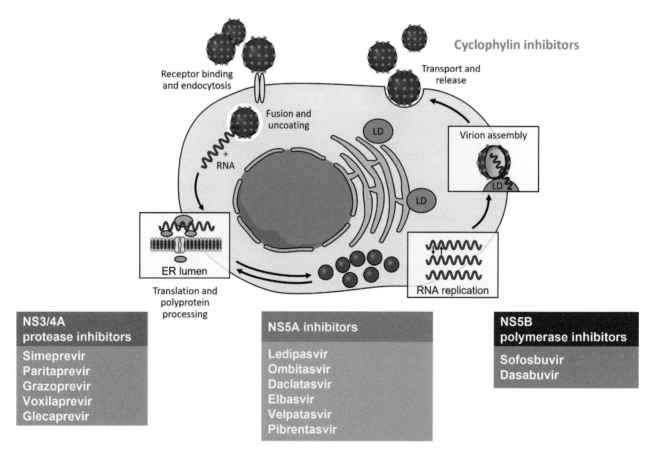

Figure 24.5. **Direct-Acting Antivirals for Hepatitis C.** ER indicates endoplasmic reticulum; LD, lipid droplet. (Courtesy of Stacy A. Rizza, MD, Department of Infectious Diseases, Mayo Clinic, Rochester, Minnesota; used with permission.)

Table 24.8.   Combinations of Direct-Acting Antivirals Used for Hepatitis C Therapy

Drug class (combination includes drugs in same row)

NS3/4A protease inhibitor (*suffix* previr)	NS5A inhibitor (*suffix* asvir)	NS5B non-nucleoside polymerase inhibitor (*suffix* buvir)	NS5B-nucleotide polymerase inhibitor (*suffix* buvir)	Trade name of combination (*manufacturer*)
Grazoprevir	Elbasvir			Zepatier (Merck & Co, Inc)
Paritaprevir	Ombitasvir	Dasabuvir		Viekira[a] (AbbVie, Inc)
Simeprevir (Olysio; Janssen Therapeutics)			Sofosbuvir (Sovaldi; Gilead Sciences, Inc)	None
	Daclatasvir		Sofosbuvir	Daklinza (Bristol-Myers Squibb Co)
	Ledipasvir		Sofosbuvir	Harvoni (Gilead Sciences, Inc)
	Velpatasvir		Sofosbuvir	Epclusa (Gilead Sciences, Inc)
Voxilaprevir	Velpatasvir		Sofosbuvir	Vosevi (Ameripharma Specialty Care)
Glecaprevir	Pibrentasvir			Mavyret (AbbVie Inc)

[a] Viekira also includes ritonavir.

Genotypes 4, 5, and 6 are less common in the US and are unlikely to be tested, so they are not discussed here.

Although 2 regimens are effective for all genotypes (glecaprevir-pibrentasvir and sofosbuvir-velpatasvir), only regimens containing sofosbuvir are safe in patients who have decompensated cirrhosis. Regimens that contain an NS3/4A protease inhibitor are not safe to use in patients who have decompensated cirrhosis because of the risk of worsening jaundice and worsening hepatic decompensation. All regimens are safe in patients who have chronic kidney disease stage 4 or 5 or who are receiving hemodialysis. Many of the DAAs interact with statins and calcineurin inhibitors. The most important drug-drug interaction with DAA therapy is between sofosbuvir-containing regimens and amiodarone, which can cause life-threatening bradycardia and, in some patients, has resulted in pacemaker implantation and even death.

Generally, in patients with decompensated cirrhosis, treatment of hepatitis C should be overseen by an experienced hepatologist or a transplant hepatologist. The best candidates are usually those with a Model for End-stage Liver Disease (MELD) score that is no higher than 15 to 18 and those who are aware that their MELD score may improve, but they may have persistent symptoms such as ascites. Recent data have suggested that patients with HCC who derive survival benefit from DAA therapy for hepatitis C have had interval follow-up studies that show no residual disease after ablative or surgical therapy.

Resistance-associated substitution (RAS) is indicated in a few scenarios: 1) Patients who have genotype 1a hepatitis C with or without cirrhosis should have RAS testing before therapy is initiated with sofosbuvir-ledipasvir. If results from RAS testing are positive, a different regimen should be selected. 2) Patients who have genotype 1a hepatitis and who will undergo therapy with grazoprevir-elbasvir, whether they are treatment naïve or experienced, should be tested for NS5A RAS; if results are positive, an alternative regimen should be used. 3) Patients who have genotype 3 hepatitis C with cirrhosis or who are treatment experienced should be tested for NS5A if they are being considered for treatment with sofosbuvir-velpatasvir or sofosbuvir-daclatasvir. If the *Y93H* substitution is detected, ribavirin can be added. The preferred treatment, however, is to use sofosbuvir-velpatasvir-voxilaprevir, which is highly effective against baseline or treatment-emergent RAS.

Patients with hepatitis C and decompensated cirrhosis (including those with HCC) should be considered for liver transplant.

Among patients who receive a liver transplant for hepatitis C, posttransplant viremia is nearly universal and posttransplant hepatitis C should be treated in all patients.

Patients with hepatitis C–associated type 2 mixed cryoglobulinemia usually have a vasculitic rash on the lower extremities, but they also may have a membranoproliferative glomerulonephritis or polyneuropathy. Mild cryoglobulinemia and its associated complications usually respond to the treatment of hepatitis C; more severe disease may require immunosuppressive therapy, such as corticosteroids and rituximab. Porphyria cutanea tarda is manifested as a rash on sun-exposed areas, particularly the back of the hands. Most patients also have abnormal iron test results, and phlebotomy improves the rash of porphyria cutanea tarda. The response of porphyria cutanea tarda to hepatitis C therapy is more uncertain than the response of cryoglobulinemia.

Hepatitis C and Pregnancy

The risk of hepatitis C vertical transmission ranges from 5% to 15%, and concomitant HIV infection increases the risk. The incidence between 2011 and 2014 was increasing to 29,000 cases of vertical transmission per year. Of the children born to mothers who are positive for hepatitis C, 3% to 5% have chronic infection. The recommendation is to avoid obstetric procedures if possible. The use of DAAs in pregnancy is not recommended because the data are limited. Breastfeeding does not seem to be a risk factor for transmission for a child born to a mother with hepatitis C. HCV antibody should be checked at or after 18 months of age, and if results are positive, the HCV RNA level should be checked at 3 years to confirm chronicity.

Recent recommendations from the AASLD-IDSA call for universal hepatitis C screening for mothers at the initial prenatal visit. An important point to remember for women who take ribavirin and for women whose male partners take ribavirin is that the teratogenic effects of ribavirin can persist for 6 months after the last dose. Hepatitis C poses an increased risk for intrahepatic cholestasis of pregnancy. Spontaneous clearance of hepatitis C post partum occurs in up to 10% of patients; the recommendation is to recheck the HCV RNA level before treatment.

Prevention

No vaccine is available for hepatitis C. Transmission by needlestick injury is unusual, although monitoring after inadvertent exposure is advised. Baseline anti-HCV testing is recommended with subsequent determination of the HCV RNA level 4 weeks after exposure. Antiviral therapy is more effective for acute hepatitis C than for chronic hepatitis C. For patients with documented acute hepatitis C, the current recommendation is to begin DAA therapy without waiting for spontaneous resolution.

Blood donation is prohibited for patients infected with HCV, and precaution should be taken when caring for open sores of patients infected with HCV. Sexual transmission is unusual, but condoms are advised for those with multiple sex partners. For patients in a monogamous long-term relationship, the partner should be tested and the couple counseled about the possibility of transmission. The decision about the use of condoms is left to the infected person and partner.

✓ Hepatitis C screening—recommended for persons 18 to 79 years old and for pregnant women
✓ The presence of both HCV antibody and HCV RNA indicates active infection, but HCV antibody persists even after a sustained virologic response at 24 weeks after treatment
✓ Sofosbuvir-velpatasvir and glecaprevir-pibrentasvir are pangenotypic and are used to treat most patients with HCV; sofosbuvir-velpatasvir-voxilaprevir is used predominately when other DAAs have not helped
✓ Genotype 3 hepatitis C—the most difficult to treat and most likely to lead to cirrhosis and HCC
✓ Patients with stage 3 or 4 cirrhosis should be monitored for hepatocellular carcinoma even after a sustained virologic response
✓ Patients with hepatitis C and mixed cryoglobulinemia who present with the Meltzer triad (purpura, myalgia, and weakness) or glomerulonephritis are usually cured with successful hepatitis C therapy
✓ DAAs have not been shown to be safe in pregnancy
✓ Sofosbuvir-containing regimens should never be used in patients receiving amiodarone because of the risk for lethal bradycardia

---

Hepatitis E

Hepatitis E causes large outbreaks of acute hepatitis in resource-limited countries. Infection with a different strain of hepatitis E has been identified in relatively affluent countries, including the US. Of the 4 genotypes, genotypes 1 and 2 are found outside the US and are transmitted by the fecal-oral route, and genotypes 3 and 4 are transmitted zoonotically (in contaminated food). Genotype 3 hepatitis E is identified in the US, where the prevalence of hepatitis E virus antibodies is 6% to 18%. Clinically, hepatitis E virus infection is similar to HAV infection. Spontaneous resolution of the hepatitis is typical, although prolonged cholestasis, with jaundice and pruritus for more than 3 months, can occur in 60% of patients. Chronic hepatitis E can occur in solid organ transplant recipients and is treated with immunosuppression reduction and ribavirin. Women who acquire hepatitis E during pregnancy may present with fulminant liver failure.

✓ Hepatitis E with prolonged cholestasis, with jaundice and pruritus for more than 3 months, occurs in 60% of patients

---

✓ Hepatitis E is usually acute and self-limited but can be chronic in recipients of solid organ transplants; treatment is immunosuppression reduction and ribavirin
✓ Pregnant women with hepatitis E can present with fulminant liver failure

---

Viral Hepatitis and HIV

Because of shared risk factors, patients with viral hepatitis are also at risk for infection with HIV. About 10% to 15% of patients with HIV infection are positive for HBsAg. Compared with patients who are negative for HIV, patients with HIV infection are at increased risk for chronic HBV infection after an acute HBV infection. Patients infected with HIV and HBV have higher HBV DNA levels and increased mortality from liver disease than patients infected with HBV and not with HIV.

The response to treatment of HBV infection with peginterferon in patients infected with HIV is low, and treatment with oral agents generally is advised. Tenofovir in combination with emtricitabine has an antiviral effect on both HIV and HBV and is often used. For the rare patient who requires treatment of HBV but not HIV, lamivudine, entecavir, or tenofovir should not be given as monotherapy because of the risk of resistance developing to later treatment of HIV disease.

About 45% of patients infected with HIV are also infected with HCV. Compared with patients who have HCV infection without HIV infection, patients infected with both HCV and HIV have higher HCV RNA levels and increased risks for vertical and sexual transmission of HCV, cirrhosis, and HCC. Treatment should be considered for patients infected with both HCV and HIV. The HIV disease should be controlled, and treatment generally is recommended only if the HIV level is less than 1,000 copies/mL and the CD4 cell count is more than 200/mL.

Suggested Reading

Ghany MG, Morgan TR, AASLD-IDSA Hepatitis C Guidance Panel. Hepatitis C guidance 2019 update: American Association for the Study of Liver Diseases-Infectious Diseases Society of America recommendations for testing, managing, and treating hepatitis C virus infection. Hepatology. 2020 Feb;71(2):686–721.

Morgan TR, Ghany MG, Kim HY, Snow KK, Shiffman ML, De Santo JL, et al. Outcome of sustained virological responders with histologically advanced chronic hepatitis C. Hepatology. 2010 Sep;52(3):833–44.

Nimgaonkar I, Ding Q, Schwartz RE, Ploss A. Hepatitis E virus: advances and challenges. Nat Rev Gastroenterol Hepatol. 2018 Feb;15(2):96–110.

Pungpapong S, Kim WR, Poterucha JJ. Natural history of hepatitis B virus infection: an update for clinicians. Mayo Clin Proc. 2007 Aug;82(8):967–75.

van der Meer AJ, Veldt BJ, Feld JJ, Wedemeyer H, Dufour JF, Lammert F, et al. Association between sustained virological response and all-cause mortality among patients with chronic hepatitis C and advanced hepatic fibrosis. JAMA. 2012 Dec 26;308(24):2584–93.

25

Clinical Approach to Liver Mass Lesions[a]
LEWIS R. ROBERTS, MB, CHB, PHD

The clinical approach to liver mass lesions requires attention to the clinical context within which the mass is identified, the symptoms of the patient, and the physical examination, laboratory tests, and imaging studies. With the advent of frequent ultrasonographic or cross-sectional imaging of the abdomen for various abdominal symptoms, many liver mass lesions are now discovered incidentally during imaging performed for unrelated symptoms. These incidentally discovered lesions should be evaluated fully because a large proportion of them indicate the presence of malignant or premalignant disease that requires appropriate management. This

[a] Portions previously published in Alberts SR, Gores GJ, Kim GP, Roberts LR, Kendrick ML, Rosen CB, et al. Treatment options for hepatobiliary and pancreatic cancer. Mayo Clin Proc. 2007 May;82(5):628-37; used with permission; and Roberts LR. Liver and biliary tract tumors. In: Goldman L, Schafer AI, eds. Goldman's Cecil Medicine. 24 ed. W.B. Saunders; 2012:1297-303.

Abbreviations: BCLC, Barcelona Clinic Liver Cancer; CA19-9, carbohydrate antigen 19-9; CT, computed tomography; DEB-TACE, drug-eluting bead transarterial chemoembolization; ERCP, endoscopic retrograde cholangiopancreatography; FDG, ^{18}F-fluorodeoxyglucose; FISH, fluorescence in situ hybridization; HBV, hepatitis B virus; HCA, hepatocellular adenoma; HCC, hepatocellular carcinoma; HCV, hepatitis C virus; H-HCA, *HNF1A*-inactivated hepatocellular adenoma; IL, interleukin; JAK, Janus kinase; LI-RADS, Liver Imaging Reporting and Data System; MELD, Model for End-stage Liver Disease; MODY, maturity-onset diabetes of the young; MRCP, magnetic resonance cholangiopancreatography; MRI, magnetic resonance imaging; MWA, microwave ablation; NASH, nonalcoholic steatohepatitis; PEI, percutaneous ethanol injection; PET, positron emission tomography; PSC, primary sclerosing cholangitis; PTC, percutaneous transhepatic cholangiography; RFA, radiofrequency ablation; STAT, signal transducer and activator of transcription; TACE, transarterial chemoembolization; TARE, transarterial radioembolization

chapter describes the overall approach to the evaluation and diagnosis of liver mass lesions and summarizes the clinical features and management of the most common benign and malignant liver masses (Box 25.1).

Evaluation

History

A history should be obtained of potential risk factors for different types of liver masses to inform the subsequent evaluation and to limit unnecessary testing. The age and sex of the patient, a history of oral contraceptive use, geographic residence and travel history, and comorbid illnesses often provide important clues to the diagnosis. A history of previous imaging studies should always be sought because information about whether the mass is new, previously seen and stable in size, or enlarging over time can be useful in the differential diagnosis of liver masses.

Pain can be an important presenting symptom. A rapidly enlarging liver mass tends to distend the liver capsule and cause right upper quadrant abdominal pain, whereas a slowly growing mass can reach a substantial size that almost completely occupies the liver without causing noticeable symptoms. The liver mass may come to attention only when it becomes a visible abdominal protuberance or causes mass effect on other organs such as the stomach, leading to early satiety (Figure 25.1). Pain associated with tumor growth is usually dull, relatively diffuse, and persistent. It may or may not be associated with tenderness in the epigastrium and right upper quadrant of the abdomen. Subcapsular lesions, whether benign or malignant, frequently cause a pleuritic pain syndrome of abdominal pain accompanied by right shoulder discomfort exacerbated by breathing. Lesions that have the propensity for intralesional rupture or hemorrhage can first become apparent with the sudden onset of severe abdominal pain. This is most

Box 25.1.   Clinical Classification of Liver Mass Lesions

Benign lesions typically requiring no further
    treatment
    Cavernous hemangioma
    Focal nodular hyperplasia
    Simple liver cysts
    Focal fatty change or focal sparing in a fatty liver
    Angiolipoma
Benign lesions requiring further follow-up and
    management
    Hepatic adenoma
    Pyogenic liver abscess
    Nodular regenerative hyperplasia
    Biliary cystadenoma
    Inflammatory pseudotumor
    Granulomatous abscesses
    Amebic liver abscess
    Echinococcal cysts
Malignant lesions requiring appropriate therapy
    Liver metastases
    Primary hepatocellular carcinoma
    Cholangiocarcinoma
    Mixed hepatocellular-cholangiocarcinoma
    Cystadenocarcinoma
    Hemangioendothelioma
    Epithelioid angiomyolipoma
    Mixed epithelial and stromal tumors
    Sarcomas

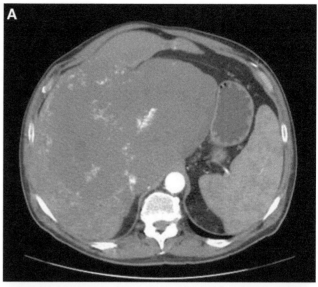

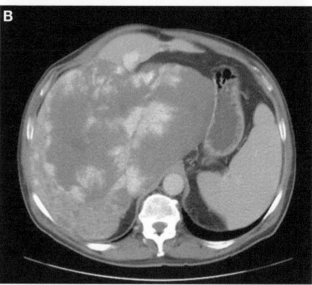

Figure 25.1. **Large Cavernous Hemangioma With the Manifestation of an Abdominal Mass.** A, Arterial phase shows peripheral nodular enhancement. B, Venous phase shows fill-in of contrast agent from the periphery toward the center of the mass.

typical of benign hepatic adenomas or hepatocellular carcinomas (HCCs), which are highly vascular. If the rupture involves the liver capsule, it can be associated with life-threatening intra-abdominal hemoperitoneum, shock, and risk of exsanguination.

A history of an underlying liver disease that predisposes to malignancy is often an important diagnostic clue. Patients with nonalcoholic steatohepatitis (NASH) or viral, alcoholic, autoimmune, metabolic, or other causes of cirrhosis are at increased risk for HCC and intrahepatic cholangiocarcinoma. These patients may have had complications of cirrhosis, including ascites, spontaneous bacterial peritonitis, bleeding esophageal varices, or hepatic encephalopathy. In addition, patients with long-standing chronic hepatitis B virus (HBV) infection are at risk for HCC even in the absence of cirrhosis. Consequently, for patients who have cirrhosis from any cause or who acquired chronic HBV infection at birth or in early life, current recommendations are to begin a regular program of surveillance with ultrasonography of the liver, with or without measurement of serum alpha fetoprotein, every 6 months. Persons with chronic HBV infection without cirrhosis who were born in sub-Saharan Africa should undergo surveillance for HCC beginning at the age of 20 years. For persons born in Asia, surveillance should be initiated at age 40 years for men and 50 years for women (Figure 25.2). Regular surveillance should also be recommended for persons with a family history of HCC, those with high HBV viral loads (HBV DNA >2,000 IU/mL), and those with a persistent or intermittent increase in the level of alanine aminotransferase.

Primary sclerosing cholangitis (PSC), which can be subclinical in patients with ulcerative colitis or other inflammatory bowel disease, is a major risk factor for cholangiocarcinoma. A history of sudden hepatic decompensation, cholangitis, or the development of a new dominant stricture in a patient with known PSC can presage the development of cholangiocarcinoma. Approximately a third of the cholangiocarcinomas that occur in patients with PSC are diagnosed within 2 years after the diagnosis of PSC; therefore, this should be a period of heightened surveillance. Current expert screening recommendations for persons with PSC are for annual magnetic resonance imaging (MRI) with MR cholangiopancreatography (MRCP) and measurement of the serum carbohydrate antigen 19-9 (CA19-9).

General, nonspecific symptoms associated with malignancy include fatigue, loss of appetite, unintended weight loss, low-grade fever, night sweats, and frailty. A recent history of iron deficiency anemia should raise suspicion of colorectal cancer with liver metastases; a long-standing history of gastroesophageal

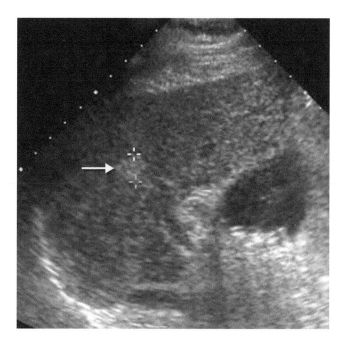

Figure 25.2. Surveillance Ultrasonography of the Liver. A small 1.3-cm mass (arrow) was identified in an at-risk patient during ultrasonographic screening for hepatocellular carcinoma.

reflux and new-onset dysphagia should prompt consideration of esophageal adenocarcinoma; the recent onset of type 2 diabetes should elicit a search for pancreatic adenocarcinoma; and a history of breast cancer should be sought and the breasts should be examined and imaged to rule out metastatic breast cancer. In the absence of other localizing symptoms, occult lymphoma should be considered.

Various paraneoplastic syndromes can be helpful in the diagnosis of liver masses. A history of flushing, hypotension, and diarrhea is classic for metastatic neuroendocrine tumors such as carcinoids. Diarrhea alone occurs most frequently with HCC as a consequence of the secretion of vasoactive intestinal polypeptide and gastrin by the tumor. HCCs can also be associated with hypoglycemia and erythrocytosis.

Physical Examination

The physical examination may provide clues to the underlying cause of a liver mass. Most frequently, patients have stigmata of chronic liver disease, including temporal muscle wasting, spider angiomas, palmar erythema, ascites, splenomegaly, and caput medusae from recanalization of the umbilical vein. The cirrhotic liver may be palpably nodular and often associated with bilobar enlargement of the liver or isolated hypertrophy of the caudate lobe. Large liver masses may give rise to palpable hepatomegaly, and subcapsular masses may be palpable if located anteriorly or inferiorly in the liver. Abdominal lymphadenopathy or peritoneal carcinomatosis may be palpable. Tumors may have associated tenderness in the epigastrium or right upper quadrant of the abdomen. Vascular masses such as primary HCCs may have an audible vascular bruit on auscultation. Pallor may be due to anemia from colon adenocarcinoma with chronic blood loss, from portal hypertensive gastropathy in patients with cirrhosis, or from anemia of chronic disease related to other malignancies. Jaundice may

be due to advanced chronic liver disease or to biliary obstruction from cholangiocarcinoma. Peripheral edema may be associated specifically with chronic liver disease or with tense ascites causing compression of the inferior vena cava and loss of intravascular oncotic pressure due to hypoalbuminemia, or it may be nonspecific from general debility. Rarely, large liver cysts will cause a mass effect on the central bile ducts and inferior vena cava, resulting in jaundice or bilateral leg edema (or both). Frequently, cancer is associated with an acute phase response syndrome, and because albumin is a negative acute phase reactant, a cancer-associated hypoalbuminemia typically contributes to peripheral edema. Many cancers are associated with a prothrombotic tendency; consequently, it is important to evaluate new-onset lower extremity edema, particularly if it is unilateral, for deep vein thrombosis.

Laboratory Tests

Laboratory tests often provide evidence of chronic liver disease or of the underlying tumor that is metastatic to the liver. A complete blood cell count may show thrombocytopenia from chronic liver disease with splenomegaly, or it may show anemia from gastrointestinal blood loss related to colon or other primary gastrointestinal cancer. Typically, aspartate aminotransferase and alanine aminotransferase levels are increased from active inflammatory liver disease or from neoplastic diseases infiltrating the liver. An increase in the bilirubin and alkaline phosphatase concentrations usually reflects either a bile duct obstruction from a primary biliary tumor or a mass effect from an intrahepatic mass or from enlarged lymph nodes in the porta hepatis. The serum albumin level is often low and the prothrombin time increased in patients with cirrhosis.

Potentially useful tests that may identify the specific cause of liver disease include tests for viral markers (antibodies to hepatitis C virus [HCV] or polymerase chain reaction for HCV RNA), hepatitis B surface antigen, antibodies to hepatitis B core antigen, antibodies to hepatitis B surface antigen, and hepatitis D antibodies or hepatitis D virus RNA in all persons who have positive results for hepatitis B surface antigen. Iron levels typically are increased in patients with hereditary hemochromatosis and low in those with anemia from colon cancer–related gastrointestinal blood loss. Tumor markers such as carcinoembryonic antigen for colon cancer, CA19-9, and alpha fetoprotein are helpful if results are positive, but they frequently are negative if patients have early-stage cancer. Also, these markers are not entirely specific for the primary site. For example, the carcinoembryonic antigen level is often increased in cholangiocarcinomas and pancreatic cancers, and the alpha fetoprotein level can be increased in patients with primary cancers of the upper gastrointestinal tract outside the liver, such as esophageal adenocarcinoma. With advances in genomics, proteomics, and metabolomics, there is substantial ongoing innovation in cancer biomarker development, including several new models that integrate clinical variables with biomarker levels and a new generation of multicancer early detection tests that are being deployed in clinical practice. Primary hepatic lymphomas or secondary lymphoma metastases can masquerade as primary liver cancers; the serum level of lactate dehydrogenase usually is increased and can be an important clue to the diagnosis. The urine 24-hour 5-hydroxyindoleacetic acid concentration is helpful in cases of suspected carcinoid syndrome.

Imaging Studies

The imaging studies most frequently helpful in the differential diagnosis of liver mass lesions include abdominal ultrasonography, cross-sectional imaging modalities such as computed tomography (CT) and MRI, ^{18}F-fluorodeoxyglucose (FDG)–positron emission tomography (PET), and fused PET/CT (most useful for imaging metastatic disease). More specialized contrast agents are now available, particularly for MRI. For example, both gadoxetate disodium (Eovist; Bayer HealthCare Pharmaceuticals Inc) and gadobenate dimeglumine (MultiHance; Bracco Diagnostics Inc) undergo biliary and kidney excretion, behaving as nonspecific gadolinium chelates in the first minutes after administration and as liver-targeted agents in later phases. This allows further delineation of lesion characteristics in MRI scans obtained 20 minutes after injection of gadoxetate disodium or 60 to 120 minutes after injection of gadobenate dimeglumine and can be particularly helpful for distinguishing between focal nodular hyperplasias and adenomas and for identifying small HCC nodules. The use of nuclear imaging studies, including tagged red blood cell studies (for cavernous hemangiomas) and technetium Tc 99m sulfur colloid imaging (to distinguish focal nodular hyperplasias from adenomas), has been largely replaced by MRI with gadoxetate or gadobenate. For neuroendocrine tumors, newer imaging tests that can illuminate tumor somatostatin receptors throughout the body include gallium Ga 68 dotatate PET and copper Cu 64 dotatate PET. These are superior to the earlier generation of octreotide scans, which used indium In 111 pentetreotide as the standard of care.

✓ Most common solid tumors in the liver: hepatic hemangioma, focal nodular hyperplasia, hepatic adenoma, HCC, cholangiocarcinoma, liver metastases

---

✓ **Hepatic hemangioma**—benign tumor consisting of a 3-dimensional network of blood-filled spaces (much like a sponge); on contrast-enhanced images it fills in gradually from the outside toward the middle, similar to how a squeezed sponge absorbs water from the edges toward the center when placed in water

✓ **Focal nodular hyperplasia**—benign tumor thought to arise around a malformed artery in the liver; has all the elements of the normal portal triad, including hepatocytes, biliary ductules, and stromal cells and no tendency to transform into a cancer

✓ **Hepatic adenoma**—benign tumor within the liver, histologically consisting of sheets of cells supplied by arterial branches (ie, "naked arteries") without bile ductules; some subtypes, particularly those with oncogenic β-catenin variants, can transform into HCCs

✓ **Hepatocellular carcinoma**—cancer arising in primary liver cells or hepatocytes, which are the primary cells that carry out the key functions of the liver

✓ **Cholangiocarcinoma**—cancer arising in the bile ducts that collect bile produced by the hepatocytes and transport it to the gallbladder and ultimately to the intestines; cholangiocarcinomas are subclassified anatomically as intrahepatic, perihilar, and distal

✓ **Liver metastases**—malignant masses in the liver that originated in a cancer at a different site but have spread through the bloodstream to the liver

---

Benign Liver Masses

Cavernous Hemangioma

Cavernous hemangiomas are the most common benign liver tumors, occurring in 7% of adults in autopsy series. They are seen predominantly in women, with a female to male ratio ranging from 1.5:1 to 5:1; they are diagnosed most frequently in multiparous women in their third to fifth decades. Cavernous hemangiomas are multicentric in up to 30% of cases and frequently coexist with focal nodular hyperplasia.

Histologic Features

Cavernous hemangiomas are characterized by an extensive network of vascular spaces lined by endothelial cells and separated by thin, fibrous stroma. Large hemangiomas may have areas of thrombosis, scarring, and calcification.

Clinical Features

Patients with hemangiomas are most often asymptomatic. Large, subcapsular hemangiomas may cause abdominal pain or discomfort. Giant hemangiomas (>10 cm) may cause systemic features of inflammation such as fever, weight loss, and anemia. Kasabach-Merritt syndrome may occur with disseminated intravascular coagulation, most commonly in children. Cavernous hemangiomas do not undergo malignant transformation, and rupture is exceedingly rare.

Imaging Characteristics

Ultrasonography. On ultrasonography, hemangiomas are well-circumscribed, homogeneously hyperechoic lesions with smooth margins.

Dynamic Contrast-Enhanced Multiphasic CT. On CT, there is peripheral nodular enhancement during the arterial phase, with later fill-in toward the center of the lesion (Figure 25.3).

MRI With Gadolinium Contrast. On contrast-enhanced MRI, hemangiomas are typically homogeneous, with low signal intensity on T1-weighted images and sharply demarcated, hyperintense lesions on T2-weighted images. As in other contrast imaging studies, there is peripheral enhancement in the arterial phase, with later fill-in toward the center of the lesion.

Technetium Tc 99m–Labeled Red Blood Cell Scintigraphy. Scintigraphy can be used to confirm the diagnosis of lesions that are atypical on other imaging studies. There is low perfusion on early images, and the isotope gradually accumulates to a high concentration within the lesion on late images. With the advances in dynamic cross-sectional imaging CT and MRI, scintigraphy is rarely used now in the diagnosis of hemangiomas.

Biopsy

Biopsy seldom is needed. It may be useful for small lesions that show uniform enhancement and resemble primary tumors or metastases and also for large lesions that have pronounced scarring and atypical imaging features. Biopsy specimens are typically a relatively acellular "dry aspirate," with occasional vascular elements seen on histologic study.

Management

Most cavernous hemangiomas do not require intervention and can be observed. Symptomatic giant cavernous hemangiomas require surgical enucleation or resection.

Hepatic Adenoma

Hepatic adenomas are benign tumors of the liver that occur predominantly in young women between the third and fourth decades of life. Key features of hepatic adenomas are that they can

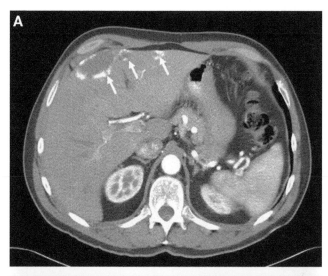

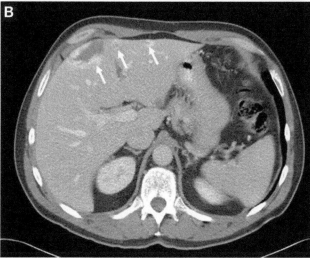

Figure 25.3. **Cavernous Hemangioma on Computed Tomography.** A, Arterial phase shows peripheral nodular enhancement of 1 large and 2 small cavernous hemangiomas (arrows). B, Venous phase shows fill-in toward the center of the 3 masses, with almost complete contrast enhancement of the 2 small hemangiomas (arrows).

undergo malignant transformation or hemorrhage and sometimes rupture, leading to hemoperitoneum. Epidemiologically, hepatic adenomas have been associated with long-term use of oral contraceptive pills. In the past, when oral contraceptives contained relatively high amounts of estrogens, studies estimated the relative risk for hepatic adenomas as 2.5 times greater for women who had taken oral contraceptive pills for 3 to 5 years compared with women who had taken them for 1 year or less. After 5 years of oral contraceptive use, the risk increased sharply to 25 times greater after 9 or more years of use. The epidemiology of hepatic adenomas is changing. Newer oral contraceptives contain less estrogen and are probably associated with a lower risk of hepatic adenomas; however, the overall incidence of hepatic adenomas does not appear to have decreased concurrently.

With increasing rates of obesity worldwide, the prevalence of obesity and the metabolic syndrome is high among patients with hepatic adenomas, particularly the inflammatory or telangiectatic variant, suggesting that obesity and the metabolic syndrome increase the risk for adenomas. Further, patients with obesity are

more likely to have multiple adenomas and to have progressive growth of adenomas if they do not lose weight. Excessive use of alcohol has been associated with the development of inflammatory hepatocellular adenomas (HCAs). Hepatic adenomas also occur in a familial pattern associated with the variety of type 2 diabetes known as maturity-onset diabetes of the young (MODY) type 3, which is associated with germline variations in the *HNF1A* gene (OMIM 600496); however, in patients with glycogen storage disease type 1A or 3, most genetic variations in HCAs appear to be somatic alterations. Persons who take the androgenic hormones methandrostenolone and methyltestosterone also have an increased risk for adenomas with subsequent malignant transformation. Adenomas are usually single, but they may be multiple, especially in patients with MODY3 or glycogen storage disease.

Advances in molecular classification have identified hepatic adenomas as clonal tumors that are molecularly heterogeneous, with different subtypes having particular etiologies and different underlying genomic features, clinical presentations, radiologic findings, histopathologic features, and risks of malignant transformation or hemorrhage. Adenomas are subclassified into 5 molecular subgroups:

1. *HNF1A*-inactivated HCAs (H-HCAs) are characterized by inactivation of the *HNF1A* transcription factor and a highly steatotic morphology. H-HCAs carry a low risk of hemorrhage or transformation into HCC.
2. Telangiectatic or inflammatory HCAs are characterized by activating variants of the interleukin (IL)-6/Janus kinase (JAK)/ signal transducer and activator of transcription (STAT) pathway, such as the IL-6 signal transducer gene (*IL6ST*; OMIM 600694) or the guanine nucleotide-binding protein alpha-stimulatory subunit complex locus (*GNAS*; OMIM 139320). Inflammatory HCAs are more common in persons who have obesity, inflammatory cell infiltration on histology, and a tendency to malignant transformation.
3. β-Catenin–activated HCAs encompass both noninflammatory and inflammatory subgroups. These are subdivided into exon 3 mutated adenomas and exon 7/8 mutated adenomas. Exon 3 mutated adenomas show stronger β-catenin–pathway activation and are more prone to malignancy, while exon 7/8 mutated adenomas show weak β-catenin–pathway activation and no increase in risk for malignancy, although they may carry an increased risk for bleeding.
4. Sonic hedgehog pathway–activated HCAs are characterized by the presence of a fusion between the inhibin beta E subunit gene (*INHBE*; OMIM 612031) and the *GLI1* gene (OMIM 165220) and appear to carry a higher risk for bleeding.
5. Unclassified HCAs comprise small groups with less clearly defined characteristics.

Male sex, size greater than 5 cm, and strong β-catenin activation as assessed by increased nuclear β-catenin staining are the major risk factors for transformation to HCC.

Histologic Features

Adenomas are characterized by the presence of sheets of hepatocytes supplied by "naked" arteries (ie, arteries unaccompanied by bile ductules, fibrous septa, portal tracts, or central veins).

Clinical Features

Patients with hepatic adenomas are most often asymptomatic. However, they may present with pain or discomfort of the upper abdomen or the right upper quadrant of the abdomen. Because these tumors have a propensity to rupture, patients may present with intrahepatic hemorrhage and pain or with hemoperitoneum and shock.

Imaging Characteristics

Adenomas frequently have nonspecific imaging characteristics. Most often, they are heterogeneous because of the presence of intralesional necrosis or hemorrhage, but frequently they are homogeneous when small. The tumors typically take up the contrast agent rapidly in the arterial phase of contrast CT or MRI studies and then almost immediately become isointense with the surrounding liver in the early portal phase. If contrast studies are not optimally timed, this important imaging feature may be missed. Adenomas often cannot be differentiated definitively from HCC or hypervascular metastases with ultrasonography, CT, or MRI. Adenomas can be differentiated from focal nodular hyperplasias in the delayed phase after MRI with gadobenate dimeglumine or gadoxetate disodium, in which adenomas show decreased retention of the contrast agent in the biliary phase when compared with the surrounding liver (Figure 25.4). On technetium Tc 99m sulfur colloid scintigraphy, there usually is no uptake because adenomas do not contain Kupffer cells.

Biopsy

Because of the frequent uncertainty about the diagnosis after a thorough noninvasive evaluation, biopsy often is required for diagnosis. Biopsy is also helpful for immunohistochemical and molecular classification to assess the risk of malignant transformation. H-HCAs show loss of staining for liver fatty acid–binding protein, indicating the functional loss of the *HNF1A* gene; inflammatory HCAs show uniform expression of the inflammatory markers serum amyloid A protein or C-reactive protein; and β-catenin–exon 3 mutated adenomas show uniform immunohistochemical staining for glutamine synthetase and nuclear staining for β-catenin, which is sometimes focal, while β-catenin–exon 7/8 mutated adenomas show only faint glutamine synthetase staining and no nuclear staining for β-catenin. A sonic hedgehog pathway–activated HCA may develop areas of hemorrhage within the adenoma and show staining for prostaglandin D2 synthase (*PTGDS*; OMIM 176803) and argininosuccinate synthetase 1 (*ASS1*; OMIM 603470).

Management

Because of the risks of rupture or transformation to HCC, surgical resection is recommended for large hepatic adenomas (>5 cm), for hepatic adenomas of any size occurring in men, for hepatic adenomas with β-catenin activation, and for hepatic adenomas that are histologically difficult to distinguish from well-differentiated HCCs.

Patients generally are advised to discontinue the use of oral contraceptive pills. Adenomas may decrease in size after withdrawal of oral contraceptives, but they usually do not; sometimes they increase in size. If the adenoma is larger than 5 cm, most experts advise against pregnancy until the lesion can be resected, although the evidence that pregnancy is associated with a higher rate of complications is scant. Pregnancy in patients with smaller adenomas can be managed by careful observation with intermittent ultrasonography. Small adenomas located in the liver where they are technically difficult to resect can be treated with radiofrequency ablation. Observation is recommended for smaller adenomas or for those that regress

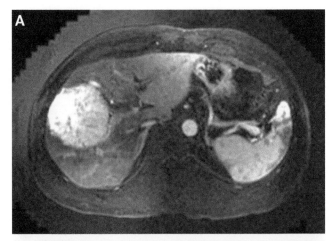

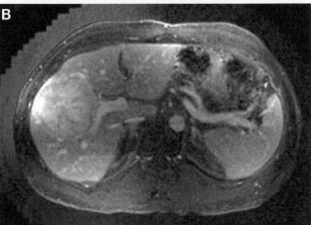

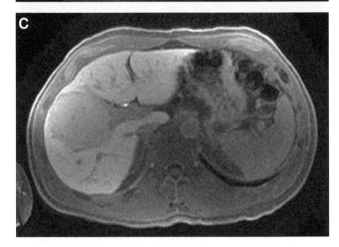

Figure 25.4. Hepatic Adenoma. A, Arterial phase after intravenous injection of gadobenate dimeglumine shows heterogeneous hyperenhancement. B, Venous phase shows the adenoma almost isoenhancing with the surrounding liver. C, Delayed hepatobiliary phase shows the adenoma excluding the contrast agent and hypoenhancing compared with the surrounding liver.

after withdrawal of estrogen, particularly in patients who do not plan any future pregnancies.

Focal Nodular Hyperplasia

Focal nodular hyperplasia is thought to develop as a reaction of the liver to an intrahepatic arterial malformation. The arterial malformation forms a vascular stellate scar that contains connective

tissue and bile ductules. The surrounding mass contains a proliferation of hepatocytes separated by fibrous septa. Unlike hepatic adenomas, focal nodular hyperplasias are polyclonal and do
not have a tendency for malignant transformation. Focal nodular
hyperplasia occurs predominantly in women of childbearing age
and is not considered to be related to oral contraceptive use. Focal
nodular hyperplasias may be multiple (10% of patients) or associated with cavernous hemangiomas (20% of patients).

Histologic Features

Focal nodular hyperplasia is characterized by benign-appearing
hepatic parenchyma, with bile ductules in septal fibrosis.

Clinical Features

Most patients with focal nodular hyperplasia are asymptomatic.
Patients with large lesions may present with abdominal discomfort or an abdominal mass.

Imaging Characteristics

Ultrasonography. Focal nodular hyperplasia has a variable
ultrasonographic appearance, with lesions being hypoechoic,
hyperechoic, or isoechoic. Most commonly, the tumors are
hypoechoic except for the central scar. Color flow Doppler imaging may show increased blood flow in the central stellate scar.

Multiphasic CT. On multiphasic CT, the presence of an
avascular central scar or a feeding artery to the mass is highly
suggestive of focal nodular hyperplasia. The lesion shows rapid
and intense contrast enhancement during the arterial phase and
isointensity during the venous phase.

Contrast-Enhanced MRI. Contrast-enhanced MRI shows
a rapid, intense contrast enhancement similar to the pattern
with multiphasic CT. Typically, focal nodular hyperplasia is
isointense on T1-weighted images and either isointense or
slightly hyperintense on T2-weighted images. The central scar
is usually hypointense on T1-weighted images but hyperintense
on T2-weighted images. Gadobenate dimeglumine or gadoxetate
disodium is taken up by the hepatocytes and partially excreted
into the immature bile ductules of focal nodular hyperplasias;
thus, they retain contrast medium in the biliary phase of imaging
(Figure 25.5).

Technetium Tc 99m Sulfur Colloid Scintigraphy. With
scintigraphy, 50% to 60% of cases of focal nodular hyperplasia
show hyperintense or isointense uptake, unlike the hypointensity
of adenomas, because of the presence of Kupffer cells.

Biopsy

Focal nodular hyperplasia can be difficult to distinguish from adenoma because fine-needle aspirates from both lesions may show
only benign-appearing hepatocytes. Immunohistochemically,
focal nodular hyperplasia typically shows a patchy "map-like"
glutamine synthetase staining, which distinguishes it from hepatic adenoma.

Management

Asymptomatic focal nodular hyperplasia can be monitored over
time, and surgery rarely is indicated. Some groups recommend

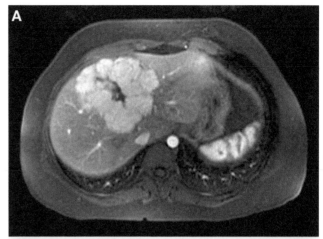
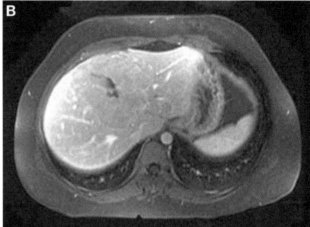
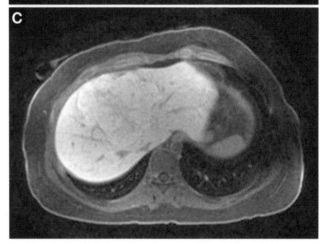

Figure 25.5. Focal Nodular Hyperplasia. A, Arterial phase shows
homogeneous hyperenhancement and a central scar. B, Venous phase
shows the tumor isoenhancing with the surrounding liver. C, Delayed
phase after intravenous injection of gadobenate dimeglumine shows the
contrast agent concentrated within the tumor.

discontinuation of oral contraceptives, although this has not been
shown to result in regression of the tumor.

Simple Liver Cysts

Solitary or multiple liver cysts are common and usually asymptomatic, and they often coexist with other mass lesions in the liver.

The female to male ratio is 4:1. Liver cysts occur in 3.6% of the population, and the prevalence increases with age.

Histologic Features

Cysts are thin-walled structures lined by cuboidal bile duct epithelium and filled with isotonic fluid.

Clinical Features

Cysts are usually asymptomatic unless they are large and causing symptoms through pressure on adjacent structures. Rarely, large cysts may cause pain, produce biliary obstruction and present with jaundice, or exert pressure on the inferior vena cava, leading to lower extremity edema.

Imaging Characteristics

Ultrasonography. Ultrasonography is the best imaging method for cysts. Classically, cysts are anechoic and have smooth, round margins; a distinct far wall; and posterior acoustic enhancement (Figure 25.6). Ultrasonography clearly shows the wall thickness and, if present, internal septations. Thick-walled cysts with nodularity or irregular septations suggest the diagnosis of cystadenoma or, rarely, cystadenocarcinoma.

Computed Tomography. On CT, cysts have the same density as water and do not change with contrast imaging.

Magnetic Resonance Imaging. On MRI, cysts are hyperintense on T2-weighted images. Small cysts may be difficult to differentiate from a cavernous hemangioma.

Biopsy

Biopsy usually is not necessary because of the distinctive imaging characteristics of simple cysts.

Management

Smaller symptomatic simple cysts can be treated with percutaneous aspiration and instillation of ethanol or 3% sodium

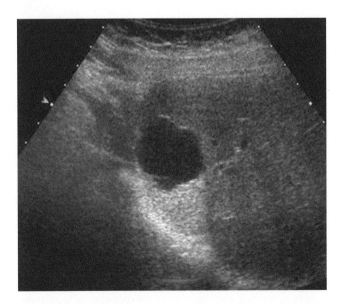

Figure 25.6. Simple Liver Cyst. Ultrasonogram shows the characteristic changes of absence of echoes within the lesion, a distinct far wall, and increased echogenicity posterior to the cyst.

tetradecyl sulfate as a sclerosant to ablate the cyst. Large symptomatic cysts or smaller cysts that recur after aspiration and attempted ablation should be treated with laparoscopic or open surgical fenestration.

Focal Fat or Fat Sparing

Fatty infiltration of the liver is common. Focal fatty infiltration can give the appearance of a mass lesion on imaging studies; conversely, focal sparing in a liver with diffuse fatty infiltration also can have the appearance of a mass. Fatty infiltration typically occurs in obese persons and in patients with type 2 diabetes, high alcohol consumption, or altered nutritional status because of chemotherapy regimens.

Histologic Features

Histologic specimens show areas of fatty infiltration with fat-laden cells.

Clinical Features

Focal fat or fat sparing is asymptomatic and is usually discovered on abdominal imaging performed for other reasons.

Imaging Characteristics

Focal fat does not distort the contour of the liver. If normal vessels, especially veins, can be seen coursing through the region, the diagnosis of focal fat is likely. Also, focal fat typically occurs in vascular watersheds, particularly along the falciform ligament. "Skip areas" of normal liver in diffuse fatty infiltration typically occur adjacent to the gallbladder fossa, in subcapsular areas, or in the posterior aspect of segment 4 of the liver.

Ultrasonography. Areas of fatty infiltration are hyperechoic.

Computed Tomography. On CT, fat is hypodense compared with the spleen, but because the fat is dispersed in normal tissue, it is not as low in density as adipose tissue. Venous structures coursing through the areas of focal fat are seen on venous phase studies.

Magnetic Resonance Imaging. On MRI, fat is occasionally hyperintense on T1- and T2-weighted images. Decreased signal intensity on out-of-phase gradient imaging is diagnostic of focal fat.

Biopsy

Biopsy can be used to exclude other lesions if the diagnosis cannot be established confidently.

Management

No therapy is needed. Areas of focal fat may resolve if patients lose weight or achieve better control of diabetes.

Malignant Liver Masses

Hepatocellular Carcinoma

The major risk factors for HCC include cirrhosis from chronic HBV or HCV infection, alcohol use, nonalcoholic fatty liver disease, hereditary hemochromatosis, other causes of liver injury such as α_1-antitrypsin deficiency, autoimmune hepatitis, primary biliary cirrhosis, and tyrosinema. Fungal aflatoxins that contaminate grains and legumes also have a synergistic effect with other causes of liver injury and contribute to the development of liver cancer in parts of sub-Saharan Africa and Asia. Approximately 80% to 90% of HCCs occur with cirrhosis. The other 10% to 20% comprise 3 groups.

One group includes patients who have chronic HBV infection and HCC in the absence of cirrhosis, presumably because of the oncogenic effects of HBV proteins and HBV integration, inherited familial tendency, and, in certain areas of the world, the synergistic effect of exposure to dietary aflatoxin. These patients are often young, between 20 and 50 years old.

Another group of patients without cirrhosis is characterized by older persons who live in countries where the incidence of HBV infection is low and who present with sporadic-onset HCC occurring in a histologically normal liver in the absence of discernible risk factors. In a proportion of these persons the adeno-associated virus type 2 is integrated in their HCCs.

The third group consists of an increasing number of people with NASH who have HCC without cirrhosis. Although the risk for HCC in this NASH population without cirrhosis is relatively low, since NASH is so prevalent in the population and has now become the most common cause of chronic liver disease in industrial countries in North America and Europe, it contributes substantially to the overall number of HCC cases. Without surveillance, most HCCs are diagnosed at an advanced stage, when radical treatment for cure is no longer feasible. Therefore, it is important that persons who are at risk for HCC be enrolled in a surveillance program for early detection of new tumors.

Surveillance and Diagnosis With Imaging, Biomarkers, or Biopsy

The best outcomes for treatment of HCC are achieved with liver transplant, surgical resection, or local ablative therapies such as microwave ablation, radiofrequency ablation, laser ablation, or percutaneous ethanol injection. Because these therapies are most effective when applied to early-stage HCC, there is a strong rationale for emphasizing a regular surveillance program to screen for the tumor in at-risk persons. Current guidelines of the American Association for the Study of Liver Diseases recommend that patients who have cirrhosis be evaluated with liver ultrasonography with or without measurement of serum alpha fetoprotein every 6 months to screen for HCC. For those who have chronic hepatitis B without cirrhosis, screening should begin at age 20 years for African-born persons, 40 years for Asian-born men, and 50 years for Asian-born women, and for patients with a family history of HCC, high HBV DNA level, and a persistent or intermittent increase in the level of alanine aminotransferase. The high body mass index and central obesity of many US patients frequently render full ultrasonographic visualization of the liver difficult; hence, there is increasing interest in the development of additional blood-based biomarkers for surveillance for HCC.

Once a new mass is identified with ultrasonography or suspected by biomarker elevation, it should be confirmed with cross-sectional imaging with multiphasic contrast-enhanced CT or MRI. The Liver Imaging Reporting and Data System (LI-RADS) was developed by the American College of Radiology for systematic evaluation and reporting of liver lesions suspected of being malignant that are imaged with CT or MRI. Combinations of arterial enhancement with washout in the portal venous phase and an enhancing capsule in the delayed phase with or without threshold growth of the lesion over time are used as diagnostic criteria for early-stage HCC and are highly specific (Figure 25.7 and Figure 25.8).

✓ Persons eligible for HCC surveillance
  • Patients with cirrhosis from any cause who would be a candidate for therapy
  • Patients with decompensated cirrhosis and end-stage liver disease only if they are eligible for liver transplant
✓ Other persons eligible for HCC surveillance are those who have chronic hepatitis B without cirrhosis
  • If African born, begin surveillance at age 20 years
  • If Asian-born male, begin surveillance at age 40 years
  • If Asian-born female, begin surveillance at age 50 years
  • Patient with high HBV DNA level
  • Patient with family history of HCC
  • Patient with active inflammation and increased alanine aminotransferase level

---

CT/MRI Diagnostic Table

Arterial phase hyperenhancement (APHE)		No APHE		Nonrim APHE		
Observation size, mm		<20	≥20	<10	10-19	≥20
Count additional major features: • Enhancing "capsule" • Nonperipheral "washout" • Threshold growth	0	LR-3	LR-3	LR-3	LR-3	LR-4
	1	LR-3	LR-4	LR-4	LR-4 / LR-5	LR-5
	≥2	LR-4	LR-4	LR-4	LR-5	LR-5

Observations in this cell are categorized based on 1 additional major feature:
• LR-4 if enhancing "capsule"
• LR-5 if nonperipheral "washout" *or* threshold growth

Figure 25.7. Liver Imaging Reporting and Data System (LI-RADS). LI-RADS was developed for systematic evaluation and reporting of liver lesions suspected of being malignant. CT indicates computed tomography; LR-3, indeterminate for malignancy; LR-4, suspicious for malignancy; LR-5, definite for malignancy; MRI, magnetic resonance imaging. (Adapted from Cerny M, Chernyak V, Olivié D, Billiard J-S, Murphy-Lavallée J, Kielar AZ, et al. LI-RADS version 2018 ancillary features at MRI. Radiographics. 2018 38[7]:1973-2001; used with permission.)

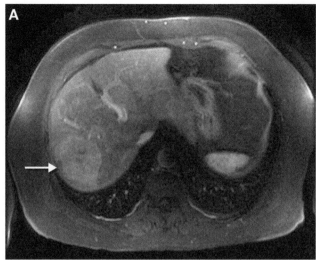

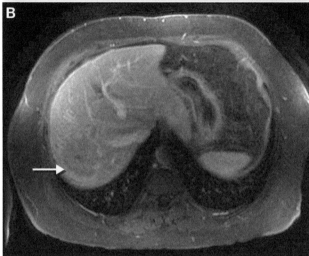

Figure 25.8. Hepatocellular Carcinoma. A, Arterial phase shows vascular enhancement (arrow). B, Portal phase shows venous washout (arrow).

HCC can be diagnosed noninvasively if a new nodule larger than 1 cm is found in a cirrhotic liver during surveillance and shows typical arterial enhancement and venous washout on triphasic CT or MRI. Additional MRI features of HCC include contrast exclusion in the delayed biliary phase of imaging with gadoxetate disodium and hyperintensity on diffusion-weighted imaging. The main rationale for noninvasive diagnosis in early-stage HCC is to prevent tumor seeding and recurrence after potentially curative treatment, including liver transplant. Patients who present with newly discovered liver masses in the absence of cirrhosis should have a biopsy study to histologically confirm HCC because conditions such as lymphomas and metastases from other primary sites may appear to be HCC in a noncirrhotic liver. Determination of the alpha fetoprotein level may obviate the need for biopsy if the level is markedly increased, but it is important to consider that malignancies at other primary sites, notably esophageal and gastric carcinomas, also can be associated with a high level of alpha fetoprotein. HCCs diagnosed at intermediate or advanced stages should be biopsied without hesitation because genomic and immunohistochemical characterization of these tumors may provide valuable information to confirm the diagnosis and guide optimal therapy.

✓ LI-RADS criteria for noninvasive diagnosis of HCC
  • Arterial phase enhancement
  • Portal and delayed venous phase washout
  • Rim enhancement in the delayed phase
  • Threshold growth of mass
  • Diffusion-weighted imaging on MRI

Management

The most comprehensive staging algorithm with associated treatment strategy used in Western countries is the Barcelona Clinic Liver Cancer (BCLC) staging and treatment system, which incorporates assessment of the physical and biomarker characteristics of the tumor, degree of underlying liver dysfunction, and cancer-related performance status to help with developing an optimal strategy for patient management (Figure 25.9). The BCLC strategy is revised regularly and has an appropriate bias toward therapies that have been proved effective in phase 3 studies; it therefore provides robust, evidence-based guidance for clinicians. The 2022 update of the BCLC system incorporates the use of transarterial radioembolization (TARE) for single tumors up to 8 cm in size. Therapies that are almost certainly effective for some patients with HCC, but which need a confirmatory base of evidence, include stereotactic body radiation therapy, proton beam therapy, and carbon ion therapy. In the past few years, the number of systemic therapy options for patients with HCC has greatly increased.

Liver Transplant. Liver resection and transplant offer the greatest chance of cure for patients with HCC. The decision to choose resection or transplant is based on a careful evaluation of the comorbid conditions of the patient, liver function, tumor size, number of tumors, vascular invasion, candidacy for transplant, and organ availability. Transplant is an effective treatment option for HCC in patients with cirrhosis because it addresses both the neoplasm and the underlying liver disease. Initially, the outcomes of transplant for HCC were poor. However, with advances in patient selection using the Milan criteria (1 tumor ≤5 cm or 2 or 3 tumors ≤3 cm, without vascular invasion or extrahepatic spread), the 5-year survival rate is 70% to 80% and the recurrence rate is less than 15%. Despite the favorable results of transplant, organ availability is less than the demand, and up to 15% of patients listed for transplant drop out because of tumor progression before an organ becomes available. With treatment, intermediate-stage HCC can be downstaged to within the Milan criteria, and patients can undergo transplant successfully with excellent outcomes.

Surgery. Liver resection is the preferred treatment of HCC in patients without cirrhosis and in those with cirrhosis who have well-preserved liver function and little or no portal hypertension. For patients without cirrhosis, major liver resection carries a low mortality rate (<5%) and a 5-year survival rate of 30% to 50%. Bleeding and liver failure are the major causes of perioperative mortality among patients with cirrhosis who undergo liver resection. Limited liver resections are safe in patients with cirrhosis who have preserved liver function (Child-Pugh class A) and no portal hypertension. Multiple methods of assessing liver function, liver reserve, and perioperative mortality have been described and are important in selecting patients for resection. The Model for End-stage Liver Disease (MELD) has been shown to predict perioperative mortality after liver resection. Patients with a MELD score less than 9 have a perioperative mortality rate of 0%, compared with 29% for those with a score of 9 or more. The albumin-bilirubin score, based on albumin and bilirubin levels,

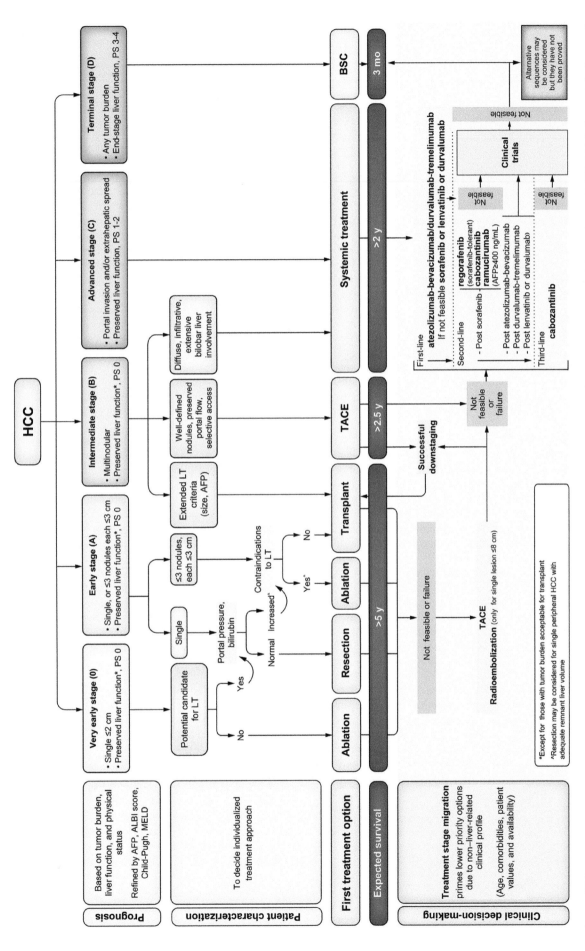

Figure 25.9. Barcelona Clinic Liver Cancer System. This system provides staging and treatment recommendations for patients with hepatocellular carcinoma (HCC). AFP indicates alpha fetoprotein; ALBI, albumin-bilirubin; BSC, best supportive care; LT, liver transplant; MELD, Model for End-stage Liver Disease; PS, performance status; TACE, transarterial chemoembolization. (Adapted from Reig M, Forner A, Rimola J, Ferrer-Fabrega J, Burrel M, Garcia-Criado A, et al. BCLC strategy for prognosis prediction and treatment recommendation: the 2022 update. J Hepatol. 2022 Mar;76(3):681-93; used with permission.)

provides another objective measure of underlying liver function. After liver resection, the tumor recurs in approximately 70% of patients within 5 years and reflects both intrahepatic metastases and the development of de novo tumors in the diseased liver. Predictors of recurrence and survival after resection include tumor size and number and vascular invasion. The 5-year survival rate after liver resection is 30% to 50%. For ideal candidates (ie, they have a single tumor, preserved liver function, and absence of portal hypertension), the 5-year survival rate is as high as 50% to 70%.

Local Ablation. Local therapies for treating HCC include ablative methods such as microwave ablation (MWA), radiofrequency ablation (RFA), and percutaneous ethanol injection (PEI). MWA and RFA are more effective ablative treatments and are used more often than PEI in clinical practice. Both MWA and RFA have similar efficacy as surgical resection in treating single, small (<2 cm) HCCs, but MWA can be used to treat a larger volume in less time. Ablation is generally used for treatment of small HCCs (≤3 cm) in patients who are not candidates for liver transplant or when liver transplant is not available. In MWA, electromagnetic energy is applied at 915 MHz or 2.45 GHz; in RFA, the frequency ranges from 375 to 500 KHz. RFA typically produces complete necrosis of a 3- to 4-cm radius of tissue during a single 10- to 15-minute treatment, while MWA can create a larger area of necrosis within a 5-minute treatment. RFA can be applied to overlapping fields to treat lesions larger than 3 cm, but it is not as effective for these lesions. RFA is not effective for the treatment of tumors close to major blood vessels because a heat-sink effect causes rapid conduction of heat away from the tumor. MWA achieves more rapid and homogeneous heating of the tumor and higher intratumoral temperatures, rendering it more effective and less susceptible to the heat sink effect from nearby blood vessels. Both modalities can damage the biliary tree or other extrahepatic structures such as the diaphragm, stomach, or bowel if applied too close to the structures. Several early studies raised concerns about increased risks of tumor seeding after ablation. Advances in the ablation technique have lowered this risk substantially. Most often, surface lesions are approached through the liver parenchyma rather than through direct puncture of the liver surface. In addition, the probe track is cauterized as the probe is being removed; this destroys and prevents dissemination of any residual HCC cells.

PEI is performed under ultrasonographic guidance. Ethanol induces tumor necrosis and is particularly effective in the cirrhotic liver because the surrounding fibrotic tissue limits the diffusion of the injected ethanol. Usually 2 or 3 injection sessions are needed for complete ablation of the tumor. The low cost of this treatment makes it attractive for use where resources are limited.

Alternative means of local ablation that are being used more frequently include laser ablation and irreversible electroporation. Cryoablation can be useful when the extent of tissue injury must be closely monitored in real-time, such as for tissue near nerves in the pelvis.

✓ HCC treatments that have the potential for cure of the disease
  • Local ablation—usually uses microwave energy applied to the tumor tissue to destroy the tissue with heat energy; is usually most effective for tumors less than 3 cm in diameter
  • Surgical resection—operative removal of a section of liver containing a tumor along with a surrounding rim of uninvolved liver to ensure removal of the whole tumor; if the tumor is large, the remaining portion of liver must have sufficient functional reserve to prevent development of liver failure

---

  • Liver transplant—for persons with underlying liver disease (eg, cirrhosis) who would not have sufficient liver function after surgical resection, the entire liver is removed and replaced with the liver from a deceased donor or with a portion of the liver from a living donor

---

Locoregional Therapies. Locoregional therapies include transarterial chemoembolization (TACE), TARE, stereotactic body radiation therapy, and proton beam therapy. TACE involves the angiographic injection of a combination of chemotherapy agents with absorbable gelatin sponge particles (Gelfoam; Pfizer Inc) into the branch of the hepatic artery that supplies the tumor. The goal is to deliver high concentrations of antitumor agents and, simultaneously, to induce tumor necrosis by occluding the arterial supply to the tumor. The chemotherapy agents typically used for TACE include cisplatin, doxorubicin, and mitomycin C. Some centers use chemotherapy agents dissolved in iodized oil (Lipiodol; Guerbet LLC); however, this iodinated contrast agent can interfere with subsequent detection of arterial enhancement in residual tumor nodules. TACE is particularly effective in the treatment of HCC because almost all the blood supply to the tumor is from branches of the hepatic artery. In contrast, the benign liver has a dual blood supply, with 70% to 80% of the blood supply provided by the portal vein and 20% to 30% by the hepatic artery. Consequently, occlusion of the branches of the hepatic artery to the tumor can be achieved without substantially compromising the blood supply to the surrounding cirrhotic liver. The major contraindication to TACE is complete obstruction of the portal vein, in which case concomitant obstruction of the arterial supply can lead to hepatic ischemia and induce liver decompensation. Randomized controlled trials have shown that TACE improves survival of patients with unresectable intermediate-stage HCC. TACE is an alternative treatment option for patients with early-stage HCC when ablative treatment cannot be performed safely because of the location of the tumor. TACE also is used frequently for downsizing the tumor or as a bridging treatment before liver transplant.

Drug-eluting bead TACE (DEB-TACE) uses porous DEBs loaded with doxorubicin for chemoembolization. The beads lodge in the tumor capillaries and gradually release doxorubicin into the local environment. Theoretically, treatment of intrahepatic tumors with DEB-TACE is more sustained and causes fewer systemic adverse effects. Most studies suggest that its efficacy is similar to that of conventional TACE.

TARE delivers intratumoral radiation by transarterial injection of yttrium 90 radioactive microspheres following the principles of TACE. TARE has been confirmed to be effective for the treatment of unresectable unifocal HCCs up to 8 cm in size, and safety and tolerability have been acceptable.

Systemic or Targeted Therapy. For more than a decade, the multitargeting kinase inhibitor sorafenib was the mainstay of therapy for patients with advanced unresectable HCC. However, for patients with advanced HCC, the current standard of care, which is more effective than sorafenib, is 1) the immune checkpoint inhibitor atezolizumab in combination with the anti–vascular endothelial growth factor A antibody bevacizumab or 2) the immune checkpoint inhibitor durvalumab, an anti–programmed cell death ligand 1 monoclonal antibody, in combination with the anti–cytotoxic T-lymphocyte antigen-4 inhibitor ipilimumab. Bevacizumab is contraindicated in persons who are at risk for variceal bleeding. These persons can have variceal banding to completion or should use a regimen that does not contain bevacizumab.

If 1 of these combinations cannot be used, acceptable options for first-line treatment are sorafenib, lenvatinib, or durvalumab. Second-line therapy includes 1) regorafenib, which can be used for patients who have tolerated sorafenib; 2) cabozantinib, which has been shown to be effective; and 3) ramucirumab, which can be used in patients who have an alpha fetoprotein level of at least 400 ng/mL. Cabozantinib is recommended for third-line therapy for patients who have not yet been exposed to this agent and who could alternatively be entered into clinical trials.

Cholangiocarcinoma

Cholangiocarcinomas are malignancies that arise from the bile duct epithelium. In Western countries, PSC is the primary identified risk factor for cholangiocarcinoma. In several countries in Asia, liver fluke infestations of the biliary tract are an important risk factor. Choledochal and other cystic disorders of the biliary tract also are associated with cholangiocarcinoma. Patients with cirrhosis due to chronic viral hepatitis, alcoholic liver disease, nonalcoholic fatty liver disease, or other chronic liver diseases are also at increased risk for cholangiocarcinoma. However, most patients with cholangiocarcinoma have no known risk factors. For patients with PSC, the risk of diagnosis of cholangiocarcinoma is highest within the first 2 years after the diagnosis of PSC, suggesting that the development of cancer may be the event that triggers the diagnosis of PSC.

Cholangiocarcinomas are classified as intrahepatic or extrahepatic tumors. The manifestation of intrahepatic cholangiocarcinomas is typically a large intrahepatic mass with or without intrahepatic or regional lymph node metastases. Extrahepatic cholangiocarcinomas may be perihilar tumors, which arise in the distal right or left hepatic duct or at the common hepatic duct bifurcation, or distal bile duct tumors arising in the common bile duct. The laboratory test most often used to confirm the diagnosis of cholangiocarcinoma is measurement of the CA19-9 level. CA19-9 (also called monosialylated Lewis) is a sialyl-Lewis[A] blood group antigen that is used clinically as a tumor marker. A CA19-9 value greater than 100 U/mL is about 65% to 75% sensitive and 85% to 95% specific for the diagnosis of cholangiocarcinoma. CA19-9 also can be increased in pancreatic adenocarcinomas and other upper gastrointestinal tract malignancies. CA19-9 values greater than 1,000 U/mL usually are predictive of extrahepatic metastatic disease. During evaluation for diagnosis or posttreatment follow-up of patients with cholangiocarcinoma, those who test negative for Lewis antigen (7%-10% of the general population) cannot synthesize CA19-9 and may erroneously be presumed to lack the tumor marker.

Histologic Features

Histologically, cholangiocarcinomas are adenocarcinomas. This frequently leads to confusion about the primary site of the tumor. Thus, cholangiocarcinoma can be misdiagnosed as metastatic adenocarcinoma of unknown primary site.

Clinical Features

The clinical features of cholangiocarcinoma depend on its location. Approximately 60% of these tumors are perihilar tumors located around the bifurcation of the hepatic duct; the rest occur in the distal extrahepatic (20%) or intrahepatic (20%) biliary tree. While the incidence of extrahepatic cholangiocarcinomas has been stable over time, in most industrial countries the incidence

of intrahepatic cholangiocarcinomas has been increasing over the past 30 years. The most common symptom of extrahepatic cholangiocarcinoma is painless jaundice due to obstruction of biliary ducts. With tumors of the intrahepatic bile ducts, patients often have pain without jaundice. With perihilar or intrahepatic tumors, jaundice often occurs later in the disease course and is a marker of advanced disease. Other common symptoms include generalized itching, abdominal pain, weight loss, and fever. Pruritis usually is preceded by jaundice, but it may be the initial presenting symptom of cholangiocarcinoma. The pain associated with cholangiocarcinoma is usually a constant dull ache in the right upper quadrant of the abdomen. Biliary obstruction results in clay-colored stools and dark urine. Physical signs include jaundice, hepatomegaly, and a palpable right upper quadrant mass. Patients with intrahepatic cholangiocarcinoma most often present with dull right upper quadrant discomfort and weight loss.

Imaging Characteristics

Abdominal Ultrasonography. Cholangiocarcinomas are typically hypoechoic on ultrasonography and sometimes are first visualized during an ultrasonographic examination of the liver for suspected gallstone disease causing right upper quadrant abdominal discomfort.

Multiphasic CT. Intrahepatic cholangiocarcinomas are usually hypodense on noncontrast imaging, often with a rounded, smooth, nodular appearance. During the arterial phase, there is minimal enhancement that progressively increases through the venous phase, often more prominent peripherally than centrally. Perihilar cholangiocarcinomas that preferentially affect 1 lobe of the liver often lead to unilobar biliary obstruction for an extended period, during which the patient has a normal bilirubin level because of adequate biliary drainage from the unaffected lobe of the liver. Eventually, the affected lobe undergoes atrophy, with prominent biliary dilatation, while the unaffected lobe undergoes compensatory hypertrophy. This syndrome is called the atrophy-hypertrophy complex (Figure 25.10). Cross-sectional imaging is particularly helpful for assessing the degree of encasement of the

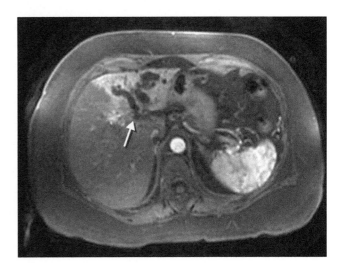

Figure 25.10. Cholangiocarcinoma With Atrophy-Hypertrophy Complex. Note cholangiocarcinoma with obstruction of the left biliary ductal system (arrow) and consequent marked dilatation of the bile ducts in the left lobe, with associated atrophy of the left lobe parenchyma. The right lobe shows compensatory hypertrophy.

hilar vasculature, a critically important part of the evaluation for surgical resectability.

MRI With Gadolinium. With contrast-enhanced MRI, intrahepatic cholangiocarcinomas are hypointense on T1-weighted images and hyperintense on T2-weighted images. There is peripheral contrast enhancement that progresses into the venous phase, similar to the pattern seen with multiphasic CT. MRCP is performed concomitantly with MRI and is now recommended as the optimal initial investigation for assessing the luminal extent and resectability of suspected cholangiocarcinoma. MRCP is noninvasive and as accurate as direct cholangiography for assessing the level of biliary tract obstruction. Often, the biliary tract peripheral to a biliary stenosis can be demonstrated better with MRCP than with endoscopic retrograde cholangiopancreatography (ERCP).

Cholangiography. With the advent of MRI and MRCP, direct cholangiography by means of ERCP and percutaneous transhepatic cholangiography (PTC) are becoming less important as initial diagnostic methods; however, the resolution provided by PTC and ERCP is still better in some cases than that of MRCP. In addition to providing tissue samples by brush cytology or biopsy, PTC and ERCP allow placement of therapeutic stents for biliary decompression if needed and also can be used to deliver photodynamic therapy or RFA to unresectable tumors. In patients with PSC, PTC may be challenging technically because of peripheral strictures; for these patients, ERCP is the preferred method. A completely occluded distal biliary tract may preclude the use of ERCP, and either PTC or a combined approach of PTC and ERCP may be needed for successful passage through a difficult stricture to accomplish internal biliary drainage, which is preferred to external drainage.

Biopsy and Cytology

Intrahepatic mass-forming cholangiocarcinomas usually are biopsied under ultrasonographic or CT guidance. Often, ductal cholangiocarcinomas are less amenable to percutaneous needle biopsy. Also, immune-associated cholangitis can mimic a malignant biliary stricture, rendering the accurate diagnosis of biliary strictures even more difficult. Transpapillary forceps biopsies and cytologic brushings usually are obtained at ERCP or PTC to help establish the diagnosis. Because many cholangiocarcinomas are highly desmoplastic, with a prominent fibrous stromal component separating small islands of malignant epithelium, histologic and cytologic confirmation of their malignancy can be challenging. Advanced cytologic tests for chromosomal polysomy such as fluorescence in situ hybridization (FISH) have been shown to improve substantially the sensitivity of brush cytology for diagnosing malignancy in biliary strictures. Cytology samples with cells that show polysomy of 2 or more relevant chromosomal loci—from chromosomal bands 1q21, 7p12, 8q24, and 9p21 in the pancreatobiliary FISH probe set—are highly specific for cancer (Figure 25.11). The combination of transpapillary forceps biopsy, cytology, and pancreatobiliary FISH has been shown to have the highest sensitivity for diagnosing malignancy in biliary strictures.

Endoscopic Ultrasonography. Endoscopic ultrasonography with an ultrasound probe at the tip of a duodenoscope allows

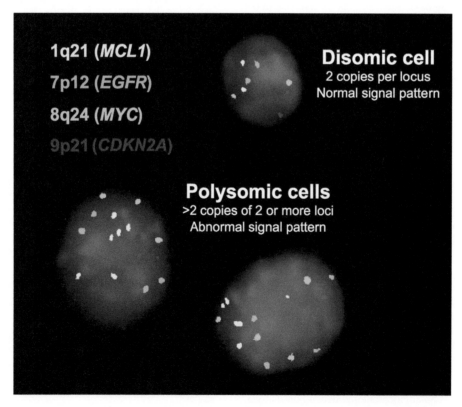

Figure 25.11. Pancreatobiliary Fluorescence In Situ Hybridization (PB-FISH) for Diagnosis of Malignancy in Biliary Strictures. Fluorescent DNA probes for chromosomal bands 1q21/*MCL1* in yellow, 7p12/*EGFR* in green, 8q24/*MYC* in aqua, and 9p21/*CDKN2A* in red are hybridized to brush cytology specimens obtained from biliary strictures at endoscopic retrograde cholangiopancreatography. The normal disomic cell has 2 copies of each of the probes. The malignant polysomic cells have 6 copies of chromosomes 1q21/*MCL1*, 4 copies of 7p12/*EGFR*, 3 or 4 copies of 8q24/*MYC*, and 2 copies of 9p21/*CDKN2A*. (Courtesy of Emily G. Barr Fritcher, CT[ASCP], MB[ASCP], and Benjamin R. Kipp, PhD, Department of Laboratory Medicine and Pathology, Mayo Clinic; used with permission.)

high-resolution evaluation of the left lobe of the liver and fine-needle aspiration of lymph nodes at the hepatic hilum. This technique is extremely useful for assessing the presence and malignancy of regional lymph nodules during staging of cholangiocarcinomas.

Management

Surgery. Hilar cholangiocarcinoma accounts for two-thirds of all cases of extrahepatic cholangiocarcinoma. Intrahepatic cholangiocarcinoma is treated with surgical resection when feasible. Tumors in the mid bile duct can be treated with resection and anastomosis of the bile duct. Distal extrahepatic cholangiocarcinomas are treated with pancreaticoduodenectomy. For hilar cholangiocarcinomas, surgical planning is more complex and preoperative evaluation of the local and regional extent of the tumor is critical. Cross-sectional imaging and cholangiography (either direct or MRCP) are necessary for appropriate patient selection and surgical planning. Current criteria that preclude resection include 1) bilateral ductal extension to secondary radicles; 2) encasement or occlusion of the main portal vein; 3) lobar atrophy with involvement of the contralateral portal vein, hepatic artery, or secondary biliary radicles; 4) peripancreatic (head only), periduodenal, posterior pancreatoduodenal, periportal, celiac, or superior mesenteric regional lymph node metastases; and 5) distant metastases. The perioperative mortality rate of hepatic resection for hilar cholangiocarcinoma is between 5% and 10% in major centers. The operation of choice for hilar cholangiocarcinoma is cholecystectomy, lobar or extended lobar hepatic and bile duct resection, regional lymphadenectomy, and Roux-en-Y hepaticojejunostomy. With surgical resection, the 5-year survival rate is 20% to 25%. Patients with PSC often have cirrhosis and are not candidates for surgical resection because of concerns about postoperative hepatic decompensation.

Liver Transplant. A protocol of neoadjuvant chemoradiotherapy with subsequent liver transplant for patients with de novo hilar cholangiocarcinoma or cholangiocarcinoma arising in association with PSC has been developed at Mayo Clinic in Rochester, Minnesota. The protocol is limited to patients who have a mass with a radial diameter up to 3 cm and excludes patients who have intrahepatic peripheral cholangiocarcinoma, metastases, or gallbladder involvement. Endoscopic ultrasonography is performed with directed aspiration to rule out involvement of regional hepatic lymph nodes. Patients are treated initially with preoperative radiotherapy (40.5-45 Gy, given as 1.5 Gy twice daily) and 5-fluorouracil. This is followed by 20- to 30-Gy transcatheter irradiation with iridium. Capecitabine is then administered until transplant. Before transplant, patients undergo staging abdominal exploration. Regional lymph node metastases, peritoneal metastases, or locally extensive disease preclude transplant. At the time of the last published review of patients treated since 1993, overall 5-year survival was 74% for patients with PSC and 58% for those with de novo perihilar cholangiocarcinoma. These results exceed those achieved with surgical resection even though all the transplant protocol patients have unresectable cholangiocarcinoma or cholangiocarcinoma arising in association with PSC.

Attempts have been made to implement liver transplant protocols for patients who have limited-stage intrahepatic cholangiocarcinoma. The rationale is that long-term outcomes

appear to be acceptable for patients who have early-stage intrahepatic cholangiocarcinoma that has been mistaken for HCC and who are enrolled in liver transplant protocols for HCC.

Systemic Chemotherapy

Various chemotherapy agents have been evaluated for the treatment of cholangiocarcinoma, but for many years there was only a limited response to these agents. Until recently, the standard of care was gemcitabine given in combination with either cisplatin or oxaliplatin. In a phase 3 clinical trial, the regimen of gemcitabine in combination with cisplatin produced tumor control (complete or partial response or stable disease) in 81.4% of patients, but this response was not sustained, with a median survival of 11.7 months compared to 8.1 months for treatment with gemcitabine alone. Recently, the use of durvalumab in combination with gemcitabine and cisplatin was approved as first-line treatment. The addition of durvalumab in a phase 3 trial (TOPAZ-1) led to a 12.8-month median overall survival compared to an 11.5-month overall survival with gemcitabine and cisplatin alone.

Over the past few years, genomic analyses of cholangiocarcinomas have shown that intrahepatic cholangiocarcinomas have a relatively high prevalence of targetable mutations or alterations, including fibroblast growth factor receptor 2 gene fusions in 10% to 20% and sequence variations in the isocitrate dehydrogenase 1 gene (*IDH1*; OMIM 147700) in 15% to 20%. The fibroblast growth factor receptor inhibitors pemigatinib and infigratinib and the inhibitor of isocitrate dehydrogenase 1, ivosidenib, are approved for treatment of intrahepatic cholangiocarcinomas that have the relevant sequence variations. Approximately 1% to 2% of cholangiocarcinomas also have a defective mismatch repair system, microsatellite instability, increased levels of tumor neoantigens, and a highly immune-infiltrative tumor microenvironment, rendering them highly sensitive to treatment with immune checkpoint inhibitors. Neurotrophic tyrosine receptor kinase gene (*NTRK*) fusions of the C-terminal of the tropomyosin receptor kinase with an N-terminal fusion partner, leading to ligand-independent phosphorylation and activation, occur in less than 1% of cholangiocarcinomas, and the tropomyosin receptor kinase inhibitors entrectinib and larotrectinib show meaningful responses in these tumors.

Maintenance of Biliary Patency. For patients with unresectable tumor causing biliary obstruction, the maintenance of biliary patency is required for substantial survival. This usually is achieved with the use of plastic endobiliary stents, which generally remain patent for 8 to 12 weeks, or metal stents, which may remain patent for more than a year. Unilateral drainage is generally sufficient for palliation of biliary obstruction and is associated with fewer complications than bilateral stenting. Photodynamic therapy is applied endoscopically through a glass fiber inserted to the site of the malignant biliary stricture. The therapy is administered by intravenous infusion of the photosensitizer porfimer sodium (Photofrin; Pinnacle Biologics, Inc) that preferentially accumulates in the proliferating tumor tissue, followed 48 hours later with endoscopic or percutaneous application of a laser light tuned to the appropriate wavelength. Overall, photodynamic therapy appears to be associated with increased survival, improved biliary drainage, and enhanced quality of life. However, the quality of evidence is low and additional randomized trials are warranted. More recently, RFA has also been used in the bile duct to palliate unresectable biliary tract cancer.

Liver Metastases

Liver metastases from other primary cancer sites are the most frequent malignant liver masses. Metastases are most commonly from colorectal adenocarcinomas but also frequently occur in patients with lung, pancreatic, esophageal, gastric, neuroendocrine, or breast cancer. Other potential primary tumors include lymphomas, melanomas, thyroid cancers, and renal cell carcinomas. Most often, liver metastases are multiple and distributed throughout both lobes of the liver. They tend not to have a large dominant lesion with multiple smaller satellite lesions, a feature that is more characteristic of primary liver tumors such as HCC and cholangiocarcinoma. Liver metastases have various imaging characteristics, depending on the degree of vascularity. Most commonly, they show persistent enhancement in the portal venous and venous phases of multiphasic cross-sectional CT or MRI studies. Some metastases also have a characteristic "halo" of nonenhancing tissue around the nodule. For certain tumor types, such as colorectal adenocarcinomas, FDG-PET CT is extremely valuable for characterizing the burden of metastatic disease. Limited disease with only a few metastatic nodules can be treated with surgical resection, local ablation, stereotactic body radiotherapy, or proton beam therapy. For metastases that are more diffuse within the liver, locoregional therapy with TARE can be administered in combination with systemic chemotherapy appropriate for the primary tumor.

Summary

A wide range of liver mass lesions initially may or may not produce symptoms. Many masses are found incidentally during imaging for nonspecific abdominal symptoms. Accurate differentiation of benign lesions from malignant lesions depends on obtaining a complete history and performing a physical examination and appropriate laboratory tests. Most benign lesions require no intervention, but an important subset requires multidisciplinary evaluation with subsequent surgical resection or other treatments.

Suggested Reading

Abou-Alfa GK, Sahai V, Hollebecque A, Vaccaro G, Melisi D, Al-Rajabi R, et al. Pemigatinib for previously treated, locally advanced or metastatic cholangiocarcinoma: a multicentre, open-label, phase 2 study. Lancet Oncol. 2020 May;21(5):671–84.

Alberts SR, Gores GJ, Kim GP, Roberts LR, Kendrick ML, Rosen CB, et al. Treatment options for hepatobiliary and pancreatic cancer. Mayo Clin Proc. 2007 May;82(5):628–37.

Asrani SK, Ghabril MS, Kuo A, Merriman RB, Morgan T, Parikh ND, et al. Quality measures in HCC care by the Practice Metrics Committee of the American Association for the Study of Liver Diseases. Hepatology. 2022 May;75(5):1289–99.

Atassi B, Bangash AK, Bahrani A, Pizzi G, Lewandowski RJ, Ryu RK, et al. Multimodality imaging following 90Y radioembolization: a comprehensive review and pictorial essay. Radiographics. 2008 Jan-Feb;28(1): 81–99.

Azad AI, Rosen CB, Taner T, Heimbach JK, Gores GJ. Selected patients with unresectable perihilar cholangiocarcinoma (pCCA) derive long-term benefit from liver transplantation. Cancers (Basel). 2020 Oct;12(11)

Banales JM, Marin JJG, Lamarca A, Rodrigues PM, Khan SA, Roberts LR, et al. Cholangiocarcinoma 2020: the next horizon in mechanisms and management. Nat Rev Gastroenterol Hepatol. 2020 Sep;17(9):557–88.

Baroud S, Sahakian AJ, Sawas T, Storm AC, Martin JA, Abu Dayyeh BK, et al. Impact of trimodality sampling on detection of malignant biliary strictures compared with patients with primary sclerosing cholangitis. Gastrointest Endosc. 2022 May;95(5):884–92.

Barr Fritcher EG, Voss JS, Brankley SM, Campion MB, Jenkins SM, Keeney ME, et al. An optimized set of fluorescence in situ hybridization probes for detection of pancreatobiliary tract cancer in cytology brush samples. Gastroenterology. 2015 Dec;149(7):1813–24.

Bioulac-Sage P, Taouji S, Possenti L, Balabaud C. Hepatocellular adenoma subtypes: the impact of overweight and obesity. Liver Int. 2012 Sep;32(8):1217–21.

Bokemeyer A, Matern P, Bettenworth D, Cordes F, Nowacki TM, Heinzow H, et al. Endoscopic radiofrequency ablation prolongs survival of patients with unresectable hilar cholangiocellular carcinoma: a case-control study. Sci Rep. 2019 Sep 23;9(1):13685.

Bunchorntavakul C, Bahirwani R, Drazek D, Soulen MC, Siegelman ES, Furth EE, et al. Clinical features and natural history of hepatocellular adenomas: the impact of obesity. Aliment Pharmacol Ther. 2011 Sep;34(6):664–74.

Chaiteerakij R, Yang JD, Harmsen WS, Slettedahl SW, Mettler TA, Fredericksen ZS, et al. Risk factors for intrahepatic cholangiocarcinoma: association between metformin use and reduced cancer risk. Hepatology. 2013 Feb;57(2):648–55.

Choi BY, Nguyen MH. The diagnosis and management of benign hepatic tumors. J Clin Gastroenterol. 2005 May-Jun;39(5):401–12.

El-Serag HB, Rudolph KL. Hepatocellular carcinoma: Epidemiology and molecular carcinogenesis. Gastroenterology. 2007 Jun;132(7):2557–76.

Finn RS, Qin S, Ikeda M, Galle PR, Ducreux M, Kim TY, et al. Atezolizumab plus bevacizumab in unresectable hepatocellular carcinoma. N Engl J Med. 2020 May;382(20):1894–905.

Forner A, Vilana R, Ayuso C, Bianchi L, Sole M, Ayuso JR, et al. Diagnosis of hepatic nodules 20 mm or smaller in cirrhosis: prospective validation of the noninvasive diagnostic criteria for hepatocellular carcinoma. Hepatology. 2008 Jan;47(1):97–104.

Javle M, Roychowdhury S, Kelley RK, Sadeghi S, Macarulla T, Weiss KH, et al. Infigratinib (BGJ398) in previously treated patients with advanced or metastatic cholangiocarcinoma with FGFR2 fusions or rearrangements: mature results from a multicentre, open-label, single-arm, phase 2 study. Lancet Gastroenterol Hepatol. 2021 Oct;6(10):803–15.

La Bella T, Imbeaud S, Peneau C, Mami I, Datta S, Bayard Q, et al. Adeno-associated virus in the liver: natural history and consequences in tumour development. Gut. 2020 Apr;69(4):737–47.

La Vecchia C, Tavani A. Female hormones and benign liver tumours. Dig Liver Dis. 2006 Aug;38(8):535–6.

Lammert C, Toal E, Mathur K, Khungar V, House M, Roberts LR, et al. Large hepatic adenomas and hepatic adenomatosis: a multicenter study of risk factors, interventions, and complications. Am J Gastroenterol. 2022 Jul;117(7):1089–96.

Leggett CL, Gorospe EC, Murad MH, Montori VM, Baron TH, Wang KK. Photodynamic therapy for unresectable cholangiocarcinoma: a comparative effectiveness systematic review and meta-analyses. Photodiagnosis Photodyn Ther. 2012 Sep;9(3):189–95.

Llovet JM, Ricci S, Mazzaferro V, Hilgard P, Gane E, Blanc JF, et al. Sorafenib in advanced hepatocellular carcinoma. N Engl J Med. 2008 Jul;359(4):378–90.

Moreno-Luna LE, Yang JD, Sanchez W, Paz-Fumagalli R, Harnois DM, Mettler TA, et al. Efficacy and safety of transarterial radioembolization versus chemoembolization in patients with hepatocellular carcinoma. Cardiovasc Intervent Radiol. 2013 Jun;36(3):714–23.

Nault JC, Bioulac-Sage P, Zucman-Rossi J. Hepatocellular benign tumors-from molecular classification to personalized clinical care. Gastroenterology. 2013 May;144(5):888–902.

Oseini AM, Chaiteerakij R, Shire AM, Ghazale A, Kaiya J, Moser CD, et al. Utility of serum immunoglobulin G4 in distinguishing immunoglobulin G4-associated cholangitis from cholangiocarcinoma. Hepatology. 2011 Sep 2;54(3):940–8.

Parra-Robert M, Santos VM, Canis SM, Pla XF, Fradera JMA, Porto RM. Relationship between CA 19.9 and the Lewis phenotype: options to improve diagnostic efficiency. Anticancer Res. 2018 Oct;38(10):5883–8.

Razumilava N, Gores GJ. Classification, diagnosis, and management of cholangiocarcinoma. Clin Gastroenterol Hepatol. 2013 Jan;11(1):13–21.

Reig M, Forner A, Rimola J, Ferrer-Fabrega J, Burrel M, Garcia-Criado A, et al. BCLC strategy for prognosis prediction and treatment recommendation: the 2022 update. J Hepatol. 2022 Mar;76(3):681–93.

Salem R, Johnson GE, Kim E, Riaz A, Bishay V, Boucher E, et al. Yttrium-90 radioembolization for the treatment of solitary, unresectable HCC: the LEGACY study. Hepatology. 2021 Nov;74(5):2342–52.

Sempoux C, Chang C, Gouw A, Chiche L, Zucman-Rossi J, Balabaud C, et al. Benign hepatocellular nodules: what have we learned using the patho-molecular classification. Clin Res Hepatol Gastroenterol. 2013 Sep;37(4):322–7.

Valle J, Wasan H, Palmer DH, Cunningham D, Anthoney A, Maraveyas A, et al. Cisplatin plus gemcitabine versus gemcitabine for biliary tract cancer. N Engl J Med. 2010 Apr;362(14):1273–81.

Valls C, Iannacconne R, Alba E, Murakami T, Hori M, Passariello R, et al. Fat in the liver: diagnosis and characterization. Eur Radiol. 2006;16(10):2292–308.

Yang JD, Kim B, Sanderson SO, Sauver JS, Yawn BP, Larson JJ, et al. Biliary tract cancers in Olmsted County, Minnesota, 1976-2008. Am J Gastroenterol. 2012 Aug;107(8):1256–62.

Zhu AX, Macarulla T, Javle MM, Kelley RK, Lubner SJ, Adeva J, et al. Final overall survival efficacy results of ivosidenib for patients with advanced cholangiocarcinoma with IDH1 mutation: the phase 3 randomized clinical ClarIDHy trial. JAMA Oncol. 2021 Nov 1;7(11):1669–77.

26

Alcohol-Related Liver Disease[a]

ROBERT C. HUEBERT, MD
VIJAY H. SHAH, MD

Epidemiology and Clinical Spectrum

Public Health Significance

Alcohol-related liver disease is a major cause of morbidity and mortality worldwide. Globally, approximately 2 billion people consume alcohol, and alcohol use disorder is diagnosed in more than 75 million people—and these numbers are probably underestimates. In the US, chronic liver disease is the 12th leading cause of death, and alcohol is implicated in approximately 50% of these deaths. Also, alcohol-related liver disease is a major source of health care expenditures, accounting for nearly $5 billion annually. Alcohol-related liver disease is the leading indication for liver transplant in the US. Recent increases in deaths due to alcohol-related liver disease are skewed toward younger age groups (25-34 years), and deaths due to alcohol-related liver disease are projected to increase in the coming years, particularly among women.

Clinical Spectrum

The clinical spectrum of alcohol-related liver disease includes 1) simple macrovesicular steatosis (fatty liver), with or without abnormal results on liver tests; 2) severe acute steatohepatitis (alcoholic hepatitis); and 3) end-stage chronic liver disease (alcohol-related cirrhosis). Fatty liver can develop in response to short, transient periods (ie, days) of alcohol misuse. It is generally asymptomatic or associated with nonspecific symptoms and is usually reversible with abstinence. This type of simple steatosis develops in 90% to 100% of regular users of alcohol. More advanced liver injury usually requires prolonged alcohol misuse over a period of years. Of note, more advanced lesions of alcohol-related liver disease do not develop in the majority of people who misuse alcohol for extended periods. However, alcohol-related steatohepatitis develops in 20% of these people, and in approximately half of those the disease progresses further to alcohol-related cirrhosis. Overall, accounting for some improvement during periods of abstinence, end-stage alcohol-related liver disease develops in about 20% of people with alcohol use disorder.

✓ **Steatosis**—simple fatty infiltration of the liver (most commonly caused by metabolic disease)
✓ **Steatohepatitis**—fatty infiltration of the liver and associated inflammation with or without fibrosis
✓ **Nonalcohol-related fatty liver disease**—liver disease in a person who consumes less than 20 g alcohol daily

Risk Factors

Alcohol Ingestion

The most obvious and important factors in the development of alcohol-related liver disease are dose and duration of alcohol misuse. Although alcohol-related fatty liver may develop in response to short periods of alcohol misuse, such as for only a few days, more advanced and morbid liver injury requires prolonged misuse of alcohol. In general, the amount of ethanol consumption required

---

[a] Portions previously published in Menon KV, Gores GJ, Shah VH. Pathogenesis, diagnosis, and treatment of alcoholic liver disease. Mayo Clin Proc. 2001 Oct;76(10):1021-9; used with permission of Mayo Foundation for Medical Education and Research.

Abbreviations: ALT, alanine aminotransferase; AST, aspartate aminotransferase; AUDIT, Alcohol Use Disorders Identification Test; CYP2E1, cytochrome P450 2E1 isozyme; GGT, γ-glutamyltransferase; HCV, hepatitis C virus; MDF, Maddrey discriminant function; MELD, Model for End-stage Liver Disease; MEOS, microsomal ethanol-oxidizing system; TNF, tumor necrosis factor

for the development of advanced forms of alcohol-related liver disease is 60 to 80 g of alcohol daily for men, or the approximate equivalent of 6 to 8 drinks daily for several years. In women, half this amount may cause clinically significant alcohol-related liver disease. The quantity of alcohol necessary for liver injury probably does not depend on the type of alcohol consumed. However, there is considerable individual variability in the threshold of alcohol necessary for advanced alcohol-related liver disease to develop. Clearly, factors other than sex and absolute quantities of ethanol consumption are important in determining which persons develop alcohol-related liver disease, including ethnicity (eg, American Indians and Alaskan natives), metabolic comorbidities (eg, obesity, iron overload, and type 2 diabetes), coexisting liver disease (eg, viral hepatitis), postsurgical anatomy (eg, Roux-en-Y gastric bypass), and genetic factors (eg, *PNPLA3* gene [OMIM 609567] alterations and α₁-antitrypsin heterozygosity).

Sex

Alcohol-related liver disease occurs more commonly in men than in women, since men are statistically more likely to misuse alcohol. However, women are predisposed to the development of this disease, and more severe disease develops in women with less alcohol consumption than in men. The reason for this greater risk in women is multifactorial, but a similar level of alcohol consumption results in higher blood alcohol levels in women than in men. Contributors to this phenomenon include a relative deficiency of gastric alcohol dehydrogenase in women, sex differences in alcohol bioavailability, and female hormone–related effects.

Genetic and Hereditary Factors

The interindividual variability in the correlation between alcohol consumption and development of liver disease emphasizes that genetic factors may predispose a person to alcohol-induced liver toxicity. Specific genetic alterations have been detected in patients who have alcohol-related liver disease, notably variations in the *HSD17B13* gene (OMIM 612127), the *TM6SF2* gene (OMIM 606563), the alcohol-metabolizing enzyme systems, and the *PNPLA3* gene. It also appears that milder phenotypes of diseases known to cause chronic liver disease may predispose individuals to alcohol-induced liver damage. Examples of this effect include compound heterozygosity at the hereditary hemochromatosis locus or an MZ α₁-antitrypsin phenotype. In addition to the genetic factors predisposing certain persons who misuse alcohol to liver disease, there also is strong evidence that genetic factors predispose persons to alcohol use disorder itself. Currently, however, no single genetic polymorphism has been shown definitively to contribute to alcohol-related liver disease.

> ✓ The global burden of alcohol-related liver disease is high, accounting for considerable morbidity, mortality, and cost, and its prevalence is probably underestimated
> ✓ Alcohol-related liver disease encompasses a clinicohistologic spectrum that includes fatty liver, alcohol-related hepatitis, and cirrhosis
> ✓ Although fatty liver occurs nearly uniformly with excessive alcohol consumption, more advanced liver injury occurs in only 15% to 20% of persons who continue to misuse alcohol
> ✓ While there is considerable variability among persons, the quantity of alcohol necessary for advanced liver injury to develop is probably 60 to 80 g (6-8 drinks) daily for several years, with a much lower threshold for women
> ✓ Genetic factors contribute to alcohol-related liver disease by predisposing a person to alcohol use disorder and to alcohol-induced liver injury

Ethanol Metabolism and Pathophysiology

More than 1 enzyme system is capable of metabolizing alcohol in the liver. Enzymes that have received the most attention include alcohol dehydrogenase, aldehyde dehydrogenase, and the microsomal ethanol-oxidizing system (MEOS) (Figure 26.1). Although the peroxisomal catalase enzyme is also capable of ethanol metabolism, its physiologic role in alcohol metabolism appears to be minor.

When physiologic circumstances are normal and blood levels of alcohol are low, the most important enzyme is alcohol dehydrogenase. This enzyme catalyzes the conversion of alcohol to acetaldehyde, and aldehyde dehydrogenase subsequently catalyzes the conversion of acetaldehyde to acetate. Alcohol dehydrogenase catalysis changes the oxidation-reduction state in the cell by increasing the ratio of reduced nicotinamide adenine dinucleotide to the oxidized form, which has important implications for other cellular processes, including the generation of free radicals, inhibition of other enzyme systems, and accumulation of fat. Also, an isoform of alcohol dehydrogenase occurs within the gastric mucosa. Although the clinical importance of the gastric component of alcohol metabolism is debated, up to a quarter of alcohol metabolism may occur there, and sex-based differences in the activity of this isoform may help to explain why women have a lower threshold for alcohol-induced liver damage.

The MEOS is localized in the endoplasmic reticulum of the hepatocyte, whereas the alcohol dehydrogenase system operates in the cytosol. The MEOS appears to be more important in alcohol metabolism when blood levels of alcohol are moderate to high. Under normal conditions when alcohol levels are low, the role of the MEOS is much smaller than that of the alcohol dehydrogenase system. As explained by its enzyme kinetics, the MEOS has a greater role in cases of chronic alcohol

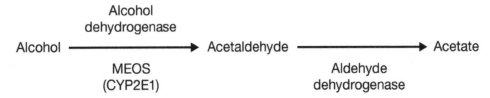

Figure 26.1. Alcohol Metabolism. Alcohol is metabolized to acetaldehyde by alcohol dehydrogenase and cytochrome P450 2E1 isozyme (CYP2E1). In most persons, the alcohol dehydrogenase pathway is dominant; however, in persons with alcohol use disorder and those with high blood levels of alcohol, CYP2E1 is induced and has a major role in metabolism. Acetaldehyde derived from both these pathways is metabolized by aldehyde dehydrogenase to acetate. MEOS indicates microsomal ethanol-oxidizing system.

use because it is induced by alcohol, thereby progressively increased ethanol metabolism in people with alcohol use disorder. The MEOS also converts alcohol to acetaldehyde, requiring aldehyde dehydrogenase for further metabolism. Importantly, the specific MEOS enzyme cytochrome P450 2E1 isozyme (CYP2E1) is responsible for the metabolism of various other compounds. The induction of CYP2E1 by alcohol affects blood levels of these compounds and accounts for the increased tolerance to sedatives for persons who have alcohol use disorder. Other compounds that are metabolized rapidly by this process in persons with alcohol use disorder include isoniazid and, importantly, acetaminophen.

Nearly half the people in eastern and southeastern Asia are deficient in aldehyde dehydrogenase activity because of the inheritance of an allelic variation. This can result in excess accumulation of aldehyde, accounting for alcohol-induced flushing symptoms in these persons. A similar flushing syndrome is observed in response to alcohol consumption when a person ingests disulfiram, which is the basis for its use in the treatment of alcoholism.

Experimental evidence suggests that the alcohol metabolite acetaldehyde may be a toxic mediator of alcohol-induced liver injury. The mechanism by which alcohol and acetaldehyde cause liver injury is being investigated. The initiation of fat accumulation within the liver appears to occur in response to the decreased oxidation and increased accumulation of fatty acids. These events may be linked to changes in the liver oxidation-reduction state induced by ethanol metabolism. Other important physiologic events that mediate liver injury include increased oxidative stress, hepatocyte apoptosis and necrosis, and deposition of collagen, with ensuing fibrosis through activation of hepatic stellate cells. Various cytokines, transcription factors, and intracellular signaling pathways have been implicated in these events.

✓ Alcohol dehydrogenase is the primary alcohol-metabolizing pathway, particularly when blood alcohol levels are low
✓ The microsomal ethanol-oxidizing system is important in persons with alcohol use disorder, especially when blood levels of alcohol are high, and induction of this system affects the metabolism of various xenobiotics, including sedatives and acetaminophen
✓ Diminished activity of aldehyde dehydrogenase accounts for the flushing syndrome detected in a large proportion of Asians who consume alcohol and in patients who take disulfiram

Fatty Liver

Clinical Presentation

A 22-year-old male college student has a series of laboratory tests performed during a routine checkup at the student health clinic. He is asymptomatic, and the physical examination findings are normal. He takes no medications and has no family history of liver disease. He is not sexually active and says he does not use intravenous or intranasal drugs, has not traveled recently, and has not had blood transfusions. Laboratory findings include the following: aspartate aminotransferase (AST) 65 U/L (reference range, 8-48 U/L); alanine aminotransferase (ALT) 43 U/L (reference range, 7-55 U/L); γ-glutamyltransferase (GGT) 336 U/L (reference range, 9-31 U/L); mean corpuscular volume, normal; and total bilirubin and alkaline phosphatase levels, normal. On further questioning, the patient admits to having had 6 to 10 drinks daily over the past week during student orientation.

This patient has clinical features suggestive of alcohol-related fatty liver. The diagnosis and treatment are discussed below.

History and Physical Examination

Bland macrovesicular hepatic steatosis, without necroinflammatory activity, may develop in response to only a transient alcohol insult over a period of days. The most salient historic feature is an alcohol binge. Liver steatosis results almost universally in those who consume alcohol regularly. Patients with fatty liver may be entirely asymptomatic or may complain of mild, nonspecific symptoms, including fatigue, malaise, abdominal discomfort, and anorexia. On physical examination, tender hepatomegaly may be prominent. Stigmata of chronic liver disease are absent, and in many patients, the physical examination findings are normal.

Laboratory and Radiographic Features

Laboratory studies may show mild to moderate increases in the serum levels of aminotransferases, predominantly an increase in AST. The classic 2:1 ratio of AST to ALT is not pathognomonic, but since AST exists both in the cytosol and in the mitochondria and since alcohol is a mitochondrial toxin, the AST level is typically higher than the ALT level. In addition, ALT production requires vitamin B$_6$, which is depleted during alcohol metabolism. Minor increases in alkaline phosphatase or bilirubin (or both) may also be observed. Prothrombin time is generally normal. As in the above case, laboratory abnormalities often are noted incidentally in an asymptomatic person.

Histologic Features

Generally, liver biopsy is not necessary to establish the diagnosis of alcohol-related fatty liver because the condition is benign and reversible. However, biopsy may be performed to determine whether the patient has more advanced alcohol-related liver disease or another condition. The principal feature of alcohol-related fatty liver in biopsy specimens is macrovesicular steatosis within hepatocytes (Figure 26.2). There are no inflammatory cells or collagen deposition. Because biopsy specimens from patients with other causes of chronic liver disease can also feature steatosis, an evaluation for these entities is sometimes advocated. It is noteworthy that certain classic causes of microvesicular steatosis and macrovesicular steatosis can be identified in addition to a mixed macrovesicular-microvesicular pattern (Box 26.1). An evaluation of ceruloplasmin (to screen for Wilson disease), hepatitis C status, α$_1$-antitrypsin phenotype, and iron stores is reasonable for young patients who have steatosis and abnormal levels of enzymes.

Prognosis and Treatment

No specific treatment other than abstinence is required for management of alcohol-related fatty liver. If abstinence is achieved, alcohol-related fatty liver is usually reversible. However, 20% to 30% of patients who continue to drink excessive amounts of alcohol chronically develop more advanced forms of alcohol-related liver disease, including alcohol-related hepatitis or cirrhosis (or both).

✓ Alcohol-related fatty liver may develop in response to short periods of alcohol misuse, although it is more common with chronic alcohol use disorder
✓ Treatment—abstinence or more judicious consumption of alcohol

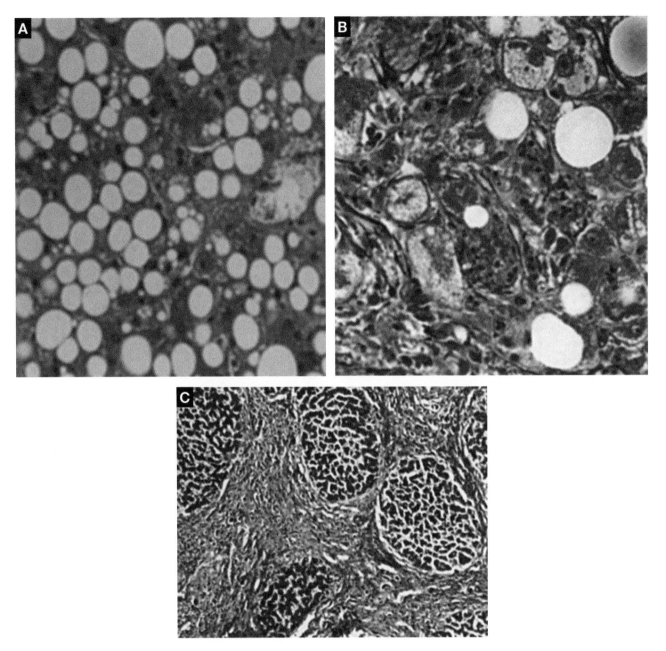

Figure 26.2.   Histopathologic Features of Alcohol-Related Liver Disease. A, Fatty liver. Note the macrovesicular steatosis and lack of inflammation and collagen deposition (hematoxylin-eosin). B, Alcohol-related hepatitis. Note the polymorphonuclear infiltrates, hepatocyte necrosis, steatosis, Mallory bodies, and variable amounts of fibrosis (hematoxylin-eosin). C, Alcohol-related cirrhosis. Note the characteristic micronodular cirrhosis, although a mixed nodularity pattern is often observed (trichrome). Frequently, there is prominent secondary hemosiderosis. (Adapted from Kanel GC, Korula J. Liver biopsy evaluation: histologic diagnosis and clinical correlations. Philadelphia [PA]: WB Saunders Company; 2000:39, 89, 94; used with permission.)

Severe Alcohol-Related Hepatitis

Clinical Presentation

A 36-year-old man describes having fatigue, dark urine, and abdominal swelling. He admits to drinking a few beers daily since his teen years, but he has never had a major medical problem. Recently, he has been drinking more heavily while unemployed. He states that he has not had blood transfusions and does not use intravenous drugs. Physical examination findings are remarkable for tachycardia and low-grade fever. He has prominent scleral icterus, and the abdominal examination shows shifting dullness. The liver span is increased on percussion.

This patient has the clinical features typical of severe alcohol-related hepatitis. The diagnosis and treatment are discussed below.

History and Physical Examination

A constellation of clinical symptoms, often nonspecific, are frequently present in patients with more advanced lesions, such as alcohol-related hepatitis. Men who drink more than 60 to 80 g of alcohol daily for a period of years are at risk for alcohol-related hepatitis; the threshold is approximately half this amount for women. Also, alcohol-related hepatitis may develop in the presence or absence of underlying liver cirrhosis. The clinical

Box 26.1. Causes of Macrovesicular and Microvesicular Steatosis

Causes of macrovesicular steatosis

Alcohol

Metabolic disease–associated fatty liver

Hepatitis C (especially genotype 3)

Wilson disease

Lysosomal acid lipase deficiency

Starvation or rapid weight loss

Long-term total parenteral nutrition

Medications: amiodarone, methotrexate, diltiazem, tamoxifen, corticosteroids, highly active antiretroviral therapy (HAART)

Causes of microvesicular steatosis

Reye syndrome

Acute fatty liver of pregnancy

Inborn errors of metabolism

Medications: valproate, tetracycline

presentation of patients with alcohol-related hepatitis includes constitutional symptoms such as weakness, anorexia, and weight loss and other nonspecific symptoms such as nausea and vomiting. Patients with severe alcohol-related hepatitis may have more advanced symptoms related to portal hypertension, including gastrointestinal bleeding, ascites, hepatorenal syndrome, and hepatic encephalopathy. It is important to identify risk factors for concomitant or other forms of acute and chronic hepatitis, such as viral hepatitis, Wilson disease, and drug-induced hepatitis.

The diagnosis of alcohol-related hepatitis is contingent on determining whether the patient is misusing alcohol. This is not always easy because patients with alcohol use disorder and their family members often minimize or hide their alcohol use. An independent history from multiple family members is often necessary to corroborate the patient's alcohol history, and different caregivers may obtain a different history from the same interviewee. It is also critical to obtain this history early in the course of the disease since the information is critical to subsequent decisions, such as those related to transplant candidacy, and since encephalopathy may develop later and limit the ability to obtain these historic details.

Questionnaires have been used to clarify alcohol use and misuse syndromes; however, because of their length, many of them are limited to research purposes. One useful screening questionnaire in clinical practice is the CAGE questionnaire, which includes the following inquiries: Has the patient felt the need to *cut down* on alcohol use? Has the patient become *annoyed* with other persons' concerns about the patient's alcohol use? Does the patient feel *guilty* about the patient's alcohol use? Does the patient use alcohol in the morning as an *eye-opener*? Although 2 positive responses have a high sensitivity and positive predictive value for alcohol dependency, any positive response to these inquiries requires a more detailed investigation and should increase suspicion for alcohol use disorder. The Alcohol Use Disorders Identification Test (AUDIT) is a 10-item screening tool developed by the World Health Organization to assess alcohol drinking behaviors and related problems.

In patients with alcohol-related hepatitis, physical examination findings are most notable for tender hepatomegaly, fever, and

hyperdynamic circulation. Other findings depend on the severity of liver insult, the presence or absence of concomitant cirrhosis, and the presence or absence of portal hypertension. These findings may include jaundice, splenomegaly, collateral vessels, hypogonadism, palmar erythema, hepatic bruit, asterixis, and ascites in patients with severe alcohol-related hepatitis and portal hypertension. Concern for concomitant infection is common because of overlapping features of alcohol-related hepatitis and infections (eg, fever, tachycardia, abdominal pain, and leukocytosis).

Laboratory and Radiographic Features

Laboratory abnormalities reflect the extrahepatic adverse effects of alcohol and alcohol-induced liver injury (Box 26.2). Mean corpuscular volume usually is increased, reflecting the adverse effect of alcohol on erythrocytes. The levels of triglycerides and uric acid also are frequently increased. Patients are prone to ketoacidosis. Peripheral polymorphonuclear leukocytosis is prominent, and in some cases, a dramatic leukemoid reaction may be present with strikingly high white blood cell counts. Aminotransferase levels are usually increased less than 5 to 10 times normal, but they may be higher with concomitant acetaminophen toxicity. Also, the level of AST is almost always higher than that of ALT, which is opposite of the pattern seen in nonalcohol-related steatohepatitis. This in combination with other variables determines the alcohol-related liver disease—nonalcohol-related fatty liver disease index (https://www.mayoclinic.org/medical-profes sionals/transplant-medicine/calculators/the-alcoholic-liver-dise ase-nonalcoholic-fatty-liver-disease-index-ani/itt-20434726). The index is a tool that helps distinguish metabolic fatty liver disease from alcohol-related liver disease.

Abnormal results of some laboratory tests, including prothrombin time and bilirubin concentration, reflect the severity of alcohol-induced liver dysfunction and are prognostically useful (in contrast to aminotransferase levels). Attempts have been made

Box 26.2. Abnormal Results of Laboratory Tests in Alcohol-Related Hepatitis

Hematology

Macrocytic anemia (increased MCV)

Leukocytosis

Thrombocytopenia

General chemistry

Hyperglycemia

Hyperuricemia

Hypertriglyceridemia

Ketosis

Liver function and injury

Hypoalbuminemia

Hyperbilirubinemia

Increased prothrombin time

Increased AST:ALT ratio (ratio, 1.5 to 2.5; total increase <10-fold)

Increased γ-glutamyltransferase

Increased alkaline phosphatase (mild increase)

Abbreviations: ALT, alanine aminotransferase; AST, aspartate aminotransferase; MCV, mean corpuscular volume.

Box 26.3.   Maddrey Discriminant Function (MDF)

MDF = 4.6 × (PT – Control PT) + Serum Bilirubin
Concentration (mg/dL)

Abbreviation: PT, prothrombin time.

---

to use bilirubin concentration, prothrombin time, and other laboratory variables to assess the prognosis of patients who have alcohol-related hepatitis. Of those assessments, the most historically noted is the Maddrey discriminant function (MDF) (Box 26.3). An MDF value greater than 32 effectively identifies patients whose short-term risk of death exceeds 50% and for whom consideration of treatment with corticosteroids is justified.

Among patients with alcohol-related hepatitis, a Model for End-stage Liver Disease (MELD) score of 21 or more appears to predict short-term risk of death as well as or better than the MDF threshold of 32. The MELD score and corresponding 90-day survival can be calculated on the basis of the patient's international normalized ratio and bilirubin, creatinine, and sodium values at the following website: https://www.mayoclinic.org/medical-professionals/transplant-medicine/calculators/meld-score-and-90-day-mortality-rate-for-alcoholic-hepatitis/itt-20434719. The general familiarity with MELD, the general availability of its components, and the ease of its calculation have led to an increased use of MELD over MDF.

The Lille score is another clinical prediction tool, driven largely by the change in bilirubin levels after 1 week of medical therapy, that can help in the decision to discontinue corticosteroid therapy for patients who are not having a response. Other frequently observed laboratory abnormalities that may cause diagnostic confusion or suggest multifactorial liver disease include increases in iron saturation indices and ferritin, hepatitis C virus (HCV) antibody positivity, and increased levels of autoimmune markers, such as antinuclear antibody and anti–smooth muscle antibody. Rather than reflecting the concomitant presence of hereditary hemochromatosis or autoimmune hepatitis, increases in iron indices and autoimmune markers more commonly reflect the pathogenic role of iron deposition and autoimmunity in the development of alcohol-related hepatitis. If the alcohol history is questionable, a Doppler ultrasonographic study is useful to exclude alternative diagnoses, such as cholecystitis, biliary obstruction, and hepatic vein thrombosis, which may manifest like alcohol-related hepatitis. The false diagnosis of gallstone disease can be catastrophic because of the high surgical morbidity and mortality of patients with alcohol-related hepatitis.

With the inherent difficulties in obtaining a reliable history of alcohol use, several biochemical markers have been evaluated for the detection of surreptitious misuse of alcohol. Many traditional serologic tests of alcohol misuse assess it indirectly by examining markers of liver injury such as AST, ALT, the AST:ALT ratio, and GGT. However, because these tests assess alcohol misuse indirectly by detecting liver injury, their sensitivity and specificity generally are less than 70%. Mean corpuscular volume also indirectly assesses alcohol misuse by evaluating the bone marrow toxicity of alcohol. Carbohydrate-deficient transferrin reflects the desialylation of transferrin that occurs in response to high alcohol use, and mitochondrial AST is a specific isoform of the enzyme that is released from hepatocytes injured by alcohol. However, these tests have not been shown universally to be more effective than the less expensive AST:ALT ratio, GGT, and mean corpuscular volume. More recently, various sensitive alcohol biomarkers, including ethyl glucuronide and phosphatidylethanol, are being used to detect surreptitious alcohol use in patients.

Histologic Features

With recent advances in noninvasive liver diagnostic capabilities, the diagnosis of alcohol-related hepatitis is often made without liver biopsy. However, liver biopsy is indicated if the diagnosis is in question after noninvasive evaluation. In particular, histologic examination may be useful in distinguishing coexisting or alternative liver disorders, such as hereditary hemochromatosis in persons with high iron saturation levels, Wilson disease in younger persons with low to low-normal ceruloplasmin levels, autoimmune hepatitis in persons with high titers of autoimmune markers, and hepatitis C in persons with positive results for HCV antibody. Liver biopsy, if pursued, may require a transjugular route rather than a percutaneous route, depending on the degree of coagulopathy and thrombocytopenia.

In alcohol-related hepatitis, liver biopsy specimens show several characteristic features, including centrilobular and sometimes periportal polymorphonuclear infiltrates, centrilobular hepatocyte swelling, ballooning degeneration, macrovesicular steatosis, and Mallory bodies (Figure 26.2). Often, pericentral and perisinusoidal fibrosis is detected with a trichrome stain. The terminal hepatic venules frequently are obliterated, and indeed the zone 3 region of the liver acinus shows the most prominent injury. Mallory bodies (eosinophilic-staining condensed cytoskeletal structures) are not specific for alcohol-related hepatitis. However, their presence in association with other salient biopsy features strongly suggests alcohol-related hepatitis. Prominent neutrophilic infiltration of hepatocytes containing Mallory bodies is termed *satellitosis*. Giant mitochondria (*megamitochondria*) are another characteristic feature. In up to 50% of cases, concomitant cirrhosis may be present. Importantly, metabolic disease–associated steatohepatitis cannot be differentiated reliably from alcohol-related hepatitis with liver biopsy specimens because of the overlap of histologic features.

Prognosis and Treatment

Abstinence

Abstinence is the most important factor in both short- and long-term survival of patients with alcohol-related hepatitis. For patients who recover and remain abstinent, the disease may continue to improve (ie, clinical sequelae and laboratory variables improve) for as long as 6 months. Although the condition of some patients continues to deteriorate even with abstinence, the 5-year survival rate for this group is more than 60%. However, for patients who continue to drink, the 5-year survival rate is less than 30%. While medications to reduce alcohol cravings, such as acamprosate or baclofen, are attractive options, their use has not been studied well, and they should be considered only in conjunction with an experienced addiction specialist. Recent trends also point to a role for cognitive behavioral therapy in maintaining abstinence.

Nutrition

Malnutrition is almost universal among patients with alcohol-related hepatitis because of concomitant poor dietary habits, anorexia, and encephalopathy. Although malnutrition was once thought to cause alcohol-related liver disease, it is no longer considered to have a major role in the pathogenesis of the disease. However, maintenance of a positive nitrogen balance and provision of adequate energy requirements through nutritional support are a vital supportive treatment approach. Patients with alcohol-related hepatitis generally have greater protein and energy needs because of the stress of illness and underlying malnutrition. Recommendations include caloric supplementation at 30 to 40 kcal/kg ideal body weight and protein supplementation at 1 to 1.5 g/kg ideal body weight. Provision of nutrients in excess of calculated requirements is unlikely to be of benefit. Every attempt should be made to provide adequate calories enterally. However, parenteral support may be necessary for some patients. Encephalopathy does not require protein restriction in most patients. For patients with severe encephalopathy that is exacerbated by dietary protein, branched-chain amino acid supplements can be considered. Increased use of dietary vegetable protein may be better tolerated than animal protein. Amino acid supplementation probably does not improve survival sufficiently for the added cost.

Corticosteroids

Corticosteroids have been studied extensively for the treatment of alcohol-related hepatitis. Although many of the initial controlled trials did not show a benefit, further analysis suggested that patients with encephalopathy and more severe disease may benefit. Therefore, follow-up studies focused on the role of corticosteroids in the treatment of patients who had an MDF function greater than 32 or hepatic encephalopathy (or both) but not kidney failure, infection, gastrointestinal tract bleeding, or, in some studies, severe type 2 diabetes. Some studies and meta-analyses that used these criteria showed that corticosteroid therapy provided a survival benefit for patients with an MDF greater than 32 or hepatic encephalopathy (or both); however, a MELD score of 21 or more appears to be an acceptable alternative threshold. In 2015, a large randomized controlled study did not show a statistically significant benefit with the use of prednisolone for alcohol-related hepatitis. Therefore, the use of corticosteroid therapy for alcohol-related hepatitis is controversial and varies among experienced hepatologists.

Pentoxifylline

Kupffer cell–derived tumor necrosis factor (TNF)-α may be important in the pathogenesis of alcohol-related hepatitis. Consequently, there has been interest historically in using the phosphodiesterase inhibitor pentoxifylline, which inhibits TNF-α transcription, for treatment of alcohol-related hepatitis. However, additional studies have not supported its use, and it is no longer considered appropriate therapy. Other anti-TNF therapies, such as infliximab and etanercept, have been studied, but the results have been similarly disappointing.

Other Pharmacotherapies Being Studied

Alcohol induces oxidative stress in the liver, resulting in an imbalance between oxidants and antioxidants. Looking for a way to decrease oxygen consumption by the liver, investigators have studied the role of propylthiouracil in treating alcohol-related hepatitis, but the results have been inconclusive. Colchicine has also been evaluated for treating alcohol-related hepatitis, but no clinical benefit has been found. Other hepatoprotective compounds, such as S-adenosyl-L-methionine, phosphatidylcholine, milk thistle, and N-acetylcysteine, have been evaluated but are not widely accepted.

Management of Portal Hypertension

Complications of portal hypertension may develop in patients with alcohol-related hepatitis regardless of the presence or absence of underlying cirrhosis. This clinical observation is supported by studies showing that alcohol directly increases portal pressure, and it emphasizes the importance of the vascular component of intrahepatic resistance and portal hypertension. Hepatic encephalopathy, bleeding esophageal varices, ascites, spontaneous bacterial peritonitis, and hepatorenal syndrome are complications of portal hypertension commonly encountered in patients with alcohol-related hepatitis. The management of these complications is discussed elsewhere in this book.

Treatment of Infection

Because of underlying malnutrition, liver cirrhosis, and iatrogenic complications, infection is one of the most common causes of death among patients with alcohol-related hepatitis. The patients must be evaluated carefully for infections, including spontaneous bacterial peritonitis, aspiration pneumonia, and lower extremity cellulitis. These infections should be treated aggressively with antibiotics. However, fever and leukocytosis are common in patients with alcohol-related hepatitis, even without infection.

Liver Transplant

Recent studies have shown that early liver transplant improves survival among highly selected groups of patients not responding to medical therapy. While many patients with alcohol-related hepatitis are not suitable candidates for liver transplant because of psychosocial reasons, abstinence for less than 6 months is not itself an absolute contraindication to liver transplant. Thus, patients who do not respond to medical therapy definitely warrant discussion with a liver transplant center team that has the expertise and resources to determine whether an evaluation for liver transplant is appropriate.

✓ Alcohol-related hepatitis may occur with or without preexisting liver cirrhosis

✓ Liver biopsy should be considered if the cause of hepatitis is questioned and specific treatments for other entities are being contemplated

✓ Histologic features cannot be used to reliably differentiate alcohol-related hepatitis from metabolic disease–associated steatohepatitis; the distinction is made best on the basis of the clinical history and the pattern of laboratory test results

✓ For most patients, the treatment of alcohol-related hepatitis includes abstinence, supportive care, and management of malnutrition, infection, and complications of portal hypertension

✓ Liver transplant evaluation can be considered for selected patients who do not respond to medical management

---

Alcohol-Related Cirrhosis

Clinical Presentation

A 56-year-old salesman is admitted to the hospital with a 2-hour history of hematemesis and dizziness. His history is remarkable for symptoms of fatigue and lower extremity edema. His wife notes that his memory has been poor recently and that he has been a "social drinker" for many years, having a few martinis with clients and during business trips. Physical examination findings are notable for orthostasis, temporal wasting, spider angiomas on the chest, and bilateral pitting edema of the lower extremities. His skin is jaundiced, and a liver edge is palpable and firm. The tip of the spleen is palpable upon inspiration. Rectal examination shows melena in the vault. There is prominent asterixis.

This patient has the clinical features typical of alcohol-related cirrhosis. The diagnosis and treatment are discussed below.

History and Physical Examination

Among persons with a clinical history of marked and prolonged misuse of alcohol, liver cirrhosis eventually develops in only about 20%. The presence or absence of symptoms is due largely to the presence or absence of liver decompensation. Patients with cirrhosis and compensated liver function may have minimal symptoms. The symptoms of patients with liver decompensation reflect the severity of portal hypertension, malnutrition, and degree of synthetic liver dysfunction and include nonspecific fatigue, weakness, and anorexia. More specific symptoms are related to the presence of specific complications of cirrhosis and portal hypertension, including gastrointestinal tract bleeding, ascites, encephalopathy, hepatorenal syndrome, and hepatocellular carcinoma. Physical examination findings may include stigmata of chronic liver disease (spider angiomas and palmar erythema), complications of portal hypertension (ascites, splenomegaly, asterixis, and pedal edema), signs of excess estrogen (gynecomastia and hypogonadism), and signs of systemic alcohol toxicity (peripheral neuropathy, dementia, and Dupuytren contracture).

Laboratory and Radiographic Features

Prominent laboratory abnormalities include an increase in the prothrombin time and bilirubin level and a decrease in the albumin level, which are reflected in an increased Child-Turcotte-Pugh score. Imaging findings may be suggestive of cirrhosis and ensuing portal hypertension, as indicated by heterogeneous liver echotexture, splenomegaly, collateralization, and ascites on ultrasonography. Computed tomography may show changes in liver contour, splenomegaly, collateralization, or ascites. Patients with cirrhosis are at risk for hepatocellular carcinoma and should be evaluated biannually with ultrasonography, with or without serum alpha-fetoprotein levels, as should patients who have had recent clinical decompensation. Patients with cirrhosis are also at risk for esophageal varices, which, when large, can cause life-threatening bleeding. Therefore, screening for esophageal varices with upper endoscopy is also indicated for patients who have cirrhosis.

Histologic Features

Traditionally, alcohol-related cirrhosis is classified as a micronodular cirrhosis (Figure 26.2). However, in many patients, larger nodules also develop, leading to mixed micro-macronodular cirrhosis. The earliest collagen deposition occurs around the terminal hepatic venules, and progression to pericentral fibrosis portends irreversible architectural changes. Hemosiderin deposition is often prominent. In patients with alcohol-related cirrhosis who continue to drink actively, many of the histologic features of alcohol-related hepatitis also are present.

Prognosis and Treatment

A good prognosis depends on the absence of liver decompensation and complications of portal hypertension and on the patient's ability to maintain abstinence. The prognosis for patients with cirrhosis who are well compensated and able to maintain abstinence is reasonably good (5-year survival rate >80%). Even for patients with decompensation, the 5-year survival rate with abstinence is more than 50%. However, patients who continue to drink have a much worse prognosis (5-year survival rate <30%).

The only established effective therapy for alcohol-related cirrhosis is liver transplant. Currently, alcohol-related liver disease is the most common indication for liver transplant in adults in the US. However, less than 20% of patients with end-stage alcohol-related liver disease undergo transplant. Despite perceptions to the contrary, survival rates after transplant for alcohol-related liver disease are comparable to those after transplant for other indications. In fact, the risk of acute cellular rejection is actually lower for persons undergoing transplant for alcohol-related liver disease than for those with other conditions.

A major issue in maintaining excellent outcomes for this population focuses on identifying candidates with a low risk for recidivism after transplant. Alcohol relapse after transplant varies among centers and is difficult to quantify accurately, but it is probably about 15% to 30%. Although detecting surreptitious alcohol use after transplant can be difficult, the low incidence of graft loss from recurrent alcohol-related liver disease suggests that most patients who return to drinking after transplant do not drink to the point of endangering the graft. However, heavy use of alcohol after liver transplant can cause rapid development of cirrhosis in the graft. Alcohol use also may interfere with compliance in taking immunosuppressive medications and alter the perception of the general public toward liver transplant, thus adversely affecting potential organ donors. Therefore, selecting patients who are appropriate for liver transplant requires a multidisciplinary team involving a hepatologist, transplant surgeon, addiction specialist, psychiatrist, and social worker. Currently, many transplant centers advocate 6 months of abstinence, appropriate addiction treatment, aftercare with Alcoholics Anonymous attendance and sponsorship, and demonstrated family and social support before performing a liver transplant for alcohol-related cirrhosis.

✓ Alcohol causes micronodular or mixed micro-macronodular cirrhosis in about 20% of people with prolonged, excessive use of alcohol
✓ Alcohol-related cirrhosis is currently the most common indication for liver transplant, which is the only curative treatment
✓ Only a small proportion of patients with alcohol-related cirrhosis undergo transplant, because of various psychosocial barriers
✓ Transplant outcomes for alcohol-related liver disease are comparable to those for most other indications

---

Alcohol and Acetaminophen

Patients who regularly use alcohol are at increased risk for acetaminophen-induced hepatotoxicity. An acetaminophen dosage of as little as 2.5 to 3 g daily may result in pronounced hepatotoxicity in patients who use alcohol. The reason for this is that both alcohol and acetaminophen are metabolized in part by CYP2E1, an enzyme in the MEOS. With the induction of this enzyme by alcohol, a greater proportion of acetaminophen is metabolized by this pathway than by the sulfation and glucuronidation detoxification pathways. The byproduct of acetaminophen metabolism by CYP2E1 is *N*-acetyl-*p*-benzoquinone imine, which is toxic to the liver. The accumulation of this compound in conjunction with diminished antioxidant defenses in the liver (glutathione) lowers the threshold of acetaminophen toxicity in patients using alcohol.

The clinical presentation of regular alcohol users with acetaminophen toxicity is distinct from that of patients with alcohol-related hepatitis. Aminotransferase levels are markedly increased—often exceeding 1,000 U/L—which is distinctly unusual for alcohol-related hepatitis. This situation may arise when a regular alcohol user has a minor illness, discontinues alcohol use, and takes moderate doses of acetaminophen (the so-called therapeutic misadventure). Ironically, discontinuation of alcohol perpetuates this problem since more cellular resources are then available for acetaminophen metabolism. Therefore, patients who use alcohol regularly should not use acetaminophen without the supervision of a physician and should limit their intake. In contrast, acetaminophen is the analgesic of choice for patients with cirrhosis, including alcohol-related cirrhosis, as long as the patient is not currently using alcohol. However, patients with cirrhosis should limit acetaminophen intake to a collective dosage that does not exceed 2 g every 24 hours.

Suggested Reading

Asrani S, Sanchez W. Epidemiology of alcoholic liver disease. In: Talley NJ, Locke GR, Moayyedi P, West JJ, Ford AC, Saito YA, eds. GI epidemiology: diseases and clinical methodology, 2nd ed. John Wiley & Sons; 2014:332–43.

Carithers R, McClain C. Alcoholic liver disease. In: Feldman M, Friedman LS, Sleisenger MH, eds. Sleisenger & Fordtran's gastrointestinal and liver disease: pathophysiology, diagnosis, management. 9th ed. Saunders; 2010:1383–400.

Ceccanti M, Attili A, Balducci G, Attilia F, Giacomelli S, Rotondo C, et al. Acute alcoholic hepatitis. J Clin Gastroenterol. 2006 Oct;40(9): 833–41.

Dominguez M, Rincon D, Abraldes JG, Miquel R, Colmenero J, Bellot P, et al. A new scoring system for prognostic stratification of patients with alcoholic hepatitis. Am J Gastroenterol. 2008 Nov;103(11):2747–56.

Dunn W, Angulo P, Sanderson S, Jamil LH, Stadheim L, Rosen C, et al. Utility of a new model to diagnose an alcohol basis for steatohepatitis. Gastroenterology. 2006 Oct;131(4):1057–63.

Gramenzi A, Caputo F, Biselli M, Kuria F, Loggi E, Andreone P, et al. Alcoholic liver disease: pathophysiological aspects and risk factors. Aliment Pharmacol Ther. 2006 Oct 15;24(8):1151–61.

Haber PS, Warner R, Seth D, Gorrell MD, McCaughan GW. Pathogenesis and management of alcoholic hepatitis. J Gastroenterol Hepatol. 2003 Dec;18(12):1332–44.

Hill DB, Deaciuc IV, Nanji AA, McClain CJ. Mechanisms of hepatic injury in alcoholic liver disease. Clin Liver Dis. 1998;2(4):703–21.

Julien J, Ayer T, Bethea ED, Tapper EB, Chhatwal J. Projected prevalence and mortality associated with alcohol-related liver disease in the USA, 2019–40: a modelling study. Lancet Public Health. 2020 Jun;5(6):e316–e23.

Kourkoumpetis T, Sood G. Pathogenesis of alcoholic liver disease: an update. Clin Liver Dis. 2019 Feb;23(1):71–80.

Lucey MR, Mathurin P, Morgan TR. Alcoholic hepatitis. N Engl J Med. 2009 Jun;360(26):2758–69.

Maher JJ. Alcoholic steatosis and steatohepatitis. Semin Gastrointest Dis. 2002 Jan;13(1):31–9.

Marsano LS, Mendez C, Hill D, Barve S, McClain CJ. Diagnosis and treatment of alcoholic liver disease and its complications. Alcohol Res Health. 2003; 27(3):247–56.

Menon KV, Gores GJ, Shah VH. Pathogenesis, diagnosis, and treatment of alcoholic liver disease. Mayo Clin Proc. 2001 Oct;76(10):1021–9.

Singal AK, Bataller R, Ahn J, Kamath PS, Shah VH. ACG clinical guideline: alcoholic liver disease. Am J Gastroenterol. 2018 Feb;113(2):175–94.

Tome S, Lucey MR. Current management of alcoholic liver disease. Aliment Pharmacol Ther. 2004 Apr;19(7):707–14.

Zeng MD, Li YM, Chen CW, Lu LG, Fan JG, Wang BY, et al. Guidelines for the diagnosis and treatment of alcoholic liver disease. J Dig Dis. 2008 May;9(2):113–6.

27

Vascular Diseases of the Liver[a]

TASHA B. KULAI, MD

WILLIAM SANCHEZ, MD

Vascular diseases of the liver can be divided into disorders of hepatic inflow (ie, disorders of portal venous inflow and disorders of hepatic arterial inflow) and disorders of hepatic venous outflow (Box 27.1). For a better understanding of the vascular diseases of the liver, a concise review of the vascular anatomy of the liver is important.

Anatomy of the Splanchnic Circulation

The splanchnic circulation comprises the arterial blood supply and venous drainage of the entire gastrointestinal tract from the distal esophagus to the midrectum and includes the spleen (which is why splenomegaly and thrombocytopenia develop in the presence of portal hypertension), pancreas, gallbladder, and liver. The arterial system is derived from the celiac artery and the superior and inferior mesenteric arteries. The celiac artery arises from the anterior aorta and typically gives rise to 3 major branches: the left gastric artery, the common hepatic artery, and the splenic artery. The superior mesenteric artery arises from the abdominal aorta just distal to the celiac trunk. The superior mesenteric artery gives off 3 sets of branches: 1) several small branches to the pancreas and duodenum before entering the mesentery, 2) 3 large arteries that supply the proximal two-thirds of the large bowel, and 3) during its course through the mesenteric root, an arcade of arterial branches to the jejunum and ileum. The branches given off in the mesentery form a row of arterial arcades that terminate in the arteriae rectae of the wall of the small bowel. The inferior mesenteric artery arises 3 cm above the aortic bifurcation close to the inferior border of the duodenum. It branches into the left colic artery and terminates as the superior rectal artery. The venous drainage has a similar pattern, with the venae rectae forming a venous arcade that drains the small bowel and:

The arterial routes of the splanchnic circulation, except for the hepatic artery, eventually empty into the portal venous system through the splenic vein and superior and inferior mesenteric veins. The portal vein, formed by the convergence of the splenic and superior mesenteric veins, constitutes the primary blood supply to the liver. After perfusing the liver, venous blood reenters the systemic circulation through the hepatic veins and suprahepatic inferior vena cava.

The liver receives a dual blood supply. The 2 sources are portal venous blood (derived from the mesenteric venous circulation, including the digestive tract, spleen, and pancreas) and hepatic arterial

---

[a] Portions previously published in Menon KV, Shah V, Kamath PS. The Budd-Chiari syndrome. N Engl J Med. 2004 Feb;350(6):578-85; used with permission.

Abbreviations: BCS, Budd-Chiari syndrome; HHT, hereditary hemorrhagic telangiectasia; SOS, sinusoidal obstruction syndrome; TIPS, transjugular intrahepatic portosystemic shunt

---

Box 27.1. Vascular Diseases of the Liver

Disorders of portal venous inflow
    Acute mesenteric or portal venous thrombosis
    Chronic mesenteric or portal venous thrombosis

Disorders of hepatic arterial inflow
    Hepatic artery thrombosis
    Hepatic arteriovenous fistula
    Ischemic hepatopathy

Disorders of hepatic venous outflow
    Venoocclusive disease
    Budd-Chiari syndrome

blood (usually from the celiac artery). Total hepatic blood flow constitutes nearly 30% of total cardiac output. The portal venous inflow comprises 65% to 75% of hepatic blood inflow, and the hepatic artery comprises approximately 25% to 35%. The hepatic artery is the main blood supply to the biliary tree. Approximately 50% of the liver's oxygen requirements is delivered by hepatic arterial blood.

The hepatic vascular bed is a low-pressure system that can maintain a large volume of blood. Sinusoidal blood collects within terminal hepatic venules and reenters the systemic circulation through the hepatic veins and inferior vena cava. The caudate lobe of the liver maintains a separate venous drainage, accounting for the compensatory hypertrophy of this lobe often observed in chronic liver disease associated with outflow obstruction of the major hepatic veins (Budd-Chiari syndrome [BCS]).

✓ Liver has a dual blood supply
  • Portal venous blood (derived from the mesenteric venous circulation)—70% of flow
  • Hepatic arterial blood (usually from the celiac artery)—30% of flow
✓ Hepatic vascular bed is a low-pressure system

Disorders of Portal Venous Inflow

Acute Mesenteric Venous Thrombosis

Acute mesenteric venous thrombosis is discussed in Chapter 11, "Vascular Disorders of the Gastrointestinal Tract."

Chronic Mesenteric Venous Thrombosis

Chronic mesenteric venous thrombosis is very different from the acute form. Lack of visualization of the superior mesenteric vein on computed tomography or duplex ultrasonography in conjunction with extensive collateral venous drainage suggests the diagnosis of chronic mesenteric venous thrombosis. Angiography can help confirm the diagnosis but rarely is required. Although many patients present with nonspecific symptoms of several months' duration, an increasing proportion are identified through imaging studies performed for unrelated reasons. These patients may be asymptomatic with respect to the primary event; hence, the time of the thrombotic event often is unclear. Patients in whom the thrombosis extends to involve the portal vein or splenic vein (or both) may have portal hypertension and esophageal varices, with the attendant complications of variceal bleeding. They also may have splenomegaly and hypersplenism.

Chronic mesenteric venous thrombosis should be differentiated from isolated splenic vein thrombosis due to pancreatic neoplasm or chronic pancreatitis. Splenic vein thrombosis, often called *sinistral* (or left-sided) *portal hypertension*, is related to a local effect on the splenic vein and is not usually a disorder of the thrombotic pathway. Thus, anticoagulation is not warranted for sinistral portal hypertension.

Patients with isolated chronic mesenteric venous thrombosis often remain asymptomatic because of the development of extensive venous collaterals. Occasionally, some patients have gastrointestinal tract hemorrhage, and the use of a nonselective β-blocker is recommended to prevent variceal bleeding. Endoscopic therapy is used both to control active bleeding and to prevent rebleeding. Surgical intervention (eg, portosystemic shunts) is restricted to patients whose bleeding cannot be controlled with conservative measures and who have a patent central vein for shunting. When thrombosis is extensive and no large vein is suitable for anastomosis, nonconventional shunts (eg, anastomosis of a large collateral vein with a systemic vein) may be considered. Surgical expertise for such

shunts is present in a small number of referral centers. For refractory variceal bleeding, gastroesophageal devascularization may be considered. For patients with thrombophilia, anticoagulation may be initiated after the risk of bleeding has been decreased by the use of β-blockers or, if bleeding has occurred, surgical shunts.

✓ Patients with chronic mesenteric venous thrombosis—typically asymptomatic or with chronic nonspecific symptoms
✓ Propranolol or other nonselective β-blockers are recommended to prevent variceal bleeding in patients who have associated portal hypertension
✓ Endoscopic therapy—to control active bleeding and to prevent rebleeding
✓ Surgical shunts—only for patients whose bleeding cannot be controlled with conservative measures and who have a patent central vein

---

Disorders of Hepatic Arterial Inflow

Hepatic Artery Thrombosis

Aside from patients who have had liver transplant, the prevalence of hepatic artery thrombosis is not certain. Hepatic artery thrombosis is the cause of considerable morbidity and mortality in approximately 3% to 7% of adult recipients of deceased donor transplants, in up to 10% of adult recipients of living donor transplants, and in perhaps as many as 40% of pediatric patients undergoing orthotopic liver transplant. The problem is more extensive in pediatric patients because of the smaller caliber of the vessels involved and the probably greater fluctuation in the concentration of coagulation factors.

Several risk factors are related to the development of hepatic artery thrombosis in adults, with the type of transplant (living donor or deceased donor) and the technical aspects of the arterial anastomosis being the most important risk factors for early thrombosis. Other risk factors are older recipients, clotting abnormalities, tobacco use, and infections by agents such as cytomegalovirus. Late hepatic artery thrombosis has been associated with chronic rejection and blood type–incompatible grafts.

The clinical presentation of hepatic artery thrombosis can vary from a mild increase in the serum level of aminotransferases to fulminant hepatic necrosis. Early hepatic artery thrombosis has a more severe clinical course, and late hepatic artery thrombosis generally has a milder course. There is no agreement about a time that distinguishes *early* from *late* hepatic artery thrombosis. However, the later that hepatic artery thrombosis develops after liver transplant, the less severe the clinical presentation.

Early hepatic artery thrombosis results in massive injury to hepatocytes and bile duct epithelial cells. Ischemic damage to the bile ducts can lead to dehiscence of the biliary anastomosis, bile duct strictures (typically nonanastomotic), and intrahepatic abscesses. Thus, biliary sepsis may be a common presentation of early hepatic artery thrombosis. However, one-third of patients with early hepatic artery thrombosis may be asymptomatic.

Hepatic artery thrombosis can be diagnosed with duplex ultrasonography, but angiography may be necessary to confirm the diagnosis. When hepatic artery thrombosis is detected early after liver transplant, surgical correction usually is recommended. Patients who have early hepatic artery thrombosis with graft dysfunction should be listed for retransplant.

✓ Hepatic artery thrombosis is primarily a complication related to liver transplant
✓ Hepatic artery thrombosis that occurs early after transplant usually requires surgical correction, and relisting the patient for transplant is necessary if acute graft dysfunction develops

Hepatic Artery Aneurysm

Although aneurysm of the hepatic artery (Figure 27.1) is rare, it is the fourth most common abdominal aneurysm. The aneurysms are usually small (<2 cm in diameter) and involve the main hepatic artery. Causes of hepatic artery aneurysms include atherosclerotic vascular diseases, infections (eg, bacterial endocarditis, liver abscess, syphilis, and tuberculosis), and trauma from liver biopsy. The hepatic artery commonly is involved in polyarteritis nodosa, manifested as symptoms related to thrombosis, rupture, or dissection of the aneurysm.

Most hepatic artery aneurysms are discovered incidentally. If they are symptomatic, the first and dominating symptom is severe abdominal pain, suggesting dissection. Vague abdominal pain in these patients is related to compression of surrounding structures. Rupture of a hepatic artery aneurysm causes massive intraperitoneal hemorrhage or hemobilia manifested as abdominal pain, jaundice, and gastrointestinal tract bleeding. Hemobilia is usually a manifestation of an intrahepatic aneurysm.

The treatment of a ruptured aneurysm is emergency surgery or embolization of the aneurysm in patients who are not optimal candidates for surgery. For asymptomatic patients, treatment is debated. Clearly, aneurysms larger than 2 cm in diameter require treatment, and those between 1 and 2 cm in diameter may be treated. For aneurysms smaller than 1 cm in diameter, follow-up at 6-month intervals is reasonable. Treatment includes interventional radiologic approaches to embolize and occlude the aneurysm, ligation at surgery, or excision of the aneurysm and reconstruction of the artery. Intrahepatic aneurysms may also be treated with liver resection.

✓ Hepatic artery aneurysms
- If smaller than 1 cm—monitor with imaging every 6 months
- If 1 to 2 cm, consider surgical repair
- If larger than 2 cm, surgical intervention is required

✓ Ruptured hepatic artery aneurysms
- Patient has severe abdominal pain
- Emergency surgery is required
- Embolization can be considered if patient is not a surgical candidate

---

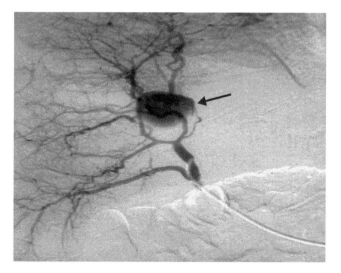

Figure 27.1. Aneurysm of the Hepatic Artery. Selective hepatic angiogram shows an aneurysm (arrow) of the intrahepatic portion of the hepatic artery.

Hepatic Artery–Portal Vein Fistulas

Hepatic artery–portal vein fistulas are rare causes of portal hypertension. Although fistulas within the liver usually are iatrogenic (the result of liver biopsy), they may be related to neoplasms or hereditary hemorrhagic telangiectasia (HHT) (Osler-Weber-Rendu disease). A hepatic artery–portal vein fistula should be suspected in a patient who has acute onset of abdominal pain and ascites, especially if associated with gastrointestinal tract bleeding, because rupture of the artery into the portal vein causes an acute increase in portal pressure. These fistulas may be accompanied by abdominal bruits in most patients. Hepatic artery–portal vein fistulas are treated with coil embolization or surgical ligation. If untreated, a hepatic artery–hepatic vein fistula may result in high-output congestive heart failure. The best treatment is embolization and occlusion of the fistula, except in the presence of HHT, when embolization is absolutely contraindicated. A hepatic artery–portal vein fistula can also result in high-output congestive heart failure. Antibody therapy against vascular endothelial growth factor (bevacizumab) has been shown to be beneficial in patients who have HHT-related bleeding, but its utility in patients with HHT-related liver disease is evolving.

Ischemic Hepatopathy

In patients with congestive heart failure, portal blood flow is minimal; thus, the major contribution of oxygenated blood to the liver is from the hepatic artery. In congestive heart failure, episodes of hypotension, as associated with arrhythmias, diminish hepatic arterial input and result in ischemic necrosis of the liver. Typical manifestations of ischemic hepatopathy are rapid increases (ie, within 24-48 hours) in the serum levels of aminotransferases (aspartate aminotransferase and alanine aminotransferase) to several thousand units per liter (sometimes >10,000 U/L). These values rapidly return to less than 100 U/L in 5 to 7 days. No specific treatment is required other than control of the cardiac condition. Extensive ischemic hepatopathy may result in acute liver failure.

Ischemic hepatopathy may also result from hypovolemic shock from any cause and obstructive sleep apnea. Postoperatively, patients are especially prone to ischemic liver damage because they often have coexisting arterial hypotension and hypoxemia. Furthermore, hepatic blood flow may be reduced by anesthetic agents. This problem may be of particular concern for patients who have open heart surgery. The typical histologic finding in these patients with ischemic liver damage is centrilobular hepatic necrosis (zone 3). The severity of liver damage is related to the duration of hypotension and the degree of hypoxemia.

Hereditary Hemorrhagic Telangiectasia

Three of the following criteria are required for the diagnosis of HHT: 1) a history of epistaxis, 2) a family history of HHT, 3) mucocutaneous telangiectasia, and 4) visceral involvement, which can be hepatic, gastrointestinal, neurologic, or pulmonary.

The vascular malformation within the liver of patients with HHT results in fistulas in 1 or more of the following locations: 1) between the hepatic artery and the hepatic vein (the most common abnormality), 2) between the hepatic artery and the portal vein, or 3) between the portal vein and the hepatic vein. Previously, the most common liver disease in patients with HHT was transfusion-related viral hepatitis, but now the most common manifestation is high-output cardiac failure resulting from hepatic artery–hepatic vein fistulas or hepatic artery–portal vein fistulas.

Additional abnormalities include 1) recurrent cholangitis due to the diversion of hepatic arterial blood to the hepatic vein, 2) portal hypertension as a result of hepatic artery–portal vein fistulas or nodular regenerative hyperplasia, and 3) hepatic encephalopathy due to fistulas between the portal vein and the hepatic vein. Embolization of these fistulas is not recommended because of the high risk of liver abscesses. This is probably related to most patients having some degree of a portal vein–hepatic vein fistula, and once the hepatic artery is occluded, there is neither hepatic arterial blood nor portal venous blood to the involved segment of the liver. Liver transplant has been performed to treat HHT and is best indicated for patients who have recurrent cholangitis.

Disorders of Hepatic Venous Outflow

Sinusoidal Obstruction Syndrome

Venoocclusive disease, or sinusoidal obstruction syndrome (SOS), results from occlusion of the central and sublobular hepatic veins. In the US, the most common cause of SOS is preconditioning therapy for bone marrow transplant. Other causes include radiation to the liver, antineoplastic drugs such as azathioprine and 6-mercaptopurine, and ingestion of alkaloids containing pyrrolizidine.

The following discussion is predominantly about SOS of the liver in relation to patients undergoing bone marrow transplant. For these patients, the incidence of SOS was approximately 50% when cyclophosphamide and total body radiotherapy were used as intensive conditioning therapy before transplant, and the mortality rate was 20% to 40%. Currently, the incidence of SOS is low because cyclophosphamide and high-dose radiotherapy are no longer used. Early changes are related to hemorrhage in zone 3, as seen in liver biopsy specimens. Diagnostic criteria include subendothelial thickening of at least 1 terminal hepatic venule in association with luminal narrowing.

The pathogenesis of SOS is not well defined. It probably results from a combination of endothelial injury and activation of clotting mechanisms. It has been hypothesized that the depletion of glutathione in zone 3 hepatocytes makes them more prone to damage by antineoplastic agents such as busulfan. The resulting accumulation of oxygen free radicals leads to zone 3 necrosis and subsequent endothelial damage.

The diagnostic criteria for SOS are listed in Table 27.1. Bilirubin levels greater than 15 mg/dL are associated with poor outcome. Treatment of SOS is difficult. Prophylactic strategies have included administration of heparin, prostaglandins, or ursodeoxycholic acid. Because of the lack of large, randomized studies, it is difficult to determine the benefits of any of these therapies. The treatment of established SOS is also debated. Defibrotide has been approved for use in adult and pediatric patients, and tissue plasminogen activator and heparin have been administered to patients at high risk for dying of complications of SOS. In addition, defibrotide

is a parenteral oligonucleotide mixture with fibrinolytic properties approved for the treatment of SOS. If there is no response to thrombolytic therapy, either a surgical shunt or a transjugular intrahepatic portosystemic shunt (TIPS) may be used. Although the initial results with portosystemic shunts may be beneficial, the long-term outcome for patients who require shunts is poor because these patients usually have severe SOS and intervention generally delays, but does not prevent, a fatal outcome.

✓ Hepatic SOS results from occlusion of central and sublobular hepatic veins, typically related to therapy for bone marrow transplant
✓ SOS generally resembles Budd-Chiari syndrome, but venous obstruction in SOS occurs more distally, closer to the liver
✓ SOS prophylaxis—heparin, prostaglandins, or ursodeoxycholic acid
✓ Established SOS—management is generally supportive; defibrotide is approved treatment

Budd-Chiari Syndrome

BCS is a heterogeneous group of disorders characterized by obstruction of hepatic venous outflow. The site of obstruction may be at the level of small hepatic venules, large hepatic veins, or the inferior vena cava. Obstruction at the level of the central and sublobular hepatic venules traditionally has been called SOS, as described above. In some countries, such as Japan and India, people may have obstruction of the inferior vena cava by membranes or webs or segmental narrowing of the vessel, which also may obstruct hepatic venous outflow.

✓ **Budd-Chiari syndrome**—hepatic venous outflow tract obstruction from any cause

Etiology

The main predisposing causes of BCS include a hypercoagulable state, tumor invasion of the hepatic venous outflow tract, and miscellaneous causes. In some patients, no clear etiologic factor is discernible. Increasingly, the presence of multiple underlying disorders that cause BCS is being recognized.

Hematologic abnormalities, particularly myeloproliferative disorders, are detected in up to 87.5% of patients with BCS. Overt polycythemia vera is the most common disorder encountered. Erythropoietin levels and demonstration of *JAK* variations have been used to diagnose occult primary myeloproliferative disorders in patients otherwise thought to have idiopathic BCS. Both fulminant and chronic forms of the syndrome have been described for patients with paroxysmal nocturnal hemoglobinuria. Increasingly, inherited deficiencies of protein C, protein S, and antithrombin are being reported in association with the syndrome. Protein C and protein S are vitamin K–dependent proteins that are synthesized in the liver and endothelial cells and act as fibrinolytic agents. Antithrombin is a vitamin K–independent protease inhibitor that is synthesized in the liver and neutralizes activated clotting factors by forming a complex with a specific serine protease. Deficiencies of any of these proteins can result in both arterial thrombosis and venous thrombosis, but the correlation between the levels of protein C and protein S and the risk of thrombosis is not precise. In several patients with BCS, protein C deficiency has also been associated with an underlying myeloproliferative disorder. The diagnosis is sometimes difficult because these proteins can become deficient in patients with impaired liver function. Normal levels of factors II and VII in

Table 27.1. Diagnostic Criteria for Venoocclusive Disease

Criteria	Weeks after BMT	Weight gain, %	Other required findings
Baltimore	≤3	>5	Hepatomegaly Ascites
Seattle	≤3	>2	Bilirubin >2 mg/dL Hepatomegaly RUQ pain

Abbreviations: BMT, bone marrow transplant; RUQ, right upper quadrant.

patients with BCS or deficiencies of protein C and protein S in family members may point toward an inherited disorder.

The factor V Leiden variant has been reported in approximately 23% of patients with BCS. This alteration, caused by the substitution of an arginine residue by glutamine at position 506 in the factor V molecule, abolishes a protein C cleavage site in factor V and prolongs the thrombogenic effect of factor V activation. The term *resistance to activated protein C* is another name for this condition. Although about 2.9% to 6% of people of European descent are believed to be heterozygous for this alteration, the relative risk of thrombosis is thought to be low. In addition to being a sole cause of BCS, this alteration has been reported to occur also in combination with other prothrombotic disorders.

Clinical Manifestations

The underlying pathophysiologic abnormality in BCS is an increase in sinusoidal pressure caused by obstruction of hepatic venous outflow. This results in hypoxic damage to the hepatocytes and increased portal venous pressure. Continued obstruction of hepatic venous outflow leads to further hepatic necrosis, ultimately resulting in cirrhosis. Because the caudate lobe drains directly into the inferior vena cava, it is not damaged. In fact, the caudate lobe hypertrophies, and this may, to various degrees, obstruct the inferior vena cava. The clinical presentation of BCS depends on the extent and rapidity of the occlusion of the hepatic vein and whether collateral circulation has developed to decompress the liver. Vague right upper quadrant abdominal pain is the most common presenting symptom of the syndrome, and ascites is the most common abnormality noted on physical examination. Some patients with hepatic vein thrombosis are asymptomatic, presumably as a result of occlusion of only 1 or 2 hepatic veins and decompression of the portal system through the development of large intrahepatic and portosystemic collaterals.

Investigations

Doppler ultrasonography of the liver is the initial investigation of choice for patients with suspected BCS; it provides visualization of the hepatic veins, splenic vein, portal vein, and inferior vena cava. Areas of necrosis are seen better with contrast-enhanced computed tomography and magnetic resonance imaging.

Venography or liver biopsy is not necessary after BCS has been diagnosed with noninvasive studies. However, if clinical suspicion is high for a diagnosis of BCS, especially if a patient has a fulminant or acute presentation, contrast venography may be necessary if noninvasive imaging is not diagnostic. The characteristic appearance of the hepatic veins in BCS is that of a spiderweb, with an extensive collateral circulation. Also, the inferior vena cava may be compressed by an enlarged caudate lobe, or it may show thrombus.

In addition to establishing the diagnosis of hepatic vein thrombosis, it is important to identify an underlying cause to determine management strategies. An appropriate hematologic evaluation should be performed to exclude the various disorders outlined in Box 27.2, including evaluation for *JAK2* alterations to determine whether the patient has a myeloproliferative disorder.

Management

The aims of treatment of BCS are to relieve obstruction of the hepatic outflow tract, to identify and treat the underlying cause,

---

Box 27.2. Causes of Budd-Chiari Syndrome

Common causes
  Hypercoagulable states
    Inherited
      Factor V Leiden alteration
      Prothrombin gene alteration
    Acquired
      Myeloproliferative disorders
      Cancer
      Pregnancy
      Oral contraceptive use
Uncommon causes
  Hypercoagulable states
    Inherited
      Antithrombin deficiency
      Protein C deficiency
      Protein S deficiency
    Acquired
      Paroxysmal nocturnal hemoglobinuria
      Antiphospholipid syndrome
  Tumor invasion
    Hepatocellular carcinoma
    Renal cell carcinoma
    Adrenal carcinoma
  Miscellaneous
    Aspergillosis
    Behçet syndrome
    Inferior vena cava webs
    Trauma
    Inflammatory bowel disease
    Dacarbazine therapy
  Idiopathic

Adapted from Menon KV, Shah V, Kamath PS. The Budd-Chiari syndrome. N Engl J Med. 2004 Feb;350(6):578-85; used with permission.

---

and to relieve symptoms. Treatment options include medical management, surgical portosystemic shunting, TIPS, and liver transplant (Table 27.2). Although most patients who have BCS can be offered some form of definitive therapy, those in whom the syndrome is due to extensive malignant disease are offered only palliative care because of the extremely poor prognosis with this condition.

Medical management consists of diuretic therapy for the treatment of ascites, anticoagulation to prevent extension of venous thrombosis, and treatment of the underlying cause. Approximately 20% of patients can be managed with this approach. If this approach fails, intervention to enhance hepatic venous outflow is the next step. Ideal candidates for angioplasty include patients with inferior vena cava webs or focal hepatic vein stenosis; thrombolytic therapy is used infrequently but is administered best by direct infusion to the site of the clot.

The aim of portosystemic shunting is to use the portal vein to provide a venous outflow tract for the liver in order

Table 27.2. Management of Budd-Chiari Syndrome (BCS)

Treatment	Indication	Advantages	Disadvantages
Thrombolytic therapy	Acute thrombosis	Reverses hepatic necrosis No long-term sequelae	Risk of bleeding Limited success
Angioplasty with and without stenting	IVC webs IVC stenosis Focal hepatic vein stenosis	Averts need for surgery	High rate of restenosis or shunt occlusion
TIPS	Possible bridge to transplant in fulminant BCS Acute BCS Subacute BCS if portacaval pressure gradient <10 mm Hg or IVC is occluded	Low mortality Useful even with compression of IVC by caudate lobe	High rate of shunt stenosis Extended stents may interfere with liver transplant
Surgical shunt	Subacute BCS Portacaval pressure gradient >10 mm Hg	Definitive procedure for many patients Low rate of shunt dysfunction with portacaval shunt	Risk of procedure-related death Limited applicability Limited availability of surgical expertise
Liver transplant	Fulminant BCS Presence of cirrhosis Failure of portosystemic shunt	Reverses liver disease May reverse underlying thrombophilia	Risk of procedure-related death Need for long-term immunosuppression

Abbreviations: IVC, inferior vena cava; TIPS, transjugular intrahepatic portosystemic shunt.

Adapted from Menon KV, Shah V, Kamath PS. The Budd-Chiari syndrome. N Engl J Med. 2004 Feb 5;350(6):578-85 with data from Ganguli SC, Ramzan NN, McKusick MA, Andrews JC, Phyliky RL, Kamath PS. Budd-Chiari syndrome in patients with hematological disease: a therapeutic challenge. Hepatology. 1998 Apr;27(4):1157-61; used with permission.

to reverse hepatic necrosis and to prevent chronic sequelae of obstruction of hepatic venous outflow. The optimal candidates for surgical shunting are patients with a subacute presentation in whom ascites is not severe, liver function is preserved, and the disease course is smoldering. Patients with acute BCS may need a less invasive procedure, such as TIPS. Covered stents have increased the long-term patency of TIPS, making this the preferred method of performing a portosystemic shunt in most patients. Indications for liver transplant in patients with BCS include 1) end-stage chronic liver disease, 2) fulminant liver failure, and 3) deterioration of liver function in spite of portosystemic shunting.

✓ Budd-Chiari syndrome
  • Usually due to hematologic abnormalities (in >85% cases), most commonly polycythemia vera
  • Clinical presentation—depends on acuity and severity of occlusion (most common is vague right upper quadrant abdominal pain)
  • Ascites—most common abnormality on physical examination
  • Doppler ultrasonography—initial investigation of choice
✓ When Budd-Chiari syndrome has been confirmed, evaluation should focus on possible causes (Box 27.2) and management (Table 27.2)

Suggested Reading

Darwish Murad S, Kamath PS. Liver transplantation for Budd-Chiari syndrome: when is it really necessary? Liver Transpl. 2008 Feb;14(2):133–5.

Darwish Murad S, Plessier A, Hernandez-Guerra M, Fabris F, Eapen CE, Bahr MJ, et al. Etiology, management, and outcome of the Budd-Chiari syndrome. Ann Intern Med. 2009 Aug;151(3):167–75.

Ganguli SC, Ramzan NN, McKusick MA, Andrews JC, Phyliky RL, Kamath PS. Budd-Chiari syndrome in patients with hematological disease: a therapeutic challenge. Hepatology. 1998 Apr;27(4):1157–61.

Garcia-Tsao G. Liver involvement in hereditary hemorrhagic telangiectasia (HHT). J Hepatol. 2007 Mar;46(3):499–507.

Kumar S, DeLeve LD, Kamath PS, Tefferi A. Hepatic veno-occlusive disease (sinusoidal obstruction syndrome) after hematopoietic stem cell transplantation. Mayo Clin Proc. 2003 May;78(5):589–98.

Kumar S, Sarr MG, Kamath PS. Mesenteric venous thrombosis. N Engl J Med. 2001 Dec;345(23):1683–8.

McDonald GB. Hepatobiliary complications of hematopoietic cell transplantation, 40 years on. Hepatology. 2010 Apr;51(4):1450–60.

Menon KV, Shah V, Kamath PS. The Budd-Chiari syndrome. N Engl J Med. 2004 Feb;350(6):578–85.

Northup PG, Garcia-Pagan JC, Garcia-Tsao G, Intagliata NM, Superina RA, Roberts LN, et al. Vascular liver disorders, portal vein thrombosis, and procedural bleeding in patients with liver disease: 2020 practice guidance by the American Association for the Study of Liver Diseases. Hepatology. 2021 Jan;73(1):366–413.

Norton ID, Andrews JC, Kamath PS. Management of ectopic varices. Hepatology. 1998 Oct;28(4):1154–8.

Pasha SF, Gloviczki P, Stanson AW, Kamath PS. Splanchnic artery aneurysms. Mayo Clin Proc. 2007 Apr;82(4):472–9.

Plessier A, Darwish-Murad S, Hernandez-Guerra M, Consigny Y, Fabris F, Trebicka J, et al. Acute portal vein thrombosis unrelated to cirrhosis: a prospective multicenter follow-up study. Hepatology. 2010 Jan;51(1):210–8.

Seeto RK, Fenn B, Rockey DC. Ischemic hepatitis: clinical presentation and pathogenesis. Am J Med. 2000 Aug;109(2):109–13.

28

Portal Hypertension–Related Bleeding[a]

MOIRA HILSCHER, MD

DOUGLAS A. SIMONETTO, MD

Portal hypertensive bleeding encompasses a spectrum of conditions that include esophageal, gastric, and ectopic varices and portal hypertensive gastroenteropathy. Esophageal variceal hemorrhage occurs through a combination of increased portal pressure and local factors within the varix itself. Management of esophageal varices includes primary prophylaxis of variceal hemorrhage, treatment of actively bleeding varices, and prevention of variceal rebleeding (secondary prophylaxis). The choice of therapy for primary prophylaxis depends on patient preferences and includes pharmacologic therapy with nonselective β-blockers (NSBBs) or variceal band ligation, especially if NSBB therapy fails or is not tolerated by the patient. Active bleeding is best treated endoscopically. Pharmacologic therapy in combination with endoscopic therapy is preferred for secondary prophylaxis. Surgical shunts or transjugular intrahepatic portosystemic shunts (TIPSs) are second-line therapy. Liver transplant is a treatment option aimed at the underlying cause of portal hypertension but does not have a role in the management of acute bleeding.

Pathogenesis of Portal Hypertension

An increase in the hepatic venous pressure gradient (HVPG)— the difference between the wedged hepatic venous pressure and the free hepatic venous pressure—of at least 10 mm Hg is required for the development of esophageal varices, and an HVPG of 12 mm Hg or more is required for the rupture of esophageal varices. Wedged hepatic venous pressures can be measured directly by a transjugular route, but expertise in this procedure is usually available only at large referral centers.

In cirrhosis, portal hypertension occurs through an increase in resistance to portal venous outflow early in the disease process. This increase is due to mechanical factors related to fibrotic distortion of liver architecture. However, approximately 30% of the increase in intrahepatic resistance occurs through reversible vascular factors that are potential targets of pharmacotherapy. Portal hypertension is maintained through the development of systemic hyperdynamic circulation and peripheral vasodilatation. Physical examination findings in a patient in the hyperdynamic state include relative hypotension and relative tachycardia; a cardiac outflow murmur may be present. The hyperdynamic circulation is characterized in the splanchnic circulation by vasodilatation and increased flow at the level of the splanchnic arterioles. This leads to increased portal venous inflow, which in turn exacerbates the existing portal hypertension. Drugs such as octreotide and vasopressin reduce splanchnic hyperemia and portal venous inflow. Portal hypertension results in the development of collateral circulation, which may decrease portal pressure. In addition to esophageal and gastric varices, gastric and intestinal vascular ectasia and portal hypertensive gastropathy occur in patients with portal hypertension.

Esophageal Varices

Pathogenesis

Local factors that determine the risk of hemorrhage from esophageal varices include the radius of the varix, the thickness of the varix wall, and the pressure gradient between the varix and the esophageal lumen. Factors that determine the severity of bleeding are the degree of liver dysfunction, the portal pressure, and the

[a] The authors thank Patrick S. Kamath, MD, and William Sanchez, MD, who authored previous versions of this chapter.

Abbreviations: BRTO, balloon-occluded retrograde transvenous obliteration; GOV, gastroesophageal varix; HVPG, hepatic venous pressure gradient; IGV, isolated gastric varix; NSBB, nonselective β-blocker; TIPS, transjugular intrahepatic portosystemic shunt

size of the rent in the varix. Band ligation is an attempt to decrease flow through the varix by inducing thrombosis and, ultimately, to obliterate the varix.

Therapy

The current recommendations for treatment of esophageal variceal bleeding are summarized in Table 28.1.

Primary Prophylaxis

Most patients with cirrhosis should undergo upper endoscopy to screen for the presence and size of esophageal varices. Patients with a platelet count greater than 150×10^9/L and liver stiffness less than 20 kPa according to transient elastography have a low risk for varices and thus can avoid screening endoscopy. Capsule endoscopy and computed tomography are promising methods for detecting varices but, currently, are not recommended for screening. Varices should be characterized as either small (≤5 mm in diameter) or large (>5 mm in diameter). Large varices are seen in 16% of patients who undergo screening by endoscopy. In approximately 25% of patients with large varices, variceal hemorrhage will develop within the ensuing 2 years. For patients with large varices and advanced liver disease (Child-Pugh class C), the risk of hemorrhage can be as high as 75%. Thus, prophylactic therapy is indicated for patients with large varices. The absence of endoscopic signs that indicate high risk (eg, red wales) does not influence the decision to initiate therapy. Prophylactic treatment may also be considered for patients with Child-Pugh class C status and small varices. If only small varices are detected at endoscopy, the procedure should be repeated in 1 year to assess for progression in size. If no varices are detected at endoscopy, the procedure should be repeated in 2 or 3 years to screen for newly formed varices in patients who have compensated cirrhosis and annually in those who have decompensated disease.

The established primary prophylaxis is treatment with NSBBs, such as propranolol and nadolol, or with endoscopic variceal band ligation. Only nonselective agents should be used rather than β_1-selective agents (eg, metoprolol). β_1-Blockade decreases cardiac output and splanchnic blood flow, whereas the additional β_2-blockade allows unopposed α_1-adrenergic constriction in the splanchnic circulation. This decreases portal blood flow and, consequently, portal pressure. Therapy is started at a low dose, with slow upward titration of the dose until a resting pulse rate of 55 to 60 beats/min is achieved or hypotension develops (systolic blood pressure <90 mm Hg).

A long-acting preparation of propranolol administered as a single dose in the early evening is preferred. This allows adequate β-blockade at night, when the risk of bleeding is higher. With the long-acting preparation administered in the evening, β-blockade is less during the following day, thus decreasing the side effect of fatigue. At the same time, the risk of bleeding is lower during

the day, and the lesser degree of β-blockade is not deleterious to the patient.

Carvedilol, an NSBB with additional α_1-blocking properties, is another agent that might be used for primary prophylaxis. Because it has vasodilating effects, carvedilol can exacerbate arterial hypotension and sodium retention, so it should be used with caution in patients who have decompensated cirrhosis. Nitrates have no place in primary prophylaxis, either when administered as single agents or in combination with NSBBs.

The goal of therapy is to decrease the HVPG to less than 12 mm Hg or by 20% when compared with baseline. However, determination of the HVPG to assess the hemodynamic response is invasive and is not recommended in routine practice.

Although sclerotherapy is no longer used as a form of primary prophylaxis, variceal band ligation may be an alternative approach to primary prophylaxis because it carries a lower rate of esophageal ulceration and provides more effective obliteration of variceal structures compared with sclerotherapy. Currently, esophageal variceal ligation is recommended for patients who have contraindications to therapy with NSBBs, who have not had a decrease in the HVPG (if obtained), or who have had adverse effects from NSBB therapy. A network meta-analysis of 32 studies that compared NSBBs and endoscopic variceal ligation showed a potential decrease in mortality risk with NSBB therapy compared to band ligation, while both were effective in decreasing the risk of first variceal bleeding. Patient preference is often the factor that determines which therapy is used.

Control of Esophageal Variceal Hemorrhage

Active esophageal variceal bleeding is managed best by endoscopic means, preferably variceal band ligation. After gastrointestinal tract bleeding has been detected in patients with cirrhosis, immediate initiation of pharmacologic therapy is beneficial—even before endoscopy has demonstrated variceal bleeding. Pharmacologic therapy is continued for up to 5 days after endoscopic treatment of varices to reduce the risk of immediate rebleeding.

Vasopressin is a potent splanchnic vasoconstrictor that decreases portal venous inflow, thereby decreasing portal pressure, but it is seldom used. Nitroglycerin is used only in conjunction with vasopressin to further decrease portal pressure and reduce the ischemic adverse effects of vasopressin, which are pronounced and limit therapy in up to 30% of patients. Octreotide, a long-acting synthetic somatostatin analogue, is the pharmacologic agent most commonly used in the US. It appears to decrease portal pressure by inhibiting the release of glucagon and the ensuing postprandial hyperemia and by having a direct vasoconstrictive effect on splanchnic arteriolar smooth muscle. Octreotide is recommended for acute variceal bleeding and for prevention of early rebleeding. It is administered as an initial bolus of 50 μg, with a subsequent infusion at 50 μg hourly for up to 5 days, in conjunction with endoscopic variceal band ligation. NSBBs should not be used in the

Table 28.1. Recommendations for Treatment of Esophageal Variceal Bleeding

Type of treatment	First-line therapy	Second-line therapy	Other therapy
Primary prophylaxis	NSBBs or endoscopic variceal band ligation		
Control of bleeding	Variceal band ligation and octreotide (or other vasoactive pharmacologic agents)	TIPS	
Secondary prophylaxis	Variceal band ligation and NSBBs	TIPS	Liver transplant

Abbreviations: NSBB, nonselective β-blocker; TIPS, transjugular intrahepatic portosystemic shunt.

presence of acute bleeding since they will worsen hypotension, but use of NSBBs should be initiated once octreotide therapy is discontinued and before hospital discharge.

Supportive and resuscitative care includes early elective intubation for airway protection, cautious volume replacement, and vigorous surveillance and treatment of concomitant infection. Maintenance of the hemoglobin level at 7 to 9 g/dL is appropriate because aggressive transfusion of blood products may precipitate further bleeding by increasing portal pressure (transfusion threshold hemoglobin <7 g/dL). Antibiotic prophylaxis for 7 days with a fluoroquinolone or third-generation cephalosporin is recommended to decrease the incidence of bloodstream infection and spontaneous bacterial peritonitis, which commonly accompany variceal hemorrhage. Antibiotic therapy is probably the most important reason why the mortality rate among patients with variceal bleeding has decreased from 50% to about 20%. Lactulose therapy may be instituted to treat hepatic encephalopathy.

TIPS may be used as preemptive, rescue, or salvage therapy for variceal bleeding. Preemptive use of TIPS, placed within 72 hours of presentation, has been shown to decrease the risk of therapy failure or early rebleeding in high-risk patients; thus, it may benefit those who have Child-Pugh class C or Child-Pugh class B status with active bleeding on index endoscopy. Risk of hepatic encephalopathy and 1-year mortality have not been shown to increase; however, the routine use of preemptive TIPS has not been recommended because of the potential for liver deterioration and the uncertain effects on long-term survival. Salvage TIPS is indicated for patients with refractory bleeding, while rescue TIPS is recommended when bleeding recurs despite variceal band ligation and vasoactive therapy. The use of TIPS is preferred to surgical intervention, particularly in patients with Child-Pugh class B or C status. Since expertise with performing surgical shunts is limited to large referral centers, surgical intervention is impractical for acute bleeding. However, surgical shunts may be considered for recurrent bleeding in patients with Child-Pugh class A status and for patients for whom continued medical surveillance will be unlikely. TIPS requires close ultrasonographic follow-up of the shunt to evaluate for restenosis, although the rate of TIPS stenosis has decreased with the adoption of covered stents. All potential transplant candidates who have variceal hemorrhage should be referred to a transplant center for evaluation.

Secondary Prophylaxis

Secondary prophylaxis involves therapies to prevent rebleeding in patients who have already bled from esophageal varices. Intervention is essential because up to 80% of patients who have already bled from varices will bleed again within 2 years. Treatments include pharmacotherapy with NSBBs, endoscopic band ligation, TIPS, and surgical shunts. The use of variceal band ligation in combination with NSBB therapy is first-line therapy to prevent recurrent bleeding. After acute bleeding has been controlled with variceal ligation, the next ligation session should be scheduled in approximately 10 to 14 days. Subsequent sessions should be scheduled every 3 to 4 weeks. Varices usually can be obliterated over several sessions.

Portal Hypertension Manifestations in the Stomach

Gastric consequences of portal hypertension that may lead to bleeding include gastric varices, portal hypertensive gastropathy, and gastric vascular ectasia. Because no evidence-based management strategies are available for gastric sources of portal hypertensive bleeding, therapy often requires an empirical approach.

Gastric Varices

The most common gastric varices are gastroesophageal varices (GOVs) that extend into the lesser curve of the cardia of the stomach (type 1 [GOV1]) and are readily treated with variceal band ligation. The most common sources of gastric variceal bleeding are cardiofundal varices, located in the greater curvature of the cardia and the fundus of the stomach, that are either extensions of esophageal varices (type 2 [GOV2]) or are isolated gastric varices (IGVs) (cardiofundal varices; type 1 [IGV1]). Recent data have suggested that the frequency of bleeding from gastric varices is similar to that from large esophageal varices. Gastric varices are more likely to be found in patients who have had bleeding from esophageal varices than in those who have not had prior bleeding. The risk of bleeding from gastric varices is related to the size of the varix, the liver function according to the Child-Pugh classification, and the presence of red signs on the varix.

NSBBs are recommended for primary prophylaxis of gastric varices, although data are limited. Acute gastric variceal bleeding is treated best endoscopically. GOV1 varices, like esophageal varices, can be treated with band ligation, while cardiofundal varices are treated best with injection of cyanoacrylate glue. Currently, however, cyanoacrylate glue injection is not widely available in the US, and its use is considered off-label. Other options include sclerotherapy with ethanolamine oleate or thrombin, but the success rate has varied. Thus, TIPS is still considered the treatment of choice for bleeding cardiofundal varices.

Although pharmacologic therapy (eg, NSBBs) may be used to prevent gastric variceal rebleeding, no studies support this practice. Thus, portosystemic shunt creation should be considered for the prevention of rebleeding in patients with documented cardiofundal variceal bleeding if variceal obturation with cyanoacrylate glue is not possible. TIPS is used for patients with poor liver function, while patients with Child-Pugh class A status may also be considered for portosystemic shunt surgery. Also, gastric varices can be obliterated concomitantly with TIPS placement through the injection of gel foam or coils into the gastroesophageal collateral vessels. Balloon-occluded retrograde transvenous obliteration (BRTO) may be an option for treatment of cardiofundal varices in patients with spontaneous gastrorenal or splenorenal shunts; it involves sclerosant injection through cannulation of the left renal vein to obliterate the cardiofundal varix and the shunt.

Portal Hypertensive Gastropathy

Portal hypertensive gastropathy is a source of gastrointestinal tract bleeding in some patients with cirrhosis and portal hypertension. The elementary lesion is a mosaic-like pattern of the gastric mucosa, but this is not specific. The more specific lesion is the red marking, which may be either a red point lesion less than 1 mm in diameter or a cherry-red spot larger than 2 mm in diameter. The presence of a mosaic-like pattern alone indicates mild portal hypertensive gastropathy, whereas red markings superimposed on the mosaic pattern suggest severe portal hypertensive gastropathy. Portal hypertensive gastropathy tends to be more common in the proximal stomach, in patients who have advanced stages of liver disease according to the Child-Pugh classification, and in those with gastric or esophageal varices. Approximately 3% of patients who have severe gastropathy may

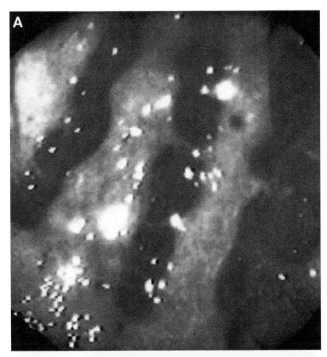

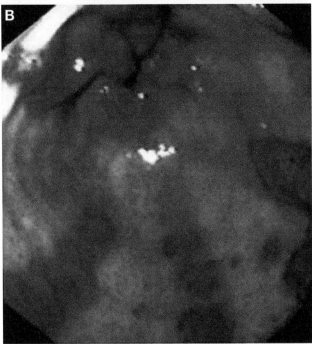

Figure 28.1. Gastric Antral Vascular Ectasia. A and B, Note the linear aggregates of red markings in the antrum and the absence of an underlying mosaic-like pattern.

present with acute upper gastrointestinal tract bleeding, and approximately 15% have chronic bleeding.

Anecdotally, acute bleeding from portal hypertensive gastropathy has been treated with vasoactive drugs such as vasopressin, somatostatin, and octreotide, and the success rate has been high. Portosystemic shunts should be considered as rescue treatment if vasoactive drug therapy fails. Patients who present with chronic bleeding may be treated with iron supplementation and NSBBs. For these patients, treatment should be continued indefinitely or until liver transplant is performed. Portosystemic shunts may be used as rescue treatment in patients who continue to be transfusion-dependent in spite of adequate NSBB therapy.

Gastric Vascular Ectasia

A less common gastric mucosal lesion in portal hypertension is gastric vascular ectasia. In contrast to portal hypertensive gastropathy, gastric vascular ectasia is characterized by red markings in the absence of a mosaic-like pattern. The red markings may be arranged in linear aggregates in the antrum, for which the term *gastric antral vascular ectasia* (or watermelon stomach) is used (Figure 28.1). If the red markings do not have a typical linear arrangement, the lesion is designated *diffuse gastric vascular ectasia*. Diffuse lesions that also involve the proximal stomach may be difficult to differentiate from severe portal hypertensive gastropathy. When the diagnosis is uncertain, gastric mucosal biopsy, which usually is safe, may be helpful. Liver dysfunction seems to be necessary for the pathogenesis of vascular ectasia because these lesions may resolve with liver transplant.

Treatment of gastric vascular ectasia is difficult. Some patients may be managed with only iron replacement therapy. NSBBs do not seem to be effective for these lesions. Therapy may be tried with thermoablation such as argon plasma coagulation, radiofrequency ablation, and cryotherapy. Antrectomy is effective, but the mortality and morbidity related to the operation can be substantial for patients with cirrhosis. These lesions do not respond to portosystemic shunts, either surgical or TIPS, but occasionally they respond to estrogen-progesterone combinations or intravenous bevacizumab.

Suggested Reading

Garcia-Tsao G, Abraldes JG, Berzigotti A, Bosch J. Portal hypertensive bleeding in cirrhosis: risk stratification, diagnosis, and management: 2016 practice guidance by the American Association for the Study of Liver Diseases. Hepatology. 2017 Jan;65(1):310–35.

Garcia-Tsao G, Bosch J. Management of varices and variceal hemorrhage in cirrhosis. N Engl J Med. 2010 Mar 4;362(9):823–32.

Kamath PS, Lacerda M, Ahlquist DA, McKusick MA, Andrews JC, Nagorney DA. Gastric mucosal responses to intrahepatic portosystemic shunting in patients with cirrhosis. Gastroenterology. 2000 May;118(5):905–11.

Primignani M, Carpinelli L, Preatoni P, Battaglia G, Carta A, Prada A, et al. Natural history of portal hypertensive gastropathy in patients with liver cirrhosis: The New Italian Endoscopic Club for the study and treatment of esophageal varices (NIEC). Gastroenterology. 2000 Jul;119(1):181–7.

Shah V, Kamath P. Portal hypertension and variceal bleeding. In: Feldman M, Friedman LS, Brandt LJ, Sleisenger MH, Fordtran JS, eds. Sleisenger and Fordtran's gastrointestinal and liver disease: pathophysiology, diagnosis, management. 11th ed. Elsevier; 2020:1442–70.

Simonetto DA, Liu M, Kamath PS. Portal hypertension and related complications: diagnosis and management. Mayo Clin Proc. 2019 Apr;94(4):714–26.

29

Ascites, Hepatorenal Syndrome, and Encephalopathy[a]

TASHA B. KULAI, MD
DOUGLAS A. SIMONETTO, MD

The portal hypertension and hepatic synthetic dysfunction of cirrhosis cause 3 main complications as liver disease progresses from compensated to decompensated disease: variceal bleeding, ascites, and hepatic encephalopathy (HE). Variceal bleeding is discussed in Chapter 27.

Ascites

Ascites is the most common major complication of cirrhosis and occurs within 10 years in about 50% of patients who have compensated cirrhosis. The development of ascites denotes the transition from compensated to decompensated cirrhosis as it is often the first decompensating event. Ascites is associated with morbidity from abdominal distention and increased mortality from complications such as spontaneous bacterial peritonitis (SBP) and kidney dysfunction, with 15% of patients dying in 1 year and 44% in 5 years.

Pathogenesis of Ascites

Persons with cirrhosis have increased hydrostatic pressure in the liver. About 70% of this increased pressure is due to structural

changes from architectural distortion by fibrosis and nodular regeneration, and 20% to 30% of the increased pressure is related to increased intrahepatic vascular tone due to vasoactive factors. Increased hepatic sinusoidal pressure appears to be the primary event that leads to splanchnic (and eventually systemic) vasodilatation, which in turn causes underfilling of the vascular compartment and baroreceptor-mediated stimulation of the renin-angiotensin-aldosterone system, the sympathetic nervous system, and antidiuretic hormone (ADH) release. The net result is retention of sodium and water by the kidneys. Nitric oxide appears to be an important factor in the regulation of intrahepatic vascular tone. Considerable evidence shows that in persons with cirrhosis, the decreased availability of hepatic vascular nitric oxide impairs relaxation and increases hepatic perfusion pressure. However, the splanchnic and systemic vasculature markedly overproduce endothelial nitric oxide, which results in arterial vasodilatation and, subsequently, hyperdynamic circulation, which is characterized by tachycardia, increased cardiac output, and decreased arterial pressure.

Compared with other capillary beds, the hepatic sinusoids are a very low-pressure hydrostatic system (vascular inflow is partly portal venous blood that has a hydrostatic pressure only slightly higher than the systemic venous pressure). However, with portal hypertension, increased pressure in the hepatic sinusoids causes fluid to move into the tissue and to "weep" from the surface of the liver as ascites. A minimum hepatic venous pressure gradient of 10 to 12 mm Hg is necessary for ascites to develop.

Evaluation of Patients With Ascites

The first step in the diagnostic approach to patients with ascites is to determine the cause (Box 29.1). In 85% of patients, ascites is due to cirrhosis and the diagnosis is usually obvious. About 15%

[a] The authors thank J. Eileen Hay, MB, ChB, who authored previous versions of this chapter.

Abbreviations: AASLD, American Association for the Study of Liver Disease; ADH, antidiuretic hormone; AKI, acute kidney injury; CTP, Child-Turcotte-Pugh; HE, hepatic encephalopathy; HRS, hepatorenal syndrome; MELD, Model for End-stage Liver Disease; NAKI, nonacute kidney injury; PMN, polymorphonuclear neutrophil; PPCD, postparacentesis circulatory dysfunction; SAAG, serum-ascites albumin gradient; SBP, spontaneous bacterial peritonitis; TIPS, transjugular intrahepatic portosystemic shunt

Box 29.1. Diagnostic and Therapeutic Algorithm for Patients With Ascites

Does the patient have cirrhosis?

If yes, are there any other complications of cirrhosis—spontaneous bacterial peritonitis, portal vein thrombosis, active liver disease, or malignancy?

Prognostic factors for therapy—urinary sodium excretion and kidney function

Consideration of therapeutic options

have nonhepatic causes (malignancy, tuberculosis, constrictive pericarditis, right-sided heart failure, myxedema, and kidney-related causes), and these must be differentiated from cirrhosis and treated appropriately.

Diagnostic paracentesis is mandatory and should be performed in all patients who present with new-onset ascites. If patients have cirrhosis and ascites, diagnostic paracentesis should also be performed if they are hospitalized or if they have a change in clinical status, such as deterioration in liver function, fever, worsening encephalopathy, or kidney failure. Because bleeding is uncommon, the routine prophylactic use of fresh frozen plasma or platelets before paracentesis is not recommended. For all patients, ascitic fluid analysis should include a cell count, with both a total nucleated cell count and a polymorphonuclear neutrophil (PMN) count, and bacterial culture by bedside inoculation of blood culture bottles. Ascitic fluid protein and albumin levels are measured simultaneously with the serum albumin level to calculate the serum-ascites albumin gradient (SAAG). The albumin concentration in ascitic fluid is inversely proportional to portal pressure. Usually, a high SAAG value (≥1.1 g/dL) confirms, with greater than 95% accuracy, the clinical suspicion of portal hypertension–related ascites. The other main cause for a high SAAG value is portal hypertension related to cardiac failure, but in cardiac failure the total protein concentration in the ascitic fluid is usually 2.5 g/dL or more (<2.5 g/dL in cirrhosis-related portal hypertension) (Table 29.1).

Other tests should be performed only if a specific diagnosis is suspected clinically. Lactate dehydrogenase and glucose levels should be determined if secondary peritonitis is suspected. Other tests to consider are amylase (>1,000 U/L suggests pancreatic ascites), cytology (at least at the initial tap), and triglycerides (if the ascitic fluid is cloudy; results are usually <100 mg/dL in cirrhosis). Mycobacterial culture should be performed only if tuberculosis is strongly suspected. Other ascitic fluid indexes (eg, lactate and pH) generally offer little or no additional information. Gram staining is rarely positive.

In addition to SBP, other complications of cirrhosis that may worsen ascites, including malignancy, portal or hepatic venous thrombosis, and active liver disease, should be sought with liver tests or imaging studies. Any active liver disease (alcohol-related, autoimmune, or hepatitis B) must be treated appropriately. Kidney function and kidney sodium excretion should be assessed because they are clinical predictors of a therapeutic response: Patients with normal serum urea nitrogen and creatinine levels and sodium excretion of more than 10 mEq/L (without taking diuretics) generally are very sensitive to sodium restriction and diuretic therapy. Patients with marked sodium retention, particularly those with abnormal urea and creatinine levels, require much higher doses of diuretics.

✓ Evaluation for new or worsening ascites
- Diagnostic paracentesis with cell count, including differential cell count, and bacterial cultures
- Albumin levels of serum and ascitic fluid (for calculation of serum-ascites albumin gradient) and total protein level of ascitic fluid for evaluation of new-onset ascites in patients who do not have a clear diagnosis of cirrhosis
- Doppler ultrasonography to rule out hepatocellular carcinoma and portal or hepatic vein thrombosis
- Evaluation for active liver disease (eg, consider alcohol use and autoimmune hepatitis)
- Serum sodium and creatinine levels
- Measurement of 24-hour urinary sodium excretion

Therapy for Cirrhosis-Associated Ascites

Sodium Restriction and Diuretic Therapy

Cirrhosis-associated ascites is perpetuated by retention of sodium and water by the kidneys. Therefore, treatment must produce a negative sodium balance. About 10% of patients have a response to salt restriction alone. Reversible factors that contribute to sodium retention should be identified and corrected (Box 29.2). Ascites is controlled in 65% of patients with the initiation of spironolactone therapy and in another 25% with the addition of a loop diuretic. Thus, ascites can be managed in 90% of patients, often as outpatients, with the sequential introduction of sodium restriction, generally to 2 g daily (88 mEq), and then diuretic therapy.

Spironolactone, an aldosterone antagonist, is an effective diuretic in most patients who have nonazotemic cirrhosis with ascites and is more effective than furosemide for single-agent therapy. Combination therapy with furosemide is generally used to achieve natriuresis more rapidly and to maintain normokalemia. Spironolactone is given at an initial dose of 100 mg daily, with increases in 100-mg increments as appropriate to 400 mg daily,

Table 29.1. Ascitic Protein and Serum-Ascites Albumin Gradient (SAAG)

Total protein, g/dL	SAAG, g/dL	
	≥1.1	<1.1
<2.5	Cirrhosis	Nephrotic syndrome
	Acute liver failure	Myxedema
≥2.5	Congestive heart failure	Peritoneal carcinomatosis
	Constrictive pericarditis	Tuberculous peritonitis
	Budd-Chiari syndrome	Pancreatic ascites
	Veno-occlusive disease	Chylous ascites

Box 29.2. Reversible Factors for Lack of Response to Diuretic Therapy in Cirrhosis-Associated Ascites

Inadequate sodium restriction

Inappropriate use of diuretics or other medications (eg, β-blockers)

Nephrotoxic medications

Spontaneous bacterial peritonitis

Portal or hepatic vein thrombosis

Untreated active liver disease

according to the clinical response and adverse effects (particularly hyperkalemia). Furosemide usually is started at a dose of 40 mg daily in combination with spironolactone and increased in 40-mg increments to 160 mg daily until the desired effect is achieved or adverse effects occur.

Diuretic therapy is titrated to achieve optimal weight loss without complications, which include 1) deterioration in kidney function, 2) excessive weight loss in relation to ascites or edema, 3) orthostatic symptoms, 4) encephalopathy, and 5) dilutional hyponatremia unresponsive to fluid restriction. Generally, a daily weight loss of 0.5 to 1.0 kg is optimal to avoid adverse effects because only 750 to 900 mL of fluid can be mobilized daily from the abdomen into the general circulation. After the fluid is mobilized by whatever method, diuretic therapy should be adjusted to keep the patient free of ascites.

Therapeutic Paracentesis

In randomized studies of patients with tense ascites and avid sodium retention, repeated large-volume paracentesis (with intravenous infusions of albumin), compared with diuretic therapy, is 1) more effective in eliminating ascites; 2) associated with a lower incidence of hyponatremia (5% vs 30%), kidney impairment (3.4% vs 27%), and HE (10.2% vs 29%); and 3) associated with shorter hospital stay and reduced cost of therapy without any differences in survival, SBP, or causes of death.

Intravenous infusion of 25% albumin is an important measure to prevent postparacentesis circulatory dysfunction (PPCD) in patients with cirrhosis and tense ascites who are treated with large-volume (>5 L) or total paracentesis. Complete mobilization of ascites without plasma volume expansion causes a deterioration in systemic hemodynamics in 75% of patients; in 20%, hyponatremia or kidney dysfunction develops, which may be irreversible. Generally, 6 to 8 g of albumin infused for every 1 L of ascitic fluid removed decreases the risk of PPCD to less than 20%. Dextran 70 and polygeline are less effective than albumin as plasma volume expanders and are not recommended.

Drugs to Avoid in Cirrhosis-Associated Ascites

For patients with cirrhosis-associated ascites, nonsteroidal antiinflammatory drugs are contraindicated and aminoglycosides are generally avoided if alternative antibiotics may be effective. Drugs that decrease arterial pressure or kidney blood flow should be avoided (eg, angiotensin-converting enzyme inhibitors, angiotensin II receptor blockers, and α-adrenergic blockers). Pharmacologic acid suppression, which may increase the incidence of SBP, should also be avoided.

> ✓ Ascites can usually be managed with sodium restriction and diuretic therapy
> ✓ For patients with tense ascites, regular large-volume paracentesis is best; if more than 5 L of fluid is removed, administer albumin (6-8 g for every 1 L fluid removed)

Refractory Ascites

Definition

Refractory ascites is due to avid retention of sodium by the kidneys and occurs in about 10% of patients with decompensated cirrhosis. Clinically, ascites is considered to be refractory when a patient has adequate sodium restriction and receives maximal,

tolerable doses of diuretics but does not lose the desired weight (ie, 24-hour urine sodium is less than intake). Patients who have not had a response to spironolactone 400 mg daily and furosemide 160 mg daily have *diuretic-resistant ascites*. Ascites is termed *diuretic-intolerant* when therapy is prevented by diuretic-related complications.

> ✓ **Refractory ascites**—ascites unresponsive to sodium restriction and diuretic therapy
> ✓ **Diuretic-resistant ascites**—ascites unresponsive to the maximal dose of diuretics
> ✓ **Diuretic-intolerant ascites**—ascites in patients who cannot tolerate diuretic therapy because of adverse effects or related complications

Treatment Options

For patients who have refractory ascites, the long-term prognosis is dismal (1-year mortality rate >70%), and the only therapy capable of improving both quality of life and patient survival is liver transplant. Consequently, liver transplant should always be considered for an otherwise acceptable candidate who has ascites that cannot be controlled with adequate sodium restriction and diuretic therapy.

Until a patient undergoes liver transplant or if a patient cannot undergo liver transplant, therapeutic options for refractory ascites are limited to repeated therapeutic paracentesis or insertion of a transjugular intrahepatic portosystemic shunt (TIPS). According to the treatment recommendations of the American Association for the Study of Liver Diseases (AASLD), first-line therapy for refractory ascites is therapeutic paracentesis, and TIPS is reserved for patients who cannot tolerate paracentesis or who require large-volume paracentesis for refractory ascites for more than 2 or 3 months. Peritoneovenous shunting may be considered as a last resort for patients who are not candidates for repeated large-volume paracentesis, liver transplant, or TIPS. Diuretic therapy should be discontinued for patients who have refractory ascites when urine sodium excretion is less than 30 mmol daily. Discontinuation of nonselective β-blockers may be considered if any of the following develops: circulatory dysfunction (systolic blood pressure <90 mm Hg), hyponatremia (<130 mmol/L), or kidney injury (serum creatinine >1.5 mg/dL).

TIPS in Refractory Ascites

The hemodynamic effects of TIPS have been well described. Increased cardiac output (due to increased venous return) and a further decrease in systemic vascular resistance occur temporarily for 1 to 3 months, but increased urinary excretion of sodium starts 7 to 28 days after the procedure. At the same time, renin activity and aldosterone levels decrease. Resolution of ascites is slow, and diuretic therapy should be continued initially.

TIPS effectively decreases ascites in about 50% of patients but increases the incidence of encephalopathy by 20%. Overall patient survival is unchanged by TIPS, although a potential benefit has been suggested in recent studies. TIPS should be used with caution in patients older than 70 years and in patients who have clinically significant cardiopulmonary dysfunction, severe kidney failure, or advanced liver disease. Mortality increases for patients with a pre-TIPS Child-Turcotte-Pugh (CTP) score greater than 11 or a Model for End-stage Liver Disease (MELD) score greater than 18. For patients with refractory ascites, survival after TIPS is lower than survival after TIPS for variceal bleeding. Predictors of worsening encephalopathy are age older than 65 years, pre-TIPS encephalopathy, sarcopenia, hyponatremia, or a TIPS gradient less than 5 mm Hg. The use of expanded polytetrafluoroethylene–covered stents is preferred to bare stents because patients have less shunt dysfunction and better survival. However, the optimal hepatic venous pressure gradient for control of ascites is not known. Expansion-controlled stents, which are now available, allow for a gradual increase in the stent diameter (starting at 8 mm).

Hepatic Hydrothorax

Hepatic hydrothorax is a complication of cirrhosis-associated ascites in 5% to 10% of patients. Management is the same as for patients with ascites (sodium restriction and diuretic therapy). TIPS is effective in some patients. Thoracentesis is recommended only if the diagnosis is uncertain, if infection is strongly suspected, or if symptomatic relief is needed. The use of chest tubes and pleurodesis should be avoided.

Spontaneous Bacterial Peritonitis

SBP occurs in 10% to 30% of patients with cirrhosis-associated ascites and frequently is recurrent (1-year recurrence rate, 70%). In the past, the infecting organisms were normal bowel flora, with 70% of cases caused by gram-negative bacilli (especially *Escherichia coli* and *Klebsiella*) and 30% by gram-positive cocci (mainly *Streptococcus* and *Enterococcus* species), with anaerobes being very uncommon (<5% of cases). Most infections

(92% of cases) are caused by a single organism, and 8% are polymicrobial. The use of norfloxacin prophylaxis has caused epidemiologic changes in the bacterial flora, with a shift toward more gram-positive infections. The main pathogenic mechanism leading to SBP is generally considered to be intestinal bacterial translocation, by which bacteria move from the gut to mesenteric lymph nodes and, hence, into the systemic circulation before infecting the peritoneal membranes.

The clinical presentation and severity of SBP can be extremely variable and range from chills, fever, and abdominal pain to no symptoms. Unless paracentesis is performed, the diagnosis may be missed. Often, the clinical picture is a lack of response to diuretics, deteriorating kidney function, or worsening portosystemic encephalopathy. Patients with cirrhosis who are at particular risk for SBP are those with more advanced cirrhotic-stage liver disease, a low concentration of ascitic fluid protein (<1 g/dL), bilirubin level higher than 3.2 mg/dL, or gastrointestinal tract hemorrhage. Kidney impairment is common in these patients and is a clinical predictor of poor outcome.

Diagnosis

Ascitic fluid analysis is essential for the diagnosis of SBP (Figure 29.1). However, the clinical presentation of this condition can be subtle and easily missed clinically. Diagnostic paracentesis should be performed in all hospitalized or emergency department patients who have cirrhosis-associated ascites and in patients who present with signs of infection, encephalopathy, deteriorating kidney function, or gastrointestinal tract bleeding. Bedside

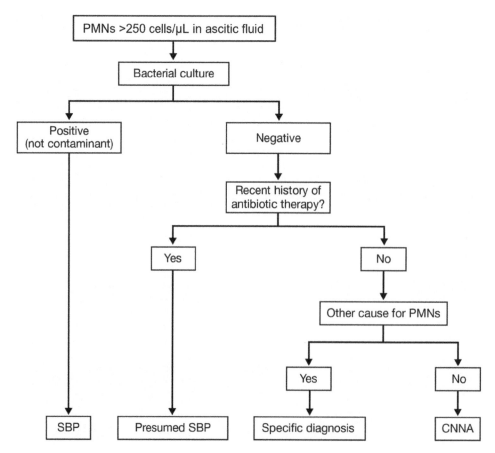

Figure 29.1. Diagnostic Algorithm for Spontaneous Bacterial Peritonitis (SBP). CNNA indicates culture-negative neutrocytic ascites; PMN, polymorphonuclear neutrophil.

inoculation of blood culture bottles with 10 mL of ascitic fluid is essential for maximizing the likelihood of positive cultures.

A presumptive diagnosis of SBP is made if the ascitic fluid PMN count is more than 250 cells/μL in a patient who has cirrhosis-associated ascites and no secondary source of infection. Blood cultures are performed before antibiotic therapy is started. A positive bacterial culture of the ascitic fluid confirms the diagnosis; if the bacterial culture is negative, the diagnosis of *culture-negative neutrocytic ascites* is made if there is no recent history of antibiotic therapy and no other cause of neutrocytic ascites (cholecystitis, pancreatitis, hemorrhage, recent abdominal surgery, or carcinomatosis). Patients with culture-negative neutrocytic ascites have clinical and biochemical features identical to those of patients with microbiologically confirmed SBP, and they are assumed to have SBP that was missed with current culture techniques. *Bacterascites* is defined by ascitic fluid with a PMN count less than 250 cells/μL and a positive bacterial culture. It usually indicates the transient residence of bacteria in the ascitic fluid. Patients with bacterascites generally have less severe liver disease than those with SBP. Although bacterascites may progress to SBP, it usually clears spontaneously without antibiotic therapy.

✓ **Culture-negative neutrocytic ascites**—ascitic fluid PMN count greater than 250 cells/μL and a negative culture; treatment should be as for SBP
✓ **Monomicrobial nonneutrocytic bacterascites**—ascitic fluid PMN count less than 250 cells/μL and a positive culture; most resolve spontaneously, but follow-up paracentesis should be performed within 72 hours or, for symptomatic patients, antibiotic therapy may be considered

---

✓ SBP often occurs without symptoms
✓ PMN count greater than 250 cells/μL in a patient with cirrhosis-associated ascites and no secondary source of infection is sufficient for a diagnosis of SBP (culture-negative neutrocytic ascites)

Treatment

Antibiotic Therapy

With the finding of a high PMN count in ascitic fluid, empirical therapy for SBP must be instituted and directed against aerobic enteric bacteria. Cefotaxime, 2 g intravenously every 8 hours, is the first choice of antibiotic for empirical therapy and is started when the PMN count in ascitic fluid is more than 250 cells/μL. This therapy is more effective (86%) than ampicillin in combination with an aminoglycoside and is associated with less kidney toxicity in patients with cirrhosis. Aztreonam is less effective because of its lack of activity against gram-positive organisms; parenteral amoxicillin-clavulanic acid and quinolones have been clinically effective. After the organism has been identified, antibiotic therapy can be adjusted accordingly. Uncomplicated SBP in patients not already receiving quinolones may be treated effectively in an outpatient setting with oral ciprofloxacin. Patients with an ascitic fluid PMN count less than 250 cells/μL but with signs of infection (fever, abdominal pain, or tenderness) should receive antibiotic therapy until culture results are available.

Epidemiologic changes in bacterial infections have occurred with norfloxacin prophylaxis, and these must be considered for each patient. In a recent study of bacterial infections in patients with cirrhosis who received norfloxacin prophylaxis, 53% of infections were due to gram-positive cocci, especially in nosocomial infections with invasive procedures and in patients in intensive care units. In 50% of patients who received norfloxacin prophylaxis and in 16% of patients who did not receive prophylaxis, SBP was caused by quinolone-resistant gram-negative bacilli; these organisms often are resistant also to trimethoprim-sulfamethoxazole therapy.

Albumin Infusions

About 30% of patients with cirrhosis who have SBP develop kidney impairment, an important predictor of mortality for these patients. In a randomized trial, albumin infusion on day 1 (1.5 g/kg) and day 3 (1 g/kg) prevented this complication; a meta-analysis of 4 randomized trials (288 patients) confirmed that albumin infusion prevented acute kidney injury (AKI) and reduced mortality. AASLD guidelines state that albumin infusions should be reserved for very ill patients who are most at risk (ie, serum creatinine >1 mg/dL, serum urea nitrogen >30 mg/dL, or total bilirubin >4 mg/dL).

Follow-up Paracentesis

Diagnostic paracentesis after 48 hours of antibiotic therapy in a recovering patient is often considered unnecessary. However, follow-up paracentesis is mandatory for patients who do not show clinical improvement. If the PMN count is greater than the baseline, the patient must be reexamined carefully for secondary sites of infection, including follow-up abdominal radiography for free air, computed tomography of the abdomen, and surgical consultation.

Differential Diagnosis

The main differential diagnosis for SBP is secondary bacterial peritonitis (5%-10% of cases of bacterial peritonitis in patients with cirrhosis), most commonly from a perforated viscus or occasionally an abscess. Secondary bacterial peritonitis appears to be a chance occurrence but is suspected in patients with liver disease less severe than SBP. The operative mortality rate for patients with cirrhosis who have infected ascites is about 85%, but for patients with secondary bacterial peritonitis who do not have surgery, mortality is close to 100%.

SBP and secondary bacterial peritonitis cannot be distinguished on the basis of clinical features. Factors that suggest a secondary infection are a high leukocyte count in ascites (>10,000 cells/μL), multiple or unusual organisms (fungi or anaerobes) in ascitic fluid culture, ascitic fluid protein less than 1 g/dL, glucose level less than 50 mg/dL, lactate dehydrogenase level more than the upper limit of the reference range for serum, and an increase in the number of PMNs in ascitic fluid despite antibiotic therapy. Radiologic imaging is mandatory.

Primary Prophylaxis

Episodes of bleeding in patients with CTP class C cirrhosis or recurrent bleeding in patients with cirrhosis are factors that predict infection and SBP, which are often severe. Intravenous ceftriaxone is the prophylactic antibiotic of choice and should be given for 7 days to all patients with advanced cirrhosis who have an episode of gastrointestinal tract bleeding. Patients with less severe liver disease and bleeding may receive an oral quinolone.

Long-term oral antibiotic prophylaxis is recommended for patients with cirrhosis who have a very low ascitic fluid protein level (<1.5 g/dL), especially if they also have a serum creatinine level of 1.2 mg/dL or more, serum urea nitrogen 25 mg/dL or more, serum sodium level 130 mmol/L or less, or a CTP score of 9 or higher with a bilirubin level of 3 mg/dL or more.

Secondary Prophylaxis

Because SBP has a 1-year recurrence rate of more than 50%, prophylactic measures are warranted for patients who have survived an episode of SBP. Rarely can the underlying liver disease be treated (except with liver transplant), and only occasionally does diuretic therapy completely clear the ascites. Treatment with ciprofloxacin can be used to eliminate the gram-negative flora (and reduce gram-negative infection), but it will not affect the other aerobic and anaerobic flora. Trimethoprim-sulfamethoxazole has also been effective for prophylaxis. Daily dosing is preferable to intermittent dosing.

Bacterascites

When diagnostic paracentesis shows no evidence of neutrocytic ascites (PMNs <250 cells/μL), but the ascitic fluid culture grows organisms that are not contaminants, the diagnosis is bacterascites. Paracentesis should be repeated within 72 hours and a decision about therapy should be based on the following: 1) if PMNs are more than 250 cells/μL, treat as SBP; 2) if PMNs are fewer than 250 cells/μL but again culture-positive, treat with antibiotics; and 3) if PMNs are fewer than 250 cells/μL but cultures are negative, do not treat.

✓ Treatment of SBP
  • Cefotaxime 2 g intravenously every 8 hours for 5 days
  • If serum creatinine is greater than 1 mg/dL, serum urea nitrogen is greater than 30 mg/dL, or total bilirubin is greater than 4 mg/dL, patients should also receive albumin infusion on day 1 (1.5 g/kg) and day 3 (1.0 g/kg)
✓ Patients who survive an episode of SBP should be treated with secondary prophylactic antibiotics
✓ Indications for primary prophylaxis for SBP (≥1 of the following):
  • Ascitic fluid protein less than 1.5 g/dL
  • Impaired kidney function (creatinine ≥1.2 mg/dL, serum urea nitrogen ≥25 mg/dL, or serum sodium ≤130 mmol/L)
  • Liver dysfunction (CTP score ≥9 and bilirubin ≥3 mg/dL)

Kidney Function Abnormalities in Cirrhosis and Hepatorenal Syndrome

Kidney dysfunction, a common complication of cirrhosis, is frequently progressive and severe and is an important predictor of mortality, especially when AKI develops after hospitalization. In 1 series, about half of all patients had volume-responsive prerenal azotemia, with acute tubular necrosis in 32% and hepatorenal syndrome (HRS) in 20%. Infection is a common precipitant in many patients. The hemodynamic changes in chronic liver disease increasingly worsen, with the progression from compensated cirrhosis to ascites (with a high incidence of AKI) to HRS.

Mild to severe sodium retention by the kidneys, mainly due to increased tubular resorption of sodium, is a key factor in the pathogenesis of ascites in patients with cirrhosis. This occurs with activation of the renin-angiotensin-aldosterone system and the sympathetic nervous system and increased secretion of ADH. As liver disease worsens, the activity of the renin-angiotensin-aldosterone and sympathetic systems increases and the secretion

of ADH increases. The increased secretion of ADH eventually impairs water excretion, resulting in increased total body water and dilutional hyponatremia. Splanchnic vasodilatation also continues to increase as liver disease worsens. As ascites progresses to type 2 HRS (HRS–non-AKI [NAKI]), arterial hypotension begins to affect blood flow to the kidneys, brain, liver, and adrenals.

Initially, cardiac output increases in cirrhosis. However, as hemodynamic changes worsen, cardiac output decreases because of cirrhotic cardiomyopathy with systolic and diastolic dysfunction, further worsening the blood flow to extrasplanchnic organs and potentiating kidney impairment.

Hyponatremia

The severity of water retention varies considerably among patients, but dilutional hyponatremia occurs in about 30% of hospitalized patients who have cirrhosis-associated ascites and is associated with increased morbidity and mortality. However, symptoms are rare until sodium levels are very low (<110-115 mmol/L). Treatment is fluid restriction, which should be implemented if serum sodium levels are less than 125 mmol/L. Rarely, patients need infusion of hypertonic (3%) saline, which is administered only to patients with severe, symptomatic hyponatremia. The vaptans are new aquaretic drugs (selective vasopressin V2 receptor antagonists) and may be considered for severe hypervolemic hyponatremia. Oral tolvaptan is now available and causes marked increases in kidney water excretion and serum sodium levels. Therapy with tolvaptan, which must be started when the patient is in the hospital, requires close monitoring and slow titration of the dose to avoid a rapid increase in serum sodium; fluid restriction is avoided, and doses of other diuretics are adjusted accordingly. The safety and efficacy of long-term tolvaptan use are undefined.

Major Diagnostic Criteria for HRS

The International Club of Ascites proposed that all the following major criteria must be present for the diagnosis of HRS:

• Cirrhosis with ascites
• Serum creatinine level >1.5 mg/dL
• No improvement after diuretic withdrawal and plasma volume expansion with 25% albumin (1 g/kg of dry body weight daily; maximum 100 g daily) for 2 days
• Absence of shock
• No current or recent nephrotoxic drugs or vasodilators
• Absence of parenchymal kidney disease, with proteinuria <500 mg/dL, and no ultrasonographic evidence of obstructive uropathy or microhematuria

The diagnosis is usually made on the basis of the serum creatinine level, which is a specific but relatively insensitive index of kidney function in this situation. Additional supportive features, which may help in making the diagnosis but are not considered essential, are low urine volume (<500 mL daily), low urine sodium level (<10 mEq/L), urine osmolality greater than plasma osmolality, and low serum sodium level (<130 mmol/L).

HRS Types 1 and 2

Type 2 HRS (HRS-NAKI) is kidney failure that progresses slowly over a long time, and the main consequence is refractory ascites; the creatinine level generally increases less than 0.5 mg/dL daily. In comparison, type 1 HRS (HRS-AKI) is rapidly progressive kidney failure. It usually occurs in patients with refractory ascites and results from a precipitating factor such as infection or gastrointestinal tract bleeding.

> ✓ **Hepatorenal syndrome**—functional kidney failure that develops in persons who have cirrhosis and ascites with no identified kidney pathologic changes

Treatment

Kidney dysfunction in cirrhosis-associated ascites is more easily prevented than treated. All factors that may potentiate kidney dysfunction should be avoided, including nephrotoxic drugs (especially nonsteroidal anti-inflammatory drugs and aminoglycosides), excessive use of diuretics or lactulose, and large-volume paracentesis without intravenous albumin. Complications such as bacterial infection, gastrointestinal tract bleeding, dehydration, or hypotension must be treated aggressively. SBP should be treated with antibiotics and intravenous albumin when indicated. Sepsis is a strong risk factor for AKI in a person with cirrhosis and is associated with arterial underfilling and kidney vasoconstriction. To reduce the risk of HRS, ciprofloxacin is recommended for patients with low-protein ascites and a CTP score of 9 or higher, bilirubin level 3 mg/dL or more, serum creatinine level 1.2 mg/dL or more, or serum sodium level 130 mmol/L or less.

The only therapy proven effective for HRS is liver transplant. In HRS-NAKI, discontinuation of diuretics and plasma volume expansion are usually effective, at least temporarily. Ongoing use of nonselective β-blockers for prophylaxis against variceal bleeding is controversial, but increasing evidence supports their discontinuation in patients who have hypotension, AKI, or hyponatremia. These patients require an expedited referral for liver transplant.

There is increasing evidence for the efficacy of vasoconstrictor therapy in combination with plasma volume expansion with 25% albumin (20-40 g daily) in HRS-AKI. Terlipressin is the most widely studied drug; it is safe, and it has been administered in doses of 0.5 mg every 4 hours, up to 12 mg daily. Terlipressin is superior to placebo for partial or complete reversal of HRS-AKI. Response to terlipressin is more likely when the bilirubin level is less than 5 mg/dL and there is an early sustained increase in arterial pressure with therapy. Norepinephrine, an α_1-adrenergic agonist, has also been used with similar benefit to terlipressin, although it requires intensive care unit admission for monitoring in most centers. In a small number of patients, the use of midodrine in combination with octreotide showed potential benefit in HRS-AKI; however, this has not been demonstrated in placebo-controlled trials. Therapy for HRS should be introduced as soon as the diagnosis is suspected, before the creatinine is markedly increased or the urine output is low.

A few small studies have suggested that kidney function improved in select patients with HRS-AKI after TIPS; however, in line with AASLD guidelines, controlled trials are required before TIPS can be recommended for this indication. Kidney replacement therapy, either hemodialysis or continuous venovenous hemofiltration, is used, especially in patients awaiting liver transplant.

Hepatic Encephalopathy

HE is a debilitating complication of cirrhosis for which therapies are still limited and nonspecific. Furthermore, no weight is given for this complication in the MELD system for organ allocation, resulting in considerable morbidity for patients and a burden for families and the health care system.

In chronic liver disease, noxious substances, presumed nitrogenous compounds from protein breakdown, are ineffectively detoxified or bypassed (or both) by the diseased liver; they affect the brain and cause HE, a neuropsychiatric syndrome. The pathophysiologic mechanism is not well understood, but ammonia is thought to be of central importance.

Clinical Features

HE is a constellation of neuropsychiatric features (dominated by considerable psychomotor slowing) that fluctuate greatly over time and range from a trivial impairment in cognition to frank confusion, drowsiness, and coma.

The 4 stages of overt HE (West Haven criteria) are well known:

- Grade 1—Confused; altered mood or behavior; psychometric defects
- Grade 2—Drowsy; inappropriate behavior
- Grade 3—Stuporous but with inarticulate speech and able to obey simple commands; marked confusion
- Grade 4—Coma; unable to be roused

For patients with advanced coma (grade 3 or 4), the Glasgow Coma Scale allows more accurate assessment of progression. Patients with cirrhosis who have no overt HE can be classified as those with normal cognitive function and those with minimal HE characterized by changes in psychomotor speed, visual perception, and attention. Studies have shown that even minimal HE can greatly affect a patient's functioning both at home and at work; recent evidence confirms attention deficit, impaired driving skills with an increased accident rate, and increased risk of falls with increased morbidity.

No laboratory test can confirm the diagnosis, which rests on typical neuropsychiatric features in patients with established chronic liver disease. Other causes of encephalopathy in patients with cirrhosis must be excluded. If a diagnosis is difficult, magnetic resonance imaging of the head is useful to identify alternative diagnoses, and imaging of the portosystemic circulation may identify large portosystemic shunts.

Neuropsychometric testing is necessary to diagnose minimal HE, which is particularly important for patients at risk for accidents and may be useful to monitor cognitive decline in patients with low-grade HE. No superior method of cognitive assessment has been identified. Testing may include paper-pencil psychomotor tests (eg, number connection tests), computerized psychomotor tests (eg, inhibitory control test), and neurophysiologic performance tests (eg, critical flicker frequency, mismatch negativity analysis, and electroencephalography). The psychometric HE score combines clinical impression with neuropsychologic performance and may prove more sensitive than the West Haven criteria. Asterixis is a nonspecific clinical sign, which generally, but not invariably, occurs in the early stages of HE. Although asterixis is associated with an increased arterial level of ammonia, there is no correlation between the degree of encephalopathy and the ammonia level. Recent studies have suggested that electroencephalographic alterations are associated with severity of liver disease and HE.

Management

Identification of Precipitants

To treat HE and to avoid precipitants of HE in patients who have advanced cirrhosis, the following general measures must be considered:

1. Avoid use of analgesics, sedatives, and tranquilizers.

2. Control gastrointestinal tract bleeding and purging of blood from the gastrointestinal tract.
3. Screen and initiate early aggressive therapy for any infection; this is especially important in advanced coma.
4. Correct acidosis, alkalosis, hypoxia, or electrolyte abnormalities (especially hyponatremia).
5. Prevent constipation and intravascular volume depletion; dehydration secondary to aggressive diuretic or lactulose therapy is a common precipitant. Diuretic use must be stopped, and albumin infusion has been found to be beneficial.
6. Ensure adequate intake of glucose to treat hypoglycemia and prevent endogenous protein breakdown.
7. Correct nutritional deficiencies, and provide adequate vitamin supplementation, including thiamine and folate.
8. Screen and correct for sarcopenia.

Treatment

Lactulose. Lactulose is the mainstay of therapy for most patients for treatment of an acute episode; it has been shown to reduce the recurrence of HE. Lactulose is a nonabsorbable synthetic disaccharide metabolized by colonic bacteria to organic acids. It decreases the absorption of ammonia by acting as an osmotic laxative, altering colonic pH, and trapping ammonia as ammonium in the gastrointestinal tract. The starting dose is 30 mL 2 or 3 times daily, titrated to produce 2 to 4 loose stools daily. If patients are comatose, lactulose is given by feeding tube or rectally. Excessive therapy can cause dehydration and hypernatremia. Lactitol is equivalent to lactulose but is not available in the US.

Antibiotics. Rifaximin is a minimally absorbable antibiotic with broad-spectrum antimicrobial activity that presumably modulates the bacterial flora. It has shown efficacy in the treatment of HE, and multicenter randomized controlled trials have shown that, at doses of 550 mg twice daily (with lactulose in many patients), it reduced the risk of recurrent episodes of HE better than lactulose alone. In 2 small randomized trials of patients with minimal HE, rifaximin improved driving simulator performance in 1 trial and psychometric testing in the other. It is as effective as, and safer than, neomycin or metronidazole. Neomycin can be absorbed to some extent (1%-3%) and may lead to ototoxicity and nephrotoxicity.

Dietary Protein. Recent studies have shown improvements in HE in patients who have better nutritional status and increased protein intake. Thus, patients with HE should avoid protein restriction. In patients with advanced coma, protein may be withheld for a short time while an adequate level of glucose is maintained with intravenous infusion; the precipitating cause for the HE can then be identified and lactulose therapy initiated. It is critical, however, to maintain a positive nitrogen balance long-term in these patients, particularly if they already have muscle wasting. Protein intake of 1.0 to 1.5 g/kg (based on ideal or dry weight) is essential. Protein is best tolerated if the amount is distributed evenly throughout the day rather than given in large doses. Also, the composition of the protein may make a difference: Vegetable proteins may be more beneficial (less ammoniagenic) than animal proteins. Furthermore, toxicity increases among animal proteins in ascending order as follows: dairy proteins, fish proteins, meat proteins, and blood proteins (red meat). Despite the absence of proven clinical benefit in trials, some patients appear to tolerate preparations of branched-chain amino acids better than other proteins.

Therapies With Indeterminate Efficacy. Zinc is a cofactor of urea cycle enzymes, and its deficiency is implicated in HE. Trials of zinc therapy in HE have been inconclusive, but therapy benefits some patients. Substrate for urea and glutamine synthesis (the 2 major routes of ammonia clearance) is provided by L-ornithine-L-aspartate, which lowers plasma ammonia levels and improves HE in patients with cirrhosis. Ammonia levels are reduced by sodium benzoate and phenylacetate, and some studies have shown benefit in HE; however, limitations of their use have prevented US Food and Drug Administration approval for HE. Probiotics, especially with lactobacilli and bifidobacteria, have shown some efficacy in HE, but their therapeutic role has not been defined. Fecal transplant is emerging as a potential therapy for HE; however, large randomized trials are still needed to confirm efficacy and safety.

Portosystemic Encephalopathy After TIPS. Most post-TIPS HE is maximal during the first 3 months and can be controlled by the above measures. For the approximately 8% of patients who have no response to medical treatment, the options are liver transplant and occluding the stent or decreasing its diameter. Stent manipulation is not without morbidity (recurrent variceal bleeding, ascites, and even death) and should be considered only for severely refractory cases. Decreasing the diameter of the stent is safer than occluding it.

Liver Support Devices. The molecular adsorbent recirculating system (MARS; Gambro) has been used to treat patients who have acute decompensation of cirrhosis and HE. A US multicenter trial showed that the treated patients had earlier and more frequent improvement in HE but no mortality benefit.

Liver Transplant. Liver transplant is the ultimate therapy for HE. Recurrent or difficult-to-treat HE is but one manifestation of deteriorating liver function and is an indication to consider orthotopic liver transplant.

HE and Spontaneous Portosystemic Shunts. Large spontaneous portosystemic shunts have been identified in some patients who have recurrent or persistent HE out of proportion to the severity of their liver disease. These shunts may be amenable to embolization with improvement in HE.

✓ HE occurs in persons with hepatic dysfunction or portosystemic shunting (or both)
✓ Management of overt HE
  • Identification and mitigation of precipitating factors
  • Lactulose as first-line therapy and for ongoing secondary prophylaxis after overt HE has resolved
  • Rifaximin can be added to prevent recurrence

Suggested Reading

Bass NM, Mullen KD, Sanyal A, Poordad F, Neff G, Leevy CB, et al. Rifaximin treatment in hepatic encephalopathy. N Engl J Med. 2010 Mar;362(12):1071–81.

Belcher JM, Garcia-Tsao G, Sanyal AJ, Bhogal H, Lim JK, Ansari N, et al. Association of AKI with mortality and complications in hospitalized patients with cirrhosis. Hepatology. 2013 Feb;57(2):753–62.

Cordoba J. New assessment of hepatic encephalopathy. J Hepatol. 2011 May;54(5):1030–40.

European Association for the Study of the Liver. EASL clinical practice guidelines on the management of ascites, spontaneous bacterial peritonitis, and hepatorenal syndrome in cirrhosis. J Hepatol. 2010 Sep;53(3):397–417.

Garcia-Tsao G. The transjugular intrahepatic portosystemic shunt for the management of cirrhotic refractory ascites. Nat Clin Pract Gastroenterol Hepatol. 2006 Jul;3(7):380–9.

Gifford FJ, Morling JR, Fallowfield JA. Systematic review with meta-analysis: vasoactive drugs for the treatment of hepatorenal syndrome type 1. Aliment Pharmacol Ther. 2017 Mar;45(5):593–603.

Gines P, Guevara M. Hyponatremia in cirrhosis: pathogenesis, clinical significance, and management. Hepatology. 2008 Sep;48(3):1002–10.

Gluud LL, Christensen K, Christensen E, Krag A. Systematic review of randomized trials on vasoconstrictor drugs for hepatorenal syndrome. Hepatology. 2010 Feb;51(2):576–84.

Lucero C, Verna EC. The role of sarcopenia and frailty in hepatic encephalopathy management. Clin Liver Dis. 2015 Aug;19(3):507–28.

Martin-Llahi M, Guevara M, Torre A, Fagundes C, Restuccia T, Gilabert R, et al. Prognostic importance of the cause of renal failure in patients with cirrhosis. Gastroenterology. 2011 Feb;140(2):488–96.

Moller S, Henriksen JH. Cirrhotic cardiomyopathy. J Hepatol. 2010 Jul;53(1):179–90.

Riggio O, Ridola L, Angeloni S, Cerini F, Pasquale C, Attili AF, et al. Clinical efficacy of transjugular intrahepatic portosystemic shunt created with covered stents with different diameters: results of a randomized controlled trial. J Hepatol. 2010 Aug;53(2): 267–72.

Salerno F, Navickis RJ, Wilkes MM. Albumin infusion improves outcomes of patients with spontaneous bacterial peritonitis: a meta-analysis of randomized trials. Clin Gastroenterol Hepatol. 2013 Feb;11(2):123–30.

Singh V, Singh A, Singh B, Vijayvergiya R, Sharma N, Ghai A, et al. Midodrine and clonidine in patients with cirrhosis and refractory or recurrent ascites: a randomized pilot study. Am J Gastroenterol. 2013 Apr;108(4):560–7.

Sola E, Gines P. Renal and circulatory dysfunction in cirrhosis: current management and future perspectives. J Hepatol. 2010 Dec;53(6):1135–45.

Wiest R, Schoelmerich J. Secondary peritonitis in cirrhosis: "oil in fire." J Hepatol. 2010 Jan;52(1):7–9.

30

Metabolic Liver Diseases[a]

ANGELA C. CHEUNG, MD

WILLIAM SANCHEZ, MD

Metabolic liver disease refers to inherited disorders of metabolism that manifest prominently with liver disease. The 3 major inherited disorders that cause liver disease in adults are α_1-antitrypsin (A1AT) deficiency (A1ATD), Wilson disease (WD), and hereditary hemochromatosis. All are multisystem disorders that cause liver injury by various mechanisms but which can ultimately lead to cirrhosis and complications of liver failure. Also, various inborn errors of metabolism that cause liver disease manifest during childhood (Box 30.1). These inborn errors of metabolism are, in aggregate, a major indication for pediatric liver transplant. As more patients who have childhood syndromes with liver involvement survive into adulthood, gastroenterologists who treat adults will need to become familiar with their care; however, the childhood syndromes rarely manifest initially in adulthood.

α_1-Antitrypsin Deficiency

A1ATD is an inherited disorder characterized by the development of liver disease or lung disease (or both) in children and adults. Clinical manifestations include cirrhosis and emphysematous obstructive lung disease. The presence of emphysema—especially among nonsmokers—in conjunction with chronic liver disease should prompt an evaluation for A1ATD.

---

[a] David J. Brandhagen, MD (deceased), John B. Gross Jr, MD, and John J. Poterucha, MD, are gratefully acknowledged as authors of this chapter in the previous editions of the book (parts of which appear in this edition).

Abbreviations: A1AT, α_1-antitrypsin; A1ATD, α_1-antitrypsin deficiency; ATPase, adenosine triphosphatase; PAS, periodic acid-Schiff; UNOS, United Network for Organ Sharing; WD, Wilson disease

---

Box 30.1. Metabolic Liver Diseases

Inborn errors of carbohydrate metabolism
  Glycogen storage disease
Inborn errors of protein metabolism
  Tyrosinemia
  Urea cycle defects
Inborn errors of lipid metabolism
  Gaucher disease
  Niemann-Pick disease
Inborn errors of bile acid metabolism
  Byler disease
  Benign recurrent cholestasis
Inborn errors of copper metabolism
  Wilson disease
Inborn errors of iron metabolism
  Hereditary hemochromatosis
  Non-*HFE* hereditary iron overload disorders
Unclassified
  α_1-Antitrypsin deficiency
  Cystic fibrosis

Adapted from Ghishan FK. Inborn errors of metabolism that lead to permanent liver injury. In: Boyer TD, Manns MP, Sanyal AJ, eds. Zakim and Boyer's Hepatology: a textbook of liver disease. 6th ed. Saunders; 2012: 1155-201; used with permission.

Inheritance and Gene Function

A1AT is a member of the serine protease supergene family. The function of A1AT is to protect tissues from the proteolytic activity of serum proteases such as neutrophil elastase. The gene for A1AT *(SERPINA1; OMIM 107400)* is located on the long arm of chromosome 14.

A1ATD is inherited as an autosomal codominant disorder. This deficiency is characterized on the basis of phenotype rather than genotype. The normal protein is labeled *M*, and abnormal phenotypes include *S, Z,* and *null*. Phenotypes are reported as the combination of alleles present; therefore, the wild-type phenotype is Pi*MM (*Pi* indicates protease inhibitor), and abnormal phenotypes include Pi*MZ, Pi*SS, and Pi*ZZ.

For liver disease, the Z phenotypes are the most clinically relevant. The normal Pi*MM phenotype is present in 95% of the population and is associated with normal serum levels of A1AT. Patients with the Pi*MZ phenotype have an intermediate deficiency, and patients with Pi*ZZ have a severe deficiency. The Z allele has a heterozygote frequency of 1:30 (Pi*MZ) and a homozygote frequency of 1:2,000 (Pi*ZZ).

Pathophysiology

It is important to recognize that A1ATD causes disease by different mechanisms in the lung and liver. Pulmonary disease is caused by unopposed activity of neutrophil elastase and other proteolytic enzymes that produce tissue damage. In contrast, in the liver, A1ATD is a storage disease. The abnormally folded A1AT protein cannot be exported from hepatocytes into the circulation, so globules of A1AT accumulate in the endoplasmic reticulum of hepatocytes, resulting in cell injury and death.

Clinical Features

The classic presentation of A1ATD is premature emphysema (especially in nonsmokers) and liver disease. This deficiency is also an important cause of childhood liver disease, often presenting as a neonatal hepatitis. The clinical manifestations of the deficiency are affected by the phenotype and by environmental factors, such as tobacco exposure and alcohol use.

In the only population-based study performed, the Swedish neonatal screening study identified 127 children deficient for A1AT who were followed prospectively through age 18 years. Neonatal cholestasis developed in 11%, and 6% had other liver disease without jaundice. Liver test results were abnormal 1 to 2 months after birth and usually normalized by 6 months. A small proportion of children either had end-stage liver disease or presented with acute liver failure in infancy. Most of the children (83%) were healthy throughout childhood, although most had abnormal liver test results in early life.

In adolescents and adults, A1ATD may cause chronic hepatitis or cirrhosis. This deficiency should be considered as a cause of abnormal liver enzyme levels in patients for which other common causes of liver disease, such as viral hepatitis, have been excluded. For adults with the Pi*ZZ phenotype, it has been estimated that cirrhosis will develop in 2% of those between 20 and 50 years old and in 19% of those older than 50 years. Patients with the Pi*MZ phenotype, which produces an intermediate degree of deficiency, are at some risk for chronic liver disease. It is more likely, however, that the Pi*MZ phenotype is a cofactor for the development of liver disease, along with other forms of liver injury such as nonalcohol-related fatty liver disease. Several studies have noted an increased prevalence of the Pi*MZ phenotype among those undergoing orthotopic liver transplant for cryptogenic cirrhosis compared with those having orthotopic liver transplant for other indications. Adults with cirrhosis due to A1ATD have a greatly increased risk for hepatocellular carcinoma, with some studies reporting a prevalence of primary liver cancer of up to 30%.

Diagnosis and Evaluation

The diagnosis of A1ATD is made by A1AT phenotyping or genotyping. Serum levels of A1AT are not useful for diagnosing the deficiency because they may be falsely increased (in inflammatory conditions, malignancy, or pregnancy or with estrogen supplementation) or spuriously decreased (in nephrotic syndrome or protein-losing enteropathy). Also, the serum levels of A1AT do not correlate with liver damage, although they do predict lung damage.

Liver disease due to A1ATD is confirmed by characteristic findings in liver biopsy samples. Biopsy is also useful in staging the degree of hepatic fibrosis. The characteristic finding is the presence of eosinophilic, periodic acid-Schiff (PAS)-positive, diastase-resistant (ie, PAS-diastase–positive) globules in the endoplasmic reticulum of periportal hepatocytes. Because these globules may be present also in persons who are heterozygous or homozygous without liver disease, their presence alone does not imply liver disease. Furthermore, because the globules may be distributed variably throughout the liver, their absence does not exclude the diagnosis of A1ATD. The histologic features of the liver in A1ATD are shown in Figure 30.1.

Patients with cirrhosis due to A1ATD should be enrolled in a surveillance program for hepatocellular carcinoma (typically with ultrasonography every 6 months). Patients with diagnosed liver disease due to A1ATD should be evaluated also for the presence of coexisting lung disease, especially if they have phenotype Pi*ZZ or are smokers. Baseline pulmonary function testing and chest radiography are recommended.

Treatment

No effective medical therapy is available for liver disease due to A1ATD. Although recombinant A1AT infusions are available, their use is limited to patients with A1ATD-related lung disease (because infusions of A1AT do not help decrease the accumulation of abnormal A1AT protein globules within hepatocytes). The mainstay of therapy is avoidance of alcohol and other hepatotoxins and maintenance of a healthy weight. Furthermore, patients should be advised to refrain from smoking to decrease their risk for obstructive lung disease.

✓ A1ATD—an autosomal codominant disease with phenotypes ranging from Pi*MM (wild-type) to Pi*ZZ (severe deficiency)
✓ Typically, Pi*MZ causes liver disease only in the presence of other risk factors (eg, nonalcohol-related fatty liver disease, alcohol-related liver disease, and viral hepatitis)
✓ A1ATD can cause hepatic abnormalities at any age, including neonatal cholestasis, neonatal hepatitis, and liver failure and end-stage liver disease in childhood
✓ Liver transplant—the only curative therapy for cirrhosis due to A1ATD

Once advanced liver disease develops, liver transplant is the only definitive therapy. A1ATD is the most common metabolic indication for liver transplant in adults. Liver transplant corrects the

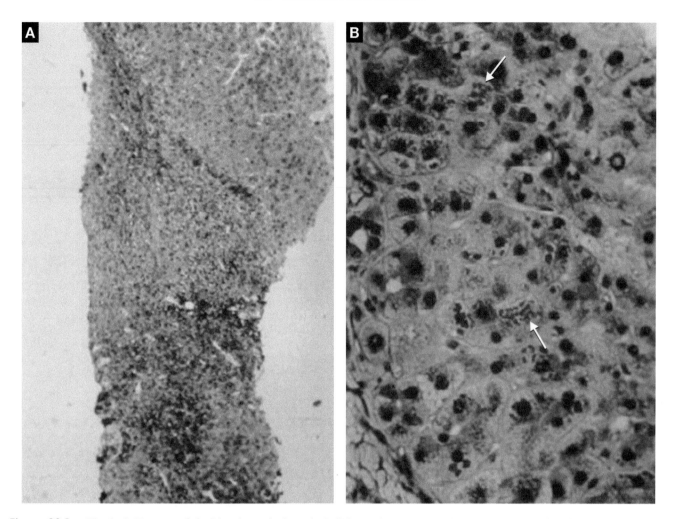

Figure 30.1. Histologic Features of the Liver in α₁-Antitrypsin Deficiency. A, Low-power view. B, High-power view. Characteristic periodic acid-Schiff–positive, diastase-resistant globules (arrows) have accumulated in hepatocytes.

consequences of portal hypertension, and the recipient assumes the *Pi* phenotype of the donor. Long-term outcomes for A1ATD after liver transplant are excellent.

A1ATD may be amenable to somatic gene therapy. Gene therapy probably would be beneficial for only the lung disease unless a method of delivering the corrected gene product to the endoplasmic reticulum of hepatocytes were available. Gene therapy continues to be an area of research, but it is not routinely clinically available.

Wilson Disease

WD is an inherited disorder of intrahepatic copper metabolism characterized by the deposition of excess copper in the liver, brain, cornea, and other organs. This rare disorder typically manifests in children, adolescents, and young adults. Patients with WD may present with various disease manifestations, including acute liver failure, chronic liver disease, hemolytic anemia, or neuropsychiatric symptoms (or a combination of these).

Inheritance and Gene Function

WD is an autosomal recessive disorder. The gene (*ATP7B*; OMIM 606882) associated with the disease is on chromosome 13 and codes for a copper-transporting P-type adenosine triphosphatase (ATPase) located predominantly in the endoplasmic reticulum and

biliary canalicular membrane of hepatocytes. Although WD is a rare disorder, it is probably underdiagnosed. Approximately 1 per 30,000 persons are homozygous and 1 per 100 are heterozygous carriers of a WD gene alteration. To date, more than 600 variants of *ATP7B* have been described. Attempts to correlate genotype with phenotype have not shown a consistent pattern and are not clinically useful. Approximately 30% to 40% of North American and European patients with WD have the *H1069Q* gene (OMIM 277900) variant.

Unlike hereditary hemochromatosis, in which approximately 90% of persons are homozygous for the C282Y alteration (see the Hereditary Hemochromatosis section below), the majority of patients with WD are compound heterozygous (ie, they have 1 copy of 2 different alterations). The number of clinically important alterations makes genetic testing less useful for this disease than for hereditary hemochromatosis. Genetic testing is most valuable for screening the siblings of an affected proband in whom the specific alterations are known.

Copper Metabolism and Pathophysiology

Copper is an essential trace element that is necessary as a cofactor for many proteins. Dietary copper is absorbed in the proximal small bowel. Copper homeostasis is maintained through the biliary excretion of excess copper by active transport with a metal-transporting ATPase. Any disease that impairs biliary excretion (eg, chronic cholestatic biliary disorders such as primary biliary cholangitis or primary sclerosing cholangitis) can cause increases in the level of hepatic copper. In WD, intestinal copper absorption is normal but biliary excretion of copper is decreased, leading to marked copper overload and ultimately end-organ toxicity.

Copper toxicity has a major role in the pathogenesis of the disease. Copper accumulates in the liver and eventually appears in other organs, particularly the brain and the eye (specifically, the cornea). Excess copper exerts its toxic effect by the generation of free radicals that result in lipid peroxidation, similar to the mechanism proposed for iron-induced damage in hereditary hemochromatosis. Deficiency of ceruloplasmin is not the cause of WD; rather, it is an effect of the abnormal cellular trafficking of copper.

Clinical Features

WD has various clinical manifestations ranging from patients who are asymptomatic to those who have crippling neurologic symptoms or acute liver failure. WD is a disease of young persons; the typical age at presentation is 12 to 23 years. Hepatic manifestations tend to be more common in childhood, whereas neurologic symptoms tend to appear in the second and third decades of life. Although age alone should not be used to exclude WD, its initial presentation in patients older than 40 years is extremely rare.

The 5 main categories of clinical presentation are hepatic, neurologic, psychiatric, hematologic, and ophthalmologic. In a large clinical series, the initial clinical manifestations were hepatic in 42% of patients, neurologic in 34%, psychiatric in 10%, and hematologic in 12%.

Hepatic Manifestations

Patients with WD can present with any form of liver disease, including asymptomatic abnormalities in liver test results, chronic hepatitis, and cirrhosis. Reports of hepatocellular cancer in patients with WD are rare even though many patients have advanced fibrosis at a young age. Although WD should be considered in all young patients with liver disease, it is responsible for less than 5% of cases of chronic hepatitis in persons younger than 35 years.

Acute liver failure is a catastrophic manifestation and may be the initial presentation of patients with WD. Acute liver failure due to this disease is 4 times more common in female patients than male patients. Fulminant WD should be suspected in any young patient with acute liver failure, especially if it is associated with hemolytic anemia. Patients with fulminant WD require urgent liver transplant because there is no other effective therapy. In the US, patients with fulminant WD awaiting liver transplant are given a high priority for deceased donor organ allocation (United Network for Organ Sharing [UNOS] status 1).

Neuropsychiatric Manifestations

The typical neurologic manifestations of WD are dominated by extrapyramidal motor symptoms, including rigidity or spasticity, tremor, ataxia, dysarthria, drooling, and involuntary movements. Dementia and seizures are rare. Psychiatric problems may be dramatic, with psychosis or depression, or they may be subtle and manifested as behavioral problems or declining school

performance for children and adolescents. Children are often classified as having behavioral problems or learning disabilities until progressive and sometimes irreversible neurologic symptoms begin to develop.

Hematologic Manifestations

Patients may present first with a Coombs-negative hemolytic anemia, frequently seen in association with acute, severe, or fulminant hepatitis. A young patient with severe liver dysfunction and hemolytic anemia should be assumed to have WD until proved otherwise.

Ocular Manifestations

Occasionally, WD is identified because of incidental eye findings, or the ocular manifestations may be noted during the evaluation of patients with suspected WD. Kayser-Fleischer rings result from copper deposition in the periphery of the cornea. These rings are frequently present in patients with neurologic manifestations of WD, but the absence of the rings does not exclude the disease. Prominent Kayser-Fleischer rings may be seen on direct examination, but more subtle rings may require slit-lamp examination. Sunflower cataracts are seen only with a slit lamp and do not interfere with vision. The ocular manifestations in WD are shown in Figure 30.2.

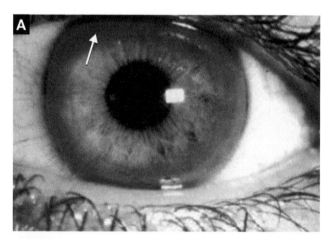

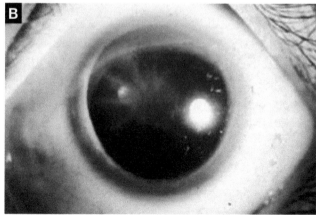

Figure 30.2. Ocular Manifestations in Wilson Disease. A, Kayser-Fleischer ring (arrow). B, Sunflower cataract. (Adapted from Zucker SD, Gollan JL. Wilson's disease and hepatic copper toxicosis. In: Zakim D, Boyer TD, eds. Hepatology: a textbook of liver disease. 3rd ed. WB Saunders; 1996:1405-39; used with permission.)

Other Manifestations

WD is associated also with proximal or distal renal tubular acidosis and nephrolithiasis. Another manifestation is azure lunulae, a blue discoloration of the base of the fingernails that is an uncommon but characteristic finding.

Diagnosis and Evaluation

The diagnosis of WD requires a strong clinical suspicion because of the multitude of potential manifestations. The disease should be considered in any person younger than 30 years who has liver disease. The presence of liver disease in combination with extrapyramidal motor abnormalities should strongly suggest WD, and the presence of severe liver disease in combination with nonimmune hemolytic anemia should be considered WD until definitively proved otherwise.

Liver chemistry values are frequently abnormal in patients with WD, and characteristic patterns may serve as a clinical clue, but they are not consistent enough to be confirmatory. The alkaline phosphatase level is often low, and the serum aminotransferase levels tend to be increased less than would be expected from other causes of liver necrosis. Uric acid levels are usually low or undetectable, often because of concomitant proximal renal tubular acidosis. Serum copper levels are of limited usefulness because they may be low, normal, or increased—normal serum copper levels do not exclude WD.

The initial evaluation for suspected WD should include 1) determination of the serum ceruloplasmin level, 2) 24-hour urine collection for copper quantification, and 3) slit-lamp examination for Kayser-Fleischer rings. The serum level of ceruloplasmin is less than 20 mg/dL in 95% of patients with WD. Even though the level of ceruloplasmin can be increased nonspecifically as an acute phase reactant or as a result of estrogen administration, a level higher than 30 mg/dL essentially excludes the diagnosis of WD except in rare patients who present with fulminant hepatitis. Low ceruloplasmin levels must be interpreted with caution because any chronic liver disease with synthetic dysfunction or protein-losing states may be associated with a ceruloplasmin level that is lower than normal. Urinary copper excretion can be increased in other liver diseases; however, a value less than 100 μg daily in a patient with clinical disease would be very unusual in a symptomatic patient with WD. A low rate of urinary copper excretion may indicate acquired copper deficiency. This may be confusing because cases of severe copper deficiency may be associated with neurologic symptoms. The neurologic syndrome in these cases is myelopathy with weakness and ataxia.

In most cases, liver biopsy is necessary to confirm the diagnosis of WD, particularly in the absence of Kayser-Fleischer rings or characteristic neurologic symptoms. Liver morphologic features are nonspecific in WD. Often, steatosis is present, and glycogenated nuclei are common. The gold standard for confirming the diagnosis of the disease is quantitative tissue copper analysis. A normal liver concentration of copper (<35 μg/g dry weight) excludes the diagnosis. Most patients with the disease have liver copper concentrations greater than 250 μg/g dry weight, but this finding is not specific and may occur in chronic cholestatic conditions or, rarely, in autoimmune hepatitis. Unlike hereditary hemochromatosis, children with WD may already have marked liver fibrosis; thus, in children, liver biopsy should be strongly considered to stage the liver disease.

Treatment

Treatment of WD is lifelong. Because many patients with WD are adolescents or young adults, adherence to therapy can be challenging, especially among asymptomatic patients. Therapies for WD can be divided broadly into 2 categories: chelating agents that remove copper from the body and agents that inhibit intestinal absorption of dietary copper. Liver transplant also is indicated as a treatment of fulminant WD (acute liver failure often associated with hemolysis) or for patients with complications of cirrhosis from the disease.

Chelating Agents

Patients with symptomatic or clinically evident disease should be treated initially with chelating agents. Penicillamine and trientine are metal chelators that induce the urinary excretion of copper. Both agents have been approved for the treatment of WD. Penicillamine is effective therapy and historically has been considered as first-line treatment, but it has numerous adverse effects. Up to 20% of patients experience drug toxicity, including hypersensitivity reactions, bone marrow suppression, proteinuria, autoimmune disorders, and dermatologic conditions. Importantly, as many as 20% of patients with neurologic symptoms may experience worsening of their symptoms during the first month of treatment. This deterioration is irreversible in some patients. Therefore, trientine should be considered as initial therapy for patients with neurologic symptoms from WD.

Trientine was introduced as an alternative to penicillamine. However, because of a lower incidence of adverse effects, trientine should be the first choice for treatment. It is given in doses similar to those for penicillamine and also has satisfactory long-term efficacy. The cupruresis is less pronounced than with penicillamine, but an initial increase is expected. Occasionally, iron deficiency may develop because of sideroblastic anemia. Dosing of agents and monitoring for patients with WD are outlined in Table 30.1.

Response to chelator therapy is demonstrated by an acute increase in urinary copper excretion that gradually plateaus at a lower level over 6 to 12 months. Initially, urinary copper output is often more than 2,000 μg daily, decreasing to 400 to 500 μg daily in the maintenance phase. The urinary and serum levels of copper and the ceruloplasmin level should be measured and a complete blood cell count should be performed weekly during the first month and then every 1 or 2 months during the first 6 months. Patients whose condition is stable can then be followed annually. A slit-lamp examination should be repeated annually to document the disappearance of Kayser-Fleischer rings (if present).

Inhibition of Copper Absorption

In the intestinal epithelium, zinc acetate induces the synthesis of metallothionein, which preferentially binds copper and prevents its absorption. Zinc therapy is indicated for patients who are presymptomatic or pregnant. It also may be used as maintenance therapy for patients who present with symptomatic disease after initial chelation therapy to remove excess copper (typically after 6-12 months). Treatment is monitored by checking urinary levels of zinc and copper. The urinary excretion of zinc should be at least 2,000 μg daily.

For pregnant women with WD, penicillamine is probably safe, but zinc is a better choice if their condition is stable. The teratogenicity of trientine is unknown, and it should not be given during pregnancy.

Table 30.1. Treatment of Wilson Disease

Agent	Daily dose by mouth		Monitoring	Comments
	Initial	Target		
Penicillamine	250-500 mg	1-2 g, divided into 2-4 doses	CBC, ceruloplasmin, and urinary and serum copper levels should be measured weekly during first month, then every 1 or 2 mo during first 6 mo; once stable, follow annually. Slit-lamp examination to document disappearance of K-F rings, if present	Administer with pyridoxine because penicillamine can deplete vitamin B_6. Do not administer to patients with neurologic symptoms because will worsen symptoms in 20%
Trientine	250-500 mg	1-2 g, divided into 2-4 doses	CBC, ceruloplasmin, and urinary and serum copper levels should be measured weekly during first month, then every 1 or 2 mo during first 6 mo; once stable, follow annually. Slit-lamp examination to document disappearance of K-F rings, if present	First-line therapy for most patients. Dosing and monitoring as with penicillamine. May cause sideroblastic anemia
Zinc acetate	50 mg, 3 times	50 mg, 3 times	Urinary copper and zinc excretion should be >2,000 μg daily	Initial therapy for presymptomatic patients and pregnant patients. Can be used as maintenance therapy after copper depletion with trientine or penicillamine

Abbreviations: CBC, complete blood cell count; K-F, Kayser-Fleischer.

Liver Transplant

The indications for liver transplant include acute liver failure, end-stage liver disease unresponsive to medical therapy, and chronic deterioration of liver function despite long-term therapy. Medical therapy is not effective in reversing fulminant WD; patients with fulminant disease require urgent liver transplant and are given high priority for donor organ allocation in the US (UNOS status 1). Outcomes for liver transplant in patients with fulminant disease are good, with a 1-year survival rate of 73%. Among those with chronic liver failure, the 1-year survival rate is about 90%. Liver transplant performed solely for refractory neurologic symptoms is still considered experimental because of the limited experience and uncertain clinical improvement.

Family Screening

After WD has been diagnosed, family members should have screening tests for the disease. Testing should be directed at siblings because each has about a 25% chance of having the disease. If treatment is begun in the presymptomatic phase of the disease before cirrhosis is established, disease progression can be prevented. Because copper metabolism in infancy and early childhood may simulate WD, children should not be tested before 5 years of age. Screening should include aminotransferase and ceruloplasmin levels and a slit-lamp examination for Kayser-Fleischer rings. If the results are normal, screening should be repeated every 5 years until age 20. If the ceruloplasmin level is less than 20 mg/dL but there are no Kayser-Fleischer rings or convincing neurologic symptoms, liver biopsy may be necessary. Genetic testing generally is used for screening once the pattern in the index case is known. This may be of value if standard copper test results are equivocal.

✓ Wilson disease
- Typical age at presentation: 12 to 23 years
- Characteristic laboratory findings: 1) normal or low alkaline phosphatase level, 2) modestly increased aminotransferases levels, and 3) Coombs-negative hemolytic anemia

- Diagnostic findings: 1) low serum level of ceruloplasmin (<20 mg/dL), 2) increased 24-hour urinary copper excretion, and 3) the presence of Kayser-Fleischer rings
- Gold standard confirmatory test: quantitative liver copper concentration (typically >250 μg/g dry weight, but a similarly high concentration may also occur in chronic cholestatic liver diseases)
✓ Treatment of WD
- Chelating agents: penicillamine (which can worsen the neurologic sequelae of WD) or trientine
- Zinc therapy to inhibit copper absorption for patients who are presymptomatic or pregnant or as maintenance therapy for patients after 6 to 12 months of chelation therapy
- Liver transplant for patients with acute liver failure or progression of end-stage liver disease despite therapy

Hereditary Hemochromatosis

Hereditary hemochromatosis is an inherited disorder of iron metabolism characterized by the deposition of excess iron in the liver, heart, joints, pancreas, skin, testes, and other organs. Patients with hereditary hemochromatosis may present with chronic liver disease, cardiomyopathy, or arthropathy.

Inheritance and Gene Function

Hereditary hemochromatosis is an autosomal recessive disorder. The gene associated with this disorder is the *HFE* gene (OMIM 613609) on the short arm of chromosome 6. In contrast to the large number of alterations of the *ATP7B* gene for WD, the *HFE* gene has 2 common point variants, C282Y and H63D. Other alterations have been described, but they probably are not of major clinical importance. About 90% of patients with iron overload consistent with hereditary hemochromatosis are homozygous for the C282Y alteration. The *HFE* gene is involved in regulating dietary iron absorption. The HFE protein binds to the transferrin receptor and acts as a signal when body iron stores are adequate. When the *HFE* variant is present, iron absorption is not downregulated from enterocytes despite adequate iron levels, leading to iron overload.

Unlike WD, hereditary hemochromatosis is not a rare disorder. It is the most common single-gene, inherited disorder in the US White population. Approximately 1 in every 200 to 300 White persons in the US is homozygous for the hemochromatosis alteration, and at least 1 in every 10 is a heterozygous carrier.

Iron Metabolism and Pathophysiology

Iron metabolism is relatively complex. The pathophysiology of hereditary hemochromatosis can be summarized as the failure to downregulate dietary iron absorption in the presence of adequate or excess body iron stores. However, not all iron overload is due to hereditary hemochromatosis; excess iron administration, multiple blood transfusions, or hematopoietic disorders can result in secondary iron overload states.

Dietary iron absorbed by enterocytes is transported through the basolateral membrane into the bloodstream by the transmembrane transporter ferroportin. *HFE* and transferrin receptor 1 are involved in signaling adequate iron stores. This, in turn, leads to increased expression of the hepcidin protein, which inhibits iron release from ferroportin into the bloodstream. In the presence of the *HFE* variant, hepcidin is not upregulated, leading enterocytes to detect a state of iron deficiency and continue to avidly transport dietary iron into the bloodstream. This uninhibited iron absorption leads to iron excess and eventually end-organ toxicity.

Clinical Features

Because persons with hereditary hemochromatosis absorb only a few more milligrams of iron each day than needed, clinical manifestations generally do not occur until after the fifth decade of life, when 15 to 40 g of iron have accumulated (normal body iron stores are approximately 4 g). Among those who are homozygous for C282Y, approximately 30% of men and 2% to 10% of women have biochemical or clinical evidence of iron overload. The frequency of clinical iron overload is lower among women than men most likely because of menstrual and pregnancy-related blood loss. Additional factors that influence disease expression include age, dietary iron intake, and unknown factors, including alterations in genes other than *HFE*. Liver disease is also affected by alcohol consumption and comorbid liver disease (eg, hepatitis C), which accelerate hepatic fibrosis.

In the past, hereditary hemochromatosis usually was diagnosed at an advanced stage. The classic description of hereditary hemochromatosis as "bronze diabetes" resulted from cutaneous hyperpigmentation, type 2 diabetes, and cirrhosis. Currently, the disease is diagnosed in most patients at an asymptomatic stage through laboratory studies. Clinical manifestations of the disease include fatigue, hepatomegaly, abnormal liver enzyme levels, cirrhosis, hepatocellular carcinoma, cardiomyopathy, cardiac conduction disorders, hypothyroidism, hypogonadism, erectile dysfunction, and arthropathy. An example of hemochromatosis arthropathy is shown in Figure 30.3. Most, if not all, clinical manifestations are preventable if the disease is diagnosed early and treated appropriately. Hepatomegaly, abnormal liver test results, skin bronzing, cardiomyopathy, and cardiac conduction disorders may reverse after iron depletion, although most other clinical manifestations are not reversible.

The development of hepatocellular carcinoma is a major consequence of hereditary hemochromatosis. In up to one-third

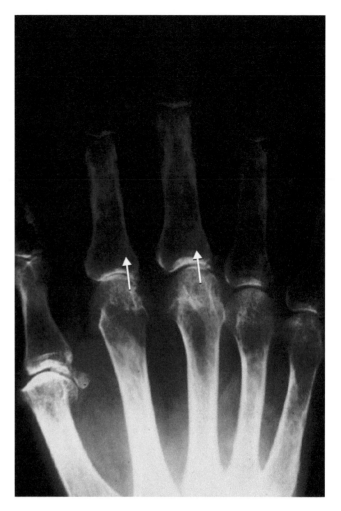

Figure 30.3. Hemochromatosis Arthropathy. A radiograph of the hand shows cartilage loss, marginal sclerosis, and osteophyte formation in the second and third metacarpophalangeal joints (arrows) without involvement of the fourth and fifth joints. Involvement of the second and third metacarpophalangeal joints is characteristic of hemochromatosis arthropathy. Occasionally, calcium pyrophosphate dihydrate crystals are present (chondrocalcinosis). (Adapted from Riely CA, Vera SR, Burrell MI, Koff RS. The gastroenterology teaching project, unit 8: inherited liver disease; used with permission.)

of patients with hereditary hemochromatosis and cirrhosis, hepatocellular carcinoma develops and often is the cause of death. The presence of hemochromatosis imparts a roughly 200-fold increased risk of liver cancer, with most cases involving patients with cirrhosis. The increased risk of hepatocellular carcinoma does not improve after iron depletion. Patients with hereditary hemochromatosis–related cirrhosis should have abdominal ultrasonography every 6 months to screen for hepatocellular carcinoma.

Diagnosis and Evaluation

Hereditary hemochromatosis is diagnosed on the basis of a combination of clinical, laboratory, and pathology criteria. Iron studies should show increased serum transferrin saturation (100×[serum iron concentration/total iron-binding capacity]) and an increased serum ferritin level. An increase in transferrin saturation is the earliest laboratory abnormality in hereditary hemochromatosis.

The serum concentration of ferritin is usually a reasonable estimate of total body iron stores. However, because ferritin is also an acute phase reactant, it is increased in various infectious and inflammatory conditions without any iron overload. This is a common pitfall in the diagnosis of hereditary hemochromatosis. Ferritin may be increased in 30% to 50% of patients who have viral hepatitis, nonalcohol-related fatty liver disease, or alcohol-related liver disease. For these reasons, ferritin should not be used as the initial screening test to detect hereditary hemochromatosis. A diagnostic algorithm for hereditary hemochromatosis is provided in Figure 30.4.

HFE Gene Testing

The *HFE* gene test is most useful for surveillance of adult first-degree relatives of an identified proband. *HFE* gene testing is also often useful in cases of diagnostic uncertainty, such as iron overload associated with hepatitis C, alcohol-related liver disease, or other causes of end-stage liver disease. *HFE* gene testing usually is not recommended for anyone younger than 18 years.

The 2 most common *HFE* variants are C282Y and H63D, which account for approximately 85% of cases of hereditary hemochromatosis. Patients homozygous for C282Y are the most likely to present with clinically evident iron overload. Patients who are compound heterozygous (C282Y/H63D) have a much lower rate of clinically evident iron overload (approximately 20%). Patients who are heterozygous (single copy of C282Y or H63D) typically do not have iron overload, but some do have slightly high (or high-normal) values on serum iron tests.

Liver Biopsy

Before the *HFE* gene test was routinely available, liver biopsy was important in the diagnosis of hereditary hemochromatosis. Currently, however, liver biopsy is used only to assess cases with diagnostic uncertainty and to assess for the presence of advanced fibrosis or cirrhosis. In patients with iron overload who are homozygous for C282Y, liver biopsy is not necessary to confirm the diagnosis. Qualitative assessments of hepatic iron may be made with an iron stain (eg, Perls Prussian blue). In hereditary hemochromatosis, iron accumulates initially in periportal hepatocytes and eventually is distributed throughout the liver. This is in

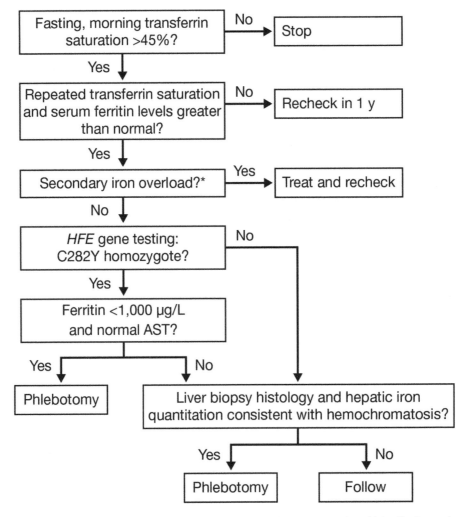

Figure 30.4. Diagnostic Algorithm for Hereditary Hemochromatosis. Asterisk indicates anemias with ineffective erythropoiesis, multiple blood transfusions, or oral or parenteral iron supplementation. AST indicates aspartate aminotransferase. (Adapted from Brandhagen DJ, Fairbanks VF, Batts KP, Thibodeau SN. Update on hereditary hemochromatosis and the *HFE* gene. Mayo Clin Proc. 1999 Sep;74[9]:917-21; used with permission of Mayo Foundation for Medical Education and Research.)

contrast to secondary iron overload in which iron often occurs predominantly in Kupffer cells. In severe iron overload, this distinction cannot be made reliably. The histologic features of the liver in hereditary hemochromatosis and secondary iron overload are shown in Figure 30.5.

Quantitative measurement of liver iron is an adjunctive diagnostic test for hereditary hemochromatosis. Liver iron stores increase progressively with age, and this has led to the development of the hepatic iron index, which is calculated as the hepatic iron concentration in micromoles per gram dry weight of liver divided by the patient's age in years. A hepatic iron index greater than 1.9 is strongly suggestive of hereditary hemochromatosis.

Identifying patients who have hereditary hemochromatosis–related cirrhosis is critical because of the need to screen for complications of cirrhosis, including esophageal varices and the increased risk for hepatocellular cancer. Age and ferritin levels can be used to predict which patients with hereditary hemochromatosis have a minimal risk for cirrhosis. Cirrhosis is unlikely and liver biopsy would be unnecessary in patients who are homozygous for C282Y, with serum ferritin levels less than 1,000 µg/L and normal aspartate aminotransferase values. Consequently,

liver biopsy is advisable to definitively assess for the presence of cirrhosis in patients older than 40 years who have abnormal aminotransferase concentrations or a ferritin concentration greater than 1,000 µg/L.

Secondary Iron Overload

Not all iron overload is due to hereditary hemochromatosis, which should be distinguished from iron overload caused by other conditions. Secondary iron overload should be suspected in patients with chronic anemia who have ineffective erythropoiesis or have had multiple blood transfusions. In rare instances, prolonged iron supplementation can produce abnormal iron test results and, even more rarely, tissue iron overload.

A commonly encountered cause of abnormal iron test results is acute or chronic liver disease. Acute liver disease may be accompanied by a high ferritin level, usually with normal transferrin saturation. Chronic liver disease, particularly if advanced, may result in abnormalities in ferritin and iron saturation that can mimic hereditary hemochromatosis. However, severe iron overload from hereditary hemochromatosis may be indistinguishable

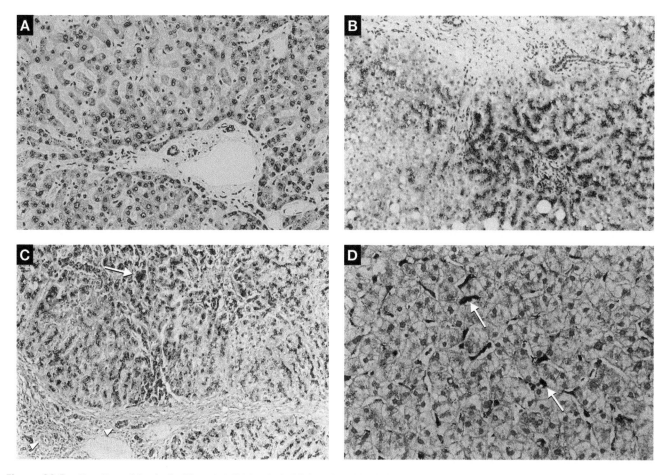

Figure 30.5. **Iron Deposition in the Liver.** A, Mild (grade 1 of 4) iron deposition in hepatocytes. B, Moderate hemosiderin deposition in precirrhotic homozygous hemochromatosis. Zone 1 hepatocytes are predominantly involved, biliary hemosiderin is not evident, and fibrosis has not yet occurred—all indicating relatively early precirrhotic disease (liver iron concentration, 10,307 µg/g dry weight; iron index, 3.2) (original magnification ×133). C, Marked hemosiderosis and cirrhosis in homozygous hemochromatosis. Although most iron is in hepatocytes, some Kupffer cells (arrow) and biliary iron (arrowheads) are also present (original magnification ×133). D, Kupffer cell hemosiderosis. The presence of hemosiderin in Kupffer cells alone (arrows) is typical of mild transfusion hemosiderosis, is nonspecific, and should not prompt further consideration of hemochromatosis (original magnification ×240). (A-D, Perls Prussian blue stain). (A, adapted from Brandhagen DJ. Liver transplantation for hereditary hemochromatosis. Liver Transpl. 2001;7[8]:663-72, and B-D, adapted from Baldus WP, Batts KP, Brandhagen DJ. Liver biopsy in hemochromatosis. In: Barton JC, Edwards CQ, eds. Hemochromatosis: genetics, pathophysiology, diagnosis, and treatment. Cambridge University Press; 2000:187-99; used with permission.)

from that due to secondary causes. Patients with alcohol-related steatohepatitis may present with markedly increased ferritin levels. If the diagnosis is in doubt, these patients can be observed because alcohol-related increases in ferritin will decrease remarkably over a short period (3 months) with abstinence from alcohol. Patients with nonalcohol-related fatty liver disease often present with increased liver enzyme and ferritin levels. This is clinically relevant because it is a frequent cause for referral and confusion. Despite hereditary hemochromatosis being a common disease, most patients with abnormal iron test results (particularly isolated elevated ferritin levels) do not have the disease.

Treatment

Hemochromatosis is a simple and satisfying disease to treat, and treatment before the development of end-organ damage can prevent serious morbidity and death. Treatment is iron depletion by therapeutic phlebotomy, which is the preferred treatment because it is simple, relatively inexpensive, and effective. Dietary modifications are not advised because iron depletion cannot be achieved with dietary changes alone. Patients should be counseled to refrain from taking iron supplements, including multivitamins with iron, and high-dose vitamin C supplements. Although iron chelators such as the parenteral agent deferoxamine and oral agent deferasirox are often administered to patients with secondary iron overload (particularly those with hematologic disorders who may not tolerate phlebotomy), they are associated with more adverse effects and are much less effective than phlebotomy.

Treatment of hereditary hemochromatosis is usually reserved for patients who have evidence of iron overload as indicated by an increase in the serum concentration of ferritin. Patients with *HFE* gene alterations without iron overload do not need phlebotomy, but they should be monitored periodically. Therapeutic phlebotomy is divided into 2 phases: 1) During the initial phase, phlebotomy is performed frequently to deplete excess iron stores. 2) This is followed by lifelong maintenance phlebotomy to prevent the reaccumulation of excess iron.

The initial phase of phlebotomy begins with removal of 500 mL of blood weekly. The hemoglobin concentration should be measured just before each phlebotomy. Weekly phlebotomy should continue as long as the hemoglobin concentration is higher than a preselected value (usually 12-13 g/dL). If the concentration is less than the preselected value, phlebotomy should not be performed. Once the hemoglobin concentration remains below the preselected value for 3 consecutive weeks without phlebotomy, the serum concentration of ferritin and transferrin saturation should be determined again. Iron depletion is confirmed if the ferritin level is not more than 50 µg/L, with a low-normal transferrin saturation. When iron depletion has been achieved, most patients require maintenance phlebotomies about every 3 to 4 months to keep the ferritin level less than 50 µg/L. Once iron is depleted, patients should have iron stores checked every 1 to 2 years to adjust the frequency of maintenance phlebotomy as necessary.

Despite being common, hereditary hemochromatosis only rarely causes complications of cirrhosis and is an uncommon indication for orthotopic liver transplant, accounting for less than 1% of all liver transplants performed in the US. Patients with hepatocellular carcinoma complicating hereditary hemochromatosis–related cirrhosis should be referred for consideration of liver transplant (the tumors must meet liver transplant criteria). The survival rate of patients with hereditary

hemochromatosis undergoing liver transplant has improved in recent years and is now similar to that of liver transplant for other indications. The death of many liver transplant recipients who have hereditary hemochromatosis is caused by cardiac or infectious complications.

✓ Hereditary hemochromatosis—approximately 90% arise from 2 sequence variants in the *HFE* gene, C282Y and H63D

✓ Typically, patients who present with hereditary hemochromatosis are older than 50 years (men typically present at a younger age than women)

✓ Clinical manifestations of hereditary hemochromatosis
  • Largely reversible conditions: hepatomegaly and fibrosis, skin bronzing, cardiomyopathy, and cardiac conduction disorders
  • Irreversible conditions: advanced cirrhosis and risk of hepatocellular carcinoma, arthropathy, primary or secondary hypogonadism, hypothyroidism, and type 2 diabetes

✓ Diagnosis of hereditary hemochromatosis
  • Increased ferritin level with increased transferrin saturation (>45%)
  • Exclusion of other causes of liver disease and iron overload
  • Liver biopsy for patients who have a ferritin concentration greater than 1,000 µg/L

✓ Goal of hereditary hemochromatosis treatment with phlebotomy—maintain ferritin concentration less than 50 µg/L and hemoglobin greater than 12 to 13 g/dL

Family Screening

Currently, experts disagree about the usefulness of screening for hereditary hemochromatosis in the general population. Despite the disease fulfilling many of the criteria of a condition appropriate for population screening, some public health experts do not advocate screening. Screening for the disease in family members of affected individuals is crucial because 25% of siblings and 5% of children of a proband will have the disease. *HFE* gene testing should be considered also for siblings of patients who are heterozygous for C282Y.

Table 30.2. Non-*HFE* Hereditary Iron Overload Disorders

Disorder	Laboratory test findings	Clinical features
TFR2 hemochromatosis	High transferrin saturation High ferritin level	Patients present at younger age (30-40 y) than patients with *HFE* hemochromatosis Hepatic, endocrine, and cardiovascular involvement
HAMP or *HJV* alterations	High transferrin saturation High ferritin level	Severe iron overload phenotype Patients present at young age (15-20 y) Cardiomyopathy
Ferroportin disease	Low or normal transferrin saturation High ferritin level	Broad age range at presentation Splenic iron deposition Liver biopsy shows iron in Kupffer cells

Abbreviations: *HAMP*, hepcidin gene (OMIM 606464); *HJV*, hemojuvelin gene (OMIM 608374); *TFR2*, transferrin receptor 2 gene (OMIM 604720).

Table 30.3. Comparison of Hereditary Hemochromatosis, Wilson Disease, and α$_1$-Antitrypsin Deficiency

Feature	Hereditary hemochromatosis	Wilson disease	α$_1$-Antitrypsin deficiency
Inheritance	Autosomal recessive	Autosomal recessive	Autosomal codominant
Homozygote frequency	1:200 to 1:300	1:30,000	1:2,000
Heterozygote frequency	1:10	1:100	1:30
Gene	*HFE*	*ATP7B*	NA
No. of clinically significant variants	2 (C282Y, H63D)	>600	NA
Chromosome	6	13	14
Diagnosis	Transferrin saturation, ferritin level, liver iron concentration, *HFE* gene test	Ceruloplasmin, slit-lamp examination for Kayser-Fleischer rings, urinary and liver copper quantification	α$_1$-Antitrypsin phenotype
Treatment	Phlebotomy	Penicillamine, trientine, or zinc	None or orthotopic liver transplant

Abbreviation: NA, not applicable.

Non-*HFE* Hereditary Iron Overload Disorders

With the expanding understanding of the pathogenesis of hemochromatosis, several non-*HFE* forms of hereditary iron overload disorders have been identified. These should be considered when iron overload is documented in the absence of a secondary cause (eg, hemolysis) and *HFE* gene testing is negative. Patients often present at an earlier age than those with typical *HFE* hemochromatosis. The clinical features are listed in Table 30.2.

Summary

The features of hereditary hemochromatosis, WD, and A1ATD are summarized and compared in Table 30.3.

Suggested Reading

Adams PC. Review article: The modern diagnosis and management of haemochromatosis. Aliment Pharmacol Ther. 2006 Jun;23(12):1681–91.

Ala A, Walker AP, Ashkan K, Dooley JS, Schilsky ML. Wilson's disease. Lancet. 2007 Feb;369(9559):397–408.

American Thoracic Society, European Respiratory Society. American Thoracic Society/European Respiratory Society statement: standards for the diagnosis and management of individuals with alpha-1 antitrypsin deficiency. Am J Respir Crit Care Med. 2003 Oct;168(7):818–900.

Bacon BR, Adams PC, Kowdley KV, Powell LW, Tavill AS, American Association for the Study of Liver Diseases. Diagnosis and management of hemochromatosis: 2011 practice guideline by the American Association for the Study of Liver Diseases. Hepatology. 2011 Jul;54(1):328–43.

Beutler E, Felitti VJ, Koziol JA, Ho NJ, Gelbart T. Penetrance of 845g--> a (c282y) HFE hereditary haemochromatosis mutation in the USA. Lancet. 2002 Jan;359(9302):211–8.

Ferenci P. Wilson's disease. Clin Gastroenterol Hepatol. 2005 Aug;3(8):726–33.

Ferrarese A, Morelli MC, Carrai P, Milana M, Angelico M, Perricone G, et al. Outcomes of liver transplant for adults with Wilson's disease. Liver Transpl. 2020 Apr;26(4):507–16.

Morrison ED, Brandhagen DJ, Phatak PD, Barton JC, Krawitt EL, El-Serag HB, et al. Serum ferritin level predicts advanced hepatic fibrosis among US patients with phenotypic hemochromatosis. Ann Intern Med. 2003 Apr;138(8):627–33.

Palmer WC, Vishnu P, Sanchez W, Aqel B, Riegert-Johnson D, Seaman LAK, et al. Diagnosis and management of genetic iron overload disorders. J Gen Intern Med. 2018 Dec;33(12):2230–6.

Perlmutter DH, Brodsky JL, Balistreri WF, Trapnell BC. Molecular pathogenesis of alpha-1-antitrypsin deficiency-associated liver disease: a meeting review. Hepatology. 2007 May;45(5):1313–23.

Pietrangelo A. Non-HFE hemochromatosis. Hepatology. 2004 Jan;39(1):21–9.

Pietrangelo A. Hereditary hemochromatosis: a new look at an old disease. N Engl J Med. 2004 Jun;350(23):2383–97.

Pietrangelo A. Hereditary hemochromatosis: pathogenesis, diagnosis, and treatment. Gastroenterology. 2010 Aug;139(2):393–408.

Roberts EA, Schilsky ML, American Association for Study of Liver Diseases. Diagnosis and treatment of Wilson disease: an update. Hepatology. 2008 Jun;47(6):2089–111.

Silverman EK, Sandhaus RA. Clinical practice: alpha1-antitrypsin deficiency. N Engl J Med. 2009 Jun;360(26):2749–57.

Yamashita C, Adams PC. Natural history of the C282y homozygote for the hemochromatosis gene (HFE) with a normal serum ferritin level. Clin Gastroenterol Hepatol. 2003 Sep;1(5):388–91.

Yu L, Ioannou GN. Survival of liver transplant recipients with hemochromatosis in the United States. Gastroenterology. 2007 Aug;133(2):489–95.

31

Cholestatic Liver Disease[a]

JOHN E. EATON, MD

Cholestatic liver disease in adults may or may not show evidence of large bile duct obstruction. Drug-induced cholestasis may be the most common explanation for cholestasis, which is often self-limiting. Primary biliary cholangitis is the most common chronic cholestatic liver disease in adults, and primary sclerosing cholangitis is about half as common as primary biliary cholangitis. In contrast to primary sclerosing cholangitis, the cause of secondary sclerosing cholangitis can often be identified.

Differential Diagnosis

The differential diagnosis for cholestasis in adults without biliary obstruction is listed in Box 31.1; key causes of secondary sclerosing cholangitis are outlined in Box 31.2.

Primary Biliary Cholangitis

Diagnosis

Primary biliary cholangitis (formerly called primary biliary cirrhosis) has a prevalence of about 150 to 300 per million people, involves women in 90% of cases, and is characterized by positive results on the serum antimitochondrial antibody (AMA) test in 95% of patients. These patients present with biochemical features of cholestasis and may be asymptomatic. Fatigue is the most common symptom. Pruritus is less common but may occur in 30% of patients. Laboratory tests show increased serum alkaline phosphatase levels; aminotransferase levels are usually less than

5 times the upper limit of the reference ranges. Total bilirubin levels are often normal at diagnosis but can increase in more advanced stages of the disease, and serum levels of cholesterol and immunoglobulin M can be abnormally high. Comorbid

---

Box 31.1. Differential Diagnosis for Cholestasis in Adults Without Large-Duct Biliary Obstruction

Drug or TPN-induced cholestasis
Primary biliary cholangitis
Small-duct primary sclerosing cholangitis
Idiopathic adulthood ductopenia
Intrahepatic cholestasis of pregnancy
Cystic fibrosis
Progressive familial intrahepatic cholestasis
Alagille syndrome
Infiltrative disorders (eg, sarcoidosis, amyloidosis)
Nonalcoholic fatty liver disease[a]
Right-sided heart failure
Sepsis
Paraneoplastic (Stauffer syndrome)
Diabetic hepatosclerosis
Sickle cell intrahepatic cholestasis
Nodular regenerative hyperplasia
Macro–alkaline phosphatase

Abbreviation: TPN, total parental nutrition.

[a] May present with slightly increased, isolated alkaline phosphatase levels.

---

[a] The author thanks Jayant A. Talwalkar, MD, MPH, who authored previous versions of this chapter.

Abbreviation: AMA, antimitochondrial antibody

Box 31.2. Differential Diagnosis for Secondary
Sclerosing Cholangitis in Adults

Mechanical
    Iatrogenic or traumatic
    Choledocholithiasis or hepatolithiasis
    Chronic pancreatitis
    Portal hypertensive biliopathy
Infectious
    Recurrent bacterial cholangitis
    Biliary parasitic infection
    Cryptosporidium parvum, Microsporidia,
        cytomegalovirus in AIDS cholangiopathy
Ischemia
    Hepatic artery occlusion
    Vascular trauma
    Liver transplant
    Vasculitis
Malignancy
    Cholangiocarcinoma
    Advanced gallbladder adenocarcinoma
    Lymphoma
    Intrahepatic or biliary metastases
Inflammatory or infiltrative
    Immunoglobulin G4–associated cholangitis with or
        without concurrent autoimmune pancreatitis
    Sarcoidosis
    Amyloidosis
    Eosinophilic cholangitis
    Mast cell cholangiopathy
    Histiocytosis X
    Graft-vs-host disease
    Chronic allograft rejection
    Hepatic inflammatory pseudotumor
Toxic
    Ketamine
    Immunotherapy (eg, pembrolizumab, nivolumab)
    Intra-arterial chemotherapy (eg, fluorouracil)
    Intraductal ethanol, formaldehyde, or
        hypertonic saline
Congenital
    Biliary atresia after Kasai portoenterostomy
    Cystic fibrosis
    Congenital biliary cysts
    Turner syndrome

cholangitis, the diagnosis can be confirmed by the presence of other specific autoantibodies, including Sp100 and gp210, or by compatible histologic features on liver biopsy. A classic histologic finding in a subset of patients with primary biliary cholangitis is a florid duct lesion, which is characterized as a destructive cholangitis with granulomatous and lymphocytic inflammation centered on the interlobular bile duct (Figure 31.1). The prognosis and treatment of AMA-negative primary biliary cholangitis are the same as for AMA-positive primary biliary cholangitis. Increases in aminotransferase levels greater than 5-fold the upper limit of the reference range may indicate concurrent autoimmune hepatitis, which is present among 5% of patients with primary biliary cholangitis.

Treatment

Currently, the accepted standard of care is ursodeoxycholic acid, 13 to 15 mg/kg daily in divided doses, for patients with any stage of primary biliary cholangitis who have abnormal liver test findings. Approximately 70% of patients have an adequate biochemical response to ursodeoxycholic acid. Among those responders, survival is similar to that in the general population. The various response criteria center around decreases in the alkaline phosphatase level to less than 2 times the upper limit of the reference range.

If patients cannot tolerate ursodeoxycholic acid (a rare situation that can occur because of adverse effects related to the gastrointestinal tract), or if they have an incomplete response to ursodeoxycholic acid after 1 year, adjunctive therapy should be considered. Obeticholic acid is a farsenoid X receptor agonist that was approved by the US Food and Drug Administration because it decreases the alkaline phosphatase level, a surrogate marker associated with improved outcomes. However, it is unclear whether its use will result in improved clinical outcomes. The use of obeticholic acid is limited by dose-dependent pruritus, and it is contraindicated in patients with compensated cirrhosis and signs of portal hypertension and in patients with prior hepatic decompensation.

There is also emerging evidence that fibrates may be used to effectively treat primary biliary cholangitis. In particular, bezafibrate has been shown to decrease alkaline phosphatase levels and improve pruritus among patients who do not have a response to ursodeoxycholic acid. Some data suggest that fenofibrate may help to achieve a biochemical response among patients who do not have a response to ursodeoxycholic acid.

✓ Primary biliary cholangitis
  • Typical presentation—middle-aged woman with fatigue, pruritus, and increased level of alkaline phosphatase
  • Positive result on serum AMA test allows diagnosis for more than 90% of patients
  • If serum AMA test results are negative, diagnosis requires liver biopsy with compatible histology or the presence of specific autoantibodies (eg, gp210 and Sp100)
  • Treatment with ursodeoxycholic acid improves survival
  • Patients with inadequate response to ursodeoxycholic acid may benefit from adjunctive therapy

---

autoimmune diseases are frequently present (eg, Sjögren syndrome, sicca syndrome, or autoimmune thyroid diseases).

The most characteristic finding is a positive result on the serum AMA test, which recognizes the lipoic acid binding site on an enzyme in the pyruvate dehydrogenase complex. The diagnosis of primary biliary cholangitis can be established in the presence of an increased level of alkaline phosphatase with a positive AMA titer. Among patients with AMA-negative primary biliary

Primary Sclerosing Cholangitis

Diagnosis

Primary sclerosing cholangitis is associated with chronic inflammation and fibrosis of the biliary tree (intrahepatic or extrahepatic or both) (Figure 31.2). It can progress to cirrhosis and is

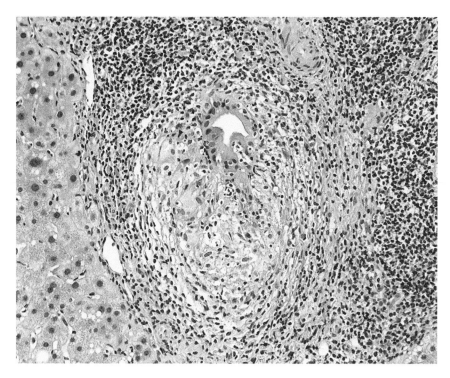

Figure 31.1. **Histologic Features of Primary Biliary Cholangitis.** Chronic nonsuppurative destructive cholangitis around the bile duct with mononuclear and granulomatous inflammation is consistent with a florid duct lesion.

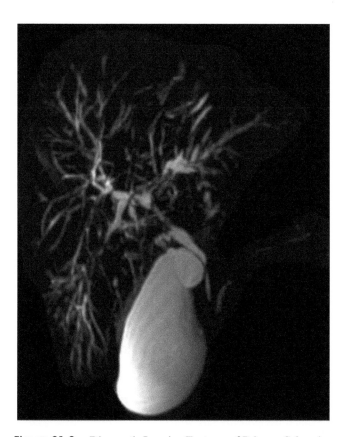

Figure 31.2. **Diagnostic Imaging Features of Primary Sclerosing Cholangitis.** Three-dimensional magnetic resonance cholangiopancreatography shows multifocal intrahepatic and extrahepatic biliary strictures.

associated with a heightened risk of hepatobiliary and colonic malignancies. Approximately 70% of patients have inflammatory bowel disease, which can develop at any time during the disease (even after liver transplant). Unlike primary biliary cholangitis, primary sclerosing cholangitis is more common in men. The typical age of onset is about 40 years.

The chief biochemical abnormality in primary sclerosing cholangitis is an increased level of serum alkaline phosphatase with transaminase levels typically less than 5 times the upper limit of the reference range (in the absence of acute biliary obstruction or overlap with autoimmune hepatitis). However, approximately 40% to 50% of patients have a normal alkaline phosphatase level sometime during the disease course. Hence, an abnormal alkaline phosphatase level is not required for a diagnosis of primary sclerosing cholangitis. Magnetic resonance cholangiography is the diagnostic method of choice for detection of multifocal biliary strictures associated with large-duct primary sclerosing cholangitis. Causes of secondary sclerosing cholangitis may generally be excluded clinically. A liver biopsy is needed only if the cholangiogram is normal and there is concern for small-duct primary sclerosing cholangitis or if there is a suspicion for concurrent autoimmune hepatitis. The classic biopsy findings of periductal fibrosis (so-called onion skin fibrosis) are not universally present (Figure 31.3). Autoantibodies such as antinuclear antibodies or perinuclear antineutrophil cytoplasmic antibodies may be present but are not specific or helpful in establishing the diagnosis. Frequently patients are asymptomatic, but they may have manifestations of biliary strictures (jaundice, pruritus, ascending cholangitis, or abdominal pain); fatigue; or signs of liver failure.

Given the prevalence of inflammatory bowel disease, typically ulcerative colitis, all patients with a diagnosis of primary sclerosing cholangitis should have a screening colonoscopy with

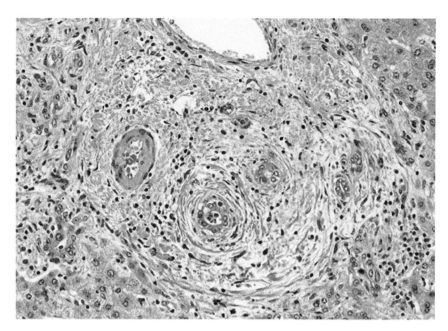

Figure 31.3.   Histologic Features of Primary Sclerosing Cholangitis. Concentric rings of collagen and fibroblasts surrounding bile ducts are consistent with onion skin fibrosis.

random biopsies to assess for underlying inflammatory bowel disease. The risk of colorectal cancer when inflammatory bowel disease is present is approximately 5-fold that of patients with inflammatory bowel disease alone. Patients with a concomitant diagnosis of inflammatory bowel disease with colonic involvement should have annual screening with surveillance biopsies for colorectal cancer screening.

Primary sclerosing cholangitis is also associated with an increased risk of hepatobiliary neoplasia. Cholangiocarcinoma is the leading cause of death in this population and may occur in 10% to 15% of patients with primary sclerosing cholangitis. The risk of cholangiocarcinoma is highest within the first year after the diagnosis of primary sclerosing cholangitis. However, cholangiocarcinoma is rare in pediatric patients or in patients who have small-duct primary sclerosing cholangitis. In addition, gallbladder cancer risk is increased, and gallbladder adenocarcinoma may develop in approximately 2% to 4% of patients. Most experts recommend annual imaging to screen for cholangiocarcinoma and gallbladder cancer. Hepatocellular carcinoma occasionally occurs with cirrhosis.

Treatment

There is no approved medical therapy for primary sclerosing cholangitis. Ursodeoxycholic acid has not been shown to be effective at decreasing the risk of death or the need for transplant. Higher doses of ursodeoxycholic acid (28-30 mg/kg) may be associated with adverse events. For patients with advanced disease, transplant has been shown to improve survival.

Patients may have evidence of rapidly progressive jaundice, they may suddenly become pruritic, or they may have fever with right upper quadrant pain. Indications for an endoscopic retrograde cholangiopancreatography are a symptomatic biliary stricture or stricture that is concerning for underlying cholangiocarcinoma. Magnetic resonance cholangiopancreatography before endoscopic intervention is often useful for detecting an underlying malignant stricture, for informing the endoscopist of the

underlying anatomy or atrophic segments that should be avoided, and for helping to triage patients who may not benefit from an invasive interventional endoscopic approach. Endoscopic retrograde cholangiopancreatography allows for biliary brushings for biliary cytology and fluorescence in situ hybridization analyses, extrication of biliary stones, or dilation of flow-limiting strictures. Biliary stenting is typically performed when balloon dilation alone does not achieve adequate decompression.

✓ Primary sclerosing cholangitis
- Typical presentation—young man with inflammatory bowel disease
- Concomitant inflammatory bowel disease in more than 70% of patients
- Magnetic resonance cholangiopancreatography—diagnostic test of choice
- Concurrent inflammatory bowel disease increases risk of hepatobiliary cancers (cholangiocarcinoma, gallbladder cancer, and hepatocellular carcinoma) and colorectal cancer

---

Secondary Sclerosing Cholangitis

Diagnosis

Secondary sclerosing cholangitis is associated with chronic inflammation and stricturing of the biliary tree (intrahepatic or extrahepatic or both) that arise as a response to an identifiable cause (Box 31.2). Frequently encountered benign causes of secondary sclerosing cholangitis include iatrogenic or postoperative causes (eg, hepatic artery thrombosis after liver transplant), recurrent infections, and chronic obstruction due to choledocholithiasis. A disease such as sarcoidosis can cause cholestasis with or without a large-duct biliary stricture. A biliary stricture (anastomotic or nonanastamotic) is a common complication after liver transplant. Over time, anastomotic strictures can lead to recurrent episodes of cholangitis, recurrent hepatolithiasis, and multifocal nonanastamotic strictures. Patients with secondary sclerosing cholangitis may present with jaundice, pruritus, or ascending cholangitis. Over time, cirrhosis may develop. The diagnosis can be established with cholangiography, although additional, specific testing may be required to identify the underlying cause.

Treatment

Management involves addressing the underlying cause when feasible (eg, institution of antiviral therapy for AIDS cholangiopathy); providing endoscopic or percutaneous therapy for flow-limiting biliary strictures or obstructions; and treating concurrent complications (eg, ascending cholangitis). Some patients may require liver transplant.

Management of Complications of Cholestasis

Vitamin Deficiency

Malabsorption and deficiency of fat-soluble vitamins may occur with cholestasis, especially if cholestasis is severe and cirrhosis develops. Serum levels of vitamins A, E, and D can be measured directly, and the serum level of vitamin K can be inferred from the prothrombin time. Replacement with water-soluble forms of the vitamins can be offered (vitamin A, 50,000 IU twice weekly; vitamin E, 200 mg twice daily; vitamin D, 50,000 IU twice weekly; and vitamin K, 5 mg daily). Adequacy of replacement can be reassessed by measuring levels after 6 to 12 months of therapy.

Hypercholesterolemia

Hypercholesterolemia, common in patients with cholestasis, is not associated with atherosclerosis. Treatment should be limited to patients who have risk factors for coronary heart disease and who may safely begin pharmacologic therapies (eg, statins) to improve lipid profiles.

Pruritus

Pruritus can be one of the most troublesome symptoms of patients with cholestasis. The severity of pruritus does not correlate closely with the severity of the underlying liver disease, and pruritus may resolve as the disease progresses. Ursodeoxycholic acid decreases pruritus in some patients with primary biliary cholangitis, but for those who remain symptomatic, antihistamines (eg, diphenhydramine 25-30 mg by mouth at bedtime) may permit sleep, although they rarely have much effect on pruritus. Cholestyramine and other bile acid–binding resins may help relieve itching and are first-line therapy. Rifampin (150-300 mg twice daily) has a rapid onset of action and may be useful long-term, although liver toxicity may develop (<15% of patients). Sertraline (75-100 mg daily) has also been shown to improve symptoms of pruritus. Naltrexone (50 mg daily) may be useful for some patients, although there is less experience with this drug than with the others. UV phototherapy and the molecular adsorbent recirculating system have also been shown to be effective for limited durations. Finally, liver transplant is available for patients who have severe, refractory pruritus.

Bone Disease

Although the insufficient delivery of bile acids to the gut lumen in advanced cholestasis may lead to fat-soluble vitamin deficiency, osteomalacia due to vitamin D deficiency occurs in less than 5% of patients with osteopenic bone disease and cholestasis. Almost all bone disease evaluated in North American patients with cholestasis is due to osteoporosis, which is the result of insufficient bone matrix rather than a mineralization defect as in osteomalacia. The cause of the osteoporosis is uncertain. These patients lose bone at a rate of about twice that of the normal population. About 33% of patients with primary biliary cholangitis and about 20% of those with primary sclerosing cholangitis have osteopenia at the time of diagnosis, and about 10% of them have vertebral fractures within a few years after diagnosis. Management of the bone disease includes exercise and adequate calcium intake with 1 to 1.5 g of elemental calcium daily in combination with vitamin D supplementation if needed to correct a deficiency. Postmenopausal women may have a response to hormone replacement therapy, which is usually given as patch therapy. Treatment with bisphosphonates and newer monoclonal antibodies has been shown to be effective.

✓ Complications of cholestatic liver disease
- Deficiencies of fat-soluble vitamins (vitamins A, D, E, and K)
- Hypercholesterolemia
- Pruritus
- Osteopenia and osteoporosis

Suggested Reading

Abdalian R, Heathcote EJ. Sclerosing cholangitis: a focus on secondary causes. Hepatology. 2006 Nov;44(5):1063–74.

Chapman R, Fevery J, Kalloo A, Nagorney DM, Boberg KM, Shneider B, et al. Diagnosis and management of primary sclerosing cholangitis. Hepatology. 2010 Feb;51(2):660–78.

Chen XM, LaRusso NF. Cryptosporidiosis and the pathogenesis of AIDS-cholangiopathy. Semin Liver Dis. 2002 Aug;22(3):277–89.

Corpechot C, Carrat F, Bahr A, Chretien Y, Poupon RE, Poupon R. The effect of ursodeoxycholic acid therapy on the natural course of primary biliary cirrhosis. Gastroenterology. 2005 Feb;128(2):297–303.

Corpechot C, Chazouilleres O, Rousseau A, Le Gruyer A, Habersetzer F, Mathurin P, et al. A placebo-controlled trial of bezafibrate in primary biliary cholangitis. N Engl J Med. 2018 Jun;378(23):2171–81.

Hilscher MB, Kamath PS, Eaton JE. Cholestatic liver diseases: a primer for generalists and subspecialists. Mayo Clin Proc. 2020 Oct;95(10):2263–79.

Lammers WJ, Hirschfield GM, Corpechot C, Nevens F, Lindor KD, Janssen HL, et al. Development and validation of a scoring system to predict outcomes of patients with primary biliary cirrhosis receiving ursodeoxycholic acid therapy. Gastroenterology. 2015 Dec;149(7):1804–12

Lewis JH. Drug-induced liver disease. Med Clin North Am. 2000 Sep;84(5):1275–311.

Lindor KD, Bowlus CL, Boyer J, Levy C, Mayo M. Primary biliary cholangitis: 2018 practice guidance from the American Association for the Study of Liver Diseases. Hepatology. 2019 Jan;69(1):394–419.

Lindor KD, Kowdley KV, Luketic VA, Harrison ME, McCashland T, Befeler AS, et al. High-dose ursodeoxycholic acid for the treatment of primary sclerosing cholangitis. Hepatology. 2009 Sep;50(3):808–14.

Nevens F, Andreone P, Mazzella G, Strasser SI, Bowlus C, Invernizzi P, et al. A placebo-controlled trial of obeticholic acid in primary biliary cholangitis. N Engl J Med. 2016 Aug 18;375(7):631–43.

Olsson R, Boberg KM, de Muckadell OS, Lindgren S, Hultcrantz R, Folvik G, et al. High-dose ursodeoxycholic acid in primary sclerosing cholangitis: a 5-year multicenter, randomized, controlled study. Gastroenterology. 2005 Nov;129(5):1464–72.

Poupon RE, Lindor KD, Cauch-Dudek K, Dickson ER, Poupon R, Heathcote EJ. Combined analysis of randomized controlled trials of ursodeoxycholic acid in primary biliary cirrhosis. Gastroenterology. 1997 Sep;113(3):884–90.

Talwalkar JA, Angulo P, Johnson CD, Petersen BT, Lindor KD. Cost-minimization analysis of MRC versus ERCP for the diagnosis of primary sclerosing cholangitis. Hepatology. 2004 Jul;40(1): 39–45.

Villa NA, Harrison ME. Management of biliary strictures after liver transplantation. Gastroenterol Hepatol (N Y). 2015 May;11(5):316–28.

Zein CO, Jorgensen RA, Clarke B, Wenger DE, Keach JC, Angulo P, et al. Alendronate improves bone mineral density in primary biliary cirrhosis: a randomized placebo-controlled trial. Hepatology. 2005 Oct;42(4):762–71.

32

Drug-Induced Liver Injury[a,b]

OMAR Y. MOUSA, MBBS, MD

MICHAEL D. LEISE, MD

Despite increased awareness through the efforts of public and regulatory agencies, the syndrome known as *drug-induced liver injury* (DILI) is still a major public health problem in the US and the world. Moreover, it is the single most common reason for US Food and Drug Administration (FDA) regulatory actions, including the removal of drugs from the marketplace. Although the frequency of this clinical syndrome is low within populations, DILI causes a significant clinical and economic burden. This chapter highlights new developments in the field of idiosyncratic DILI and provides information about DILI from acetaminophen.

✓ DILI—an adverse drug reaction with presentations ranging from asymptomatic increases in liver values to hepatocellular injury, cholestasis, chronic hepatitis, or liver failure
✓ DILI—one of the common and most challenging disorders faced by gastroenterologists and hepatologists

---

[a] The authors thank John J. Poterucha, MD, and Jayant A. Talwalkar, MD, who coauthored previous versions of this chapter.

[b] Portions of this chapter were adapted from Ghabril M, Chalasani N, Björnsson E. Drug-induced liver injury: a clinical update. Curr Opin Gastroenterol. 2010 May;26(3):222-6 and Daly AK. Drug-induced liver injury: past, present and future. Pharmacogenomics. 2010 May;11(5): 607–11; used with permission.

Abbreviations: ALP, alkaline phosphatase; ALT, alanine aminotransferase; AST, aspartate aminotransferase; CYP, cytochrome P450; DILI, drug-induced liver injury; DILIN, Drug-Induced Liver Injury Network; DRESS, drug rash with eosinophilia and systemic symptoms; FDA, US Food and Drug Administration; GWAS, genome-wide association study; HEV, hepatitis E virus; HLA, human leukocyte antigen; Ig, immunoglobulin; NAFLD, nonalcoholic fatty liver disease; NHANES, National Health and Nutrition Examination Survey; NIH, National Institutes of Health; OR, odds ratio; ULRR, upper limit of the reference range

Overview of Drug Metabolism

Orally administered drugs are lipid soluble, which allows them to be absorbed into cells and affect biologic processes. Drug-metabolizing systems convert the parent drug into water-soluble compounds, which are excreted into bile and urine. The metabolizing systems are divided into phase 1 and phase 2 reactions. Phase 1 reactions involve the cytochrome P450 (CYP) family of enzymes (the CYP3A subfamily is the most prominent) and include the addition of polar groups by oxidation, reduction, or hydrolysis. The metabolites formed by phase 1 reactions may be toxic if not subsequently excreted or further metabolized. Activity of phase 1 reactions is influenced by age, other drugs, and toxins (Box 32.1).

Phase 2 reactions further enhance the water solubility of a compound and generally involve conjugation of glucuronide, sulfate, acetate, glycine, or glutathione to a polar group. Occasionally, phase 2 reactions may affect the parent compound directly (ie, without a previous phase 1 reaction). Dietary factors, including nutritional status, can alter the activity of phase 2 reactions. The influence of alterations in drug-metabolizing systems on DILI is incompletely understood.

Clinical Epidemiology

Worldwide, the annual incidence rate of DILI is estimated to be between 13.9 and 24 cases per 100,000 persons, and the syndrome accounts for an estimated 3% to 9% of all adverse drug reactions reported to health authorities. Epidemiologic data on DILI from prospective national registries have been published. A study from Iceland included an enumerated population and was linked to a prescription database, allowing for improved estimation of incidence. Cases of DILI were

Box 32.1.   Drugs and Conditions That Affect Activity of the Cytochrome P450 (CYP) System

Inhibit CYP Activity
  Cimetidine
  Clarithromycin
  Erythromycin
  Fluconazole
  Itraconazole
  Ketoconazole
  Older age
  Quinidine
  Ritonavir
Induce CYP Activity
  Carbamazepine
  Chronic alcohol use
  Isoniazid
  Omeprazole
  Phenobarbital
  Phenytoin
  Rifampin

✓ Amoxicillin-clavulanate—the most common cause of clinically apparent, drug-induced acute liver injury
✓ Most common classes of agents that cause DILI—antimicrobials, herbal and dietary supplements, and anticancer therapeutics

Mechanisms and Classification

DILI is largely an unsolved problem because of our limited knowledge about the mechanisms of hepatic toxicity. Traditionally, the classification of injury patterns with DILI is based on specific histologic features such as inflammation, cholestasis, sinusoidal cell injury, immune-mediated damage, mitochondrial injury, and oxidative stress. Liver biopsy samples may show pathologic features such as prominent eosinophilia, granulomas, zonal or massive necrosis, or cholestasis with hepatitis. The usefulness of histologic examination of the liver is limited by knowledge about DILI, particularly information on the patterns of injury caused by various agents. An overview of common histologic patterns seen with specific drugs is presented in Table 32.1.

DILI can be divided broadly into direct chemical toxicity and idiosyncratic hepatotoxic reactions. *Direct chemical toxicity* is dose related; the most common example is the hepatotoxicity associated with acetaminophen. Other examples include *Amanita* mushrooms and carbon tetrachloride. Direct toxicity usually occurs after a brief exposure. For a given drug, there is considerable variability in the dose required to cause toxicity, largely because of individual differences in drug metabolism. These differences can be genetic or due to exogenous effectors of drug metabolism.

collected prospectively from 2010 through 2011. Among the 96 cases identified, the crude annual incidence was 19.1 cases per 100,000 inhabitants (95% CI, 1.6-23.3 cases per 100,000 inhabitants). Amoxicillin-clavulanate was the most common drug, with an incidence of 1 in 729 users among inpatients and 1 in 2,350 among outpatients. The Regional Registry of Hepatotoxicity in Spain reported on 461 cases of DILI identified between 1994 and 2004. In this experience, hepatocellular damage was the most common pattern observed (58%), and nearly 12% of patients with jaundice at presentation died or required liver transplant, compared with only 4% of patients who did not have jaundice. The main causative medications were antibiotics (32% of cases), central nervous system drugs (17%), musculoskeletal drugs (17%), and gastrointestinal drugs (10%). Amoxicillin-clavulanate was again the most commonly implicated drug in this cohort.

Among the first 300 patients enrolled in the ongoing National Institutes of Health (NIH) Drug-Induced Liver Injury Network (DILIN) prospective study, an estimated 73% of cases resulted from use of a single prescription medication, 9% were attributed to herbal and dietary supplements, and 18% resulted from patients taking multiple agents. Among patients followed for at least 6 months, the mortality rate was 8%, although the cause of death was liver related for only 44% of patients. Among patients with DILI caused by a single prescription drug, the major classes of implicated agents were antimicrobials (46%), central nervous system agents (15%), immunomodulatory agents (5%), analgesics (5%), and lipid-lowering agents (3%). As in the Spanish and Icelandic registries, amoxicillin-clavulanate was the drug most commonly implicated.

The Acute Liver Failure Study Group reported that acetaminophen and idiosyncratic drug reactions together accounted for approximately 50% of cases of acute liver failure in the US. DILI is recognized as the most commonly identified cause of acute liver failure that requires liver transplant in the US.

Table 32.1. Histologic Patterns of Liver Injury and Associated Drugs

Liver injury	Associated drugs
Drug-induced autoimmune hepatitis	Atorvastatin, halothane, hydralazine, ipilimumab, methyldopa, minocycline, nitrofurantoin, TNF-α antagonists, vemurafenib
Steatohepatitis	Amiodarone, tamoxifen, valproic acid
Steatosis	Methotrexate, nucleoside reverse transcriptase inhibitors, tetracycline, valproic acid
Cholestasis	Amoxicillin-clavulanate, antifungal agents, chlorpromazine, erythromycin, histamine blockers, NSAIDs, oral contraceptives, trimethoprim-sulfamethoxazole
Granulomatous	Allopurinol, amiodarone, carbamazepine, diltiazem, hydralazine, penicillamine, phenytoin, procainamide, sulfonamides
Fibrosis	Methotrexate
Nodular regenerative hyperplasia	Azathioprine, bleomycin, chlorambucil, cyclophosphamide, doxorubicin, interleukin 2, trastuzumab
Sinusoidal obstruction syndrome	Actinomycin, azathioprine (occasionally), cytosine arabinoside, dacarbazine, 5-fluorouracil, oxaliplatin, plicamycin, 6-mercaptopurine (occasionally)
Hypersensitivity (immunoallergic) reaction	Abacavir, allopurinol, amoxicillin-clavulanate, fluoroquinolones, halothane, phenytoin, sulfonamides

Abbreviations: NSAID, nonsteroidal anti-inflammatory drug; TNF, tumor necrosis factor.

Adapted from Leise MD, Poterucha JJ, Talwalkar JA. Drug-induced liver injury. Mayo Clin Proc. 2014 Jan;89(1):95-106. Used with permission of Mayo Foundation for Medical Education and Research.

In contrast to the relatively predictable dose-related toxicity from acetaminophen, the more common *idiosyncratic hepatotoxic reactions* appear to be related to genetic or environmental influences, or both, that are less well understood. They affect only susceptible individuals, have less consistent relationships to dose, and are more varied in their presentations. Most drug-induced hepatotoxicity is metabolic, which involves the accumulation of toxic metabolites within hepatocytes, leading to necrosis and inflammation. Recent investigations have identified several categories of idiosyncratic DILI, as discussed below.

✓ DILI can be divided into 2 broad categories: direct chemical toxicity and idiosyncratic hepatotoxic reactions

Hypersensitivity (Immunoallergic) Reaction

Liver injury from a hypersensitivity reaction usually follows 1 to 6 weeks of exposure to the drug and is accompanied by rash, fever, eosinophilia, and autoantibodies (alone or in combination) and recurs rapidly with rechallenge. Hypersensitivity features are seen in only about 20% of all cases of idiosyncratic DILI. DILI may also be seen in the context of stereotypical hypersensitivity reactions, such as drug rash with eosinophilia and systemic symptoms (DRESS) syndrome, Stevens-Johnson syndrome, and toxic epidermal necrolysis. Examples of drugs that can result in a hypersensitivity reaction are sulfonamides, amoxicillin-clavulanate, fluoroquinolones, phenytoin, halothane, allopurinol, and abacavir.

Autoimmune Reaction

Autoimmune-mediated DILI may be caused by specific drugs, and the immune responses mimic those typically observed in de novo or idiopathic autoimmune hepatitis. Hydralazine, minocycline, and nitrofurantoin are drugs that are commonly associated with autoimmune-mediated DILI. Infliximab, statins, and α-methyldopa can also lead to autoimmune-mediated DILI. Although it is difficult to distinguish autoimmune-mediated DILI from autoimmune hepatitis on the basis of history, laboratory findings, and histologic features, the absence of relapse after the withdrawal of corticosteroid therapy is highly suggestive of a drug-induced autoimmune reaction.

✓ Drug-induced autoimmune reaction—characterized by the absence of relapse after the withdrawal of corticosteroid therapy
✓ Nitrofurantoin, infliximab, and minocycline are commonly associated with autoimmune-mediated DILI

Cholestasis

Drug-induced cholestasis may occur as an acute disorder manifesting as canalicular (bland jaundice), hepatocanalicular (cholestatic hepatitis), or ductular (cholangiolar hepatitis) disease. Chronic cholestasis often results from the vanishing bile duct syndrome. Amoxicillin-clavulanate, erythromycin, trimethoprim-sulfamethoxazole, chlorpromazine, antifungal agents, and oral contraceptives typically produce this form of DILI. Other medications include nonsteroidal anti-inflammatory drugs and histamine blockers.

Steatosis

The deposition of small or large fat droplets in the liver is another recognized form of DILI. Microvesicular steatosis generally indicates acute disease, whereas macrovesicular steatosis or the combination of both microvesicular steatosis and macrovesicular steatosis occurs with chronic exposure. Salicylate, valproate, amiodarone, highly active antiretroviral therapy, hepatitis B antiviral therapy, and tamoxifen typically have been associated with this form of DILI. Exposure to glucocorticoids, methotrexate, or diltiazem can be associated with macrovesicular steatosis. Amiodarone hepatoxicity is typically associated with microvesicular steatosis, ballooning degeneration, and Mallory bodies.

Sinusoidal Obstruction Syndrome

Sinusoidal obstruction syndrome (formerly called venoocclusive disease) is diagnosed most often in patients who have received a myeloablative chemotherapeutic conditioning regimen (cyclophosphamide, busulfan, and melphalan) before undergoing stem cell transplant for malignancy. This syndrome is seen also after exposure to 5-fluorouracil, oxaliplatin, cytosine arabinoside, actinomycin, dacarbazine, or plicamycin and, occasionally, azathioprine, 6-mercaptopurine, or 6-thioguanine. The pyrrolizidine alkaloids found in many plants and shrubs are well-known causes, and the exposure is linked usually to bush tea. Other risk factors include preexisting liver disease and previous radiotherapy to the abdomen. The diagnosis usually is based on the findings of hepatomegaly, weight gain, and hyperbilirubinemia. In some cases, histologic examination of the liver may be required. Management is largely supportive. The mortality rate is as high as 20%.

Nodular Regenerative Hyperplasia

Nodular regenerative hyperplasia is a rare disease that can lead to noncirrhotic portal hypertension with possible variceal hemorrhage but usually not ascites, hepatic encephalopathy, or synthetic dysfunction. While it can be seen with hematologic and rheumatologic conditions, it can also be found in association with several medications, including azathioprine, bleomycin, chlorambucil, cyclophosphamide, didanosine, and interleukin 2. The diagnosis should be made from liver histologic findings. Nodular regenerative hyperplasia is often overlooked since it is not easily appreciated with routine hematoxylin-eosin staining and requires a reticulin stain. The key histologic finding is small nodules around the portal tract with hypertrophied hepatocytes centrally and atrophic hepatocytes peripherally.

✓ Patients with DILI may present with noncirrhotic portal hypertension secondary to nodular regenerative hyperplasia

Peliosis Hepatis

Peliosis hepatis is a rare condition that manifests with multiple, dilated, blood-filled cavities in the liver and is associated with the following drugs: anabolic steroids, azathioprine, 6-mercaptopurine, danazol, tamoxifen, hydroxyurea, and oral contraceptives.

Risk Factors

Older age is associated with DILI caused by several common drugs, including isoniazid, erythromycin, amoxicillin-clavulanate, and nitrofurantoin. The reason that age affects the risk of DILI is not clear because phase 1 and phase 2 metabolizing enzyme activities are not altered markedly in older people. In contrast to earlier data, data from recent studies have not confirmed an increased predisposition to DILI among women in comparison with men. However, men and women might have differences in susceptibility to particular agents that cause DILI. For example, the majority of patients who have acute liver failure or require liver transplant because of DILI are women.

Recent studies also suggest that the daily dose of a drug might influence the development of DILI, which is in contrast to previous concepts. Among US prescription medicines, daily doses greater than 50 mg have been associated significantly with liver failure, liver transplant, and death from DILI. In the Swedish and Spanish registries, 77% of the DILI cases were seen with oral medication doses of 50 mg or more. Lipophilicity has recently been shown to be an important medication risk factor. Although not an independent risk factor, it has synergism with increased medication dose: high drug lipophilicity (logP ≥3) and high medication dosage (>100 mg daily) increase the risk of DILI by as much as 14 times. Drugs with hepatic metabolism and hepatobiliary excretion are also associated with a higher risk of serious DILI. The role of alcohol in idiosyncratic DILI is debated; however, chronic alcohol consumption upregulates several CYP system enzymes, which leads to increased metabolism of different medications to potentially toxic metabolites. The influence of underlying chronic liver disease as a risk factor for DILI is not fully understood. Clearly, patients with underlying liver disease have a higher risk for adverse outcomes than those without liver disease.

There is growing evidence that obesity and nonalcoholic fatty liver disease (NAFLD) can increase the risk of DILI, at least with some drugs, either by aggravating NAFLD (eg, methotrexate and tamoxifen) or by causing acute hepatitis (eg, acetaminophen, halogenated anesthetic halothane, and isoflurane). Patients with a history of DILI have a higher risk of DILI from other medications. Other risk factors include malnutrition, tobacco use, and polypharmacy. The understanding of genetic risk factors for DILI is still emerging.

Clinical Presentation

The clinical presentation of patients with DILI varies with the severity of injury to the liver. Patients with mild DILI may have an increase in the level of aspartate aminotransferase (AST), alanine aminotransferase (ALT), or alkaline phosphatase (ALP) (or a combination of these) and normal levels of total bilirubin and have no symptoms or nonspecific symptoms such as fatigue and nausea. Moderate to severe DILI is accompanied often by abdominal pain, jaundice, and pruritus. Rash, fever, facial edema, and lymphadenopathy, in combination with eosinophilia or atypical lymphocytosis, may be present with hypersensitivity-type reactions. Coagulopathy, kidney dysfunction, and mental status changes, when present, are seen typically when patients have fulminant DILI.

Many drugs cause mild, clinically insignificant, and transient increases in liver enzyme levels within a few months. These increased levels usually indicate an adaptive response to the drug and do not necessitate withdrawal of treatment with the agent. For example, isoniazid increases the ALT level more than 3 times the upper limit of the reference range (ULRR) in 15% of patients, but the enzyme levels usually normalize despite continued treatment. Generally, clinically significant DILI may be present when liver enzyme levels increase more than 3 to 5 times the ULRR, when the bilirubin level is 2.5 mg/dL or more, or when

the patient has symptoms or impaired liver function. Under these circumstances potentially causative medications should be discontinued immediately.

✓ Careful medication history is crucial in establishing the diagnosis of DILI

✓ DILI can be characterized biochemically as specific patterns of injury, such as hepatocellular, cholestatic, or mixed

---

Diagnosis

There is no specific test for DILI. The maxim that "almost any drug can do almost anything" is important to consider when evaluating patients who have abnormal liver test results. Although the time between the initiation of medication use and the onset of hepatotoxicity varies, most cases of DILI occur within a year after treatment is started with the drug. DILI should be suspected when liver injury occurs soon (within 4 weeks) after the initiation of treatment with an agent or after an increase in the dose of an agent that had been administered previously.

Generally, other causes of liver disease must be excluded before the diagnosis of DILI can be made. Screening is required for hepatitis (hepatitis A, B, C, and E), alcoholic or autoimmune hepatitis, and hemodynamic derangement. Although infections are less common, testing to exclude cytomegalovirus and Epstein-Barr virus infections is helpful. The possibility of hepatitis E involvement in suspected DILI cases was recently evaluated. Hepatitis E virus (HEV) immunoglobulin (Ig) G serologies were positive in 16% of patients (50 of 318) in the NIH DILIN series, with 3% testing positive for HEV IgM, which suggests acute HEV infection. Of the participants in a National Health and Nutrition Examination Survey (NHANES) study (N=18,695), 21% were HEV seropositive, suggesting that HEV should no longer be considered a disease found only in resource-limited countries. If a patient is suspected of having DILI with a hepatocellular pattern, HEV serology should be checked. Also, biliary abnormalities, through obstruction or infection, can injure the liver, as in cholangitis. If the liver injury pattern is cholestatic, the biliary tree should be imaged, initially with ultrasonography and then with computed tomography or magnetic resonance imaging (Figure 32.1). Also, resolution of the injury after withdrawal of the drug ("dechallenge") is helpful in confirming the diagnosis of DILI, although the timing of improvement after the withdrawal varies.

DILI can be characterized biochemically as specific patterns of injury, such as hepatocellular, cholestatic, or mixed (Box 32.2), with the use of the R ratio, defined by the following equation:

$$R = \frac{\text{ALT (Reported as Multiple of ULRR)}}{\text{ALP (Reported as Multiple of ULRR)}}$$

The liver injury pattern is *hepatocellular* when, at presentation, R exceeds 5, *cholestatic* when R is less than 2, and *mixed* when R is between 2 and 5. An important issue in calculating the R ratio is which values to use during the course of illness. For example, in the NIH DILIN study, R was calculated for 192 patients in whom DILI was thought to be due to a single agent. When R was calculated from the values obtained initially in the study, 57% of patients had the hepatocellular pattern of injury, 21% the mixed pattern, and 22% the cholestatic pattern. However, when R was calculated from the values at the time of the peak serum levels of bilirubin, 45% of patients had the hepatocellular pattern, 37% the cholestatic pattern, and 17% the mixed pattern.

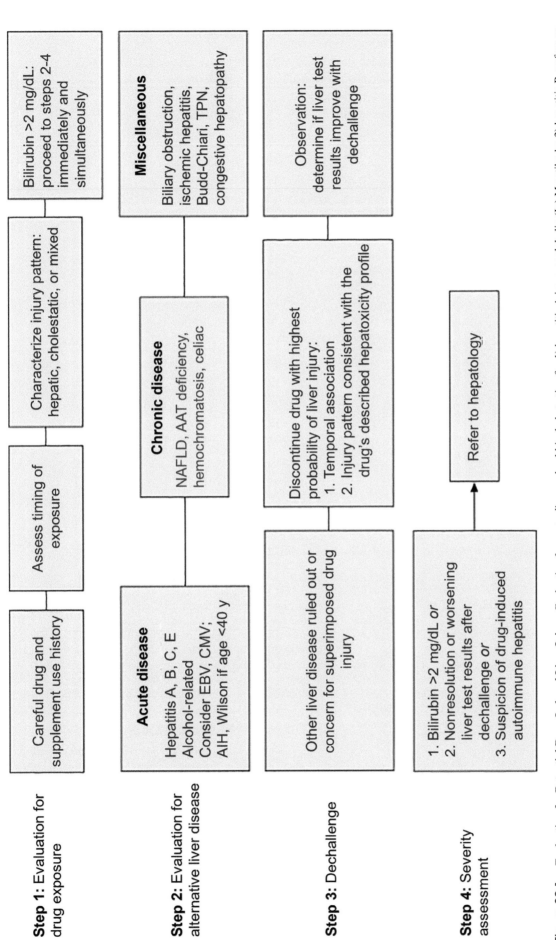

Figure 32.1. Evaluation for Potential Drug-Induced Liver Injury. *Evaluation for acute disease* should include testing for 1) hepatitis A immunoglobulin (Ig) M antibody; 2) hepatitis B surface antigen and hepatitis B core antibody IgM; 3) hepatitis C antibody (and subsequent hepatitis C virus RNA testing if antibody result is positive); 4) hepatitis E IgM antibody; 5) cytomegalovirus (CMV) (IgM antibody or polymerase chain reaction or both); 6) Epstein-Barr virus (EBV) (heterophile antibody or EBV-specific antibody); 7) autoimmune hepatitis (AIH) (anti–smooth muscle antibody, antinuclear antibody, and serum IgG level—there is no specific blood test for diagnosis); and 8) Wilson disease (ceruloplasmin, and consider ophthalmologic examination and 24-hour urine copper test—there is no specific blood or urine test for diagnosis). *Evaluation for chronic disease* should include testing for 1) nonalcoholic fatty liver disease (NAFLD) with a combination of historic and imaging features with or without histology (there is no specific blood test for diagnosis); 2) α₁-antitrypsin (AAT) deficiency (AAT phenotype); 3) hemochromatosis (transferrin saturation and ferritin level); and 4) celiac disease (tissue transglutaminase IgA). *Evaluation for miscellaneous diseases* should include testing for 1) biliary obstruction (ultrasonography or magnetic resonance cholangiopancreatography); 2) ischemic hepatitis (clinical diagnosis); 3) Budd-Chiari syndrome (ultrasonography with Doppler studies of hepatic veins); 4) total parental nutrition (TPN) (clinical diagnosis with or without histology); and 5) congestive hepatopathy (transthoracic echocardiography). (Adapted from Leise MD, Poterucha JJ, Talwalkar JA. Drug-induced liver injury. Mayo Clin Proc. 2014 Jan;89[1]:95-106. Used with permission of Mayo Foundation for Medical Education and Research.)

Box 32.2. Biochemical Patterns of Liver Injury With Certain Drugs

Hepatocellular (increased ALT)	Cholestatic (increased ALP)	Mixed (increased ALP and ALT)
Acarbose	Amoxicillin-clavulanate	Amitriptyline
Acetaminophen	Anabolic steroids	Azathioprine
Allopurinol	Chlorpromazine	Captopril
Amiodarone	Clopidogrel	Carbamazepine
Baclofen	Erythromycins	Clindamycin
Bupropion	Estrogens	Cyproheptadine
Fluoxetine	Fluconazole	Enalapril
HAART drugs	Histamine blockers	Flutamide
Isoniazid	Irbesartan	Nitrofurantoin
Ketoconazole	Mirtazapine	Phenobarbital
Lisinopril	NSAIDs	Phenytoin
Losartan	Oral contraceptives	Sulfonamides
Methotrexate	Phenothiazines	Trazodone
NSAIDs	Phenytoin	Trimethoprim-sulfamethoxazole
Omeprazole	Terbinafine	Verapamil
Paroxetine	Tricyclic antidepressants	
Pyrazinamide		
Rifampin		
Risperidone		
Sertraline		
Statins		
Tetracyclines		
Trazodone		
Trovafloxacin		
Valproic acid		

Abbreviations: ALP, alkaline phosphatase; ALT, alanine aminotransferase; HAART, highly active antiretroviral therapy; NSAID, nonsteroidal anti-inflammatory drug.

Adapted from Navarro VJ, Senior JR. Drug-related hepatotoxicity. N Engl J Med. 2006 Feb;354(7):731-9; used with permission.

Consequently, during DILI, a shift occurs in the ALP levels in relation to the ALT levels, and the later in the course of disease that values are obtained for calculating R, the more likely the patient is to have a cholestatic pattern of injury.

Ultimately, the level of certainty for making a diagnosis of DILI is related to the clinical history, chronology of exposure and injury, exclusion of competing causes, and previous knowledge of DILI with a specific agent through clinical experience and published data. Several causality assessment systems have been developed to identify the likelihood of suspected DILI and an implicated agent in research settings. Recent studies have shown that the results from these assessment systems are not well reproduced among multiple users, thus limiting their usefulness in research and clinical settings. More precise algorithms and ones that are easier to use in clinical practice are being developed.

Recent progress has been made related to biomarkers for DILI. MicroRNAs produced by the liver were evaluated in patients with acetaminophen liver injury or nonacetaminophen liver injury and in healthy controls. MicroRNA 122 was significantly elevated in patients with acetaminophen or nonacetaminophen liver injury compared with controls. Day 1 microRNA 122 levels correlated with the peak ALT level and were 2-fold higher in patients meeting King's College criteria, but these relationships were not statistically significant. The clinical utility of microRNA requires

further study. Protein adducts have also been investigated, and acetaminophen-cysteine adducts were found in 18% of 110 patients with indeterminate cases in the US Acute Liver Failure Study Group series as compared with 95% of the 199 patients with established acetaminophen-related acute liver failure. A recent proteomic analysis suggested that apolipoprotein E may be helpful in the diagnosis of DILI, but that will require further study.

Histologic Patterns

No unique histologic patterns unequivocally confirm the diagnosis of DILI. Notably, the results of histologic examination of the liver may vary with the timing of biopsy because hepatocellular injury is more prominent in the initial few weeks of injury; cholestatic features, however, are more prominent later in the course of disease. The 2 main categories of histologic change that can be observed are 1) acute and chronic hepatitis and 2) acute and chronic cholestasis/mixed hepatocellular-cholestatic injury.

Acute and Chronic Hepatitis

In the acute and chronic hepatitis pattern, the dominant feature is expansion of the portal area by a mononuclear infiltrate in the presence of interface hepatitis. Also, involvement of bile ducts by inflammation or reactive changes may be seen. The paren-chyma has scattered foci of inflammation and usually apoptotic hepatocytes. At the severe end of liver injury, lobular disarray, areas of confluent necrosis, and central venulitis without true venoocclusive changes may be observed. Microgranulomas are common in cases of DILI due to allopurinol and phenytoin. Fibrin ring granulomas have been described in allopurinol-related DILI, but this is a nonspecific finding that can be seen in Q fever, hepa-titis A, leishmaniasis, and Hodgkin lymphoma.

Acute and Chronic Cholestasis/Mixed Hepatocellular-Cholestatic Injury

The acute or intrahepatic cholestatic pattern is defined as hepatocellular or canalicular bile stasis (or both) in the ab-sence of marked inflammation. If intrahepatic cholestasis is as-sociated with one of the necroinflammatory patterns described for hepatocellular injury, the pattern is categorized as *mixed hepatocellular-cholestatic injury* or *cholestatic hepatitis*. Bile duct injury is usually present, although pronounced duct loss suggests a chronic disorder such as primary biliary cholangitis, primary sclerosing cholangitis, or vanishing bile duct syndrome. The combination of cholestasis with inflammation and hepatic injury is a common histologic pattern of injury in DILI.

Liver Biopsy

Liver biopsy is not mandatory in the evaluation of DILI. However, the findings can be helpful for confirming a clinical suspicion of DILI, assessing disease severity, and excluding other competing causes of liver injury. Biopsy should be considered if autoim-mune hepatitis remains a possible cause and if immunosuppres-sive therapy is considered. Biopsy may be considered if liver biochemistry results or liver function are worsening even though use of the suspected offending agent was stopped, or if continued use of the agent or reexposure to it is expected. In addition, a reasonable consideration would be a biopsy at 60 days for unre-solved acute hepatocellular DILI (if the peak ALT level has not decreased by >50%) and 180 days for cholestatic DILI (if the peak ALP level has not decreased by >50%) despite stopping the suspected offending agent. Biopsy may also be considered in the evaluation of chronic DILI if abnormalities in liver biochemistry persist beyond 180 days.

Examples of Drugs Associated With DILI

Acetaminophen

The most common cause of acute liver failure in the US and Europe is acetaminophen toxicity. The metabolism of acetamino-phen is shown in Figure 32.2. Decreases in glutathione in patients with chronic liver disease predispose the patients to production of the toxic metabolite. Also, patients with chronic excessive intake of alcohol produce more of the toxic intermediate because of the induction of CYP2E1 activity.

Acetaminophen hepatotoxicity is characterized by very high levels of aminotransferases (often >5,000 U/L). Kidney failure is also common. The degree of increase in the AST level at the time of presentation after an acetaminophen overdose is helpful in predicting hepatotoxicity. Hepatotoxicity rarely develops in patients with AST levels less than 50 U/L at presentation, whereas 16% of those with AST levels more than 1,000 U/L at presentation die or need liver transplant. Patients with acetamin-ophen hepatotoxicity and poor prognostic markers should be

hospitalized and their condition monitored. The King's College criteria for liver transplant are listed in Box 23.2 in Chapter 23. When *N*-acetylcysteine is administered soon after acetamino-phen has been ingested, it acts by enhancing the conjugation and, thus, the water solubility and excretion of *N*-acetyl-*p*-quinone imine. When administered later, after liver injury has devel-oped, *N*-acetylcysteine acts by antioxidant and anti-inflammatory mechanisms that are not well understood. *N*-acetylcysteine also may enhance liver perfusion through inotropic and vasodilatory effects. Although the efficacy of *N*-acetylcysteine diminishes when it is given more than 8 hours after acetaminophen has been ingested, it nonetheless should be administered up to 24 hours after ingestion because of its putative hepatoprotective effects.

✓ Acetaminophen hepatotoxicity is characterized by very high levels of aminotransferases (often >5,000 U/L)
✓ Recommended treatment of acetaminophen hepatotoxicity: *N*-acetylcysteine

---

Antibiotics

The drug class that most commonly causes nonfulminant liver in-jury is antibiotics. Amoxicillin-clavulanate is the most frequently reported antibiotic that causes hepatotoxicity. Liver injury usually manifests within 1 to 4 weeks after treatment with the drug has been stopped, but it can occur even later. The clinical presentation of patients with DILI can be either hepatocellular or cholestatic. Similar to other forms of drug-induced cholestatic liver injury, the cholestasis due to amoxicillin-clavulanate may take weeks or months to resolve. Other classic antibiotics associated with DILI are nitrofurantoin, minocycline, isoniazid, trimethoprim-sulfamethoxazole, erythromycin, and the fluoroquinolones. Telithromycin, a ketolide antibiotic, has been reported to cause severe hepatotoxicity, including the development of ascites. In 2007, the FDA required a label change and a boxed warning about hepatotoxicity.

The NIH DILIN series has also reported on 12 patients with fluoroquinolone-related DILI, of which 7 had features of hyper-sensitivity. The biochemical pattern of liver injury was evenly split between hepatocellular, mixed, and cholestatic types. The median latency was 2.5 days. Serious outcomes occurred: 3 patients had hepatic or other organ failure, 1 patient required liver transplant for vanishing bile duct syndrome, and another died of acute liver failure. Antifungal agents such as ketoconazole can lead to cholestasis as well.

Antiretroviral Agents

Drugs for HIV cause hepatotoxicity in 2% to 18% of patients. Most episodes of DILI are asymptomatic, and in most cases, increases in ALT levels resolve spontaneously.

Of the protease inhibitors, ritonavir (especially at high doses) carries the highest risk of liver toxicity, with an incidence of 3% to 9%. The newer protease inhibitor tipranavir has been associ-ated with severe hepatotoxicity, especially when used in combi-nation with ritonavir and particularly in patients with hepatitis B or C.

Newer nucleoside reverse transcriptase inhibitors, such as emtricitabine, abacavir, and tenofovir, are associated with a low incidence of increased ALT levels. The major toxic effect of nucleoside reverse transcriptase inhibitors (especially didan-osine and stavudine) is lactic acidosis due to mitochondrial tox-icity, which generally occurs after several weeks or months of

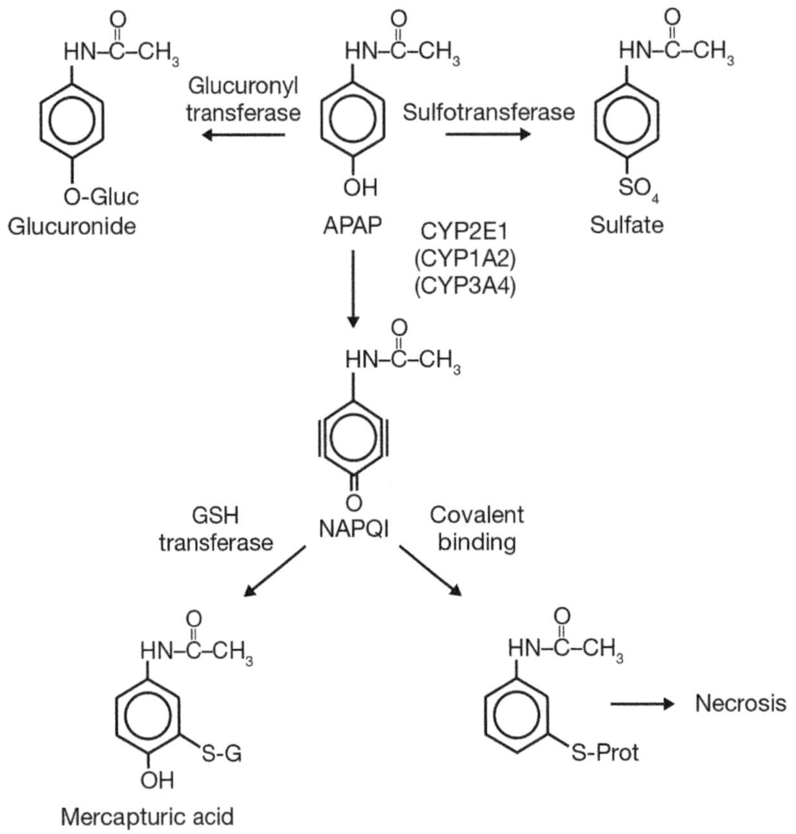

Figure 32.2.   Metabolism of Acetaminophen (APAP). Most APAP is conjugated to either glucuronide or sulfate. The portion that is oxidized to *N*-acetyl-*p*-benzoquinone imine (NAPQI) is further detoxified by glutathione (GSH) transferase. If this system is overwhelmed, NAPQI binds to cellular targets, leading to hepatocellular necrosis. CYP indicates cytochrome P450. (Adapted from Zimmerman HJ. Acetaminophen hepatotoxicity. Clin Liver Dis. 1998 Aug;2[3]:523-41; used with permission.)

treatment. Histologic examination of the liver usually shows steatosis, and the mortality rate is high. Among patients with hepatitis C, the administration of ribavirin to those also receiving didanosine or stavudine has been associated with mitochondrial toxicity.

A hypersensitivity DILI reaction due to the nonnucleoside reverse transcriptase inhibitor nevirapine occurs in 2.3% of patients and has also been seen with abacavir and efavirenz. This form of liver injury tends to develop within a few weeks after the start of therapy. A different pattern of drug injury has emerged with the use of nevirapine: Liver enzyme levels begin to increase after more than 16 weeks of therapy, consistent with direct or idiosyncratic host-mediated liver injury. Patients who have chronic viral hepatitis are likely at increased risk for toxicity with nevirapine therapy. In a large group of 8,851 patients studied by the AIDS Clinical Trials Group, baseline elevations of aminotransferases, hepatitis C, and regimens containing didanosine or nevirapine were associated with severe hepatoxicity.

Herbal and Dietary Supplements

Herbal and dietary supplements are commonly used in the US and throughout the world. The clinical patterns of presentation and severity of hepatotoxicity associated with these supplements can be highly variable, even for the same product. Box 32.3 lists some of the most common herbal and dietary supplements associated with DILI. The FDA assigned warnings to several Hydroxycut (Iovate Health Sciences, Inc) and Herbalife (Herbalife International of America, Inc) products on the basis of

documented reports of severe liver injury, transplant, and death associated with these compounds. Hydroxycut products were recalled, and new formulations were released.

According to the NIH DILIN prospective study, herbal and dietary supplements were implicated in approximately 10% of consecutively enrolled cases of DILI. Furthermore, in the Spanish registry, 2% of cases of DILI were attributed to herbal remedies or dietary supplements. In Asian countries, the proportion of DILI caused by herbal supplements can be as high as 19% to 63%.

Herbal and dietary supplements should be considered in the differential diagnosis of liver injury. Many patients do not consider over-the-counter, nutritional, or herbal supplements as medicine; thus, these agents may not be included when patients are asked about medicines taken before the episode of liver injury. Careful, repeated, and directed questioning is required.

Lipid-Lowering Agents

Because of the frequency with which statins are prescribed, there has been much interest in the potential liver toxicity of these agents. Determining whether patients receiving statins have DILI is difficult because mild increases in liver enzyme levels are common within 1 month after the initiation of statin therapy, but the levels nearly always improve despite continued administration of these agents. Furthermore, mildly fluctuating liver enzyme levels occur also in hyperlipidemic patients not receiving statin therapy. The presence of nonalcoholic fatty liver disease in many

Box 32.3. **Selected Herbal and Dietary Supplements Associated With Hepatoxicity**

Aloe vera

Atractylis gummifera

Black cohosh

Callilepsis laureola (impila)

Camphor oil

Cascara (cascara sagrada)

Centella asiaticus (gotu kola)

Chaparral (*Larrea tridentata*)

Dai-saiko-to (Sho-saiko-to, TJ-19, Da-Chai-Hu-Tang, Xiao-Chai-Hu-Tang)

Geniposide (*Gardenia jasminoides*)

Germander (*Teucrium chamaedrys* and other *Teucrium* species)

Greater celandine (*Chelidonium majus*)

Green tea (*Camellia sinensis*)

Herbalife products[a]

Hydroxycut products[b] (first-generation formulation production was halted in 2009)

Jin bu huan (*Lycopodium serratum*)

Kava (*Piper methysticum*)

Ma huang (*Ephedra sinica*)

Mistletoe (*Viscum album*)

Noni juice (*Morinda citrifolia*)

Pennyroyal (squawmint oil)

Pyrrolizidine alkaloids (*Crotalaria, Heliotropium, Senecio, Symphytum* [comfrey])

Saw palmetto (*Serenoa repens*)

Senna (*Cassia angustifolia* and *Cassia acutifolia*)

Skullcap (*Scutellaria*)

Valerian (*Valeriana officinalis*)

[a] Herbalife International of America, Inc.

[b] Iovate Health Sciences, Inc.

patients who are candidates for statin therapy further confounds the issue, although it has been well demonstrated that statin drugs are safe for patients with nonalcoholic fatty liver disease.

Serious DILI from statin agents is rare. The risk of acute liver failure associated with lovastatin, the first of the statins to be approved for treatment of hypercholesterolemia, is about 1 in 1 million patient-treatment years. From 1990 to 2002, only 3 of more than 51,000 liver transplants in the US were performed for presumed statin-induced liver injury. In a study from Sweden (1998-2010), 73 cases of DILI from statins were identified; 19% were considered probable, and 10% highly probable. One patient required liver transplant, and 2 patients died. The median latency was 3 months. Patients taking atorvastatin were more likely to present with a cholestatic or mixed profile (57%) compared with patients taking simvastatin (25%). Although atorvastatin and simvastatin were the most frequent culprits responsible for DILI, patients taking fluvastatin had the highest incidence of DILI compared with patients taking any other statin. The estimated incidence of DILI from statins was estimated to be 1.6 per 100,000 person-years.

The FDA labeling for statins has changed. Patients should have baseline liver tests before treatment is initiated. Routine posttreatment monitoring is not recommended, although symptoms, such as jaundice, that suggest liver disease should be investigated with liver tests. Statins rarely have been associated with the development of autoimmune hepatitis, although the association may be only coincidental.

Ezetimibe, which blocks the intestinal absorption of cholesterol, has been associated with increased liver enzyme levels and, when administered in combination with statins, may rarely cause clinically significant hepatoxicity. Sustained-release niacin also may produce symptomatic hepatotoxicity.

✓ Slight increases in transaminase levels after treatment with statins are expected as part of an adaptive response and do not necessitate treatment withdrawal

Tumor Necrosis Factor α Antagonists

In the NIH DILIN study, 6 patients who had DILI from tumor necrosis factor antagonists were evaluated with 28 other cases from the DILI literature. All reported cases were caused by infliximab (n=26), adalimumab (n=4), and etanercept (n=4). Interestingly, 67% of patients had positive autoantibodies, and for 15 of 17 patients who underwent liver biopsy, the histologic findings included autoimmune features. The median latency was 13 weeks, but patients with autoimmune features tended to present later than those without. Most cases of DILI were either mild or moderate; 1 patient with preexisting cirrhosis required liver transplant.

Vedolizumab has been linked to a low rate of increased liver enzyme levels during therapy, but it has not been linked to cases of idiosyncratic clinically apparent liver injury with jaundice.

Immunotherapy with immune checkpoint inhibition is a recent advancement in the management of various solid tumors. Checkpoint inhibitors have been shown to initiate an antitumor immune response directed against melanoma. Pembrolizumab and nivolumab are antibodies directed against programmed cell death receptor 1, and ipilimumab is an antibody directed against the cytotoxic T-lymphocyte antigen-4 receptor on T lymphocytes. They can cause various autoimmune adverse effects, including immune-mediated hepatitis. Increased levels of ALT and AST (with either value >3 up to 5 times the ULRR), ALP, and total bilirubin (>1.5 up to 3 times the ULRR) have been reported, most commonly 8 to 12 weeks after initiating treatment.

Treatment

For most patients with DILI, treatment is based on withdrawal of the agent and general support (Figure 32.1). For acetaminophen toxicity, *N*-acetylcysteine should be given. Carnitine may be helpful for valproate-induced microvesicular steatosis. Drug-induced autoimmune hepatitis that does not improve spontaneously can be treated with corticosteroids.

The US Acute Liver Failure Study Group reported the results of a randomized controlled trial examining intravenous *N*-acetylcysteine for the treatment of acute liver failure from causes other than acetaminophen. In this prospective, double-blind trial, patients with acute liver failure (nonacetaminophen) were randomly assigned to receive *N*-acetylcysteine or placebo infusion for 72 hours. Patients with acute liver failure caused by DILI (n= 45) represented the single largest group among the 173 patients. Although the overall survival at 3 weeks was not significantly different between the groups, transplant-free survival was significantly better for patients in the *N*-acetylcysteine group (40% vs 27%, *P*=.43). The benefits of *N*-acetylcysteine were seen primarily in patients with early-stage disease and coma grade I or II (52% vs 30% transplant-free survival) but not in those with advanced coma grade (III or IV) at randomization. When the overall and transplant-free survival of the 4 largest etiologic groups was considered, patients with DILI and hepatitis B virus infection showed improved outcome compared with patients in the autoimmune hepatitis indeterminate groups. For the DILI patients, the transplant-free survival was 58% for those receiving *N*-acetylcysteine and 27% for those receiving placebo. The study results suggest that therapy with intravenous *N*-acetylcysteine should be considered for patients with acute liver failure due to idiosyncratic DILI.

Compared with hepatocellular drug injury, cholestatic liver injury is less likely to be serious but more likely to be prolonged. Ursodiol has been used in cases of drug-induced cholestasis, with a prolonged recovery phase. Responses have been reported, but the lack of controlled data makes it difficult to draw conclusions about the efficacy of ursodiol.

Management of checkpoint inhibitor–related liver injury should follow the American Society of Clinical Oncology guidelines. For asymptomatic patients with an ALT or AST level that is abnormal but less than 3 times the ULRR or an abnormal bilirubin level less than 1.5 times the ULRR, the checkpoint inhibitor can be continued with biweekly laboratory monitoring. For asymptomatic patients with persistently increased AST or ALT (>3 up to 5 times the ULRR) or increased total bilirubin levels (>1.5 to ≤3 times the ULRR) or both, the checkpoint inhibitor should be withheld and prednisone should be initiated at a dose of 0.5 to 1 mg/kg daily. For patients with symptoms, fibrosis detected by biopsy, cirrhosis, or high levels of AST or ALT (>5 times the ULRR) or bilirubin (>3 times the ULRR), the checkpoint inhibitor should be permanently discontinued and intravenous methylprednisone should be initiated at 1 to 2 mg/kg daily.

Prognosis

The prognosis for patients with DILI varies. According to the Hy rule (named after the hepatologist Hyman Zimmerman), patients with jaundice due to drug-induced hepatocellular injury have a 10% mortality rate without transplant even if treatment with the drug is discontinued promptly. This rule has been confirmed by recent studies from Spain, Sweden, and the US that reported mortality rates between 9% and 12% for patients with hepatocellular jaundice. Patients with acute liver failure due to idiosyncratic drug injury have an 80% mortality rate without transplant. Thus, patients who have hepatocellular DILI and jaundice in whom encephalopathy or coagulopathy develops should be referred for consideration of liver transplant.

Whether chronic DILI will develop after a patient recovers from an acute injury is not clear. Most patients with DILI who survive have complete biochemical and histologic recovery. Yet, a small proportion of patients may have chronically increased serum levels of liver enzymes that may signify chronicity. A recent follow-up study of DILI patients from Sweden (mean duration of follow-up, 10 years) concluded that the development of clinically important liver disease after severe DILI was highly uncommon. A prospective follow-up of DILI patients in the Spanish hepatotoxicity registry showed a 5% incidence of chronic DILI; in comparison, 14% of patients in the NIH DILIN study had persistent laboratory test result abnormalities. The most recent data from Iceland showed chronicity in 7% of patients. Further study is needed to determine the frequency and impact of chronic DILI.

✓ Without liver transplant, acute liver failure due to idiosyncratic drug injury carries a high mortality rate (up to 80%)
✓ If encephalopathy or coagulopathy develops in patients who have hepatocellular DILI and jaundice, they should be referred to a liver transplant center

---

Pharmacogenetics

There is considerable interest in identifying the genes that contribute to DILI. Before the year 2000, little information was available on genetic susceptibility to DILI. However, both genome-wide association studies (GWASs) and candidate gene studies have confirmed an important role for human leukocyte antigen (HLA) class I and class II genes in some but not all forms of DILI. An identified association between DILI due to flucloxacillin and the HLA-B*5701 allele is the strongest reported association between any gene and DILI (odds ratio [OR], 80). The HLA-B*5701 allele is also associated with the thrombin inhibitor ximelagatran (OR, 45) and lapatinib-related DILI. The second replicated HLA association is between amoxicillin-clavulanate–related DILI and the HLA class II allele DRB1*1501. The same risk allele is associated with DILI due to lumiracoxib. Also, evidence for the association between a polymorphism in the gene encoding *N*-acetyltransferase 2 (*NAT2*), an enzyme important in isoniazid metabolism, and susceptibility to DILI has been confirmed. Persons who have *NAT2* variants associated with slow acetylation appear to have an increased risk of isoniazid-related DILI. Common variants in the *SLCO1B1* gene were found to be strongly associated with an increased risk of statin-induced myopathy. This demonstrated that GWASs can successfully identify genetic risk factors for adverse drug reactions.

In recent studies, HLA-A*33:01 was associated with DILI due to ticlopidine (OR, 163.1), methyldopa (OR, 97.8), fenofibrate (OR, 58.7), terbinafine (OR, 40.5), enalapril (OR, 34.8), sertraline (OR, 29), and erythromycin (OR 10.2) in GWASs of persons of European descent. HLA-B*35:02 carriers were found to have an increased risk for minocycline-induced DILI (OR, 29.6). *ERN1* was associated with efavirenz-related DILI (OR, 18.2), and DRB1*16:01-DQB1*05:02 was associated with the nonopioid analgesic flupirtine (OR, 18.7). Genetic polymorphisms associated with statin-related DILI were found on chromosome 18.

However, not all genetic effects relevant to DILI will necessarily be of the magnitude identified in GWASs, and larger studies may be needed to detect genes with smaller effects. Emerging techniques, such as whole-genome sequencing, will be needed for further progress in this area of study.

Suggested Reading

Bell LN, Chalasani N. Epidemiology of idiosyncratic drug-induced liver injury. Semin Liver Dis. 2009 Nov;29(4):337–47.

Bjornsson E, Talwalkar J, Treeprasertsuk S, Kamath PS, Takahashi N, Sanderson S, et al. Drug-induced autoimmune hepatitis: Clinical characteristics and prognosis. Hepatology. 2010 Jun;51(6):2040–8.

Bjornsson ES, Bergmann OM, Bjornsson HK, Kvaran RB, Olafsson S. Incidence, presentation, and outcomes in patients with drug-induced liver injury in the general population of iceland. Gastroenterology. 2013 Jun;144(7):1419–25, 25 e1–3; quiz e19–20.

Chalasani N, Bjornsson E. Risk factors for idiosyncratic drug-induced liver injury. Gastroenterology. 2010 Jun;138(7):2246–59.

Chalasani N, Fontana RJ, Bonkovsky HL, Watkins PB, Davern T, Serrano J, et al. Causes, clinical features, and outcomes from a prospective study of drug-induced liver injury in the United States. Gastroenterology. 2008 Dec;135(6):1924–34, 34 e1–4.

Chalasani NP, Hayashi PH, Bonkovsky HL, Navarro VJ, Lee WM, Fontana RJ, et al. ACG clinical guideline: the diagnosis and management of idiosyncratic drug-induced liver injury. Am J Gastroenterol. 2014 Jul;109(7):950–66; quiz 67.

Chalasani NP, Maddur H, Russo MW, Wong RJ, Reddy KR, Practice Parameters Committee of the American College of Gastroenterology. ACG clinical guideline: diagnosis and management of idiosyncratic drug-induced liver injury. Am J Gastroenterol. 2021 May 1;116(5):878–98.

Daly AK. Drug-induced liver injury: Past, present and future. Pharmacogenomics. 2010 May;11(5):607–11.

Jones M, Nunez M. Liver toxicity of antiretroviral drugs. Semin Liver Dis. 2012 May;32(2):167–76.

Kaliyaperumal K, Grove JI, Delahay RM, Griffiths WJH, Duckworth A, Aithal GP. Pharmacogenomics of drug-induced liver injury (DILI): Molecular biology to clinical applications. J Hepatol. 2018 Oct;69(4):948–57.

Kleiner DE. The pathology of drug-induced liver injury. Semin Liver Dis. 2009 Nov;29(4):364–72.

Kullak-Ublick GA, Andrade RJ, Merz M, End P, Benesic A, Gerbes AL, et al. Drug-induced liver injury: Recent advances in diagnosis and risk assessment. Gut. 2017 Jun;66(6):1154–64.

Larson AM, Polson J, Fontana RJ, Davern TJ, Lalani E, Hynan LS, et al. Acetaminophen-induced acute liver failure: Results of a united states multicenter, prospective study. Hepatology. 2005 Dec;42(6):1364–72.

Leise MD, Poterucha JJ, Talwalkar JA. Drug-induced liver injury. Mayo Clin Proc. 2014 Jan;89(1):95–106.

Navarro VJ, Senior JR. Drug-related hepatotoxicity. N Engl J Med. 2006 Feb 16;354(7):731–9.

Nicoletti P, Aithal GP, Bjornsson ES, Andrade RJ, Sawle A, Arrese M, et al. Association of liver injury from specific drugs, or groups of drugs, with polymorphisms in HLA and other genes in a genome-wide association study. Gastroenterology. 2017 Apr;152(5):1078–89.

Search Collaborative Group, Link E, Parish S, Armitage J, Bowman L, Heath S, et al. SLCO1B1 variants and statin-induced myopathy: a genomewide study. N Engl J Med. 2008 Aug 21;359(8):789–99.

Urban TJ, Nicoletti P, Chalasani N, Serrano J, Stolz A, Daly AK, et al. Minocycline hepatotoxicity: Clinical characterization and identification of HLA-B *35:02 as a risk factor. J Hepatol. 2017 Jul;67(1):137–44.

33

Autoimmune Hepatitis

JOHN E. EATON, MD[a]

Epidemiology

Autoimmune hepatitis is a chronic inflammatory disorder of the liver that is associated with formation of autoantibodies, hypergammaglobulinemia, plasma cell infiltrate, and interface hepatitis seen on histologic examination. Autoimmune hepatitis affects patients of all ages and both sexes but occurs more commonly in women (female to male ratio, 3.6:1). The global annual incidence of autoimmune hepatitis ranges from 0.7 to 2 cases per 100,000 persons. Among White people of northern European ancestry, the mean annual incidence of autoimmune hepatitis is 1.9 per 100,000, and the point prevalence is 16.9 per 100,000. The annual incidence of autoimmune hepatitis in children is 0.4 cases per 100,000 persons with a prevalence of 3 cases per 100,000 persons. Autoimmune hepatitis occurs in 100,000 to 200,000 persons in the US annually and accounts for approximately 6% of liver transplants performed in the US.

Originally described from White patients of northern European ancestry and North Americans, autoimmune hepatitis is now recognized to occur worldwide. Ethnic background may affect the clinical presentation: African American patients have a higher frequency of cirrhosis at presentation than White North Americans; Alaskan natives have a higher occurrence of acute icteric disease than nonnative patients; Asian patients tend to have late-onset, mild disease; and South American patients are more commonly young children with severe disease.

Etiology

The cause of autoimmune hepatitis is unknown, and the vast majority of cases are not preceded by an inciting exposure. However, several potential triggers of the disease have been suggested, such as hepatitis A, hepatitis B, hepatitis C, Epstein-Barr, herpes simplex, and measles viruses. Medications can cause drug-induced autoimmune hepatitis. Key examples include immunotherapy (eg, pembrolizumab), antimicrobials (eg, minocycline, nitrofurantoin, moxifloxacin, and isoniazid), antihypertensive medications (eg, hydralazine and α-methyldopa), complementary and alternative medications or supplements (eg, black cohosh, khat, and Chinese herbal teas), and others (eg, diclofenac, propylthiouracil, atorvastatin, infliximab, and adalimumab). Hepatitis A virus infection (and hepatitis A vaccine) and minocycline have been implicated most often worldwide. In 1 series, drug-induced autoimmune hepatitis accounted for 9% of all autoimmune hepatitis cases; nitrofurantoin and minocycline were the leading culprits.

Distinguishing drug-induced autoimmune hepatitis from classic autoimmune hepatitis can be challenging. However, several key features can assist clinicians: 1) Drug-induced autoimmune hepatitis has a temporal relationship with the offending agent. 2) The presence of cirrhosis in patients with drug-induced autoimmune hepatitis is rare. Otherwise, histologic features can look similar. 3) Cessation of the offending agent and short-term use of prednisone is sufficient to treat drug-induced autoimmune hepatitis. 4) Drug-induced autoimmune hepatitis is characterized by a low rate of relapse and better outcomes when compared to classic autoimmune hepatitis. 5) Up to a quarter of patients with drug-induced autoimmune hepatitis may have a concurrent

[a] The author thanks Albert J. Czaja, MD, who authored previous versions of this chapter.

Abbreviations: ALT, alanine aminotransferase; ANA, antinuclear antibody; anti-LKM1, antibody to liver-kidney microsome type 1; Ig, immunoglobulin; PBC, primary biliary cholangitis; PSC, primary sclerosing cholangitis; SMA, smooth muscle antibody; TPMT, thiopurine methyltransferase

fever, rash, and eosinophilia, which is rare in classic autoimmune hepatitis.

Presentation

Autoimmune hepatitis is characterized by a phenotypic spectrum. Most patients with autoimmune hepatitis have normal findings on physical examination despite having severe inflammatory activity (Table 33.1). Women constitute at least 70% of cases, and 50% are younger than 40 years (Table 33.1). Onset is usually between the third and fifth decades but can occur at any age. Children are less likely to have sustained remission and are more likely to have disease relapse after treatment withdrawal, particularly if they have antibodies to liver-kidney microsome type 1 (anti-LKM1).

There are 2 subtypes of autoimmune hepatitis (Table 33.2). Type 2 occurs in children, is rarely associated with remission after drug withdrawal, and has varied disease associations and autoantibodies when compared to type 1 autoimmune hepatitis.

Nearly 30% of patients may present with asymptomatic increases in liver test results. Of those asymptomatic patients, 25% have inactive autoimmune hepatitis with advanced fibrosis when their diagnosis is established. Nonspecific symptoms such as fatigue, arthralgias, and malaise are common. Jaundice, pruritus, and manifestations of portal hypertension can be present in severe or advanced disease. Approximately 30% of patients have cirrhosis at presentation. Although many patients have a long history of increased liver test results, 25% to 75% of patients have an acute presentation with variable severity. At their initial presentation, less than 6% of patients have acute severe autoimmune hepatitis with jaundice and coagulopathy or, more rarely, acute liver failure.

Concurrent Immune-Mediated Diseases

Concurrent immune-mediated diseases are present in 30% to 48% of patients with autoimmune hepatitis (Box 33.1). Autoimmune thyroid disease, synovitis, and ulcerative colitis are the most common concurrent immune diseases. Autoimmune hepatitis is present in 15% of patients with autoimmune polyendocrinopathy-candidiasis-ectodermal dystrophy.

A subset of patients with autoimmune hepatitis may also have primary sclerosing cholangitis (PSC) or primary biliary cholangitis (PBC). Of the patients who have autoimmune hepatitis and ulcerative colitis, 41% have PSC. In children, this has historically been referred to as *autoimmune sclerosing cholangitis*. Approximately 5% of patients with PSC and PBC have an overlap syndrome with concurrent autoimmune hepatitis. An overlap syndrome should be considered if patients have pronounced cholestasis on presentation or a persistently increased level of alkaline phosphatase after the aminotransferase levels have improved with therapy directed to autoimmune hepatitis. The diagnosis of concurrent PSC can be established when multifocal biliary strictures are seen on magnetic resonance cholangiography or when characteristic histologic features are found on liver biopsy. Concurrent PBC can be diagnosed when the serum alkaline phosphatase level is increased with either positive results for antimitochondrial antibodies or compatible histologic changes.

Diagnosis

There is no specific diagnostic biomarker for autoimmune hepatitis. Instead, the diagnosis of autoimmune hepatitis can be established with compatible histologic features along with typical laboratory and clinical features after excluding other causes of liver disease such as viral hepatitis and drug-induced liver injury. Diagnostic scoring systems have been created, such as the simplified scoring system shown in Table 33.3. However, their use has been limited by a lack of prospective validation and uncertain accuracy with severe presentations of autoimmune hepatitis and by situations when concurrent PSC, PBC, or nonalcoholic fatty liver disease is present and testing involves autoantibody quantification with indirect immunofluorescence titers rather than enzyme-linked immunoassay units. Clinicians should always reconsider a previous diagnosis of autoimmune hepatitis when patients do not have an expected response to medical therapy.

Laboratory Features

In patients with active autoimmune hepatitis, abnormalities in serum aminotransferase levels are essential for the diagnosis (Table 33.1). The serum aminotransferase levels at presentation are often 500 U/L or less but occasionally exceed 1,000 U/L in a severe presentation. Increased levels of serum alkaline phosphatase occur in 81% of patients, but the values are typically less than 2-fold the upper limit of the reference range. Mild hyperbilirubinemia is present in 83% of patients with severe inflammatory activity. The serum γ-globulin level is often increased and is usually a polyclonal increase that involves serum immunoglobulin (Ig) G.

Antinuclear antibody (ANA), smooth muscle antibody (SMA), and anti-LKM1 are often increased in autoimmune hepatitis. Among adults with autoimmune hepatitis, ANA is detected in 80% and SMA is detected in 63%. However, anti-LKM1 is seen in only 3% of adults but is more common in children and is associated with type 2 autoimmune hepatitis (Table 33.2). Autoantibodies such as ANA and SMA are frequently seen in other conditions such as nonalcoholic fatty liver disease. Moreover, anti-LKM1 is found in as many as 10% of European patients with chronic hepatitis C. Hence, the presence of these autoantibodies is not pathognomonic, and ANA or SMA titers

Table 33.1. Typical Features of Autoimmune Hepatitis

Feature	Patients, %
Clinical features	
Female sex	70
Age <40 y	50
Acute onset	25-75
Asymptomatic	25-34
Common symptoms	
Fatigue	85
Arthralgia	30
Myalgia	30
Development after asymptomatic presentation	26-70
Frequent physical examination findings	
Normal	80
Hepatomegaly	20
Typical laboratory abnormalities	
Increased serum levels of AST and ALT	100
Increased serum levels of γ-globulin and IgG	90
Mild hyperbilirubinemia (bilirubin <3 mg/dL)	83
Serum ALP increased <2-fold ULRR	67
ANA, SMA, or anti-LKM1 present	80

Abbreviations: ALP, alkaline phosphatase; ALT, alanine aminotransferase; ANA, antinuclear antibody; anti-LKM1, antibody to liver-kidney microsome type 1; AST, aspartate aminotransferase; IgG, immunoglobulin G; SMA, smooth muscle antibody; ULRR, upper limit of the reference range.

Table 33.2. Comparison of Types 1 and 2 Autoimmune Hepatitis

Feature	Autoimmune Hepatitis	
	Type 1	Type 2
Characteristic autoantibodies	ANA, SMA	Anti-LKM1
Associated autoantibodies	pANCA	Anti-LC1
	Anti-SLA	Anti-ASGPR
	Anti-actin	Anti–parietal cell
	Anti-ASGPR	
Age at onset	Any age	Mainly pediatric (2-14 y)
Common concurrent immune diseases	Autoimmune thyroiditis	Vitiligo
	Synovitis	Type 1 diabetes
	Ulcerative colitis	Autoimmune thyroiditis
Overlap syndrome with PSC	Varies (6%-11%); more common in children	Rare
Overlap syndrome with PBC	Varies (7%-11%); seen in adults	Not reported
Cirrhosis at time of diagnosis	Approximately 30%	Rare
Implicated genetic factors	DRB1*0301 (northern Europe)	DQB1*02
	DRB1*0401 (northern Europe)	DRB1*03 (anti-LKM1)
	DRB1*1501 (protective)	DRB1*07 (anti-LC1)
	DRB1*1301 (South America)	
Autoantigen	Uncertain	CYP2D6
Remission after drug withdrawal	Possible in select cases	Rare

Abbreviations: ANA, antinuclear antibody; anti-ASGPR, antibody to asialoglycoprotein receptor; anti-LC1, antibody to liver cytosol type 1; anti-LKM1, antibody to liver-kidney microsome type 1; anti-SLA, antibody to soluble liver antigen; CYP2D6, cytochrome P450 2D6; pANCA, perinuclear antineutrophil cytoplasmic antibody; PBC, primary biliary cholangitis; PSC, primary sclerosing cholangitis; SMA, smooth muscle antibody.

Adapted from Czaja AJ. Autoimmune liver disease. In: Zakim D, Boyer TD, editors. Hepatology: a textbook of liver disease. Vol 2. 4th ed. Philadelphia (PA): Saunders; c2003. p. 1163-202; used with permission.

do not have prognostic significance. They may be absent in approximately 20% of patients with autoimmune hepatitis (ie, seronegative autoimmune hepatitis). Therefore, low or undetectable titers should not dissuade a clinician from the diagnosis if other features implicate the disorder.

Several other autoantibodies are used less frequently in clinical practice. Atypical perinuclear antineutrophil cytoplasmic antibodies are often seen in type 1 autoimmune hepatitis but have limited specificity. Conversely, antibodies to soluble liver antigen have high specificity for type 1 autoimmune hepatitis but poor sensitivity. Additional autoantibodies that can be present are shown in Table 33.2.

Histologic Features

A liver biopsy that shows compatible histologic features is essential. *Interface hepatitis* is the histologic hallmark of autoimmune hepatitis (Figure 33.1). Plasma cell infiltration of the hepatic parenchyma or portal tracts (or both) is apparent in 66% of tissue specimens, but its presence is neither specific nor required for the diagnosis (Figure 33.2). A lobular, or panacinar, hepatitis frequently accompanies interface hepatitis, and a centrilobular (zone 3) necrosis has also been described. Successive examinations of liver tissue have shown transition of the centrilobular (zone 3) necrosis to interface hepatitis, and it may be an early form of the disease. Emperipolesis can be present in 65% of specimens; hepatocyte rosettes in 33%. While these histologic features are typical for autoimmune hepatitis, they are not pathognomonic and can be seen in other conditions.

Treatment

Therapy for autoimmune hepatitis involves immunosuppression to achieve remission and subsequent long-term maintenance

therapy. When therapy is successful, improvement can be expected in transaminase values, histologic findings, and survival.

Autoimmune hepatitis can be treated effectively with immunosuppression with glucocorticoids alone or at a lower dose in combination with azathioprine. Treatment induces clinical, laboratory, and histologic remission in 65% of patients within 18 months and in 80% within 3 years (Figure 33.3). Medical therapy also enhances survival expectations. For example, the life expectancy of successfully treated patients exceeds 80% after 20 years of observation and is akin to that of the general population. Improvement in hepatic fibrosis occurs in conjunction with decreases in liver inflammation, and corticosteroids suppress inflammatory activity.

Patients who have autoimmune hepatitis with active disease are candidates for therapy. Dosages for adults are prednisone alone at 40 to 60 mg daily (prednisolone is frequently used in Europe) or at 20 to 40 mg daily in combination with azathioprine (50-150 mg daily in the US; 1-2 mg/kg daily in many European centers). For most patients, combination therapy is preferred because it is associated with fewer corticosteroid-related adverse effects. However, azathioprine is not recommended in the following situations: 1) when patients have complete deficiency of thiopurine methyltransferase (TPMT); 2) when oral or intravenous corticosteroid monotherapy is used in the initial treatment of hospitalized patients who have acute severe autoimmune hepatitis; 3) when patients have drug-induced autoimmune hepatitis, where treatment with prednisone for less than 6 months is generally sufficient; 4) when patients have decompensated cirrhosis; and 5) when patients have active malignancy (eg, lymphoma) that could be exacerbated by azathioprine.

In many centers, the introduction of azathioprine is delayed for 2 weeks after initiation of corticosteroids. This delay is used to confirm a response to corticosteroids, to verify TPMT status, and to decrease the rare likelihood of azathioprine-associated

Box 33.1. Key Immune-Mediated Diseases Associated With Autoimmune Hepatitis

Autoimmune thyroiditis[a]

Celiac disease

Coombs-positive hemolytic anemia

Cryoglobulinemia

Dermatitis herpetiformis

Erythema nodosum

Fibrosing alveolitis

Focal myositis

Gingivitis

Glomerulonephritis

Graves disease[a]

Idiopathic thrombocytopenic purpura

Intestinal villous atrophy

Iritis

Lichen planus

Myasthenia gravis

Neutropenia

Pericarditis

Peripheral neuropathy

Pernicious anemia

Primary biliary cholangitis

Primary sclerosing cholangitis

Pyoderma gangrenosum

Rheumatoid arthritis[a]

Sjögren syndrome

Synovitis[a]

Systemic lupus erythematosus

Type 1 diabetes

Ulcerative colitis[a]

Vitiligo[a]

---

[a] Most common associations.

Adapted from Czaja AJ. Autoimmune liver disease. In: Zakim D, Boyer TD, editors. Hepatology: a textbook of liver disease. Vol 2. 4th ed. Philadelphia (PA): Saunders; c2003. p. 1163-202; used with permission.

Table 33.3. Diagnostic Criteria for Autoimmune Hepatitis (AIH)

Variable	Points[a]
ANA or SMA ≥1:40	1
ANA or SMA ≥1:80 *or*	2[b]
Anti-LKM1 ≥1:40 *or*	
Anti-SLA positive	
IgG >1×ULRR	1
IgG >1.10×ULRR	2
Histology *compatible with* AIH	1
Histology *typical of* AIH	2
Absence of viral hepatitis	2

Abbreviations: ANA, antinuclear antibody; anti-LKM1, antibody to liver-kidney microsome type 1; anti-SLA, antibody to soluble liver antigen; IgG, immunoglobulin G; SMA, smooth muscle antibody; ULRR, upper limit of the reference range.

[a] Score ≥6 points = probable AIH (sensitivity, 88%; specificity, 97%). Score ≥7 points = definite AIH (sensitivity, 81%; specificity, 99%).

[b] Maximum of 2 points for all autoantibodies.

Data from Hennes EM, Zeniya M, Czaja AJ, Pares A, Dalekos GN, Krawitt EL, et al; International Autoimmune Hepatitis Group. Simplified criteria for the diagnosis of autoimmune hepatitis. Hepatology. 2008 Jul;48(1):169-76.

Alternatively, other smaller studies have suggested that patients treated with budesonide are more likely to have an incomplete response, which suggests that prednisone is a more potent agent for induction of remission. Hence, there is limited quality of evidence to suggest that either is superior for inducing remission. For patients with more mild disease and those at risk for corticosteroid-related adverse effects, budesonide may be a pragmatic option. Budesonide has a 90% first-pass effect on the liver and should not be used in patients who have cirrhosis or portosystemic shunting. Moreover, it has not been studied in patients with severe disease and should be avoided in those with acute severe autoimmune hepatitis.

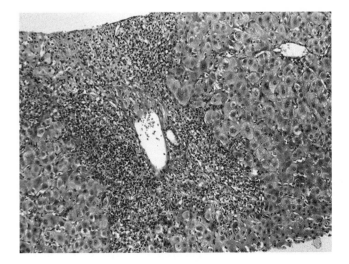

Figure 33.1. Interface Hepatitis. The limiting plate of the portal tract is disrupted by an inflammatory infiltrate that extends into the acinus. Interface hepatitis is a requisite for the diagnosis of autoimmune hepatitis, but it is not specific for the diagnosis (hematoxylin-eosin, original magnification ×200). (Adapted from Czaja AJ. Current concepts in autoimmune hepatitis. Ann Hepatol. 2005 Jan-Mar;4[1]:6-24; used with permission.)

liver injury as a confounding factor in the determination of whether there is biochemical improvement with corticosteroids. For most outpatients without severe disease, laboratory values are typically checked every 2 to 4 weeks. After biochemical remission is achieved, a response-guided approach to corticosteroid tapering is recommended, where the prednisone dosage is gradually decreased to 5 to 10 mg daily (or budesonide to 3 mg daily) over the next 6 months. Thereafter, patients with biochemical remission are candidates for a trial of withdrawal of corticosteroids and continuation of azathioprine monotherapy long-term for maintenance of remission.

Budesonide has been used to avoid the short- and long-term adverse effects associated with prednisone. In a randomized controlled trial, budesonide was more likely to be associated with biochemical remission compared to prednisone.

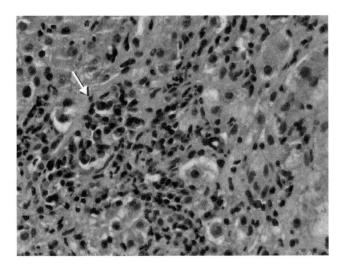

Figure 33.2. Plasma Cell Infiltration of the Hepatic Parenchyma. Plasma cells (arrow) are characterized by a cytoplasmic halo adjacent to a deeply basophilic nucleus. Plasma cells typically are abundant at the interface and throughout the acinus, but their presence does not have diagnostic specificity (hematoxylin-eosin, original magnification ×400). (Adapted from Czaja AJ. Current concepts in autoimmune hepatitis. Ann Hepatol. 2005 Jan-Mar;4[1]:6-24; used with permission.)

Patients with normalization of alanine aminotransferase (ALT) levels at 6 months after diagnosis have improved outcomes. Histologic improvement lags behind clinical and laboratory resolution by 3 to 8 months (Figure 33.3). A decrease in liver stiffness, measured by elastography, is associated with biochemical remission, fibrosis regression, and an enhanced prognosis. Examination of a liver biopsy specimen before initial withdrawal of drug therapy is the only method for confirming histologic resolution, but biopsy is infrequently performed in clinical practice. Before withdrawal of drug therapy is considered, treatment should be continued for at least 2 years after normalization of transaminase and IgG levels and clinical remission.

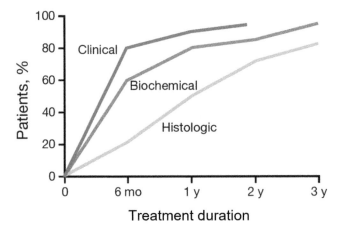

Figure 33.3. Frequencies of Clinical, Biochemical, and Histologic Remission During Conventional Corticosteroid Treatment of Autoimmune Hepatitis. Histologic improvement lags clinical and biochemical improvement by 3 to 8 months. (Data from Czaja AJ. Treatment strategies in autoimmune hepatitis. Clin Liver Dis. 2002 Aug;6[3]:799-824.)

Patients with overlap syndromes should receive the standard medical therapy for autoimmune hepatitis along with the typical treatment and management of PBC or PSC.

Relapse

Relapse connotes the exacerbation of disease activity after withdrawal of drug therapy. It is characterized by an increase in serum levels of liver enzymes (ALT or AST) and reappearance of characteristic hepatic inflammation (although biopsy is not often required in this situation). Normalization of the serum levels of aminotransferases and IgG in conjunction with histologic resolution decreases the relative risk of relapse after drug withdrawal by 3- to 11-fold. However, it is noteworthy that among non–drug-induced autoimmune hepatitis cases, only a minority of patients have disease that stays in remission without maintenance therapy. For example, among 131 patients with autoimmune hepatitis who had clinical and biochemical remission for 2 years, nearly 90% had a relapse within 5 years after withdrawal of immunosuppression. In a smaller study with 28 patients who had prolonged biochemical remission, 46% had a relapse within 2 years of stopping immunosuppression. Hence, relapse is common and long-term monitoring is required. Moreover, multiple relapses can be associated with progression to cirrhosis and shorter transplant-free survival.

The initial step in treating relapse is reinstitution of the original corticosteroid. The second step is reintroduction of azathioprine as the dose of prednisone is gradually decreased and then stopped. In more than 80% of patients treated in this fashion the disease remains in clinical and laboratory remission for 10 years.

Suboptimal Response and Treatment Failure

Incomplete resolution of inflammation with therapy (according to biochemical markers and histologic findings) is considered a suboptimal response, which occurs in 13% of patients. A lack of a biochemical response to prednisone should prompt considerations of alternative diagnoses. Approximately 9% of patients have a deterioration in their condition despite their adherence to the drug regimen (ie, treatment failure). The use of a high dose of prednisone (60 mg daily) or prednisone at a lower dose (30 mg daily) in conjunction with a high dose of azathioprine (150 mg daily) is the regimen for treatment failure that induces laboratory remission in 75% of patients within 2 years. Intolerable adverse effects (ie, drug toxicity) develop in 13% of patients, who stop taking the medication prematurely.

Data supporting second- and third-line treatment options (after exclusion of azathioprine and corticosteroids) are largely from uncontrolled and retrospective studies. Mycophenolate mofetil is the most widely studied second-line agent, which can be used instead of azathioprine. Response rates to mycophenolate mofetil appear to be higher among patients who have an intolerance to azathioprine rather than an incomplete response. Use of mycophenolate mofetil should be avoided during pregnancy. Calcineurin inhibitors such as tacrolimus have also been examined. For example, in an international multicenter retrospective study, 57% of patients who had an inadequate response to standard therapy had a complete biochemical response 6 months after initiation of tacrolimus. Small case series and anecdotal reports from specialized centers have also reported the successful use of rituximab and mammalian target of rapamycin inhibitors (eg, sirolimus and everolimus) in patients who have had difficulty with other therapies.

Liver Transplant

Autoimmune hepatitis accounts for 5% of all liver transplants in the US. Liver transplant is effective in the treatment of patients who have acute liver failure, severe acute hepatitis that is unresponsive to conventional therapies, or cirrhosis-related complications. The 5-year survival rate of patient and graft ranges from 83% to 92%. Autoimmune hepatitis recurs in approximately one-third of patients after 5 years. Rejection occurs more frequently in patients who underwent liver transplant for autoimmune hepatitis compared to other indications. In some studies, long-term use of prednisone (5-10 mg daily) in addition to the standard immunosuppression regimen (typically a calcineurin inhibitor) has decreased the risk of recurrent autoimmune hepatitis without increasing the risk of infections or osteoporosis. In contrast, other studies have shown that corticosteroid withdrawal is not associated with disease recurrence, episodes of rejection, or shortened survival of patient or graft. Hence, management of immunosuppression should be individualized. Autoimmune hepatitis can develop in 2.5% to 3.4% of allografts of children and adults who received liver transplants for liver diseases other than autoimmune hepatitis.

Suggested Reading

Czaja AJ. Overlap syndromes. Clin Liver Dis (Hoboken). 2014 Jan;3(1): 2–5.

Efe C, Hagstrom H, Ytting H, Bhanji RA, Muller NF, Wang Q, et al. Efficacy and safety of mycophenolate mofetil and tacrolimus as second-line therapy for patients with autoimmune hepatitis. Clin Gastroenterol Hepatol. 2017 Dec;15(12):1950–6.

Kalra A, Burton JR, Jr., Forman LM. Pro: Steroids can be withdrawn after transplant in recipients with autoimmune hepatitis. Liver Transpl. 2018 Aug;24(8):1109–12.

Mack CL, Adams D, Assis DN, Kerkar N, Manns MP, Mayo MJ, et al. Diagnosis and management of autoimmune hepatitis in adults and children: 2019 practice guidance and guidelines from the American Association for the Study of Liver Diseases. Hepatology. 2020 Aug;72(2):671–722.

Theocharidou E, Heneghan MA. Con: Steroids should not be withdrawn in transplant recipients with autoimmune hepatitis. Liver Transpl. 2018 Aug;24(8):1113–8.

Trivedi PJ, Hubscher SG, Heneghan M, Gleeson D, Hirschfield GM. Grand round: Autoimmune hepatitis. J Hepatol. 2019 Apr;70(4):773–84.

van Gerven NM, Verwer BJ, Witte BI, van Hoek B, Coenraad MJ, van Erpecum KJ, et al. Relapse is almost universal after withdrawal of immunosuppressive medication in patients with autoimmune hepatitis in remission. J Hepatol. 2013 Jan;58(1):141–7.

34

Nonalcoholic Fatty Liver Disease[a]

GOPANANDAN PARTHASARATHY, MBBS
HARMEET MALHI, MBBS

Nonalcoholic fatty liver disease (NAFLD) refers to a spectrum of disorders defined by accumulation of fat in hepatocytes and includes isolated hepatic steatosis, also known as *nonalcoholic fatty liver* (NAFL), and *nonalcoholic steatohepatitis* (NASH), which is characterized by the presence of inflammation and hepatocyte injury (including ballooning), with or without fibrosis. NAFLD is the most common chronic liver disease in the Western world, affecting a quarter of the population. NAFL, defined by steatosis without inflammation, is generally benign, whereas NASH may progress to cirrhosis, liver failure, and hepatocellular carcinoma. Hence, distinguishing between NAFL and NASH has important prognostic and management implications. Recently, to improve the nomenclature, experts have proposed the use of the term *metabolic dysfunction–associated fatty liver disease* (MAFLD). This terminology better captures the underlying obesity-associated or obesity-independent metabolic dysfunction, which is often a prerequisite for the development of hepatic steatosis. However, neither term, *NAFLD or MAFLD*, captures the heterogeneous pathogenesis and progression; ideally terms related to molecular phenotypes will replace them in the future. This chapter uses the existing nomenclature: *NAFLD, NAFL,* and *NASH*.

Hepatic steatosis may be categorized as primary or secondary, depending on the underlying pathogenesis (Table 34.1). Primary steatosis, the more common type, is associated with insulin-resistant states, such as obesity, type 2 diabetes, and dyslipidemia. Other conditions associated with insulin resistance, such as polycystic ovarian syndrome and hypopituitarism, have also been described in association with NAFLD; however, the exact prevalence and significance of NAFLD in these conditions is not clear. The differentiation of primary steatosis from secondary types is important because the treatments and prognoses are different.

Table 34.1. Causes of Hepatic Steatosis

Type of cause	Characteristics
Primary	Obesity, glucose intolerance, type 2 diabetes, hypertriglyceridemia, low HDL cholesterol, hypertension
Nutritional	Protein-calorie malnutrition, rapid weight loss, gastrointestinal bypass surgery, total parental nutrition
Pharmacologic	Glucocorticoids, estrogens, tamoxifen, amiodarone, methotrexate, diltiazem, zidovudine, valproate, aspirin, tetracycline, cocaine
Metabolic	Lipodystrophy, hypopituitarism, dysbetalipoproteinemia, Weber-Christian disease
Toxic	Poisoning from *Amanita phalloides* (a mushroom), phosphorus, petrochemicals, *Bacillus cereus* toxin
Infectious	HIV, hepatitis C, small-bowel diverticulosis with bacterial overgrowth

Abbreviation: HDL, high-density lipoprotein.

Adapted from Aithal GP, Das A, Chowdhury A. Epidemiology of nonalcoholic fatty liver disease (NAFLD). In: Talley NJ, Locke GR, Moayyedi P, West J, Ford AC, Saito YA, eds. GI epidemiology: diseases and clinical methodology. 2nd ed. John Wiley & Sons; 2014:357-72; used with permission.

[a] The authors thank Kymberly D. Watt, MD, who authored previous versions of this chapter.

Abbreviations: ALT, alanine aminotransferase; AST, aspartate aminotransferase; BMI, body mass index; CT, computed tomography; FXR, farnesoid X receptor; GLP-1, glucagon-like peptide-1; HCC, hepatocellular carcinoma; MAFLD, metabolic dysfunction–associated fatty liver disease; MR, magnetic resonance; MRI, magnetic resonance imaging; NAFL, nonalcoholic fatty liver; NAFLD, nonalcoholic fatty liver disease; NASH, nonalcoholic steatohepatitis; PPAR, peroxisome proliferator-activated receptor; ULRR, upper limit of the reference range

✓ **Nonalcoholic steatohepatitis (NASH)**—hepatic steatosis with evidence of inflammation and hepatocyte injury, such as ballooning, with or without fibrosis
✓ **Nonalcoholic fatty liver disease (NAFLD)**—spectrum of disorders ranging from isolated accumulation of fat in the liver (nonalcoholic fatty liver [NAFL]) to NASH and NASH cirrhosis
✓ **Metabolic dysfunction–associated fatty liver disease (MAFLD)**—hepatic steatosis in the presence of obesity, type 2 diabetes, or metabolic dysfunction

Epidemiology

NAFLD has reached epidemic proportions in many countries, as shown by several population-based studies. In the US, an estimated 30% to 40% of the adult population (75 million to 100 million persons) has NAFLD. The prevalence of NAFLD in the general population in the US is almost 14-fold higher than the prevalence of hepatitis C, which affects about 4 million people. It also is almost 3-fold higher than alcohol-associated liver disease. Although the majority of patients with NAFLD have NAFL, an estimated 15 million to 20 million have NASH, and in approximately 10% to 30% of those patients, NASH progresses to cirrhosis (Table 34.2).

NAFLD is more prevalent in men than in women, especially premenopausal women (men, 31%; premenopausal women, 16%), and prevalence is higher among Hispanic patients (45%) compared to White patients who are not Hispanic (33%) and African American patients (24%).

✓ An estimated one-third of adults in the US have NAFLD; about 5% have NASH, and advanced fibrosis may develop in a third of them
✓ Prevalence of NAFLD is greater in men, Hispanic persons, and patients with obesity or type 2 diabetes

Pathogenesis

The pathogenesis of NAFLD is complex and includes contributions from many genetic, environmental, and lifestyle factors. Since the recognition of the initial "2-hit pathogenesis" in the late 1980s, several additional factors have been identified that contribute to the development of NAFLD (eg, lipotoxicity, bile acid metabolism, genetic polymorphisms, and intestinal dysbiosis).

Hepatic steatosis, the hallmark feature of NAFLD, is the net result of altered lipid homeostasis in the liver. Insulin resistance is pathogenically linked to hepatic steatosis. Increased adipose tissue lipolysis in insulin-resistant states results in the delivery of excess free fatty acids to the liver. These free fatty acids provide substrate for triglyceride accumulation. In addition, contributors to steatosis include increased de novo lipogenesis in the liver, which persists in selective insulin resistance in the liver, and increased diet-derived fatty acids. Several additional mechanistic processes are recognized as contributors or modifiers of steatosis. These include bile acid metabolism, intestinal dysbiosis, defects in lipidation or secretion of very low-density lipoprotein, and genetic variations.

Bile acid metabolism is predominantly regulated through the nuclear hormone receptor farnesoid X receptor (FXR), which is found in the hepatocyte. Activation of the FXR decreases lipogenesis and increases fatty acid oxidation. The bile acid metabolism pathway has been a key target in clinical trial development. Several other nuclear hormone receptors have also been associated with NAFLD, and studies are ongoing.

Research into the genetics behind the pathogenesis has been prompted by differences in the prevalence of NAFLD among ethnic groups and clustering in families and in twin cohorts. The protein PNPLA3 (also called adiponutrin) is important in lipid metabolism, and patients who have the I148M variant of *PNPLA3* (OMIM 609567) have a greater risk for increased incidence and severity of disease. *TM6SF2* (OMIM 606563) is a risk allele associated with dyslipidemia and hepatic steatosis. A variant in *MBOAT7* (OMIM 606048) is associated with NAFLD. Conversely, a recently recognized variant in *HSD17B13* (OMIM 612127) decreases the risk of NAFLD development.

Sophisticated sequencing of the gut microbiome has shown that patients with NAFLD have lower gut microbial diversity (ie, dysbiosis) compared with healthy persons. Separate studies have shown that differences in the gut microbiome are correlated with the presence of obesity and the degree of fibrosis. This dysbiosis is thought to alter the function of the intestinal barrier and allow for the translocation of more bacterial components and microbial

Table 34.2. Definitions of Liver Diseases

Term	Definition	Prevalence	Prognosis
NAFLD	Spectrum of fatty liver disease without excessive alcohol consumption	Estimated 25%-52% of global population Estimated 30%-40% of US population	
NAFL	Liver fat ≥5% (hepatic steatosis) without evidence of hepatocellular injury (hepatocyte ballooning) or fibrosis	>80% of patients with NAFLD	Minimal risk for progression to cirrhosis
NASH	Liver fat ≥5% (hepatic steatosis) *and* inflammation *and* hepatocellular injury with ballooning *with or without* fibrosis	≤20% of patients with NAFLD; estimated 1.5%-6.45% of general population	10%-30% of patients have progression to cirrhosis over 15 y
NASH cirrhosis	Presence of cirrhosis with current or past histologic evidence of steatosis	10%-30% of patients with NASH	About 31% of patients have decompensation over 8 y; in about 7%, hepatocellular carcinoma develops over 6.5 y
Cryptogenic cirrhosis	Presence of cirrhosis without a specific cause; often with similar risk factors as for NAFLD		

Abbreviations: NAFL, nonalcoholic fatty liver; NAFLD, nonalcoholic fatty liver disease; NASH, nonalcoholic steatohepatitis.

metabolites, including short-chain fatty acids and bile acids, which contributes to hepatic steatosis and inflammation.

In addition to hepatic steatosis, the pathogenesis of NASH is characterized by hepatocyte injury, inflammation, and fibrosis. The accumulation of toxic lipids, a process referred to as *lipotoxicity*, results in direct injury and cell death of hepatocytes. Danger signals released from hepatocytes, translocation of microbial products from the intestine, and direct effects of lipids on the innate immune system contribute to the sterile inflammatory response that occurs in the liver in NASH. *Hepatocyte ballooning*, a key feature of NASH and a component of the histologic NAFLD activity score, refers to enlarged hepatocytes with accumulation of fat droplets, loss of keratin 8 and 18 staining, and the presence of Mallory-Denk bodies. Ballooned hepatocytes are thought to be bioactive and secrete inflammatory mediators, which also contribute to the inflammatory response in NASH. Fibrosis occurs in response to ongoing hepatocyte injury and inflammation.

✓ Steatosis results from increased free fatty acid delivery from the gut and adipose tissue lipolysis and from increased de novo synthesis of free fatty acid in the liver; the result is hepatocyte injury and death, which perpetuates inflammation and fibrosis

✓ Genetic variants and risk of NAFLD
  • Increased risk of NAFLD: variants in *PNPLA3*, *TM6FSF2*, and *MBOAT7*
  • Decreased risk of NAFLD: variants in *HSD17B13*

✓ Histologic features of NASH are assessed with the NAFLD activity score, which includes severity of steatosis, lobular inflammation, and hepatocyte ballooning

---

Clinical Manifestations

The clinical, laboratory, histologic, and diagnostic features of NAFLD are listed in Table 34.3. The majority of patients are asymptomatic, but they may complain of fatigue or malaise and a sensation of fullness or discomfort in the right upper abdomen. In children and adolescents, hepatomegaly and acanthosis nigricans are common physical findings, but stigmata of chronic liver disease, which would suggest cirrhosis, are uncommon.

The most common clinical scenario leading to the diagnosis of NAFLD is an asymptomatic increase in alanine aminotransferase (ALT) and aspartate aminotransferase (AST) not due to viral hepatitis, autoimmune processes, iron overload, or alcohol use. Aminotransferase levels can be increased in up to 50% to 90% of hospitalized patients who have NASH but are less commonly increased in patients in the general population who have NAFLD. The increase is usually mild (1-4 times the upper limit of the reference range [ULRR]) with the AST:ALT ratio less than 1:1. This ratio increases as fibrosis advances but is almost never greater than 2. Fatty infiltration of the liver is detected with ultrasonography or computed tomography (CT) (as described below) and often is an incidental finding, prompting further investigation or referrals.

Because a patient with NAFLD is commonly asymptomatic, fibrosis can progress silently over many years, and the patient may then present with cirrhosis, termed *NASH cirrhosis*. With its asymptomatic nature, NASH is a leading cause of "cryptogenic" cirrhosis. In support of this, the prevalence of metabolic risk factors such as type 2 diabetes and obesity is similar among patients with cryptogenic cirrhosis and NAFLD but is less frequent among patients with cirrhosis of other causes, suggesting that NASH may account for a substantial proportion of cases of cryptogenic cirrhosis. Histologic hepatic steatosis has been

Table 34.3. Principal Clinical, Laboratory, Histologic, and Diagnostic Characteristics of Patients With Nonalcoholic Fatty Liver Disease (NAFLD)

Type of feature	Characteristics
Clinical	Usually asymptomatic; sometimes mild right upper quadrant discomfort, hepatomegaly, acanthosis nigricans, or "cryptogenic" cirrhosis
	Often associated with features of metabolic syndrome: type 2 diabetes, obesity, dyslipidemia (hypertriglyceridemia, low HDL cholesterol, hypobetalipoproteinemia), and cardiovascular disease
Biochemical	Increased AST and ALT levels (usually <5-fold ULRR)
	Increased levels of alkaline phosphatase and γ-glutamyltransferase (usually <3-fold ULRR)
	AST:ALT ratio <1:1
	Hyperinsulinemia and insulin resistance
	Dyslipidemia and increased ferritin level
Histologic	Steatosis (fatty infiltration >5% hepatocytes)
	Necroinflammation (lobular or portal inflammation, Mallory-Denk bodies, ballooning)
	Fibrosis (perisinusoidal, perivenular, bridging, cirrhosis)
Imaging	Imaging indicative of fatty infiltration of the liver (ultrasonography, computed tomography, magnetic resonance imaging, magnetic resonance spectroscopy)
Exclusion of other causes (alcohol use, secondary causes)	Alcohol intake <140 g weekly for women and <210 g weekly for men
	Absence of liver disease of viral, autoimmune, or genetic origin

Abbreviations: ALT, alanine aminotransferase; AST, aspartate aminotransferase; HDL, high-density lipoprotein; ULRR, upper limit of the reference range.

Adapted from Moscatiello S, Manini R, Marchesini G. Diabetes and liver disease: an ominous association. Nutr Metab Cardiovasc Dis. 2007 Jan;17(1):63-70; used with permission.

observed to resolve over time in patients with NASH-related cirrhosis, potentially masking the diagnosis. Not infrequently, NAFL occurs in patients who received a liver transplant for cryptogenic cirrhosis, suggesting that NASH is the cause of what was previously thought to be cryptogenic cirrhosis. Rarely, NASH could be a consideration for patients who have subacute liver failure because they may have a background of asymptomatic NASH and an unknown stimulus that precipitates liver failure (in an already metabolically stressed liver). The clinical spectrum of NAFLD is summarized in Table 34.2.

✓ Most patients with NAFLD and NASH are asymptomatic and have an incidental finding of fatty liver on imaging or slightly increased levels of serum alanine aminotransferase (ALT)

✓ Cardiovascular disease—the leading cause of death among patients with NAFLD

Comorbidities Associated With NAFLD

The comorbidities most commonly associated with NAFLD are the components of metabolic syndrome. The most commonly used definition is from the 2005 recommendations of the National Cholesterol Education Program (Adult Treatment Panel III) (Table 34.4). An associated condition not included in this definition is obstructive sleep apnea. Of patients with NAFLD, 50% to 90% have obesity (body

Table 34.4. National Cholesterol Education Program (Adult Treatment Panel III) Criteria for Metabolic Syndrome

Criterion[a]	Definition
Impaired glucose tolerance	Fasting plasma glucose ≥100 mg/dL
Abdominal obesity[b]	Waist circumference >102 cm for men and >88 cm for women
Hypertriglyceridemia	≥150 mg/dL or drug treatment for high triglyceride level
Low levels of HDL	<40 mg/dL in men, <50 mg/dL in women, or drug treatment for low HDL
High blood pressure	≥130/85 mm Hg or drug treatment for hypertension

Abbreviation: HDL, high-density lipoprotein.

[a] Patient must meet 3 or more of these criteria.

[b] The International Diabetes Federation uses the same criteria but defines the waist circumference criteria by ethnicity: South Asian, Chinese, and South or Central American, 90 cm for men and 80 cm for women; Japanese, 85 cm for men and 90 cm for women; and all others, 94 cm for men and 80 cm for women.

Adapted from National Cholesterol Education Program (NCEP) Expert Panel on Detection, Evaluation, and Treatment of High Blood Cholesterol in Adults. Third Report of the National Cholesterol Education Program (NCEP) Expert Panel on Detection, Evaluation, and Treatment of High Blood Cholesterol in Adults (Adult Treatment Panel III) final report. Circulation. 2002 Dec 17;106(25):3143-421; used with permission.

mass index [BMI] ≥30 [calculated as weight in kilograms divided by height in meters squared]), 55% to 65% have dyslipidemia, and 60% to 70% have hypertension. Type 2 diabetes is present in 30% to 60% of patients with NAFLD, and, if tested, up to 50% of patients with nondiabetic NAFLD may have insulin resistance. Conversely, up to 70% of patients with type 2 diabetes have ultrasonographic evidence of NAFLD (86% have normal levels of liver enzymes). A separate study showed that 87% of patients with type 2 diabetes and fatty infiltration who underwent biopsy had histologic confirmation of NAFLD. Almost 50% of patients with NAFLD have metabolic syndrome (ie, ≥3 features of the syndrome). Also, about 75% of lean patients (BMI <25) with NAFLD have at least 1 feature of metabolic syndrome. More than 80% of patients with metabolic syndrome have steatosis on ultrasonography.

Most patients with NAFLD who have a BMI of 30 or more also meet the criteria for central obesity, as defined by waist circumference (Table 34.4). The presence and severity of NAFLD correlate more strongly with central obesity than with BMI, which emphasizes the importance of visceral adiposity in steatosis development. BMI is not an accurate measure of visceral obesity; some patients with NAFLD have a BMI less than 30 and still have central obesity.

The degree of obesity can be difficult to quantify in patients with liver disease. BMI can be affected also by the fluid volume status of a patient with cirrhosis where the presence of ascites and edema must be accounted for clinically in the weight used for calculation. Although waist circumference is a better measure than BMI in patients without cirrhosis, it is of limited value in patients with ascites.

NAFLD is not only intricately tied to metabolic syndrome but also to overt cardiovascular disease (and vice versa), which is the leading cause of death among patients with NAFLD. NAFLD has been linked to increased cardiovascular disease that is independent of metabolic syndrome in populations of patients without obesity and without type 2 diabetes. Among patients who have diabetes, those who have NAFLD have higher prevalence rates of cardiovascular disease than those who do not have NAFLD. Among

patients undergoing coronary angiography, whether they do or do not have diabetes, ultrasonographically confirmed presence of NAFLD is the strongest predictor of positive results on angiography (even stronger than diabetes or smoking). Patients with carotid artery disease seen on imaging were more likely to have not only increased steatosis but also more necroinflammation and fibrosis, as confirmed with liver biopsy specimens.

NAFLD is associated with an increased risk of incident cancers, including hepatocellular carcinoma (with or without cirrhosis), colon cancer, and history of colon polyps on prior colonoscopy.

Biochemical Features

The level of serum liver enzymes (ALT or AST or both) may be increased. The increase is usually less than 5-fold the ULRR. Aminotransferase levels in patients with NAFLD fluctuate; with any 1 measurement, 70% to 80% of patients have levels less than the ULRR, but with repeated measurements, increased levels are detected in most patients with NAFLD. However, the finding of transaminase levels less than the ULRR does not exclude NAFLD because disease along the entire histologic spectrum can still be present with those values. Alkaline phosphatase and γ-glutamyltransferase levels may be increased modestly (generally <3-fold the ULRR) in one-third of patients; rarely, the level of either or both enzymes has been reported to be increased without an increase in aminotransferase levels. Hyperbilirubinemia, low albumin levels, or an increase in the international normalized ratio usually indicates advanced liver disease and cirrhosis.

Serum iron test results are commonly abnormal. Ferritin levels are increased in up to 50% of patients, and transferrin saturation is increased in up to 10%. These findings may lead to confusion about a diagnosis of hemochromatosis. The presence of heterozygous *HFE* gene variants does not appear to be associated with hepatic iron loading or liver fibrosis. Testing for antinuclear antibody or anti–smooth muscle antibody (or both) is recommended for screening for autoimmune hepatitis in patients with chronically increased enzyme levels. Although serum autoantibodies are present in 23% to 36% of patients with NAFLD, liver biopsy features help to exclude the diagnosis of autoimmune hepatitis in most patients with NAFLD who have a positive test for antinuclear antibody or anti–smooth muscle antibody (or both).

Imaging Features

Ultrasonography, CT, and magnetic resonance imaging (MRI) can be used to noninvasively diagnose fatty infiltration of the liver. Hepatic steatosis causes increased echogenicity on ultrasonography, which can be compared with the lower echogenicity of the spleen or kidney cortex (Figure 34.1). The use of ultrasonography for detecting hepatic steatosis (≥30% of hepatocytes must be steatotic) has a sensitivity of 80% to 94% and a specificity of 88% to 95%. If patients have morbid obesity, the sensitivity decreases to 49% and the specificity decreases to 75%. If detected with ultrasonography, fatty infiltration is highly likely to be present, but if fatty infiltration is not detected with ultrasonography, the diagnosis should not be ruled out.

On noncontrast CT images, hepatic steatosis has a low attenuation and appears darker than the spleen (Figure 34.2). The sensitivity of CT for detection of hepatic steatosis of more than 33% is as high as 93%, with a positive predictive value of 76%. Both phase-contrast MRI techniques and magnetic resonance (MR) spectroscopy are reliable for detecting steatosis and offer good

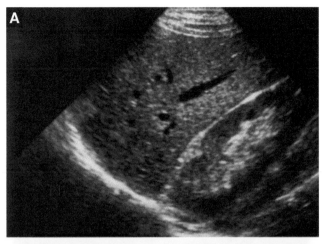

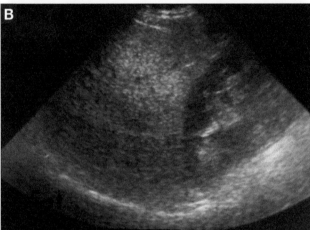

Figure 34.1. **Ultrasonographic Findings in Hepatic Steatosis.** A, Normal liver has distinctive vascular features. B, Liver with fatty infiltration has a diffuse bright echotexture and blurring of hepatic vessels.

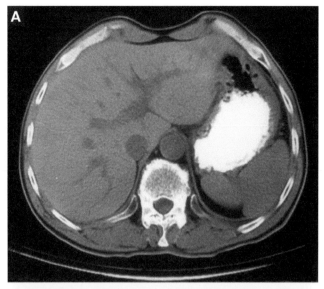

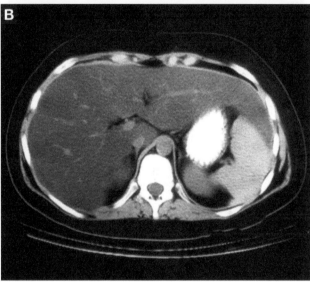

Figure 34.2. **Features of Hepatic Steatosis Visualized With Computed Tomography.** A, Normal liver has no attenuation of the signal compared with the spleen. B, Liver with fatty infiltration has an attenuated signal compared with the spleen.

correlation with the volume of liver fat. A liver fat content of more than 5% apparent on MR spectroscopy indicates steatosis. MRI-derived proton density fat fraction allows for fat mapping of the entire liver with results closely correlated to those of liver biopsies. Studies have shown superiority to biopsy, which is subject to heterogeneity of the tissue, in evaluating liver fat content. Routine application of MRI is limited by cost and lack of availability.

Histologic Features

Histologically, NAFLD is indistinguishable from liver damage that results from alcohol-induced liver injury. Liver biopsy features include steatosis, mixed inflammatory cell infiltration, hepatocyte ballooning and necrosis, glycogenated nuclei, Mallory-Denk bodies, and fibrosis. The presence of steatosis alone or in combination with the other features accounts for the wide spectrum of NAFLD (Figure 34.3). Steatosis is present predominantly as macrovesicular fat, although some hepatocytes may show an admixture with microvesicular steatosis. Fatty infiltration that is mild is concentrated typically in acinar zone 3; moderate to severe fatty infiltration shows a more diffuse distribution. Inflammation in NASH is predominantly lobular and consists of mixed inflammatory cell infiltrates (neutrophils, lymphocytes, eosinophils, and infiltrating macrophages). Neutrophils can surround ballooned

hepatocytes, forming a lesion termed *satellitosis*, which is more commonly seen in alcohol-related hepatitis. Portal inflammation is also seen but is generally mild and lymphocyte predominant. Severe portal inflammation should prompt a search for concomitant liver disease, including hepatitis C and autoimmune hepatitis.

Ballooned hepatocytes are characterized by ubiquitination and subsequent destruction of keratin cytoskeleton (forming keratin-empty cells), the accumulation of fat droplets, and Mallory-Denk bodies. These hepatocytes are typically noted in zone 3 and are 2 to 3 times larger than surrounding steatotic hepatocytes. In about half the adult patients who have NAFLD, Mallory-Denk bodies are found in ballooned hepatocytes in zone 3, but they are neither unique nor specific for NAFLD. The pattern of fibrosis is a characteristic feature of NAFLD. Collagen is laid down first in the pericellular space around the central vein and in the perisinusoidal region in zone 3. In some areas, the collagen fibers invest single cells with a pattern referred to as chicken-wire fibrosis, as described in alcohol-induced liver damage. This pattern

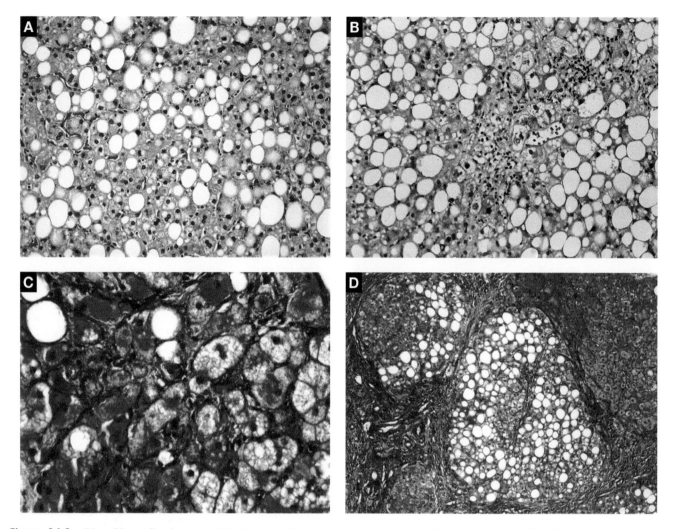

Figure 34.3. Liver Biopsy Specimens. A, Bland steatosis. Steatosis is present predominantly as macrovesicular fat, although some hepatocytes may show an admixture with microvesicular steatosis (hematoxylin-eosin, original magnification ×100). B, Nonalcoholic steatohepatitis with steatosis, inflammatory infiltrate, Mallory-Denk bodies, and hepatocyte ballooning (hematoxylin-eosin, original magnification ×100). C, Pericellular and perisinusoidal fibrosis in zone 3 (Masson trichrome, original magnification ×400). D, Cirrhotic stage of nonalcoholic fatty liver disease (Masson trichrome, original magnification ×100).

of fibrosis helps to distinguish NAFLD and alcohol-related liver disease from other forms of liver disease in which fibrosis shows an initial portal distribution (Figure 34.3).

Portal tracts are relatively spared from inflammation, although children with NAFLD may show a predominance of portal-based injury instead of a lobular pericentral injury. Mallory-Denk bodies are notably sparse or absent in children with NAFLD. In some patients with cirrhotic-stage NAFLD, the features of steatosis and necroinflammatory activity may no longer be present. Although liver biopsy is the gold standard for diagnosing NASH and staging fibrosis, sampling variability may underestimate the severity of liver injury in up to 30% of patients.

> ✓ Liver biopsy is the gold standard for diagnosis of NASH, and a careful evaluation of the patient's history is crucial to look for secondary causes of steatohepatitis, especially alcohol intake

Diagnosis

The gold standard for diagnosing NAFLD is clinicopathologic correlation, which is based on the confirmation of steatosis by

liver biopsy or imaging tests and the appropriate exclusion of other causes (Table 34.3). Alcohol should be excluded as the cause of fatty liver. Fatty liver can be induced with a minimal amount of alcohol—20 g daily (1-2 standard drinks) for women and 30 g daily (2-3 standard drinks) for men—and these limits are commonly used to distinguish between alcohol-related fatty liver and NAFL. Secondary causes of steatosis (Table 34.1) should be excluded because steatosis associated with these conditions has a different course and treatment.

For patients with persistently increased serum levels of liver enzymes, other causes of steatosis and other common causes of liver disease should be excluded by clinical review and laboratory testing. With the increasing prevalence of NAFLD, more patients may have a second cause of liver disease superimposed on a background of steatosis. Thus, it is essential to exclude viral hepatitis, drug-induced liver disease, celiac disease, autoimmune disease, vascular disease, and metabolic diseases such as α_1-antitrypsin deficiency. In a young person, Wilson disease can manifest with steatohepatitis findings on biopsy, requiring hepatic copper quantification, slit-lamp examination, and 24-hour urine studies to rule it out. The need for a liver biopsy to establish the diagnosis of

NAFLD should be determined on an individual basis. Liver biopsy may be useful for diagnosing NAFLD when a potential differential diagnosis is suggested by clinical, serologic, or biochemical testing. These situations include the presence of autoantibodies or increased iron index results, a history of recent medication change, or the absence of detectable hepatic steatosis on cross-sectional imaging. Also, the persistence of increased levels of aminotransferases after 3 to 6 months of lifestyle intervention with appropriate weight loss and control of lipid and glucose levels may suggest another diagnosis and dictate the need for liver biopsy.

Staging

Liver biopsy is the gold standard investigation that can be used to help differentiate NASH from NAFL and to stage the extent of fibrosis. Standard imaging studies such as ultrasonography, CT, and MRI cannot be used to distinguish between steatosis and NASH nor to stage the degree of hepatic fibrosis. Elastography with either ultrasound-based shear waves (transient elastography) or MR-based technology (MR elastography) can be used to estimate liver stiffness as a noninvasive surrogate for fibrosis. Obesity and abdominal wall thickness can limit the effectiveness of ultrasound-based elastography because the depth of penetration is limited, but they do not seem to have a major effect on MR-based elastography. Vibration-controlled transient elastography is more sensitive for distinguishing between mild and advanced fibrosis (and results have a good correlation with histologic findings) than for distinguishing between mild and moderate fibrosis. The sensitivity of MR elastography is better than that of transient elastography, but cost and availability limit its widespread use.

The potential benefits of liver biopsy must be weighed against the small risk of complications, including pain, bleeding, and, rarely, death. Several clinical and laboratory features are recognized in association with NASH or advanced fibrosis (or both) in patients with NAFLD, including older age, presence of type 2 diabetes, higher BMI, higher AST:ALT ratio, low albumin level, and low platelet count. Several calculators incorporate those features and provide an estimate of the risk of advanced fibrosis; they include the fibrosis-4 index for liver disease, the AST to Platelet Ratio Index, and the NAFLD fibrosis score. Among these, the NAFLD fibrosis score has the best validation for predicting liver-related outcomes.

Advanced fibrosis in patients with NAFLD has been associated with levels of serum markers of fibrogenesis, including hyaluronic acid, propeptide of type III collagen, and tissue inhibitor of matrix metalloproteinase 1. These serum markers have been combined in the Enhanced Liver Fibrosis score, which is a numerical value that is used to predict the presence and severity of liver fibrosis in NAFLD. Similarly, the FibroTest (BioPredictive; FibroSURE in the US [LabCorp]), which has been studied extensively for viral hepatitis to predict the severity of fibrosis, has been evaluated for NAFLD. A combination of several other markers is used in the SteatoTest (BioPredictive). In addition, caspase-3–generated cytokeratin-18 fragments, a marker of apoptosis measured in plasma, showed initial promise for distinguishing between simple steatosis and NASH that could not be confirmed in large meta-analyses. Other noninvasive test results have been studied, but overall, additional validation is required before the markers can be used routinely in clinical practice. (For a summary of these tests, see the article by Anstee et al in the Suggested Reading list.)

✓ Advanced fibrosis—the most important predictor of liver-related death
✓ Diagnosis of liver fibrosis—noninvasive modalities such as scores based on blood tests (eg, FIB-4) or imaging (eg, vibration-controlled transient elastography or magnetic resonance elastography) can be used

---

Prognosis

Knowledge of the histologic subtype of NAFLD (NAFL vs NASH) and the stage of fibrosis is useful in determining prognosis and may alter clinical management. The natural history of uncomplicated hepatic steatosis is relatively benign; followup of 342 patients for over 15 years showed progression to cirrhosis and liver-related mortality in less than 1% of patients. In contrast, NASH may progress to cirrhosis in up to 11% of patients, and about 7% of patients with NASH die of liver-related complications within 15 years after diagnosis. Therefore, the diagnosis of NASH, particularly when associated with any fibrosis, may prompt a more aggressive therapeutic approach toward metabolic risk factors and participation of patients in clinical trials with novel agents, if available. The presence of advanced fibrosis or cirrhosis should initiate screening for hepatocellular carcinoma and esophageal varices, with closer monitoring for disease-related complications.

Prevention

No studies have been aimed at preventing the development of NAFLD. Achieving and maintaining appropriate weight control would be expected to prevent the development of metabolic syndrome, and thus NAFLD, in many people. The treatment of established glucose and lipid abnormalities may decrease the likelihood of NAFLD or NASH, but no data exist that specifically validate this. However, data from the Diabetes Prevention Program in the US showed that both lifestyle intervention and the insulin-sensitizing drug metformin significantly decreased the development of metabolic syndrome, which, intuitively, may prevent the development of NAFLD.

Treatment

Weight Loss

Weight loss, particularly if gradual, may lead to improvement in the histologic features of the liver in NAFLD. Rapid weight loss or very low-calorie diets may cause worsening of the histologic features and, thus, should be avoided. Weight loss of as little as 5% of the baseline weight has been shown to improve or normalize ALT levels in NASH, and a 7% to 10% decrease in weight produced histologic improvement at 1 year. Studies have shown that a rigorous lifestyle modification program is necessary for patients to achieve successful weight loss. These modifications include the following: 1) *dietary restrictions*, depending on the baseline weight (1,000-1,200 kcal daily if the baseline weight is ≤91 kg, or 1,200-1,500 kcal daily if the baseline weight is >91 kg), and a daily goal for grams of fat of 25% of caloric requirements; 2) *physical activity* (goal of 10,000 steps daily and 200 minutes weekly of moderate-intensity activity); and 3) *weekly group sessions* for behavioral modifications. With rigorous programs, which usually are accomplished through the work of a multidisciplinary team, successful weight loss and histologic improvement are possible.

Box 34.1.   **Therapeutic Interventions for Nonalcoholic Fatty Liver Disease**

Sufficient evidence of benefit

> Weight loss of 7%-10% of body weight
>
> > Nonsurgical—caloric restriction, 10,000 steps daily, and 200 min weekly of moderate-intensity exercise
> >
> > Surgical—bariatric surgery
>
> Vitamin E
>
> Pioglitazone

Insufficient evidence but possible benefit

> Rosiglitazone
>
> Metformin
>
> Statins
>
> Fish oil
>
> Angiotensin-converting enzyme inhibitors
>
> Angiotensin II receptor blockers
>
> Pentoxifylline
>
> Coffee (regular, not espresso)
>
> Milk thistle
>
> Probiotics with or without prebiotics

Ongoing select clinical drug trials

> Obeticholic acid
>
> Tropifexor
>
> Lanifibranor
>
> Semaglutide
>
> Aramchol
>
> NGM282 (engineered human hormone FGF19)
>
> Pegbelfermin (pegylated recombinant analogue of human FGF21)
>
> Resmetirom (MGL-3196; oral selective THR-β agonist)

No benefit

> Ursodiol
>
> Betaine

Abbreviations: FGF, fibroblast growth factor; THR, thyroid hormone receptor.

---

syndrome measures and improvement in or resolution of steatosis. The severity of inflammation and fibrosis seen in liver biopsy specimens often improves 5 years after bariatric surgery, but both inflammation and fibrosis worsen in some patients. For medically complicated obesity, bariatric surgery should be considered.

In addition to weight loss, treatment of patients with NAFLD should include management of cardiovascular comorbidities and obstructive sleep apnea and age-appropriate cancer screening. 3-Hydroxy-3-methylglutaryl coenzyme A reductase inhibitors are safe to use in patients with NAFLD. Patients with comorbid diabetes may benefit from glucagon-like peptide-1 (GLP-1) agonist therapy for glycemic control, reduction in liver fat, and histologic improvement in NASH.

> ✓ First-line management of NAFLD—lifestyle interventions that include dietary restriction and regular physical activity with or without weight loss
> ✓ Bariatric surgery improves all histologic features of NASH and liver fibrosis

Nonpharmacologic Treatment

Caffeine from regular coffee (not espresso) has been associated with reduced fibrosis progression in patients with established NASH. Two studies confirmed that more than 2 cups of coffee daily potentially affected disease progression favorably. In a meta-analysis of 8 randomized controlled trials evaluating silymarin, an active ingredient extracted from the seeds of milk thistle, AST and ALT levels improved in the treatment groups compared to control groups and compared to other interventions, which included simvastatin, vitamin E, pioglitazone, and gankangyin.

Results were also favorable from the use of probiotics with or without prebiotics in 3 small, randomized studies. Thus far, their use has been associated with lower values for liver enzymes, but histologic effects are not known. Studies are ongoing in the use of nutraceuticals and in targeting the microbiome as its contribution in the development of NAFLD is better understood.

Pharmacologic Treatment

Achieving and maintaining appropriate weight control is difficult for most patients who have obesity. The use of medications to directly decrease the severity of liver damage independently of weight loss is an attractive alternative. Medical management of metabolic syndrome is important, but pharmacologic therapy also may benefit patients who do not have metabolic syndrome (Box 34.1). Until recently, the results of only pilot studies suggested that insulin-sensitizer medications, antioxidants, lipid-lowering medications, and some hepatoprotective medications may be of potential benefit. Most of these studies were uncontrolled, open-label studies that lasted 1 year or less, and only a few evaluated the effect of treatment on the histologic features of the liver. More data from phase 2 and phase 3 clinical trials are available now for several classes of agents, including oral hypoglycemics, vitamin E, GLP-1 agonists, and nuclear receptor agonists.

A collaboration of investigators, the NASH Clinical Research Network, has found histologic benefit with vitamin E therapy (800 IU daily) or pioglitazone therapy (30 mg once daily) over placebo for patients who have NASH but not diabetes. This study, with approximately 80 patients in each treatment group followed for more than 2 years, showed improvement in the serum levels of aminotransferases and biopsy evidence of improved steatosis and

Weight loss agents such as orlistat and sibutramine produce only modest weight loss (generally 3-5 kg more than placebo) at the expense of adverse effects. Orlistat can cause diarrhea, gastrointestinal pain, and vitamin deficiencies, and sibutramine can cause hypertension and drug interactions. Rimonabant (a cannabinoid type-1 receptor antagonist) produced clinically meaningful weight loss and improvement in metabolic syndrome measures, but it has been withdrawn from the market because of its psychiatric adverse effects. Newer agents recently approved by the US Food and Drug Administration for weight loss (phentermine-topiramate and lorcaserin) have not been studied for NAFLD.

Bariatric surgery has become one of the most common surgical procedures performed in the US. Several surgical procedures are available to decrease the size of the gastric reservoir (restrictive procedures) and to decrease intestinal absorption of nutrients (malabsorptive procedures). Because weight loss after these procedures can be extreme and rapid, careful monitoring is required. Several studies have shown improvement in metabolic inflammation scores in both treatment groups compared with placebo. Improvement in the vitamin E group showed greater statistical significance, but fibrosis scores did not improve in any treatment group. Although improvement in aminotransferase levels and biopsy findings was greater in the treatment groups, only 36% to 47% of the patients had histologic resolution of definite NASH. More importantly, 30% of patients in the placebo group had elements of histologic improvement and 21% had histologic resolution of definite NASH, as seen in biopsy specimens. The beneficial effects of vitamin E and pioglitazone in NASH should be weighed against the risk of serious adverse events, such as increased mortality or increased risk of prostate cancer associated with vitamin E at a daily dose of 400 IU or more, and weight gain, bone fractures, heart failure, and bladder cancer associated with pioglitazone.

Several drugs are currently undergoing clinical trial testing for efficacy in NAFLD. Obeticholic acid, an FXR agonist administered at 25 mg daily, has been shown in trials to improve liver histology, including steatosis, inflammation, and fibrosis, and to improve NAFLD activity scores without worsening fibrosis. This effect size was similar to that achieved with vitamin E. Adverse effects of this medication include pruritus, which is dose dependent, and dyslipidemia, which can be treated with statins.

In recent years, several lead agents did not meet predetermined primary end points in phase 3 clinical trials. These include elafibranor, a dual agonist of peroxisome proliferator-activated receptor (PPAR)-α and PPAR-δ; selonsertib, an inhibitor of apoptosis signal-regulating kinase 1; simtuzumab, an anti–lysyl oxidase-like 2 monoclonal antibody; and emricasan, a pan-caspase inhibitor. Despite these setbacks, the drug pipeline for NASH is robust with several agents in phase 2 or phase 3 clinical trials. Some of the mechanisms include FXR agonists, pan-PPAR agonists, fibroblast growth factor analogues, GLP-1 agonists, inhibitors of fatty acid synthesis, and thyroid receptor-β agonists. Trial designs incorporate both single agents and combinations of agents. The heterogeneity in drug mechanisms of action that may be effective in NASH underscores the heterogeneity in the pathogenesis.

A meta-analysis of all NASH placebo-controlled trials reported that up to 30% of patients receiving placebo may have had modest histologic improvement. Previously, it was determined that up to 20% to 30% of liver biopsy specimens may be understaged by sampling error. Thus, it cannot be overstated that NASH studies need to be placebo-controlled to assess the true benefit of any agent studied.

For patients with cirrhotic-stage NAFLD and decompensated disease, liver transplant is a potentially life-extending therapeutic alternative. However, some patients with cirrhotic-stage NAFLD have comorbid conditions, including type 2 diabetes, cardiovascular disease, hepatocellular carcinoma (HCC), and other cancers, that may limit their candidacy for liver transplant.

✓ Therapy for NASH
  - No US Food and Drug Administration–approved pharmacotherapies
  - Oral vitamin E can be used in patients without type 2 diabetes who have biopsy-proven NASH
  - Pioglitazone (PPAR-γ agonist) or liraglutide (GLP-1 agonist) can be considered for patients with type 2 diabetes who have biopsy-proven NASH
✓ For any patient with NAFLD, statins are safe to use, and intake of regular coffee (not espresso) may have a favorable effect on disease progression

---

Hepatocellular Carcinoma Screening

NAFLD is an important contributor to the burden of HCC globally and the third most common cause of HCC in the US. In observational studies, the reported annual incidence of HCC ranges from 0.5% to 2.4%. Most HCC arises secondary to NASH cirrhosis, and routine screening for HCC is recommended for patients with NASH cirrhosis. The small reported increase in HCC risk in patients with noncirrhotic NAFLD does not meet the threshold to justify population-based screening, although advanced fibrosis can increase patients' risk for HCC.

Suggested Reading

Adams LA, Lymp JF, St Sauver J, Sanderson SO, Lindor KD, Feldstein A, et al. The natural history of nonalcoholic fatty liver disease: A population-based cohort study. Gastroenterology. 2005 Jul;129(1):113–21.

Angulo P, Hui JM, Marchesini G, Bugianesi E, George J, Farrell GC, et al. The NAFLD fibrosis score: A noninvasive system that identifies liver fibrosis in patients with NAFLD. Hepatology. 2007 Apr;45(4):846–54.

Anstee QM, Lawitz EJ, Alkhouri N, Wong VW, Romero-Gomez M, Okanoue T, et al. Noninvasive tests accurately identify advanced fibrosis due to NASH: Baseline data from the STELLAR trials. Hepatology. 2019 Nov;70(5):1521–30.

Chalasani N, Younossi Z, Lavine JE, Charlton M, Cusi K, Rinella M, et al. The diagnosis and management of nonalcoholic fatty liver disease: Practice guidance from the American Association for the Study of Liver Diseases. Hepatology. 2018 Jan;67(1):328–57.

Cotter TG, Rinella M. Nonalcoholic fatty liver disease 2020: The state of the disease. Gastroenterology. 2020 May;158(7):1851–64.

Ekstedt M, Franzen LE, Mathiesen UL, Thorelius L, Holmqvist M, Bodemar G, et al. Long-term follow-up of patients with NAFLD and elevated liver enzymes. Hepatology. 2006 Oct;44(4):865–73.

Eslam M, Sanyal AJ, George J, International Consensus P. MAFLD: A consensus-driven proposed nomenclature for metabolic associated fatty liver disease. Gastroenterology. 2020 May;158(7): 1999–2014.

Friedman SL, Neuschwander-Tetri BA, Rinella M, Sanyal AJ. Mechanisms of NAFLD development and therapeutic strategies. Nat Med. 2018 Jul;24(7):908–22.

Kang JH, Cho KI, Kim SM, Lee JY, Kim JJ, Goo JJ, et al. Relationship between nonalcoholic fatty liver disease and carotid artery atherosclerosis beyond metabolic disorders in non-diabetic patients. J Cardiovasc Ultrasound. 2012 Sep;20(3):126–33.

Lassailly G, Caiazzo R, Buob D, Pigeyre M, Verkindt H, Labreuche J, et al. Bariatric surgery reduces features of nonalcoholic steatohepatitis in morbidly obese patients. Gastroenterology. 2015 Aug;149(2):379–88.

Newsome PN, Buchholtz K, Cusi K, Linder M, Okanoue T, Ratziu V, et al. A placebo-controlled trial of subcutaneous semaglutide in nonalcoholic steatohepatitis. N Engl J Med. 2021 Mar 25;384(12):1113–24.

Sanyal AJ, Chalasani N, Kowdley KV, McCullough A, Diehl AM, Bass NM, et al. Pioglitazone, vitamin e, or placebo for nonalcoholic steatohepatitis. N Engl J Med. 2010 May 6;362(18):1675–85.

Sanyal AJ, Van Natta ML, Clark J, Neuschwander-Tetri BA, Diehl A, Dasarathy S, et al. Prospective study of outcomes in adults with nonalcoholic fatty liver disease. N Engl J Med. 2021 Oct 21;385(17):1559–69.

Welsh JA, Karpen S, Vos MB. Increasing prevalence of nonalcoholic fatty liver disease among United States adolescents, 1988-1994 to 2007-2010. J Pediatr. 2013 Mar;162(3):496–500.

35

Liver Disease in Pregnancy[a,b]

PROWPANGA UDOMPAP, MD

ALINA M. ALLEN, MD

Because most pregnant women are young and healthy, liver disease is uncommon in this population. Also, the presence of liver disease must not be confused with some of the physiologic changes of pregnancy that mimic features commonly associated with liver dysfunction (Table 35.1). Examples of physiologic changes include spider angioma and palmar erythema, which may occur in half the pregnant women because of the hyperestrogenic state, increased serum alkaline phosphatase level from placental production, and decreased albumin and hemoglobin levels with volume expansion. Increased bilirubin and transaminase levels, hepatomegaly, splenomegaly, liver tenderness, and bruits do not occur in normal pregnancy, and the clinical finding of jaundice is always abnormal. Abnormal liver test results occur in about 3% to 5% of pregnant women, and jaundice occurs in about 0.1%,

with a clinical significance that varies from self-limiting to rapidly fatal.

For diagnostic purposes, it is useful to divide liver diseases in pregnant women into 3 main categories (Box 35.1): 1) liver diseases unique to pregnancy, 2) preexisting liver disease before pregnancy, and 3) coincidental liver diseases that are discovered during pregnancy.

Within the framework of these 3 categories, the gestational age is used as a guide in the differential diagnosis of liver disease in pregnancy. Coincidental liver disease and preexisting liver diseases can occur at any point in pregnancy. However, the liver diseases unique to pregnancy are related to gestational age (Figure 35.1). Liver enzyme levels are variable in all diseases and

[a] Portions of this chapter were adapted from Shams M. Update in liver diseases with pregnancy. J Gastroenterol Hepatol Res. 2013 2(2):391-8; used under Creative Commons Attribution License (https://creative commons.org/licenses/by/3.0/)

[b] The authors thank J. Eileen Hay, MB, ChB, who authored the previous version of this chapter.

Abbreviations: AFLP, acute fatty liver of pregnancy; ALT, alanine aminotransferase; AST, aspartate aminotransferase; CMV, cytomegalovirus; DAA, direct-acting antiviral; DIC, disseminated intravascular coagulation; DILI, drug-induced liver injury; EBV, Epstein-Barr virus; HBeAg, hepatitis B e antigen; HBIG, hepatitis B immunoglobulin; HBV, hepatitis B virus; HCV, hepatitis C virus; HELLP, hemolysis, elevated liver enzymes, and low platelet count; HG, hyperemesis gravidarum; HSV, herpes simplex virus; ICP, intrahepatic cholestasis of pregnancy; LCHAD, long-chain 3-hydroxyacyl–coenzyme A dehydrogenase; LDH, lactate dehydrogenase; MELD, Model for End-stage Liver Disease; UDCA, ursodeoxycholic acid; ULRR, upper limit of the reference range

Table 35.1. Physiologic Changes in Liver-Related Laboratory Test Results During Pregnancy

Test	Change
Bilirubin	Unchanged
AST and ALT	Unchanged
Alkaline phosphatase	Increased
Prothrombin time	Unchanged
Fibrinogen	Increased
Globulin	
α-Globulin	Increased
β-Globulin	Increased
γ-Globulin	Unchanged
Alpha fetoprotein	Increased
Leukocytes	Increased
Ceruloplasmin	Increased
Cholesterol	Increased
Triglyceride	Increased

Abbreviations: ALT, alanine aminotransferase; AST, aspartate aminotransferase.

Box 35.1. Liver Diseases Occurring During Pregnancy

Diseases unique to pregnancy
    Hyperemesis gravidarum
    ICP
    Preeclamptic liver dysfunction
    HELLP syndrome
    Acute fatty liver of pregnancy
Preexisting diseases
    Viral hepatitis
    Autoimmune liver disease
    Primary biliary cholangitis
    Primary sclerosing cholangitis
    Wilson disease
    Cirrhosis from any cause
Coincidental diseases
    Viral hepatitis
    Gallstone-related disease
    DILI
    Budd-Chiari syndrome

Abbreviations: DILI, drug-induced liver injury; HELLP, hemolysis, elevated liver enzymes, and low platelet count; ICP, intrahepatic cholestasis of pregnancy.

---

are generally not helpful in identifying the cause. The details of each liver disease in pregnancy are discussed below. Medications commonly used for liver diseases are listed in Table 35.2.

Liver Diseases Unique to Pregnancy

Five diseases unique to pregnancy primarily or secondarily affect the liver. Each has characteristic clinical features and timing of onset in relation to pregnancy: hyperemesis gravidarum (HG); intrahepatic cholestasis of pregnancy (ICP); acute fatty liver of pregnancy (AFLP); preeclampsia; and hemolysis, elevated liver enzymes, and low platelet count (HELLP) syndrome.

Hyperemesis Gravidarum

About half of pregnant women have mild nausea and vomiting, which is transient and does not cause weight loss. However, HG is defined as excessive intractable nausea and vomiting in the first trimester or the first part of the second trimester that result in dehydration and weight loss.

Pathogenesis

The etiology of HG is multifactorial. It occurs more commonly in parous sisters. It is also associated with a molar pregnancy, a multiple pregnancy, hyperthyroidism, and hypoadrenalism. An animal study showed that the genes *GDF15* (OMIM 605312) and *GFRAL* (OMIM 617837) contribute to HG.

Clinical Features and Diagnosis

Patients with HG typically present with persistent vomiting for more than 1 week during the first or second trimesters, usually

between 4 and 10 weeks of gestation. This condition usually resolves by the 20th week of gestation, although up to 20% of pregnant women can have symptoms throughout the pregnancy.

The diagnosis of HG is made on clinical grounds primarily. According to the UK Royal College of Obstetricians and Gynaecologists guidelines, the diagnosis should be based on the triad of weight loss of at least 5%, electrolyte imbalance, and dehydration. Increased transaminase values are present in approximately 50% of patients, yet the degree of transaminase abnormalities is not diagnostic for this condition and can be as high as 20-fold above the upper limit of the reference range (ULRR). If transaminase levels are high, serologic testing for viral hepatitis should be performed. Rarely a patient requires a liver biopsy to exclude more severe disease; the histologic appearance of the liver is generally normal but may show necrosis, steatosis, and bile plugs. Despite high transaminase levels, no inflammation or notable necrosis is observed.

Management

Supportive and symptomatic management is a mainstay of therapy for this condition. Pyridoxine or alternative medicine (eg, acupressure, ginger capsule, antihistamine, antiemetics, and dopamine agonists) can be used for nausea control. Hospitalization might be necessary for treatment with intravenous hydration, thiamine, corticosteroids, or, in severe cases, total parenteral nutrition. Thiamine should be given to all women admitted with prolonged vomiting. Referral to a psychiatrist could be considered for mental health support because of a high rate of suicidal ideation.

Prognosis and Complications

HG contributes to maternal morbidity mainly through the consequences of electrolyte abnormality (eg, arrhythmia from hypokalemia and encephalopathy). In addition, Wernicke encephalopathy can result from thiamine deficiency. HG can also heighten the suicidal ideation.

For infants, HG is not associated with adverse prenatal or fetal outcomes. However, it could lead to low gestational weight gain, which is associated with low birth weight and premature delivery. In addition, the recurrence rate is high (approximately 64% in subsequent pregnancies).

Intrahepatic Cholestasis of Pregnancy

ICP is characterized by severe pruritus, mild jaundice, and cholestasis in the second half of pregnancy, and it disappears after delivery. However, these features typically recur in subsequent pregnancies. ICP is second only to viral hepatitis as a cause of jaundice in pregnant women.

Pathogenesis

The pathogenesis of ICP is thought to be related to impaired secretion and transport of bile acids into biliary canaliculi when estrogen and progesterone levels are high, as evidenced by the temporal relationship to hormone levels in late pregnancy and by the fact that estrogens may cause cholestasis in nonpregnant women who have ICP when they are pregnant. These and other observations suggest that ICP is due to a genetically abnormal or exaggerated metabolic response by the liver to the physiologic increase in estrogens during pregnancy. Impaired sulfation

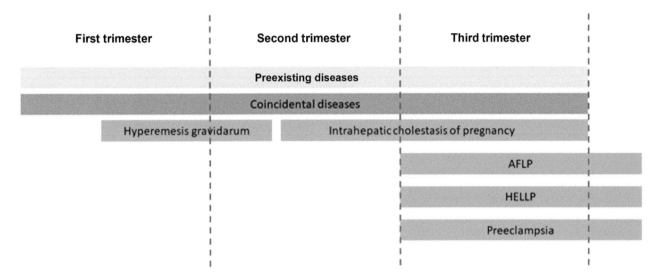

Figure 35.1. **Liver Diseases Occurring During the Trimesters of Pregnancy.** AFLP indicates acute fatty liver of pregnancy; HELLP, hemolysis, elevated liver enzymes, and low platelet count.

(an important detoxification pathway) has been identified in some patients with ICP. Abnormalities in progesterone metabolism may occur from genetic or exogenous causes. Exogenous progesterone therapy administered in the third trimester of pregnancy increases the serum levels of bile acid and alanine aminotransferase (ALT). Progesterone given to prevent premature delivery can precipitate ICP in some women. Also, the clear seasonal variability of ICP suggests that the disease is modified by exogenous factors. Dietary factors, such as selenium deficiency, have been implicated in some studies from Chile.

Genetic predisposition is probably important because ICP occurs more frequently in some ethnic groups (eg, the Mapuche population of the Andean nations and Hispanics). Variants of *ABCB4* (*MDR3*) (OMIM 171060), the transporter for phospholipids across the canalicular membrane, and *ABCB11* (*BSEP*) (OMIM 603201) have been shown to be associated with ICP. Variants of other genes (eg, *ATP8B1* [OMIM 602397], *FXR* [OMIM 603826], and *TJP2* [OMIM 607709]) have also been reported to be associated with ICP.

Clinical Features and Diagnosis

ICP should be a strong consideration if pruritus begins at 25 to 32 weeks of gestation without other signs of liver disease. This is especially true if pruritus occurred in other pregnancies and then resolved immediately after delivery. In the first pregnancy, diagnosis is generally made on clinical grounds alone and can be confirmed with the rapid postpartum disappearance of pruritus. Serum bile acid concentration can be used to help diagnose ICP.

The pruritus affects all parts of the body, worsens at night, and may be so severe that the patient has suicidal ideation. Excoriations are usually obvious, and occasionally cholestasis is complicated by diarrhea or steatorrhea. Jaundice occurs but is less common and usually occurs after the onset of pruritus by 2 to 4 weeks. Jaundice without pruritus is rare. Biliary tract obstruction must be excluded first. After biliary obstruction is excluded, ICP is confirmed if the bile acid level is high.

Variable levels of transaminases occur in ICP (from 10- to 20-fold increases). The concentration of bilirubin usually increases by less than 5 mg/dL. The serum level of alkaline phosphatase is less helpful during pregnancy. The most specific and sensitive

marker of ICP is a serum level of bile acid, which is always increased in this condition (eg, 100 times above the ULRR) and may correlate with fetal risk. A liver biopsy is needed only if a more serious liver disease is strongly suspected clinically. In ICP, the appearance of the liver is nearly normal, with mild cholestasis and minimal or no hepatocellular necrosis.

Management

Management strategies center around controlling maternal pruritus and decreasing the bile acid levels to improve the pregnancy outcome. Ursodeoxycholic acid (UDCA) is the most commonly used agent for the treatment of ICP. Therapy with UDCA (10-20 mg/kg daily; 500-2,000 mg daily) decreases the levels of liver enzymes and bile acid and improves pruritus, although not all pregnant women have remarkable improvement with UDCA. UDCA has no adverse maternal or fetal effects. Other agents that can control pruritus include rifampicin (US Food and Drug Administration pregnancy category C) and topical emollients. Plasma exchange is reserved for severe cases when other options have been exhausted.

Elective early delivery can be considered. The decision can be based on the bile acid levels: Delivery should be considered at 37 weeks if the bile acid level is greater than 40 μmol/L; otherwise, delivery should be considered at 39 weeks.

Prognosis and Complications

Pruritus and liver dysfunction resolve immediately after delivery without maternal mortality, although some data show that ICP may lead to increased risk for future development of hepatobiliary diseases and liver cancer. In addition, after ICP has occurred, the recurrence rate is remarkably high (63%-90% in subsequent pregnancies).

Fetal complications in ICP include placental insufficiency, premature labor, asphyxia, and sudden fetal death, which most likely result from the increased fetal levels of bile acid due to increased maternal levels of bile acid and the immaturity of the fetal bile acid transport system across the placental membranes, which may all contribute to increased fetal levels of bile acid in ICP. Fetal monitoring for chronic placental insufficiency is

Table 35.2.   Commonly Used Medications for Liver-Related Conditions and Their Compatibility With Pregnancy and Lactation

Medication	FDA category	Pregnancy	Lactation
Anti-copper agents			
D-penicillamine	D	May continue with dose adjustments during pregnancy	Compatible but limited data
Trientine	C	Compatible with dose adjustments during pregnancy	Compatible but limited data
Zinc	C	Compatible	Compatible
Antivirals			
DAAs	Ledipasvir-sofosbuvir: B Glecaprevir-pibrentasvir and sofosbuvir-velpatasvir: not assigned	Not recommended (no data)	Not recommended (no data)
Entecavir	C	Not recommended	Not recommended
Lamivudine	C	Compatible on the basis of HIV data	Compatible on the basis of HIV data
Pegylated interferon alfa	C	Use if potential benefit outweighs potential risk	Use if potential benefit outweighs potential risk
Ribavirin	X	Avoid	Avoid
Telbivudine	B	Compatible	Compatible
Tenofovir	Tenofovir disoproxil fumarate: B Tenofovir alafenamide: not assigned	Compatible	Compatible
Antihistamines			
Chlorpheniramine	B	Compatible	Compatible (lowest dose possible)
Diphenhydramine	B	Compatible	Compatible (lowest dose possible)
Hydroxyzine	C	Compatible	Compatible (lowest dose possible)
Antimicrobials			
Acyclovir	B	Compatible	Compatible
Cephalosporins (eg, cefotaxime, ceftriaxone)	B	Compatible	Compatible
Fluoroquinolones	C	Not recommended (toxic effects on cartilage development in animal studies; arthralgias and tendonitis in adolescents)	Compatible, but need close monitoring of infant GI infections (*Clostridioides difficile*, *Candida*)
Rifampin	C	Compatible	Compatible
Rifaximin	C	Not recommended (no data)	Not recommended (no data)
β-Blockers			
Carvedilol	C	Not recommended (no data)	Not recommended (no data)
Nadolol	C	Compatible (but propranolol is preferred for its shorter half-life)	Compatible (but propranolol is preferred for its shorter half-life)
Propranolol	C	Compatible (some risks of intrauterine growth restriction, neonatal respiratory depression, and infant hypoglycemia)	Compatible
Bile acid–related			
Cholestyramine	C	Compatible	Compatible
UDCA	B	Compatible	Compatible
Vasoactive			
Octreotide	B	Appropriate when benefits outweigh the risk (eg, acute variceal bleeding); otherwise, data are limited	Appropriate when benefits outweigh the risk (eg, acute variceal bleeding); otherwise, data are limited
Diuretics			
Furosemide	C	Use lowest effective dose; risk of decreasing uteroplacental circulation	Use lowest effective dose; may suppress lactation
Spironolactone	C	Not recommended	Compatible
Immunosuppressives			
Azathioprine	D	Compatible (benefits of controlling the disease, especially autoimmune hepatitis, outweigh the risks of the disease flare)	Compatible
Cyclosporine	C	Compatible	Compatible
Methylprednisolone	C	Can be used if benefits outweigh the risk	Can be used if benefits outweigh the risk
Mycophenolate mofetil	D	Avoid	Not recommended (limited data)
Prednisone	B	Compatible	Compatible
Tacrolimus	C	Compatible	Compatible
Laxatives			
Lactulose	B	Compatible	Compatible

Abbreviations: DAA, direct-acting antiviral; FDA, US Food and Drug Administration; GI, gastrointestinal tract; UDCA, ursodeoxycholic acid.

essential but does not prevent adverse outcomes. Acute anoxic injury can be prevented only by delivery as soon as the fetus is mature. A bile acid level greater than 40 μmol/L at any time during pregnancy is usually associated with worse fetal outcomes.

Acute Fatty Liver of Pregnancy

AFLP is a rare catastrophic illness that occurs almost exclusively in the third trimester. The incidence of AFLP is approximately 1 in 10,000 to 1 in 20,000 deliveries. AFLP occurs with microvesicular fatty infiltration of the liver that results in encephalopathy and liver failure. Although the pathogenesis of AFLP is different from that of preeclampsia and HELLP syndrome, preeclampsia can be present in about 50% of the patients, making the diagnosis of AFLP particularly challenging.

Pathogenesis

The pathogenesis of AFLP involves abnormalities in mitochondrial fatty acid oxidation. Autosomally inherited genetic variations affect the enzyme long-chain 3-hydroxyacyl–coenzyme A dehydrogenase (LCHAD) (eg, *G1528C*), resulting in LCHAD deficiency, and are associated with AFLP. AFLP tends to occur among persons who have the heterozygous LCHAD-related variants and whose babies may or may not have homozygous LCHAD-related variants. It has been speculated that maternal heterozygosity for LCHAD deficiency decreases the maternal capacity to oxidize long-chain fatty acids in the liver and the placenta.

Clinical Features and Diagnosis

Unlike patients with HELLP syndrome, 50% of patients with AFLP are nulliparous. Patients usually present with nonspecific symptoms (eg, vomiting, abdominal pain, polydipsia and polyuria, and jaundice). Laboratory results may show increased levels of transaminases and bilirubin (usually up to 5 mg/dL), leukocytosis, thrombocytopenia, and acute kidney injury. These signs and symptoms can be seen in patients with preeclampsia or HELLP syndrome. However, several other features that are highly suggestive of AFLP include encephalopathy, hypoglycemia, coagulopathy, increased urate level, ascites or bright liver on ultrasonography, and microvesicular steatosis on liver biopsy (but liver biopsy is not required for the diagnosis). At least 6 of the features mentioned above, in the absence of another explanation, support the diagnosis of AFLP (according to the Swansea criteria). In addition, liver test abnormalities are common in AFLP. Therefore, patients should undergo testing for other causes of acute liver injury unrelated to pregnancy (eg, viral hepatitis and drug-induced liver injury).

Management

AFLP is an obstetric emergency. Early recognition of AFLP, with immediate delivery of the newborn and intensive supportive care, is essential for the survival of both the mother and the newborn. Recovery before delivery has not been reported. Transaminase levels and encephalopathy usually start to improve by 2 to 3 days after delivery. However, full recovery can take months. Patients should be transferred to a liver transplant center for consideration of liver transplant if they are critically ill at presentation, if they have complications (eg, encephalopathy, hypoglycemia, coagulopathy, or bleeding), or if their clinical condition deteriorates despite emergency delivery.

Prognosis and Complications

The major causes of maternal morbidity and death are hemorrhage, liver failure, and acute kidney injury. The maternal mortality rate has decreased considerably over the past several decades. It is best predicted by the Model for End-stage Liver Disease (MELD) score. However, the long-term maternal consequences of AFLP remain unclear. Women with a history of AFLP should be closely monitored in a subsequent pregnancy because of the risk of recurrence, particularly among women who are heterozygous for genetic variants involved in LCHAD deficiency.

Fetal and neonatal deaths are related to maternal decompensation or preterm birth (or both). Infants are at risk for hypoketotic hypoglycemia, neuromyopathy, and sudden death, and they should be evaluated for fatty acid oxidation disorders. If results are positive, the parents should also be tested, and genetic counseling should be pursued. No long-term consequence is expected in persons who do not have defects in fatty acid oxidation disorders.

Preeclamptic Liver Dysfunction and HELLP Syndrome

Preeclampsia is the triad of hypertension, edema, and proteinuria from the third trimester of pregnancy through the first several weeks post partum. The prevalence varies from 3% to 10% of pregnancies. Liver involvement occurs in approximately 10% to 20% of patients with preeclampsia. Preeclamptic liver dysfunction and HELLP syndrome are the most common causes of abnormal liver test results in pregnancy, and both conditions are within the spectrum of preeclampsia.

Pathogenesis

The pathophysiology of preeclampsia appears to involve placental hypoperfusion (from shallow placental implantation), which affects the remodeling of spiral arteries and leads to hypoperfusion and increased placental oxidative stress. The result is systemic vasoconstriction and endothelial dysfunction, which cause fibrin thrombi deposition and ischemic necrosis.

Clinical Features

Patients with preeclampsia tend to present with nonspecific symptoms, such as headache, nausea and vomiting, flulike illness, and abdominal pain. Jaundice is uncommon (≤5% of patients). Aspartate aminotransferase (AST) and ALT can be mildly elevated or extremely high (>1,000 U/L). Total bilirubin is usually less than 5 mg/dL. Disseminated intravascular coagulation (DIC) is uncommon in patients who have preeclampsia or eclampsia alone, but it occurs more frequently in patients with HELLP. Liver biopsy is not required for the diagnosis, but, if performed, it would be expected to show periportal hemorrhage and fibrin deposition.

Hepatic infarction or hematoma can occur and should be suspected in patients with severe abdominal pain in the right upper quadrant or sudden increases in transaminase levels. Imaging should be performed. Liver rupture, a rare but life-threatening condition, usually is preceded by an intraparenchymal hemorrhage that progresses to a contained subcapsular hematoma and then intraperitoneal rupture.

Criteria for Diagnosis

Preeclamptic liver dysfunction is diagnosed when the criteria for preeclampsia are fulfilled (hypertension with systolic blood pressure ≥140 mm Hg or diastolic blood pressure ≥90 mm Hg; edema; and proteinuria after gestational age of 20 weeks or within the first several weeks post partum) and the patient has increased levels of liver enzymes or bilirubin.

The degree of increase in the level of liver enzymes or bilirubin does not help distinguish between preeclamptic liver dysfunction and HELLP syndrome because the ranges are wide, and there are no specific cutoffs. The Tennessee Classification System for the diagnosis of HELLP syndrome uses the following criteria: 1) lactate dehydrogenase (LDH) 600 IU/L or greater; 2) AST 70 U/L or greater; and 3) platelets 100×10^9/L or less. Patients could be considered to have partial HELLP if they have 1) LDH 600 IU/L or greater; 2) AST 40 U/L or greater; and 3) platelets 150×10^9/L or less. Prothrombin time, activated partial thromboplastin time, and fibrinogen levels are usually normal, but DIC may occur even with these normal values. If patients meet the criteria for HELLP syndrome, liver imaging is indicated to screen for liver rupture, subcapsular hematomas, intraparenchymal hemorrhage, or liver necrosis. These abnormalities may be consistent with the platelet count but not with abnormal liver values.

Management

The recommended preventive approach is to start low-dose aspirin (81 mg) at a gestational age of approximately 12 to 16 weeks and continue until delivery. However, once preeclampsia occurs, the mainstay management is blood pressure control, seizure prevention, DIC treatment if indicated, and prompt delivery if the patient meets the criteria for severe preeclampsia or HELLP. If hepatic infarction or hematoma occurs, it is managed conservatively in hemodynamically stable patients, but all patients need close hemodynamic monitoring in an intensive care unit. If liver necrosis or hepatic rupture eventually leads to liver failure, liver transplant should be considered.

In most patients, HELLP syndrome resolves rapidly after delivery. The platelet count usually normalizes within 5 days. If improvement is not apparent within 72 hours after delivery, plasmapheresis could be considered, particularly if the patient's condition worsens.

Prognosis and Complications

Preeclampsia leads to high rates of maternal and fetal complications. Serious maternal complications are common in HELLP syndrome, including DIC, abruptio placentae, acute kidney failure, pulmonary edema, and liver failure. Fetal complications include preterm delivery and fetal loss. However, once delivered, most babies do well.

Survival depends on rapid and aggressive medical management and immediate surgery, although the best surgical management is still debated. Preoperatively, aggressive supportive management is essential for hypovolemia, thrombocytopenia, and coagulopathy. Maternal mortality from liver rupture is high (50%), and perinatal mortality rates are 10% to 60%, mostly from placental rupture, intrauterine asphyxia, or prematurity. Recurrent preeclampsia is common, particularly in patients with early-onset preeclampsia. The risks of preterm delivery, intrauterine growth retardation, and abruptio placentae are also heightened in subsequent pregnancies. In addition, women with preeclampsia have an increased lifetime risk of cardiovascular disease, including major adverse cardiovascular events and stroke.

Preexisting Liver Disease Before Pregnancy

Chronic Hepatitis B

Pregnancy does not increase the maternal risk of complications from hepatitis B if the infection is well controlled. Transmission of hepatitis B virus (HBV) is not transplacental but occurs at delivery. The risk of maternal-fetal transmission is approximately 90% if the mother tests positive for hepatitis B e antigen (HBeAg) and 10% to 40% if the mother tests negative. Whether the mother tests positive or negative for HBeAg, immunoprophylaxis with hepatitis B immunoglobulin at birth for the baby decreases the risk of maternal-fetal transmission to approximately 26%, and hepatitis B vaccination as well as hepatitis B immunoglobulin (HBIG) at birth could decrease the risk further to as low as 3%.

The risk for vertical transmission varies with the level of HBV DNA. If the maternal HBV DNA level is greater than 10^6 copies/mL (>200,000 IU/mL), antiviral therapy should be initiated because the risk of vertical transmission will remain high despite the use of immunoprophylaxis. In addition, antiviral treatment should be started in patients with liver injury, including advanced fibrosis or cirrhosis, despite the lower level of HBV DNA. Antiviral treatment (eg, tenofovir, telbivudine, or lamivudine) should be started in the third trimester or by approximately 28 weeks of gestation, and consideration should be given to stopping therapy 3 months after delivery if patients do not have cirrhosis, with close monitoring for flare (Figure 35.2). The data on mode of delivery are limited. The benefits of cesarean delivery for decreasing vertical transmission are controversial. All infants require the HBV vaccination series and HBIG within 12 hours of birth. Breastfeeding is not contraindicated for mothers with chronic hepatitis B.

Chronic Hepatitis C

In a woman who has chronic hepatitis C and is pregnant, liver enzyme levels may decrease during pregnancy, while hepatitis C virus (HCV) RNA levels may increase. The risk of vertical transmission is approximately 5%, but the risk increases to 10% to 15% for mothers who have HIV coinfection or who are active intravenous drug users. Recent data showed that no vertical transmission occurred in patients with HCV RNA less than 3.5 $\log_{10}$ IU/mL, while the odds of vertical transmission increased at least 3-fold in those with HCV RNA of 6 $\log_{10}$ IU/mL or more. In addition, HCV viremia was associated with adverse pregnancy outcomes (eg, preterm delivery, ICP, and postpartum hemorrhage). Treatment of hepatitis C with direct-acting antivirals (DAAs) is recommended before or after pregnancy. Breastfeeding is not contraindicated for mothers with chronic hepatitis C.

Autoimmune Hepatitis

Autoimmune liver disease can flare during or after pregnancy because of changes in the activity of the immune system. Therefore, pregnant women must continue therapy to maintain remission. Azathioprine therapy in pregnancy has not been associated with increased fetal risk, and patients should continue treatment to maintain remission. Mycophenolate mofetil, however, is contraindicated during pregnancy because it has teratogenic

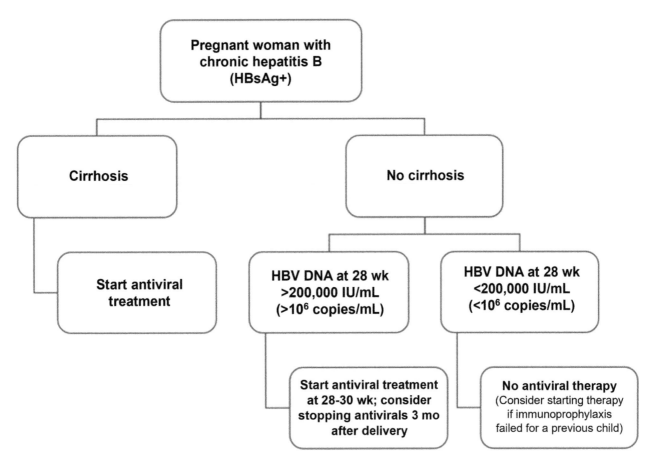

Figure 35.2. **Management of Hepatitis B in a Pregnant Woman.** For patients without cirrhosis, testing should include tests for hepatitis B e antigen, hepatitis B e antibody, hepatitis B virus (HBV) DNA, and alanine aminotransferase at baseline and at 28 weeks. HBsAg+ indicates positive results for hepatitis B surface antigen. (Data from Ayoub WS, Cohen E. Hepatitis B management in the pregnant patient: an update. J Clin Transl Hepatol. 2016 Sep;4[3]:241-7.)

effects, so the therapy should be switched to other agents before a patient is pregnant. The best pregnancy outcomes are associated with autoimmune hepatitis that has been adequately controlled for at least 12 months.

Wilson Disease

Patients with Wilson disease must receive adequate treatment before pregnancy and continue receiving therapy throughout pregnancy. Cessation of treatment during pregnancy can lead to fulminant Wilson disease and acute liver failure. Although data showed teratogenic effects in animal studies, D-penicillamine and trientine are safe in clinical practice. The dosages of both medications should be decreased by 25% to 50% (750-1,000 mg daily of D-penicillamine or trientine during the first and second trimesters; 500 mg daily during the third trimester). Patients should not breastfeed while they are receiving D-penicillamine.

Cholestatic Liver Disease

Pregnant women with a history of primary biliary cholangitis or primary sclerosing cholangitis generally do well throughout pregnancy. They may have a worsening of pruritus, jaundice, and cholangitis because of gallstones or biliary strictures. Preterm delivery and ICP that occurred in a cohort study seemed to be associated with peak maternal bile acid level. UDCA therapy is the mainstay. It is safe and should be continued throughout the pregnancy.

Other Liver Diseases

Patients with Dubin-Johnson syndrome or benign recurrent intrahepatic cholestasis may become more jaundiced during pregnancy, especially in the second and third trimesters. It is still crucial to rule out other possible causes when jaundice occurs. Also, symptomatic therapy for pruritus should be provided. Gilbert syndrome and Rotor syndrome are unaffected by pregnancy.

Pregnancy and Cirrhosis

Successful pregnancies are possible in patients with well-compensated cirrhosis. Most patients with advanced cirrhosis are amenorrheic and infertile because of hypothalamopituitary dysfunction, but if pregnancy does occur, the risk of maternal and fetal problems can be expected to increase. Plasma volume expansion and increased intra-abdominal pressure can lead to increased portal pressure and, therefore, to a heightened risk of variceal bleeding during pregnancy. MELD scores greater than 10 also predict hepatic decompensation during pregnancy.

All pregnant patients with cirrhosis should undergo upper endoscopy for esophageal variceal screening and treatment as indicated. Abdominal ultrasonography should be used to screen for splenic artery aneurysm, which could be fatal if it ruptured. Acute variceal bleeding is managed endoscopically in the same way as for nonpregnant patients, although vasoconstrictive medications may induce uterine contraction, decrease uterine blood flow, and lead to placental abruption and spontaneous abortion. Therefore, those medications should be avoided. Octreotide, however, can be used. Ascites and hepatic encephalopathy are treated similarly as in nonpregnant patients, except that the use of spironolactone, rifaximin, and prophylactic antibiotics should be avoided.

Vaginal deliveries with an assisted, short second stage are preferable because abdominal surgeries should be avoided. However, for patients who are known to have large varices, cesarean delivery is recommended to avoid labor and, thus, to prevent an increase in portal pressure and in the risk of variceal bleeding. The risk of postpartum hemorrhage and bacterial infection is decreased when the patient receives therapy to correct coagulopathy and antibiotic prophylaxis.

Pregnancy in the Liver Transplant Recipient

A pregnant liver transplant recipient requires specialized care. With the success of liver transplant, more liver transplant recipients are becoming pregnant, and a carefully planned pregnancy in a clinically stable, healthy patient at least 1 or 2 years after orthotopic liver transplant can have excellent outcomes for the fetus, mother, and graft. However, the pregnancy still has a high risk of increased fetal prematurity and dysmaturity. Also, the allograft has some risk from acute cellular rejection or recurrent viral hepatitis. Consequently, immunosuppression must be monitored closely and the calcineurin inhibitor doses must be adjusted as needed for increased blood volume in the second half of pregnancy. Mycophenolate mofetil should never be used in women contemplating pregnancy or who are pregnant. Liver biochemistry values must be monitored regularly, and all liver abnormalities must be investigated.

Coincidental Liver Diseases Discovered During Pregnancy

Viral Hepatitis

Hepatotropic Viruses

Hepatitis A, B, and C occur with the same frequency in pregnant and nonpregnant populations and during each trimester of pregnancy. Hepatitis D is rare. Hepatitis E is rare in the US, but it is endemic in large areas of Asia, Africa, and Central America, where, in the third trimester of pregnancy, the infection can become fulminant and carry a high mortality rate. The serologic course of acute hepatitis in pregnant women is the same as in nonpregnant patients with the exception of hepatitis E as mentioned above. In general, viral hepatitis does not adversely affect pregnancy. For patients who have acute viral hepatitis, management is primarily supportive care. Acute or chronic hepatitis is not an indication for termination of pregnancy. In addition, viral hepatitis itself is not an indication for cesarean delivery, and breastfeeding should not be discouraged.

Vertical transmission of hepatitis A and D is rare. In the third trimester, newborns of mothers with hepatitis A should be given passive immunoprophylaxis with immunoglobulin within 48 hours after birth. The benefits of immunoglobulin for babies of mothers who are seropositive for HCV are unknown, and there is no effective therapy for preventing transmission of HCV. The use of DAAs in pregnancy has not been studied well, and DAAs should not be used. Other details of chronic hepatitis B and hepatitis C infection are discussed above.

Nonhepatotropic Viruses

The 3 nonhepatotropic viruses most likely to affect pregnancy are herpes simplex virus (HSV), Epstein-Barr virus (EBV), and cytomegalovirus (CMV).

Herpes simplex hepatitis is a rare condition; however, it must be diagnosed because it can lead to liver failure and death. In pregnant women, it typically occurs as a primary infection in the third trimester and has systemic features with a prodrome of fever, diffuse vesicular rash, leukopenia, vulvar or oropharyngeal vesicular lesions, and coagulopathy. These patients usually do not have icterus even if they have liver failure. Serology testing, HSV polymerase chain reaction, or liver biopsy may be necessary to diagnose herpes simplex hepatitis. All patients with herpes simplex hepatitis should be treated with intravenous acyclovir.

For patients with EBV or CMV infection, serologic testing for the viruses should be performed for pregnant patients who have acute jaundice, and serologic testing should also be performed for hepatitis A, B, and C. Congenital fetal malformations tend to occur only with early CMV infection.

Gallstones and Biliary Disease

Increased lithogenicity of bile and biliary stasis during pregnancy predispose pregnant women to enhanced formation of biliary sludge and stones. Despite their prevalence, symptomatic gallstones occur in only 0.1% to 0.3% of pregnancies, and symptoms usually develop after multiple pregnancies rather than during gestation. The common clinical presentations are biliary colic and gallstone pancreatitis; less commonly, acute cholecystitis occurs. Clinical features of biliary disease and pancreatitis are the same as in nonpregnant patients. The diseases can also occur at any time during gestation, and they may recur during pregnancy.

Intractable biliary colic, severe acute cholecystitis not responding to conservative measures, and acute gallstone pancreatitis are indications for immediate cholecystectomy despite the patient's pregnant state. For acute biliary colic or acute cholecystitis, conservative therapy (bed rest, intravenous fluids, and antibiotics) is instituted initially and successfully in more than 80% of patients with no fetal or maternal mortality. However, because symptoms recur during pregnancy in about 50% of patients, cholecystectomy is indicated for all patients with symptoms in the second trimester. For these patients, the operation has minimal morbidity and mortality. Indeed, patients who undergo cholecystectomy have better pregnancy outcomes than those treated medically. Surgery is avoided in the first 10 weeks of pregnancy because of the risk of abortion with anesthesia and the potential teratogenic effect from carbon dioxide. In the third trimester, the uterus may impinge into the surgical field, and the risk of premature labor is increased. Laparoscopic cholecystectomy with precautions for the pregnant state is now the standard of care for these patients. If choledocholithiasis is suspected, endoscopic retrograde cholangiopancreatography can be performed safely in pregnant women. Radiation exposure with fluoroscopy is well below the fetal safety level. Midazolam, meperidine, and glucagon can be given safely.

Budd-Chiari Syndrome

Budd-Chiari syndrome is rare, and when it occurs in pregnancy, it is usually in the postpartum period. It has been associated with antiphospholipid syndrome, thrombotic thrombocytopenic purpura, preeclampsia, and septic abortion.

Bacterial Infection in Pregnancy

Sepsis associated with pyelonephritis or abortion can cause jaundice in early pregnancy. Severe gram-negative sepsis with jaundice has been described for patients in the third trimester. Listeriosis is an uncommon infection, but 43% of cases occur during pregnancy. Listeriosis occasionally affects the liver. Maternal symptoms are generally mild, but fetal infection is a serious condition that causes preterm birth, abortion, or death. In a murine model, listeriosis led to severe necrotizing hemorrhagic hepatitis and abortion.

Drug-Induced Liver Injury

Drug-induced liver injury (DILI) should be in the differential diagnosis for pregnant women with hepatitis. DILI is a diagnosis of exclusion in both pregnant and nonpregnant women. The hepatotoxicity is usually of the idiosyncratic form and usually resolves spontaneously. Common medications causing DILI in pregnant women include antihypertensives (eg, α-methyldopa), antithyroid medication (eg, propylthiouracil), antiretrovirals (eg, nevirapine), antituberculosis medications, and antibiotics.

Suggested Reading

Abram M, Schluter D, Vuckovic D, Waber B, Doric M, Deckert M. Effects of pregnancy-associated listeria monocytogenes infection: necrotizing hepatitis due to impaired maternal immune response and significantly increased abortion rate. *Virchows Arch.* 2002 Oct;441(4):368–79.

Ayoub WS, Cohen E. Hepatitis B management in the pregnant patient: an update. *J Clin Transl Hepatol.* 2016 Sep 28;4(3):241–7.

Bradke D, Tran A, Ambarus T, Nazir M, Markowski M, Juusela A. Grade III subcapsular liver hematoma secondary to HELLP syndrome: a case report of conservative management. *Case Rep Womens Health.* 2020 Jan;25:e00169.

Brown MC, Best KE, Pearce MS, Waugh J, Robson SC, Bell R. Cardiovascular disease risk in women with pre-eclampsia: systematic review and meta-analysis. *Eur J Epidemiol.* 2013 Jan;28(1):1–19.

Cauldwell M, Mackie FL, Steer PJ, Heneghan MA, Baalman JH, Brennand J, et al. Pregnancy outcomes in women with primary biliary cholangitis and primary sclerosing cholangitis: a retrospective cohort study. *BJOG.* 2020 Jun;127(7):876–84.

Chang MS, Gavini S, Andrade PC, McNabb-Baltar J. Caesarean section to prevent transmission of hepatitis b: a meta-analysis. *Can J Gastroenterol Hepatol.* 2014 Sep;28(8):439–44.

Kamath P, Kamath A, Ullal SD. Liver injury associated with drug intake during pregnancy. *World J Hepatol.* 2021 Jul 27;13(7):747–62.

Kushner T, Djerboua M, Biondi MJ, Feld JJ, Terrault N, Flemming JA. Influence of hepatitis C viral parameters on pregnancy complications and risk of mother-to-child transmission. *J Hepatol.* 2022 Nov;77(5):1256–64.

Lao TT. Drug-induced liver injury in pregnancy. *Best Pract Res Clin Obstet Gynaecol.* 2020 Oct;68:32–43.

Murali AR, Devarbhavi H, Venkatachala PR, Singh R, Sheth KA. Factors that predict 1-month mortality in patients with pregnancy-specific liver disease. *Clin Gastroenterol Hepatol.* 2014 Jan;12(1):109–13.

Nana M, Tydeman F, Bevan G, Boulding H, Kavanagh K, Dean C, et al. Hyperemesis gravidarum is associated with increased rates of termination of pregnancy and suicidal ideation: Results from a survey completed by >5000 participants. *Am J Obstet Gynecol.* 2021 Jun;224(6):629–31.

Pan YC, Jia ZF, Wang YQ, Yang N, Liu JX, Zhai XJ, et al. The role of caesarean section and nonbreastfeeding in preventing mother-to-child transmission of hepatitis B virus in HBsAg-and HBeAg-positive mothers: results from a prospective cohort study and a meta-analysis. *J Viral Hepat.* 2020 Oct;27(10):1032–43.

Rahim MN, Pirani T, Williamson C, Heneghan MA. Management of pregnancy in women with cirrhosis. *United European Gastroenterol J.* 2021 Feb;9(1):110–9.

Royal College of Obstetricians & Gynaecologists. *The management of nausea and vomiting of pregnancy and hyperemesis gravidarum.* Green-top guideline no 69. 2016:27.

Shames BD, Fernandez LA, Sollinger HW, Chin LT, D'Alessandro AM, Knechtle SJ, et al. Liver transplantation for HELLP syndrome. *Liver Transpl.* 2005 Feb;11(2):224–8.

Terrault NA, Williamson C. Pregnancy-associated liver diseases. *Gastroenterology.* 2022 Jul;163(1):97–117.

Wang J, Zhu Q, Zhang X. Effect of delivery mode on maternal-infant transmission of hepatitis b by immunoprophylaxis. *Chin Med J (Engl).* 2002 Oct;115(10):1510–2.

Wang Z, Tao X, Liu S, Zhao Y, Yang X. An update review on listeria infection in pregnancy. *Infect Drug Resist.* 2021 14:1967–78.

Webb GJ, Elsharkawy AM, Hirschfield GM. The etiology of intrahepatic cholestasis of pregnancy: towards solving a monkey puzzle. *Am J Gastroenterol.* 2014 Jan;109(1):85–8.

Westbrook RH, Yeoman AD, O'Grady JG, Harrison PM, Devlin J, Heneghan MA. Model for end-stage liver disease score predicts outcome in cirrhotic patients during pregnancy. *Clin Gastroenterol Hepatol.* 2011 Aug;9(8):694–9.

Wikstrom Shemer E, Marschall HU, Ludvigsson JF, Stephansson O. Intrahepatic cholestasis of pregnancy and associated adverse pregnancy and fetal outcomes: a 12-year population-based cohort study. *BJOG.* 2013 May;120(6):717–23.

Wikstrom Shemer EA, Stephansson O, Thuresson M, Thorsell M, Ludvigsson JF, Marschall HU. Intrahepatic cholestasis of pregnancy and cancer, immune-mediated and cardiovascular diseases: a population-based cohort study. *J Hepatol.* 2015 Aug;63(2):456–61.

Yang J, Zeng XM, Men YL, Zhao LS. Elective caesarean section versus vaginal delivery for preventing mother to child transmission of hepatitis B virus: a systematic review. *Virol J.* 2008 Aug 28;5:100.

36

Liver Transplantation[a]

OMAR Y. MOUSA, MBBS, MD

SUMERA I. ILYAS, MBBS

Liver transplant (LT) is highly effective for patients with liver failure to restore normal health and a normal lifestyle. Patient survival after LT is excellent, reaching 90% at 1 year and 77% at 5 years in the US according to the Scientific Registry of Transplant Recipients. The 5-year survival rate for living-donor LT (LDLT) recipients for 2008-2011 was 81.2%. Timely evaluation for transplant and optimization of pretransplant care is essential for the potential liver recipient. However, the demand for donor organs greatly exceeds supply. In 2019 in the US, 8,345 liver transplants were performed for patients 18 years or older, 442 (5.3%) of whom underwent LDLT. At the end of 2019, the liver transplant waiting list had 12,562 patients. Patient selection and organ allocation are the 2 main problems.

✓ Liver transplant is highly effective in restoring patients' health and lifestyle and in extending their lifespan

Indications for LT

Decompensated cirrhosis is the most common indication for LT (about 70% of cases) (Box 36.1). Until 2015, the most common underlying liver disease that led to LT in the US was cirrhosis due to chronic hepatitis C infection. Since 2016, however, alcohol-associated liver disease (ALD) and nonalcoholic steatohepatitis have been the leading indications for patients being added to the LT waiting list (both diagnoses accounted for over half the patients

---

Box 36.1. Indications for Liver Transplant

Cirrhosis of any cause

Cirrhotic complications

    Hepatocellular carcinoma

    Hepatopulmonary syndrome

    Portopulmonary hypertension

Acute liver failure

Fulminant Wilson disease

Primary nonfunction or early hepatic artery thrombosis of hepatic allograft

Metabolic diseases

    Hereditary hemochromatosis

    α_1-Antitrypsin deficiency

    Primary hyperoxaluria

    Familial amyloidosis

    Cystic fibrosis

    Glycogen storage disease

Perihilar cholangiocarcinoma

Severe alcoholic hepatitis not responding to medical therapy[a]

---

[a] Liver transplant may be considered for carefully selected patients who have favorable psychosocial profiles.

---

[a] The authors thank J. Eileen Hay, MB, ChB, who authored the previous version of this chapter.

Abbreviations: ALD, alcohol-associated liver disease; DAA, direct-acting antiviral; DCD, donation after cardiac death; HCC, hepatocellular carcinoma; INR, international normalized ratio; LDLT, living-donor liver transplant; LT, liver transplant; MELD, Model for End-stage Liver Disease; MELD-Na, Model for End-stage Liver Disease incorporating sodium level; mTOR, mammalian target of rapamycin; OPTN, Organ Procurement and Transplantation Network

added to the waiting list). The complications of cirrhosis that are accepted indications for LT are hepatocellular carcinoma (HCC), hepatopulmonary syndrome, and portopulmonary hypertension. In addition, unresectable perihilar cholangiocarcinoma with a mass no larger than 3 cm in radial diameter is an accepted indication for LT after neoadjuvant radiotherapy and chemotherapy. LT may be considered for carefully selected patients who have favorable psychosocial profiles and no response to medical therapy for severe alcoholic hepatitis (Model for End-stage Liver Disease [MELD] incorporating sodium level [MELD-Na] score >20). A favorable psychosocial profile includes 1) first presentation with decompensated ALD; 2) absence of severe, uncontrolled medical or psychiatric comorbidities; 3) lack of repeated, unsuccessful attempts at rehabilitation; 4) lack of other substance use or dependency; 5) acceptance of ALD diagnosis with insight; 6) commitment of the patient to lifelong sobriety; and 7) the presence of close, supportive family members or caregivers who will assist the patient with abstinence goals.

The Organ Procurement and Transplantation Network (OPTN) T2 criteria (also known as the Milan criteria) (Box 36.2) are used to select tumors suitable for LT (ie, those likely to be cured by LT): The patient should have 1 tumor with a diameter of at least 2 cm and no larger than 5 cm *or* 2 or 3 tumors with diameters of at least 1 cm and no larger than 3 cm without vascular invasion or extrahepatic spread.

About 5% of all LTs in the US are performed for acute medical emergencies: acute liver failure, fulminant Wilson disease, or early failure of a liver allograft (primary nonfunction or hepatic artery thrombosis within the first postoperative week). Acute liver failure is an uncommon condition, with only about 2,500 cases annually in the US. The most frequent causes are acetaminophen hepatotoxicity (nearly 50% of all cases), indeterminate causes (20%), and idiosyncratic drug reactions (14%). Other recognized indications for LT in adults are primary hyperoxaluria, familial amyloid polyneuropathy, cystic fibrosis, and metabolic diseases in which the metabolic defect is in the liver. For children, several other metabolic diseases are indications for LT. Controversy continues to surround several proposed indications for LT, including metastatic neuroendocrine tumors, metastatic colorectal cancer, and polycystic liver disease. Occasionally, in some regions of the US, LT is performed for these indications.

Despite the success of LT, the procedure has some absolute and relative contraindications (Box 36.3). The relative contraindications do not necessarily preclude transplant depending on the transplant center, but several relative contraindications in aggregate may result in a patient being ineligible for transplant.

✓ **Hepatic decompensation**—development of life-threatening complications, including hepatic encephalopathy, ascites, spontaneous bacterial peritonitis, esophageal variceal hemorrhage, hepatocellular carcinoma, hepatopulmonary syndrome, and hepatorenal syndrome

---

Box 36.2. Organ Procurement and Transplantation Network (OPTN) T2 Criteria (Milan Criteria)

Patient with cirrhosis or hepatocellular carcinoma is a suitable candidate for transplant

Patient has a single tumor with a diameter of 2-5 cm

Patient has 2 or 3 tumors that each have a diameter of 1-3 cm

Patient has no extrahepatic involvement

Patient has no major vessel involvement

✓ Alcohol-associated liver disease and nonalcoholic steatohepatitis are the leading indications for patients being added to the waiting list for LT
✓ Patients are eligible for LT if they have hepatocellular carcinoma that meets the OPTN T2 criteria (also known as the Milan criteria), cirrhosis, and an alpha fetoprotein level less than 1,000 ng/mL
✓ Some patients do not qualify for LT because they have absolute or relative contraindications, which are listed in Box 36.3

Allocation of Organs

In February 2002, the allocation system for deceased donor livers in the US was changed to a system based on short-term mortality; that is, an organ is allocated to the patient most likely to die in the next 3 months (Table 36.1). The most urgent indication for LT is acute liver failure, and these patients are given the highest priority for urgent organ allocation (status 1A). Unlike patients with status 1A, who should be assigned an organ quickly after activation, patients with chronic liver disease generally have a 2-step process: listing for LT and allocation of a donor organ. If otherwise suitable to be a transplant recipient, a patient with cirrhosis will be registered with the United Network for Organ Sharing on the liver transplant waiting list; however, organ allocation is prioritized for patients listed within each ABO blood group, according to their expected 3-month mortality, as defined by the MELD scoring system. In January 2016, the updated OPTN Policy 9.1 (MELD Score) incorporated the serum sodium level into calculation of the MELD score. Hyponatremia is a common problem in patients with cirrhosis, and the severity of hyponatremia is a marker of the severity of cirrhosis.

The MELD-Na score is based on serum levels of creatinine, bilirubin, and sodium and the international normalized ratio (INR). It is calculated according to the following formula:

$$\text{MELD-Na Score} = \text{MELD} + 1.32 \times (137 - \text{Na}) - [0.033 \times \text{MELD} \times (137 - \text{Na})]$$

The 4 variables (serum levels of creatinine, bilirubin, and sodium and the INR) are entered into a computer program, and the MELD-Na score is calculated (https://optn.transplant.hrsa.gov/resources/allocation-calculators/meld-calculator/). For patients with MELD scores higher than 40, the expected 3-month mortality rate is 80% without LT; for patients with scores of 20 to 29, the rate is 20% to 25%; and for patients with scores less than 10, there is no excess short-term mortality. In 2021, MELD 3.0 was proposed. To the MELD-Na variables, MELD 3.0 added serum albumin level and female sex (women received an additional 1.3 points) and updated creatinine cutoffs. MELD 3.0 resulted in fewer deaths of patients on the waiting list, but the OPTN continues to use the MELD-Na score.

HCC is an accepted indication for LT even though mortality is not reflected by the MELD score. In the US, patients with HCC within the Milan criteria and an alpha fetoprotein level less than 1,000 ng/mL are eligible for the standardized MELD score exception based on the median MELD at transplant score 6 months after being listed as an acceptable candidate. If the HCC burden extends beyond the Milan criteria, the patient needs to meet the criteria of the OPTN downstaging protocol to be eligible for a MELD exception score. In this situation, HCC should be downstaged to and maintained within the Milan criteria with a treatment modality such as locoregional therapy, and the patient must have an alpha fetoprotein level less than 1,000 ng/mL.

Table 36.1. Allocation of Deceased Donor Organs for Adult Candidates

Allocation status	Disease category
Status 1A	Acute liver failure in ICU, no preexisting liver disease, hepatic encephalopathy within 56 d of onset, and 1 of the following: ventilator dependency, receiving hemodialysis or continuous venovenous hemofiltration, or INR >2.0
	Acute decompensated Wilson disease
	Anhepatic
	Primary nonfunction of allograft within 7 d of transplant
	Hepatic artery thrombosis within 7 d of transplant
MELD-Na score, calculated	Cirrhosis from any cause
MELD-Na score exceptions	Hepatocellular carcinoma
	Perihilar cholangiocarcinoma
	Hepatopulmonary syndrome
	Portopulmonary hypertension
	Primary hyperoxaluria
	Familial amyloid polyneuropathy
	Cystic fibrosis
	Metabolic disease (urea cycle disorder or organic acidemia)
	Hepatic artery thrombosis (within 14 d of transplant but does not meet criteria for status 1A)
	Appeal to regional review board[a]

Abbreviations: ICU, intensive care unit; INR, international normalized ratio; MELD-Na, Model for End-stage Liver Disease incorporating sodium level.

[a] Any transplant program can appeal to the regional review board for an assigned MELD-Na score for any patient to allow the patient to receive an organ.

Box 36.3. Contraindications to Liver Transplant

Absolute contraindications

Extrahepatic malignancy unless tumor-free for ≥2 y and low probability of recurrence

Untreated alcoholism

Uncontrolled sepsis

Severe multiorgan failure

Severe psychologic disease likely to affect adherence to therapy

Severe pulmonary hypertension

Advanced cardiopulmonary disease

AIDS

Hepatocellular carcinoma or perihilar cholangiocarcinoma with metastasis

Fulminant liver failure with sustained ICP >50 mm Hg or CPP <40 mm Hg

Relative contraindications

General debility

Persistent nonadherence to therapy

Social isolation

Advanced age

Extensive, previous abdominal surgery

Extensive portal or mesenteric thrombosis

Abbreviations: CPP, cerebral perfusion pressure; ICP, intracranial pressure.

In addition, adult patients with any of the following diagnoses are eligible for the standardized MELD score exception based on the median MELD at transplant policy: hepatopulmonary syndrome, primary hyperoxaluria, familial amyloidosis, perihilar cholangiocarcinoma, cystic fibrosis, and portopulmonary hypertension. For all these MELD exceptions, there are strict inclusion and exclusion criteria (https://unos.org/).

The only ways for patients to be guaranteed consideration for allocation of a deceased donor organ are to have status 1A, have a calculated MELD-Na score, or have an assigned MELD score (ie, standardized MELD exceptions). For controversial indications for LT or for patients who are more symptomatic than suggested by their MELD score, transplant programs may appeal to the national review board to be given an assigned MELD score.

> ✓ Each liver transplant candidate is assigned a score that reflects the probability of death within a 3-month period as determined with the calculated MELD score
> ✓ A candidate can also be assigned a priority status if the candidate meets the requirements for that status

Immunosuppression

Five main groups of immunosuppressive medications are used in LT (Table 36.2). Each immunosuppressive drug has its own site of action and adverse effects. The risk of rejection is highest in the first weeks after LT, when immunosuppression is at its highest level. Tacrolimus has replaced cyclosporine as the calcineurin inhibitor of choice in most liver transplant programs. Frequently, corticosteroids with or without mycophenolate mofetil are administered in the first postoperative weeks. Immunosuppression is tapered by 4 months, often to tacrolimus monotherapy, with lower serum levels. Long-term calcineurin inhibitor monotherapy is ideal, but if nephrotoxicity develops in response to the treatment, a low dose of calcineurin inhibitor *and* mycophenolate mofetil or a mammalian target of rapamycin (mTOR) inhibitor may be used. Overall, the trend now is to tailor immunosuppression to each patient, depending on the time from LT, rejection history, and adverse effects from individual drugs. Newer agents are being sought to avoid kidney and metabolic dysfunction.

> ✓ Risk of rejection is highest in the first weeks after LT, when immunosuppression is at its highest level
> ✓ Calcineurin inhibitors (tacrolimus and cyclosporine) can lead to nephrotoxicity and neurotoxicity
> ✓ mTOR inhibitors (sirolimus and everolimus) can lead to cytopenias, hepatic artery thrombosis, and poor wound healing

Complications After LT

Primary Nonfunction of the Liver Allograft

The worst early complication is primary nonfunction of the allograft. This starts immediately with the appearance of clear bile or no output of bile, high aminotransferase levels, and an increase in bilirubin concentration. The main identified risk factor is high fat content of the allograft. Grafts may be biopsied to assess this before implantation. No therapy is available for primary nonfunction, and the patient's status needs to be reactivated as status 1A for the patient to receive a second graft.

Table 36.2. Immunosuppressive Drugs and Their Adverse Effects

Drug class	Drug	Adverse effects
Corticosteroids[a]	Methylprednisolone	Hypertension, type 2 diabetes, neurotoxicity, hyperlipidemia, bone loss, myopathy
	Prednisone	
Purine antagonists	Azathioprine	Cytopenias
	Mycophenolate mofetil	Adverse effects in the gastrointestinal tract (mycophenolate mofetil only)
Calcineurin inhibitors[a,b]	Tacrolimus	Nephrotoxicity, hypertension, type 2 diabetes, neurotoxicity (headache, tremors,
	Cyclosporine	seizures, posterior reversible encephalopathy syndrome), hair loss (tacrolimus), hair gain (cyclosporine)
mTOR inhibitors	Sirolimus (rapamycin)	Cytopenias, hypertriglyceridemia, poor wound healing, hepatic artery thrombosis, oral
	Everolimus	and gastrointestinal tract ulcers, edema, proteinuria
Antibody therapy (intravenous)[a]	Antithymocyte globulin (thymoglobulin)	Profound immunosuppression, opportunistic infections
	Basiliximab	

Abbreviation: mTOR, mammalian target of rapamycin.

[a] Used for treatment and prevention of rejection (others used only for prevention).

[b] Interactions can occur with drugs that affect the cytochrome P450 enzyme system: Drugs inhibiting the cytochrome P450 system (eg, fluconazole) increase the levels of calcineurin inhibitors, and drugs stimulating the cytochrome P450 system (eg, phenytoin) decrease calcineurin inhibitor levels and thus increase the risk of rejection.

Hepatic Artery Thrombosis

Another dreaded early complication of LT is hepatic artery thrombosis. This is most common in children, size-mismatched grafts, and LDLT. It usually occurs in the first week after LT, but it can develop later. The clinical manifestations may be subtle, and patients may be asymptomatic or have mild fever or increased aminotransferase levels. In the majority of adults with hepatic artery thrombosis, the grafts fail because of hepatic necrosis or ischemic cholangiopathy. When hepatic artery thrombosis occurs in the first 7 days after LT and there is evidence of severe graft dysfunction, the patient will be listed for retransplant as status 1A. If graft dysfunction is not severe or hepatic artery thrombosis occurs 7 to 14 days after transplant, the patient can be listed with a MELD exception score of 40.

Cellular Rejection

Acute cellular rejection occurs in up to 50% of liver recipients and usually is associated with mild to moderate biochemical abnormalities and, occasionally, fever. Although the diagnosis can be suspected by the timing in the early weeks after LT, definitive diagnosis requires histologic examination of the liver and the following findings: 1) portal infiltrates with activated lymphocytes and some eosinophils, 2) lymphocytic cholangitis, and 3) venous endotheliitis. Ninety percent of cases of rejection occur in the first 2 postoperative months. Most rejections are treated with intravenous corticosteroids, and 85% of patients with rejection have a response to corticosteroids. Of the patients with corticosteroid-resistant rejection, 90% respond to intravenous antibody therapy with antithymocyte globulin. Acute cellular rejection soon after LT generally has no effect on long-term graft outcome, except for patients with hepatitis C, and very few grafts are lost to chronic rejection.

> ✓ Acute cellular rejection is associated with mild to moderate biochemical abnormalities and, occasionally, fever
> ✓ Definitive diagnosis of acute cellular rejection requires a liver biopsy that shows: 1) portal infiltrates with activated lymphocytes and some eosinophils, 2) lymphocytic cholangitis, and 3) venous endotheliitis

Biliary Strictures

The biliary anastomosis, either duct-to-duct or biliary-enteric anastomosis, is the most common site of biliary strictures, which usually form in the first month. Most strictures respond to endoscopic dilatation, with or without stents, but occasionally surgical revision of the anastomosis is needed.

Nonanastomotic or ischemic-type biliary strictures may form at any time, but the median time is about the eleventh postoperative week. The most commonly identified cause is hepatic artery thrombosis, either early or late. Other associations are with ABO incompatibility, long warm (>90 minutes) or cold (>12 hours) ischemia time, and graft donation after cardiac death (DCD). Some of these strictures can be managed with endoscopic or percutaneous biliary stenting, although ischemic-type biliary stricturing leads to death or a need for retransplant in about 50% of patients.

Infections

A systemic fungal, viral, or bacterial infection develops in 1 in 5 LT recipients during the first postoperative month. Cytomegalovirus infection is the most common viral infection. Its incidence peaks in the first 3 to 5 postoperative weeks, and it is rare after the first year. Its presence is suggested by fever and leukopenia. Treatment is with intravenous ganciclovir or oral valganciclovir. *Candida* infection is the most common fungal infection, although opportunistic infections can also be seen with *Aspergillus*, *Nocardia*, *Cryptococcus*, and *Pneumocystis*. Many transplant programs provide prophylaxis for *Pneumocystis* in the early postoperative months when immunosuppression is at its highest level.

Late Complications

The main late complications after LT are recurrent disease, complications of immunosuppression, and de novo malignancies.

When late allograft dysfunction occurs in a patient who is well and receiving stable, therapeutic immunosuppression, recurrent disease is the most likely diagnosis. The diagnosis is histologic, and liver biopsy is needed. The incidence and potential severity of recurrent disease in an allograft is greatest with hepatitis C. In the past, treatment of recurrent hepatitis C with peginterferon and ribavirin resulted in a sustained virologic response in about 30% of patients. Since 2014, introduction of interferon-free regimens with direct-acting antiviral (DAA) regimens provided LT recipients with efficacious hepatitis C treatment and sustained virologic response rates of up to 83% to 100%. The safety profile of these agents is favorable. The DAA regimen for LT recipients—regardless of the hepatitis C genotype, the recipient being treatment naïve or experienced with peginterferon and ribavirin, or the presence or absence of cirrhosis—includes the following for 12 weeks: glecaprevir-pibrentasvir or sofosbuvir-velpatasvir. Ledipasvir-sofosbuvir can be used for 12 weeks in patients with hepatitis C genotypes 1, 4, 5, or 6. Patients with decompensated cirrhosis require treatment with ledipasvir-sofosbuvir *and* a low initial dose of ribavirin (genotypes 1, 4, 5, or 6) or sofosbuvir-velpatasvir *and* a low initial dose of ribavirin (all genotypes) for 12 to 24 weeks. DAA-experienced patients with genotype 1 to 6 infection in the allograft with or without compensated cirrhosis can be treated with sofosbuvir-velpatasvir-voxilaprevir for 12 weeks (https://www.hcvguidelines.org/). Recurrent hepatitis B is prevented in more than 90% of patients with hepatitis B immunoglobulin and antiviral therapy. Other liver diseases, including primary biliary cholangitis and primary sclerosing cholangitis, autoimmune hepatitis, nonalcoholic fatty liver disease, and HCC, may also recur. The incidence of immune-mediated liver disease recurrence is 10% to 20%.

Most LT recipients have normal cardiac function, but increasingly patients who are obese or have type 2 diabetes or hypertension are undergoing LT. In addition, even in those with no risk factors for coronary artery disease before LT, treatment with immunosuppressive drugs may lead to hypertension, type 2 diabetes, kidney failure, dyslipidemia, and obesity in a high percentage of patients. This predisposes many LT recipients to a high risk for cardiovascular disease, with cyclosporine having more metabolic effects than tacrolimus. LT recipients must receive adequate screening and therapy for these risk factors.

LT recipients have multiple potential risk factors for cancer: immunosuppression, viruses (hepatitis C virus, hepatitis B virus, human papillomavirus, human herpesvirus 6, Epstein-Barr virus), alcohol use, and smoking. Furthermore, many recipients are older than 60 years at the time of LT and, thus, have the increased cancer risk of aging. The effect of immunosuppression probably is related to the degree of immunosuppression rather than to individual agents. Depending on the series, the reported overall incidence of cancer varies from 2.9% to 14%; the reported cancer-related mortality rate is 0.6% to 8%. Malignancies are an important cause of long-term mortality.

Malignancies that occur frequently in LT recipients are skin cancers and posttransplant lymphoproliferative disease in addition to cervical, vulvar, and anal squamous cancers. The incidence of colorectal cancer is increased only for recipients with primary sclerosing cholangitis, likely related to ulcerative colitis.

Increasingly, data show notable mortality at 5 to 10 years after LT from upper aerodigestive cancers in recipients who continue to smoke and drink.

Expansion of the Donor Pool

Adult-to-adult LDLT uses the right, and less frequently the left, lobe of the donor for implant into the recipient. For pediatric recipients, the left lobe may be used, depending on size. The major advantages of LDLT over deceased donor transplant are availability of the organ and expansion of the donor pool. LDLT is associated with more vascular and biliary complications but not less rejection. The donor morbidity rate is 8% to 26%, and the mortality rate is 0.3%. In addition, expanding the donor pool can be achieved by using grafts from older donors (higher rate of primary nonfunction); split livers (higher complication rate, labor-intensive procedure, and disadvantage for the primary recipient); marginal donors (eg, fatty liver with an increased risk of primary nonfunction); DCD graft (increased risk of biliary complications; 5-year graft survival among adult deceased donor liver transplant recipients, 73%); and high-risk donors (high-risk lifestyle or medical history).

Suggested Reading

Burra P, Freeman R. Trends in liver transplantation 2011. J Hepatol. 2012 56 Suppl 1:S101–11.

Burton JR, Jr, Everson GT. Management of the transplant recipient with chronic hepatitis C. Clin Liver Dis. 2013 Feb;17(1):73–91.

Cholankeril G, Ahmed A. Alcoholic liver disease replaces hepatitis C virus infection as the leading indication for liver transplantation in the United States. Clin Gastroenterol Hepatol. 2018 Aug;16(8):1356–8.

Crabb DW, Im GY, Szabo G, Mellinger JL, Lucey MR. Diagnosis and treatment of alcohol-associated liver diseases: 2019 practice guidance from the American Association for the Study of Liver Diseases. Hepatology. 2020 Jan;71(1):306–33.

Kwong AJ, Kim WR, Lake JR, Smith JM, Schladt DP, Skeans MA, et al. OPTN/SRTR 2019 annual data report: liver. Am J Transplant. 2021 Feb;21 Suppl 2:208–315.

Limaye AR, Firpi RJ. Management of recurrent hepatitis C infection after liver transplantation. Clin Liver Dis. 2011 Nov;15(4):845–58.

Lucey MR, Terrault N, Ojo L, Hay JE, Neuberger J, Blumberg E, et al. Long-term management of the successful adult liver transplant: 2012 practice guideline by the American Association for the Study of Liver Diseases and the American Society of Transplantation. Liver Transpl. 2013 Jan;19(1):3–26.

Marrero JA, Kulik LM, Sirlin CB, Zhu AX, Finn RS, Abecassis MM, et al. Diagnosis, staging, and management of hepatocellular carcinoma: 2018 practice guidance by the American Association for the Study of Liver Diseases. Hepatology. 2018 Aug;68(2):723–50.

Tan HH, Martin P. Care of the liver transplant candidate. Clin Liver Dis. 2011 Nov;15(4):779–806.

Weber ML, Ibrahim HN, Lake JR. Renal dysfunction in liver transplant recipients: evaluation of the critical issues. Liver Transpl. 2012 Nov;18(11):1290–301.

Wiesner RH, Fung JJ. Present state of immunosuppressive therapy in liver transplant recipients. Liver Transpl. 2011 Nov;17 Suppl 3:S1–9.

Questions and Answers

Questions

Abbreviations used:

AFP,	alpha fetoprotein
ALP,	alkaline phosphatase
ALT,	alanine aminotransferase
AMA,	antimitochondrial antibody
ANA,	antinuclear antibody
anti-HAV,	antibody to hepatitis A virus
anti-HBc,	antibody to hepatitis B core antigen
anti-HBs,	antibody to hepatitis B surface antigen
anti-HCV,	antibody to hepatitis C virus
anti-LKM,	antibody to liver-kidney microsome type 1
ASMA,	anti–smooth muscle antibody
AST,	aspartate aminotransferase
BCLC,	Barcelona Clinic Liver Cancer
BCS,	Budd-Chiari syndrome
BMI,	body mass index
CBC,	complete blood cell count
CT,	computed tomography
DAA,	direct-acting antiviral
DILI,	drug-induced liver injury
EGD,	esophagogastroduodenoscopy
ERCP,	endoscopic retrograde cholangiopancreatography
FISH,	fluorescence in situ hybridization
GAVE,	gastric antral vascular ectasia
HAV,	hepatitis A virus
HBsAg,	hepatitis B surface antigen
HBV,	hepatitis B virus
HCC,	hepatocellular carcinoma
HCV,	hepatitis C virus
HE,	hepatic encephalopathy
IBD,	inflammatory bowel disease
Ig,	immunoglobulin
INR,	international normalized ratio
LDL,	low-density lipoprotein
MCV,	mean corpuscular volume
MELD,	Model for End-stage Liver Disease
MRCP,	magnetic resonance cholangiopancreatography
MRI,	magnetic resonance imaging
NAFLD,	nonalcoholic fatty liver disease
NASH,	nonalcoholic steatohepatitis
NSBB,	nonselective β-blocker
PBC,	primary biliary cholangitis
PMN,	polymorphonuclear neutrophil
PSC,	primary sclerosing cholangitis
SMA,	smooth muscle antibody
TIPS,	transjugular intrahepatic portosystemic shunt
WBC,	white blood cell count

Multiple Choice (choose the best answer)

VI.1. **A 20-year-old man is referred with abnormally high liver test results. He felt well until 2 weeks ago when he noted fatigue and sore throat. His primary care provider cultured his throat; results were negative. The symptoms continued, and jaundice developed. The patient has no prior history of liver disease. He drinks 3 or 4 alcoholic beverages weekly. Medications include minocycline for 2 months for acne and acetaminophen 2 g daily for the past 2 weeks. Physical examination findings are notable for a relatively well-appearing man in no distress. His temperature is 38.2 °C. He has mild scleral icterus, enlarged and soft cervical lymph nodes, and mild splenomegaly. Notable laboratory test results are shown below:**

Component	Result
Hemoglobin, g/dL	14
WBC count, /µL	3,300
Neutrophils, %	20
Lymphocytes, %	60
Monocytes, %	20
Platelet count, ×10³/µL	130
ALP, U/L	100
AST, U/L	202
ALT, U/L	217
Total bilirubin, mg/dL	3.4
Direct bilirubin, mg/dL	2.1
ANA, U	1.4
Smooth muscle antibody	Negative
Gammaglobulin, g/dL	1.2
Hepatitis B surface antigen	Negative
Hepatitis B core antibody	Negative
Hepatitis C antibody	Negative
Hepatitis A antibody	Negative

Which of the following is the most likely diagnosis?

a. Minocycline-induced liver disease
b. Wilson disease
c. Lymphoma
d. Infectious mononucleosis
e. Acetaminophen hepatotoxicity

VI.2. A 63-year-old woman presents with a 4-hour history of abdominal pain, fever, and nausea. She has no prior history of liver disease. Physical examination findings are notable for blood pressure 110/60 mm Hg, heart rate 104 beats/min, and temperature 38.7 °C. She has jaundice and mild epigastric tenderness. Notable laboratory test results are shown below:

Component	Result
WBC count, /µL	18,000
Polymorphonuclear cells, %	80
Band cells, %	10
ALP, U/L	150
AST, U/L	745
ALT, U/L	650
Total bilirubin, mg/dL	5.0
Amylase, U/L	270

Ultrasonography shows gallbladder stones, no bile duct dilatation, and a pancreas that appears normal. The patient is prescribed antibiotics. Blood cultures 12 hours later are positive for *Escherichia coli*. Which of the following would you advise next?

a. Endoscopic ultrasonography
b. MRCP
c. ERCP
d. Laparoscopic cholecystectomy
e. Doppler ultrasonography of the hepatic vasculature

VI.3. A 39-year-old asymptomatic man presents with a high ALP level that was initially discovered when he had blood tests done to assess symptoms that turned out to be due to a COVID-19 infection. The ALP level has been persistently high for a year. He drinks 1 or 2 alcoholic beverages weekly. He has no family history of liver disease. Physical examination findings are unremarkable. Notable laboratory test results are shown below:

Component	Result
Hemoglobin, mg/dL	14.2
Platelet count, ×10³/µL	160
Total bilirubin, mg/dL	1.0
Direct bilirubin, mg/dL	0.3
ALP, U/L	343
AST, U/L	64
ALT, U/L	79

Ultrasonography of the liver shows mild hepatosplenomegaly and slightly enlarged abdominal lymph nodes. Chest radiography shows mild hilar adenopathy and changes consistent with interstitial lung disease. Which of the following is the most likely diagnosis?

a. Amyloidosis
b. Sarcoidosis
c. PSC
d. PBC
e. Celiac disease

VI.4. You are asked to evaluate a 53-year-old man who has high liver test results. He was admitted 4 days ago when he was found on his apartment floor. Initial examination findings were notable for a tongue laceration, so it was thought that he might have had a seizure. Blood work on admission was notable for the following: AST 4,120 U/L, ALT 714 U/L, and normal levels of ALP and bilirubin. An acetaminophen level was undetected. Results from yesterday were AST 1,024 U/L and ALT 434 U/L. The patient has a history of heavy alcohol use. He does not use medications. Examination findings are notable for obesity with a normal liver and spleen. Which of the following is the most likely diagnosis?

a. Muscle injury
b. Alcoholic hepatitis
c. Acute viral hepatitis
d. Acetaminophen hepatotoxicity
e. Hepatic ischemia

VI.5. Which of the following agents can be used to treat HCV genotype 1a in a patient with decompensated cirrhosis?

a. Grazoprevir-elbasvir
b. Glecaprevir-pibrentasvir
c. Sofosbuvir-velpatasvir-voxilaprevir
d. Sofosbuvir-ledipasvir

VI.6. A 23-year-old woman presents with jaundice that she noticed 1 week ago. The transplant service is aware of her admission. On examination she is oriented, and she has jaundice but no asterixis. Laboratory test results are shown below:

Component	Result
ALT, U/L	1,648
Total bilirubin, mg/dL	5.5
Direct bilirubin, mg/dL	3.4
INR	1.2
HBsAg	Positive
IgM anti-HBc	Positive
HBV DNA, IU/mL	35,000
Anti-HCV	Negative
Anti-HAV	Negative

Which of the following should you advise now?

a. Urgent liver transplant

b. Peginterferon and entecavir

c. Entecavir

d. *N*-acetylcysteine

e. Serial monitoring

VI.7. A 58-year-old man, a former user of intravenous drugs, is evaluated for treatment of infection with HCV genotype 1 with stage 2 fibrosis. Baseline laboratory tests include normal results for the following: CBC, creatinine, total bilirubin, ALP, and albumin. Other results are ALT 64 U/L, AST 54 U/L, HIV negative, HBsAg positive, and HBV DNA less than 20 IU/mL. He is not taking any medications. He begins treatment with an interferon-free DAA regimen. At week 4, he presents to the clinic and says that his eyes are yellow. Which of the following should be evaluated next?

a. HAV RNA

b. HBV DNA

c. HCV RNA

d. Lactate

e. Smooth muscle antibody

VI.8. Which antiviral regimen is contraindicated in patients receiving amiodarone?

a. Glecaprevir-pibrentasvir

b. Entecavir

c. Tenofovir

d. Sofosbuvir-ledipasvir

VI.9. A 55-year-old woman with type 2 diabetes has abdominal pain. On abdominal ultrasonography that was performed to rule out cholecystitis, the gallbladder appears normal, but an indeterminate 5-cm mass is apparent in the right lobe of the liver. No previous imaging studies of the liver have been performed. Multiphasic MRI is performed with gadoxetate as a contrast agent to characterize the mass. The MRI shows rapid homogeneous enhancement of the mass with a prompt return to isointensity with the surrounding liver in the portal venous phase. The mass retains contrast material in the biliary phase of the study. What is the most likely diagnosis?

a. Hepatic adenoma

b. Hepatic hemangioma

c. Focal nodular hyperplasia

d. Intrahepatic cholangiocarcinoma

VI.10. A 36-year-old man who was born in South Korea and was adopted to live in the US at the age of 5 years had a positive test result for HBsAg at the time of adoption. His hepatitis B status has been monitored periodically. Results are now negative for hepatitis B e antigen and positive for hepatitis B e antibody. His baseline ALT level ranges from 20 to 28 U/L. The hepatitis B virus DNA level is 1,000 IU/mL. He has no known family history of HCC. Laboratory tests show no evidence of cirrhosis or complications of chronic liver disease. Transient elastography shows no increase in liver stiffness. On physical examination he has no evidence of cirrhosis or chronic liver disease. At what age should surveillance begin for liver cancer?

a. 20 years

b. 30 years

c. 40 years

d. 50 years

VI.11. A 55-year-old woman presents with a 3-month history of progressive right upper quadrant abdominal pain, jaundice, and bilateral leg swelling. She slipped and fell on her side during the winter and has had progressively worse abdominal pain since then. About a week ago her daughter noticed that she appeared to have a yellow tint to her skin. Two days ago, the patient noticed increased puffiness of her feet and ankles. On abdominal ultrasonography, a large 15-cm cyst is in the central right lobe of the liver. The bile ducts are compressed centrally in the liver with bilateral peripheral biliary dilatation. The cyst appears to compress the intrahepatic inferior vena cava. The cyst wall shows no nodularity or increased vascularity on Doppler evaluation. Echogenic densities in the cyst suggest prior hemorrhage. The ultrasonographic findings are confirmed on multiphasic contrast MRI. After the cyst was aspirated and sclerosis was performed with 3% sodium tetradecyl sulfate, the symptoms resolved. However, the abdominal pain returned after 2 months and ultrasonography showed reaccumulation of the cyst fluid with no evidence of increased nodularity or vascularity of the cyst wall. What is the best next step in management?

a. A second cyst aspiration and sclerosis with 3% sodium tetradecyl sulfate

b. Laparoscopic decompression and unroofing of the cyst

c. Initiation of diuretic therapy

d. Evaluation for liver transplant

VI.12. A 44-year-old man with ulcerative colitis has an increased ALP level during a follow-up evaluation for ulcerative colitis. MRI with MRCP suggests that he has cirrhotic-stage PSC with a dominant stricture in the left hepatic duct. MRI does not show a definite enhancing mass. The carbohydrate antigen 19-9 value is high (150 U/mL). ERCP evaluation with brushings and biopsies provides cytologic confirmation of malignancy, and pancreatobiliary FISH shows polysomy. Transpapillary forceps biopsy findings are negative. Endoscopic ultrasonography shows no evidence of lymph node metastasis. What is the best next step in management?

a. Surgical resection for cure

b. Referral for evaluation for liver transplant

c. Radiofrequency ablation of the area of the dominant stricture

d. Photodynamic therapy

VI.13. A 73-year-old woman who has cirrhosis secondary to NAFLD received a diagnosis of BCLC stage C multifocal advanced HCC. EGD showed large varices with red wale signs, which were banded until all varices had been successfully treated. She has Child-Pugh class A cirrhosis. The serum AFP value was 1,500 ng/mL, and she is not a candidate for surgical resection. Her performance status at the time of diagnosis was 0. She had 1 session of transarterial chemoembolization without evidence of benefit, and the AFP value increased to 2,500 ng/mL 3 months after chemoembolization. What is the best next step in management?

a. Atezolizumab in combination with bevacizumab

b. Sorafenib

c. Best supportive care

d. Ramucirumab

VI.14. A 39-year-old woman who has a history of obesity (treated with Roux-en-Y gastric bypass), hypertension, and hyperlipidemia is referred for evaluation of abnormal liver biochemistry results. She drinks 2 glasses of wine each evening. Laboratory test results are shown below:

Component	Result
ALT, U/L	75
AST, U/L	144
ALP, U/L	125
Bilirubin, mg/dL	0.7
INR	1.1
ANA, U	Negative
SMA	Negative
HBV and HCV antibodies	Negative

Her BMI is 33. Ultrasonography of the liver shows fatty infil-tration. What should be your initial management approach?

a. Recommend that she lose 7% to 10% of her body weight
b. Recommend that she abstain from drinking alcohol
c. Begin treatment with ursodiol (13-15 mg/kg daily)
d. Refer her for evaluation for liver transplant

VI.15. A 32-year-old man who had been well now has fatigue, jaun-dice, and dark urine. He typically drinks 6 cans of beer daily. He has been drinking more heavily recently while he is unem-ployed. Examination findings are as follows: blood pressure 130/86 mm Hg, heart rate 102 beats/min, temperature 38.5 °C, scleral icterus, hepatomegaly with an abdominal bruit, and no splenomegaly. Laboratory test results include the following: WBC count 20×10^9/L, platelet count 232×10^9/L, and albumin 4.5 g/dL. Which of the following is the most likely cause of the bruit?

a. Splenorenal shunting
b. Dilation of the hepatic artery
c. HCC
d. Cruveilhier-Baumgarten murmur

VI.16. A 45-year-old woman drinks 2 alcoholic beverages daily. She decreased her consumption when she recently received a diag-nosis of COVID-19–related pneumonia. She was treated ini-tially with azithromycin and later with COVID-19 monoclonal antibody therapy. She recently completed a 10-day quaran-tine period. On follow-up evaluation with her primary care physician, test results included the following: AST 1,000 U/L, ALT 1,100 U/L, CBC normal, total bilirubin 0.5 mg/dL, and INR 1.0. She does not take herbal supplements, but she took over-the-counter cold medications while she was ill. What is the most likely cause of the increased liver test results?

a. COVID-19–related hepatitis
b. Drug-induced autoimmune-like hepatitis
c. Acetaminophen hepatotoxicity
d. Severe alcohol-related hepatitis

VI.17. A 62-year-old man with alcohol-related cirrhosis is being evaluated for liver transplant. His blood type is B, and his MELD score with determination of sodium is 25. His cir-rhosis is complicated by ascites that requires diuretic therapy, mild hepatic encephalopathy that requires lactulose, and small, nonbleeding esophageal varices. He has abstained from drinking alcohol for 1 year, he has completed primary addiction treatment, and he attends Alcoholics Anonymous meetings regularly. On the 6-minute walk test, he had a total of 200 m, which was limited by knee pain due to severe osteo-arthritis. What is the best management for his knee pain?

a. Acetaminophen 500 mg 4 times daily
b. Ibuprofen 400 mg 4 times daily
c. Oxycodone 10 mg 4 times daily
d. Knee replacement surgery

VI.18. A 32-year-old woman presents to the emergency depart-ment with sudden onset of abdominal pain and distention. Previously, she had been healthy, and her only medication is an oral contraceptive. She smokes 1 pack of cigarettes daily. On examination she has tender hepatomegaly with moderate ascites. Laboratory studies are notable for the following: INR 1.8, AST 780 U/L, ALT 890 U/L, and total bilirubin 5.6 mg/dL. The hepatic veins are not apparent on ultrasonography of the abdomen. The patient is hospitalized, and therapy is started with unfractionated heparin. The next morning, she is disoriented and somnolent, and she has asterixis. What is the most appropriate next step?

a. Continue therapy with intravenous unfractionated heparin
b. Switch therapy to subcutaneous low-molecular-weight heparin

c. Begin diuretic therapy with furosemide and spironolactone
d. Refer for an urgent TIPS
e. Refer for urgent liver transplant

VI.19. A 64-year-old man presents to the emergency department with hematemesis that began this morning. He has no known history of chronic liver disease. His past medical history is notable for controlled hypertension, hyperlipidemia, and a previous episode of severe gallstone pancreatitis. After he receives fluid resuscitation, his condition is stabilized. On upper endoscopy, esophageal varices are not seen, but there are large gastric fundic varices with red signs, and there is altered blood in the stomach. What is the most appropriate next step?

a. Therapy with propranolol
b. CT of the abdomen with an intravenous contrast agent
c. Endoscopic band ligation of the gastric varices
d. TIPS
e. Referral for liver transplant

VI.20. A 48-year-old woman underwent a liver biopsy during evalu-ation of abnormal liver test results 1 week ago. Liver biopsy showed mild autoimmune hepatitis with minimal hepatic fi-brosis. This morning she had sudden onset of abdominal pain and distention, with light-headedness and diaphoresis; subse-quently she had a large bowel movement with melenic stool. Which of the following is the most likely cause of the patient's clinical presentation?

a. Hepatic vein thrombosis
b. Portal vein thrombosis
c. Hepatic artery thrombosis
d. Hepatic artery aneurysm
e. Hepatic artery–portal vein fistula

VI.21. A 29-year-old woman is brought to the emergency depart-ment by ambulance after being found unresponsive. She has a history of polysubstance use with multiple hospitalizations for intoxication. After fluid resuscitation she is alert but disoriented. Physical examination findings are notable for signs of injection drug use. Laboratory test results are no-table for markedly increased aminotransferase levels (AST 8,500 U/L; ALT 9,700 U/L). After she is admitted to the hospital, her condition improves. The next day, her liver enzyme values have improved (AST 3,000 U/L; ALT 4,500 U/L). Urine drug screening is positive for alcohol and meth-amphetamine. She feels better and is requesting to leave the hospital. What is the most likely cause of her abnormal liver tests?

a. Alcohol-associated hepatitis
b. Ischemic hepatopathy
c. Acute hepatitis A
d. Acute hepatitis B
e. Acute hepatitis C

VI.22. A 52-year-old woman is referred for evaluation of high liver test values. She has obesity (BMI 36) and type 2 diabetes. She consumes 2 or 3 alcoholic beverages a week. Laboratory test results are shown below:

Component	Result
Hemoglobin, g/dL	11.2
MCV, fL	92.3
Platelet count, $\times 10^9$/L	187
ALT, U/L	62
AST, U/L	53
ALP, U/L	117
INR	1.0

Liver stiffness is 15 kPa on transient elastography, and hepatic steatosis is apparent on ultrasonography. What should you advise for variceal screening?

a. Perform CT of the abdomen and pelvis with an intravenous contrast agent
b. Proceed with EGD now
c. Monitor platelet count and transient elastography annually
d. Start primary prophylaxis with NSBB therapy

VI.23. A 63-year-old woman presents for evaluation of compensated cirrhosis secondary to NASH. Her medical history is significant for hypertension, type 2 diabetes, hyperlipidemia, and obesity (BMI 33). Laboratory test results are shown below:

Component	Result
Platelet count, ×10⁹/L	130
AST, U/L	52
ALT, U/L	58
INR	1.3
Total bilirubin, mg/dL	1.9

Ultrasonography shows hepatic steatosis, and EGD findings are normal. Which of the following should you recommend to screen for varices?

a. Repeat EGD in 3 years
b. Repeat EGD in 2 years
c. Start NSBB therapy to prevent development of varices
d. Recommend annual transient elastography and follow-up EGD if liver stiffness exceeds 20 kPa

VI.24. A 42-year-old man with cirrhosis due to alcohol use presents with hematemesis. He has hypotension (blood pressure 83/56 mm Hg) and a heart rate of 112 beats/min. Laboratory test results include the following: hemoglobin 7.2 g/dL, platelet count 59×10⁹/L, INR 1.9, and total bilirubin 3.1 mg/dL. He is intubated and admitted to the intensive care unit. Which of the following is the best next step in management of this patient's bleeding?

a. Transfusion of packed red blood cells
b. Urgent TIPS
c. Fresh frozen plasma and then EGD
d. Proton pump inhibitor, octreotide, and antibiotics

VI.25. A 68-year-old woman with cirrhosis due to α₁-antitrypsin deficiency presents for evaluation of anemia. Laboratory test results are shown below:

Component	Result
Hemoglobin, g/dL	7.1
MCV, fL	77.7
Platelet count, ×10⁹/L	67
INR	1.4
Total bilirubin, mg/dL	1.8
Creatinine, mg/dL	1.1

On EGD, antral red spots in a linear pattern suggest GAVE. Which of the following should you recommend to stop the bleeding?

a. TIPS
b. NSBB
c. Surgical portosystemic shunt
d. Argon plasma coagulation

VI.26. A 52-year-old man with alcohol-related cirrhosis presents to the emergency department with confusion. He has a history of esophageal variceal hemorrhage, ascites, and a prior episode of overt HE. His medications include furosemide,

spironolactone, lactulose, nadolol, and zinc. Laboratory test results are shown below:

Component	Result
Hemoglobin, g/dL	8.0
WBC count, ×10⁹/L	4.5
Platelet count, ×10⁹/L	70
Albumin, g/dL	2.5
Total bilirubin, mg/dL	2.0
INR	1.7
Creatinine, mg/dL	0.8

On paracentesis, the WBC count is 700 cells/μL, with 40% PMNs. What is the best next step in management?

a. Discontinue nadolol
b. Perform EGD to evaluate for recurrent bleeding in the gastrointestinal tract
c. Start rifaximin 550 mg orally every 12 hours
d. Start cefotaxime 2 g intravenously every 8 hours

VI.27. A 62-year-old woman with cirrhosis secondary to primary biliary cholangitis reports ongoing abdominal distention. For 5 months she has had ascites, which was previously drained, and she does not have a history of gastrointestinal tract bleeding or HE. She reports that her ascites has improved only partially with diuretics that her primary care doctor prescribed 3 months ago. Her medications include furosemide 80 mg daily and spironolactone 200 mg daily. On examination, she has no jaundice or asterixis. She has bulging flanks, shifting dullness, and peripheral edema but no fluid wave or tense ascites. Laboratory test results include the following: creatinine 0.8 mg/dL, sodium 132 mmol/L, and potassium 5.1 mmol/L. What is the best next step in management?

a. Refer the patient to a dietitian
b. Increase furosemide to 120 mg daily
c. Refer the patient to a tertiary center to consider TIPS
d. Perform large-volume paracentesis

VI.28. A 74-year-old man presents with new-onset ascites. He has not received regular care from a medical professional throughout his adult life, and he has a history of untreated hypertension and obstructive sleep apnea. The serum albumin level is 3 g/dL. Ascitic fluid analysis shows the following: albumin 1.4 g/dL, total protein 2.8 g/dL, and WBC count 200 cells/μL with 40% PMNs. What is the best next step in his management?

a. Initiate therapy with furosemide and spironolactone
b. Order a transthoracic echocardiographic examination
c. Start cefotaxime 2 g intravenously every 8 hours
d. Order an upper endoscopic examination for variceal screening

VI.29. A 66-year-old woman has alcohol-associated cirrhosis with diuretic-responsive ascites. She presents to the emergency department feeling dehydrated. Her medications include levothyroxine 88 μg daily, furosemide 100 mg daily, and spironolactone 40 mg daily. Her heart rate is 78 beats/min, and her blood pressure is 105/50 mm Hg. Laboratory test results are shown below:

Component	Result
Hemoglobin, g/dL	9.2
WBC count, ×10⁹/L	4.8
Platelet count, ×10⁹/L	88
Albumin, g/dL	2.5
Total bilirubin, mg/dL	2.0
INR	1.3
Creatinine, mg/dL	1.9

The creatinine value (1.9 mg/dL) was increased from 0.6 mg/dL 1 week ago. On diagnostic paracentesis, the WBC count is 100 cells/μL with 10% PMNs. Urinalysis shows no proteinuria or other abnormality. What is the best next step in management?

a. Fluid resuscitation with normal saline (0.9% sodium chloride) 1 L intravenously
b. Midodrine and octreotide
c. Urgent evaluation for liver transplant
d. Administration of 25% albumin 1 g/kg intravenously daily and discontinuation of diuretics

VI.30. A 63-year-old woman is referred for further evaluation of high liver enzyme values, which were identified during routine health screening. Laboratory test results include the following: CBC normal, total and direct bilirubin levels normal, AST 103 U/L, ALT 49 U/L, and ALP 112 U/L. Her medical history is notable for hypothyroidism, hypertension, and obstructive sleep apnea. She does not have a family history of liver disease or iron storage disorders. She consumes approximately 2 or 3 alcoholic beverages daily on most days. On physical examination she has central obesity without stigmata of chronic liver disease. Additional laboratory studies include negative results for hepatitis B and hepatitis C serologies, normal α$_1$-antitrypsin genotype, transferrin saturation 39%, and serum ferritin 480 μg/L. What is the most likely diagnosis?

a. Hereditary hemochromatosis
b. NAFLD
c. Alcohol-related liver disease
d. Wilson disease
e. Ferroportin disease

VI.31. A 19-year-old college student is brought to the emergency department by his roommate because of jaundice and altered mental status. He had been feeling unwell with nonspecific symptoms for the past 3 or 4 days. He has no previous medical history. He typically consumes 2 or 3 beers on weekend nights but has not had anything to drink since he began feeling unwell. The patient has not used recreational drugs, but he does have a new sexual partner. He has not traveled outside the state this semester. On examination, he is drowsy and difficult to arouse, he has intense jaundice, and he has asterixis. He does not have palpable ascites. Notable laboratory test results are shown below:

Component	Result
Hemoglobin, g/dL	8.6
INR	2.8
Total bilirubin, mg/dL	13.2
Direct bilirubin, mg/dL	4.5
AST, U/L	109
ALT, U/L	128
ALP, U/L	75

Results of abdominal ultrasonography and additional serologies, including laboratory tests for viral hepatitis, are pending. What is the most likely diagnosis?

a. Acute BCS
b. Acute hepatitis A
c. Acute hepatitis B
d. Wilson disease
e. Alcohol-related hepatitis

VI.32. A 54-year-old man presents for evaluation because his older brother recently received a diagnosis of cirrhosis secondary to hemochromatosis. The patient has no symptoms and does not consume alcohol. He is an avid runner and has been training for a marathon without any cardiopulmonary symptoms. Laboratory tests are notable for normal CBC results and normal levels of bilirubin and albumin; increased values for AST (204 U/L), ALT (284 U/L), and transferrin saturation (64%); and a ferritin level of 692 μg/L. *HFE* gene testing confirms 2 copies of the C282Y alteration. What should you advise next?

a. Begin therapeutic phlebotomy weekly
b. Begin therapeutic phlebotomy every 3 months
c. Advise the patient to follow a strict low-iron diet
d. Initiate treatment with deferasirox
e. Initiate treatment with trientene

VI.33. A 21-year-old man is being evaluated for recently diagnosed cardiomyopathy. Liver test results were high (AST 185 U/L and ALT 215 U/L). Results of serologic evaluation show the following: normal CBC and normal levels of bilirubin, albumin, and ceruloplasmin level; and elevated results of iron tests (transferrin saturation 75% and ferritin 893 μg/L). What is the most likely diagnosis?

a. Acute viral hepatitis
b. Wilson disease
c. Hereditary hemochromatosis (*HFE* alteration)
d. Juvenile hemochromatosis (*HJV* alteration)
e. Ferroportin disease

VI.34. A 55-year-old man presents with high levels of liver enzymes (ALT 68 U/L, AST 97 U/L, ALP 165 U/L, and total bilirubin 0.8 mg/dL). His BMI is 31, and during the past 10 years he has been drinking 2 or 3 beers daily. Results from the other laboratory investigations are unremarkable, except for the iron studies (iron 250 μg/dL, ferritin 988 μg/L, and transferrin saturation 95%). Ultrasonography shows hepatomegaly and normal spleen size. What is the best next step in management?

a. Liver biopsy for iron quantification
b. MRI with elastography for measurement of hepatic iron concentration
c. *HFE* genetic testing
d. Counseling for 10% weight loss and alcohol abstinence

VI.35. You are examining a 16-year-old adolescent boy, who is accompanied by his parents, for right upper quadrant pain. An incidental finding is increased values for liver enzymes. The ceruloplasmin level is 20 mg/dL, and the 24-hour urine copper level is 120 μg. What is the best next step in management?

a. Ophthalmologic referral for assessment for Kayser-Fleischer rings
b. Liver biopsy for copper quantification
c. Testing for serum copper level
d. Genetic testing for *ATP7B* variants

VI.36. You have made a definitive diagnosis of Wilson disease in a patient and want to start treatment. What are the potential complications from treatment?

a. Acute liver failure
b. New-onset extrapyramidal symptoms
c. Sideroblastic anemia
d. Myelopathy with weakness and ataxia

VI.37. A patient with increased liver enzyme levels has been referred to you for evaluation. The laboratory test results include the following: ALT 68 U/L, AST 78 U/L, ALP 115 U/L, and total bilirubin 0.7 mg/dL. The other results are unremarkable. You perform a complete evaluation for causes of chronic liver disease. The α$_1$-antitrypsin level is low

(75 mg/dL). What is the most likely diagnosis and the best next step in management?

a. Pi*ZZ phenotype; liver biopsy to assess for globules with periodic acid-Schiff–diastase staining and for staging of fibrosis
b. Pi*ZZ phenotype; pulmonary function tests to assess for emphysema
c. Pi*MZ phenotype; noninvasive testing for fibrosis
d. Pi*MZ phenotype; screening ultrasonography for HCC

VI.38. A 52-year-old woman presents with pruritus and fatigue. She is otherwise healthy and does not use medications or supplements. Liver test results are as follows: ALT 134 U/L, AST 72 U/L, ALP 653 U/L, and total bilirubin 1.1 mg/dL. Abdominal ultrasonographic findings are normal. What is the best next step in management?

a. ERCP
b. AMA testing
c. Liver biopsy
d. MRCP

VI.39. A 22-year-old man recently received a diagnosis of PSC. He is asymptomatic and has 1 formed, nonbloody bowel movement daily. Laboratory test results are shown below:

Component	Result
ALT, U/L	155
AST, U/L	172
ALP, U/L	1,053
Total bilirubin, mg/dL	0.8
INR	1.1
Hemoglobin, g/dL	9.0
WBC count, ×10⁹/L	4.5
Platelet count, ×10⁹/L	356

MRCP shows multifocal biliary strictures involving the intrahepatic ducts. What is the best next step?

a. Refer for liver transplant evaluation
b. Start therapy with ursodeoxycholic acid (28-30 mg/kg in divided doses)
c. Perform abdominal ultrasonography
d. Perform colonoscopy with random biopsies

VI.40. A 67-year-old woman with PBC was recently referred to your clinic. Three months ago, she tripped on carpet in her home, fell, and fractured her right hip. She underwent an uncomplicated right hip replacement. What is the best next step in management?

a. Start supplementation with calcium (1,500 mg daily) and vitamin D (800 IU daily)
b. Check ionized calcium levels
c. Begin therapy with a bisphosphonate
d. Perform bone densitometry

VI.41. You are evaluating a 32-year-old man with asymptomatic cholestasis and a history of ulcerative colitis. Liver test results are as follows: ALT 52 U/L, AST 47 U/L, ALP 563 U/L, and total bilirubin 1.0 mg/dL. AMA test results are negative and MRCP findings are normal. What is the most likely diagnosis?

a. HIV-related cholangiopathy
b. Large-duct PSC
c. Small-duct PSC
d. PBC

VI.42. A 28-year-old woman has a known history of seasonal allergies. She received a diagnosis of peritonsillar abscess 1 month ago when she presented to the primary care clinic with acute cough, fever, and severe sore throat. She received a 10-day course of amoxicillin-clavulanate, and her symptoms improved. However, jaundice, generalized itching, low-grade fever, fatigue, and nausea developed over the past 2 days. She does not have abdominal pain or confusion. Laboratory tests show abnormal values for ALP (650 U/L) and total bilirubin (10 mg/dL) and normal values for AST, ALT, albumin, INR, and the CBC. Results were negative for ANA, AMA, and ASMA. Viral hepatitis serology results were unremarkable. What is the best next step in management?

a. Initiate a short course of prednisone 40 mg daily with taper dosing
b. Proceed with a liver biopsy
c. Proceed with evaluation for liver transplant
d. Provide conservative management with close monitoring of her liver profile

VI.43. A 62-year-old woman has a known history of hypertension, type 2 diabetes, obesity, and recurrent urinary tract infections requiring several courses of antibiotics over the past year. She presented to her primary care physician with dysuria and lower abdominal discomfort for 3 days. Urinalysis confirmed a urinary tract infection, and she was prescribed nitrofurantoin 100 mg twice daily for 7 days. She also took acetaminophen 325 mg twice daily as needed. She continued to take metformin and amlodipine as her regular home medications. A few weeks later, she presents with fatigue, jaundice, and nausea. Blood work results include serum ALT, 1,250 U/L; ALP, 142 U/L; and total bilirubin, 3.3 mg/dL. ANA is present (1:160), and globulin levels are mildly elevated. Viral hepatitis serology results are unremarkable. What is the best next step in management?

a. Recommend a liver biopsy
b. Initiate prednisone 40 mg daily
c. Stop nitrofurantoin
d. Recommend abdominal Doppler ultrasonography

VI.44. A 50-year-old man presents with a known history of coronary artery disease, hypertension, type 2 diabetes, and hyperlipidemia. He takes lisinopril, metoprolol, and metformin. He began taking atorvastatin 1 month earlier. He has adhered to his medical therapy, and he does not have any new symptoms. He drinks alcohol 4 times a week. At an annual evaluation, he had increased values for AST (70 U/L) and ALT (74 U/L). Otherwise, results were unremarkable for ALP, total bilirubin, a CBC, and a kidney profile. Abdominal ultrasonography showed a hyperechoic liver consistent with fatty liver but otherwise no liver masses or biliary ductal dilatation. What is the best next step in management?

a. Withhold atorvastatin and monitor the liver enzymes
b. Stop alcohol consumption and recommend liver biopsy to confirm the diagnosis of steatohepatitis
c. Continue atorvastatin
d. Recommend magnetic resonance elastography to assess the stage of fibrosis

VI.45. A 40-year-old man presents to the emergency department of a community hospital with abdominal pain, nausea, and vomiting. A year ago, he had acute cholecystitis, for which he underwent laparoscopic cholecystectomy; however, he states that his current symptoms are different. Earlier this week, he had flulike symptoms and myalgia. He has been taking 2 extra-strength acetaminophen tablets 3 or 4 times daily to help him finish an important project he is working on. The last dose of acetaminophen was before his presentation to the emergency department. He also states that he has been drinking a couple beers each night to help with his stressful job. On physical examination, he appears ill but is awake and alert. Blood work results at presentation showed an unremarkable CBC but increases in AST (3,500 U/L), ALT

(2,500 U/L), INR (3.5), and total bilirubin (2.2 mg/dL). The creatinine level is 2 mg/dL. Results for the acetaminophen level and viral hepatitis serology are pending. Findings from abdominal ultrasonography are unremarkable. What is the best next step in management?

a. Wait for the acetaminophen level results before considering intravenous *N*-acetylcysteine
b. Administer penicillin G
c. Recommend intravenous corticosteroids for 7 days
d. Administer activated charcoal and intravenous *N*-acetylcysteine, and monitor the patient in the hospital

VI.46. A 55-year-old man with a past medical history of type 2 diabetes and hypertension presents for evaluation of increased liver enzyme levels detected during a routine annual visit. He does not consume alcohol. His medications include lisinopril and metformin. On physical examination, his blood pressure is 132/89 mm Hg, and he appears well. His BMI is 36. He has obesity, but abdominal examination findings are otherwise normal. Laboratory test results are shown below:

Component	Result
ALT, U/L	55
AST, U/L	40
ALP, U/L	90
Total bilirubin, mg/dL	1.0
Hemoglobin A$_{1c}$,%	8.5
Lipid profile	Normal
Hepatitis A and C serology	Negative
Hepatitis B core and surface antibodies	Positive
Hepatitis B surface antigen	Negative
Serum IgG	Normal
ANA	1:160

Ultrasonography of the liver showed increased echogenicity consistent with hepatic steatosis. What is the most likely diagnosis?

a. Chronic hepatitis B
b. NAFLD
c. Autoimmune hepatitis
d. PBC

VI.47. A 19-year-old woman presents with recent-onset fatigue and scleral icterus. She has a history of acne and recently completed a course of minocycline 2 weeks before the onset of symptoms. On examination she has scleral icterus and jaundice without other abnormal findings. Laboratory tests 6 months ago showed normal liver values. Current laboratory test results are shown below:

Component	Result
Total bilirubin, mg/dL	6.1
Direct bilirubin, mg/dL	5.0
ALT, U/L	624
AST, U/L	510
ALP, U/L	180
IgG, mg/dL	1,400
INR	1.2
Epstein-Barr virus	Negative
Hepatitis A, B, and C	Negative
ASMA, ANA, and anti-LKM	Normal

Abdominal ultrasonographic findings are normal. Liver biopsy shows mild interface hepatitis and plasma cell infiltration of the hepatic parenchyma. There is no evidence of fibrosis. What is the best next step?

a. Avoid use of minocycline in the future, and start prednisone therapy with subsequent taper
b. Start therapy with prednisone and azathioprine
c. Refer the patient for liver transplant evaluation
d. Assess AMA

VI.48. A 28-year-old woman presents with fatigue, scleral icterus, and mild constant discomfort in the right upper quadrant of her abdomen. The symptoms began 6 months earlier. At that time ALT was 500 U/L, ALP was 125 U/L, and total bilirubin was 3.1 mg/dL. No additional testing was performed at that time. One year earlier she recalled being told that her aminotransferase levels were high, but they had been normal on routine testing when she was 25 years old. Five years ago, when she received a diagnosis of hypothyroidism and celiac sprue, she began therapy with levothyroxine; since then, she has adhered to a gluten-free diet. She does not use alcohol, supplements, or other medications. On examination she has scleral icterus and jaundice. Current laboratory test results are shown below:

Component	Result
ALT, U/L	567
AST, U/L	450
ALP, U/L	189
Total bilirubin, mg/dL	4.5
Direct bilirubin, mg/dL	4.0
INR	1.2
Albumin, g/dL	3.6
Ferritin, µg/L	300
Transferrin saturation, %	22
IgG, mg/dL	7,620

Results for the following are normal or negative: thyrotropin, hepatitis B surface antigen, hepatitis C antibody, ANA, SMA, AMA, ceruloplasmin, tissue transglutaminase IgA, serum IgA, and α$_1$-antitrypsin. Abdominal ultrasonography shows nonspecific coarsening of the liver parenchyma without ductal dilation or splenomegaly. A liver biopsy shows moderate inflammation with a lymphoplasmacytic infiltrate and interface hepatitis with stage 3 fibrosis. What is the most likely cause of the increased liver test values?

a. Celiac sprue
b. Hemochromatosis
c. Drug-induced liver injury
d. Autoimmune hepatitis

VI.49. A 48-year-old woman presents to your office for routine follow-up and reports no problems. She received a diagnosis of autoimmune hepatitis 7 months ago when she presented with jaundice. Test results at that time showed the following:

Component	Result
Total bilirubin, mg/dL	8.5
ALT, U/L	1,005
AST, U/L	905
ALP, U/L	200
ANA	1:1,280
SMA	1:320
IgG, mg/dL	7,620

Results from laboratory investigations for other causes of chronic liver disease were unremarkable. At that time, she did not use medications or supplements, and a liver biopsy showed severe inflammation with lymphoplasmacytic infiltrate, areas of necrosis, and interface activity. Bridging fibrosis was also present. Prednisone therapy was initiated, and the laboratory

test results improved. Azathioprine was added several weeks later, and the prednisone dose was slowly tapered as the liver test results improved. Three months ago, the liver test results were normal, and prednisone was decreased to 10 mg daily. Now she takes azathioprine 50 mg daily and prednisone 5 mg daily. Results of the physical examination, CBC, and blood glucose and liver tests are normal. What is the best next step?

a. Stop prednisone therapy and continue use of azathioprine 50 mg daily
b. Discontinue use of azathioprine but continue prednisone therapy
c. Start mycophenolate mofetil therapy (1,000 mg twice daily) and discontinue use of azathioprine and prednisone
d. Discontinue use of azathioprine and prednisone and monitor laboratory results for relapse

VI.50. A 50-year-old man is referred to you for evaluation of unexplained elevated liver enzymes for the past 6 months. Laboratory test results are shown below:

Component	Result
AST, U/L	70
ALT, U/L	84
ALP, U/L	90
Total bilirubin, mg/dL	0.9
Serum albumin, g/dL	4.0
CBC	Normal
Hepatitis B surface antigen	Negative
Hepatitis B surface antibody	Positive
Hepatitis B core antibody, total	Negative
Hepatitis C antibody	Negative
ANA	1:40
ASMA	Negative
AMA	Negative
Iron studies	Normal
α_1-Antitrypsin phenotype	MM

Ultrasonography of the liver shows an enlarged, echogenic liver with patent portal and hepatic veins and no radiographic signs of portal hypertension or cirrhosis. Physical examination findings are notable for central obesity (BMI, 39) in a man who appears well otherwise. His past medical history includes diagnoses of type 2 diabetes, hypertension, and obstructive sleep apnea. His medications include metformin and hydrochlorothiazide. He has not used any alcohol since his 20s. What is the best next step in management?

a. Prescribe prednisone for autoimmune hepatitis
b. Perform EGD to look for varices
c. Perform liver biopsy
d. Reassure the patient and repeat the tests in 4 weeks

VI.51. A 60-year-old man with obesity and type 2 diabetes receives a diagnosis of NASH with stage F3 fibrosis according to liver biopsy results. What is the most common cause of death among patients with NASH?

a. Liver cancer
b. Other malignancies
c. Cardiovascular disease
d. Infection

VI.52. A 60-year-old woman underwent a liver biopsy for persistent, slightly increased liver test values. Biopsy findings showed histologic features typical of NASH with stage 1 fibrosis. Her past medical history is notable for obesity (BMI, 32), hypertension, and hyperlipidemia (LDL cholesterol, 90 mg/dL). Her hemoglobin A_{1c} is 5.9%, and she drinks 2 or 3 glasses of wine weekly. In addition to adopting lifestyle interventions to achieve a weight loss of 5% to 10%, she wants to know

what treatments are available for her condition. Which of the following statements is true?

a. Initiation of statin therapy is safe despite the increased liver test values
b. Alcohol cessation counseling should be considered
c. Prophylactic use of metformin is beneficial for NASH
d. A ketogenic diet is recommended for NASH

VI.53. In which of the following genes are variants protective against the development of advanced fibrosis in NAFLD?

a. *PNPLA3*
b. *MBOAT7*
c. *TM6SF2*
d. *HSD17B13*

VI.54. A 25-year-old woman who is pregnant for the first time presents during the 35th week of gestation with abdominal pain, nausea, and vomiting for 2 days. Her blood pressure is 140/90 mm Hg. She is somnolent; she does not have jaundice. Pertinent laboratory test results are shown below:

Component	Result
Hemoglobin, g/dL	11.3
Platelet count, ×10⁹/L	140
AST, U/L	180
ALT, U/L	238
Bilirubin, mg/dL	0.9
INR	2.0
Creatinine, mg/dL	1.5
Lactate dehydrogenase, U/L	250
Glucose, mg/dL	55

What is the best next step for management?

a. Test for viral hepatitis
b. Continue to monitor with liver tests and other laboratory tests
c. Control the patient's blood pressure
d. Proceed with a prompt delivery

VI.55. A 30-year-old pregnant woman with a gestational age of 14 weeks presents to the emergency department with a new onset of right upper quadrant abdominal pain for the past 2 hours. The pain started approximately 1 hour after her dinner. Laboratory results are unremarkable except for ALT of 78 U/L. Abdominal ultrasonography shows cholelithiasis without biliary duct dilatation. The pain subsided in the emergency department during evaluation. What is the best next step for management?

a. Proceed with cholecystectomy
b. Conservative management
c. Proceed with MRCP to rule out biliary obstruction given the abnormal value for ALT
d. Proceed with ERCP

VI.56. A 28-year-old woman was found to have hepatitis B infection about 1 year ago. She does not have cirrhosis and has not received any antiviral treatment. She is pregnant with a gestational age of 14 weeks. She was referred from her primary care provider to you for advice. Her mother and her other 2 siblings also have chronic hepatitis B. She feels well. She is aware that her newborn child should receive both HBV vaccine and hepatitis B immunoglobulin. Her laboratory test results include a platelet count of 300×10⁹/L and ALT of 12 U/L. Results are positive for hepatitis B surface antigen, hepatitis B core antibody, and hepatitis B e antigen. The level of HBV DNA is 10⁶ IU/mL. What should you advise this patient?

a. Start lamivudine now
b. Start tenofovir now

c. Repeat the tests for HBV DNA and ALT in 3 months and decide whether antiviral treatment is indicated at that time

d. No further testing is indicated until after pregnancy

VI.57. **A 26-year-old woman with a history of autoimmune hepatitis has just found out that she is pregnant. Her gestational age is approximately 8 weeks. She does not have cirrhosis, and her autoimmune hepatitis has been in remission during the past year. Her current treatment is monotherapy with azathioprine 150 mg once daily. She feels well. Laboratory test results include AST 15 U/L and ALT 20 U/L. She presents to your clinic to discuss medication management during her pregnancy. What should you advise this patient?**

a. Continue therapy with azathioprine

b. Change the therapy from azathioprine to prednisone, and plan to continue use of prednisone throughout the pregnancy

c. Stop the azathioprine therapy, and do not use any medication during the pregnancy because autoimmune diseases tend to become less active during pregnancy

d. Stop the azathioprine therapy and restart it during the second trimester

VI.58. **A 66-year-old man has a known history of chronic hepatitis C cirrhosis. When he received direct-acting antiviral therapy for chronic hepatitis C infection, genotype 1, he had a sustained virologic response. He is asymptomatic and has no ascites, encephalopathy, or evidence of bleeding in the gastrointestinal tract. He is presenting for routine follow-up for HCC screening. His MELD score is 10. Recent upper endoscopy showed grade 2 esophageal varices. The alpha fetoprotein level is 320 ng/mL. Ultrasonography of the abdomen shows a liver mass. CT of the abdomen provided confirmation of a 4-cm mass in the right hepatic lobe. The mass shows arterial enhancement with portal venous washout. Hepatic vessels are patent without thrombosis. CT of the chest and a bone scan show no evidence of metastatic disease. What is the best next step in management?**

a. Biopsy of the lesion under ultrasonographic guidance to confirm the diagnosis

b. Administration of sorafenib 400 mg orally twice daily

c. Evaluation for liver transplant

d. Interventional radiology consultation for transarterial embolization of the tumor before surgical consultation for resection

VI.59. **A 62-year-old woman with a known history of PBC presents to the general hepatology clinic for a scheduled follow-up. Her liver biopsy 2 years ago showed cirrhosis. She has not had hepatic encephalopathy, variceal bleeding, or ascites. Her main symptoms are fatigue, pruritus, and leg edema. Her current MELD score is 17. What is the best next step in management?**

a. Recommend ultrasonography of the abdomen every 6 months for HCC screening because she has PBC

b. Recommend an annual bone density scan

c. Postpone liver transplant evaluation until her MELD score is greater than 20

d. Proceed with liver transplant evaluation

VI.60. **A 70-year-old man underwent deceased-donor liver transplant 1 year ago for NASH. He has been receiving immunosuppressive therapy with tacrolimus. Odynophagia developed recently, and upper endoscopy showed candidal esophagitis, for which he was prescribed fluconazole. He called the transplant clinic this morning and reported an acute, worsening headache and vomiting but no light-headedness or presyncope. On presentation the physical examination findings were remarkable for new tremors in both hands, and he appeared anxious. Results from liver profile testing were unremarkable, but the creatinine level increased to 2.0 mg/dL from 1.2 mg/dL 1 month before. Results for tacrolimus trough level are pending. What is the best next step in management?**

a. Liver biopsy

b. Doppler ultrasonography of the abdomen

c. CT of the head

d. Withhold tacrolimus therapy

VI.61. **A 54-year-old man underwent deceased-donor liver transplant for cirrhosis secondary to chronic hepatitis C. He received chronic hepatitis C therapy before liver transplant and had a sustained virologic response. He was discharged home within a week with no immediate complications. He presents to the liver transplant clinic 4 weeks after liver transplant. His CBC results are similar to previous results. Liver test results, which are increased compared to results from 1 week before, are as follows: total bilirubin, 2.2 mg/dL; ALT, 195 U/L; AST, 210 U/L; and ALP, 305 U/L. Findings from Doppler ultrasonography of the liver were unremarkable except for mild steatosis. The patient describes adherence to the tacrolimus regimen, and his current tacrolimus trough level is 3.0 ng/mL. What is the most likely diagnosis?**

a. Recurrent hepatitis C infection

b. Acute cellular rejection

c. Hepatic artery thrombosis

d. Cytomegalovirus infection

Answers

VI.1. Answer d.

The patient presents with increased liver test results and symptoms compatible with a recent viral infection. The symptoms and lymphocytosis would be compatible with infectious mononucleosis, most likely due to Epstein-Barr virus. Minocycline can cause a drug-induced liver injury that mimics autoimmune hepatitis, but that would be less likely than an infection to explain the sore throat, fever, and enlarged lymph nodes. Wilson disease should always be considered when a patient presents with acute liver disease, but that would not explain the symptoms, which suggest infection. Lymphoma can result in fever and abnormal liver test results but would be less likely than infectious mononucleosis for explaining an acute syndrome that includes sore throat. Acetaminophen hepatic toxicity produces much higher liver enzyme levels than present in this patient. In addition, 2 g of acetaminophen daily is unlikely to cause liver injury.

VI.2. Answer c.

Acute biliary obstruction, usually from a stone, can produce markedly increased levels of aminotransferases, and the clinical presentation, gallbladder stones, and positive blood cultures would be compatible with acute cholangitis. According to guidelines, the patient should undergo ERCP directly. Both endoscopic ultrasonography and MRCP are reasonable options, but when clinical suspicion is high, as in this case, it is best to proceed directly with ERCP. Laparoscopic cholecystectomy should be considered after her episode of acute cholangitis resolves. In the absence of clinical features suggestive of portal hypertension, Doppler ultrasonography of the hepatic vasculature would be unnecessary.

VI.3. Answer b.

This asymptomatic patient has a cholestatic liver disease and evidence of lymphadenopathy with interstitial lung disease. This constellation of findings suggests sarcoidosis. Amyloidosis can present as intrahepatic cholestasis, but patients usually are more ill with abnormalities of the CBC. PSC would be a consideration if the patient had a history of ulcerative colitis. PBC is more common in women than in men. Celiac disease should be excluded in patients with chronic liver disease but would be unlikely to explain the pulmonary findings.

VI.4. Answer a.

The marked AST out of proportion to the ALT is suggestive of muscle injury. Severe muscle injury, as can occur with polymyositis or rhabdomyolysis, may produce enough muscle injury to cause an increase in ALT. ALT has a longer half-life than AST; therefore, improvements occur less rapidly than for AST. Liver disease associated with alcohol produces an increased AST to ALT ratio, but the AST is rarely over 400 U/L and would certainly not be increased to this extent. Acute viral hepatitis would produce an ALT that is generally the same or slightly higher than the AST. Acetaminophen hepatic toxicity and hepatic ischemia produce markedly increased levels of aminotransferases, but the ALT is elevated to a similar range as the AST.

VI.5. Answer d.

Grazoprevir, glecaprevir, and voxilaprevir are all NS3/4A protease inhibitors, which are contraindicated in patients with decompensated cirrhosis because of the risk of worsening hepatic decompensation. Sofosbuvir and the NS5A inhibitors (including ledipasvir) are safe to use in patients with decompensated cirrhosis, although they are most often used in patients who have MELD scores of 20 or less.

VI.6. Answer e.

The positive findings for HBsAg and IgM anti-HBc are consistent with acute hepatitis B infection. This patient has acute liver injury but not acute liver failure given the absence of hepatic encephalopathy and coagulopathy. Therefore, neither liver transplant nor *N*-acetylcysteine is appropriate. Treatment of hepatitis B is not indicated given that more than 95% of adults with acute hepatitis B recover spontaneously and do not require specific treatment. Oral antiviral drugs are recommended (in addition to urgent listing for liver transplant) for patients who have acute HBV infection with acute liver failure or severe, protracted (>4 weeks) symptoms.

VI.7. Answer b.

This patient has evidence of chronic hepatitis B with a positive surface antigen. Hepatitis B has been reported to reactivate during treatment of hepatitis C with DAA therapy. Although 29 cases of HBV reactivation, including 2 patients who died and 1 patient who required liver transplant, were initially reported to the US Food and Drug Administration, this is not unique to a particular DAA regimen and occurs at 4 to 8 weeks. Most of the patients had positive results for HBsAg and a low level of HBV DNA. One patient had an isolated anti-HBc. The recommendation is to test for HBsAg, anti-HBs, and anti-HBc at baseline and to check HBV DNA in patients who have positive results for HBsAg. Hepatitis B treatment or vaccination should be determined according to standard guidelines. HBV DNA should be monitored about every 4 weeks if results are positive for HBV DNA at baseline. Antiviral treatment should be initiated if the HBV DNA level increases more than 10 times or exceeds 1,000 IU/mL in a patient who has undetectable or unquantifiable levels of HBV DNA before DAA treatment.

VI.8. Answer d.

The interaction between amiodarone and sofosbuvir-containing regimens can result in serious bradycardia requiring a pacemaker or in death. Amiodarone therapy is an absolute contraindication for the use of sofosbuvir-containing regimens.

VI.9. Answer c.

Masses that show rapid arterial phase enhancement and a return to the isointensity of the surrounding liver in the portal venous phase are most likely either a focal nodular hyperplasia or a hepatic adenoma. Because they contain biliary elements, focal nodular hyperplasias retain contrast material in the biliary phase of MRI with gadoxetate. Because hepatic adenomas consist of sheets of hepatocytes with naked arteries but no biliary elements, they do not retain contrast material in the biliary phase of multiphasic imaging. Hepatic hemangiomas show peripheral nodular enhancement of the mass that fills in during the portal venous and delayed phases of the imaging study. Intrahepatic cholangiocarcinomas show moderate enhancement in the arterial phase that increases progressively during the portal venous and delayed phases of imaging.

VI.10. Answer c.

The recommended age for starting surveillance for HCC in persons with chronic hepatitis B without cirrhosis depends on the person's region of birth and sex. For Asian men, the recommended age for initiation of surveillance is 40 years. For persons (male or female) born in Africa, 20 years is the recommended age for surveillance initiation, and for women born in Asia, 50 years is the recommended age. Age 30 years is not a recommended age for surveillance initiation for any group of persons.

VI.11. Answer b.

Laparoscopic decompression and unroofing or fenestration of a cyst wall is usually definitive therapy for a large or recurrent simple cyst. A second cyst aspiration and sclerosis is less likely to succeed as the sclerosant causes thickening of the cyst walls, and it becomes more difficult to completely empty and collapse the cyst. Diuretic therapy typically has no effect on the cyst volume. Liver transplant may be required for patients with progressive adult polycystic liver disease whose functional status is severely compromised, but it typically is not indicated for a patient with a recurrent simple cyst.

VI.12. Answer b.

This patient has cirrhotic-stage PSC. The evidence of malignancy is conclusive from positive results on cytology, and FISH shows polysomy. Liver transplant after combined chemoradiation therapy (the protocol at Mayo Clinic) would offer the best chance of long-term survival. Surgical resection is generally not advised for patients with cirrhotic-stage PSC because of the likelihood of liver decompensation after surgery. Radiofrequency ablation is considered palliative therapy for patients who have inoperable biliary tract cancer. Similarly, photodynamic therapy is used as a palliative treatment.

VI.13. Answer a.

Patients who have advanced BCLC stage C HCC and are not at risk for variceal bleeding are candidates for first-line systemic therapy with atezolizumab and bevacizumab. Sorafenib is a reasonable choice for first-line treatment of patients who are not candidates for treatment with atezolizumab and bevacizumab or with the alternative first-line treatment of durvalumab in combination with tremelimumab. Best supportive care is not appropriate for this patient who still has several treatment options available. Ramucirumab is approved for second-line treatment of patients whose condition has progressed after use of first-line sorafenib and whose AFP level is 400 ng/mL or more.

VI.14. Answer b.

This patient has alcohol-related steatohepatitis. Risk factors include female sex and a history of weight loss surgery. In this scenario, considerable liver injury can occur at a lower threshold of alcohol intake, so she should abstain from drinking alcohol. The high AST:ALT ratio supports the diagnosis. Weight loss would be reasonable but is not the best answer among the choices provided. None of the information about this patient suggests that she has cholestatic liver disease or a need for ursodiol. Her liver synthetic function is preserved, so evaluation for transplant is not needed.

VI.15. Answer b.
This patient has severe alcohol-related hepatitis without cirrhosis. Patients with alcohol-related hepatitis can have a profound hepatic bruit related to dilation of the hepatic artery. The other answer choices are also causes of hepatic bruits, but they are less likely in this patient. Splenorenal shunting is unlikely without splenomegaly. HCC is unlikely in the absence of cirrhosis. A Cruveilhier-Baumgarten murmur is caused by recanalization of the umbilical vein in a person with chronic portal hypertension, which this patient does not have.

VI.16. Answer c.
This is an example of therapeutic misadventure, in which a regular user of alcohol has an intercurrent illness, stops drinking, and begins taking over-the-counter medications containing acetaminophen. Chronic alcohol exposure induces the cytochrome P450 2E1 isozyme system that also metabolizes acetaminophen to acetaldehyde, allowing for acetaminophen hepatotoxicity to occur at lower doses. Ironically, stopping alcohol use accentuates this problem. Even moderate doses of acetaminophen can cause hepatotoxicity in this scenario. COVID-19–related hepatitis is possible, but the transaminase values are increased out of proportion. Azithromycin is not a typical cause of drug-induced autoimmune-like hepatitis, and this entity also rarely causes transaminase values to increase to more than 1,000 U/L. Severe alcohol-related hepatitis is unlikely with this quantity of alcohol consumption, and other features of alcohol-related hepatitis are not present.

VI.17. Answer a.
Although acetaminophen can be hepatotoxic, acetaminophen is the analgesic of choice for patients with cirrhosis. This is true even in alcohol-related cirrhosis as long as the patient is not currently drinking alcohol. The total cumulative daily dose of acetaminophen should remain less than 2,000 mg. Nonsteroidal anti-inflammatory drugs such as ibuprofen can precipitate gastrointestinal bleeding and hepatorenal syndrome in people with cirrhosis. Opiates such as oxycodone can precipitate or worsen hepatic encephalopathy. Elective surgery would be contraindicated because of the high risk of hepatic decompensation with general anesthesia.

VI.18. Answer e.
This woman has BCS and acute (fulminant) liver failure characterized by the acute onset of jaundice, coagulopathy, and hepatic encephalopathy. For a patient with acute liver failure, the most appropriate next step is referral for urgent liver transplant. Although anticoagulation is critical in the management of BCS, this patient's condition has progressed despite anticoagulation therapy. TIPS can be used in patients who have BCS that is not responsive to anticoagulation, but it is not the best treatment if a patient has acute liver failure.

VI.19. Answer b.
This patient had an episode of upper gastrointestinal bleeding from isolated gastric varices, but he did not have a history of cirrhosis or chronic liver disease. The prior episode of pancreatitis

is a risk factor for splenic vein thrombosis, which can lead to sinistral portal hypertension. CT with a contrast agent would be the next step to assess for splenic vein thrombosis. For patients with gastric varices due to splenic vein thrombosis, splenectomy can be curative. Nonselective β-blockers such as propranolol are used for prophylaxis against bleeding in patients with portal hypertension but not for an acute situation. Gastric fundic varices are typically not amenable to endoscopic band ligation. TIPS is the treatment of choice for bleeding gastric fundic varices from cirrhosis. Liver transplant is not indicated for patients with sinistral portal hypertension.

VI.20. Answer e.
This patient had delayed gastrointestinal bleeding after a liver biopsy. The most likely cause is an iatrogenic fistula between a branch of the hepatic artery and a branch of the portal vein. Rupture of the hepatic artery branch leads to an acute increase in portal pressure with ascites and gastrointestinal tract bleeding. Although both hepatic vein thrombosis (as in BCS) and portal vein thrombosis could occur acutely, the recent liver biopsy makes the fistula more likely. The patient does not have risk factors for hepatic artery thrombosis. Patients with hepatic artery aneurysms are typically asymptomatic until the aneurysms rupture, but then hemoperitoneum and hemorrhagic shock would be the presenting signs.

VI.21. Answer b.
The pattern of extremely high liver test results (several thousand units per liter) with rapid improvement after supportive care suggests ischemic hepatopathy. The most likely cause in this patient is global hypotension and vasoconstriction from methamphetamine intoxication. The laboratory pattern does not suggest alcohol-associated hepatitis (in which aminotransferase levels are typically 200-300 U/L). Although the patient has risk factors for acute viral hepatitis, a rapid improvement in the liver tests would not be expected.

VI.22. Answer c.
This patient is presenting for evaluation of increased aminotransferase values. She does not have thrombocytopenia (platelet count >150×10⁹/L), and transient elastography does not suggest that she has clinically significant portal hypertension (liver stiffness <20 kPa). Therefore, according to the American Association for the Study of Liver Diseases guidelines, she has a low risk for large esophageal varices, and screening endoscopy can be deferred. Transient elastography and platelet count should be repeated annually. Although portosystemic collaterals can be incidentally noted on cross-sectional imaging, CT scans are not recommended to screen for varices. NSBBs have been shown to reduce the risk of first decompensation in patients with clinically significant portal hypertension; however, this patient does not have features that suggest clinically significant portal hypertension.

VI.23. Answer b.
Continued screening for varices is indicated in 2 years. The presumed cause of the cirrhosis is NASH, and this patient has obesity with features of the metabolic syndrome. For patients who have compensated cirrhosis and quiescent injury, such as hepatitis C infection that has been eradicated, the screening interval can be decreased to every 3 years. Studies suggest that NSBBs are not effective in preventing the development of varices; therefore, initiation of NSBB therapy is not warranted. This patient has thrombocytopenia, so continued endoscopic surveillance for varices is indicated.

VI.24. Answer d.
This patient's presentation is concerning for variceal bleeding. In patients with suspected variceal bleeding, after intubation and establishment of intravenous access, hemodynamic resuscitation is warranted. Guidelines recommend a conservative transfusion strategy with a hemoglobin goal of 7 g/dL to prevent portal pressure increases associated with excessive volume resuscitation. Studies have not shown benefit after transfusion of clotting factors; thus, fresh frozen plasma transfusion is not warranted. Therapy with an intravenous proton pump inhibitor and octreotide should be started without delay. Antibiotics are also warranted to prevent sepsis and have been shown to decrease mortality associated with variceal bleeding. EGD for band ligation is recommended within 12 hours of admission and after the patient is hemodynamically stable.

VI.25. Answer d.
This patient presents with microcytic anemia due to gastrointestinal blood loss. EGD shows GAVE. In contrast to portal hypertensive gastropathy, GAVE does not typically respond to portosystemic shunts, regardless of whether they are done surgically or as a TIPS. NSBBs have also not shown efficacy in reducing blood loss due to GAVE. Thermoablation therapies such as argon plasma coagulation can decrease bleeding and are often first-line therapy in the management of GAVE.

VI.26. Answer d.
This patient has spontaneous bacterial peritonitis, and antibiotic therapy with cefotaxime must begin immediately to reduce mortality. Nadolol does not need to be discontinued in patients with spontaneous bacterial peritonitis unless the sodium level is less than 130 mmol/L, systolic blood pressure is less than 90 mm Hg, or acute kidney injury develops; however, the maximum dose should be 80 mg daily in patients with ascites. Gastrointestinal tract bleeding can precipitate HE, but there is no indication that this patient has been overtly bleeding, and he has a clear diagnosis of infection that merits expedited treatment. This patient's lactulose dose could be increased if the current dose is inadequate, and initiation of rifaximin could be considered to prevent further recurrent HE, but the primary management of HE in this patient would be to treat the precipitating cause (spontaneous bacterial peritonitis).

VI.27. Answer a.
This patient has moderate ascites despite diuretic therapy. Most patients with ascites can achieve good control with sodium restriction and diuretics alone. Before increased diuretic dosages are considered, she should be assessed by a dietitian to ensure that she is adhering to a strict, low-sodium diet (<2,000 mg daily). If ascites persists despite adherence to a sodium-restricted diet, it would be reasonable to increase the furosemide dose to 120 mg and the spironolactone dose to 300 mg while monitoring her electrolytes and kidney function. TIPS could be considered if she had clearly defined refractory ascites and a low MELD score. Large-volume paracentesis should not be necessary because she does not have tense ascites; however, a diagnostic paracentesis would be recommended if it was not done when ascites was diagnosed.

VI.28. Answer b.
This patient appears to have postsinusoidal portal hypertension related to a hepatic venous outflow obstruction as indicated by the high serum-ascites albumin gradient (≥1.1) and the high ascitic fluid protein level (≥2.5 g/dL). The best next step would be an investigation with transthoracic echocardiography to rule out a cardiac cause, which could include constrictive pericarditis or right-sided heart failure. Doppler abdominal ultrasonography would also be a reasonable option to rule out BCS, although a cardiac cause appears more likely given his history. Furosemide and spironolactone could be considered to help manage the ascites, but the underlying diagnosis should be clarified first. The patient does not have spontaneous bacterial peritonitis, so he does not require antibiotics. Upper endoscopy is recommended for variceal screening if patients have cirrhosis when the first decompensating event occurs, but it is not clear that this patient has cirrhosis.

VI.29. Answer d.
This patient has acute kidney injury and cirrhosis with ascites. Before a diagnosis of hepatorenal syndrome–acute kidney injury is made, she must first have no improvement in kidney function after 2 days of diuretic withdrawal and plasma volume expansion with 25% albumin. In patients with cirrhosis, normal saline should generally be avoided, and albumin is the preferred volume expander. She does not have a confirmed diagnosis of hepatorenal syndrome, so midodrine and octreotide and urgent evaluation for liver transplant are not yet necessary.

VI.30. Answer c.
This patient has an isolated increase in the serum ferritin level. This is a common clinical pitfall, which can lead to confusion. This patient's alcohol consumption is above the threshold for causing liver injury in a woman (ie, >1 standard alcoholic beverage daily), and she has laboratory evidence of alcohol-related liver disease (AST-ALT ratio 2:1). Hemochromatosis is unlikely because the transferrin saturation is not increased. NAFLD is less likely because of the pattern of alcohol use. Patients with Wilson disease can present with various laboratory findings, but they would be unlikely to present initially in their 60s. Ferroportin disease is a non-*HFE* iron overload state in persons with increased ferritin levels; however, the clinical pattern makes alcohol-related liver disease more likely.

VI.31. Answer d.
This patient has acute liver failure with sudden onset of jaundice, coagulopathy, and hepatic encephalopathy. For a patient in this age group, fulminant Wilson disease (Wilsonian crisis) is an important diagnostic consideration. Although the patient has a new sexual partner, it is unclear whether there are other risk factors for viral hepatitis. Patients with acute BCS can present with acute liver failure but will often present with ascites. The presence of hemolytic anemia (low hemoglobin), unconjugated (indirect) hyperbilirubinemia, and a low ALP level make Wilson disease the most likely diagnosis.

VI.32. Answer a.
This patient has hereditary hemochromatosis with biochemical evidence of iron overload. The mainstay of treatment is phlebotomy, which is typically recommended at an initial frequency of every 1 to 2 weeks until iron stores are depleted. Patients are then treated with maintenance phlebotomy approximately every 3 months. Dietary restriction is insufficient to treat this patient's iron overload. Chelation therapy, such as with deferasirox, is more commonly used with secondary iron overload (eg, for patients who have hematopoietic disorders). Trientene is a chelation agent used to treat Wilson disease.

VI.33. Answer d.
This patient has clinical and biochemical evidence of severe iron overload at a young age, which would be unusual for typical

(*HFE*) hemochromatosis. This clinical presentation (early onset, severe iron overload, and cardiomyopathy) is more characteristic of disease caused by *HJV* alteration. Patients with ferroportin disease typically have splenic iron deposition and high ferritin levels but normal transferrin saturation. Wilson disease can occur in patients in this age group, and atypical viruses can cause cardiomyopathy, but the clinical and laboratory features are not consistent with these diagnoses.

VI.34. Answer c.

This patient may have hereditary hemochromatosis, but confirmatory testing is required as other conditions (eg, NASH and alcohol-related steatohepatitis) may also cause increased values for iron indices. Additional testing would include viral hepatitis serologies. Liver biopsy is generally not required for diagnostic purposes unless hereditary hemochromatosis is a strong possibility and genetic testing is negative or advanced fibrosis or cirrhosis is a concern (eg, ferritin level >1,000 µg/L or aminotransferase levels are high or both). Similarly, there is no need to use MRI with elastography to measure hepatic iron concentration for the diagnosis of hereditary hemochromatosis unless cirrhosis is a concern. Counseling for weight loss and alcohol abstinence is indicated but would not be the best next step.

VI.35. Answer a.

A definitive diagnosis of Wilson disease can be made if the patient has a markedly low ceruloplasmin level, a high 24-hour urine copper level, and Kayser-Fleischer rings. Liver biopsy would be performed if the patient did not have evidence of Kayser-Fleischer rings or if the ceruloplasmin and 24-hour urine copper results were conflicting. Testing for serum copper levels and *ATP7B* variants would not be helpful.

VI.36. Answer c.

Trientene may be associated with sideroblastic anemia. Acute liver failure occurs as a result of a fulminant presentation of Wilson disease rather than the treatment itself. The only therapy for fulminant Wilson disease is liver transplant. Penicillamine can worsen the neurologic symptoms of Wilson disease if they are preexisting. Myelopathy is associated with copper deficiency rather than with Wilson disease or its treatment.

VI.37. Answer b.

With the low α_1-antitrypsin level, this patient most likely has the PI*ZZ phenotype. The patient is at risk for emphysema and should undergo baseline chest radiography and pulmonary function testing. Liver biopsy can be nondiagnostic because globules that stain with periodic acid-Schiff–diastase can be present throughout the liver, so liver biopsy would not be necessary to confirm the diagnosis for this patient. Noninvasive fibrosis assessment is useful if patients have α_1-antitrypsin deficiency, and screening for HCC is useful if patients have α_1-antitrypsin deficiency and cirrhosis; however, this patient has a low level of α_1-antitrypsin, so the Pi*MZ phenotype is unlikely.

VI.38. Answer b.

The most likely diagnosis is PBC in this patient, a middle-aged woman presenting with pruritus and cholestasis. Given the clinical presentation and normal findings on ultrasonography, the likelihood of a large bile duct obstruction is low. Therefore, neither MRCP or ERCP would be an appropriate next step. Moreover, ERCP is invasive. Liver biopsy would not be indicated until a complete serologic and imaging evaluation has been performed.

VI.39. Answer d.

This patient with newly diagnosed PSC should undergo colonoscopy, regardless of his symptoms, because of the high prevalence of IBD in patients with PSC. Patients with PSC and IBD have an increased risk for colorectal neoplasia and require colonoscopies with surveillance biopsies annually. The patient has no clear indications for liver transplant. High doses of ursodeoxycholic acid have been shown to be harmful. Abdominal ultrasonography would not be indicated because recent MRCP findings supported the diagnosis of PSC.

VI.40. Answer d.

Patients with PBC, particularly postmenopausal women, are at risk for osteoporosis. Bone densitometry should be performed to assess for osteopenia or osteoporosis. Calcium supplementation is recommended if dietary consumption of calcium is inadequate. Likewise, vitamin D supplementation is recommended, particularly if vitamin D levels are low. There is no reason to check ionized calcium levels, and there is no reason to start a bisphosphonate without evidence of bone disease.

VI.41. Answer c.

This patient has cholestasis and a history of IBD, but AMA test results are negative and imaging findings are normal. Therefore, the most likely diagnosis is small-duct PSC, but a biopsy would be required to confirm the diagnosis. In the era of highly active antiretroviral therapy, HIV-related cholangiopathy is quite rare and manifests with large-duct abnormalities. With large-duct PSC, imaging findings would be abnormal. In a young man who has a history of IBD, AMA-negative PBC is less likely.

VI.42. Answer d.

Amoxicillin-clavulanate is the most common cause of clinically apparent acute DILI in the US and Europe. The onset of injury is typically a few days to 8 weeks after initiation of therapy, and a patient may present with liver injury days or weeks after cessation of therapy. Patients commonly present with fatigue, low-grade fever, nausea, abdominal pain, jaundice, and pruritus. The pattern of injury is typically cholestatic, but some patients may present with liver biochemistry results that suggest a mixed or hepatocellular pattern. As in other forms of cholestatic DILI, the cholestasis due to amoxicillin-clavulanate may take weeks or months to resolve. Conservative management is recommended at this time. Amoxicillin-clavulanate does not lead to autoimmune-mediated DILI; therefore, initiating prednisone or proceeding with a liver biopsy would not be indicated. The patient does not have evidence of liver failure (ie, hepatic encephalopathy or coagulopathy) and therefore does not require evaluation for liver transplant.

VI.43. Answer c.

Autoimmune-mediated DILI may be caused by specific drugs, and the immune responses mimic those typically observed in de novo or idiopathic autoimmune hepatitis. Nitrofurantoin is commonly associated with autoimmune-like DILI. Other medications include hydralazine, minocycline, diclofenac, and anti–tumor necrosis factor agents. Although it is difficult to distinguish autoimmune-like DILI from autoimmune hepatitis on the basis of history, laboratory findings, and histologic features, the absence of relapse after the withdrawal of corticosteroid therapy is highly suggestive of a drug-induced autoimmune-like reaction. The clinical pattern is more similar to chronic hepatitis, and recovery may be delayed. The best next step for this patient is discontinuation of the suspected offending agent. Autoantibodies (including ANA or ASMA) may persist after withdrawal of nitrofurantoin. Drug-induced autoimmune hepatitis that does not improve spontaneously can be treated with corticosteroids. Ultrasonography and liver biopsy would be useful if the patient did not improve upon withdrawal of nitrofurantoin and initiation of prednisone.

VI.44. Answer c.

Because of the frequency with which statins are prescribed, there has been much interest in the potential liver toxicity of these agents. Determining whether patients receiving statins have DILI is difficult because mild increases in liver enzyme levels are common within 1 month after the initiation of statin therapy, but the levels nearly always decrease despite continued administration of the agents. The increased levels usually result from an adaptive response to the drug and do not necessitate withdrawal of treatment. Patients should have baseline liver tests before treatment is initiated. Routine posttreatment monitoring is not recommended, although signs and symptoms that suggest liver injury or disease (eg, jaundice) should be investigated with liver tests. Serious DILI from statins is rare. Patients taking atorvastatin are more likely to present with a cholestatic or mixed profile (57%) compared with patients taking simvastatin (25%). Statins rarely have been associated with the development of autoimmune-like hepatitis, although the association may be only coincidental. It would be premature to consider a liver biopsy or magnetic resonance elastography at this time.

VI.45. Answer d.

Acetaminophen hepatotoxicity is characterized by very high levels of aminotransferases (often >5,000 U/L). Of the patients who have AST levels greater than 1,000 U/L at presentation, 16% will die or require liver transplant. Patients with acetaminophen hepatotoxicity and poor prognostic markers should be hospitalized and their condition monitored. N-acetylcysteine enhances the conjugation and excretion of N-acetyl-p-quinone imine, and when administered after liver injury has developed, N-acetylcysteine acts by antioxidant and anti-inflammatory mechanisms. It may enhance liver perfusion through inotropic and vasodilatory effects. Although the efficacy of N-acetylcysteine diminishes when it is given more than 8 hours after acetaminophen ingestion, it nonetheless should be administered up to 24 hours after ingestion because of its putative hepatoprotective effects. To maximize the potential benefit of N-acetylcysteine, it should be used to treat any patient who has high serum transaminase concentrations and a history consistent with acetaminophen exposure regardless of the serum acetaminophen concentration. Treatment with activated charcoal is recommended as well for all patients who present within 4 hours of a known or suspected acetaminophen ingestion unless there are contraindications to its administration. This patient does not need penicillin G, which is used to treat poisoning from the mushroom *Amanita phalloides*. He does not have alcoholic hepatitis, and corticosteroids are not indicated at this time.

VI.46. Answer b.

NAFLD is common and is the most likely diagnosis given this patient's metabolic risk factors and the imaging finding consistent with steatosis. Up to one-third of patients with NAFLD have slight increases in ANA, but titers greater than 1:320 are rare. With the negative result for hepatitis B surface antigen, chronic hepatitis B is unlikely. In contrast to NAFLD, autoimmune hepatitis is uncommon. Approximately 80% of patients

with autoimmune hepatitis have a positive ANA titer. While autoimmune hepatitis can occur in men, the prevalence is higher in women, and comorbid autoimmune conditions are frequently present. PBC is a rare cholestatic liver disease characterized by increases in ALP values and positive results for AMA, and more than 90% of affected patients are women.

VI.47. Answer a.

This patient has drug-induced autoimmune hepatitis related to minocycline. Drug-induced autoimmune hepatitis accounts for about 9% of autoimmune hepatitis cases and can resemble classic autoimmune hepatitis both biochemically and histologically. However, cirrhosis is rarely present in drug-induced autoimmune hepatitis, which should respond to discontinuation of the offending agent and a limited duration for the use of glucocorticoids (<6 months) without azathioprine. Recurrent increases in liver test results after cessation of corticosteroids is unusual for drug-induced autoimmune hepatitis and may suggest classic autoimmune hepatitis. The patient has no indication for liver transplant at this time. PBC is a chronic cholestatic liver disease characterized by positive AMA titers. This patient has a hepatocellular-predominant injury pattern that was acute in onset and liver biopsy findings that were not consistent with PBC.

VI.48. Answer d.

This clinical presentation is typical for seronegative autoimmune hepatitis in a young woman with comorbid immune-mediated disease. She has chronic hepatocellular-predominant injury. The biopsy shows typical features of autoimmune hepatitis with advanced fibrosis. Other causes of liver disease have been excluded, so autoimmune hepatitis is the most likely cause. Approximately 20% of patients may have seronegative autoimmune hepatitis without increased titers of ANA or SMA. Initiation of prednisone therapy should result in improvement in her liver test results within several weeks. If the expected response to medical therapy does not occur, the diagnosis should be reconsidered. Celiac sprue can lead to mild aminotransferase elevations with nonspecific histologic features, which can improve with gluten avoidance. Although ferritin was slightly increased (most likely from underlying inflammation), the normal result for transferrin saturation, the biopsy findings, and her clinical presentation would not be consistent with hemochromatosis. Drug-induced liver injury is less likely given the lack of temporal relationship between the increase in liver test results and the use of a medication. Drug-induced liver injury from levothyroxine, a frequently prescribed medicine, would be unusual. Moreover, advanced fibrosis in drug-induced autoimmune hepatitis is uncommon.

VI.49. Answer a.

The patient presented with acute autoimmune hepatitis and has features of advanced fibrosis. With the disease in biochemical remission with prednisone and azathioprine, she has had persistently normal liver test results while taking low doses of prednisone and azathioprine. For most patients the recommended strategy is to withdraw the corticosteroid, thereby decreasing its adverse effects, while remission is maintained with azathioprine. Mycophenolate mofetil is a second-line agent that can be used instead of azathioprine if a patient has a drug intolerance or an incomplete response to standard therapy. Discontinuing therapy completely would not be recommended. After liver test results become normal, histologic remission may take months to occur. The recommendation is to treat and maintain remission for at least 2 years before withdrawal of immunosuppression is considered for select patients. Even when patients have had biochemical re-mission for 2 years, relapse after stopping immunosuppression is common. This patient already has advanced fibrosis and would be at higher risk for complications of repeated disease flares and uncontrolled disease activity.

VI.50. Answer c.
This patient has metabolic syndrome and the evaluation has been negative for other causes of increased liver values. A low-positive ANA test result is common in patients with NAFLD and does not have diagnostic significance. With normal findings on ultra-sonography and the CBC, the likelihood of advanced fibrosis is low, so EGD is not indicated at this time. A liver biopsy would help confirm the diagnosis of NASH, assess for fibrosis, and jus-tify the use of pharmacotherapy for NASH and type 2 diabetes. Given the persistent increases in the liver test results, subsequent testing would not be appropriate at this time.

VI.51. Answer c.
NAFLD is a well-established risk factor for NASH and progres-sion to cirrhosis. Risk of liver-related death is greater for patients with NASH than isolated steatosis, and the most common causes of death are cardiovascular disease (15.5%), nonliver cancer (5.6%), and liver cancer (2.8%). Among patients with NASH, the stage of fibrosis is the most important predictor of death.

VI.52. Answer a.
Patients with NASH have an increased risk of cardiovas-cular events; thus, optimal management of cardiovascular risk with lipid-lowering treatment if indicated, is appropriate. This patient's high score for atherosclerotic cardiovascular disease risk and high LDL cholesterol level justify the use of statin therapy. Statins are safe to use in patients with NAFLD, NASH, and compensated NASH-related cirrhosis. Although statins are not indicated for treatment of NASH, several studies have suggested a hepatoprotective effect from statins. The patient's low alcohol intake does not justify therapy for cessation. Although no data suggest benefit, limited data do suggest that a low amount of al-cohol (average of <2 drinks daily for a man and <1 drink daily for a woman) is associated with increased risk of NASH progression. Although prophylactic use of metformin may be considered for patients with prediabetes, it is not recommended for management of NASH. Weight loss of even 5% to 10% of body weight is the cornerstone of NASH therapy and is associated with improve-ment in all histologic features of NASH. A Mediterranean diet is recommended for patients who have NASH and metabolic syndrome.

VI.53. Answer d.
Published genome-wide and exome-wide association studies have led to the identification of loci in *PNPLA3*, *TM6SF2*, *HSD17B13*, *MBOAT7*, and *MTARC1* that are associated with NASH, progres-sion of fibrosis, and hepatocellular carcinoma in patients with NAFLD. Of these, a variant in *HSD17B13* is associated with a decreased risk of progression from NAFL to NASH and chronic liver disease; the others are associated with an increased risk of disease progression.

VI.54. Answer d.
This patient has abdominal pain, nausea, vomiting, increased transaminase levels, impaired kidney function, coagulopathy, and hypoglycemia. She most likely has acute fatty liver of pregnancy, with more than 6 features of the Swansea criteria, and prompt de-livery is the best management option.

VI.55. Answer b.
This patient's presentation is most consistent with biliary colic. Gallstones are common in pregnancy. The first episode of biliary colic can be managed conservatively and successfully in most patients. If patients have recurrent biliary colic, laparoscopic cho-lecystectomy should be considered in the second trimester. ERCP can be safely performed during pregnancy if indicated (eg, con-cern for choledocholithiasis) with limited fluoroscopic exposure and fetal shielding. Nothing in this patient's history or laboratory findings suggests choledocholithiasis or biliary obstruction.

VI.56. Answer c.
The level of HBV DNA should be checked at baseline and at approximately 28 weeks of gestation. If the HBV DNA level at 28 weeks of gestation is greater than 200,000 IU/mL (>10^6 copies/mL), antiviral treatment with category B medications (eg, tenofovir) should be initiated at 28 to 30 weeks of pregnancy and continued until delivery. All babies should receive hepatitis B vaccination and hepatitis B immunoglobulin at birth. There is no contraindication for vaginal delivery or breastfeeding.

VI.57. Answer a.
Patients who have autoimmune hepatitis that has been adequately controlled for at least a year before conception can expect to have desirable outcomes and a successful pregnancy. The treatment of autoimmune hepatitis should be continued without cessation or interruption during the pregnancy to avoid flares. The use of azathioprine is safe and should be continued, but mycophenolate mofetil is contraindicated during pregnancy. Patients of child-bearing age who are receiving mycophenolate mofetil should have a preconception discussion with their clinician, and mycophenolate mofetil should be changed to an alternative therapy. Treatment of flares in pregnant patients is the same as in nonpregnant patients.

VI.58. Answer c.
For patients who have hepatocellular carcinoma and cirrhosis, transplant is an effective option because it addresses both the ne-oplasm and the underlying liver disease. In the past, outcomes were poor with transplant for hepatocellular carcinoma. However, with advances in patient selection and use of the Milan criteria (1 tumor ≤5 cm *or* 2 or 3 tumors ≤3 cm, without vascular invasion or extrahepatic spread), the 5-year survival rate is 70% to 80% and the recurrence rate is less than 15%. A patient with hepatocellular carcinoma within the Milan criteria is assigned a MELD score to allow orthotopic liver transplant in 3 to 12 months (called a MELD exception). Biopsy of the lesion is not recommended be-cause arterial enhancement with portal venous washout on CT is diagnostic for HCC. Chemotherapy is indicated for advanced, unresectable HCC. Transarterial embolization is not indicated before completion of a liver transplant evaluation for poten-tial listing on the liver transplant waiting list. Liver resection is the preferred treatment of hepatocellular carcinoma in patients without cirrhosis and in those with cirrhosis who have well-preserved liver function and little or no portal hypertension.

VI.59. Answer d.
Patients with cirrhosis are typically candidates for liver trans-plant when their biologic MELD score is 15 or more. This is im-portant because for patients with a MELD score less than 15, the 3-month mortality after transplant exceeds the 3-month mortality without a transplant. However, some patients may be candidates for liver transplant evaluation when they have Child-Pugh class B cirrhosis with portal hypertension despite having a low MELD score. This permits the patient to meet the transplant team before the

development of end-stage liver disease and its complications (eg, hepatic encephalopathy). It ensures adequate time for the patient to complete the pretransplant evaluation and the necessary education. Patients may also qualify for liver transplant if they have a complication or condition that qualifies for standard MELD exception points. Ultrasonographic screening for hepatocellular cancer should be performed every 6 months in patients with cirrhosis and in men with PBC. Bone mineral density should be assessed every 2 years, depending on baseline density and severity of cholestasis.

VI.60. Answer d.

Clinicians should be aware of drug interactions with drugs affecting cytochrome P450 enzymes. Drugs that inhibit the cytochrome P450 system (eg, fluconazole for candidal esophagitis) increase the levels of calcineurin inhibitors, and drugs that stimulate the cytochrome P450 system (eg, phenytoin) decrease calcineurin inhibitor levels and thus increase the risk of rejection. The patient likely had a drug-drug interaction between tacrolimus and fluconazole, which was recently prescribed for candidal esophagitis. Tacrolimus should be withheld while the tacrolimus level results are pending. Classic adverse effects of increased tacrolimus levels include nephrotoxicity and neurotoxicity. At this time a liver biopsy would not be useful, and findings from Doppler ultrasonography of the liver would most likely be unremarkable. CT of the head would be reasonable because of the acute headache, but both medications should be withheld first.

VI.61. Answer b.

Acute cellular rejection occurs in up to 50% of liver recipients and usually is associated with mild to moderate biochemical abnormalities (mixed hepatocellular-cholestatic pattern) and, occasionally, fever. The tacrolimus level is low for 4 weeks after transplant. Although the diagnosis can be suspected by the timing in the early weeks after liver transplant, definitive diagnosis requires histologic examination of the liver, and the following findings: 1) portal infiltrates with activated lymphocytes and some eosinophils, 2) lymphocytic cholangitis, and 3) venous endotheliitis. Most cases of rejection (90%) occur in the first 2 months postoperatively. Acute cellular rejection soon after liver transplant generally has no effect on long-term graft outcome, except for patients with hepatitis C, and very few grafts are lost to chronic rejection. The patient had a sustained virologic response before transplant, and recurrent hepatitis C would be unlikely. Although hepatic artery thrombosis usually occurs in the first week after orthotopic liver transplant, it can develop later, but that would be unlikely in this patient given the normal findings from Doppler ultrasonography of the allograft. Cytomegalovirus infection is the most common viral infection. Its incidence peaks in the first 3 to 5 postoperative weeks, and it is rare after the first year. Its presence is suggested by fever, malaise, and leukopenia, and patients tend to appear sicker than the patient described above. Cytomegalovirus infection is less common than acute cellular rejection.

VII

Pancreas and Biliary Tree

37

Acute Pancreatitis[a]

DANIEL B. MASELLI, MD

VINAY CHANDRASEKHARA, MD

Acute pancreatitis is an inflammatory condition characterized by severe abdominal pain and both locoregional and systemic inflammatory complications. More than 200,000 new cases of acute pancreatitis occur in the US each year, and the incidence is increasing. The disease is severe in 20% of patients with acute pancreatitis, and approximately 5% of all patients with pancreatitis die of the disease. Hence, key management principles include prompt diagnosis, triage of patients with severe pancreatitis to aggressive care, and identification of the underlying cause to prevent recurrence. Necrotizing pancreatitis accounts for most of the morbidity and nearly all the mortality associated with acute pancreatitis.

Pathophysiology

The pathophysiology of acute pancreatitis begins with inappropriate activation of trypsin within the acinar cell. Activated intracellular trypsin, in turn, activates a cascade of digestive enzymes that leads to autodigestion and cellular injury. Acinar cell injury leads to inflammation by recruitment of inflammatory cells through cytokines and other mediators. In 80% of cases, acute pancreatitis is mild and self-limited, with little or no long-term sequelae to the pancreatic parenchyma or systemic toxicity. In

[a] The authors thank Bret T. Petersen, MD, and Randall K. Pearson, MD, who authored previous versions of this chapter.

Abbreviations: APACHE, Acute Physiology and Chronic Health Evaluation; CT, computed tomography; ERCP, endoscopic retrograde cholangiopancreatography; EUS, endoscopic ultrasonography; ICU, intensive care unit; MRI, magnetic resonance imaging; SIRS, systemic inflammatory response syndrome; ULRR, upper limit of the reference range; WON, walled-off necrosis

20% of cases, severe acute pancreatitis develops, leading in the early phase to the systemic inflammatory response syndrome (SIRS), organ failure (hypotension, kidney failure, and acute respiratory distress syndrome), and pancreatic necrosis.

Clinical Presentation and Diagnosis

The clinical presentation of patients with acute pancreatitis ranges from mild, nonspecific epigastric pain to catastrophic, unstable acute medical illness. Typically, the pain of acute pancreatitis is located in the epigastrium and, in approximately half the patients, radiates into the back. The onset of pain is usually swift, reaching maximum intensity within an hour. Pain is frequently unbearable and generally persists without episodic improvement for at least 24 hours in the absence of intervention. Pain often is accompanied by nausea and vomiting. In severe episodes of acute pancreatitis, SIRS dominates and patients appear systemically ill, with fever, tachycardia, tachypnea, and hypotension.

It is now understood that there are 2 overlapping phases of acute pancreatitis. The *early phase*, characteristically lasting 1 to 2 weeks, manifests as cytokine-mediated systemic inflammation as a host response to pancreatic injury. The *late phase* is typified by 1 or more of the following (described later in this chapter): persistence of systemic inflammation, diminished immune function, and the evolution of local complications. Consequently, most of the morbidity and mortality that occur early in the course of severe acute pancreatitis is due to systemic toxicity and organ failure secondary to SIRS, whereas late mortality (ie, beyond 10-14 days) is typically related to pancreatic necrosis and infection.

The differential diagnosis of acute pancreatitis is broad and includes most of the important causes of abdominal pain, including mesenteric ischemia and infarction, perforated peptic ulcer, symptomatic cholelithiasis, dissecting aortic aneurysm, intestinal obstruction, and inferior wall myocardial infarction.

By consensus, the diagnosis of acute pancreatitis requires 2 of the following 3 findings:

1. Abdominal pain features consistent with acute pancreatitis
2. Serum level of amylase or lipase >3 times the upper limit of the reference range (ULRR)
3. Findings of acute pancreatitis seen on cross-sectional imaging with computed tomography (CT), ultrasonography, or magnetic resonance imaging (MRI)

These criteria indicate that the diagnosis of acute pancreatitis can be based on classic pain symptoms and diagnostic levels of amylase and lipase, obviating the need for imaging in many cases. If the serum levels of amylase or lipase are only modestly elevated (<3 times the ULRR), the lack of specificity dictates the need for imaging, most commonly CT, to establish the diagnosis. The definition also provides means to diagnose acute pancreatitis when a patient cannot give a clinical history because of altered mental status or the severity of the acute presentation. When performed more than 48 hours after presentation, CT with contrast enhancement also provides important prognostic information, as discussed below.

Both amylase and lipase levels are usually increased during the acute phase of pancreatitis. Amylase elevations are more than 90% sensitive for acute pancreatitis, and 3-fold elevations are more than 90% specific (but with lower sensitivity). The serum lipase level generally is preferred to the serum amylase level because lipase is more specific to the pancreas. Therefore, increased lipase levels tend to reflect pancreatic pathology for a longer interval compared with amylase levels, which become lost in the noise of normal basal amylase from multiple sources. Amylase and lipase levels can be abnormally high from bowel ischemia, obstruction, or perforation leading to enteric leakage and systemic absorption of intraluminal pancreatic enzymes. The amylase level is also increased nonspecifically in various nongastrointestinal conditions (Box 37.1), including macroamylasemia, diseases of the parotid glands, and some carcinomas.

Macroamylasemia is a benign condition that may cause confusion when present with other causes of abdominal pain. Macroamylase is a macromolecular aggregation of amylase molecules that are poorly excreted by the kidney, yielding chronically fluctuating increases in serum amylase, which are generally less than twice the ULRR. Infrequent disease associations have been reported. The diagnosis of macroamylasemia may be suggested by a low ratio of amylase to creatinine clearance and is easily established by immunologic assay.

Importantly, the degree of increase of either lipase or amylase beyond diagnostic criteria for acute pancreatitis is not predictive of disease severity. After the diagnosis of acute pancreatitis has been made, serial measurements of lipase and amylase levels have no prognostic value in guiding management and should be avoided. Resolution of high enzyme levels may lag clinical improvement, and thus reassessment of enzyme levels has a diminishingly limited role in acute pancreatitis, although reassessment may be useful in selected patients when clinical relapse is suspected.

Plain abdominal radiographs are frequently normal at presentation with acute pancreatitis, but they are useful in excluding bowel perforation. A nonspecific ileus may be present along with a focally dilated small-bowel loop, the so-called sentinel loop.

Abdominal ultrasonography is frequently nondiagnostic in acute pancreatitis because overlying bowel gas may obscure the pancreas. However, ultrasonography is sensitive for detecting

---

Box 37.1. Differential Diagnosis of High Levels of Pancreatic Enzymes

Amylase: cleared by reticuloendothelial system excretion *and* kidney filtration

- Pancreatic inflammation (acute and chronic pancreatitis) or trauma; ERCP
- Salivary inflammation, obstruction, or trauma
- GI inflammation, obstruction, perforation, or ischemia
- Ovarian disease or cysts; ectopic pregnancy
- Cancer of the ovary, prostate, lung, breast, or thymus; multiple myeloma; pheochromocytoma
- Macroamylasemia: rarely associated with celiac disease, ulcerative colitis, rheumatoid arthritis, lymphoma, HIV infection, or monoclonal gammopathy
- Other causes, including kidney failure, burns, acidosis, anorexia nervosa, bulimia, cerebral trauma, and drugs

Lipase: kidney filtration and tubular resorption (increased half-life)

- Pancreatic inflammation (acute and chronic pancreatitis), trauma, or tumors
- GI: acute cholecystitis, bowel obstruction or infarction, duodenal ulcer, or celiac disease

Abbreviations: ERCP, endoscopic retrograde cholangiopancreatography; GI, gastrointestinal tract.

---

gallstones and, thus, adds clinical information about the underlying cause of the pancreatitis and should be used for patients with an intact gallbladder.

Etiology

Once a diagnosis of acute pancreatitis is established, characterization of the underlying cause is critical for prevention of future episodes (Box 37.2). Gallstones are the most common cause of acute pancreatitis in middle and upper socioeconomic groups in the US. Gallstones cause acute pancreatitis by mechanical obstruction of the common channel shared by the bile duct and pancreatic duct, with increased intraductal pressure in the pancreas and possibly pancreatic reflux of bile acids in some cases. When they present with acute pancreatitis, patients often have a history of biliary-type pain, ultrasonographic evidence of cholelithiasis, and abnormal liver test results.

Alcohol, which induces a direct toxic injury to the pancreas, is the predominant cause of acute pancreatitis in resource-limited populations in the US. Development of acute pancreatitis from alcohol typically requires prolonged consumption of a considerable amount of alcohol (usually >50 g daily), but acute pancreatitis develops in less than 5% of those who drink this heavily.

An important metabolic cause of acute pancreatitis is hypertriglyceridemia; a threshold triglyceride level of 1,000 mg/dL has been established as being causative, although lower levels, especially in combination with other pancreatic insults, are now thought to precipitate acute pancreatitis. Severity corresponds to the degree of increase in the triglyceride level. Hypertriglyceridemia can arise from inherited disorders of lipoprotein metabolism or from

Box 37.2. Etiology of Acute Pancreatitis

- Mechanical: gallstones, biliary sludge, ascariasis, periampullary diverticulum, pancreatic or periampullary cancer, ampullary or papillary stenosis, duodenal stricture or obstruction
- Toxic: ethanol, methanol, scorpion venom, organophosphate poisoning
- Metabolic: hypertriglyceridemia, hypercalcemia
- Drugs: numerous (see Box 37.3)
- Infection
  Viruses: mumps, coxsackievirus, hepatitis B virus, cytomegalovirus, varicella-zoster virus, herpes simplex virus, HIV
  Bacteria: *Mycoplasma, Legionella, Leptospira, Salmonella*
  Fungi: *Aspergillus*
  Parasites: *Toxoplasma, Cryptosporidium, Ascaris*
- Trauma: post-ERCP, blunt or penetrating abdominal injury, iatrogenic injury, surgery
- Congenital or anatomical: choledochocele, pancreas divisum
- Vascular: ischemia, atheroembolism, vasculitis (polyarteritis nodosa, systemic lupus erythematosus)
- Genetic: *CFTR* and other genetic alterations
- Miscellaneous: pregnancy, kidney transplant, α_1-antitrypsin deficiency, sphincter of Oddi dysfunction (possibly)
- Idiopathic

Abbreviation: ERCP, endoscopic retrograde cholangiopancreatography.

Box 37.3. Drugs Reliably Associated With Acute Pancreatitis[a]

- Antimicrobials: erythromycin, clarithromycin, isoniazid, metronidazole, nitrofurantoin, ceftriaxone, trimethoprim-sulfamethoxazole, **pentamidine**, ampicillin, rifampin, **tetracycline**
- HIV agents: **didanosine**, nelfinavir
- Diuretics: **furosemide**, chlorothiazide, **hydrochlorothiazide**
- GI agents: omeprazole, cimetidine, ranitidine, **sulfasalazine**, hydrocortisone, lamivudine, interferon, ribavirin, octreotide
- Cardiac agents: procainamide, α-methyldopa, captopril, enalapril, lisinopril, amiodarone, losartan
- Immunosuppressives or chemotherapeutics: **azathioprine**, **6-mercaptopurine**, **L-asparaginase**, cytosine arabinoside, dexamethasone, ifosfamide, paclitaxel, tacrolimus, cyclosporine
- Neuropsychiatric agents: **valproic acid**, clozapine, carbamazepine, risperidone, sertraline
- Other common drugs: bezafibrate, carbimazole, codeine, pravastatin, simvastatin, all-*trans* retinoic acid, acetaminophen, **estrogens**, alendronate, indomethacin, metformin, naproxen, diclofenac, sulindac, orlistat, danazol, ergotamine, propofol

Abbreviation: GI, gastrointestinal tract.

[a] Boldface type indicates medications that have strong associations.

changes in lipid homeostasis, such as those that occur in obesity, type 2 diabetes, hypothyroidism, or pregnancy or with the use of certain medications (eg, tamoxifen or estrogen). Distinct clinical features include eruptive xanthomas, hepatosplenomegaly from fatty infiltration, and lipemia retinalis.

Medications are implicated in 0.1% to 2% of cases of acute pancreatitis (Box 37.3), although the range may be as high as 5% to 10%. Less than half the cases of drug-induced pancreatitis are recognized by clinicians because there are no unique clinical features, and most cases are mild. Historically, case reports and small series have enabled drugs to be classified as *definite*, *probable*, or *possible* causes of acute pancreatitis. An important diagnostic clue is the rapid onset of acute pancreatitis after rechallenging with the offending medication. Medications associated with pancreatitis are classified into 5 risk classes according to the strength of the supporting literature, temporal relationships between drug use and onset of pancreatitis, and reaction with rechallenge. Patients at heightened risk for drug-induced pancreatitis include pediatric and elderly patients, female patients, and those with inflammatory bowel disease or HIV infection.

Pancreatitis occurs as an adverse event of endoscopic retrograde cholangiopancreatography (ERCP) in 3% to 10% of patients undergoing ERCP. In up to 90% of patients, the severity of post-ERCP is mild or moderate. Risk factors for post-ERCP pancreatitis include 1) operator-related factors (eg, relatively less experience); 2) patient-related factors (eg, younger age, female sex, recurrent pancreatitis, previous episode of post-ERCP

pancreatitis, and evaluation for sphincter of Oddi dysfunction); and 3) procedure-related factors (eg, difficult cannulation, pancreatic duct injection, and pancreatic sphincterotomy). Pancreatic stent placement and periprocedural rectal administration of nonsteroidal anti-inflammatory drugs are reasonably effective for prevention of post-ERCP pancreatitis.

Genetic causes are increasingly recognized as etiologic factors in acute pancreatitis. Loss of the *PRSS1* gene (OMIM 276000) or gain-of-function alterations in the *CFTR* (OMIM 602421) and *SPINK1* (OMIM 167790) genes are notable examples. Other causes of acute pancreatitis include hypercalcemia, trauma, postoperative state, and infections by various agents.

About 15% to 20% of acute pancreatitis cases are classified as idiopathic because no cause is found even after extensive testing. Several clues to the cause should be kept in mind (Box 37.4). Most useful is early characterization of the serum transaminase levels, since they are often increased transiently in biliary pancreatitis, reflecting liver injury associated with the obstruction of the bile duct. In patients with pancreatitis, an increase in the alanine aminotransferase level greater than 3-fold has a positive predictive value greater than 90% for a biliary source and a sensitivity of about 50%.

If the cause of acute pancreatitis is unclear, the diagnostic approach should include investigations for neoplasm (eg, intraductal papillary mucinous neoplasm of the main duct, neuroendocrine tumor, or pancreatic ductal adenocarcinoma). Dedicated pancreatic imaging with CT, MRI, or endoscopic ultrasonography (EUS) should be performed if patients are older than 40 years or have unintentional weight loss, new-onset type 2 diabetes, or a family history of pancreatitis, particularly in a first-degree relative.

Box 37.4. Etiologic Clues in Acute Pancreatitis (AP)

- Early transaminase elevations (>3 times ULRR) are the best laboratory indicators of biliary AP.
- Normal gallbladder ultrasonographic findings do not exclude biliary AP.
- Finding gallbladder sludge at presentation is equivalent to finding gallstones; subsequent development of sludge is common in patients who are fasting or ill.
- In hypertriglyceridemic AP (usually triglycerides >1,000 mg/dL), amylase levels may be artificially normal.
- Triglyceride values decrease rapidly when a patient is taking nothing by mouth. Levels should be checked soon after diagnosis, and, if normal, they should be rechecked again after resolution of AP.
- Serum calcium level may normalize in severe AP, and it should be rechecked after resolution if a cause is not identified.
- Cancer should be considered in patients older than 50 years; cancer causes 2% of AP, and up to 5% of patients with pancreatic cancer present with AP.
- Genetic causes should be considered if a patient is young and AP is idiopathic or recurrent.

Abbreviation: ULRR, upper limit of the reference range.

Box 37.5. Ranson Criteria for Assessing the Severity of Acute Pancreatitis

Measured at admission

　Age >55 y

　Leukocytes >16.0×10⁹/L

　Blood glucose >200 mg/dL

　Serum lactate dehydrogenase >350 U/L

　Serum aspartate aminotransferase >250 U/L

Measured during initial 48 h

　Hematocrit decreases >10%

　Serum urea nitrogen increases >5 mg/dL

　Serum calcium <8 mg/dL

　Arterial Pao₂ <60 mm Hg

　Base deficit >4 mEq/L

　Fluid sequestration >6 L

Adapted from Banks PA. Practice guidelines in acute pancreatitis. Am J Gastroenterol. 1997 Mar;92(3):377-86; used with permission.

Severity Stratification

After acute pancreatitis has been diagnosed, patients most likely to have severe disease should be identified promptly for early triage to aggressive monitoring and supportive care. Most patients (approximately 80%) have interstitial or edematous pancreatitis with a mild self-limited course and very low mortality. In 20% of patients the disease is moderate to severe with considerable local morbidity and a mortality rate of about 20%. Most patients with severe disease have necrotizing pancreatitis. Several severity-of-illness scoring systems have been devised to identify patients at risk for complications; some systems are remarkably simple, while others are more complex or require serial investigations over 48 hours. Owing to the cumbersome nature of many of the scoring systems, the revised Atlanta classification has been adopted by many centers to provide a simplified schema of degree of illness in acute pancreatitis (discussed below).

Patient Characteristics

Risk factors for a severe course can be understood as 1) patient characteristics (age >55 years, body mass index >30, and altered mental status); 2) the presence of SIRS; 3) abnormal laboratory values (serum urea nitrogen >20 mg/dL, hematocrit >44%); and 4) abnormal imaging findings (pleural effusion, pulmonary infiltrates, and peripancreatic collections). Organ failure at admission, particularly kidney or pulmonary, is an especially foreboding feature of severe acute pancreatitis. Patients with these findings require close observation and often warrant admission to an intensive care unit (ICU).

The *Ranson criteria* consist of 11 clinical signs with prognostic significance: 5 criteria are measured at admission, and 6

are measured between admission and 48 hours later (Box 37.5). The number of Ranson criteria correlates with the incidence of systemic complications and the presence of pancreatic necrosis. The main disadvantage of the Ranson criteria is that they may not be evaluated until 48 hours after admission.

The *Acute Physiology and Chronic Health Evaluation (APACHE) II* scoring system is based on 12 physiologic variables, patient age, and previous history of severe organ system insufficiency or immunocompromised state (Table 37.1). It allows stratification of the severity of illness on admission and may be recalculated daily. Although the APACHE II scoring system has the advantage of being completed at the initial presentation and being repeated daily, it is cumbersome to use.

To simplify prognostication, clinical investigators have sought a single biochemical marker for severity. The acute-phase reactant C-reactive protein level has been used to predict severity, but it generally must increase to more than 150 mg/L over 36 to 72 hours after admission before it is useful. Other simple markers have included serum glucose and creatinine, but all have poor specificity.

Hemoconcentration due to extravasation of fluid into third spaces, reflected by an increase in the serum hematocrit, has been proposed as a simple reliable predictor of necrotizing pancreatitis. This is particularly true if the hematocrit does not decrease after 24 hours, which likely reflects inadequate volume resuscitation. According to other reports, hemoconcentration, although quite sensitive, is nonspecific in that it overpredicts severity. This is the problem with most of the single biochemical markers determined on admission.

The *harmless acute pancreatitis score* is designed to identify patients who will have a mild, self-limited course rather than severe disease. Its 3 components, which can be measured within 30 minutes, include 1) an absence of rebound tenderness on physical examination, 2) a normal hematocrit, and 3) a normal serum creatinine level. The presence of all 3 components was found to predict a mild course with 96% specificity and a 98% positive predictive value. This has been validated in several European studies and may guide clinicians in at least identifying patients who do not need aggressive early management.

Table 37.1. Acute Physiology and Chronic Health Evaluation (APACHE) II Scoring System[a,b]

	Physiology points								
Variable	4	3	2	1	0	1	2	3	4
Rectal temperature, °C	≥41.0	39.0-40.9	NA	38.5-38.9	36.0-38.4	34.0-35.9	32.0-33.9	30.0-31.9	≤29.9
Mean blood pressure, mm Hg	≥160	130-159	110-129	NA	70-109	NA	50-69	NA	≤49
Heart rate, beats/min	≥180	140-179	110-139	NA	70-109	NA	55-69	40-54	≤39
Respiratory rate, breaths/min	≥50	35-49	NA	25-34	12-24	10-11	6-9	NA	≤5
Oxygenation, kPa[c]									
F_{IO_2} ≥50% A_{aDO_2}	66.5	46.6-66.4	26.6-46.4	NA	<26.6	NA	NA	NA	NA
F_{IO_2} >50% Pa_{O_2}	NA	NA	NA	NA	>9.3	8.1-9.3	NA	7.3-8.0	<7.3
Arterial pH	≥7.70	7.60-7.69	NA	7.50-7.59	7.33-7.49	NA	7.25-7.32	7.15-7.24	<7.15
Serum sodium, mmol/L	≥180	160-179	155-159	150-154	130-149	NA	120-129	111-119	≤110
Serum potassium, mmol/L	≥7.0	NA	6.0-6.9	NA	5.5-5.9	3.5-5.4	3.0-3.4	2.5-2.9	<2.5
Serum creatinine, mg/dL	≥3.5	2.0-3.4	1.5-1.9	NA	0.6-1.4	NA	<0.6	NA	NA
Packed cell volume, %	≥60	NA	50-59.9	46-49.9	30-45.9	NA	20-29.9	NA	<20
White blood cell count, ×10⁹/L	≥40.0	NA	20.0-39.9	15.0-19.9	3.0-14.9	NA	1.0-2.9	NA	<1.0

Abbreviations: A_{aDO_2}, alveolar-arterial oxygen difference; F_{IO_2}, fraction of inspired oxygen; NA, not applicable.
[a] APACHE II score = acute physiology score + age points + chronic health points.
[b] Other points are determined as follows:
- Glasgow Coma Scale: score is subtracted from 15 to obtain points.
- Age: <45 y = 0 points; 45-54 y = 2 points; 55-64 y = 3 points; 65-75 y = 5 points; >75 y = 6 points.
- Chronic health points (must be present before hospital admission): 5 points are added for an emergency surgical or nonsurgical patient, and 2 points are added for an elective surgical patient who has chronic liver disease with hypertension or previous liver failure, encephalopathy, or coma; chronic heart failure (New York Heart Association class IV); chronic respiratory disease with severe exercise limitation, secondary polycythemia, or pulmonary hypertension; dialysis-dependent kidney disease; or immunosuppression (eg, radiotherapy, chemotherapy, recent or long-term therapy with high-dose corticosteroid therapy, leukemia, AIDS).
[c] If F_{IO_2} ≥50%, the alveolar-arterial gradient is assigned points. If F_{IO_2} <50%, partial pressure of oxygen is assigned points.
Adapted from Banks PA. Practice guidelines in acute pancreatitis. Am J Gastroenterol. 1997 Mar;92(3):377-86; used with permission.

Revised Atlanta Classification

Adopted in 2012, the *revised Atlanta classification* is the most widely used clinical system for characterizing acute pancreatitis. It is principally helpful in 3 ways: phenotyping acute pancreatitis, describing severity of acute pancreatitis, and describing local complications of acute pancreatitis.

Acute pancreatitis is divided into 2 phenotypes according to imaging findings: 1) *interstitial edematous pancreatitis*, which has uniform enhancement of the gland on contrast-enhanced imaging, and 2) *necrotizing pancreatitis*, which is seen in about 5% to 10% of patients with acute pancreatitis and is identified by unenhanced (ie, necrotic) pancreatic parenchyma on contrasted-enhanced imaging. Necrosis may involve the pancreatic tissue or the peripancreatic tissue (or both); the presence of either implies necrotizing pancreatitis. Notably, this impaired enhancement may take several days to be appreciated, so lack of necrosis on presentation should not obviate the need for reappraisal with subsequent imaging if the patient's condition does not improve with appropriate care.

The revised Atlanta classification describes illness severity as *mild*, *moderately severe*, or *severe* depending on the presence or absence of organ failure or local complications (Table 37.2). *Organ failure* typically refers to respiratory, cardiovascular, and kidney function and can be identified with the *modified Marshall scoring system*. Local complications manifest as immature or mature (ie, organized) fluid collections, which can cause pain, nausea, and luminal or biliary obstruction.

Four distinct subtypes of these local complications may arise from acute pancreatitis. They are based primarily on the presence or absence of necrosis and whether they have matured into defined collections (Table 37.3). *Interstitial edematous pancreatitis* can have peripancreatic fluid collections that mature into encapsulated collections called *pseudocysts*, which contain homogeneous fluid. Conversely, *necrotizing pancreatitis* may have pancreatic or peripancreatic acute necrotic collections that mature into defined, encapsulated collections called walled-off necrosis (WON), which contain both fluid and debris. Maturation in either presentation typically occurs over a 4-week period after disease onset. WON is often associated with signs of persistent systemic inflammation. Importantly, none of these terms implies infection, and any sterile mature or immature fluid collection can be secondarily infected, although infection is far more frequently

Table 37.2. Summary of Revised Atlanta Criteria for Severity of Acute Pancreatitis

	Severity of acute pancreatitis		
Feature	Mild	Moderately severe	Severe
Organ failure	Absent	Transient (<48 h)	Persistent (>48 h)
Local complications	Absent	May be present	Often present

Table 37.3. Summary of Revised Atlanta Criteria for Pancreatic Collections

Type of pancreatitis	Time after disease onset, wk	
	≤4	>4
Interstitial edematous	**Acute peripancreatic fluid collection** Homogeneous Confined by normal fascial planes Adjacent to pancreas	**Pseudocyst** Homogenous, without nonliquid content Well-circumscribed, well-defined
Necrotizing	**Acute necrotic collection** Heterogeneous (liquid and nonliquid component) No definable capsule Intrapancreatic and/or extrapancreatic	**Walled-off necrosis** Heterogeneous (liquid and nonliquid component) Well-defined capsule Intrapancreatic and/or extrapancreatic

encountered in necrotic collections. Infection of a fluid collection often has internal gas, although this feature does not reliably differentiate infected collections from WON.

Abdominal Imaging Studies

Disruption of pancreatic perfusion causes pancreatic necrosis and is detectable when an intravenous contrast agent is given during CT imaging (Figures 37.1, 37.2, and 37.3). The *Balthazar score* is a CT classification system for estimating the severity of acute pancreatitis according to the proportion of pancreas that is not perfused (reflecting necrosis) and the number of fluid collections. High mortality can be expected if the Balthazar CT severity index is 7 or more. Patients with acute pancreatitis who have normal CT findings have a good prognosis. The correlation is good between the lack of enhancement of more than 30% of the pancreas on contrast-enhanced CT and the finding of pancreatic necrosis at surgery or autopsy. As the degree of necrosis increases, morbidity and mortality also increase.

Features of poor perfusion are often lacking in the first 48 to 72 hours after the onset of acute pancreatitis. Hence, CT performed early in the course of disease may be falsely reassuring when necrosis is not identified. In definite cases of acute pancreatitis, contrast-enhanced CT can be deferred for 2 to 3 days and then—only if the patient's clinical condition is deteriorating or not responding to supportive care—performed to confirm the presence of necrosis and guide appropriate therapy. MRI has been compared prospectively with CT in the context of severe pancreatitis and found to be reliable for staging severity, to have predictive value for the prognosis of the disease, and to have fewer contraindications than CT. It may also detect disruption of the pancreatic duct, which can occur early in the course of acute pancreatitis.

Treatment

Keys to management of all cases of acute pancreatitis are 1) early estimation of severity (as outlined above), 2) aggressive initial fluid administration, 3) antiemetics and analgesia, and 4) elucidation and treatment of the underlying cause.

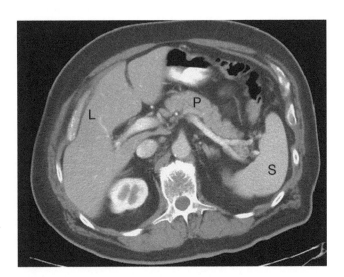

Figure 37.1.   Normal Pancreas. Contrast-enhanced computed tomography shows the pancreas (P) with a uniform enhancement intermediate between that of the liver (L) and the spleen (S).

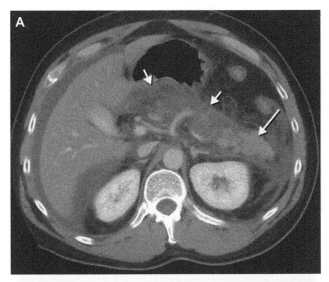

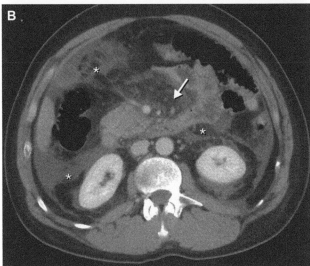

Figure 37.2.   Acute Necrotizing Pancreatitis. A, The patient had severe biliary pancreatitis. The density of the necrotic portion of the pancreas (short arrows) is less than that of the normal enhancement in the tail (long arrow). B, Note the necrosis in the body (arrow) and the peripancreatic edema (asterisks). The pancreatic head is well perfused.

In the absence of heart failure or chronic oliguria, lactated Ringer solution or normal saline should be administered intravenously at a rate of at least 200 to 300 mL hourly and titrated according to urine output (goal >1.5-3 mL/kg/h) and change in the serum urea nitrogen or creatinine level. In patients with severe volume depletion, an intravenous fluid bolus of 10 to 20 mL/kg over 1 to 2 hours may be required before continuous intravenous infusion. Lactated Ringer solution, with its calcium content, should not be used in patients with acute pancreatitis because of possible hypercalcemia. After the hematocrit decreases, the adequacy of fluid resuscitation must be monitored carefully at 12 and 24 hours, with more frequent serial checking of vital signs and measurement of urinary output. Serum levels of electrolytes, calcium, magnesium, and glucose and oxygenation should be monitored and supported or corrected as indicated. These issues may require admission to an ICU. To prevent volume overload and abdominal compartment syndrome, aggressive fluid resuscitation should be limited to the first 24 to 48 hours after the onset of acute pancreatitis (not hospital admission).

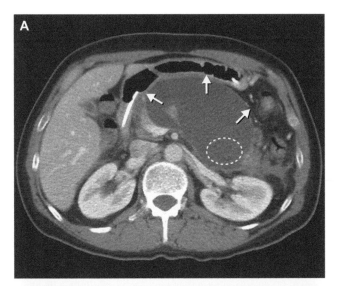

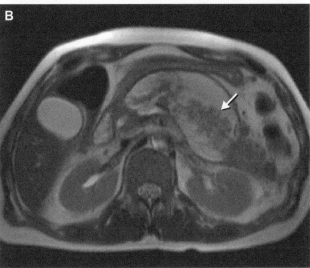

Figure 37.3. Walled-off Pancreatic Necrosis. A, Computed tomographic scan from the same patient as in Figure 37.2 shows that, 6 weeks later, most of the peripancreatic edema has resolved. The necrosis and fluid collection are well contained in the lesser sac, with a discrete wall or rind (arrows). The scan does not show the necrotic debris contained within the fluid collection (broken circle indicates area void of material). B, Magnetic resonance imaging of the same collection shows clear evidence of solid debris (arrow) within the fluid collection, a result of necrosis of the pancreatic body.

The need for early and adequate fluid resuscitation in patients with acute pancreatitis cannot be overstated. Aggressive intravenous fluid replacement counteracts intravascular volume depletion caused by third space losses, vomiting, fever, and the vascular permeability related to SIRS. Intravascular volume depletion causes hemoconcentration, low urine output, azotemia, tachycardia, and hypotension, thus compromising the blood supply of the pancreas, which contributes to the development of pancreatic necrosis with its attendant complications. Evidence from experimental models and from large clinical databases supports the concept that early aggressive fluid resuscitation minimizes or aborts pancreatic necrosis and improves survival. In a retrospective comparative study of 39 patients with acute pancreatitis of various severities, pancreatic necrosis developed in all patients who had evidence of hemoconcentration

(according to the hematocrit) that did not decrease with fluid resuscitation in 24 hours, underscoring the importance of sufficient volume resuscitation early in the disease course. Although our understanding of optimal fluid selection for treatment has considerable gaps, hydration with lactated Ringer solution, compared with normal saline, has been associated with less inflammation (as measured with C-reactive protein), shorter length of hospital stay, and fewer ICU admissions. Thus, in many centers lactated Ringer solution is the fluid of choice for patients with acute pancreatitis without contraindications to its use. Analgesia requires narcotic-strength agents (typically fentanyl or morphine) administered as patient-controlled analgesia. Although in animal experiments, morphine has caused spasm of the sphincter of Oddi, there is no definite evidence that morphine worsens the disease in humans.

Interstitial edematous pancreatitis can be managed with supportive care in a general hospital ward without the need for monitoring in an ICU. Generally, nasogastric tubes are not indicated because they do not improve disease outcome and they increase patient discomfort. However, nasogastric tubes may decrease symptoms in patients with extreme nausea, vomiting, and ileus. Empirical use of antibiotics should be avoided in patients with interstitial pancreatitis because these agents do not alter the outcome. Nutritional support (discussed below) is indicated only if the patient is expected to receive nothing by mouth for 1 or more weeks. For mild interstitial pancreatitis, recent studies have shown that early oral feeding, as tolerated, is safe.

Specific therapy for identified causes of acute pancreatitis should be instituted early to prevent recurrence of acute episodes. This includes discontinuation of suspected medications that might have induced pancreatitis, initiation of therapy for hypertriglyceridemia, and performance of cholecystectomy for suspected biliary pancreatitis. Cholecystectomy should be performed during the index hospital admission to prevent early recurrence of acute pancreatitis—and other gallstone-related complications—among patients who delay their return or do not return for follow-up. If the patient is a poor surgical candidate because of severe coexisting medical illness, ERCP with biliary sphincterotomy may be a good alternative to cholecystectomy, especially if ultrasonography shows only sludge or small stones.

If biliary stone disease, hyperlipidemia, and medications are excluded as causes, abdominal CT should be performed to exclude anatomical causes of pancreatic ductal obstruction, such as a pancreatic or ampullary mass lesion or intraductal papillary mucinous neoplasm, especially in patients older than 40 years. For elderly patients with negative CT findings, consideration should be given to performing EUS or MR cholangiopancreatography after the acute changes have resolved.

Severe acute pancreatitis, with or without pancreatic necrosis, requires aggressive medical management, with greater emphasis on fluid supplementation and the prevention and early diagnosis of infection. In recent years, the management of severe acute pancreatitis has shifted from early surgical débridement (necrosectomy) to intensive medical care.

Early mortality during the first 1 to 2 weeks of acute pancreatitis is primarily due to multisystem organ failure resulting from SIRS. Systemic complications include adult respiratory distress syndrome, acute kidney failure, shock, coagulopathy, hyperglycemia, and hypocalcemia. These complications are managed with endotracheal intubation, aggressive fluid resuscitation, fresh frozen plasma, insulin, and calcium as needed.

Nutritional Support

Nutritional support is often indicated to meet increased metabolic demands and to rest the pancreas during the prolonged fasting state of acute pancreatitis. Multiple randomized prospective studies of severe acute pancreatitis have compared total parenteral nutrition with enteral feeding through a nasoenteric feeding tube placed under endoscopic or radiographic guidance. Enteral feeding yields significantly fewer total and infectious complications, a 3-fold decrease in the cost of nutritional support, and improvement in the acute-phase response and disease severity scores, compared with parenteral (intravenous) nutrition. Enteral nutrition helps preserve the mucosal barrier of the gut and reduces translocation of bacteria from the gut, thus decreasing the rate of infected necrosis. A recent meta-analysis of nutritional therapy for patients with acute pancreatitis reported that, compared with parenteral nutrition, enteral nutrition was associated with a significantly lower incidence of infections, fewer surgical interventions to control pancreatitis, and a decrease in mortality. Enteral nutrition should be considered the standard of care for patients with severe acute pancreatitis.

For patients who have mild disease (ie, no organ failure or necrosis) and no symptoms of nausea or vomiting, and for whom ileus is not a concern, oral feeding can be initiated within 24 hours and advanced as tolerated. For patients who have more severe disease (ie, with failure of 1 or more organs or the presence of necrosis), emphasis should still be placed on aggressive, early nutritional support to reduce the risk of further organ failure, infection, and need for operative intervention.

For patients who have moderately severe or severe pancreatitis who cannot tolerate oral feeding, enteral tube feeding should be considered by days 3 to 5. Ideally, enteral nutrition is delivered to the jejunum or at least to the postpyloric gut. Placement of the feeding tube into the jejunum theoretically decreases stimulation of the inflamed pancreas, but radiologic or endoscopic guidance adds expense and is not readily available in all facilities. From studies with contradictory results, nasogastric feeding may or may not be as safe and beneficial as nasojejunal feeding, but this issue requires further study. Enteral feeding with a high-protein, low-fat, semielemental formula should be initiated even in severe cases unless the patient has bowel obstruction. If this enteral feeding does not help, a transition to total parental nutrition should be initiated promptly.

Prophylactic Antibiotics

Prophylactic antibiotics are not recommended in patients with acute pancreatitis, regardless of severity or presence of necrosis. Clinically, patients with severe pancreatitis often have features of sepsis, including fever, leukocytosis, and organ failure in the first 7 to 10 days, which may be clinically difficult to distinguish from infection. Furthermore, patients may have extrapancreatic infections (eg, pneumonia or bacteremia). Therefore, patients who are thought to have an infection may begin appropriate antimicrobial therapy; however, if the evaluation and blood cultures are negative for infection, antibiotic therapy should be discontinued.

Detection of Pancreatic Infection

Sterile or infected acute necrotizing pancreatitis can be difficult to distinguish clinically because either may produce fever, leukocytosis, and severe abdominal pain. Infection of pancreatic necrosis is rare during the first week of acute pancreatitis, a period characterized by overactivation of the immune system, and is more often recognized by the third or fourth week. Nevertheless, without intervention, the mortality rate for patients with infected acute necrotizing pancreatitis is nearly 100%; thus, early empirical use of antibiotics is warranted while the infection is investigated. Predisposing factors for the development of infection include necrosis (90% of infections in acute pancreatitis occur in the presence of necrosis) and an increased number of fluid collections. The bacteriologic status of the pancreas can be determined with CT-guided fine-needle aspiration of pancreatic and peripancreatic tissue or fluid. This aspiration method is safe, accurate (96% sensitivity and 99% specificity), and recommended for patients with acute necrotizing pancreatitis whose clinical condition deteriorates or does not improve despite aggressive supportive care. Ultrasonographically guided aspiration may have lower sensitivity and specificity, but it can be performed at the bedside. If CT-guided sampling documents the presence of gram-negative organisms, appropriate choices for antibiotics include a carbapenem, a fluoroquinolone with metronidazole, or a third-generation cephalosporin with metronidazole. If Gram stains show gram-positive organisms, the addition of vancomycin is appropriate. In all cases, antibiotic coverage can be narrowed or expanded once the identity and sensitivities of the organism are known. An evolving understanding implicates fungal organisms as also having a pivotal role in infected pancreatic necrosis.

Therapy for Pancreatic Fluid Collections

As mature, encapsulated collections, pancreatic pseudocysts and WON can be targeted through endoscopic, percutaneous radiologic, or surgical means. In addition to their inherent risks, any such procedure threatens infection of a sterile fluid collection; thus, intervention on fluid collections should be pursued only if they are causing symptoms (eg, pain, nausea, or anorexia), causing luminal or biliary obstruction, contributing to SIRS (as is often the case with WON), or becoming infected. Ideally, interventions should be delayed until fluid collections have become organized, a process that typically takes 4 weeks. Pseudocysts may require only simple drainage, whereas WON with a considerable amount of solid necrotic material is likely to require mechanical débridement (ie, necrosectomy), often necessitating multiple procedures over time. Minimally invasive endoscopic drainage is now the first-line therapy for symptomatic pseudocysts and WON at many centers. Asymptomatic and sterile pancreatic fluid collections can be managed through observation and serial imaging alone.

Role of ERCP

Early ERCP with biliary sphincterotomy improves outcomes among patients who have severe gallstone pancreatitis with associated cholangitis. Studies that exclude patients with biliary obstruction have shown limited or no benefit from early ERCP in patients predicted to have severe acute pancreatitis. Hence, improved outcome after ERCP and sphincterotomy in gallstone pancreatitis appears to be the result of reduced biliary sepsis rather than improvement in pancreatitis. Ideally, when performed for concomitant cholangitis, ERCP should be undertaken in the first 24 to 48 hours, since later cholestasis often reflects pancreatic edema rather than stone obstruction and biliary infection; moreover, associated duodenal edema compromises the success of ERCP after this interval.

Additional Complications

Disconnected pancreatic duct syndrome is characterized by complete discontinuity of the pancreatic duct that occurs in up to 30% of persons with necrotizing pancreatitis. It typically results from inflammation and swelling in the pancreatic neck, which leads to failure of the viable distal pancreas to drain through the proximal pancreas into the duodenum. This causes pancreatic secretions to leak into the retroperitoneum, where they may eventually coalesce into a pseudocyst or WON. CT or MRI findings may suggest the presence of a disconnected pancreatic duct, but confirmation may require pancreatography to show extravasation of contrast material injected into the main pancreatic duct, most often with ERCP or EUS. Management of disconnected pancreatic duct syndrome may require surgical resection of the disconnected but functional upstream portion of the gland (distal pancreatectomy) or surgical cyst enterostomy for prolonged diversion of leaking pancreatic juice. In some cases, a chronic fistula can be maintained to the stomach or the duodenum by endoscopic long-term placement of transmural stents. A *disrupted* pancreatic duct leads to a similar clinical presentation from lack of duct continuity without a complete disconnected segment. Continuity may be reestablished by endoscopic stent placement through the papilla and across the disrupted duct segment; endoscopic management becomes considerably more challenging if the disruption is closer to the tail.

Beyond local duct and parenchymal pancreatic phenomena, vascular complications can occur in patients who have acute pancreatitis; these include splanchnic vein thrombosis and splanchnic artery pseudoaneurysm. Treatment of *splanchnic vein thrombosis* focuses on managing the underlying pancreatitis. While the majority of splanchnic vein thromboses resolve spontaneously, anticoagulation is needed if the clot extends into the portal or superior mesenteric vein, as this could lead to hepatic or enteric ischemia. *Pseudoaneurysm* develops in approximately 10% of patients with a pancreatic fluid collection, typically occurring in the wake of inflammation and erosion of the gastroduodenal or splenic arteries. Pseudoaneurysm can manifest as bleeding—which may be catastrophic—into the gastrointestinal tract or into a pancreatic fluid collection. Evaluation for pseudoaneurysm and treatment with interventional radiology-based embolization therapies is critical before the use of endoscopic therapy for pancreatic fluid collections.

Prognosis

The overall mortality rate for patients with severe acute pancreatitis has decreased to approximately 15% as a result of improved ICU therapies, antibiotics, and deferral of surgery. Early deaths (1-2 weeks after the onset of pancreatitis; approximately 50% of all deaths) are primarily due to multisystem organ failure, and late deaths result from local or systemic infections. The overall mortality rate for patients with sterile acute necrotizing pancreatitis is approximately 10%. The mortality rate is at least 3 times higher if infected necrosis occurs. Patients with sterile necrosis and severe disease accompanied by multisystem organ failure, shock, or kidney insufficiency have a significantly higher mortality rate.

The long-term clinical endocrine and exocrine consequences of acute necrotizing pancreatitis appear to depend on several factors: the severity of necrosis, the cause of pancreatitis (alcoholic or nonalcoholic), the continued use of alcohol, and the degree of pancreatic débridement. Sophisticated exocrine function studies have shown persistent subclinical exocrine insufficiency in many patients up to 2 years after severe acute pancreatitis. Treatment with pancreatic enzymes should be restricted to patients with symptoms of steatorrhea and weight loss due to fat malabsorption. Although subtle glucose intolerance is frequent, overt type 2 diabetes is uncommon.

Suggested Reading

Abu Dayyeh BK, Topazian M. Endoscopic management of pancreatic necrosis. Am J Gastroenterol. 2018 Sep;113(9):1269–73.

ASGE Standards of Practice Committee, Chandrasekhara V, Khashab MA, Muthusamy VR, Acosta RD, Agrawal D, et al. Adverse events associated with ERCP. Gastrointest Endosc. 2017 Jan;85(1):32–47.

Crockett SD, Wani S, Gardner TB, Falck-Ytter Y, Barkun AN, American Gastroenterological Association Institute Clinical Guidelines Committee. American Gastroenterological Association Institute guideline on initial management of acute pancreatitis. Gastroenterology. 2018 Mar;154(4):1096–101.

Forsmark CE, Vege SS, Wilcox CM. Acute pancreatitis. N Engl J Med. 2016 Nov;375(20):1972–81.

Lee A, Ko C, Buitrago C, Hiramoto B, Hilson L, Buxbaum J, et al. Lactated ringers vs normal saline resuscitation for mild acute pancreatitis: a randomized trial. Gastroenterology. 2021 Feb;160(3):955–7.

Sandrasegaran K, Heller MT, Panda A, Shetty A, Menias CO. MRI in acute pancreatitis. Abdom Radiol (NY). 2020 May;45(5):1232–42.

Schepers NJ, Hallensleben NDL, Besselink MG, Anten MGF, Bollen TL, da Costa DW, et al. Urgent endoscopic retrograde cholangiopancreatography with sphincterotomy versus conservative treatment in predicted severe acute gallstone pancreatitis (APEC): a multicentre randomised controlled trial. Lancet. 2020 Jul 18;396(10245):167–76.

Tenner S, Baillie J, DeWitt J, Vege SS, American College of Gastroenterology. American College of Gastroenterology guideline: management of acute pancreatitis. Am J Gastroenterol. 2013 Sep;108(9):1400–15; 16.

Vaughn VM, Shuster D, Rogers MAM, Mann J, Conte ML, Saint S, et al. Early versus delayed feeding in patients with acute pancreatitis: a systematic review. Ann Intern Med. 2017 Jun 20;166(12):883–92.

Vege SS, DiMagno MJ, Forsmark CE, Martel M, Barkun AN. Initial medical treatment of acute pancreatitis: American Gastroenterological Association Institute technical review. Gastroenterology. 2018 Mar;154(4):1103–39.

Wan J, He W, Zhu Y, Zhu Y, Zeng H, Liu P, et al. Stratified analysis and clinical significance of elevated serum triglyceride levels in early acute pancreatitis: a retrospective study. Lipids Health Dis. 2017 Jun;16(1):124.

38

Chronic Pancreatitis[a]

LAURENS P. JANSSENS, MD

SHOUNAK MAJUMDER, MD

Chronic pancreatitis is an inflammatory condition of the pancreas characterized by progressive fibrosis that leads to irreversible destruction of exocrine and endocrine tissue, resulting eventually in exocrine and endocrine insufficiency. There is considerable heterogeneity in the manifestation and natural history of the condition. Chronic pancreatitis is classified broadly into chronic calcifying pancreatitis, chronic obstructive pancreatitis, and chronic autoimmune pancreatitis.

Chronic calcifying pancreatitis is usually characterized by recurrent bouts of clinically acute pancreatitis early in the course of the disease and development of intraductal stones later in the disease course. Steatorrhea and diabetes mellitus eventually develop in most patients. This is the clinical profile of the disease that readily comes to mind when the term *chronic pancreatitis* is used in clinical practice. However, about 10% of patients may be asymptomatic, and the disease is incidentally detected on cross-sectional imaging; nearly half the patients with chronic pancreatitis have not had previous episodes of acute pancreatitis.

Chronic obstructive pancreatitis results from obstruction of the pancreatic duct due to any cause. The disease affects only the portion of the organ that is upstream of the obstruction. It is usually not associated with pancreatic duct stone formation. Although patients are often asymptomatic, partial obstruction can lead to recurrent bouts of clinically acute pancreatitis

involving the obstructed part of the gland. Obstructive pancreatitis commonly occurs distally to pancreatic tumors (ductal adenocarcinoma and intraductal papillary mucinous tumor), anastomotic strictures related to pancreaticojejunostomy, and postinflammatory strictures after acute or traumatic pancreatitis. The preferred treatment of symptomatic disease is resection of the obstructed upstream portion of the pancreas, but pancreatic duct stenting may be an alternative in carefully selected patients who have benign strictures.

Chronic autoimmune pancreatitis, simply known as *autoimmune pancreatitis* (AIP), is a unique form of chronic pancreatitis that is characterized histologically by lymphoplasmacytic infiltrate and storiform fibrosis and therapeutically by a dramatic response to corticosteroids. When so defined, AIP has 2 subtypes, type 1 and type 2 (Table 38.1.).

Type 1 AIP is considered the pancreatic manifestation of a multiorgan fibroinflammatory syndrome known as immunoglobulin (Ig)G4-related disease. This syndrome affects not only the pancreas but also other organs and tissues, including the bile duct, orbital tissue, salivary glands, retroperitoneum, and lymph nodes. Type 1 AIP is a disease of older men. Serum IgG4 levels are often elevated in type 1 AIP, and organs and tissues affected by AIP have a lymphoplasmacytic infiltrate that is rich in IgG4-positive cells. In type 1 AIP, the pancreas has a typical histologic pattern called *lymphoplasmacytic sclerosing pancreatitis*, characterized by a dense lymphoplasmacytic infiltrate around medium-sized ducts, a peculiar swirling (storiform) fibrosis, and an intense inflammation that surrounds veins (obliterative phlebitis) and spares adjacent arteries.

Most commonly, patients presenting with this form of chronic pancreatitis have obstructive jaundice that mimics pancreatic cancer; they rarely present with clinically acute or painful chronic pancreatitis. Pancreatic calcification is uncommon in

---

[a] The authors thank Suresh T. Chari, MD, who was the author of the previous version of this chapter (parts of which appear in this edition).

Abbreviations: AIP, autoimmune pancreatitis; CT, computed tomography; ERCP, endoscopic retrograde cholangiopancreatography; EUS, endoscopic ultrasonography; FE1, fecal elastase-1; Ig, immunoglobulin; MRCP, magnetic resonance cholangiopancreatography; MRI, magnetic resonance imaging

Table 38.1. Demographic, Clinical, and Histologic Features of Autoimmune Pancreatitis (AIP)

Feature[a]	AIP type	
	Type 1 (LPSP)	Type 2 (IDCP)
Age at diagnosis, y	60-70	40-50
Sex predominance	Male	Equivalent
Acute pancreatitis	Rare	Most common presentation
Extrapancreatic disease	Frequently present, involving bile ducts, orbit, salivary gland, kidney, and retroperitoneum	Absent
Association with IBD	Weak	Strong
IgG4 increased	60%-70% of patients	Uncommon
Relapses	30%-50% of patients	<10% of patients
Storiform fibrosis	Prominent	Less prominent
Obliterative phlebitis	Typical	Rare
Granulocyte epithelial lesion	Absent	Typical
Tissue IgG4-positive cells	Abundant; usually >10/HPF	Rare; usually <10/HPF

Abbreviations: HPF, high-power field; IBD, inflammatory bowel disease; IDCP, idiopathic duct-centric pancreatitis; Ig, immunoglobulin; LPSP, lymphoplasmacytic sclerosing pancreatitis.

[a] Pancreatic imaging features are similar in both types of AIP; histologically, both types have lymphoplasmacytic infiltrate.

AIP. The inflammatory process in type 1 AIP responds to corticosteroid therapy, although relapse is common after withdrawal of treatment. If patients have a confirmed diagnosis of type 1 AIP but cannot tolerate corticosteroids, rituximab may be used for initial treatment. Patients with relapsing disease require long-term maintenance immunosuppression with either a low dose of corticosteroids or steroid-sparing agents such as azathioprine, mycophenolate mofetil, or rituximab.

Type 2 AIP occurs in younger patients and appears to be a pancreas-specific disorder. It is typically not associated with either increased serum levels of IgG4 or dense tissue infiltration with IgG4-positive cells. About 15% to 30% of patients with type 2 AIP have inflammatory bowel disease (predominantly ulcerative colitis). Histologically, type 2 AIP (also known as *idiopathic duct-centric pancreatitis*) is characterized by neutrophilic infiltrate in the pancreatic duct epithelium (ie, a granulocyte epithelial lesion), which can lead to ductal obliteration. Type 2 AIP also responds to corticosteroid therapy, and relapses, which are far less common than in type 1 AIP, are treated with corticosteroids.

The rest of the discussion in this chapter is related to chronic calcifying pancreatitis.

Etiology and Risk Factors

Several conditions are associated with chronic calcifying pancreatitis (Table 38.2). The pathogenesis of chronic pancreatitis is largely unknown. However, clinical acute pancreatitis and the eventual development of chronic pancreatitis are thought to be due to the interaction between genetic and environmental factors. The synergistic interaction between alcohol use and smoking is an increasingly recognized risk factor for chronic pancreatitis.

Genes that have been associated with chronic pancreatitis include the following: cationic trypsinogen gene (*PRSS1*; OMIM 27600); serine protease inhibitor Kazal-type 1 gene (*SPINK1*; OMIM 167790); cystic fibrosis transmembrane conductance regulator gene (*CFTR*; OMIM 602421); chymotrypsin C gene (*CTRC*; OMIM 601405); and calcium-sensing receptor gene (*CASR*; OMIM 601199). The claudin-2 gene (*CLDN2*; OMIM 300520) is associated with accelerated progression from acute pancreatitis to chronic pancreatitis in persons who have alcohol-related disease. Alterations in the *PRSS1* gene cause chronic

hereditary pancreatitis in an autosomal dominant pattern. The most frequent variations in *PRSS1* associated with pancreatitis are p.R122H and p.N29I, which have penetrance greater than 80%. *SPINK1* alterations are frequent in the general population and are associated with an increased risk for pancreatitis; however, pancreatitis develops in less than 1% of persons who have

Table 38.2. Etiologic and Risk Factors of Chronic Calcifying Pancreatitis (CP)

Etiologic or risk factor	Salient features
Alcohol	Most common cause of CP in the West
	CP develops in about 5% of persons with alcohol use disorder, usually after a long history of alcohol ingestion; occasional binge drinking alone is not sufficient to cause CP, and smoking is a strong cofactor
Smoking	Independent risk factor
	Increased risk for pancreatic calcifications, EPI, and pancreatic cancer
Hereditary	Alterations in the cationic trypsinogen gene (*PRSS1*) are associated with a high-penetrance (80%) autosomal dominant form of CP, accounting for 1% of all CP cases
	Patients present at an early age (first and second decades)
	High risk of pancreatic cancer with time, especially for smokers
Tropical	Cause unknown
	Highest prevalence in South India
	Early age at onset (first and second decades)
	High prevalence (>80%) of diabetes mellitus and calcification at diagnosis
Idiopathic	Early (juvenile) and late (senile) forms
	Juvenile form is associated with alterations in the *CFTR* and *SPINK1* genes and with other alterations in the *PRSS1* gene, which are also associated with CP (probably as disease modifiers)
	Pain is a common feature of early-onset disease
	Senile form may be painless
Hypertriglyceridemia	Triglyceride levels usually >1,000 mg/dL

Abbreviation: EPI, exocrine pancreatic insufficiency.

an alteration. In patients who have a heterozygous *SPINK1* alteration, it likely acts as a disease modifier rather than a primary cause of pancreatitis. Interactions between these genes, other unknown genetic factors, and toxic-metabolic factors (eg, alcohol, smoking, hypertriglyceridemia, and hypercalcemia) are thought to lead to recurrent acute and chronic pancreatitis.

Diagnosis

Although histologic examination is the gold standard for diagnosis of chronic pancreatitis, it often is not available. Without histologic study, a combination of morphologic findings on imaging studies, functional abnormalities, and clinical findings is used to diagnose chronic pancreatitis. The diagnosis is relatively straightforward in the later stages of the disease when calcification and steatorrhea are present, but the diagnosis is difficult when pancreatic structure and function are not unequivocally abnormal. Currently available diagnostic modalities are not adequate for making a firm diagnosis of chronic pancreatitis without obvious changes in structure and function.

Structural Evaluation

The imaging procedures commonly used to evaluate for structural changes in the pancreas are computed tomography (CT), endoscopic ultrasonography (EUS), magnetic resonance imaging (MRI), and MR cholangiopancreatography (MRCP). Endoscopic retrograde cholangiopancreatography (ERCP) is no longer recommended as a diagnostic test for chronic pancreatitis because of the risk of procedural complications and the widespread availability of high-resolution cross-sectional imaging modalities that are safe and noninvasive. Pancreatic calcification that is suggestive but not diagnostic of chronic pancreatitis can be identified on abdominal radiographs. However, CT and EUS can be used to detect small specks of calcification not visible on plain radiographs. CT, MRI, and EUS all have similar diagnostic sensitivity and specificity for chronic pancreatitis.

Abdominal CT is a good first test for the evaluation of a patient with possible chronic pancreatitis. It is noninvasive and widely available, with relatively good sensitivity for the diagnosis of moderate to severe chronic pancreatitis. The findings, however, can be normal in early chronic pancreatitis. Chronic pancreatitis is diagnosed with CT by the identification of pathognomonic calcifications within the main pancreatic duct or parenchyma or calcification within the dilated main pancreatic duct in combination with parenchymal atrophy (Figure 38.1). CT is also suitable for the evaluation of pain in a patient with known chronic pancreatitis, because most complications of chronic pancreatitis, including peripancreatic fluid collections, bile duct obstruction, and bowel obstruction, can be identified and inflammatory or neoplastic masses can be visualized.

EUS provides high-resolution images of the pancreatic parenchyma and duct. Nine ductal and parenchymal EUS features have been identified; the presence of more than 5 features strongly suggests the diagnosis of pancreatitis with structural abnormalities seen on other imaging studies. However, the diagnosis of "early" chronic pancreatitis (ie, chronic pancreatitis not evident on other imaging studies) based on EUS changes alone is still controversial. There is considerable interobserver disagreement on the presence or absence of EUS features and their interpretation. Problems with interpretation also may arise for 1) older patients who have senile changes in the pancreas, 2) patients with alcohol use in whom fibrosis may be present but not pancreatitis, 3) patients with increased intrapancreatic fat, and 4) patients who had a recent episode of acute pancreatitis. Currently, the diagnosis of chronic pancreatitis should not be based on EUS criteria alone.

ERCP is no longer recommended as a diagnostic tool in the evaluation of suspected chronic pancreatitis because of its inherent risks of complications (5%). It should be performed only when therapy is planned (eg, pancreatic duct stone extraction or dilation and stent placement for a pancreatic ductal stricture).

MRCP is noninvasive, avoids the use of ionizing radiation, and does not routinely require sedation, making it a diagnostic procedure of choice for most patients, especially when CT findings are normal and there is reasonable, continued clinical suspicion for the diagnosis of chronic pancreatitis. MRCP avoids the risks associated with ERCP while providing a detailed evaluation of the pancreatic duct. Major lesions such as grossly dilated ducts,

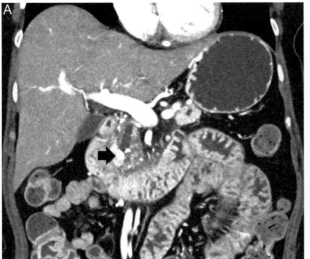 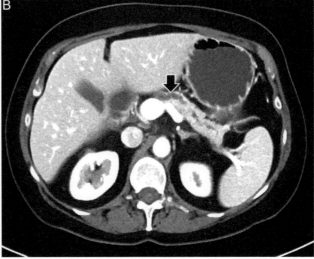

Figure 38.1. Chronic Pancreatitis. A, Contrast-enhanced computed tomography (CT) of the abdomen (coronal view) shows a stone (arrow) in the dilated main pancreatic duct in the head of the pancreas. B, Contrast-enhanced CT of the abdomen (axial view) shows a dilated main pancreatic duct in the body (arrow) and tail.

communicating pseudocysts, and even pancreas divisum can be detected, but small duct changes and calcifications are not readily visualized. Secretin administered intravenously during MRCP can further enhance pancreatic duct visualization and aid in the diagnosis of chronic pancreatitis. Secretin-enhanced MRCP can be used to identify subtle morphologic changes suggestive of chronic pancreatitis such as pancreatic duct irregularity and ectatic side branches, allow for a dynamic assessment of main pancreatic duct compliance, and assess pancreatic ductal fluid secretion as a surrogate for exocrine function.

Functional Testing

The pancreas has great functional reserve, which means it must be damaged severely before functional loss is recognized clinically. For example, 90% of the pancreas must typically be destroyed before steatorrhea occurs. Abnormal results of functional testing alone are not diagnostic of chronic pancreatitis, and diagnosis requires additional evidence from imaging studies of structural alteration consistent with chronic pancreatitis. Imaging studies by themselves usually are diagnostic by the time steatorrhea develops.

Invasive or direct tests of pancreatic function (eg, the "tubed" secretin test) show functional impairment even in the absence of steatorrhea. However, these tests are complex, invasive, and not widely available. The only direct pancreatic function test currently in use at some centers with available expertise is the endoscopic pancreatic function test, which involves a periodic collection of duodenal fluid for assessment of bicarbonate concentration after administration of intravenous secretin. Noninvasive or indirect tests of pancreatic function, such as 72-hour fecal fat estimation and fecal elastase-1 (FE1) quantification, have poor sensitivity for the detection of early disease and are not indicated as tests to establish a diagnosis of CP. However, in patients with established CP, these stool tests can be used to diagnose exocrine pancreatic insufficiency. Although an FE1 level of less than 200 μg/g of stool is considered abnormal, values less than 100 μg/g usually indicate exocrine pancreatic insufficiency, whereas mild to moderately decreased FE1 levels (ie, 100-200 μg/g of stool) may be indeterminate and require clinical context for accurate interpretation. FE1 estimation may be falsely low in watery stool samples because of dilution. In patients with diarrhea and a low pretest probability of chronic pancreatitis, the FE1 assay can have a high false-positive result, and an abnormal value should be interpreted with caution.

Clinical Features and Natural History

Abdominal pain is the dominant symptom in the early part of the natural history of chronic pancreatitis, and steatorrhea and diabetes mellitus are the prominent features of late, end-stage disease. Pain is usually related to acute inflammatory flares or local complications, although patients can have chronic persistent pain due to visceral hypersensitivity. Some authors have reported a painless "burn out" of the pancreas in the late stages of the disease, but others have reported pain occurring even in late stages. Complications can occur after acute flares of pancreatitis or from chronic fibrosis in and around the pancreas.

The clinical features and natural history of chronic pancreatitis can differ remarkably in different forms of chronic pancreatitis. The age at onset of pain is much younger (first and second decades of life) in the hereditary and tropical forms of chronic pancreatitis. Although pain is a dominant feature of most forms

of chronic pancreatitis, it may be absent in up to 10% of patients overall and more commonly in patients with late-onset (senile) idiopathic chronic pancreatitis. Diabetes mellitus and calcification may be absent at diagnosis in patients with alcoholic chronic pancreatitis, but they are present at diagnosis in more than 80% of patients with tropical pancreatitis.

For patients with alcoholic chronic pancreatitis, death often is related to smoking and nonpancreatic and alcohol-related complications (especially cancers). For patients with tropical pancreatitis, the most common cause of death is diabetes-related complications; the second most common cause is pancreatic cancer. Pancreatic cancer can complicate any form of chronic pancreatitis, but it is especially common in the hereditary and tropical forms, probably because of the long duration of disease.

Complications

Diabetes Mellitus

Progressive decrease in islet cell mass leads to diabetes mellitus in chronic pancreatitis, classified as pancreatogenic diabetes or type 3c diabetes. Whereas diabetes is common at presentation in the tropical form of chronic pancreatitis, it is usually a late complication in other forms of the disease. Diabetes eventually develops in most patients (85%), with or without pancreatic resection, and nonresective surgery such as ductal drainage does not prevent it. Even after total pancreatectomy with autologous islet transplant, most patients are insulin-dependent at 10 years after surgery.

Steatorrhea

Steatorrhea usually occurs after more than 90% of the gland has been destroyed. Persistent steatorrhea can lead to deficiencies in fat-soluble vitamins (vitamins A, D, E, and K) and other micronutrients (zinc, magnesium, and vitamin B_{12}) and malnutrition, weight loss, and osteoporosis. Treatment involves oral pancreatic enzyme replacement therapy and supplementation to correct vitamin and micronutrient deficiencies. Pancreatic enzyme replacement therapy is available as uncoated tablets or enteric-coated capsules or microspheres with pH-dependent release of enzymes. Patients with severe steatorrhea require 30,000 to 45,000 US Pharmacopeia units of lipase per meal and lesser amounts with snacks. Enzymes should be given with meals to allow proper mixing of food with the enzymes. Acid suppression may be required to prevent destruction of the enzymes by gastric acid. Fat-soluble vitamin levels should be measured at baseline and monitored periodically to correct any concomitant nutritional deficiencies. Bone mineral density testing should also be considered at baseline, especially in patients with concomitant osteoporosis risk factors.

Pseudocyst

In the early stages of the disease, pseudocysts result from pancreatic duct leakage after an attack of clinically acute pancreatitis. In later stages, ductal dilatation can lead to leakage and the formation of pseudocysts from ductal "blowout." Upstream ductal obstruction due to stricture or a large stone often results in the reformation of pseudocysts after simple enteral drainage (eg, endoscopic cyst drainage). This may require endoscopic intervention or concomitant drainage of the main pancreatic duct (usually surgically) or resection of the diseased portion of the gland (or both).

Biliary Obstruction

Biliary obstruction can result from edema of the head of the gland after an acute attack, compression from a pseudocyst, bile duct entrapment in the fibrotic process involving the head of the gland, or complicating pancreatic malignancy in patients with long-standing disease. Acute inflammatory edema of the head of the gland usually responds to conservative management, and compression of a pseudocyst responds to drainage of the pseudocyst. Fibrotic stricturing requires endoscopic intervention typically with a prolonged period of stenting with covered metal biliary stents and surgical biliary bypass if strictures persist or recur after appropriate endoscopic intervention. Pancreatic cancer complicating chronic pancreatitis can be difficult to diagnose early. The management of pancreatic cancer is described in detail in Chapter 39 ("Pancreatic Neoplasms").

Duodenal Obstruction

Potentially reversible gastric outlet obstruction can occur during an acute flare of pancreatitis when peripancreatic inflammation involves the gastroduodenal region. Nasojejunal feeding may be required to maintain nutrition during this period. Patients with a persistent fibrotic process involving the duodenum require either surgical bypass of the gastric outlet obstruction or pancreaticoduodenectomy.

Splenic Vein Thrombosis

Because of the proximity of the splenic vein to the pancreas, the vein is often affected by pancreatic inflammation or fibrosis. Patients with left-sided portal hypertension (ie, sinistral portal hypertension) can present with gastric variceal bleeding, which is treated with splenectomy.

Pancreatic Cancer

Patients with chronic pancreatitis have an increased risk for pancreatic cancer. However, screening for early detection of pancreatic cancer in these patients is not recommended because of a lack of effective screening tools. Expert consensus recommends screening in patients who have hereditary chronic pancreatitis associated with a *PRSS1* variant starting at age 40 years or 20 years after onset of pancreatitis, whichever is earlier. The carbohydrate antigen 19-9 level may be falsely high in chronic pancreatitis and is therefore not useful for pancreatic cancer screening.

Management

Abdominal pain is the most dominant and vexing problem in the management of patients with chronic pancreatitis. It can vary in severity from mild, intermittent pain to severe, chronic, debilitating pain. In addition to the addiction to alcohol and tobacco that patients with alcoholic pancreatitis often have, patients with severe pain also have a considerable potential for addiction to narcotics. It is very difficult to assess the true severity of pain if patients misuse narcotics, and therapeutic interventions often are seemingly unsuccessful because of continued dependence on narcotics. Apart from these issues, a poor understanding of the pathogenesis of pain has made it difficult to rationally manage abdominal pain in patients who have chronic pancreatitis. Despite some optimism that pancreatic pain eventually "burns out," most clinicians agree that the pain has a large negative impact on the quality of life of patients with chronic pancreatitis, and although the severity may fluctuate, it rarely disappears with time.

A stepwise approach to pain management is recommended. However, the scientific evidence to support any of the measures taken (medical, endoscopic, or surgical) is scant, and there are very few well-defined prospective trials that compare groups receiving therapy with groups receiving either no therapy or a competing therapy.

An important first step is the assessment of a patient's pain and its nature, frequency, severity, and effect on quality of life and other activities. Patients who have intermittent (eg, ≤1 episode per year), uncomplicated episodes with full function between episodes are probably better off without potentially injurious interventions. Regardless of the severity of pain, all patients with chronic pancreatitis should be counseled during each visit about abstinence from not only alcohol but also tobacco.

Patients who have more frequent or severe pain and a tendency to take narcotics for pain control need further evaluation. The initial evaluation with imaging studies (eg, CT) should be undertaken to rule out complications of pancreatitis such as persistent acute inflammation (inflammatory mass) in the pancreas, pancreatic and peripancreatic fluid collections, biliary obstruction, and duodenal stenosis. Other diagnoses to be considered in the appropriate clinical context are opioid-induced constipation, abdominal wall pain, peptic ulcer disease, gallbladder disease, and pancreatic cancer. The presence of any of these should lead to appropriate intervention.

In patients without the above conditions, medical, endoscopic, and surgical options have been attempted. Medical therapy includes avoidance of a high-fat diet, abstinence from alcohol and smoking, and use of pancreatic enzyme replacement therapy, often in association with acid suppression. Endoscopic therapy includes sphincterotomy, lithotripsy, and pancreatic duct stenting. Endoscopic interventions are appropriate before surgical therapy is considered except in patients with a heavy burden of stone disease, where surgery has been shown to result in better outcomes. Celiac plexus block (performed with EUS guidance or percutaneously) appears to have limited benefit in patients with chronic pancreatitis. Chronic pancreatitis is a complex disease and medical management needs to be individualized according to the clinical context, local expertise, and needs of the patient.

Surgical therapy is an option for patients who clearly appear to have disabling pancreas-related pain. The choice of operation, if elected, should be based on the morphology of the pancreatic duct and the distribution and character of parenchymal disease. Treatment options include decompressive surgery, such as lateral pancreaticojejunostomy for patients with a dilated pancreatic duct; partial pancreatic resection for those with a persistent inflammatory mass; or total pancreatectomy for patients with disease unresponsive to medical therapy and not suitable for other surgical options. A randomized controlled trial comparing pancreaticojejunostomy with endoscopic therapy for chronic pancreatitis with dilated ducts showed that surgery provided superior results, and a higher proportion of surgical patients reported pain relief. However, the 20% to 40% failure rate and the potential for surgical morbidity and mortality warrant reserving surgical treatment for patients who have severe pain not responsive to less invasive approaches. In a more recent randomized clinical trial, which included patients with painful chronic pancreatitis, early surgery resulted in lower pain scores over 18 months when compared to an endoscopy-first approach. However, further studies are warranted to ascertain if this difference persists over a longer period.

Suggested Reading

Gardner TB, Adler DG, Forsmark CE, Sauer BG, Taylor JR, Whitcomb DC. ACG clinical guideline: chronic pancreatitis. Am J Gastroenterol. 2020 Mar;115(3):322–39.

Hegyi P, Parniczky A, Lerch MM, Sheel ARG, Rebours V, Forsmark CE, et al. International consensus guidelines for risk factors in chronic pancreatitis: recommendations from the working group for the international consensus guidelines for chronic pancreatitis in collaboration with the International Association of Pancreatology, the American Pancreatic Association, the Japan Pancreas Society, and European Pancreatic Club. Pancreatology. 2020 Jun;20(4):579–85.

Majumder S, Chari ST. Chronic pancreatitis. Lancet. 2016 May 7;387(10031):1957–66.

Nagpal SJS, Sharma A, Chari ST. Autoimmune pancreatitis. Am J Gastroenterol. 2018 Sep;113(9):1301.

Vege SS, Chari ST. Chronic pancreatitis. N Engl J Med. 2022 Mar 3;386(9):869–78.

39

Pancreatic Neoplasms[a]

JAIME DE LA FUENTE, MD

SHOUNAK MAJUMDER, MD

Pancreatic Ductal Adenocarcinoma

Pancreatic ductal adenocarcinoma (PDAC), sometimes referred to as *pancreatic cancer*, is a leading cause of cancer death in the US. The worldwide trend shows increasing PDAC incidence and mortality. Survival has improved in recent years, but the overall 5-year survival is only about 11%; it is nearly 50% among persons with a diagnosis of localized disease. Less than 20% of patients are candidates for surgical resection, and more than 50% have metastatic disease at the time of diagnosis (Tables 39.1 and 39.2). In the US, the lifetime risk for PDAC is approximately 1.6%, and the risk increases with age. In part because of its relatively low incidence, PDAC is the only malignancy among the 5 most lethal cancers in the US for which there is no approved population screening test.

Risk Factors for Development of PDAC

Early diagnosis of PDAC is uncommon because symptoms develop at a late stage when surgical resection is often not possible.

Table 39.1. American Joint Committee on Cancer, 8th Edition, TNM Classification for Staging of Pancreatic Ductal Adenocarcinoma[a]

Category	Description
Primary tumor (T)	
TX	Primary tumor cannot be assessed
T0	No evidence of a primary tumor
Tis[b]	In situ carcinoma
T1	Tumor ≤2 cm in greatest dimension
T2	Tumor >2 cm and ≤4 cm in greatest dimension
T3	Tumor >4 cm in greatest dimension
T4	Tumor involves the celiac axis, superior mesenteric artery, or common hepatic artery, regardless of size
Regional lymph nodes (N)	
NX	Regional lymph nodes cannot be assessed
N0	No regional lymph node metastasis
N1	Metastasis in 1-3 regional lymph nodes
N2	Metastasis in ≥4 regional lymph nodes
Distant metastasis (M)	
M0	No distant metastasis
M1	Distant metastasis

[a] Stages are defined in Table 39.2.
[b] Includes intraductal papillary mucinous neoplasm with high-grade dysplasia, mucinous neoplasm with high-grade dysplasia, and high-grade intraepithelial neoplasia.

Adapted from Kakar S, Pawlik TM, Allen PJ, Vauthey J-N. Exocrine pancreas. In: Amin MB, Edge SB, Greene FL, et al., eds. AJCC cancer staging manual. 8th ed. American Joint Committee on Cancer; 2017:337-47; used with permission.

[a] Randall K. Pearson, MD, is gratefully acknowledged as the author of this chapter in previous editions of the book (parts of which appear in this edition).

Abbreviations: CA19-9, carbohydrate antigen 19-9; CEA, carcinoembryonic antigen; CT, computed tomography; ENDPAC, Enriching New-Onset Diabetes for Pancreatic Cancer; ERCP, endoscopic retrograde cholangiopancreatography; EUS, endoscopic ultrasonography; FNA, fine-needle aspiration; FOLFIRINOX, leucovorin, fluorouracil, irinotecan, and oxaliplatin; IPMN, intraductal papillary mucinous neoplasm; MCN, mucinous cystic neoplasm; MRCP, magnetic resonance cholangiopancreatography; MRI, magnetic resonance imaging; NOD, new-onset diabetes; PCL, pancreatic cystic lesion; PCN, pancreatic cystic neoplasm; PDAC, pancreatic ductal adenocarcinoma; PET, positron emission tomography; SCN, serous cystic neoplasm; SPN, solid pseudopapillary neoplasm

Table 39.2. Stage Grouping for Pancreatic Ductal Adenocarcinoma[a]

Stage	T	N	M
0	Tis	N0	M0
IA	T1	N0	M0
IB	T2	N0	M0
IIA	T3	N0	M0
IIB	T1	N1	M0
IIB	T2	N1	M0
IIB	T3	N1	M0
III	T1	N2	M0
III	T2	N2	M0
III	T3	N2	M0
III	T4	Any N	M0
IV	Any T	Any N	M1

[a] TNM staging system is defined in Table 39.1.

Adapted from Kakar S, Pawlik TM, Allen PJ, Vauthey J-N. Exocrine pancreas. In: Amin MB, Edge SB, Greene FL, et al., eds. AJCC cancer staging manual. 8th ed. American Joint Committee on Cancer; 2017:337-47; used with permission.

A specific cause of PDAC has not been identified, but several risk factors have been implicated in its development.

Lifestyle and Metabolic Risk Factors

Countries with the greatest PDAC incidence and mortality are those with a high human development index. This index considers several dimensions, including life expectancy, education, and standard of living. Certain environmental factors that are associated with a high human development index are also associated with increased risk for PDAC.

Several modifiable risk factors have been linked to PDAC. *Cigarette smoking* is an important risk factor for the development of PDAC that increases the relative risk 1.5- to 3-fold, but the risk decreases considerably if abstinence is maintained for 2 years. *Alcohol use*, especially binge drinking, has also been associated with an increased risk for PDAC. Both *obesity* and *physical inactivity* increase the risk for PDAC, and increased weight is linked to increased risk for PDAC. The association between *type 2 diabetes* and PDAC is well described in the literature. Long-standing diabetes has been reported to mildly increase risk for PDAC, whereas new-onset diabetes (NOD) may occur secondary to PDAC and be a harbinger of the disease. NOD, typically defined

as a new diagnosis of type 2 diabetes within 3 years, has been strongly associated with PDAC, especially when it is present in patients at an advanced age who have unintentional weight loss.

Hereditary Pancreatitis

Certain genetic variants have been associated with hereditary pancreatitis. Persons who have hereditary pancreatitis often have episodes of pancreatitis early in life and have a much higher lifetime risk for PDAC. In light of this increased risk for PDAC, the current expert consensus is to consider pancreatic cancer screening starting at age 40 years for patients who have hereditary pancreatitis and certain sequence variants (Table 39.3).

Chronic Pancreatitis

Chronic pancreatitis is a well-established risk factor for PDAC. The risk of PDAC for patients with chronic pancreatitis varies according to the cause of chronic pancreatitis and appears to be highest for patients with hereditary pancreatitis and for those with a history of smoking. However, despite the risk association, PDAC occurs infrequently among patients with chronic pancreatitis, and the cumulative incidence increases with the duration of the disease. The diagnosis of PDAC in a patient with chronic pancreatitis can be challenging because both diseases can occur with similar symptoms, and cross-sectional imaging and endoscopic ultrasonography (EUS) have limitations for detection of small tumors that are present with mass-forming chronic inflammation and calcification.

Pancreatic Cystic Lesions

Intraductal papillary mucinous neoplasms (IPMNs) are the most prevalent neoplastic pancreatic cystic lesions (PCLs). Depending on certain clinical and imaging characteristics, surveillance or surgical excision should be recommended (see the Pancreatic Cystic Lesions section below).

Genetic and Familial Risk

Although most PDAC cases are sporadic, 5% to 15% occur in patients with underlying genetic or familial risk. *High-risk individuals* are patients who have a family history of PDAC or pathogenic (or likely pathogenic) germline variants in

Table 39.3. Germline Variants Associated With Pancreatic Ductal Adenocarcinoma in Persons With a High Risk

Gene	Syndrome	Risk estimate for pancreatic cancer	Age to consider screening, y[a]
LKB1/STK11	Peutz-Jeghers syndrome	RR 132	35-40
PRSS1	Hereditary pancreatitis	SIR 87	40
CDKN2A	Familial atypical multiple mole melanoma	OR 12-36	40
PALB2[b]	NA	OR 14.8	50
MLH1/MSH2/MSH6[b]	Lynch syndrome	OR 6.7-7.8	50
BRCA2[b]	Familial breast and ovarian syndrome	OR 6.2-9.1	50
ATM[b]	NA	OR 5.7-9.0	50
BRCA1[b]	Familial breast and ovarian syndrome	OR 2.6-3.0	50

Abbreviations: NA, not applicable; OR, odds ratio; RR, relative risk; SIR, standardized incidence ratio.
[a] Or 10 years earlier than the youngest blood relative with pancreatic cancer.
[b] Need at least 1 affected first-degree blood relative with pancreatic cancer to consider screening.

Adapted from de la Fuente J, Kastrinos F, Majumder S. How I approach screening for pancreatic cancer. Am J Gastroenterol. 2021 Aug 1;116(8):1569-71; used with permission.

PDAC-susceptibility genes (or both of these criteria). These patients have an estimated lifetime risk for PDAC of 5% or more. *Familial pancreatic cancer kindreds* are families with 2 or more first-degree relatives with pancreatic cancer or 3 or more first- or second-degree relatives with pancreatic cancer; the lifetime risk for PDAC increases with the total number of family members affected. Certain genetic syndromes are associated with an increased risk for PDAC; these include Peutz-Jeghers syndrome (*LKB1* [*STK11*] variant; OMIM 602216) and familial atypical multiple mole melanoma syndrome (*CDKN2A* variant; OMIM 600160). Other germline variants associated with an increased risk for PDAC include *BRCA1* (OMIM 113705); *BRCA2* (OMIM 600185); *ATM* (OMIM 607585); *PALB2* (OMIM 610355); *MLH1* (OMIM 120436); *MSH2* (OMIM 609309); *MSH6* (OMIM 600678); and *TP53* (OMIM 191170). The specific variants, syndromes, and risk for PDAC are shown in Table 39.3.

Current guidelines recommend against screening for PDAC in the general population, but PDAC screening may be considered for patients with a high risk for PDAC after the risks and benefits have been discussed in detail with the patient (Table 39.3). Screening, which should be offered only at centers of pancreatic excellence, is performed with MR cholangiopancreatography (MRCP) and EUS. Typically, screening is annually if patients are asymptomatic and if no abnormalities are found on the index imaging; if abnormalities are discovered, individualized treatment should be undertaken.

- ✓ Cigarette smoking—risk factor for PDAC that increases the relative risk 1.5- to 3-fold
- ✓ New-onset diabetes
  - Defined as a new diagnosis of type 2 diabetes within 3 years
  - Strongly associated with PDAC, especially in elderly patients who have unintentional weight loss
- ✓ Most cases of PDAC are sporadic, but 5% to 15% occur in patients with underlying genetic or familial risk

---

Pathology

PDAC is the most common malignant neoplasm of the pancreas and accounts for up to 85% to 90% of malignant exocrine neoplasms in the pancreas. About 70% of PDACs occur in the head of the pancreas. Histologically, the neoplasms vary from well-differentiated tumors, which have glandular structures in a dense stroma, to poorly differentiated tumors, which have little or no glandular structure or stroma (Figure 39.1). In general, PDAC itself is thought to arise from pancreatic intraepithelial neoplasia consisting of small lesions (<0.5 cm) that can progress from low-grade dysplasia to high-grade dysplasia and eventually to invasive cancer. Lymphatic spread appears to occur earlier than vascular invasion, which is present in more advanced lesions. Metastatic disease occurs mainly in the liver and lungs, but it can also occur in the adrenals, kidneys, bone, brain, and skin.

Diagnosis

Patients with pancreatic cancer usually present with symptoms of abdominal pain, back pain, jaundice, weight loss (with or without anorexia), and early satiety; they may or may not have fatigue. The most common symptoms are abdominal pain, weight loss, and fatigue, and less than 10% of patients are asymptomatic at diagnosis. Jaundice, which occurs in about 50% of patients, is a common presentation when PDAC involves the head of the pancreas. Presentation with painless jaundice often indicates resectable disease. A small percentage of patients (<5%) present with otherwise unexplained acute pancreatitis, but most patients who present with symptoms that bring the cancer to clinical attention already have locally advanced or metastatic disease.

Tumor Markers for Diagnosis

Various tumor markers are increased in patients with pancreatic cancer, but no reliable biomarker has been identified for screening or early detection of PDAC. Carbohydrate antigen 19-9 (CA19-9) is the only blood-based biomarker that is routinely used in current clinical practice. However, CA19-9 testing has limited utility if the biliary tract is obstructed, as even benign biliary tract obstruction can cause a marked increase in CA19-9 levels. Approximately 5% to 10% of patients do not express Lewis blood group antigen (a glycosyl transferase); thus, CA19-9 would not be detectable in this subgroup, further compromising the test results. Also, CA19-9 levels are more likely to increase as the disease advances and becomes metastatic. For early-stage or resectable pancreatic cancer (stages I and II), the sensitivity of an increased CA19-9 value is reported to be as low as 50%, so

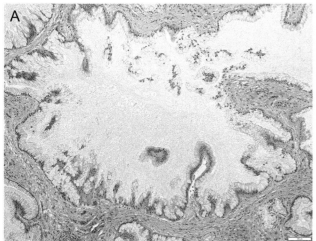
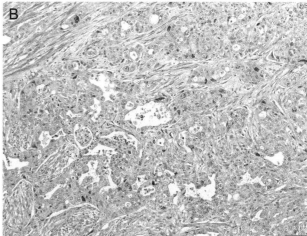

Figure 39.1. **Precursor Lesions of Pancreatic Cancer.** A, Intraductal papillary mucinous neoplasm with low-grade dysplasia (hematoxylin-eosin; scale bar =100 μm). B, Intraductal papillary mucinous neoplasm with high-grade dysplasia (hematoxylin-eosin; scale bar =100 μm).

half the patients with disease would not be identified at the stage appropriate for presymptomatic screening.

As described above, type 2 diabetes can be a consequence of PDAC. Recent epidemiologic studies have demonstrated the development of diabetes as a potential biomarker for early detection of PDAC. This NOD can be seen as early as 36 months before the clinical diagnosis of PDAC. The Enriching New-Onset Diabetes for Pancreatic Cancer (ENDPAC) model, which accounts for age at diabetes diagnosis, weight loss, and increased level of fasting blood glucose, has been proposed to further identify patients who have NOD and a substantial risk for PDAC. The ENDPAC model is undergoing prospective validation for possible use as a clinical practice tool for identifying patients who may be considered for pancreatic cancer screening. Several other promising molecular biomarkers are in various stages of validation for early detection of PDAC.

Imaging Tests for Diagnosis

Multidetector computed tomography (CT) of the abdomen with multiphase (triple-phase) contrast enhancement (pancreas protocol CT) should be the primary imaging study for the evaluation of patients with symptoms or imaging findings that suggest PDAC. PDAC typically appears as an irregular, hypodense lesion in the pancreas (Figures 39.2 and 39.3). Pancreas protocol CT is the appropriate study because it can be used to stage the tumor and provide valuable information about vascular involvement and resectability. When used for PDAC staging, the 3 phases in the protocol are 1) arterial phase, which allows for excellent visualization of the celiac and superior mesenteric arteries; 2) late arterial or pancreatic phase, which allows for optimal contrast between the normal pancreatic parenchyma and tumor; and 3) portal phase, which allows for detection of liver metastasis and PDAC involvement of the portal, superior mesenteric, and splenic veins. The sensitivity of pancreas protocol CT for detection of primary lesions is about 90%, but small (<2 cm) primary lesions may be missed. Other cross-sectional imaging modalities that can be used

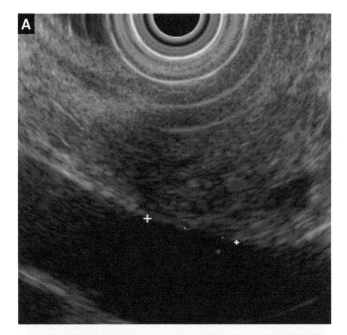

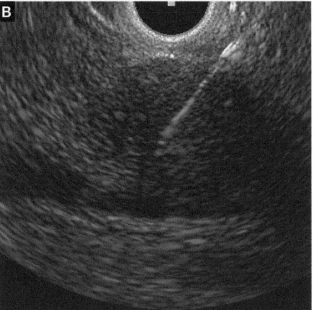

Figure 39.3. Hypoechoic Mass in Pancreas. A, Endoscopic ultrasonogram of the pancreatic head shows a poorly defined hypoechoic mass that impinges on the portal vein for a distance of 11 mm (indicated by 2 markers). Surgical resection confirmed invasion of the portal vein. B, Endoscopic ultrasonogram shows fine-needle aspiration of the mass in A.

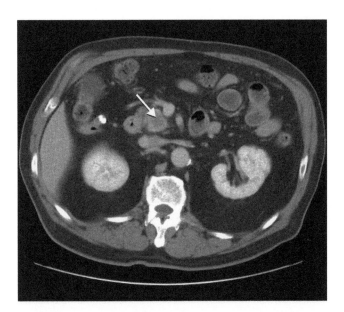

Figure 39.2.   Pancreatic Ductal Adenocarcinoma. Computed tomogram shows a small hypoattenuating lesion in the head of the pancreas (arrow). The superior mesenteric vessels are not involved by the tumor, which is resectable.

include MRI and positron emission tomography (PET). MRI may provide better evaluation of hepatic lesions when metastatic disease is suspected. The use of PET/CT and PET/MRI is an area of active study, and the data so far indicate that they are useful for determining the treatment response of resectable and borderline resectable tumors being treated with neoadjuvant therapy and in evaluating for evidence of extrapancreatic metastases.

EUS is highly sensitive for detecting small solid tumors, but with the advent of multidetector CT, EUS is usually reserved for fine-needle aspiration (FNA) and biopsy of the primary lesion or suspicious lymph nodes. For resectable PDAC, EUS with FNA is preferred over percutaneous biopsy. In patients with hepatic metastasis, percutaneous liver biopsy is often the preferred modality for diagnosis. Tissue diagnosis in PDAC is important and should be performed even for resectable disease, especially as more institutions shift away from upfront surgery toward the use of neoadjuvant chemotherapy. Not only does this ensure accurate diagnosis that rules out autoimmune pancreatitis and other neoplasms that can mimic PDAC, it may also guide the use of chemotherapeutic agents according to results of tumor genetic testing. Another recommendation is that all patients with PDAC should undergo genetic counseling and germline testing for cancer susceptibility genes. A desmoplastic response may occur in 10% to 15% of patients with PDAC, so tumor tissue may be difficult to procure with FNA, necessitating multiple biopsy attempts.

Endoscopic retrograde cholangiopancreatography (ERCP) is reserved primarily for placement of a common bile duct stent in patients who have obstructive jaundice due to PDAC involving the head of the pancreas. Although brush cytology from biliary strictures obtained during ERCP may aid in the diagnosis of PDAC, diagnostic tissue acquisition in current clinical practice is primarily performed with EUS as described above.

> ✓ Multidetector CT of the abdomen with multiphase (triple-phase) contrast enhancement (pancreas protocol CT)—the primary imaging study for evaluation of patients with symptoms or imaging findings that suggest PDAC

Staging Pancreatic Tumors

Pancreas protocol CT is the initial test not only for diagnosis but also for staging of PDAC because it can help identify distant metastases and vascular involvement. EUS is complementary for staging local extent (T staging) and nodal status (N staging). For EUS, operator experience is an important variable.

In addition, CT of the chest is recommended for staging, although lung metastasis is uncommon in the absence of liver metastasis or extensive local vascular involvement. Staging laparoscopy with peritoneal fluid cytology is also frequently performed if surgical resection is a consideration and the patient does not have overt metastatic disease. The staging method currently in use for PDAC is the TNM (tumor, node, metastasis) system from the eighth edition of the cancer staging manual of the American Joint Committee on Cancer (Tables 39.1 and 39.2). Accurate clinical staging based on imaging at diagnosis can be challenging, especially for nodal status. In addition to TNM staging, the resectability of the tumor is typically determined by a multidisciplinary team of pancreatologists, radiologists, surgeons, and oncologists who classify PDAC as *resectable*, *borderline resectable*, *locally advanced disease*, or *metastatic disease*. The findings from the pancreas protocol CT largely guide this categorization depending on which arterial and venous structures are involved and to what degree. (The specific details of this categorization are outside the scope of this chapter.) Recent evidence supports the use of PET/MRI for local tumor staging at diagnosis, detecting occult metastatic disease, and monitoring treatment response in patients undergoing neoadjuvant therapy before surgery.

Treatment

The treatment of PDAC is best provided by a multidisciplinary team of medical pancreatologists, therapeutic endoscopists, pancreatobiliary surgeons, medical oncologists, geneticists, and palliative medicine specialists, and the goals, values, and performance status of the patient must be considered. Treatment should ideally be done in centers that have a large volume of patients with PDAC and have access to clinical trials and the necessary clinical expertise. The only hope for cure involves surgical resection of the primary tumor with negative surgical margins. The decision to perform surgical resection must consider staging at diagnosis and whether the patient is a surgical candidate. In a patient with metastatic PDAC, treatment is palliative. In patients with borderline resectable disease, the current approach is to consider neoadjuvant chemoradiotherapy initially, with or without consolidative radiotherapy, with subsequent surgery depending on treatment response and performance status. Although radiologic downstaging is uncommon, chemotherapy appears to be better tolerated in the preoperative period; in carefully selected patients who undergo surgical resection after neoadjuvant therapy, more than 90% have an R0 resection.

The management of resectable PDAC is evolving. At many centers, even if PDAC is diagnosed at an early resectable stage and the tumor is confined to the pancreas, a neoadjuvant approach is considered, although an adjuvant treatment approach with upfront surgery would also be reasonable. Limited data are available for comparison of neoadjuvant and adjuvant therapies for resectable PDAC, and results of ongoing clinical trials are not yet available.

Surgery

The standard operation for PDAC at the head of the pancreas is a pancreaticoduodenectomy (Whipple procedure), which involves performing a cholecystectomy and removing a portion of the stomach (at least an antrectomy), the distal bile duct, the head of the pancreas, the duodenum, the proximal jejunum, and regional lymph nodes. Reconstruction with gastrojejunostomy, hepaticojejunostomy, and pancreaticojejunostomy is required. Results are good and mortality is low when the operation is performed at high-volume centers with experienced surgeons.

Alternative operations include a pylorus-preserving Whipple resection, which has become the surgical standard of care at most centers. This preserves the stomach and is a less extensive operation. It has been assumed that this operation, compared with the Whipple procedure, would improve outcome, especially long-term morbidity related to dumping syndrome and weight loss. Tumors in the body or tail of the pancreas can be resected with distal pancreatectomy and splenectomy. Depending on the vascular contact of the tumor, venous and arterial reconstructions can be performed by a select group of highly trained pancreatic surgeons, so patients have a chance at a cure despite vascular involvement. In some patients, especially in those with a hereditary predisposition to PDAC, total pancreatectomy may need to be considered. Although surgery provides the only chance of cure, a large proportion of patients who undergo surgical resection for pancreatic cancer ultimately die of the disease. New molecular and imaging tools for early detection of postoperative recurrence and minimal residual disease may improve future long-term outcomes of patients with this lethal disease.

Chemotherapy

In 2011, a multicenter European trial compared a combination chemotherapy regimen of leucovorin, fluorouracil, irinotecan, and oxaliplatin (FOLFIRINOX) with single-agent gemcitabine in patients who had metastatic PDAC. The patients who received

FOLFIRINOX had a better objective response rate (32% vs 9%) and increased overall survival (11.1 months vs 6.8 months), but, as expected with a multidrug regimen, they had a higher rate of toxicity (especially neutropenia). For patients with metastatic PDAC, good performance status, and normal or nearly normal liver function, FOLFIRINOX is the standard first-line chemotherapy. Alternatively, gemcitabine in combination with nanoparticle albumin-bound paclitaxel (nab-paclitaxel) can also be used and typically is better tolerated with improved median overall survival compared to gemcitabine (8.5 months vs 6.7 months). Among patients with metastatic PDAC and a germline *BRCA* variant, progression-free survival was shown to be longer with use of the poly(adenosine diphosphate–ribose) polymerase (PARP) inhibitor olaparib compared to placebo (7.4 months vs 3.8 months).

Adjuvant chemotherapy with a modified dose of FOLFIRINOX ("modified FOLFIRINOX") is the standard of care in appropriately selected patients with resected PDAC, although less than 10% of patients can complete adjuvant therapy after a pancreatic resection. In patients who can tolerate adjuvant therapy, modified FOLFIRINOX is associated with significantly longer survival compared to gemcitabine (54.4 months vs 35 months). Precision oncology with tumor molecular and genetic profiling may help individualize the choice of treatment regimen in the future.

The role of neoadjuvant chemoradiotherapy in the management of PDAC is poorly defined, although its use has been increasing in recent years. This is largely based on the idea that chemotherapy is better tolerated as part of neoadjuvant therapy, and this greater likelihood of receiving adequate chemotherapy will result in improved overall survival. However, there is no high-quality evidence to support this approach. A recent study indicated that preoperative chemoradiotherapy with gemcitabine for resectable or borderline resectable pancreatic cancer is not associated with significant improvement in overall survival. This finding has limited clinical relevance, however, since single-agent gemcitabine is rarely used in current clinical practice. Randomized controlled trials assessing the effect of neoadjuvant modified FOLFIRINOX are underway. Clinical trial participation should be strongly encouraged, especially among patients who have a diagnosis of resectable disease and are undergoing neoadjuvant therapy.

Biliary Obstruction

Biliary obstruction in PDAC typically manifests as painless jaundice. Pruritus is often the most disabling symptom, and cholangitis is rare unless instruments have been used in the biliary tract. The preferred treatment is transpapillary biliary stent placement. In patients undergoing neoadjuvant therapy or destination chemotherapy, a metal biliary stent is preferred over plastic stents. Percutaneous drainage is used if endoscopic transpapillary drainage fails. EUS-guided transgastric or transduodenal biliary drainage is a therapeutic alternative for carefully selected patients.

Duodenal Obstruction

In patients presenting with symptoms of gastric outlet obstruction such as nausea, vomiting, early satiety, and poor oral intake, a bypass procedure is often necessary. Although surgical gastrojejunostomy was the previous standard, therapeutic endoscopy options have expanded in recent years and include both duodenal stenting and EUS-guided gastrojejunostomy with a lumen-apposing metal stent.

Pain

Palliation of pain is a major problem in patients with PDAC. A palliative or pain medicine team with extensive expertise in management of cancer pain should be involved early in the patient's care to maximize quality of life. A celiac plexus neurolysis performed percutaneously or with endoscopic ultrasonography is often considered for managing pain in patients who have unresectable disease. Celiac plexus neurolysis effectively decreases pain in 40% to 80% of patients, typically for 4 to 8 weeks, with a definite but limited advantage over analgesic therapy. Although celiac plexus block is reasonably effective for short-term pain control, most published data do not show increased survival.

If oral analgesia is used to control pain related to pancreatic cancer, the type and dose of medication is determined according to the severity of pain. For example, mild pain may be controlled with acetaminophen (325 mg) in combination with oxycodone (5 mg), 1 or 2 tablets every 4 to 6 hours, whereas more severe pain may require a longer-acting opioid for durable pain control in combination with short-acting analgesics as needed to control breakthrough pain. Alternatively, a fentanyl transdermal patch, 25 to 100 mg hourly, is effective for some patients.

Nutrition

A key component of cancer treatment is to ensure that the patient's nutritional status is optimal. Patients with PDAC, especially those who have tumors in the pancreatic head and considerable pancreatic atrophy, frequently have signs of exocrine pancreatic insufficiency such as steatorrhea and weight loss. Pancreatic enzyme replacement therapy should be considered for those patients. The use of pancreatic enzyme replacement therapy improves the quality of life for patients who have unresectable PDAC.

✓ Treatment of PDAC
- Multidisciplinary team is best: medical pancreatologists, therapeutic endoscopists, pancreatobiliary surgeons, medical oncologists, geneticists, and palliative medicine specialists
- Patient's goals, values, and performance status must be considered

---

Box 39.1.   Classification of Pancreatic Cystic Lesions[a]

Benign pancreatic cystic lesions
   Benign epithelial cyst/true simple cyst
   Lymphoepithelial cyst
   Retention cyst
   Mucinous nonneoplastic cyst
Pancreatic cystic neoplasms[b]
   Serous cystic neoplasm
   Mucinous cystic neoplasm
   Intraductal papillary mucinous neoplasm
   Solid pseudopapillary neoplasm

---

[a] Excludes cystic pancreatic neuroendocrine tumor and cystic degeneration of pancreatic adenocarcinoma.

[b] Various degrees of malignant potential.

Table 39.4. Characteristics of Specific Pancreatic Cystic Neoplasms

Characteristic	Intraductal papillary mucinous neoplasm	Mucinous cystic neoplasm	Serous cystic neoplasm	Solid pseudopapillary neoplasm
Patient age at usual encounter, y	60-70	40-50	50-60	<50
Sex predilection	None	Female only	Female	Female
Imaging	Typically multifocal cysts Dilated MPD if involved Cysts communicate with MPD	Unilocular Body or tail	Typically polycystic honeycomb appearance Central stellate scar	Commonly body or tail solid component
Clinical cyst fluid analysis	Elevated CEA Mucin stain positive	Elevated CEA Mucin stain positive	Very low CEA	Cytology positive for β-catenin
Treatment[a]	Surveillance or resection	Surveillance or resection	No surveillance Resection if large or symptomatic	Resection

Abbreviations: CEA, carcinoembryonic antigen; MPD, main pancreatic duct.

[a] For surgically fit patients.

Pancreatic Cystic Lesions

The malignant potential of PCLs ranges from benign to advanced neoplasia (high-grade dysplasia or cancer). The majority of persons with PCLs are asymptomatic; therefore, PCLs are usually discovered incidentally on imaging, and the true population prevalence of PCLs is unknown. Over the past 2 decades, the increase in prevalence of PCLs has been attributed to the widespread availability and use of high-resolution abdominal cross-sectional imaging. Pooled prevalence of PCLs worldwide is about 8%, but the prevalence ranges from less than 1% to 50% depending on the ages of the patients in the population and the type of imaging (ultrasonography, CT, MRI, or EUS) used to detect the PCLs. The prevalence increases with age and is typically higher in studies that used MRI rather than CT.

Classification and Histology

PCLs can be classified according to their histology into 2 main categories: *benign PCLs*, which do not develop into cancer, and *PCLs with malignant potential*, which are also called pancreatic cystic neoplasms (PCNs). The classification of PCLs is summarized in Box 39.1.

Surgical pathology is required for definitive classification and histologic diagnosis of PCLs. Although the imaging appearance on CT, MRI, or MRCP and the location of the PCL, the age and sex of the patient, and findings from EUS with FNA for cytology and cyst fluid analysis can provide clues to the most likely type of PCL, preoperative histologic diagnosis can be inaccurate in approximately one-third of patients. PDAC, pancreatic neuroendocrine tumors, and rare forms of pancreatic cancer (eg, acinar cell cancer) can undergo cystic degeneration and thus have a cystic or solid-cystic radiologic appearance. (Pancreatic neuroendocrine tumors are discussed in Chapter 6.)

✓ PCLs can be classified histologically into 2 main categories:
- Benign PCLs
- PCLs with malignant potential (also called pancreatic cystic neoplasms)

Pancreatic Cystic Neoplasms

All PCNs have various degrees of malignant potential. They are the most commonly encountered PCLs in clinical practice, and they account for over 80% of all PCLs that are surgically resected. Although PCNs have malignant potential, the overall risk of pancreatic cancer is low, and the majority of PCNs never require surgical resection. The specific features of each PCN are used to guide management and determine whether surveillance or surgical resection is required. Table 39.4 summarizes the most common clinical and imaging features of these PCNs that can aid in their diagnosis and management.

Serous Cystic Neoplasm

Previously called serous cystic adenoma, serous cystic neoplasms (SCNs) are often present in women 50 to 60 years old. SCNs commonly occur in 2 forms: *microcytic* (cystic compartments <2 cm with a honeycomb appearance) and *macrocytic* (cystic compartments ≥2 cm) (Figure 39.4). A stellate scar is sometimes seen on cross-sectional imaging. Generally, the malignant potential of SCNs is exceptionally low, although malignant

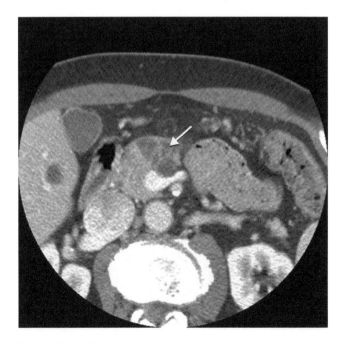

Figure 39.4. **Serous Cystic Neoplasm.** Computed tomogram shows a serous cyst. The mass lesion in the head of the pancreas consists of multiple small cystic lesions (arrow). The findings are typical of serous cystic neoplasm.

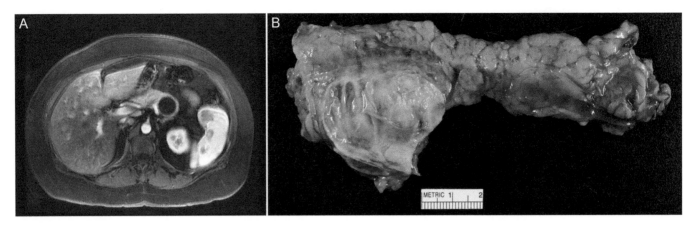

Figure 39.5. Mucinous Cystic Neoplasm. A, Magnetic resonance image of the abdomen shows a unilocular cyst in the tail of the pancreas. B, Surgical pathology gross specimen shows ovarian stroma.

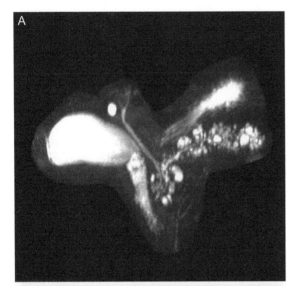

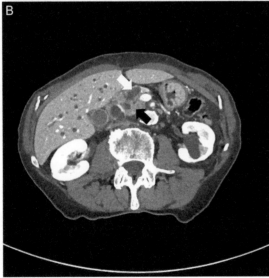

Figure 39.6. Intraductal Papillary Mucinous Neoplasm (IPMN). A, Magnetic resonance cholangiopancreatography shows multifocal pancreatic cysts communicating with a dilated main pancreatic duct suggestive of a mixed IPMN. B, A hypoattenuating mass (black arrow) in the pancreatic head is associated with a cystic lesion and dilated main pancreatic duct (white arrow) (diameter, 10 mm) with abrupt cutoff, distal pancreatic atrophy, and bile duct dilation; these imaging features are suggestive of malignant degeneration of an IPMN.

transformation has been rarely reported. Therefore, if the diagnosis is established, surveillance is typically not recommended, and SCNs should be resected only if the patient is symptomatic. Analysis of SCN cyst fluid from EUS FNA shows low levels of carcinoembryonic antigen (CEA) (<5 ng/mL) and amylase; the occasional finding of cuboidal glycogen-staining cells on EUS-guided core biopsy of the cyst wall establishes the histologic diagnosis.

Mucinous Cystic Neoplasm

Mucinous cystic neoplasms (MCNs) occur almost exclusively in women 40 to 60 years old. MCNs usually occur as a solitary unilocular cyst in the body or tail of the pancreas (Figure 39.5) and are histologically characterized by the presence of ovarian stroma. On analysis of the cyst fluid, the CEA level is high (>192

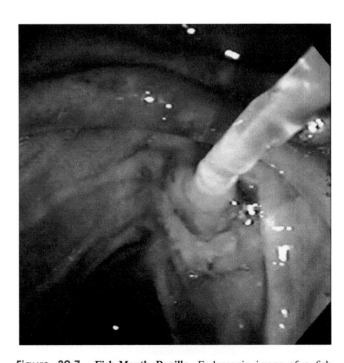

Figure 39.7. Fish-Mouth Papilla. Endoscopic image of a fish-mouth papilla with extruding mucin, which is pathognomonic for main duct intraductal papillary mucinous neoplasm. (Adapted from Levy MJ, Geenen JE. Idiopathic acute recurrent pancreatitis. Am J Gastroenterol. 2001 Sep;96[9]:2540-55; used with permission of Mayo Foundation for Medical Education and Research.)

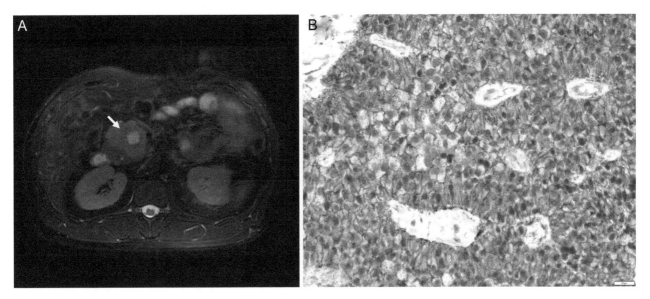

Figure 39.8. **Solid Pseudopapillary Neoplasm.** A, Magnetic resonance image of the abdomen shows a solid-cystic lesion (arrow) in the pancreatic body. B, Surgical pathology specimen shows positive β-catenin staining (scale bar =20 μm).

ng/mL); the cyst does not communicate with the main pancreatic duct. MCNs have moderate malignant potential, so resection is commonly offered for patients who are young and surgically fit, especially if they have a mural nodule, although surveillance may be considered for patients who have small asymptomatic MCNs. Surveillance may be recommended for older patients if they have comorbidities, small cysts (<4 cm), no high-risk features, and the possible need for pancreaticoduodenectomy because of the location of the MCN.

Intraductal Papillary Mucinous Neoplasm

IPMNs consist of intraductal papillary growth of mucin-producing columnar epithelium. They are the most commonly encountered PCL in clinical practice. IPMNs can be classified according to the extent of ductal involvement: branch duct, main duct, and mixed duct (affecting both branch and main pancreatic ducts) (Figure 39.6). IPMN is intrinsically a multifocal disease that often manifests as multiple cysts in different regions of the pancreas; when the main pancreatic duct is affected, the risk of advanced neoplasia is much greater than when only the branch duct is affected. Branch duct IPMNs communicate with the main pancreatic duct, although this connection may not always be readily identifiable on cross-sectional imaging. Cyst fluid analysis often shows positive mucin staining and high levels of CEA (>192 ng/mL) and amylase. The presence of a patulous papilla extruding mucus (described as a fish-mouth papilla) is considered pathognomonic for main duct IPMN (Figure 39.7). IPMNs are often encountered in patients 60 to 80 years old, and either surveillance or surgical resection is almost uniformly recommended unless the patient has a limited life expectancy or prohibitive surgical risks.

Solid Pseudopapillary Neoplasm

Solid pseudopapillary neoplasms (SPNs) are rare PCNs with malignant potential. They are typically seen in women (>80%) younger than 50 years, although they can be present at any age,

and they are typically located in the body or tail of the pancreas. As the name implies, SPNs often have a solid component that is seen on cross-sectional imaging (Figure 39.8). SPNs have malignant potential, so surgical resection is recommended for all patients who have SPN unless surgery would be contraindicated. The prognosis is typically good, although SPNs recur or metastasize in 2% to 10% of patients.

Approach to Managing PCNs

The approach to PCNs is individualized and requires shared decision-making, keeping in mind the patient's life expectancy, comorbidities, wishes, and goals. Figure 39.9 provides a summary and a general framework for approaching PCLs in clinical practice.

If a PCN is related to recurrent acute pancreatitis, gastric outlet obstruction, biliary obstruction, or abdominal pain, surgical resection may need to be considered. Most PCNs, however, are discovered incidentally. For these asymptomatic PCNs, the initial evaluation should focus on ruling out the presence of advanced neoplasia and determining whether the next step should be surgical resection or imaging-based surveillance. If a patient is not a candidate for pancreatic resection, proceeding further with the clinical investigation is typically not necessary because it probably would not change the clinical outcome.

If the diagnosis of SCN can be established and the patient is asymptomatic, further surveillance is usually not recommended. SPNs, however, should be surgically resected at diagnosis because they can harbor malignancy, commonly occur in young patients, and have metastatic potential.

Most PCNs encountered in clinical practice are asymptomatic mucinous PCNs, and IPMNs are the most commonly encountered. Owing to the risk of potential malignancy, resection is recommended for MCNs in patients who have acceptable surgical risk. Specific situations related to surveillance for patients with MCN are described above. In patients with suspected IPMNs, initial assessment aims to determine whether worrisome features or high-risk stigmata are present

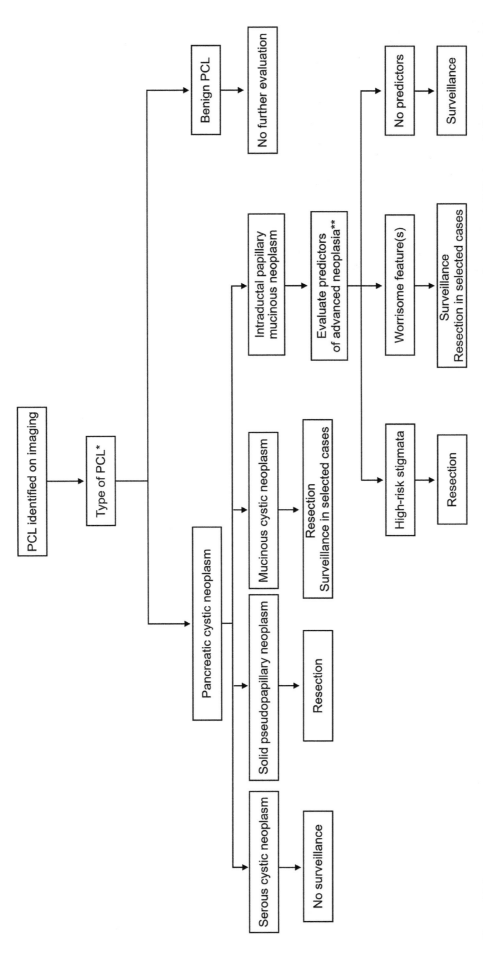

Figure 39.9. **Management of Asymptomatic Pancreatic Cystic Lesions (PCLs).** Flow diagram shows a general approach to management of asymptomatic PCLs in surgically fit patients. Asterisk indicates that the PCL subtype should be determined with clinical and imaging criteria and biopsy when available (20%–30% of PCLs are classified incorrectly with the use of only clinical and imaging criteria). Double asterisk indicates that predictors of advanced neoplasia are listed in Box 39.2.

(Box 39.2). These criteria are described in the international consensus guidelines for management of IPMNs. Patients who have IPMNs with high-risk stigmata should be considered for surgery. When worrisome features are present, further evaluation with EUS is usually pursued to assess for a mural nodule and features of main pancreatic duct involvement; FNA may be considered for the detection of advanced neoplasia, although the sensitivity is low (33%-57%). If any of these higher-risk features are detected on EUS and the patient is an appropriate surgical candidate, surgical resection should be strongly considered. In the absence of any of these high-risk features on EUS, imaging-based surveillance (typically with MRI) is often recommended at various intervals according to PCL size, with more frequent surveillance for larger IPMNs initially and then subsequently increased surveillance intervals if the IPMN has been stable.

Approximately one-third of surgically resected IPMNs have high-grade dysplasia or cancer, and the risk of morbidity and mortality with pancreatic resection must be considered. Hence, regardless of the guidelines and expert consensus recommendations, a value-congruent and evidence-based discussion must occur with the patient and incorporate input from a multidisciplinary team of experts to determine whether the best next step is immediate surgery, surveillance, or no further follow-up. Ongoing efforts to develop novel biomarkers that accurately detect advanced neoplasia in patients with IPMNs may further refine management in the future with the goal of individualizing risk stratification and improving patient outcomes.

Box 39.2. Risk Stratification of Suspected Intraductal Papillary Mucinous Neoplasms

High-risk stigmata[a]

MPD ≥10 mm

Solid malignant-appearing pancreatic mass

Cytology that suggests or is positive for HGD or cancer

Mural nodule ≥5 mm

Obstructive jaundice with cyst in pancreatic head

Main duct features that suggest involvement (intraductal mucin, fish-mouth papilla, or mural nodules in MPD)

Worrisome features[b]

Elevated CA19-9

Cyst ≥3 cm

Mural nodule <5 mm

MPD 5-9 mm

Lymphadenopathy

Cyst growth ≥5 mm in 2 y

Change in caliber of pancreatic duct with distal pancreatic atrophy

Thickened or enhancing cyst walls

Pancreatitis

Abbreviations: CA19-9, carbohydrate antigen 19-9; HGD, high-grade dysplasia; MPD, main pancreatic duct.

[a] Strong consideration for surgical treatment.

[b] Individualized monitoring typically with endoscopic ultrasonography and subsequent periodic surveillance if no high-risk stigmata are identified.

✓ PCNs in clinical practice
- Most are asymptomatic mucinous PCNs
- IPMNs are the most commonly encountered

Suggested Reading

de la Fuente J, Kastrinos F, Majumder S. How I approach screening for pancreatic cancer. Am J Gastroenterol. 2021 Aug 1;116(8):1569–71.

de la Fuente J, Majumder S. Molecular diagnostics and testing for pancreatic cysts. Curr Treat Options Gastroenterol. 2020 Jan 27.

Elta GH, Enestvedt BK, Sauer BG, Lennon AM. ACG clinical guideline: diagnosis and management of pancreatic cysts. Am J Gastroenterol. 2018 Apr;113(4):464–79.

European Study Group on Cystic Tumours of the Pancreas. European evidence-based guidelines on pancreatic cystic neoplasms. Gut. 2018 May;67(5):789–804.

Huang J, Lok V, Ngai CH, Zhang L, Yuan J, Lao XQ, et al. Worldwide burden of, risk factors for, and trends in pancreatic cancer. Gastroenterology. 2021 Feb;160(3):744–54.

Sharma A, Kandlakunta H, Nagpal SJS, Feng Z, Hoos W, Petersen GM, et al. Model to determine risk of pancreatic cancer in patients with new-onset diabetes. Gastroenterology. 2018 Sep;155(3):730–9.

Vege SS, Ziring B, Jain R, Moayyedi P, Clinical Guidelines Committee. American Gastroenterological Association institute guideline on the diagnosis and management of asymptomatic neoplastic pancreatic cysts. Gastroenterology. 2015 Apr;148(4):819–22.

40

Gallstones[a,b]

ERIC J. VARGAS VALLS, MD, MS

Introduction

Over 20 million people in the US are affected by gallbladder-related diseases, and the estimated direct annual costs exceed $6.3 billion. The formation of gallstones, *cholelithiasis*, affects people throughout the world, but the prevalence varies among different groups, ranging from 60% to 70% among American Indians to 5% among persons in sub-Saharan Africa. In the US, 20% of patients with cholelithiasis have gallstone-related complications (annual incidence rate, 1%-4%), and more than 700,000 cholecystectomies are performed annually. This chapter reviews the anatomy, development, physiology, clinical manifestations, diagnosis, and management of gallstone and gallstone-related diseases.

---

[a] The author thanks Ferga C. Gleeson, MB, BCh, who was the author of the previous version of this chapter.

[b] Portions of this chapter were adapted from Abou-Saif A, Al-Kawas FH. Complications of gallstone disease: Mirizzi syndrome, cholecysto-choledochal fistula, waand gallstone ileus. Am J Gastroenterol. 2002 Feb;97(2):249-54; Sonmez G, Ozturk E, Mutlu H, Sildiroglu O, Basekim C, Kizilkaya E. Education and imaging. Hepatobiliary and pancreatic: emphysematous cholecystitis. J Gastroenterol Hepatol. 2007 Nov;22(11):2035; and Attasaranya S, Fogel EL, Lehman GA. Choledocholithiasis, ascending cholangitis, and gallstone pancreatitis. Med Clin North Am. 2008 Jul;92(4):925-60; used with permission.

Abbreviations: ASGE, American Society for Gastrointestinal Endoscopy; AST, aspartate aminotransferase; CT, computed tomography; ERCP, endoscopic retrograde cholangiopancreatography; EUS, endoscopic ultrasonography; FXR, farnesoid X receptor; GBC, gallbladder carcinoma; HIDA, hepatobiliary iminodiacetic acid; MRCP, magnetic resonance cholangiopancreatography; TPN, total parenteral nutrition

✓ Gallbladder disease affects over 20 million people in the US
✓ Of the patients with cholelithiasis, 80% are asymptomatic; the annual rate of new biliary pain in the first 5 years is 2%
✓ Among patients with cholelithiasis, 90% of complications (cholecystitis, cholangitis, and gallstone pancreatitis) are preceded by an episode of uncomplicated biliary colic

Embryology, Anatomy, and Physiology

Gallbladder and Cystic Duct Anatomy

The gallbladder, cystic duct, and common bile duct all develop from the cystic portion of the hepatic diverticulum in utero and are fully developed by 12 weeks of gestation. Bile secretion begins at 16 weeks. The gallbladder is situated primarily in the cystic fossa on the posteroinferior aspect of the right hepatic lobe. The neck of the gallbladder is connected to the cystic duct, which is 3 to 4 cm long and joins the common hepatic duct, forming the common bile duct. The cystic duct has 5 to 12 oblique folds that create the spiral valves of Heister. The cystic artery, usually a branch from the right hepatic artery, courses superior to the cystic duct and reaches the superior aspect of the neck, where it divides into superficial and deep branches.

Anatomical variations include gallbladder agenesis, multiple gallbladders, bilobed gallbladder, and double cystic duct. A Phrygian cap is an inconsequential deformity reflecting kinking of the gallbladder fossa and is usually noted with computed tomography (CT) or radionuclide hepatobiliary imaging. In a double gallbladder, each gallbladder may have its own cystic duct, or the duct may join and form a common cystic duct before joining the common hepatic duct.

Cholesterol Metabolism, Bile, and Bile Acid Synthesis

The liver is important in regulating total body cholesterol and plasma lipid levels; bile and bile acids are especially important. In fact, the 2 main pathways for cholesterol elimination in the body are excretion into bile and synthesis of bile acid.

The major components of bile are water, inorganic solutes, and organic solutes such as bilirubin, bile acids, and biliary lipids. Bilirubin is a degradation product of heme and is usually present as conjugated water-soluble diglucuronide. Gilbert syndrome is a common condition (occurring in 10% of the White population), where an alteration in the promoter region of the *UGT1A1* gene (OMIM 191740) results in unconjugated hyperbilirubinemia. The unconjugated form of bilirubin precipitates, contributing to pigment stones (typically black) or mixed cholesterol stones. Bile acids are bipolar water-soluble molecules synthesized from cholesterol in the liver by either the classic pathway with 7α-hydroxylase (predominant) or the alternate pathways with 27-hydroxylase. The classic pathway is regulated by the level of cholesterol substrate, hepatocellular bile acid concentration, and other metabolic and hormonal factors. The primary bile acids synthesized are cholic acid and chenodeoxycholic acid. Bacteria in the gut convert them to the secondary bile acids deoxycholic and lithocholic acids. Overall bile acid synthesis is controlled by the nuclear hormone receptor farnesoid X receptor (FXR), with primary bile acids serving as the most potent natural ligands of FXR. Another important regulator of bile acid synthesis is fibroblast growth factor 19, which is secreted by ileal enterocytes (in response to luminal levels of bile acids) and inhibits the classic pathway enzyme, 7α-hydroxylase.

The other major components of bile are biliary lipids, phospholipids, and cholesterol, which are insoluble in water. They are secreted into bile as lipid vesicles and are carried in both vesicles and mixed micelles. When the concentration of bile acids exceeds the critical micellar concentration, bile acids self-associate and form micelles capable of solubilizing hydrophobic lipid molecules in bile or intestinal chyme. Through this process, many lipophilic drugs and steroid hormones are excreted from the body. However, the overall primary function of these micelles is to facilitate fat digestion and absorption.

The gallbladder concentrates bile 10 times for efficient storage during fasting and empties 25% of its contents every 2 hours. When intraduodenal protein and fat are sensed, cholecystokinin is released, stimulating contractions of the gallbladder, relaxation of the sphincter of Oddi, and flow of bile to the intestine, which facilitates fat digestion and absorption. More than 90% of bile acids are actively absorbed in the terminal ileum and recycled (termed *enterohepatic circulation*). This cycle occurs 4 to 12 times daily, slowing during fasting and accelerating greatly after a meal (Figure 40.1). Daily bile acid loss is matched by hepatic synthesis of bile; in this way, steady amounts of bile acids are maintained in the body. Several conditions that impair this recirculation lead to increased gallstone formation, malabsorption, and diarrhea.

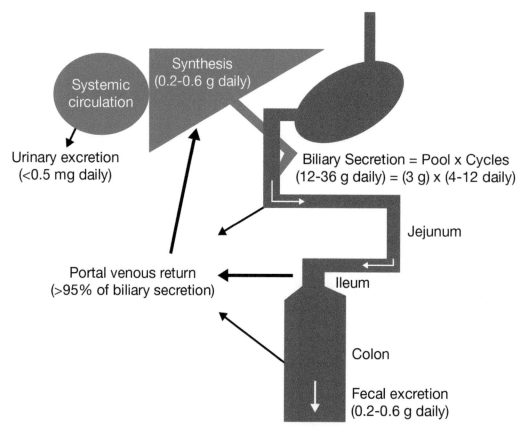

Figure 40.1. Enterohepatic Circulation. A pool of 3 g of bile acid cycles 4 to 12 times daily. Ileal absorption returns 97% of intraluminal bile acids to the circulation; 90% of bile acids are extracted from the portal system on their first pass through the liver. In health, hepatic synthesis of bile acids is equivalent to enteric losses. (Adapted from Zucker SD, Gollan JL. Physiology of the liver. In: Haubrich WS, Schaffner F, Berk JE, editors. Bockus gastroenterology. Vol 3. 5th ed. WB Saunders; 1995: 1858-904; used with permission.)

Gallstone Epidemiology and Pathogenesis

The prevalence of cholesterol gallstones varies with geography and ethnicity. Cholesterol gallstones are rare in populations in Africa and most of Asia, they are common in most Western populations (15% of women; 10% of men), and they occur almost uniformly in North and South American Indians (80% of women). For all populations, the prevalence increases with age and is approximately twice as high in women as in men.

Gallstones are categorized on the basis of composition as *cholesterol gallstones* (80% of patients) and *pigment* (black and brown) *gallstones* (20%). Each category has a unique structural, epidemiologic, and risk factor profile (Table 40.1). Cholesterol crystal formation requires the presence of 1 or more of the following: cholesterol supersaturation, accelerated nucleation, gallbladder hypomotility, bile stasis, and genetic factors.

Cholesterol gallstones contain a mixture of cholesterol (50%-99% by weight), a glycoprotein matrix, and small amounts of calcium and bilirubin. Cholesterol supersaturation can result from deficient secretion of bile acid or hypersecretion of cholesterol. Bile acid secretion may be diminished because of *decreased synthesis*, as occurs with older age or liver disease, or because of *decreased enterohepatic circulation*, as occurs with hormonal defects and increased gastrointestinal losses from bile acid sequestrant therapy or terminal ileal disease, resection, or bypass. Additionally, weight loss and decreased fat intake lead to decreased bile acid synthesis. Cholesterol secretion increases with hormonal stimuli (female sex, pregnancy [estrogen], and exogenous estrogens), obesity, hyperlipidemia, age, chronic liver disease, and sometimes with excessive dietary polyunsaturated fats or increased caloric intake. In a supersaturated environment, gallstone crystals form initially from an imbalance of nucleating effects and antinucleating effects of the various proteins in bile (Figure 40.2 and Box 40.1).

Gallbladder dysmotility results in inadequate clearance of crystals and nascent stones. Motility is decreased in the presence of supersaturated bile even before stone formation. Decreased motility is a dominant contributing factor to stone development during pregnancy because of increased levels of progestin, prolonged total parenteral nutrition (TPN) (absence of intraduodenal fat and decreased cholecystokinin release), somatostatin therapy, or a somatostatinoma.

Generally, *pigment gallstones* are formed by the precipitation of bilirubin in bile. *Black pigment gallstones* are formed in sterile gallbladder bile in association with chronic hemolytic states, cirrhosis, Gilbert syndrome, or cystic fibrosis, or they may have no identifiable cause. These stones are small, irregular, dense, and insoluble aggregates or polymers of calcium bilirubinate. *Brown pigment gallstones* occur primarily in the bile ducts, where they are related to stasis and chronic bacterial colonization, as may occur above strictures or duodenal diverticula after sphincterotomy, or in association with biliary parasites. They are composed of 20% cholesterol, they are softer than black pigment gallstones, and they may soften or disaggregate with ursodeoxycholic acid.

✓ Risk factors for stone formation
- Cholesterol stones: obesity, female sex, type 2 diabetes, ethnicity, rapid weight loss, ileal disease or resection, pregnancy, TPN, and medications (eg, estrogens, progestins, lipid-lowering agents, bile acid sequestrants, glucagon-like peptide-1 agonists, and octreotide)
- Black pigment stones: chronic hemolysis, Gilbert syndrome, TPN, cirrhosis, and old age
- Brown pigment stones: cholecystectomy, recurrent biliary infection, stasis (eg, duodenal diverticulum and biliary strictures)

Clinical Presentation and Complications

Asymptomatic Cholelithiasis

The diagnosis of asymptomatic cholelithiasis is the result of widespread use of abdominal ultrasonography to evaluate nonspecific abdominal symptoms. Approximately 20% of Western populations have cholelithiasis, and of these people, 80%

Table 40.1. Types of Stones: Characteristics and Clinical Association

Feature	Cholesterol gallstones	Black pigment gallstones	Brown pigment gallstones
Composition	50%-99% cholesterol by weight	Calcium bilirubinate Calcium phosphate	Unconjugated bilirubin, palmitate stearate, cholesterol, and mucin
Color	Yellow-brown	Black	Brown
Consistency	Crystalline	Hard	Soft, greasy
Location	Gallbladder or common bile duct (or both)	Gallbladder or common bile duct (or both)	Intrahepatic and extrahepatic bile ducts
Radiodensity	Lucent (85%)	Opaque (>50%)	Lucent (100%)
Bile culture	Sterile	Sterile	Infected (eg, *Escherichia coli*)
Recurrent stones	Rare	Rare	Frequent
Clinical associations	Increased losses through the gastrointestinal tract from bile acid sequestrant therapy	Chronic hemolytic states (eg, sickle cell disease and mechanical heart valves)	Proximal to biliary stricture
	Terminal ileal disease, resection, or bypass	Cirrhosis	Proximal to duodenal diverticulum (stasis)
	Hormonal stimuli (female sex, pregnancy, exogenous estrogens, and progestins)	Gilbert syndrome	After sphincterotomy
	Obesity	Cystic fibrosis	Biliary parasites
	Hyperlipidemia	Total parenteral nutrition	
	Older age	May have no identifiable cause	
	Chronic liver disease		
	Excessive dietary polyunsaturated fats or caloric intake		
	Pregnancy		
	Prolonged total parenteral nutrition		
	Somatostatin therapy		
	Somatostatinoma		

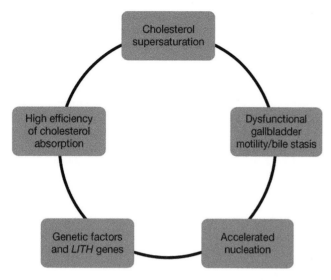

Figure 40.2. Defects Resulting in Gallstone Formation. Studies have shown that interactions of 5 defects result in nucleation and crystallization of cholesterol monohydrate crystals in bile, with eventual formation of gallstones.

Box 40.1. *LITH* Genes and Potential Mechanisms

ATP-binding cassette transporter B4: Biliary phospholipid secretion is decreased

β_3-Adrenergic receptor: Gallbladder hypomotility

Apolipoprotein A-I: Biliary cholesterol secretion is increased from an increase in reverse cholesterol transport

Apolipoprotein B: Biliary cholesterol secretion is increased from a decrease in hepatic VLDL synthesis and an increase in intestinal cholesterol absorption

Cholecystokinin 1 receptor: Gallbladder and small intestinal hypomotility

Cytochrome P450 7A1 isozyme: Bile salt synthesis is decreased

Estrogen receptor 2: Cholesterol synthesis is increased

Cholesterol ester transfer protein: Hepatic cholesterol uptake is increased from HDL catabolism

---

Abbreviations: ATP, adenosine triphosphate; HDL, high-density lipoprotein; VLDL, very low-density lipoprotein.

---

are asymptomatic when cholelithiasis is initially identified. Commonly, asymptomatic disease has a benign course and the proportion of those with disease that evolves from asymptomatic to symptomatic is relatively low (20% over a lifetime). More than 90% of gallstone disease complications are preceded by an episode of uncomplicated biliary colic. Thus, while asymptomatic stones generally do not require therapy, when they become symptomatic, cholecystectomy is indicated.

Prophylactic cholecystectomy should be considered, however, for patients who are planning extensive travel in remote areas and for American Indian populations, in whom the relative risk for stone-associated gallbladder carcinoma (GBC) is 20 times higher than for those without stones. The risk of GBC for patients who have stones larger than 3 cm is 10-fold higher than for patients with stones smaller than 1 cm. Prophylactic cholecystectomy should also be considered for patients treated with somatostatin analogues for midgut carcinoids or other neuroendocrine tumors. The adverse effects of these analogues include impairment of gallbladder function, formation of gallstones, and cholecystitis. Therefore, prophylactic cholecystectomy may be beneficial for this cohort of patients but still needs to be investigated. Concomitant cholecystectomy at the time of a Roux-en-Y gastric bypass for ultrasound-confirmed gallbladder pathology is feasible and safe and may reduce the potential for future gallbladder-related morbidity. A similar rationale may be used when prophylactic splenectomy is performed in patients with hereditary spherocytosis. However, cholecystectomy is not recommended for asymptomatic patients who have stones and type 2 diabetes or sickle cell disease if they have regular access to medical care.

Progressive gallstone dissolution by oral litholysis with hydrophilic ursodiol may be attempted in patients who have mild symptoms and small, uncalcified cholesterol gallstones in a functioning gallbladder with a patent cystic duct. This often requires at least 6 months of therapy and can be costly. Daily ursodiol may reduce the frequency of gallstone formation in patients with obesity who are eating low-calorie diets or who have had bariatric surgery.

Symptomatic Cholelithiasis

Biliary colic is a relatively specific form of pain secondary to increased pressure in the gallbladder due to hormonal or neural stimulation. This may be triggered by a fatty meal or a stone compressed against the gallbladder outlet or cystic duct opening. The pain usually develops rapidly in the epigastrium or right upper quadrant and lasts longer than 30 minutes but not longer than 4 to 6 hours. The likelihood of patients having a severe event or complication is approximately 1% per year, prompting the recommendation of surgical therapy for symptomatic gallstones. Histologically, most patients with recurrent biliary colic have chronic cholecystitis.

Cholecystitis is a syndrome that encompasses a continuum of clinicopathologic states. Patients with acute calculous cholecystitis generally present with abdominal pain that lasts longer than 6 hours and is accompanied by fever, leukocytosis, or cholestasis. The diagnostic criteria for acute cholecystitis is based on the Tokyo Guidelines 2018 (Box 40.2). Acute calculous cholecystitis is associated with age older than 60 years, male sex, type 2 diabetes, history of cardiovascular disease, and history of cerebrovascular accident or stroke. In an immune-compromised patient, it may be related to cytomegalovirus or *Cryptosporidium* infections. The most common complication is gangrene of the gallbladder (20%); therefore, early cholecystectomy is recommended for patients who have symptomatic cholelithiasis and these adverse risk factors. However, cholecystectomy is not indicated for patients who have isolated abnormal results on liver biochemical tests or cholestasis in the absence of choledocholithiasis. For patients who are not surgical candidates, gallbladder drainage can be achieved with endoscopic retrograde cholangiopancreatography (ERCP) with transpapillary drainage, endoscopic ultrasonography (EUS) for transmural drainage with a lumen-apposing metal stent, and percutaneous drainage through a cholecystostomy tube.

Acute *acalculous* cholecystitis accounts for 10% of all acute episodes, is associated with a high mortality rate, and is difficult to diagnose. It generally occurs in acutely ill, hospitalized patients. It also may develop postoperatively and in critically ill patients and may be complicated by the development of gangrene, perforation, and empyema. Type 2 diabetes, malignant disease, abdominal vasculitis, congestive heart failure, cholesterol embolization, shock, and cardiac arrest also have been associated with acute acalculous cholecystitis. The overall mortality rate is 50%. Ultrasonography, CT, and hepatobiliary iminodiacetic acid (HIDA) scans are the most useful imaging examinations. Hyperamylasemia may be a diagnostic clue. Diagnostic laparoscopy and, potentially, laparotomy have been recommended by the Society of American Gastrointestinal and Endoscopic Surgeons for acute acalculous cholecystitis. Nonsurgical approaches such as transpapillary, transmural, or percutaneous drainage are also used when necessary.

Between 5% and 40% of all laparoscopic cholecystectomy procedures are associated with spillage of gallstones. Gallstones also may be dropped during open cholecystectomy, but the larger operating field makes them easier to retrieve. Dropped gallstones may mimic colon cancer, liver abscess, subphrenic abscess, peritoneal metastases, and intra-abdominal actinomycosis. Symptoms can present years after the index cholecystectomy, and a high degree of clinical awareness is usually needed for diagnosis.

Gallbladder Polyps

Polypoid lesions of the gallbladder typically are incidental findings and indicate any projection of mucosa into the gallbladder lumen regardless of neoplastic potential. The majority are benign nonneoplastic lesions that include cholesterol polyps (usually pedunculated), adenomyomatosis, and inflammatory polyps. Cholesterol polyps are usually smaller than 10 mm in diameter and appear on ultrasonography as tiny echogenic spots or echogenic pedunculated masses without acoustic shadowing. Gallbladder polyps can also develop in patients with a congenital polyposis syndrome such as Peutz-Jeghers syndrome or familial adenomatous polyposis. Patients with solitary sessile polyps

larger than 10 mm in diameter should be considered for cholecystectomy, as should polyps of any size in patients who have cholelithiasis or primary sclerosing cholangitis. In patients older than 50 years or of Indian ethnicity, cholecystectomy should be recommended when the polyp size is greater than 6 mm given the increased risk for gallbladder cancer in this population. Polyps that are 5 to 9 mm generally require close surveillance with abdominal ultrasonography in 3 to 6 months.

Gallstones and Pregnancy

Symptomatic gallstone disease is the second most common abdominal emergency in pregnant women. Insulin resistance is a risk factor for incidental gallbladder sludge and stones during pregnancy, even after adjustment for body mass index. Insulin resistance may be a causal link between obesity and gallstones. In addition, the pregnant state impairs gallbladder motility and increases biliary cholesterol saturation. ERCP can be performed safely during pregnancy but may be associated with an increased rate of post-ERCP pancreatitis compared with the rate for the general population. Studies that compared conservative management with surgical management of cholecystitis showed no significant difference in the incidence of preterm delivery or fetal mortality. Laparoscopic cholecystectomy is safe in all trimesters. In 12 reports of gallstone pancreatitis, the fetal mortality rate was 8% for the conservative management group and 2.6% for the surgical management group, suggesting the need for earlier surgical intervention. Hospitalization for gallstone-related disease is common in the first postpartum year, most often for uncomplicated cholelithiasis. Risk factors for hospitalization include high prepregnancy body mass index, Latino ethnicity, and older maternal age.

Microlithiasis and Sludge

Microliths are a component of biliary sludge, consisting of relatively larger particles (1-3 mm) that are essential in the development of gallstones. Microscopic examination of bile under polarized light can be used to detect cholesterol crystals, which are a surrogate marker for biliary sludge and gallstones. The chemical composition of sludge includes cholesterol monohydrate crystals, calcium bilirubinate granules, calcium phosphate and calcium carbonate crystals, and calcium salts of fatty acids; the composition of sludge correlates well with the composition of stones. A higher prevalence of detectable gallbladder sludge is noted during pregnancy, TPN (secondary to gallbladder stasis), weight loss, prolonged fasting, and prolonged treatment with octreotide and after intravenous administration of ceftriaxone.

Biliary sludge or microlithiasis may cause acalculous biliary pain and may obstruct the common bile duct, manifesting as acute cholangitis or pancreatitis. Consequently, occult microlithiasis should be suspected when patients have acute pancreatitis of unknown origin, particularly if relapses are frequent. Additionally, it is a well-recognized complication after liver transplant; in 6% of patients, cholangiography shows biliary filling defects ultimately attributed to sludge-cast, gallstones, or necrotic debris. Biliary strictures and prestenotic dilatations of the bile ducts are the major reasons for sludge formation.

Expectant management is warranted for incidentally detected asymptomatic sludge. Similar to that for overt gallstone disease, treatment is necessary only if patients are symptomatic or have complications. Endoscopic sphincterotomy with either ursodiol treatment or laparoscopic cholecystectomy is a useful alternative for patients who have biliary sludge and recurrent obstruction of biliary outflow associated with recurrent cholangitis or pancreatitis. After liver transplant, biliary sludge should be treated endoscopically when biochemical evidence of obstruction or clinical signs of infection are evident to avoid graft dysfunction and other life-threatening complications.

Choledocholithiasis

Choledocholithiasis (ie, stones in the common bile duct) should be suspected in patients who have symptomatic cholelithiasis or acute biliary pancreatitis and even in patients who have had cholecystectomy. Choledocholithiasis occurs in 15% of people who have cholelithiasis. Concomitant cholelithiasis and choledocholithiasis occur more frequently in elderly Asian patients, in patients with chronic bile duct inflammation (sclerosing cholangitis or parasitic infestation), and in patients with hypothyroidism. A common bile duct stone detected on any imaging is the most reliable predictor of such stones at ERCP or surgery. The American Society for Gastrointestinal Endoscopy (ASGE) 2019 guidelines recommend 3 criteria for proceeding directly to ERCP before cholecystectomy: 1) choledocholithiasis on imaging, 2) total bilirubin greater than 4 mg/dL *and* a dilated common bile duct, and 3) ascending cholangitis (Figure 40.3). If patients do not meet these criteria but a stone is suspected, further diagnostic evaluation such as with EUS, magnetic resonance cholangiopancreatography (MRCP), or cholecystectomy with intraoperative cholangiography should be pursued. Those who do not meet any of the criteria should proceed to cholecystectomy. Endoscopic therapy (therapeutic ERCP) consists of endoscopic biliary sphincterotomy and stone removal with the use of various devices for direct extraction or lithotripsy (mechanical or electrohydraulic) when necessary. Extracorporeal shock wave lithotripsy of duct stones is clinically approved and feasible but infrequently used. It is coupled with ERCP for the removal of stone debris.

Bile duct stones recur in 15% of patients during follow-up. They may recur after cholecystectomy. This is thought to be due to bile stasis and bacterobilia. A small amount of postcholecystectomy syndromes (in symptomatic patients after cholecystectomy) are related to a residual stone in a particularly long cystic duct or to the relapse of lithiasis in a gallbladder remnant. Common bile duct dilatation (≥13 mm) and the presence of a periampullary diverticulum are risk factors for recurrent stones.

✓ Factors associated with gallstone formation—increased cholesterol excretion, bile acid loss, stasis, and imbalanced nucleation
✓ Laparoscopic cholecystectomy—treatment of choice for both acute calculous and acalculous cholecystitis
✓ Acalculous cholecystitis
  • Common in severely ill patients
  • Diagnosis requires a high degree of clinical awareness
✓ Choledocholithiasis occurs in 15% of patients with cholelithiasis

---

Ascending Cholangitis

Acute cholangitis, or biliary tree infection, occurs as a consequence of biliary tract obstruction that promotes bile stasis and bacterial growth. Bacteria ascending from the duodenum are the main bacterial entry route. Secondary and less frequent routes of entry are the portal venous system and the periportal lymphatic system. Most episodes are due to coliforms such as *Escherichia coli*, *Klebsiella* (70% of cases), *Enterococcus*, *Pseudomonas*, and anaerobes (*Clostridium* and *Bacteroides*) (10% of cases). The occurrence of bacteremia or endotoxemia correlates directly with intrabiliary pressure.

Common bile duct stones are the most common cause, and the presentation may range from a mild, self-limited process to a serious, life-threatening condition that requires urgent intervention. Ascending cholangitis also may be due to a biliary stricture from a previous biliary operation, liver transplant, primary sclerosing cholangitis, or acquired immunodeficiency syndrome–related cholangiopathy. In 1877, Charcot described a triad of fever, right upper quadrant pain, and jaundice; this triad occurs in 50% of patients who have cholangitis. The Reynolds pentad, which includes hypotension and alteration of consciousness in addition to the features of the Charcot triad, is seen less frequently (5% of patients). In clinical practice, the Tokyo Guidelines 2018 are frequently used to diagnose and grade acute cholangitis (Box 40.3).

Initial therapy should include adequate resuscitation and the empirical use of broad-spectrum antibiotics with adequate biliary excretion. Useful antibiotics include ampicillin-sulbactam, piperacillin-tazobactam, third- or fourth-generation cephalosporins, quinolones, and carbapenems. Ceftriaxone is associated with the appearance of biliary sludge due to calcium salt precipitation, but the sludge should dissipate spontaneously when use of the drug is discontinued. Elderly patients, patients with a biliary stent in situ, or those who had previous enterobiliary

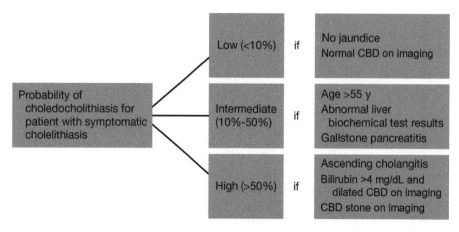

Figure 40.3. **Probability of Choledocholithiasis.** The probability of common bile duct stones is based on clinical, laboratory, and ultrasonographic variables. CBD indicates common bile duct.

Box 40.3. **The Tokyo Guidelines 2018 for Diagnosis of Acute Cholangitis**

A. Systemic inflammation
1. Fever or shaking chills (or both)
2. High white blood cell count
3. High C-reactive protein level

B. Cholestasis
1. Jaundice (bilirubin ≥2 mg/dL)
2. High ALT, AST, or ALP level

C. Imaging
1. Biliary dilatation
2. Evidence of the cause on imaging (eg, stricture, stone, or stent)

Suspected diagnosis: 1 item in A *and* 1 item in either B or C

Definite diagnosis: 1 item in A *and* 1 item in B *and* 1 item in C

Abbreviations: ALP, alkaline phosphatase; ALT, alanine aminotransferase; AST, aspartate aminotransferase.

Adapted from Kiriyama S, Kozaka K, Takada T, Strasberg SM, Pitt HA, Gabata T, et al. Tokyo guidelines 2018: diagnostic criteria and severity grading of acute cholangitis (with videos). J Hepatobiliary Pancreat Sci. 2018 25(1):17-30; used with permission.

surgery may benefit from additional enterococcal and anaerobic antimicrobial coverage. The timing of biliary decompression depends on the initial response to antibiotics, and supportive care can be provided by endoscopic, percutaneous, or surgical approaches or by multimodal therapy. The ASGE recommends ERCP within 48 hours and as soon as possible if the patient has no response to initial resuscitation and antibiotic therapy. Several reports have shown that ERCP after more than 48 hours is associated with increased mortality and increased in-hospital length of stay. ERCP with endoscopic sphincterotomy and common bile duct clearance is associated with considerably lower morbidity and mortality than traditional surgical management. If ERCP is not feasible, subsequent EUS-guided biliary drainage or percutaneous or, rarely, surgical decompression, should be pursued, depending on clinical urgency and expertise. In patients with altered anatomy (eg, Roux-en-Y gastric bypass), percutaneous drainage or EUS-guided biliary drainage may be preferred given the challenges of altered anatomy at ERCP.

Recurrent Pyogenic Cholangitis

Patients with recurrent pyogenic cholangitis present with recurrent, progressively severe, and frequent attacks of cholangitis with associated extensive stone disease, especially of the intrahepatic ducts. Secondary duct dilatation, stricture formation, and further stone formation become self-perpetuating. This form of cholangitis occurs especially in the Asian-Pacific basin. The pathogenetic mechanism is not understood completely; however, postulated causes include primary congenital biliary strictures and cysts, biliary parasitic infection (*Ascaris lumbricoides*, *Opisthorchis* species, or *Opisthorchis sinensis* [also known as the Chinese liver fluke]), and chronic intrahepatic bacterial colonization from unclear sources. Ascaris infection is also associated

with intrahepatic gallstones. Therapy is directed at duct decompression, drainage, stone clearance, and, occasionally, lobar or segmental resection for isolated intrahepatic disease. Isolated unilateral intrahepatic involvement is most common in the left hepatic ductal system. Peroral cholangioscopy, through a percutaneous tract or ERCP, can occasionally be a successful, minimally invasive approach depending on clinical expertise.

Sump Syndrome

In some patients who have had choledochoduodenostomy, sump syndrome occurs as debris (mainly food) accumulates in segments of the native biliary tree. This results in pain and cholangitis, requiring native papilla sphincterotomy. However, choledochoduodenostomy is rarely performed now, so fewer patients have sump syndrome.

Functional Gallbladder Disorder (Gallbladder Dyskinesia)

Functional gallbladder disorder is characterized by pain resembling biliary pain in patients who have an ultrasonographically normal gallbladder. Synonyms include *gallbladder dyskinesia, chronic acalculous gallbladder dysfunction, acalculous biliary disease,* and *biliary dyskinesia* (Box 40.4). The estimated prevalence is 10% for men and 20% for women, but the pathogenesis is poorly understood. Even though evidence-based recommendations cannot be made, the use of a neuromodulator is reasonable for patients with suspected functional gallbladder disorder. Anticholinergic drugs and narcotics are associated with impaired gallbladder emptying. If symptoms

Box 40.4. **Rome IV Criteria for the Diagnosis of Functional Gallbladder Disorder**

Diagnostic criteria

1. Absence of gallstones or other structural pathology *and*

2. Presence of biliary pain, defined as epigastric pain or right upper quadrant pain (or both), and *all* the following:

Pain increases to a steady level and lasts ≥30 min

Recurrent episodes occur at different intervals (not daily)

Pain is severe enough to interrupt daily functioning or leads to an emergency department visit

Pain is not related to bowel movements (<20%)

Pain is not relieved by postural change or acid suppression <20%

Supportive criteria

1. Low ejection fraction on gallbladder scintigraphy (HIDA scanning)

2. Normal levels of liver enzymes, conjugated bilirubin, and amylase and lipase

Abbreviation: HIDA, hepatobiliary iminodiacetic acid.

Adapted from Cotton PB, Elta GH, Carter CR, Pasricha PJ, Corazziari ES. Gallbladder and sphincter of Oddi disorders. Gastroenterology. 2016 150(6):1420-9; used with permission.

Box 40.5. Rome IV Criteria for the Diagnosis of Functional Biliary Sphincter of Oddi Disorder

Diagnostic criteria

1. High liver enzyme levels or dilated bile duct, but not both

   and

2. Absence of bile duct stones or other structural abnormalities

   and

3. Presence of biliary pain, defined as epigastric pain or right upper quadrant pain (or both), and *all* the following:

   Pain increases to a steady level and lasts ≥30 min

   Recurrent episodes occur at different intervals (not daily)

   Pain is severe enough to interrupt daily functioning or leads to an emergency department visit

   Pain is not related to bowel movements (<20%)

   Pain is not relieved by postural change or acid suppression (<20%)

Supportive criteria

1. Normal levels of amylase and lipase
2. Abnormal results on sphincter of Oddi manometry
3. Hepatobiliary scintigraphy

Adapted from Cotton PB, Elta GH, Carter CR, Pasricha PJ, Corazziari ES. Gallbladder and sphincter of Oddi disorders. Gastroenterology. 2016 150(6):1420-9; used with permission.

persist, oral cholecystography should be performed with and without cholecystokinin stimulation and with measurement of the gallbladder ejection fraction (a quantitative measurement of gallbladder emptying). An alternative and more frequently used investigation is the HIDA scan to evaluate functional gallbladder disorder. If the ejection fraction is less than 35%, cholecystectomy should be considered—but only for patients with classic biliary symptoms. Functional biliary sphincter of Oddi disorders are listed in Box 40.5.

Gallstone Complications

The incidence of *gallstone pancreatitis* is increased for women older than 60 years. The pathogenesis is thought to be related to increased pressure within the pancreatic duct, with biliopancreatic reflux, due to passage of a common bile duct stone or an impacted stone at the level of the papilla. Suspicion of acute gallstone pancreatitis is increased if patients have acute pancreatitis associated with abnormal results from liver function tests, evidence of cholelithiasis, or biliary tree dilatation. Transabdominal ultrasonography is the most cost-effective initial investigation to document the presence of cholelithiasis, with or without common bile duct dilatation. Bowel gas and stones smaller than 4 mm may reduce the overall sensitivity. Pancreatic parenchymal and peripancreatic inflammatory changes are best detected and evaluated with contrast-enhanced CT, which also may show pancreatic neoplasm, pancreatic calcification, or choledocholithiasis. Because patients have a high risk for recurrence within 30 days after an attack, they should undergo cholecystectomy during the index hospitalization after their symptoms have resolved. ERCP with sphincterotomy is recommended for patients who are not candidates for surgery or for patients who cannot undergo cholecystectomy within a few months.

Gallstone ileus is a disease of the elderly, with a female predominance. It frequently is preceded by an episode of acute cholecystitis. The resulting obstruction is a true mechanical phenomenon; therefore, the term *ileus* is a misnomer. The cholecystitis-related inflammation and adhesions facilitate the erosion of the offending gallstone through the gallbladder wall, forming a cholecystoenteric fistula and facilitating stone passage. The duodenal wall is the most common fistula site, but it may occur anywhere in the gastrointestinal tract (colon, stomach, or small bowel). An iatrogenic fistula can form after endoscopic sphincterotomy or a surgical choledochoduodenostomy. A stone smaller than 2 to 2.5 cm usually passes spontaneously through a normal gastrointestinal tract. Stones larger than 5 cm are more likely to become impacted. The terminal ileum and ileocecal valve are the most common locations because of the relatively narrow lumen and decreased peristalsis. Presenting symptoms may be intermittent because the passing stone may lodge at various levels of the bowel. A passing stone is responsible for 25% of all bowel obstructions in patients older than 65 years, compared with 1% to 3% in all age groups. Abdominal radiography may show bowel obstruction, pneumobilia, and an abnormally located stone. CT may be used to identify larger stones, evidence of bowel obstruction, and the level of obstruction. Surgical intervention is the treatment of choice for the majority of patients and may include biliary surgery when the intestinal obstruction is relieved.

Obstruction at the level of the gastric outlet by a gallstone is called *Bouveret syndrome*. It is an uncommon form of gallstone ileus. A single gallstone at least 2.5 cm in diameter is the most common underlying cause of this syndrome.

Mirizzi syndrome results from a common hepatic duct obstruction due to extrinsic compression from an impacted cystic duct stone. Patients present with a triad of fever, right upper quadrant pain, and jaundice, with high levels of bilirubin and alkaline phosphatase. They have an increased risk for gallbladder cancer. Mirizzi syndrome is noted in 1% of patients undergoing biliary surgery. In 10% of patients, the cystic duct courses parallel to the extrahepatic bile duct and inserts medially into it at the level of the papilla.

Emphysematous cholecystitis is a rare form of acute cholecystitis in which the gallbladder becomes infected with gas-forming organisms such as *Clostridium perfringens*, *E coli*, and *Klebsiella* species. Most patients are 50 to 70 years old and, in contrast to typical patients with acute cholecystitis, men are more likely to be affected than women. Approximately 25% of patients have type 2 diabetes. Although the initial symptoms may be relatively mild, the disorder often progresses rapidly and is associated with a high risk of gallbladder perforation. The diagnosis can be made with plain abdominal radiographs, ultrasonographic studies, or CT. CT is the most sensitive method for detecting small amounts of gas in the gallbladder wall. Treatment includes intravenous antibiotics that cover anaerobic organisms and subsequent early open or laparoscopic cholecystectomy. Another option is percutaneous drainage of the gallbladder, particularly in patients who are critically ill. Emphysematous cholecystitis has occurred in patients with gallstone cholecystitis or acalculous cholecystitis and has been associated with a mortality rate of approximately 15%. This is substantially higher than the mortality rates of 3% to 4% for patients with acute cholecystitis without gas-forming organisms.

Porcelain gallbladder is seen more frequently in women, primarily in the sixth decade. It can be identified on plain abdominal radiographs or CT and is an uncommon finding in chronic cholecystitis. Porcelain gallbladder is characterized by extensive calcification manifested as a brittle consistency of the wall and is seen in less than 1% of cholecystectomy specimens, with stones identified in 95% of pathology specimens. The diagnosis of porcelain gallbladder is important because of its association with gallbladder cancer. However, making the diagnosis may be difficult because rim calcifications in the right upper quadrant may be due to gallstones or liver, kidney, adrenal, or pancreatic cysts. The incidence of gallbladder cancer in patients with porcelain gallbladder ranges from 0% to 20%. Prophylactic cholecystectomy is the treatment of choice for porcelain gallbladder.

Clinical Investigations

Liver Biochemical Testing

Uncomplicated biliary colic usually is not accompanied by changes in hematologic and biochemical test results. However, the initial evaluation of suspected stone disease should include serum liver biochemical testing (eg, alanine aminotransferase, aspartate aminotransferase [AST], alkaline phosphatase, and total bilirubin) and transabdominal ultrasonography of the right upper quadrant. Liver biochemical tests may be most useful in excluding the presence of common bile duct stones. In a series of more than 1,000 patients undergoing laparoscopic cholecystectomy, completely normal results on liver biochemical tests had a negative predictive value of more than 97%, whereas the positive predictive value of any abnormal liver biochemical test result was only 15%, according to the current guidelines of the ASGE.

Patients with cholangitis or pancreatitis associated with abnormal results on serum liver function tests have an increased risk for bile duct stones. The conventional wisdom that the alkaline phosphatase level increases more than the AST level in obstructive jaundice holds true when jaundice is due to strictures, but in obstructive stone disease, the increase in AST may equal that in alkaline phosphatase or even exceed it during periods of maximal jaundice and painful episodes. Occasionally, serum transaminase levels may be increased dramatically, mimicking acute viral hepatitis. With biliary stones, the increased levels tend to decrease rapidly over several days rather than weeks, as with acute viral hepatitis.

Biliary Imaging

Several improvements have been made in biliary imaging. Although ultrasonography is the primary initial modality for the evaluation of the biliary tree, the advent of and improvements in CT, magnetic resonance imaging, and EUS techniques have resulted in superior detection and characterization of disease.

Plain Abdominal Radiography

Plain abdominal radiography can show radiopaque stones (about 25% of all stones) and pneumobilia due to a previous biliary sphincterotomy, a bilioenteric anastomosis or fistula, or an incompetent sphincter, as may occur with duodenal Crohn disease, duodenal diverticulum, or other periampullary disease.

Oral Cholecystography

Oral cholecystography involves standard radiographic imaging of the right upper quadrant after oral administration of an iodinated radiodense contrast agent. Thus, the agent needs to be ingested, absorbed and taken up by the liver, excreted by the biliary system, and concentrated by the gallbladder. Most gallbladders opacify after a single oral dose, and 85% to 90% opacify after a second or double dose. Nonvisualization of the gallbladder after a reinforced 1- or 2-day study is 95% predictive of gallbladder disease. The use of oral cholecystography has diminished in clinical practice because it is less sensitive (65%-90%) than ultrasonography for cholelithiasis, and it is not indicated when acute cholecystitis is suspected. Oral cholecystography may be useful when ultrasonography does not image the gallbladder and EUS is not available.

HIDA Scanning

HIDA scanning, also known as *cholescintigraphy*, may be used to diagnose acute cholecystitis or to confirm intra-abdominal bile leakage. This method involves noninvasive scanning of gamma emissions after the intravenous administration, liver uptake, and biliary excretion of technetium iminodiacetic acid derivatives. The inability to visualize the gallbladder despite excretion into the common bile duct at 4 hours after the injection is indicative of cystic duct obstruction. Nonvisualization of the gallbladder is 97% sensitive and 96% specific for acute calculous cholecystitis. False-negative results occur with acalculous cholecystitis, and false-positive results occur with chronic cholecystitis and chronic liver disease and during TPN or fasting states.

Transabdominal Ultrasonography

Ultrasonography has greater sensitivity for detecting dilatation of the common bile duct than for detecting choledocholithiasis. It is most sensitive (90%-98%) for the detection of cholelithiasis (>2 mm) identified as mobile, intraluminal, echogenic, shadowing particles. Obesity and bowel gas make interpretation challenging, but ultrasonography is relatively inexpensive and noninvasive compared with other imaging options. Cholecystitis is identified by gallbladder contraction or marked distention with surrounding fluid or wall thickening. Gallbladder thickening also may be due to portal hypertension, ascites, and hypoalbuminemia. The diameter of the common bile duct is normally 3 to 6 mm, and it may increase with older age. Biliary obstruction should be suspected when the diameter is more than 8 mm in a patient with a gallbladder in situ. Multiple small stones (<5 mm in diameter), compared with larger stones, increase the risk of common bile duct migration 4-fold. Transabdominal ultrasonographic examination of the gallbladder permits the visualization of particles in bile, usually those 2 to 3 mm or more in diameter.

Abdominal CT

CT is the best imaging method for the evaluation of possible complications of biliary stone disease if ultrasonography is suboptimal, as in patients with fever, right upper quadrant pain, and associated jaundice. Bowel gas and ribs do not interfere with CT. CT is superior to ultrasonography for patients with obesity, in whom imaging is improved by discrete fat planes. CT is not appropriate for the diagnosis of uncomplicated stone disease or evaluation of biliary colic because 50% of gallstones are radiolucent on CT.

Endoscopic Ultrasonography

Suspected Choledocholithiasis

The major advantage of EUS in suspected choledocholithiasis, as compared with transabdominal ultrasonography, is the ability to position the ultrasound transducer within the duodenal lumen,

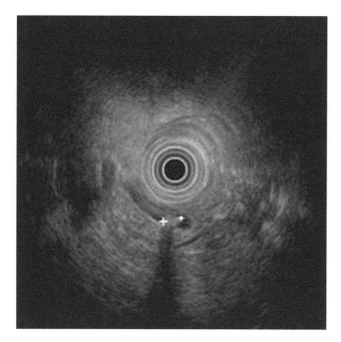

Figure 40.4. Endoscopic Ultrasonographic Image of Choledocholithiasis. Echo-rich areas with typical postacoustic shadowing are seen within the common bile duct.

thereby allowing visualization of the adjacent biliary tree without interference from intestinal gas or abdominal fat. EUS is particularly important in correctly distinguishing acute biliary pancreatitis from other causes of pancreatitis.

Choledocholiths may be mobile, multiple, and of variable size (Figure 40.4). Occasionally, stones do not show acoustic shadowing and may be associated with a thickened bile duct wall. Bile duct sludge is seen as variably shaped and easily distorted echo-rich structures without acoustic shadowing.

In suspected choledocholithiasis, EUS has a sensitivity of more than 90% for the detection of common bile duct stones. The findings compare favorably with those of ERCP and are superior to those obtained with transabdominal ultrasonography, without the associated postprocedural ERCP risk of pancreatitis. For patients with a low or intermediate risk for bile duct stones, EUS is a cost-effective initial screening study. Comparative controlled trials of EUS and MRCP have shown that the accuracy of EUS is comparable to or higher than that of MRCP for the detection of common bile duct stones.

A recent systematic review has suggested that EUS should be reserved for the evaluation of patients for whom there is an intermediate suspicion of common bile duct stones. Although EUS does not have the therapeutic capacity of ERCP for stone removal, algorithms have been developed that incorporate its use into clinical practice. Ultimately, the choice of modality should be based on clinical suspicion, availability of resources, experience, and cost.

Cholelithiasis

EUS can be used to reliably identify cholelithiasis, particularly in patients with obesity and small stones. The appearance is that of a hyperechoic structure within the gallbladder, sometimes associated with an acoustic shadow. In patients with suspected gallbladder stone disease but with negative findings on conventional transabdominal ultrasonographic examinations, EUS has

a sensitivity of 96% and a specificity of 86% compared with the corresponding cholecystectomy specimens or long-term clinical follow-up.

Microlithiasis

EUS has been shown to be as accurate as crystal analysis for the detection of microlithiasis (Figure 40.5). In approximately 20% of patients with acute pancreatitis, the cause is not established by history, physical examination, routine laboratory testing, or abdominal imaging. Recent studies suggest that microlithiasis may account for an unexplained attack of acute pancreatitis in as many as 75% of patients with a gallbladder in situ. Sphincter of Oddi

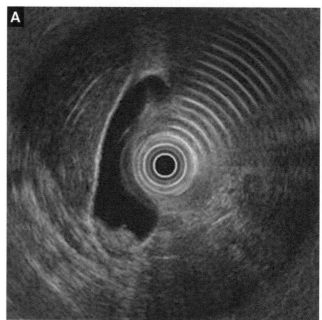

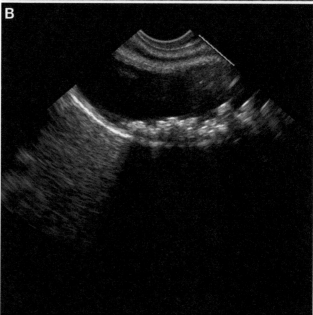

Figure 40.5. Microlithiasis on Endoscopic Ultrasonography. A, The crystals appear as floating hyperechoic foci that move when abdominal pressure is applied to the right upper quadrant and as layering material indicating sludge. B, Note the presence of a shadowing stone with layering sludge.

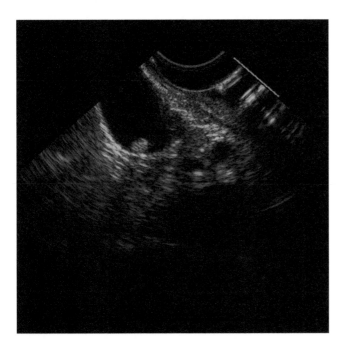

Figure 40.6. Cholesterol Polyps. Endoscopic ultrasonography shows an echogenic region without acoustic shadowing.

dysfunction is most prevalent in patients with recurrent attacks who have previously undergone cholecystectomy. Therefore, EUS is an important diagnostic tool for evaluation of patients who have unexplained biliary colic.

Polyps

With EUS, the normal gallbladder wall is seen as a 2- or 3-layer structure: The inner hypoechoic layer corresponds to the muscularis propria layer and the outer hyperechoic layer corresponds to an adipose layer. Cholesterol polyps are usually smaller than 10 mm in diameter and appear on ultrasonography as tiny echogenic spots or echogenic pedunculated masses without acoustic shadowing (Figure 40.6).

Cholangiography

Cholangiography can be performed either invasively or noninvasively. The selection of MRCP, percutaneous transhepatic cholangiography, ERCP, or EUS-guided biliary access is based largely on the clinical setting and institutional expertise.

Magnetic Resonance Cholangiopancreatography

MRCP should be the first examination of choice because it is less invasive than EUS. MRCP is favored over EUS for frail patients who are not candidates for conscious sedation and for patients who have coagulopathy or who need concurrent staging or evaluation of the liver parenchyma or other organs, especially when therapeutic intervention is unlikely. MRCP appears to be a valuable and safe technique for the evaluation of pregnant patients who have acute pancreaticobiliary disease. Especially when ultrasonography shows biliary dilatation, MRCP can be used to determine the cause and prevent unnecessary ERCP by excluding biliary abnormality. When MRCP results are negative, EUS is recommended to check for small common bile duct stones.

Hemorrhagic cholecystitis is a form of acute cholecystitis often seen in the absence of gallstones. Hemorrhage is identified by the characteristic appearance of hemoglobin breakdown products within the wall or lumen of the gallbladder. The use of MRCP in combination with CT is useful for preoperative diagnosis of Mirizzi syndrome.

Percutaneous Transhepatic Cholangiography

Percutaneous transhepatic cholangiography may be favored for patients with a proximal obstruction (hilar or more proximal) or surgically distorted gastroduodenal anatomy (especially Roux limbs but also after a Whipple or Billroth II procedure) and after failure of previous ERCP, EUS-assisted ERCP, or EUS-guided biliary drainage. It is almost uniformly successful in patients with dilated ducts and in 75% to 95% of those with nondilated ducts. The overall risk, including death, sepsis, bile leaks, and intraperitoneal bleeding, is 5%.

Endoscopic Retrograde Cholangiopancreatography

ERCP is favored for patients with ascites or coagulation defects, suspected periampullary or pancreatic neoplasia, nondilated ducts, anticipated need for therapeutic maneuvers (stone removal and stenting), or hypersensitivity to contrast agents and if use of percutaneous routes has been unsuccessful. Purely diagnostic use is diminishing rapidly because, for most patients, EUS and MRCP serve this purpose more safely. ERCP is successful in more than 95% of diagnostic applications, in 95% of sphincterotomies and complete stone extraction, and in 90% of procedures for stenting of malignant obstruction (Figure 40.7). Nonemergent ERCP in patients 80 years or older is reported to be safe and cost-effective, without significantly greater rates of complications or mortality. Intraductal shock wave lithotripsy is a therapeutic option that may be effective despite the difficulties of a large, impacted stone that cannot be captured by a basket or a stricture that prohibits delivery of

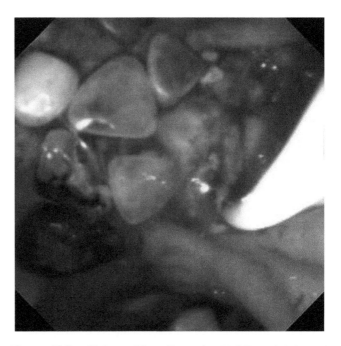

Figure 40.7. Cholesterol Stone Extraction. Multifaceted cholesterol stones are retrieved at endoscopic retrograde cholangiopancreatography.

Box 40.6. Gallstone Treatments

Indications for cholecystectomy (open or laparoscopic)

    Symptomatic cholelithiasis (with or without complications)

    Asymptomatic cholelithiasis in patients who are at increased risk for gallbladder carcinoma or gallstone complications

    Acalculous cholecystitis

    Gallstone size >3 cm

    Gallbladder polyps >10 mm in diameter (any size in PSC)

    Porcelain gallbladder

Nonsurgical treatment of gallbladder stones

    Oral bile acid dissolution therapy with ursodiol for noncalcified stones

    Extracorporeal shock wave lithotripsy

Abbreviation: PSC, primary sclerosing cholangitis.

Table 40.2. Mimics of Biliary Colic

Condition	Comments
Intravenous ceftriaxone therapy	May lead to formation of crystalline biliary precipitates of drug
	Ceftriaxone crystals can induce all potential complications of small bile duct stones, including biliary colic and pancreatitis
Erythromycin hepatotoxicity	Manifests as syndrome of pain, fever, and cholestatic hepatitis, mimicking acute cholecystitis
	Antibiotic history should be elicited during evaluation of symptoms
	Consistent history and associated eosinophilia may help identify syndrome
Leptospirosis	Weil syndrome (characterized by fever, jaundice, azotemia, and right upper quadrant pain) mimics acute bacterial cholangitis
	Clues to diagnosis include history of exposure risk, myalgias, ocular pain, photophobia, azotemia, and abnormal urinalysis findings

---

a stone beyond it. The overall risk of the procedure in patients with suspected gallstones is 5% for diagnostic procedures and 10% for therapy. Risks include death, pancreatitis, infection, sedation or cardiovascular events, hemorrhage, and perforation.

For patients who have gallstone pancreatitis and concomitant cholangitis, ERCP should be performed within 24 hours. If a persistent common bile duct stone is highly likely (ie, the patient has a visible common bile duct stone on noninvasive imaging, a persistently dilated common bile duct, and jaundice), the patient should undergo ERCP in 48 to 72 hours because data suggest that ERCP in patients with gallstone pancreatitis without cholangitis in less than 48 hours may be harmful. Although data are lacking to support the practice of endoscopic sphincterotomy in the absence of choledocholithiasis at the time of the procedure, the practice is a reasonable therapeutic option. ERCP and sphincterotomy alone may provide adequate long-term therapy for patients who are not candidates for surgery as previously mentioned. In cases of mild gallstone pancreatitis, cholecystectomy should be performed during the same hospital admission if possible and no later than 2 to 4 weeks after discharge.

Gallstone treatments are listed in Box 40.6, and mimics of biliary colic are listed in Table 40.2.

✓ Elective cholecystectomy is required for gallbladder polyps larger than 10 mm (or any size in patients with primary sclerosing cholangitis or concomitant cholelithiasis) owing to increased cancer risk

✓ Gallstones larger than 3 cm require elective cholecystectomy owing to increased cancer risk

---

Suggested Reading

ASGE Standards of Practice Committee, Buxbaum JL, Abbas Fehmi SM, Sultan S, Fishman DS, Qumseya BJ, et al. ASGE guideline on the role of endoscopy in the evaluation and management of choledocholithiasis. Gastrointest Endosc. 2019 Jun;89(6):1075–105.

Attasaranya S, Fogel EL, Lehman GA. Choledocholithiasis, ascending cholangitis, and gallstone pancreatitis. Med Clin North Am. 2008 Jul;92(4):925–60.

Buxbaum JL, Buitrago C, Lee A, Elmunzer BJ, Riaz A, Ceppa EP, et al. ASGE guideline on the management of cholangitis. Gastrointest Endosc. 2021 Aug;94(2):207–21.

O'Neill DE, Saunders MD. Endoscopic ultrasonography in diseases of the gallbladder. Gastroenterol Clin North Am. 2010 Jun;39(2):289–305.

Plecka Ostlund M, Wenger U, Mattsson F, Ebrahim F, Botha A, Lagergren J. Population-based study of the need for cholecystectomy after obesity surgery. Br J Surg. 2012 Jun;99(6):864–9.

Tang SJ, Mayo MJ, Rodriguez-Frias E, Armstrong L, Tang L, Sreenarasimhaiah J, et al. Safety and utility of ERCP during pregnancy. Gastrointest Endosc. 2009 Mar;69(3 Pt 1):453–61.

Tse F, Liu L, Barkun AN, Armstrong D, Moayyedi P. EUS: a meta-analysis of test performance in suspected choledocholithiasis. Gastrointest Endosc. 2008 Feb;67(2):235–44.

✓ Acute cholangitis requires ERCP within 24 to 72 hours according to clinical status

✓ Gallstone pancreatitis with concomitant cholangitis warrants urgent ERCP within 24 hours

Questions and Answers

Questions

Abbreviations used:

AIP,	autoimmune pancreatitis
CT,	computed tomography
ERCP,	endoscopic retrograde cholangiopancreatography
EUS,	endoscopic ultrasonography
IPMN,	intraductal papillary mucinous neoplasm
MRCP,	magnetic resonance cholangiopancreatography
MRI,	magnetic resonance imaging
PET,	positron emission tomography
PSC,	primary sclerosing cholangitis
SUN,	serum urea nitrogen
TPN,	total parenteral nutrition
ULRR,	upper limit of the reference range
WBC,	white blood cell

Multiple Choice (choose the best answer)

VII.1. A 36-year-old man with a history of heavy alcohol use presents 8 hours after the onset of acute epigastric abdominal pain that radiates to the midback. The lipase level is 370 U/L (ULRR, 13-60 U/L). Other notable laboratory test values are the following: WBC count 11.0×10^9/L, SUN 31 mg/dL, and hematocrit 46%. Triglycerides, calcium, and liver biochemistry values are all within the ULRRs. He is afebrile, tachycardic (heart rate 110 beats/min), and normotensive. He is visibly uncomfortable and describes having nausea in addition to pain. Ultrasonography does not show cholelithiasis, and the sonographic Murphy sign is absent. Which of the following is the best next step in management?

    a. Contrast-enhanced CT of the abdomen
    b. ERCP
    c. A carbapenem antibiotic

    d. Intravenous isotonic fluids
    e. Genetic testing for inherited pancreatitis

VII.2. A 45-year-old woman has been admitted for pancreatitis after having undergone ERCP for choledocholithiasis. On the first day of admission, she has mild nausea and epigastric pain, but she is not vomiting and she is passing flatus. She is afebrile and hemodynamically stable. Which of the following is the correct management strategy for nutrition in this patient?

    a. Initiate TPN
    b. Place a nasojejunal tube, and feed a low-fat formula
    c. Begin a trial of a liquid-based diet, and advance the diet as tolerated
    d. Feed nothing by mouth until the lipase value is normal
    e. Feed nothing by mouth until 3 days after admission

VII.3. A 22-year-old man with Crohn disease has been in the hospital for 5 days for acute pancreatitis after reinitiation of azathioprine therapy caused a second episode of acute pancreatitis. When he was admitted for this episode, CT with a contrast agent showed a normally enhancing pancreas with peripancreatic fluid. Although he had modest improvement on the second day of hospitalization after beginning therapy with intravenous fluids, antiemetics, and analgesics, he has not tolerated an oral diet. His abdomen is visibly more distended. His WBC count has increased in the past 2 days to 17,000/μL; his highest temperature has been 38.5 °C. Which of the following is the best next step in management?

    a. Placement of a nasojejunal tube for postpancreatic feeding
    b. Fecal calprotectin testing
    c. Contrast-enhanced CT
    d. Abdominal radiography
    e. Intravenous antibiotics

VII.4. A 52-year-old woman with decompensated alcoholic cirrhosis and portal hypertension has been hospitalized in the intensive care unit for severe, necrotizing acute pancreatitis from gallstones. On day 6 of hospitalization, she has an increased requirement for norepinephrine for blood pressure support, and she has a sudden decrease in the hemoglobin level. She is given blood products and additional intravenous fluids. CT with a contrast agent shows dilatation of the gastroduodenal artery, and contrast material is visible in a walled-off necrotic collection posterior to the duodenal bulb. Which of the following is the best next step in management?

a. Interventional radiology–based targeted coil embolization
b. Upper endoscopy with epinephrine injection and hemostatic clip
c. Upper endoscopy with band ligation
d. Surgical exploration of the abdomen
e. Monitoring for signs of further hemodynamic instability

VII.5. A 62-year-old man presents to the pancreas clinic for a follow-up visit after a recent hospitalization. He initially presented 6 weeks ago with epigastric abdominal pain and a high serum lipase level (1,270 U/L; ULRR, 13-60 U/L). At that time, CT of the abdomen showed a 5-mm stone in the head of the pancreas near the ampulla with upstream dilatation of the pancreatic duct, a few prominent side branches in the pancreatic tail, and peripancreatic fat stranding without any fluid collections. No gallstones were seen. He has no prior history of pancreatitis. He was treated with intravenous fluids and analgesics; his condition greatly improved, and he was discharged from the hospital after 4 days. What is the most likely diagnosis?

a. Gallstone pancreatitis
b. Alcoholic pancreatitis
c. Intraductal papillary mucinous neoplasm
d. Autoimmune pancreatitis

VII.6. A 72-year-old man with a history of nicotine dependance presents with painless jaundice, and MRI of the abdomen shows a mass in the pancreatic head and a distal bile duct stricture. EUS-guided biopsy of the mass shows lymphoplasmacytic infiltrate and storiform fibrosis with obliterative phlebitis without any evidence of neoplasia. What is the best next step in management?

a. Treatment with oral prednisone
b. Follow-up biopsy of the pancreas
c. Surgical consultation for pancreaticoduodenectomy
d. PET/CT

VII.7. A 66-year-old man with long-standing daily alcohol use presents with weight loss and diarrhea. CT of the abdomen with a pancreas protocol shows an atrophic pancreas with calcification and main pancreatic duct dilatation without a pancreatic mass. The fecal elastase concentration is 82 µg/g (ULRR >200 µg/g). Which of the following is the best next step in management?

a. EUS with direct pancreatic function testing
b. Secretin-enhanced MRCP
c. Pancreatic enzyme replacement therapy
d. Fat-restricted diet

VII.8. Which of the following genes has pathogenic variants that are associated with hereditary pancreatitis?

a. *PRSS1*
b. *STK11*
c. *MLH1*
d. *CDKN2A*

VII.9. Which of the following is a known risk factor for pancreatic ductal adenocarcinoma?

a. Family history of breast and ovarian cancer
b. Obesity

c. Hypertension
d. Celiac disease

VII.10. A 45-year-old woman with a family history of melanoma undergoes genetic counseling and germline genetic testing, which identifies a pathogenic germline variant in the *CDKN2A* gene. She has no personal history of cancer and no family history of pancreatic cancer. Which of the following is the best next step in management?

a. Referral for pancreatic cancer screening
b. Baseline and annual testing for serum carbohydrate antigen 19-9
c. Bilateral mastectomy
d. Total pancreatectomy with autologous islet cell transplant

VII.11. A 66-year-old man undergoes CT of the abdomen before elective umbilical hernia repair. CT shows multiple cysts in the pancreas; the largest measures 3.2 cm. The main pancreatic duct is dilated to 6 mm, and some of the cysts communicate with it in the head. He does not have abdominal pain, and he has no previous history of pancreatitis. Which of the following is the best next step in the management of these incidentally detected pancreatic cysts?

a. EUS
b. Pylorus-preserving pancreaticoduodenectomy
c. Follow-up MRI of the abdomen in 2 years
d. No need for further testing or surveillance

VII.12. A 36-year-old woman presents to the emergency department after a motor vehicle accident. CT of the abdomen incidentally shows a 3-cm solid cystic lesion in the body of the pancreas. At a subsequent follow-up, an EUS-guided biopsy is performed, and the histologic features are consistent with a solid pseudopapillary neoplasm. What is the recommended next step in management?

a. The patient has a benign cystic neoplasm that does not require further follow-up
b. Upfront surgical resection should be considered
c. Neoadjuvant therapy with subsequent surgery is the preferred approach
d. Imaging surveillance should be performed annually with MRI

VII.13. A 70-year-old woman presents with right upper quadrant abdominal pain, fever, increased WBC count, and total bilirubin of 2 mg/dL. Abdominal ultrasonography shows cholelithiasis and a common bile duct with a normal diameter. What is the best next step in management?

a. MRCP
b. Cholecystectomy
c. ERCP
d. EUS and ERCP

VII.14. A 60-year-old man with a history of PSC presents for an annual follow-up visit. His liver test results are similar to baseline, and he has not had episodes of cholangitis or infection in the past year. On abdominal ultrasonography, an 8-mm gallbladder polyp is found. What is the best next step in management?

a. Repeat ultrasonography in 3 to 6 months
b. Perform MRCP now
c. Proceed with ERCP
d. Refer for elective cholecystectomy

VII.15. A 50-year-old man with a history of class 2 obesity (body mass index 37), type 2 diabetes, hypertension, and high cholesterol levels underwent Roux-en-Y gastric bypass for weight loss. Six months after surgery, he presented with biliary colic and was referred for elective cholecystectomy. While waiting for his surgery date, he presented to the emergency department with recurrent right upper quadrant abdominal pain. On examination, he is afebrile and has jaundice. The Murphy sign is negative. Laboratory test results are notable for a WBC count of 10×10⁹/L and total bilirubin of 4 mg/dL. Abdominal ultrasonography showed cholelithiasis, and the distal common bile duct was not visualized. Which of the following is the best next step in management?

 a. Cholecystectomy
 b. MRCP
 c. EUS with ERCP
 d. Placement of a percutaneous transhepatic drain

VII.16. An 80-year-old man with a history of type 2 diabetes, obesity, and coronary artery disease presents to the medical intensive care unit in shock. He receives fluid resuscitation and begins therapy with vasopressors. On examination, he is febrile and has right upper quadrant tenderness. Laboratory test results include a WBC count greater than 18×10⁹/L, total bilirubin 5 mg/dL, aspartate aminotransferase 500 U/L, and alanine aminotransferase 650 U/L. Abdominal ultrasonography shows a distended gallbladder with multiple small stones, a trace of pericholecystic fluid, and a common bile duct diameter of 9 mm. Which of the following is the most likely diagnosis?

 a. Acute calculous cholecystitis
 b. Acute acalculous cholecystitis
 c. Acute cholangitis
 d. Choledocholithiasis

Answers

VII.1. Answer d.
Initiation of intravenous isotonic fluids is a pivotal step for organ perfusion to counteract the vasodilatory cytokine effect from the systemic inflammatory response to pancreatic injury and to help prevent organ failure. The patient's increased SUN and hematocrit suggest intravascular volume depletion. CT is not necessary at this time because the diagnosis of pancreatitis can be made from the clinical picture of pain and the lipase value that is greater than 3 times the ULRR. Prophylactic antibiotics are not recommended for acute pancreatitis and are used only when unstable systemic inflammation cannot reliably be differentiated from sepsis; use of antibiotics is then promptly stopped when results from evaluation for infection are negative for 48 hours. Genetic testing for acute pancreatitis is appropriate when patients have a family history of pancreatitis or when other causes are not identified; alcohol-induced pancreatitis is far more common and is more likely to be the cause in patients consuming more than 50 g of alcohol daily. Further, both volume resuscitation and nutritional support are more appropriate next steps for this patient, and nuanced testing for the cause can be performed later.

VII.2. Answer c.
For patients with either mild or severe acute pancreatitis, early feeding is the best nutritional strategy, and the preferred method is enteral feeding, which decreases the risk of organ failure and infection. To avoid unnecessary procedures, patients should be given a trial with an oral diet; if the oral diet is not tolerated, nasogastric or nasojejunal feeding can be attempted next. If enteral feeding is not successful, as may happen in patients with severe or necrotizing pancreatitis or in those with ileus or obstructive symptoms from local collections, TPN should be initiated. A trial of resting the pancreas is no longer thought to be of therapeutic benefit for patients with acute pancreatitis who can tolerate enteral feeding. The lipase concentration is not useful for determining the severity of pancreatitis or the timing of feeding.

VII.3. Answer c.
The patient is most likely showing signs of the evolution of necrotizing pancreatitis, which is classically associated with systemic inflammatory signs. This can be accompanied by ileus or mechanical obstruction of the luminal gastrointestinal tract, which would explain the patient's distention and inability to tolerate oral intake. Diagnosis of necrotizing pancreatitis is critical for both disease prognosis and anticipation of management strategies as the necrosis becomes organized. This is best evaluated with contrast-enhanced CT to look for areas of malperfusion of the pancreatic gland. Even though the pancreas showed normal enhancement on admission, necrotizing pancreatitis tends to develop over days after the initial presentation, so reevaluation is warranted given the worsening clinical picture. Abdominal radiography may show distended intestine but would not provide useful clinical information about the specific complications of acute pancreatitis and would delay appropriate testing. Fecal calprotectin testing is not useful for pancreatitis, but it may be used in certain situations of Crohn disease flare associated with diarrhea, which this patient does not have. Infection related to pancreatic necrosis is extremely rare in the first week of acute pancreatitis and is more common in the third or fourth week after presentation. Use of prophylactic antibiotics is not recommended even if a patient has acute necrotizing pancreatitis because it has not been shown to reliably decrease the rate of infected necrosis, systemic complications, or mortality.

VII.4. Answer a.
This patient is having a pseudoaneurysm, a vascular complication of acute pancreatitis that is most common in the gastroduodenal and splenic arteries. Bleeding can be intraluminal or into a fluid collection, as in this patient. Best care is with prompt, catheter-based elimination of the bleeding source through interventional radiology. Endoscopy provides little benefit in the management of pseudoaneurysm and would delay appropriate care. Surgical exploration can be carried out if interventional radiologic techniques are not an option but would be contraindicated in a patient with cirrhosis and portal hypertension. Unless it is within the patient-specific goals of care, monitoring would be inappropriate at this time because exsanguination from her splanchnic arterial source, particularly with this patient's comorbidities, would almost certainly be associated with a high risk of mortality.

VII.5. Answer b.
The presence of a pancreatic duct stone indicates underlying chronic pancreatitis in this patient who presented with an episode of acute pancreatitis. Alcohol use is one of the most common causes of chronic pancreatitis. Gallstone disease, a common cause of acute pancreatitis, does not lead to chronic pancreatitis. Intraductal papillary mucinous neoplasm is a pancreatic cystic neoplasm that can be associated with main pancreatic duct dilatation. However, in this case dilatation of the duct is secondary to an obstructing pancreatic duct stone. Autoimmune pancreatitis is typically not associated with pancreatic duct dilatation and rarely presents with an episode of acute pancreatitis, so it is an unlikely diagnosis for this patient.

VII.6. Answer a.
The diagnosis is type 1 AIP on the basis of the definitive histologic findings: lymphoplasmacytic infiltrate, storiform fibrosis,

and obliterative phlebitis. The appropriate treatment is oral prednisone. AIP often mimics pancreatic cancer, and follow-up biopsy and metabolic imaging may be considered if the initial biopsy shows any indication of malignancy or does not show the histologic hallmarks of AIP. Management of AIP does not involve surgery.

VII.7. Answer c.
For this patient the diagnosis is chronic pancreatitis with exocrine pancreatic insufficiency because imaging showed atrophy and calcification, and the fecal elastase concentration was very low. The appropriate next step in management is initiation of pancreatic enzyme replacement. Both EUS with endoscopic pancreatic function testing and secretin-enhanced MRCP are diagnostic modalities for chronic pancreatitis that can be used when the diagnosis is not overt on cross-sectional imaging. Although excess dietary fat is generally avoided in patients with CP, a fat-restricted diet is not necessary if exocrine pancreatic insufficiency is managed appropriately with pancreatic enzyme replacement therapy.

VII.8. Answer a.
Alterations in the cationic trypsinogen gene (PRSS1) are the most common cause of hereditary pancreatitis. Other genes that have been implicated include SPINK1 and CFTR. The other genes listed are associated with the following heritable cancer syndromes, not with hereditary pancreatitis: Peutz-Jeghers syndrome (STK11), Lynch syndrome (MLH1), and familial atypical multiple mole melanoma syndrome (CDKN2A).

VII.9. Answer b.
Obesity is associated with an increased risk for pancreatic cancer. Other risk factors include family history of pancreatic cancer, pathogenic germline variants in pancreatic cancer susceptibility genes, smoking, alcohol use, and a history of type 2 diabetes. Family history of breast and ovarian cancer could be related to a germline BRCA variant, which would increase the risk for pancreatic cancer, but confirmatory genetic testing would be necessary. Uncontrolled celiac disease has been associated with small-bowel cancer but not pancreatic cancer.

VII.10.   Answer a.
A pathogenic germline variant in the CDKN2A gene indicates the presence of familial atypical multiple mole melanoma syndrome, which greatly increases a patient's lifetime risk for pancreatic cancer. Current expert consensus recommends that pancreatic cancer surveillance be considered for those patients starting at age 40 years or at 10 years before the youngest age at onset of exocrine pancreatic cancer in the family. Serum carbohydrate antigen 19-9 is not routinely used as a screening test for pancreatic cancer. Prophylactic mastectomy is considered for patients who have a germline BRCA variant. There is no need for prophylactic pancreatectomy in patients who have a germline variant in the CDKN2A gene.

VII.11.   Answer a.
The finding of multiple cysts communicating with the main pancreatic duct suggests a diagnosis of IPMN. The finding that the main pancreatic duct is dilated to more than 5 mm is a concern that warrants further evaluation with EUS to assess for features of main duct IPMN and other high-risk features that suggest advanced neoplasia. Surgery is typically reserved for IPMNs with high-risk features, which this patient does not have according to

the CT findings described above. The interval and modality of future surveillance will depend on the EUS results. For a cyst larger than 3 cm in diameter, the surveillance interval is usually 6 months initially with increases in future intervals if the size of the IPMN remains stable. Surveillance is recommended for all patients with suspected IPMN unless age or comorbidities preclude surgical intervention.

VII.12.   Answer b.
Solid pseudopapillary neoplasms are low-grade malignant pancreatic cystic neoplasms with metastatic potential; hence, management is surgical resection in all patients who are fit to undergo surgery. Unlike therapy for pancreatic ductal adenocarcinoma, neoadjuvant therapy is not appropriate for solid pseudopapillary neoplasms.

VII.13.   Answer c.
This patient is presenting with acute cholangitis given the evidence of systemic infection, inflammation, and biochemical evidence of jaundice. MRCP would not be the best next step because cholangitis is suspected, and delaying management more than 24 hours may increase the risk of death. Cholecystectomy is indicated after treatment of cholangitis to prevent future attacks, but it is not the best next step for this patient. EUS with ERCP would be a reasonable step given the high clinical suspicion for cholangitis. However, even if the EUS were negative for a stone, ERCP would still be indicated.

VII.14.   Answer d.
With this patient's history of PSC, he has a relatively high risk for gallbladder cancer. Patients who have PSC and polyps of any measurable size should be referred for elective cholecystectomy. If the patient did not have PSC, repeating ultrasonography in 3 to 6 months would be appropriate. MRCP is not indicated at this time because the gallbladder polyp was already detected with abdominal ultrasonography; however, in some instances, an MRCP is performed instead of abdominal ultrasonography for PSC surveillance for cholangiocarcinoma. ERCP is not indicated for evaluation of gallbladder polyps.

VII.15.   Answer b.
This patient has an intermediate risk for choledocholithiasis, so proceeding to cholecystectomy directly would not be appropriate. Given his altered anatomy, both EUS and ERCP may be challenging and would not be the preferred next step. Placement of a percutaneous transhepatic drain is not indicated for this patient because acute cholangitis is not suspected at this time. MRCP is the most appropriate of the choices provided. If a stone is found on MRCP, the patient may benefit from laparoscopic-assisted ERCP at the time of cholecystectomy, balloon-assisted ERCP, or EUS-assisted ERCP.

VII.16.   Answer c.
This elderly man has severe acute cholangitis as evidenced by fever, right upper quadrant pain, hypotension, a relatively dilated common bile duct, and high levels of bilirubin, aspartate aminotransferase, and alanine aminotransferase. Although the gallbladder is distended with pericholecystic fluid, distention can be present in common bile duct obstruction and severe sepsis with hypoperfusion; therefore, neither calculous cholecystitis nor acalculous cholecystitis would be the most likely diagnosis. This patient probably has choledocholithiasis, but the most likely diagnosis is cholangitis.

Index

In the digital version, indexed terms that span 2 pages (eg, 52–53) may occasionally appear on only 1 of those pages

Tables, figures, and boxes are indicated by an italic *t*, *f*, and *b*, respectively, after the page number.

gastrojejunal anastomosis ulceration, 161–62
gastrojejunal anastomotic strictures, 161
gastroparesis
  classification of, 85*t*
  overview, 85
  presentation and diagnosis of, 87–89, 89*f*
  treatment of, 89–91
gastropathy
  chemical, 62
  definition, 57
  hypertrophic, 62–63
  portal hypertensive, 62, 63*f*, 129, 333–34
  vascular, 62, 63*f*
GAVE (gastric antral vascular ectasia), 62, 63*f*, 130
genetics
  in alcohol-related liver disease, 316
  in colorectal cancer, 225–27, 226*b*
  in drug-induced liver injury, 372
  in gastric adenocarcinoma, 67*b*, 67, 68*t*
  in IBD, 185–86
  in pancreatic ductal adenocarcinoma, 444–45, 444*t*
GERD. *See* gastroesophageal reflux disease
giant migrating complex, 84
Giardia lamblia, 211*t*, 214
giardiasis, 152
GIM (gastric intestinal metaplasia), 66
ginger, 254
GISTs (gastrointestinal stromal tumors), 71–72, 72*f*
glucagon, 253
glucagonomas, 79–80
GNETs (gastroenteric neuroendocrine tumors), 72–73, 80
golimumab, 193–94, 266
G-POEM (gastric peroral endoscopic myotomy), 91
graft-vs-host disease (GVHD), 154
granisetron, 255
granuloma, 189
granulomatous gastritis, 58*t*, 60–61, 61*f*
ground-glass hepatocytes, 290
gynecologic conditions, GI manifestations of, 157

H₂-receptor blockers, 15, 56
hamartomatous polyposis syndromes, 227
harmless acute pancreatitis score, 430
HAV (hepatitis A virus), 287–88, 288*t*, 398
HBeAg-positive chronic hepatitis B phase, 288–89
HBV. *See* hepatitis B virus
HCAs (hepatocellular adenomas), 301–2
HCC. *See* hepatocellular carcinoma
HCV. *See* hepatitis C virus
HDGC (hereditary diffuse gastric cancer), 67*b*, 67, 68
HDV (hepatitis D virus), 288*t*, 292
heartburn, 7–8, 8*b*
heart failure, 143, 144
Helicobacter pylori infection
  acute gastritis and, 57
  chronic gastritis and, 58, 59
  diagnosis of, 54–55, 54*t*
  esophageal adenocarcinoma and, 31

functional dyspepsia and, 92, 93–94
gastric adenocarcinoma and, 67
gastric lymphoma and, 70, 71
GERD and, 5
lymphocytic gastritis and, 61
and NSAIDs, 53
overview, 51
pregnancy and, 255*t*
PUD and, 52–53, 53*f*
treatment, 55–56, 55*t*
UGI bleeding and, 129
HELLP syndrome, 395–96
hemangioma, cavernous, 298*f*, 300, 301*f*
hematologic disorders, GI manifestations of, 147*b*, 147*f*, 147–49, 148*f*, 149*f*
hemobilia, 129
hemochromatosis, hereditary, 350–55, 352*f*, 353*f*, 354*t*, 355*t*
hemochromatosis arthropathy, 351*f*, 351
hemodialysis, 153
hemorrhage, after RYGB, 161
hemostasis, therapeutic agents for, 254
hemosuccus pancreaticus, 129
Henoch-Schönlein purpura (HSP), 139–40, 156*f*, 156–57
hepatic adenoma, 300–2, 302*f*
hepatic arterial inflow disorders, 325*b*, 326–28
hepatic arterial outflow disorders, 325*b*, 328–30
hepatic artery aneurysm, 140–41, 327*f*, 327
hepatic artery–portal vein fistulas, 327
hepatic artery thrombosis, 326, 404
hepatic decompensation, 402
hepatic encephalopathy, 283, 283*t*, 341–42
hepatic hemangioma, 300
hepatic hydrothorax, 337–38
hepatic steatosis, 381, 381*t*, 382, 384–85, 385*f*
hepatitis. *See also specific viruses*
  acute, 280–81, 280*t*, 287
  autoimmune, 375–80, 396–97
  cholestatic, 369
  chronic, 281, 281*t*, 287
  DILI and, 368–69
  severe alcohol-related, 318–21, 319*b*, 320*b*
  treatment in pregnancy, 257–59
hepatitis A virus (HAV), 287–88, 288*t*, 398
hepatitis B virus (HBV)
  clinical presentation and natural history, 282–89, 289*f*, 289*t*
  comparison of viruses, 288*t*
  diagnostic tests, 280–90, 290*t*, 291*f*
  epidemiology, 288
  HIV and, 296
  pregnancy and, 396, 397*f*, 398
  treatment, 280–81, 291*t*
hepatitis C virus (HCV)
  clinical presentation and natural history, 292*f*, 292–93
  comparison of viruses, 288*t*
  diagnostic tests, 293*f*, 293
  epidemiology, 292
  HIV and, 296
  pregnancy and, 295, 396, 398
  prevention, 295–96
  screening, 293
  treatment, 293–95, 294*f*, 294*t*, 295*t*

hepatitis D virus (HDV), 288*t*, 292
hepatitis E, 296
hepatobiliary manifestations of IBD, 202*b*, 202–3
hepatocellular adenomas (HCAs), 301–2
hepatocellular carcinoma (HCC)
  definition, 300
  hereditary hemochromatosis and, 351
  management of, 306–9, 307*f*
  nonalcoholic fatty liver disease and, 389
  overview, 304–5
  risk factors, 298
  surveillance and diagnosis, 305*f*, 305–6, 306*f*
hepatocellular disorders, 280–81, 280*t*, 281*t*
hepatocyte ballooning, 383, 385–86
hepatocytes, ground-glass, 290
hepatopathy, ischemic, 327
hepatorenal syndrome (HRS), 340–41
herbal supplements, liver injury from, 370, 371*b*
hereditary colorectal cancer genetic syndromes, 225–27, 226*b*
hereditary coproporphyria, 148
hereditary diffuse gastric cancer (HDGC), 67*b*, 67, 68
hereditary hemochromatosis, 350–55, 352*f*, 353*f*, 354*t*, 355*t*
hereditary hemorrhagic telangiectasia (HHT), 144*b*, 144*f*, 144, 145, 327–28
hereditary nonpolyposis colorectal cancer (HNPCC), 226*b*, 226
hereditary pancreatitis, 444, 444*t*
hernias, internal, 162
herpes simplex virus (HSV), 19, 20*f*, 398
Heyde syndrome, 143
HHT (hereditary hemorrhagic telangiectasia), 144*b*, 144*f*, 144, 145, 327–28
high-amplitude propagated contractions, 237
high-grade dysplasia (HGD), 27, 28*f*, 29–30, 30*f*
high-output heart failure, 144*b*
high-resolution manometry (HRM), 38*f*, 38, 39*f*, 41, 42*f*
histamine receptor antagonists, 255*t*
HIV, 296
HNPCC (hereditary nonpolyposis colorectal cancer), 226*b*, 226
hospitalization, small-bowel diseases in, 115
HRS (hepatorenal syndrome), 340–41
HSP (Henoch-Schönlein purpura), 139–40, 156*f*, 156–57
HSV (herpes simplex virus), 19, 20*f*, 398
hydrothorax, hepatic, 337–38
hyperbilirubinemia, 281–82
hypercholesterolemia, 361
hypercontractile esophagus, 38, 39*f*, 39*t*, 43*f*, 43
hyperemesis gravidarum, 392
hypergastrinemia, 77
hyperparathyroidism, 154
hyperplasia, focal nodular, 300, 302–3, 303*f*
hypersecretion of gastric acid, 53–54, 54*f*
hypersensitivity drug reaction, 365
hyperthyroidism, 154
hypertriglyceridemia, 428–29
hypertrophic gastropathy, 62–63, 68